COMPREHENSIVE
DENTAL HYGIENE
CARE

COMPREHENSIVE DENTAL HYGIENE CARE

FOURTH EDITION

Irene R. Woodall R.D.H., M.A., Ph.D.
Clinical Associate Professor,
Department of Dental Hygiene,
University of Colorado School of Dentistry, Denver, Colorado;
President, Connaissance Partners, Redwood City, California

with 710 *illustrations and* 5 *color plates*

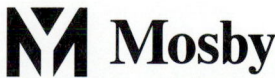 Mosby

St. Louis Baltimore Boston Chicago London Philadelphia Sydney Toronto

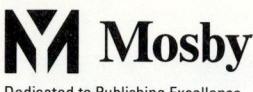

Mosby

Dedicated to Publishing Excellence

Editor: Robert W. Reinhardt
Developmental Editor: Elaine Steinborn
Assistant Editor: Jo Salway
Project Manager: John A. Rogers
Senior Production Editor: Shauna Burnett Sticht, Helen C. Hudlin
Editing: Tim O'Brien, April Naumann
Designer: Jeanne Wolfgeher
Manufacturing Supervisor: Theresa Fuchs

FOURTH EDITION

Printed in the United States of America

Mosby–Year Book Inc.
11830 Westline Industrial Drive,
St. Louis, Missouri 63146

Library of Congress Cataloging in Publication Data
Comprehensive dental hygiene care / [edited by] Irene R. Woodall.
   p.   cm.
Includes bibliographical references and index.
ISBN 0-8016-7019-5
1. Dental hygiene. I. Woodall, Irene R. (Irene Rita), 1946-
II. Title: Dental hygiene care.
   [DNLM: 1. Dental Prophylaxis.   WU 113 C737 1993]
RK60.7.C65 1993
617.6'01—dc20
DNLM/DLC
for Library of Congress   92-48466
                                                         CIP

CL/DC 9 8 7 6 5 4 3

CONTRIBUTORS

Susan Barnard, R.D.H., M.S.
Adjunct Faculty
Bergen Community College
Paramus, New Jersey

Judith C. Berry, R.D.H., M.Ed.
Private practice
Researcher, Special Projects
University of Texas Health Science Center at
 San Antonio
San Antonio, Texas

Thomas G. Berry, D.D.S., M.A.
Chairman
Department of Restorative Dentistry
University of Texas Health Science Center at
 San Antonio
San Antonio, Texas

Bonnie R. Dafoe, R.D.H., M.Ed.
Connaissance Partners
Redwood City, California

Susan J. Daniel, R.D.H., M.S.
Chair and Assistant Professor
Department of Dental Hygiene
School of Health-Related Professions
University of Mississippi Medical Center
Jackson, Mississippi

Catherine C. Davis, R.D.H., Ph.D.
Clinical Associate Professor
Department of Dental Hygiene
University of Colorado
Denver, Colorado;
Associate Clinical Professor
Department of Periodontology
Creighton University
Omaha, Nebraska;
Clinical Research Coordinator
Poudre Valley Hospital
Fort Collins, Colorado

JoAnn R. Gurenlian, R.D.H., Ph.D.
Chairman
Department of Dental Hygiene
College of Allied Health Sciences
Thomas Jefferson University
Philadelphia, Pennsylvania

Wendy A. Halowski, DIP.D.H., B.S., M.S.
Clinical Instructor
University of British Columbia
Vancouver, British Columbia

Barbara Jones
Clinical Monitor
Vipont Pharmaceutical
Fort Collins, Colorado;
Clinical/Statistical Consultant
Colgate-Palmolive Company
Piscataway, New Jersey

Donna Karras, R.D.H., M.A.
Assistant Clinical Professor
School of Dentistry
University of Colorado
Denver, Colorado

Theresa Levy, R.D.H., M.S.
Associate Professor
Director, Dental Hygiene Program
Oregon Institute of Technology
Klamath Falls, Oregon

Hermine McLeran, R.D.H., M.P.H.
Associate Professor
Preventive and Community Dentistry
University of Iowa
Iowa City, Iowa

Laura Mueller-Joseph, R.D.H., A.S., B.S.,
M.S.
Assistant Professor
Department of Dental Hygiene
State University of New York
Farmingdale, New York

Trisha E. O'Hehir, R.D.H., B.S.
Editor
Perio REPORTS
Flagstaff, Arizona

Eric E. Spohn, D.D.S.
Professor, Department of Oral Health Science
Director, Dental Auxiliary Training Programs
School of Dentistry
University of Kentucky
Lexington, Kentucky

Donna J. Stach, R.D.H.
Assistant Professor
Department of Dental Hygiene
School of Dentistry
University of Colorado
Denver, Colorado

James S. Wefel, Ph.D.
Director, Center for Clinical Studies
Associate Director
Dows Institute for Dental Research
University of Iowa
Iowa City, Iowa

Dianna Weikel, R.D.H., M.S.
Assistant Professor
Department of Oral Medicine
Baltimore College of Dental Surgery;
School of Dentistry
University of Maryland at Baltimore;
Program of Oncology University of Maryland
    Cancer Center
Baltimore, Maryland

Cheryl Wiles, R.D.H., M.S.
Assistant Professor
School of Dentistry
University of Colorado
Denver, Colorado;
Private Practice
Boulder, Colorado

Gail F. Williamson, R.D.H., M.S.
Associate Professor
Dental Diagnostic Sciences
School of Dentistry
Indiana University
Indianapolis, Indiana

Irene R. Woodall, R.D.H., M.A., Ph.D.
Clinical Associate Professor
Department of Dental Hygiene
School of Dentistry
University of Colorado
Denver, Colorado;
President, Connaissance Partners
Redwood City, California

Nancy Stutsman Young, R.D.H., M.Ed.
Assistant Professor
School of Dentistry
Indiana University
Indianapolis, Indiana

TO
My brothers,
Richard D. and William R. Zimmerman,
who taught me about competition and to have
high expectations of myself.

My mother,
Augusta V. Doktor,
who taught me how to respect my
womanhood in a man's world.

My father,
William W. Zimmerman,
who taught me how to throw a ball
and how to care.

— IRW —

PREFACE

This edition is dramatically different from previous versions of *Comprehensive Dental Hygiene Care*. We still focus on the student as a partner in learning and the patient as a partner in care. The sequencing of parts and chapters still follows the course of preparation, assessment, planning, treatment, and evaluation for each patient, and its overall goal remains the preparation of the student for the first day of clinical practice followed by skill development in complex procedures. However, the role of the dental hygienist is described more in terms of individualizing care, stepping out of rote practice modes, and relying on a solid knowledge base for assessing, diagnosing, planning, and modifying care. Thus, you will find a major emphasis on the emerging paradigm of the hygienist assuming greater responsibility for determining treatment needs and implementing a variety of educational and therapeutic approaches to meet those needs.

A plethora of research in the area of periodontics has stimulated a second major change. This text presents the position that scaling and root planing should be replaced by subgingival debridement given a revised view of the necessity for "vigorous root planing." A complete review of the literature over the past 20 years explains why vigorous root planing was adopted as the standard of care and also why it is being replaced by a more conservative approach to eliminating endotoxins and disrupting pathogens. Ultrasonic instrumentation using explorer-thin tips that reach into the depths of furcations and periodontal pockets and that are focused on this new goal of instrumentation are featured. Hand instruments are offered as important alternatives and adjuncts. There is a new section on the basics of immunology and how that relates to new diagnostic tests being developed. We have also added a section on "continuing care" strategies for patients who need to be maintained in an individualized fashion on regular recall.

Our hope is that this text will stimulate debate and cooperation among students, faculty, and even patients as we face the challenges presented to us by the knowledge gleaned from recent research. This is not a time for arbitrarily clinging to old procedures and values. It is a time for identifying which procedures have a solid basis in research, which deserve much more consideration and experimentation, and which should be discarded as no longer defensible. If we are to mature into a research-based profession, we need to develop a value for open inquiry, where challenge is expected and original thinking is rewarded. As faculty we should be delighted when students ask "why," and as students we should be grateful that our faculty want us to think on our own, develop flexibility as well as diligence, and to inquire continuously about what constitutes the best care we can provide the people who entrust themselves to us.

The previous editions laid the groundwork for some of this professional development by encouraging class activities rather than lectures and by presenting controversies to consider, as well as facts to assimilate. We also planted the seeds for the partnership relationship between faculty and students. Some of the concepts and recommendations made in this text will have a dramatic impact on the structure of dental hygiene education and clinical practice. More than ever that strong partnership among us is needed as we evolve toward the dental hygiene care of a new century.

Irene R. Woodall

Acknowledgments for first edition

Many people contributed their efforts to make the final preparation of the manuscript possible. Conrad Woodall, Phil Young, and Kuna Yankell were invaluable in our times of greatest need, not only with their support, but also with their willingness to type, duplicate, collate, proofread, and visit the post office and the office supply and photographic stores. Don Dafoe was especially helpful in his review of the chapters on health history and emergency procedures. Sally Verity's review of the chapters on comprehensive charting was also particularly helpful. Jan Griffin and Susan Muhler deserve a thank you for finding rare equipment items for our use.

The word processing staff, Catherine Redden, Delores DiCocco, Patricia DeVuono, and Julia Marguilles, were invaluable in their preparation of the final manuscript, especially in May and June, 1979. Emily Mintz deserves a thank you for her contribution in typing tables and letters for us.

We also wish to thank Michael Schwager for his advice and efforts in meeting our most critical photographic needs. We wish to acknowledge the case documentation prepared by Deborah Drazek while she was a student at the University of Pennsylvania and the role she, Dianna Mumma, and Sharon Herr played in photograph preparation. Rosemarie Valentine's leadership and efforts in developing learning materials for the department are also gratefully acknowledged. Slides prepared by Mary Robb Gross and Catherine Schifter were especially helpful in showing the use of Gracey instruments, and we thank our colleagues for sharing them with us.

Elissa Berardi, our medical illustrator, worked long and hard to prepare the many detailed drawings for the text. Her work is beautifully done and reflects a great deal of caring for the quality of the project.

We also owe thanks to all the participants in the Penn-EFDA Faculty Institute I: Periodontics/Anesthesia for their continuous support and for sharing in the excitement during the final weeks of our efforts. We shall never forget Sue Agostini, Regina Byrne, Sue Colangelo, Sue Daniel, Kandie Dautel, Mary Ann Haag, Gwen Hlava, Joyce Jenzano, JoAnne Karr, Jane Emerson Knight, Joan Madden, Pat Mulford, Lin Nassar, Joan Gluch-Scranton, Maureen Pratt Smith, and Debbie Vlanis.

Acknowledgments for second edition

Once again, many people helped us in preparing the manuscript and in ensuring that the time and moral support were there when we needed them most. We offer our heartfelt thanks and appreciation.

For their reviews of the first edition—Phyllis Beemsterboer, Debbie Brown, Sherry Castle Harfst, Ralph Lobene, Hunter Rackley, Patricia Randolph, Karen Ridley, Ellen Rogo, and Joan Gluch Scranton.

For his review of the intraoral photography chapter—Clifford L. Freehe; and for his review of the medical history and emergencies chapters—Donald C. Dafoe.

For their assistance in locating references—Sue Seeger and Ruth Cressman at the University of Michigan dental library and Kathy Marousek, Helen Itkin, and Dorothea Colburn at the Fairleigh Dickinson dental library.

For their outstanding photographic assistance—Bonnie Dafoe, William Prior, Catherine Schifter, David Sullivan, and Robert Benedon; and for the beautiful new illustrations—Elissa Berardi.

For giving permission to use the Fairleigh Dickinson School of Dentistry facilities—Richard Oglesby.

For the index preparation and service as a photographic model—Conrad Woodall.

For the much needed time to write—Michael Fonner and Dani Kazista.

For continuing support during the project—the dental hygiene faculty at the Fairleigh Dickinson University (especially Ellen Rogo and Cheryl Westphal) and at the University of Pennsylvania (Catherine Schifter, Kate Fitzgerald, Jean Byrnes, Charlotte Hangorsky, Roberta Throne, Joyce Levy, and Joanne Prifti, and Janet Yellowitz).

For their consistent, helpful presence and support in every way during this project—Conrad Woodall, Kuna Yankell, and Phil Young.

Acknowledgments for third edition

The authors wish to thank:

For outstanding photographic assistance: *Mike Halloran, Tom Berry,* and *Dennis Thompson.*

For their patient assistance as photographic models: *Philip Young, Janet Mulherin,* and *Jennifer* and *Jonathan Tilliss.*

For assistance in reviewing and revising chapters: *Michael Sabat, Lynda Sabat, Joan Gluch Scranton, Jaclyn Gleber, Pauline Spencer, Donna Stach,* and *Sherry Harfst.*

For use of beautiful clinical facilities: the Thomas Jefferson University School of Allied Health Services, Philadelphia, PA and the University of Colorado School of Dentistry, Denver, CO.

For the latest computer skills in locating references and other research assistance: *Sherry Montgomery,* Librarian, University of Pennsylvania, School of Dental Medicine, Philadelphia, PA.

For library search services: *Conrad Woodall.*

For her wonderful talents in illustration (and music): *Elissa Berardi.*

For her assistance in manuscript preparations: *Catherine Reddon.*

For moral support and assistance with a perpetual series of details: *Diane Ware, Barb Jones,* and *Lynn Brown.*

To the authors of selected chapters for their efforts, quality work and timeliness: *Eric Spohn, Tom Berry, Wendy Halowski, Jill Jaroski, Jan Brown, Donna Karras, Donna Stach, Hunter Rackley, Carol Janz, Shawn O'Neill-Hoffman, Marcia Collins,* and *Kathleen Ross.*

Acknowledgments for fourth edition

These contributing authors wish to thank the following people:

Irene Woodall: for library services; to James Robertson, for extra effort finishing the job; Bonnie Dafoe, for research assistance, love, and support; and James Dieroff.

Nancy Stutsman Young: to Phil, for his help, love, and support.

Catherine Davis: to Dr. Michael Finkelstein, Associate Professor of Oral Pathology, University of Iowa, for loaning scientific articles, information on OSHA regulations, and photographs. Also thanks to my husband, Steven Scheffel, and daughter Elizabeth.

Donna Stach: to my students and fellow dental hygienists who, by constantly seeking a better way, have encouraged and rewarded me for the efforts that went into these chapters. I especially thank Irene Woodall, Gail Cross-Poline, and Janis Keating for challenging and supporting me as a colleague and as a friend and thanks to my husband, Jim, for his love and laughter.

Judy Berry and Tom Berry: to Michele Ismail for carefully and patiently inputting and tracking numerous versions of the chapters through the computer to final draft.

Donna Karras: to my husband, Don, who always thinks I can do everything. Thank you for taking time out of your hectic schedule to type and edit my chapter. To my boys, Dane and Dillon, for making me smile everyday—you're the greatest. To the most remarkable person I know, Irene Woodall, for having confidence in me to undertake such a rewarding experience. It meant so much. Thank you all.

Susan J. Daniel: to Joseph S. Giansanti, for encouragement and assistance in reviewing and revising chapters; Dr. Louis Gangarosa, for reviewing and revising content on iontophoresis; Earline Fitzhugh, for assistance in locating references; the dental hygiene faculty of the University of Mississippi Medical Center, for understanding and patience; Brian Fitzhugh, for assistance as a photographic model; and, for the opportunity to contribute, Irene Woodall.

Gail Williamson: to Drs. Thomas Razmus and Don John Summerlin, for their assistance and review of the chapter; and Alana Barra, Mike Halloran, and Mark Dirlam, and the Indiana University School of Dentistry, Indianapolis, Indiana, for their skilled photographic assistance in the preparation of radiographic illustrations.

Barbara Jones: to Irene Woodall, for her inspiration and support.

JoAnn R. Gurenlian: to my family, Tom, Laura, and TJ; and the faculty and staff of the department of dental hygiene at Thomas Jefferson University during the preparation of the chapter on diagnostic decision making.

Bonnie Dafoe: to Gayle Schmidt, for assistance and friendship during the preparation of the chapter on intraoral photography; my family, Don, Erin, and Andy, for their support; all the CDHC authors, Helen Hudlin, and others at Mosby–Year Book for their understanding and hard work in the final days of manuscript preparation; James Robertson for editorial assistance; special thanks to Mandy and Lotte Woodall and James Dieroff for their courage and inspiration; and, of course, to Irene for her strength of character, her vision, and leadership—and forgiveness for imperfections that may have slipped by without her attention to every detail.

Trisha E. O'Hehir: to Irene Woodall for bringing together dental hygiene colleagues interested in the future of our profession. Sharing ideas, visions, insights and experiences to produce this text also built a national network of resources and friendships that will continue long after this edition is published.

CONTENTS

COMPREHENSIVE DENTAL HYGIENE CARE

PART ONE INTRODUCTION

Dental hygiene is a changing profession. The influence of compelling new research is changing the fundamental basis of our role in health care. The procedures we perform, the rationale for the care we deliver, and the emphasis we place on therapeutic and preventive care are coming under in-depth scrutiny and revision. As a result, the dental hygiene profession you have come to know through personal encounters and descriptions of what the profession does may be quite different from the way you will learn to practice.

If you are a currently practicing dental hygienist, or one returning to practice, you are probably reading this book to update your professional skills. You will find much to consider.

Chapter 1 introduces you to the forces that are driving change in the profession. It will help you focus on the characteristics dental hygienists share and help reinforce your sense of belonging. Enjoy your participation in a dynamic profession that is keeping pace with the changes in health needs and the scientific advances that help us make sense of those needs and necessary treatment.

1 DENTAL HYGIENE PRACTICE

Irene Woodall

LEARNING OUTCOMES

The dental hygienist will be able to

1. Define a philosophy of patient-centered care.
2. Identify examples of patient-hygienist interactions that reflect the philosophy of patient-centered care.
3. Recognize the major influences on the development of the dental hygiene profession over the past three decades.
4. Recognize clinical practice that can be characterized as "technical/doing" versus "scientific/thinking" versus a combination of those two approaches.
5. Define *professional culture*.
6. List at least 10 key components of dental hygiene's professional culture.

This text was written to prepare you for dental hygiene clinical practice. Its primary goal is to help you, the student, feel confident and competent on your first day of clinical practice. It also is intended to help graduate dental hygienists rethink their goals, strategies, and procedures.

The early chapters introduce the sequence of procedures typically followed in the comprehensive dental hygiene appointment plan. Later chapters address more advanced clinical skills and provide guidelines for integrating ideal principles of care into a realistic practice environment.

The philosophy of patient-centered care is integrated into each phase of care. The patient is viewed as a partner in care, involved extensively in decision making and in the self-care necessary for restoring and maintaining oral health. The mastery of technical procedures is emphasized in the individual chapters to ensure safe and effective therapy. But in each instance the *need* for the procedure and the *way* in which the *patient* is involved are critical components of developing the relative role of technical skill in dental hygiene care.

Many beginning students see the profession of dental hygiene as being founded on this service orientation, which is the philosophic basis for patient-centered care. For those students, the text should enhance that approach to learning dental hygiene care. Other new students, whose exposure to the profession has been somewhat limited, may focus largely on the technical components of dental hygiene practice. For them, the text should help develop a more comprehensive approach to dental hygiene care.

In addition, this book was written to help prepare students for future roles in health care delivery by introducing a flexible approach to patient care as well as controversies regarding the efficacy of time-honored practice procedures.

MOTIVATIONS FOR SELECTING DENTAL HYGIENE

People select dental hygiene as a career for many different reasons. The interest of some students begins with their own encounters with dentistry and dental hygiene. They may have learned as patients to respect and enjoy the people in the dental office. Factors attracting students to dental hygiene include the desire to work in preventive health; the availability of jobs; the opportunity to focus on health sciences, to enjoy a flexible work schedule, to make independent decisions, to have a good salary and opportunity for advancement, to have prestige, and to work with healthy people (Carr, 1989). Students who were visited by the school dental hygienist each year may identify with the relative independence of the person who travels from school to school helping young people improve their oral health. As with most professions, a family tradition in dentistry or dental hygiene may be a major determining factor.

Growing up around a dental office can have a significant effect on career awareness and interest. Still other students may select dental hygiene as a result of careful career counseling and information programs.

EXPECTATIONS FOR PRACTICE

When considering a career in dental hygiene, most applicants have a few common needs or expectations. When asked what special characteristics a dental hygienist should have, most students identify the ability to work well with people and the ability to use their hands. They expect to earn a reasonable income, to work in pleasant surroundings, to have flexibility in scheduling, to have the respect of the patient, and to help people. When the functional role of the dental hygienist is addressed, most see the primary duties to be "cleaning teeth" and "teaching people how to care for their teeth." Most applicants expect to work with a dentist in private practice.

There are, of course, some students whose expectations are quite different from these. Varying perceptions may result from a quite different exposure to the profession or, perhaps, from misinformation.

However, any incoming student must have clear, specific expectations and perceptions of the profession and of his or her expected performance in the educational program. Sharing these perceptions with each other and with faculty members can be an enlightening experience that can prevent or at least reduce conflict.

Usually the more extensive exposure of dental hygiene faculty members to the profession has altered their initial perceptions of it. A faculty member has had an opportunity to compare expectations with reality and to develop an educational approach that blends the ideal with the real. Faculty members may vary greatly with regard to their respective perceptions. Whereas one faculty member may relate primarily to practical applications of skill, another may strive to preserve ideal, conceptual approaches to patient care with a strong basic and behavioral science foundation. Still other faculty members may see their role as one of preparing hygienists for the future—dental hygiene as it ought to be rather than as it is.

CHANGES IN THE PROFESSION
Legal and educational changes

Many of these varying perceptions, whether among faculty or students, are the result of changes in the profession since the early 1960s. After several decades of slow—at times imperceptible—change, the profession encountered the era of "expanded functions" and the challenge of defining how its members could maintain or alter their role.

Before the flurry of debate of the 1960s, dental hygiene was for the most part practiced in solo dental practices. The role of the dental hygienist was largely defined as oral prophylaxis, patient education, and the exposing of radiographs. Particularly in the east, hygienists were employed in school systems providing dental health education, prophylaxis, and eventually fluoride treatments. (See Fig. 1-1 for a view of a school-based clinic in the early days of dental hygiene.)

The events of the 1960s and 1970s helped revise that relatively narrow scope of practice. In *Survey of Dentistry,* Hollinshead (1961) described the deplorable state of our nation's oral health at that time. Many wondered how a country that was a world leader and was investing in a major space program and providing millions of dollars in aid to foreign countries could allow its own people to have such limited access to quality dental care. President Lyndon Johnson launched his War on Poverty in the mid-1960s with a call for legislation to provide comprehensive federally funded medical care for the elderly and other needy people. Under Medicaid, states were to provide dental benefits to qualified, financially handicapped persons. In addition, numerous proposals for federally supported health care for all persons were introduced in the federal legislature, some of which included dental benefits. It seemed imminent that persons previously denied medical and dental care because of financial barriers would soon be flooding the health care delivery system.

The 1970 Carnegie Commission report predicted that there would soon be a great shortage of physicians and dentists: "With the advent of national health insurance, the shortcomings in our methods of health care delivery and the critical shortages of our health manpower and facilities will become even more glaringly apparent." The Commission's recommendation for dentistry was that "progress could be achieved through more extensive use of dentist's assistants and dental hygienists and through greater emphasis on preventive programs."

Several plans developed from this recommendation, including the allocation of federal funds to

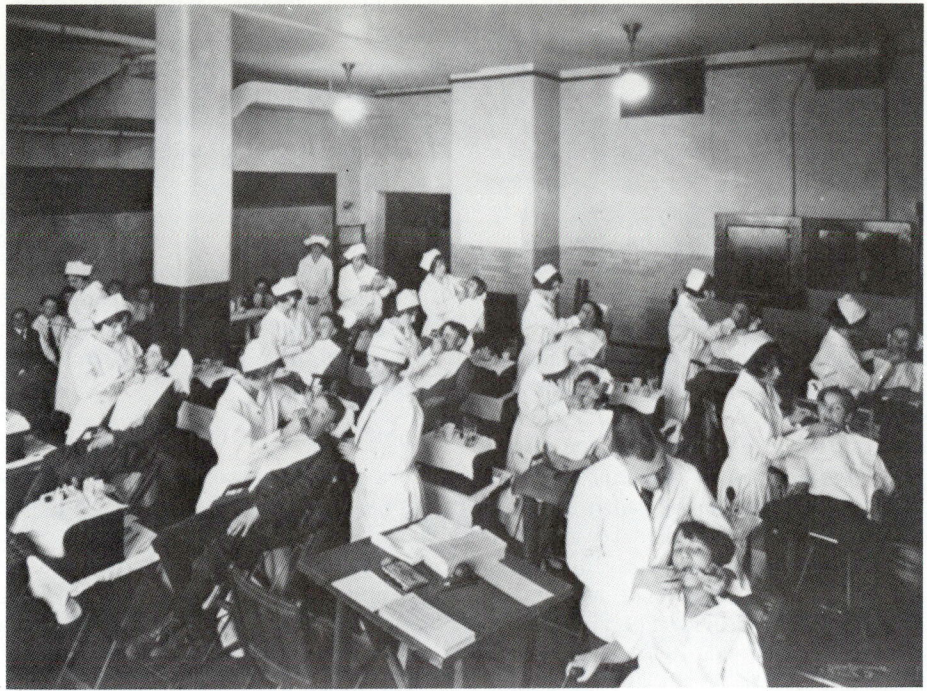

Fig. 1-1. Students in early 1900s of the Department of Oral Hygiene, University of Pennsylvania holding clinic in the S. Weir Mitchell School, 50th and Kingsessing Ave., Philadelphia.

increase the number of dentists, dental hygienists, physicians, nurses, and other health care providers being prepared in educational programs. Experiments to evaluate the delegation of functions to dental assistants and hygienists were conducted to determine whether the dentist could be relieved of some of their typical clinical functions. In many states, as the results of the research proved to be positive, laws were debated and changed to permit auxiliary personnel to perform additional services. Curricula in dental assisting and dental hygiene programs were altered to include the new skills and knowledge required to provide these services.

Although dental and medical programs expanded and support personnel for dentistry and medicine increased in number and variety, national health insurance was not enacted. In 1976 the Carnegie Council (formerly the Carnegie Commission) revised its recommendations to state that increased numbers of physicians and dentists were not needed but that the number of support personnel should continue to grow and provide greater varieties of health care services.

Along with which skills should be added to

practice, there was considerable discussion about increasing the variety of settings and the range of responsibility and decision making that a dental hygienist might assume. In the early 1970s the American Dental Hygienists' Association (ADHA) defined practice sites including hospitals, geriatric centers, penal institutions, and centers for the physically and mentally handicapped as appropriate and desirable locations for serving the public. Programs of care, that would require a great deal more expertise and responsibility whether for individuals or groups, were identified as the function of the hygienist (ADHA Resolutions, 1971, 1973, 1975, and 1976).

The number of programs rose from 70 in 1967 (American Dental Association annual report, 1969) to 187 in 1978. The number of graduates increased from 1739 to 4847 per year between 1967 and 1977 (ADA annual report, 1978). The functions taught in various programs ranged from the most limited scope to a full array of procedures.

Bachelor's and master's degree programs available to dental hygienists increased in number and variety. In addition to the several long-standing bachelor of science programs in which clinical dental hygiene training followed previous college education in the sciences and liberal arts, newer programs offered the dental hygienist with a certificate or associate (2-year) degree the opportunity to add new skills and knowledge and earn a bachelor of science degree. Just as the 2-year basic preparation in dental hygiene varies greatly from state to state and from program to program, the content and emphasis of the bachelor's and master's degree programs vary greatly. These degree programs may focus on teacher education, public health, oral medicine, expanded functions, research, administration, biocommunications, or any combination of these elements.

A survey reported in 1986 revealed the diversity in degree programs. Some programs focus on preparation for specific alternative career settings, others encourage students to explore a variety of settings while providing a wide array of educational opportunities in management and issues analysis, and still others provide liberal arts education (Rubinstein and Brand, 1986).

In the 1960s and 1970s, legally allowable clinical skills for dental hygienists changed in a variety of ways, depending on the state. At the same time, sites and roles were being reevaluated and new emphases on comprehensive care were being developed to decrease the dichotomy between the interests of the "clinical hygienist" and the "community dentistry hygienist." Conceptually, at least, dental hygiene grew not only in scope and responsibility, but also in complexity.

The scope of dental hygiene practice did not expand greatly during the early 1980s. The increased number of dentists and hygienists was not matched by the demand in the number of persons seeking care. With no national health insurance program, the cost barrier remained for many people. This was worsened by a recession that resulted in high unemployment rates, particularly in heavily industrialized regions. Suddenly dentists and hygienists working in communities where union benefits included dental insurance had barren appointment books. Workers postponed their dental care until they were back to work and benefits were reinstated. Why discuss delegating components of care to dental auxiliaries during a slow period?

The late 1980s also provided little incentive for expanded functions. Although the U.S. economy improved, dental caries was in a state of decline, particularly among young people. The emphasis turned to periodontal disease, but not with the idea of delegating its identification and treatment to dental hygienists. Rather, dentists began developing their skills to include periodontal treatment. Thus, though major strides were made to change the day-to-day practice of dental hygiene during the 1970s, there has been no continuing effort to increase the number of functions a dental hygienist can perform. Rather, the focus of the late 1980s and the agenda for the early 1990s is to secure dental hygiene as a profession that serves a vital function in identifying, treating, and preventing disease.

Length and scope of education

Issues of professionalism include defining the appropriate minimum entry criterion for licensure. Should the baccalaureate degree represent the minimum number of years of preparation? Pressure is mounting to make the 4-year degree mandatory for dental hygiene to make its case as a profession (ADHA Resolution, 1986; Kraemer, 1985; Walsh et al, 1988). Even if the dual entry system is retained, it is likely that there will be an effort to redefine the skills expected of graduates of the two levels, with greater expectations of the baccalaureate hygienist (Gluch-Scranton and Rigolizzo Gurenlian, 1985) and changes in the curriculum necessary to prepare hygienists for today's and tomorrow's employment responsibilities (Cohen et al, 1985).

Educational programs differ with regard to what the students learn, according to the legal definition of practice in the state in which the program is located. Therefore a program in a state where the laws have not changed or where the expansion of duties is limited may include only the traditional functions of scaling, polishing, fluoride treatments, exposing radiographs, and recording the medical history and intraoral findings. In another state students may learn local anesthesia, curettage, placement of restorations, and physical evaluation.

Practice roles

Dental hygiene is not what it was in 1960, or so it would seem from all this discussion of changed laws, functions, education, responsibilities, and practice sites. Yet entering students often describe dental hygienists in terms reminiscent of their pre-1960s roles.

After 30 years of debate and attempts at regional and national planning, each state still has its own definition of dental hygiene and assisting practice, with some duties disallowed and others permitted under varying degrees of supervision. The practice of dental hygiene differs from state to state (Table 1-1).

Further, dental hygiene is shifting from a procedure-based to an outcome-oriented profession that focuses on patients' needs and on combining prevention and therapy to help patients achieve jointly determined health goals. Hygienists are using a more comprehensive approach to care, especially among baccalaureate graduates (Benicewicz and Metzger, 1989). In this text, dental hygiene will be described as a continuous process of care rather than as a series of "delegated duties." Though you will learn to approach dental hygiene care from the standpoint of this new approach (or paradigm), you will encounter many clinicians who have not made this transition and who define dental hygiene as "cleaning teeth and teaching brushing and flossing."

Thus the struggle within dental hygiene may not be how to add new functions to the legal definition. Rather, it may be how to rethink clinical practice so that we select components of care based on patient need and take responsibility for providing appropriate care based on a dental hygiene diagnosis and a written treatment plan. The new paradigm will fit the appointment time and content to the specific needs of the patient rather than fitting the patient into a predetermined time and performing, almost by rote, a standard oral prophylaxis for each person who appears for care. It will be less based on mechanical therapy than on the oral medicine aspects of diagnosis and treatment. It will integrate the concept of the patient learning self-care and self-responsibility so that the relationship is a partnership.

Self-regulation

Self-regulation has emerged as the central issue of the 1990s for dental hygiene (Gurenlian, 1991). Dental hygiene has opted to define its own future rather than relying on the path chosen for it by dentistry. To do this, it is likely that the profession will need to 1) accredit its own dental hygiene education programs (currently accredited by the ADA Commission on Dental Accreditation), 2) control its licensure and regulate practice (currently under the purview of state dental boards made up largely of dentists), and 3) control the employment options available to dental hygienists (currently largely defined by employment in a dental office).

An example is increasing representation on state boards of dentistry. Forty-eight states and the District of Columbia have dental hygiene representation on state boards of dentistry (or other governing boards) in varying forms (Grady, 1988), ranging from full representation with one or more voting members to a committee that "advises" the board. This is a vast improvement from 20 years ago, when few state boards even consulted dental hygienists regarding their regulation. However, the power of dental hygiene to influence decisions is hampered by the disproportionate number of dentists on the boards and certain limitations in voting rights and privileges (Reveal, 1989). As a result, several jurisdictions are considering establishment of a dental hygiene practice act and regulatory board that functions separately from dentistry. Improving representation, whether by increasing membership on existing regulatory bodies or by earning our own board, will help dental hygiene define its own future and assume responsibility for its actions.

In Canada, over two-thirds of dental hygienists—those in Ontario, Quebec, and Alberta—have achieved self-regulatory status, and it is being considered in other provinces (Johnson, 1989). The premise behind these changes is consistent with the ideologic differences between Canada and the United States. In Canada, it was a matter of civil rights that one profession not be regulated by another; further, Canadians value equal access to health care and perceive the provision for self-regulation as creating a less restrictive system for licensing and enforcing the scope of practice.

Organized dentistry rarely supports dental hygiene self-regulation, largely because dentists interpret self-regulation as synonymous with unsupervised or independent practice. Challenges to state laws prohibiting unsupervised practice triggered a "turf war" between dental hygiene and dentistry in the 1980s (Morganstein, 1989). Dentistry's concern that dental hygienists could establish a financially and professionally independent setting for providing care carries over to the concept of self-regulation. However, self-regulation does not necessarily mean that unsupervised practice will follow.

One of the central reasons for seeking self-regulation is to ensure that accreditation standards

Table 1-1. Number of states allowing expanded functions for dental assistants and/or hygienists

	Assisting	Hygiene		Assisting	Hygiene
Inspecting the oral cavity	23/49	N/A	Carving amalgams	4/48	9/50
Exposing radiographs	47/49	50/50	Polishing amalgam restorations	15/48	49/50
Performing pulp vitality testing	12/46	17/46	Placing & finishing composite resin restorations	4/49	7/49
Making impressions for study casts	43/49	47/49	Removing excess cement from coronal surfaces of teeth	39/49	N/A
Placing periodontal dressings	23/49	43/50	Scaling coronal surfaces of teeth	1/49	N/A
Removing periodontal dressings	37/49	48/50	Polishing coronal surfaces of teeth	23/49	50/50
Placing sutures	N/A	1/50			
Removing sutures	41/49	47/50	Applying pit & fissure sealants	16/48	46/49
Placing matrices	31/46	36/49	Applying cavity liners and bases	11/49	17/49
Removing matrices	26/46	36/49	Monitoring nitrous oxide analgesia	23/49	29/49
Applying topical anesthetic agents	39/49	N/A	Administration of nitrous oxide analgesia	N/A	12/49
Administering local anesthetic agents by infiltration	N/A	15/50	Performing supragingival scaling	N/A	50/50
Administering local anesthetic agents by block	N/A	12/50	Performing subgingival scaling	N/A	50/50
Applying topical anticariogenic agents	33/49	48/50	Root planing	N/A	49/50
Placing rubber dams	43/49	48/50	Closed gingival curettage	N/A	36/50
Removing rubber dams	42/49	48/50	Cementing bands/bonding brackets	4/47	N/A
Placing temporary restorations	21/49	37/49	Bending archwires	10/47	N/A
Removing temporary restorations	21/49	30/49			
Placing amalgams for condensation by the dentist	10/49	11/49			
Placing & condensing amalgams	5/49	7/49			

NOTE: The number to the left of the (/) is the total number of jurisdictions that permit delegation of the function. The number to the right of the (/) is the total number of jurisdictions that provided information on the specific function.

N/A - Not applicable as an expanded function (either not allowed *or* not considered "expanded" for that group). For instance, administering anesthesia is not allowed anywhere for dental assistants, while scaling coronal surfaces is a long-standing function for hygienists.

are not lowered to provide for on-the-job, preceptor training for dental hygienists. Requirements specify at least 2 years of formal education. If preceptorship is approved, formal education will be restricted to a short didactic program, and clinical education will occur largely in individual dental offices with the dentist serving as the educator. This situation exists only in Alabama, although there have been numerous proposals to institute such a program in other states. Regressing to preceptor training will deter the movement from "duties" to "thinking" and will make it difficult for clinicians to see the need to move away from the rote approach to clinical care (see Studstill, 1990 and Hein, 1990 for a summary of the debate).

Unsupervised practice

Only one state, Colorado, permits unsupervised practice (Colorado, 1986). All others require some degree of supervision by a licensed dentist.

The ADA describes the concept of unsupervised practice as a major threat to the health of the public. Its leaders see this development as the establishment of two standards of care. If dental hygienists were to secure universal status as independent practitioners who could choose to work with a dentist or not, it would also have a financial impact on most practices that currently employ dental hygienists. Referring patients to a contracting or independent dental hygienist would mean lost income to the practice without a hygienist.

The option of unsupervised practice may change the way in which an employer dentist treats an employee. If the employee could become a competitor by opening a dental hygiene practice, the dentist is more likely to ensure his or her continued satisfaction. A controlled research program in California demonstrated that unsupervised practice can be financially viable and provide comparable or superior care when compared with dental practices (Kushman, 1991).

Dental hygiene research

Much of dental hygiene practice is derived from traditional approaches to care, with minimal reliance on a sound scientific base. If only principles based on solid research were included in this text, it would be much shorter. Fortunately, there has been a considerable focus on dental research in areas relating to dental hygiene. Thus we have learned much in the past 10 years about the disease processes we identify, treat, and prevent. Some of the practices we have followed for years have been proven to be sound approaches to care; others have been shown to be less useful. This text will focus on many of the changes in our beliefs about clinical procedures.

If dental hygiene is to become a self-regulated profession it must be research based. It should have a framework for planning and conducting research so that appropriate research questions are identified and answered through well-controlled trials or appropriate surveys and field studies. The profession needs to systematically develop a base for research findings that can be translated into clinical practice. It must build a bridge between research and daily patient care (Bowen, 1990).

Thus the issues facing our profession today will define what the profession will be tomorrow. These issues are challenging, exciting, and extremely important.

PREPARING FOR THE FUTURE

It is important for the beginning dental hygiene student to learn the ideal, the conceptual, and the futuristic models of dental hygiene as well as the realistic, immediately applicable models. Graduates may need to be able to function within delivery systems of the past, present, and future. For this reason, the scope of practice is broadly defined as *dental hygiene care*.

Creating change

Change should be planned rather than haphazard or the result of uncontrolled external influences. Whenever a profession is contemplating or creating dramatic change, it is important to consider what aspects of that profession's culture should be kept and which should be changed.

A key to addressing this issue was discussed at the 1987 Second National Conference on Dental Hygiene Research: defining dental hygiene's professional culture. *Professional culture* comprises those characteristics which are unique to the profession. It is defined by specifying the terms and conditions that describe and differentiate a profession from all other professions and from closely related vocations. Though dentistry and dental hygiene share many cultural elements, there must be characteristics that differentiate dental hygienists from dentists as a group. This way of defining dental hygiene becomes the "germ cell" of our profession, a reference point that helps us realize who we are, even as we diversify and grow within the profession (Dickoff and James, 1988).

Subsequent workshops with hygienists from 10 states identified these common cultural characteristics: caring, gentle, meticulous, listening, communicating, detail conscious, dedicated, prevention oriented, service oriented, motivated less by monetary gain than by service, female, persevering, healer, altruistic, cottage-industry based, and competent. The participants identified those characteristics that they believed should be retained and those that should be changed or eliminated.

This list does not completely define dental hygiene's culture; rather, it represents a first effort. In looking for and defining the characteristics of professional culture, answers to the following questions are necessary:

1. Are there times when a person should see a dental hygienist rather than a dentist for certain aspects of care? What are they?
2. What characteristics make dental hygienists more like each other than like dentists?
3. What functions do dental hygienists perform that dentists tend to disregard or treat perfunctorily?
4. What makes dental hygienists different from nurses and other health professionals?
5. When you envision a dental hygienist, what characteristics do you attribute to that person?
6. How are graduating dental hygienists different from entering dental hygiene students?
7. When a dental hygienist lists several characteristics, which ones trigger immediate group agreement among other hygienists?

As dental hygienists continue to define dental hygiene culture, the core of the profession should become apparent. The research focus emerging from that core will identify questions, hypotheses, and projects to improve our understanding of giving care. It can help us to identify appropriate practice settings, claim new technology as appropriate for dental hygiene, and create the basis for evaluating our progress in emerging as a key profession in the delivery of oral health care.

ACTIVITIES

1. Ask a dentist what he or she believes are the functions of a hygienist. Compare replies in class and see how accurately they reflect the skills and the overall role the student will learn. Identify which skills require assimilation "thinking" and/or mechanical "doing."
2. Discuss each of the phases of the dental hygiene appointment, using the program model of assessment, planning, implementation, and evaluation.
3. Review functions that are legally allowable in different states. Summarize the variety of ways in which *supervision* is defined. Select the states in which you may seek licensure. This information can be found in the American Dental Association's most recent edition of *Legal Provisions for Delegating Functions to Dental Assistants and Dental Hygienists*.
4. Review publications written by hygienists about their practice sites, particularly those that differ from traditional solo and group practices. Discuss the advantages and disadvantages of each role and what special skills or interests a hygienist would need to fulfill them.
5. Read one or more "alternative employment" profiles in Dreyer R: *Career Directions for Dental Hygienists,* Holmdel, NJ, 1991, Career Directions. Discuss how hygienists build on their basic education in dental hygiene to qualify for other career opportunities.
6. Read and discuss Darby's "Collaborative Practice Model" (Darby ML: *J Dent Educ* 47:589, 1983).
7. Review the current literature to locate other articles on the future of dental hygiene. Conduct a panel discussion on one of the major issues receiving attention.
8. Read the research report from the California experiment and discuss its results and complications.

REVIEW QUESTIONS

1. Briefly define a philosophy of patient-centered care.
2. Why may faculty members' perceptions of dental hygiene education and practice differ from students' perceptions?
3. What effect do dental practice acts have:
   a. On the scope of practice?
   b. On educational programs?
4. What impact might the legalization of independent practice have on dental hygiene?
5. Define *professional culture*.

REFERENCES

American Dental Hygienists' Association Resolutions SR-45-71; R-17-Am-73-H; SR-18-73-H; R-30-73-H; R-10-Am-75; SR-36-Am-76; R-56-1976-H; and 14-88.

Annual report on dental auxiliary education, 1968-1969. Chicago, 1969, American Dental Association, Division of Educational Measurements, Council on Dental Education.

Annual report on dental auxiliary education, 1977-1978. Chicago, 1978, American Dental Association, Division of Educational Measurements, Council on Dental Education.

Benicewicz D, Metzger C: Supervision and practice of dental hygienists: report of ADHA survey, *J Dent Hyg,* 63:173-180, 1989.

Bowen DM: Dental hygiene research: issues and challenges of the next decade, *Can Dent Hyg Probe* 24:163, 1990.

The Carnegie Commission on Higher Education: *Higher education and the nation's health: policies for medical and dental education,* New York, 1970, McGraw-Hill.

The Carnegie Council on Policy Studies in Higher Education: *Progress and problems in medical and dental education: federal support versus federal control.* San Francisco, 1976, Jossey-Bass.

Carr S: Factors influencing the career selection of first-year dental hygiene students, *J Dent Hyg* 63:266-271, 1989.

Cohen L, LaBelle A, Singer J: Educational preparation of hygienists working with special populations in nontraditional settings, *J Dent Educ* 49:592, 1985.

Colorado passes unsupervised practice, *ADA News* 17(10):5, 1986.

Darby ML: Collaborative practice model: the future of dental hygiene, *J Dent Educ* 47:589, 1983.

Dickoff J, james P: Organization and expansion of knowledge toward a constructive assault on the imperious distinction of pure from applied knowledge, of knowledge from technique, *Dent Hyg* 62:15, 1988.

Dreyer R: *Career directions for dental hygienists,* Holmdel, NJ, 1991, Career Directions.

Gluch-Scranton J, Rigolizzo, Gurenlian J: A model for two-year and baccalaureate clinical dental hygiene education, *J Dent Educ* 49:95, 1985.

Grady A: Dental hygienists and state boards of dentistry: an overview of the legislative action packet, *Dent Hyg* 62:87, 1988.

Gurenlian J: The self-regulation of dental hygiene, *J Dent Hyg,* 65:104, 1991.

Hein JW: Dental hygiene education: the case for the currently accredited model, *J Am Coll Dent* 57:14, 1990.

Hollinshead BS: *Survey of dentistry,* Washington, DC, 1961, American Council on Education.

Johnson P: Self-regulation for dental hygienist: the Canadian example, *J Dent Hyg* 63:294, 1989.

Kraemer LG: The dental hygiene entry dilemma: an issue of prestige, image and professional credibility, *Dent Hyg* 59:117, 1985.

Kushman JE: *Final report to American Dental Hygienists' Association on California Health Manpower Pilot Project 139: Independent Practice of Dental Hygienists,* University of Delaware, 1991.

Legal provisions for delegating functions to dental assistants and dental hygienists, Chicago, 1991, American Dental Association, Division of Education.

Morganstein WM: Auxiliary personnel in dentistry: an epoch of turf, trends, and territoriality. *Am J Hosp Pharm* 46:507, 1989.

Reveal M: Dental hygiene regulation and practice, *J Pub Health Dent,* 49:228, 1989.

Rubinstein L, Brand MK: A description of postcertificate dental hygiene programs, *J Dent Educ* 50:608, 1986.

Studstill ZD: Dental hygiene education: the case for the Alabama dental hygiene program, *J Am Coll Dent* 57:15, 1990.

Walsh MM et al: The bachlor's degree as the entry-level credential for dental hygiene practice, *J Dent Hyg* 62:509-513, 1988.

PREPARATION

Imagine that you are anticipating the arrival of your first dental hygiene patient. What would you need to have learned to provide meaningful, helpful care to the person looking to you with trust? This text is designed to help you, the new clinician, be ready when that day arrives. This portion of the text covers the fundamental skills you must master before you see a patient. It is important to know how to operate the equipment you will have at your fingertips. You need to know how to prevent cross-infecting your patients with microorganisms brought to your operatory and how to protect yourself from infection. You also need to know how to find your way through the preparation of a dental record.

When you have completed this portion you should be ready to move on to assessing a patient's current health status.

2 PREPARING THE CLINICAL SITE: OPERATION AND MAINTENANCE OF EQUIPMENT

Donna J. Stach

LEARNING OUTCOMES

The dental hygeniest will be able to

1. Identify, operate, and/or adjust the following operatory equipment:
   a. Dental chair, including lowering, raising, tilting, and lowering back; rotating chair; and positioning headrest, if adjustable
   b. Dental unit, including operating air-water syringe, handpiece, prophylaxis angle, saliva ejector, high-volume suction, and cuspidor (if applicable)
   c. Overhead light
   d. Clinician's and assistant's stools
   e. Sink and soap dispenser
2. Given any of the common components of the dental operatory, identify basic maintenance procedures to improve its longevity and ensure its cleanliness and satisfactory appearance.
3. Given a series of mechanical or cleanliness problems associated with equipment, identify how the problems could have been prevented.

Most dental services are more easily provided with dental equipment specifically designed for the comfort of the patient, clinician, and assistant and for housing special electrically powered or air-powered equipment. This includes a dental chair; a dental unit with overhead intraoral illumination, air, water, high- and slow-speed rotary engines, and high-volume evacuation equipment to remove fluids from the patient's mouth; and stools for the clinician and the assistant (Richardson and Barton, 1978; Snyder and Domer, 1983).

It is helpful to be completely familiar with the dental equipment and its function before seating a patient. This section describes the operation and control of various pieces of equipment. Because dental equipment varies among manufacturers and over time and because most large pieces of equipment are designed for years of productive service, dental hygienists are likely to operate many different styles of equipment during their careers. Although every operatory is different, many principles of operation and maintenance are common to most models. In addition to the generally applicable guidelines presented, a maxim to follow is to *read the directions* provided by the manufac-

turer. Once the directions have been reviewed, it is wise to follow suggestions for cleaning, lubricating, and securing periodic maintenance evaluations and to retain the brochures, warranties, and instructions for future reference.

Properly maintained equipment will break down less often and require replacement less frequently. Considering the cost of dental equipment and the importance of productive hours of "chair time," care in using and maintaining equipment results in less frustration and is an important cost-effective measure (Richardson and Barton, 1978; Young, 1991b).

As you acquaint yourself with the dental operatory, look for potential sources of cross-contamination. Disease transmission theory, sterilization, disinfection, and barrier use are discussed in detail in Chapter 3, but begin to think about the potential for contamination as you explore any new dental equipment. Depending on the material, surface configuration, and location of equipment and controls this may be easier or harder to accomplish. In general, newer equipment is designed to facilitate maintenance of an aseptic field.

THE DENTAL CHAIR

The dental chair supports the patient comfortably while allowing the operator maximum access to the oral cavity. Chair backs should be thin to allow the operator's legs to fit underneath (Chasteen, 1989).

Most modern dental chairs are of the contour or lounge type, which allow flexible patient positioning with relative ease. There are usually two or three controls located on the chair back or a foot switch (Fig. 2-1) that provide a range of adjustments. One button or switch will *raise* or *lower the back* of the chair, and a second will *tilt* the entire chair back so that the footrest rises and the headrest lowers without changing the angle between the back and the seat of the chair. An optional third button will automatically place the patient in a standard working position or return the patient to an upright seated position. The control to raise or lower the entire chair is usually located at the base of the chair and is operated by foot.

With these basic controls it is possible to (1) seat the patient in an upright position, (2) tilt the chair back so that the patient's hips are well seated at the angle of the chair, (3) lower the back of the chair so that the patient is in the supine position, and (4) raise or lower the entire chair to the correct height for the clinician (Figs. 2-2 to

2-4). The patient's back should receive full support from the chair.

Most models allow for *rotating* the chair on its axis. This control is usually located at the base of the chair. It allows the clinician to seat the patient with maximum space for patient maneuvering and then rotate the chair to approximate other stationary equipment and to facilitate the seating of the clinician and assistant. This is particularly useful for left-handed clinicians.

It is helpful to identify the full range of adjustment for each chair. This allows optimal patient positioning and saves the clinician the embarrassment of running the chair up and down when it is obviously supposed to tilt back. Some chairs have locking devices in which one press of a button

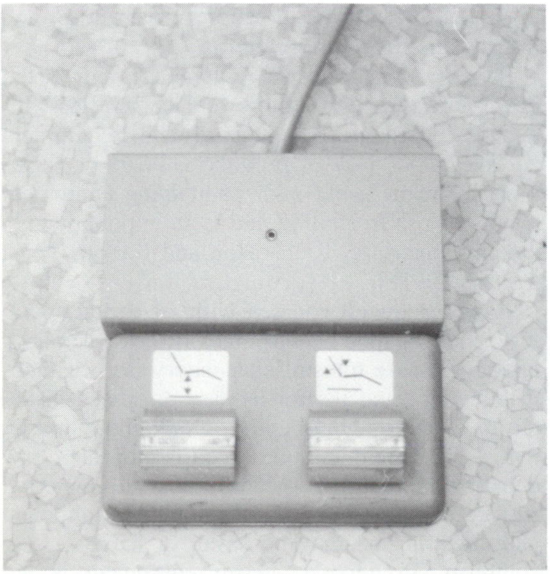

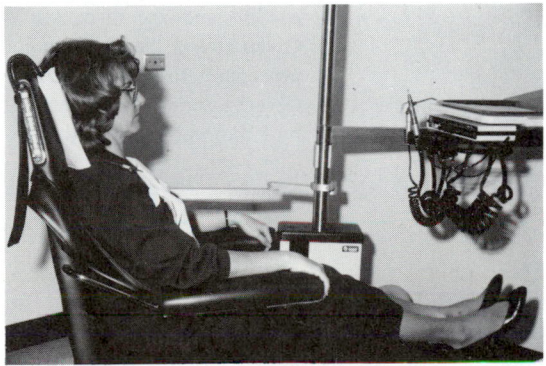

Fig. 2-2. Dental lounge chair positioned with back upright. Patient should be seated with the chair in this position as the first step in attaining the supine position.

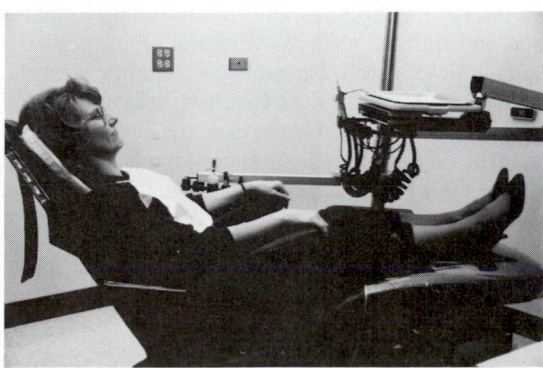

Fig. 2-3. Second step in placing patient in supine position. Chair is tilted backward so that patient's hips are well seated in angle of chair.

Fig. 2-1. Foot switch that controls positioning of the dental chair.

will move the patient to a full reclining position. The clinician who intends only a minor chair adjustment may find this "runaway chair" quite unexpected (Weinert, 1971).

With increased emphasis on asepsis, dental chairs have evolved into sleeker designs that are easier to clean. Chair surfaces should be as smooth and seamless as possible and have a sur-

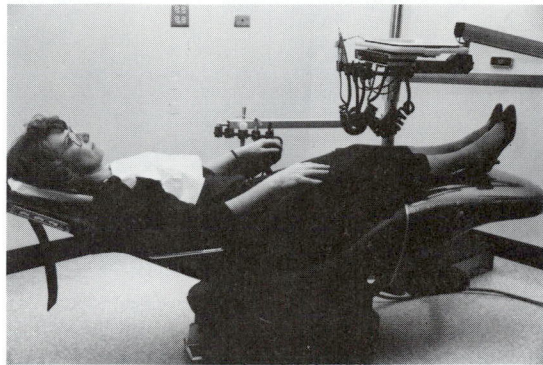

Fig. 2-4. Third step in placing patient in supine position. Back of chair is lowered until patient is in full supine position with toes and chin at approximately the same height. Overall height of chair can then be adjusted to position of seated clinician.

face that can withstand repeated cleaning and disinfection (Cottone, 1991; Young, 1991a). Hand-operated control switches have high potential for cross-contamination because of grooves and crevices. They also have the potential for electrical short circuits if spray disinfectant is used. Foot controls for all chair functions are highly desirable and can be retrofitted to most dental units (Cottone, 1991; Young, 1991a).

Headrest adjustments also vary from chair to chair. In most modern chairs the headrest is in the same plane as the back of the chair. Two common variations are a removable horseshoe- or donut-shaped piece that fits over a solid chair back (Fig. 2-5) or a slightly contoured section that may be hinged to allow adjustments in head tilt (Fig. 2-6). In some cases this top section can be extended or removed entirely from the chair back, allowing modification for very tall patients or small children (Weinert, 1971).

For chairs with the multijointed headrest, the best rule to follow in positioning the headrest is to seat the patient in the fully supine position and then adjust the headrest so that the pads, or bowl, of the headrest are located behind the occipital bone. With the patient's head in the headrest, the clinician can raise or lower the whole unit (head

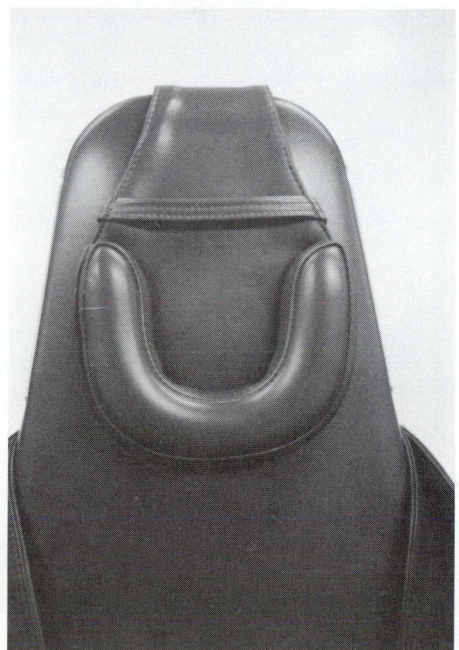

Fig. 2-5. Horseshoe-shaped headrest that positions the head on a smooth chair back.

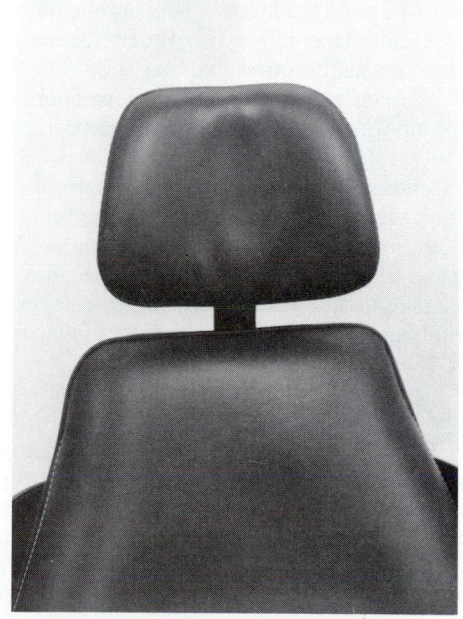

Fig. 2-6. Adjustable headrest that allows tilting and angling of the patient's head. This chair section can be extended or removed.

and headrest) until the patient's neck is in the same plane with the spine (Fig. 2-7).

THE DENTAL UNIT

The electrical circuitry for many chairs is connected to the master switches for the dental unit. If a modular cart is connected to the main circuitry for air and water flow, high-volume suction, and other systems, there may be a second master switch on the cart itself.

Because of the high potential for contamination and difficulty in cleaning, the switches for dental units are moving undercover or out of the immediate patient treatment area. Three examples of solutions used in newly designed dental units are (1) seamless touch pads, (2) remote wall-mounted control panels (Young, 1991a), and (3) infrared sensors that detect and switch on a handpiece as it is removed from its carrier.

Once all switches are located and activated, the following pieces of equipment should be tested for proper function:

Air-water syringe

Sometimes referred to as a *trisyringe* or *triplex syringe* (Fig. 2-8), the air-water syringe enables the clinician or assistant to direct a stream of water, air, or an air-water spray onto the operative site. Usually there is one button for air and one for water, with spray produced when both buttons are pushed simultaneously. The tip of the air-water syringe is usually removable and should be sterilized between patients; in a few newer units, the entire air-water syringe snaps off for sterilization.

The syringe has outdated the cup of water that for decades was the primary means for rinsing. Current practices include irrigating the oral cavity with an air-water spray and evacuating the resultant fluid and debris by high-volume suction or an efficient saliva ejector. "Cuspidor calisthenics" throughout the appointment are no longer necessary.

If a cuspidor is included with the unit and used by the patients, it is important to locate the controls for the volume of water. It is possible to overflow a cuspidor if the volume of water flow is too great. Conversely, a mere trickle is inadequate to clear away debris. The trap in the cuspidor should be removed at the completion of each appointment and freed of debris, both for appearance and to ensure proper drainage (Richardson and Barton, 1978). This task may be another reason for the popularity of high-volume suction.

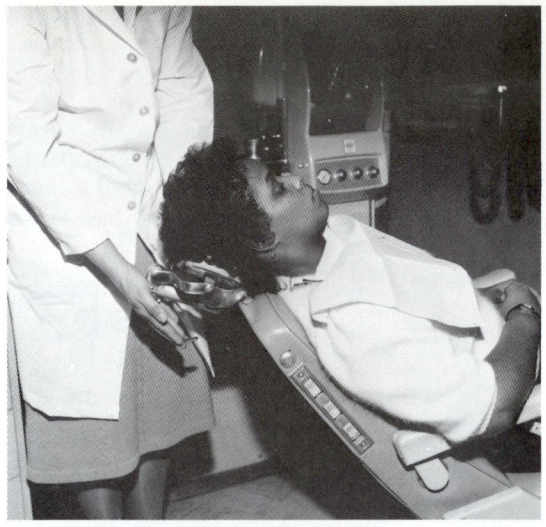

Fig. 2-7. Adjust hinged headrest so that occipital bone at base of skull is resting on padding and neck is in same plane as patient's back. When these criteria are met and patient is comfortable, lock headrest in place by pushing up on lever.

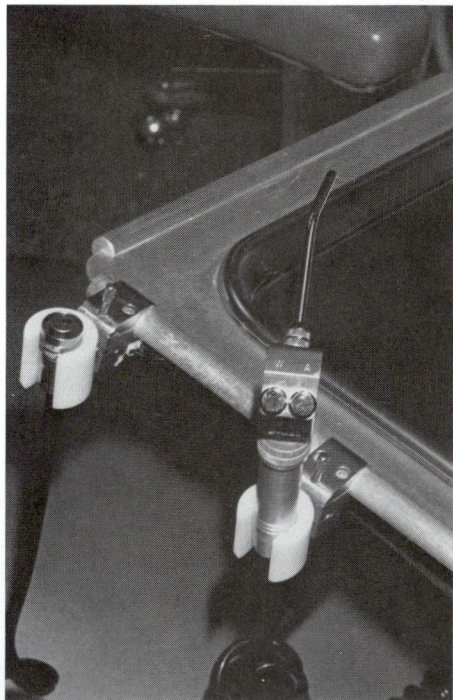

Fig. 2-8. Air-water syringe includes a button for water and a button for air; activating both buttons results in air-water spray that is ideal for flushing oral cavity. Routine use of this device eliminates the need for frequent rinsing with a cup of water.

Oral evacuation attachments

The passively gurgling saliva ejector of yesteryear has been replaced by *high-speed suction* and an efficient *saliva ejector*. High-speed or high-volume suction was introduced to dental practice to enable rapid removal of the coolant water that accompanies the high-speed drill (Richardson and Barton, 1978). It is also useful in removing the water used with the ultrasonic scaler and in evacuating the mouth with frequent use of an air-water spray. In dental hygiene procedures in which loosened deposits, polishing pastes, and necrotic tissue need to be flushed from the sulcus around each tooth, the air-water spray and the oral evacuation are close companions. Evacuation is, of course, also useful for restorative procedures and for helping remove saliva during fluoride and sealant applications.

Saliva ejector tips traditionally have been, and still may be, bent into shapes that sit comfortably in the floor of the patient's mouth during the treatment. However, modern equipment will quickly remove a great quantity of fluid. Saliva ejectors are often used like a reverse straw, with patients closing their lips around the tip and letting the fluids be drawn out of the mouth.

The evacuation lines should be flushed between patients and disinfected more thoroughly at the end of each day (Young, 1991a). Tips used intraorally should be sterilized or discarded if disposable. Many mobile carts and individual saliva ejectors contain traps to catch large particulate matter. These must be cleaned daily.

Hoses and tubing

All hoses, whether for handpieces or oral evacuation, should be smooth and seamless both inside and out to facilitate disinfection. Straight hoses are preferred over curved or coiled tubing and exposed over retractable hoses because they are easier to clean (Cottone, 1991; Young, 1991a). Straight, smooth cords can usually be retrofitted onto older units. If hoses on retractable reels are used they should be gently withdrawn from storage and carefully replaced, not stuffed back into their compartments. Another advantage of straight cords is the avoidance of tug-back, which is a factor in hand fatigue and may be a factor in carpal tunnel syndrome (Gerwatowski et al, 1992).

Rotary engine equipment

It is important to know which hoses are for high speed and which are for low speed and which handpieces are intended for each.

A complete dental operatory includes slow- and high-speed rotary equipment powered by electricity (electrotorque) or compressed air (air torque, air rotor). A slow-speed handpiece is used for finishing and polishing restorations, for some steps in cavity preparation, and for polishing teeth. It operates at approximately 6000 revolutions per minute (rpm) and offers sufficient torque power to facilitate removal of stains when an abrasive agent is applied to the tooth with a rubber cup or brush attachment. High-speed handpieces operate at over 100,000 rpm (Sockwell, 1971).

The handpieces are activated by a foot pedal, called a *rheostat*. Depending on the design, the pedal can be activated by pressing down, by moving a lever to the side, or by rotating a disk. Pushing the lever or disk in one direction causes the handpiece to move forward; moving it in the opposite direction runs it backward. Fig. 2-9 shows one type of rheostat, which is activated by downward foot pressure.

Handpieces, whether for electric, air, or belt-driven engines, require regular cleaning, lubrication and sterilization (ADA Councils, 1988; Centers for Disease Control, 1986, 1987; Young, 1991a & b). It is imperative to follow the manu-

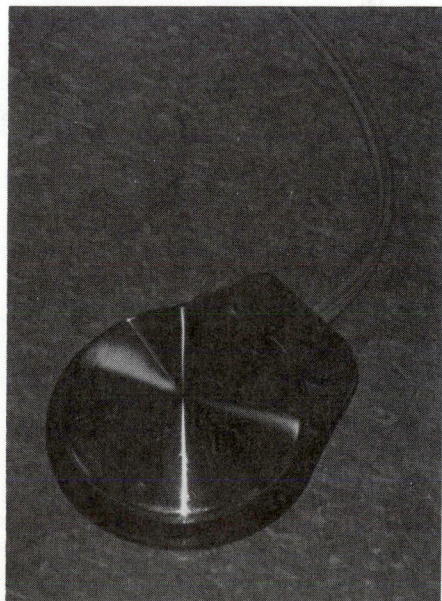

Fig. 2-9. Foot pedal adjusts speed of operation of handpiece. This style requires downward foot pressure. Other styles have a pedal that rotates with a push of the foot.

facturer's directions for each handpiece because these are complex and valuable pieces of equipment and the product warranty may be voided if instructions are not followed (Cottone, 1991; Young, 1991a). Problems with handpieces most often arise from improper air pressure or cleaning and lubrication. Manufacturer specifications must be followed carefully (Young, 1991b).

The prophylaxis "prophy" angle is attached to the slow-speed handpiece and adapts the torque power of the handpiece for the specific purpose of polishing teeth or restorations. Prophylaxis angles are either single use and disposable or reusable, in which case they must be carefully cleaned and sterilized between patients. Most reusable angles need to be completely disassembled and cleaned after each polishing procedure, since the abrasive polishing paste easily enters the gears of the device, and wears them away, usually clogging the mechanism so that it freezes shut. A few brands are sealed so that entry of debris is reduced or eliminated. These brands are accompanied by specific maintenance directions that must be followed carefully to ensure longevity of the angle.

There are a variety of methods for attaching rubber cups or brushes to prophylaxis angles to hold the polishing paste against the tooth. (See Chapter 30 for discussion of these methods.)

Overhead light

Once all the unit controls are identified and found to be functional, it is appropriate to locate and turn on the overhead, intraoral light. Usually there is a single switch on the light itself. A special high-intensity lamp shines out onto a highly reflective concave surface that focuses the light rays so that they may be directed to illuminate the oral cavity. The reflective surface should be polished at least daily to ensure brightness. This should be done at the start of the day when the lamp is cool (Williams and Williams, 1982a).

The lamp should be allowed to cool before a burned-out bulb is replaced. Because lights often fail when they are first switched on, the lamp may still be cool to the touch and not cause a schedule delay. If the dental light has a quartz halogen bulb, only the sleeve should be handled, as fingerprints can cause the bulb to explode or to burn out more quickly. Sealed-beam bulbs require that the entire unit containing the bulb be replaced. A spare bulb or unit should be kept available for replacement and reordered according to specifica-

tions on the package as soon as a bulb is used. In some units a fuse in the dental lamp will blow at the same time that the bulb fails. Extra fuses should be kept for this reason (Williams and Williams, 1982a).

Many overhead lights are covered by a plastic shield as a safety precaution against an exploding lamp or shattering reflector. A piece of metal flung from rotary equipment could easily trigger such an accident.

To diminish wear on the switch and the lamp, the overhead light should be turned on at the beginning of the appointment and left on for the duration of the visit. When not in use, it can be directed down from the patient's face. Turning the lamp on and off causes it to burn out more rapidly than leaving it on. As with any mechanical switch, each use causes wear. Many clinicians leave the overhead light on all day if a succession of patients is to receive care, turning it off only during extended periods of nonuse, such as the lunch period. It should, of course, be turned off at the end of the day, as should all switches on the unit. Leaving a dental unit on for extended periods of nonuse will burn out its electrical components.

Another precaution is to shut off the water supply so that pressure is not exerted against the tubing in the unit. Rises in water pressure occur most often at night; thus so do floods in operatories where the water is left on overnight (Williams and Williams, 1982b).

CLINICIAN'S AND ASSISTANT'S STOOLS

When all main equipment appears to be functional and the hygienist is familiar with its operation, the clinician's and assistant's stools should be adjusted for their intended occupants. The height of the operator's stool should be adjusted so that the feet are flat on the floor and the thighs are parallel to the floor. The back support should be adjusted both vertically and horizontally to support the lumbar region of the back. The height of the assistant's stool should allow an eye level about 4 to 6 inches above the clinician's. This will require a ring or platform on the stool on which the feet can rest. Because the assistant often leans forward during treatment, an abdominal rest on the assistant's stool is customary. This should be adjusted to fit below the rib cage to provide optimal body support. Neither the clinician nor the assistant should feel the pressure of the stool against the back of the thighs, because that position inhibits blood circulation to the legs (Chasteen, 1989; Harris and Crabb, 1978; Richardson and Barton, 1978).

Stool adjustments should be customized for each person. Because of the wide variety of adjustment mechanisms, read equipment instructions and experiment before the patient arrives.

THE SINK

The sink is another essential item of equipment. It should be used for thorough scrubbing at the beginning of a clinical period and for thorough hand washing before seeing each patient and after touching an item that may have microorganisms other than those specific to the patient's oral flora (cross-contaminants).

Ideally, the sink and the soap dispenser will be controlled by a foot pedal. This obviously decreases the possibility that the sink will be a fomite for transferring bacteria from patient to patient.

Towel dispensers should allow the person to grasp and remove a single paper towel without touching the dispenser itself.

STORAGE CABINETRY AND TRAY SYSTEMS

The use of a tray system for the delivery of dental instruments is almost universal. Preset trays are prepared in a support room and delivered to the operatory, where they are used either on a bracket table, attached by a hinged arm to the dental chair, or on a mobile cart. The bracket table or mobile cart should be as seamless and smooth as possible (Young, 1991a). They also have carriers for the air-water syringe, handpieces, and suction equipment (Fig. 2-10).

Most operatories allow for some storage of supplies, instruments and auxiliary equipment. The trend is to keep this to a minimum and streamline the treatment room so that all equipment not in use is covered and protected. Supplies are brought into the treatment area as needed, ideally in the amount needed per patient.

OTHER DENTAL OPERATORY EQUIPMENT

Other essential dental equipment includes the viewbox for mounting and interpreting radiographic films. It should be located at the chairside so that the exposed films are readily available

throughout a procedure. Likewise, it is convenient to have x-ray equipment in the operatory (Fig. 2-11) to expose films when indicated. The room must, of course, be lead lined and provide complete protection for the clinician. Because of the cost of lead lining and the amount of room needed to manipulate radiographic equipment, it may be located in a separate operatory for a number of clinicians to use as needed.

Ultrasonic or sonic equipment for periodontal scaling and debridement should be included in the operatory. There may also be an amalgamator for triturating metal alloys for amalgam restorations.

STERILIZATION OR EQUIPMENT SUPPORT ROOM

Sterilizing and cleaning equipment should be located in a nearby room or central laboratory area. Standard equipment should include one of the following sterilizers: (1) an autoclave (Fig. 2-12), (2) dry heat, (3) unsaturated chemical vapor, or (4) rapid heat transfer (Miller, 1992). Each sterilization system has its own advantages, precautions, and maintenance. Familiarize yourself with the ones you are likely to use. (See Chapter 3 for

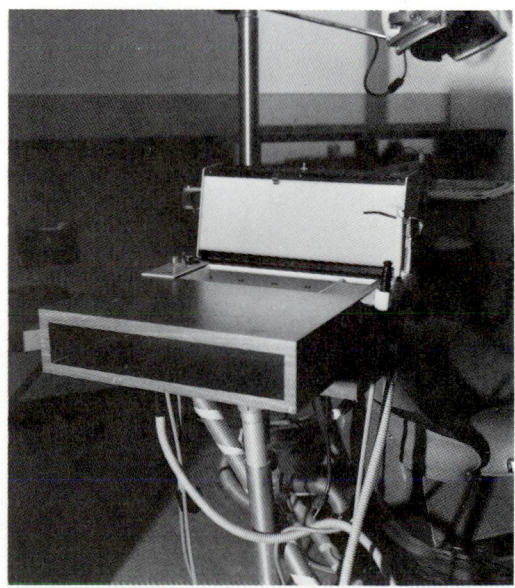

Fig. 2-10. Cart outfitted with trisyringe, evacuation system, and handpiece for slow- or high-speed use may be all that is needed as a "dental unit" for many intraoral procedures.

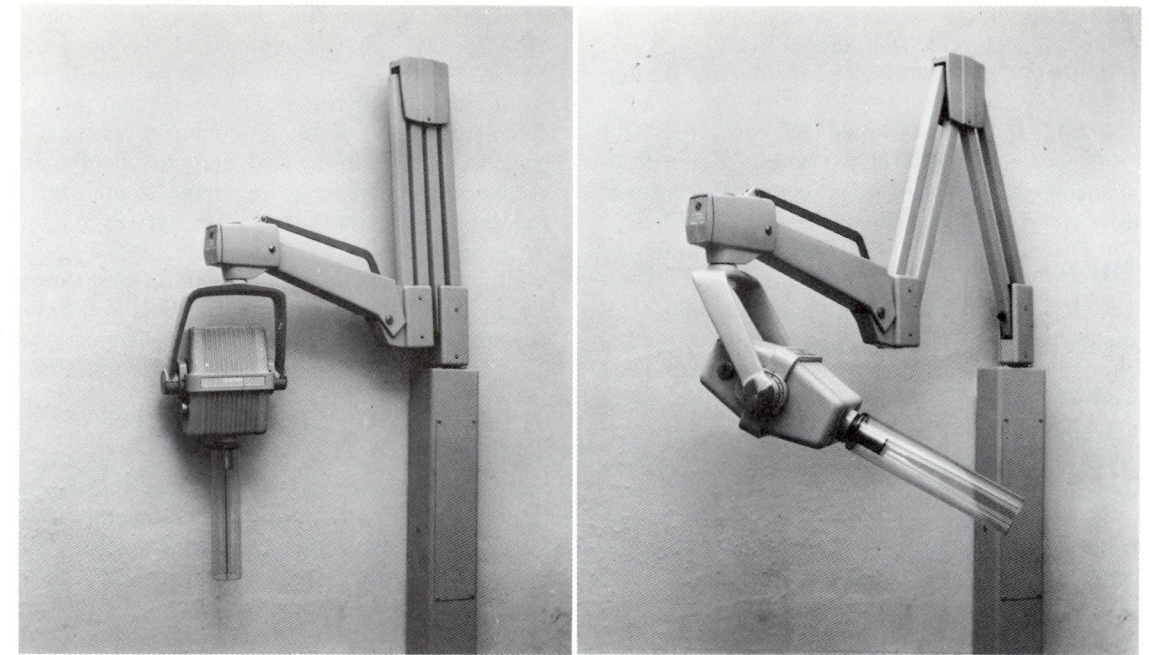
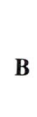

A   B

Fig. 2-11. **A,** X-ray unit should be stored so that all hinges are closed. This places less stress on hinges and helps prevent eventual "drifting" of head away from patient's face during its use. **B,** Improperly stored x-ray unit.

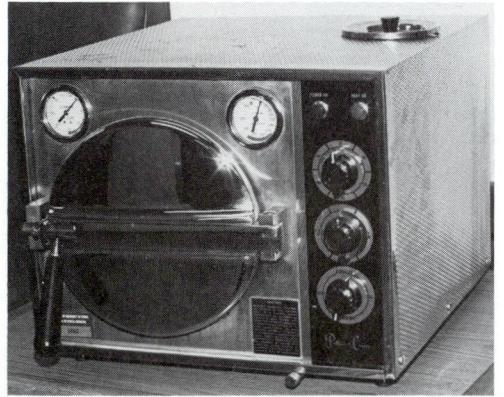

Fig. 2-12. Autoclave provides complete sterilization of instruments and other materials that are able to withstand steam under pressure.

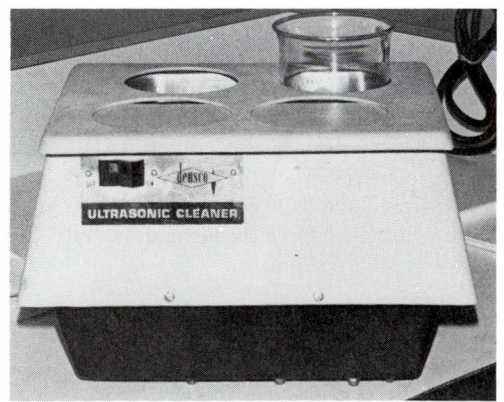

Fig. 2-13. Ultrasonic cleaner removes debris from instruments before they are packaged for sterilization.

further discussion of the use of sterilizing equipment.)

Ultrasonic cleaning tanks are recommended to remove debris from instruments (Fig. 2-13). The ultrasonic cleaner should be drained frequently (at least once a day), the tank washed, and fresh solution mixed and added. Proper proportions of solution should be used, and the level of solution must be maintained to ensure proper cavitation and cleaning.

GENERAL CARE OF EQUIPMENT

It is essential that every patient be treated in a clean, safe environment. The bulk of effort will be directed toward presenting the patient with chemically disinfected and barrier-covered surfaces and sterilized instruments and equipment whenever feasible. These processes are detailed in Chapter 3.

Beyond sanitization, dental equipment also needs maintenance to ensure longevity and good service. The owner's manual for an individual piece of equipment or direct contact with a manufacturer's representative is the best source of specific maintenance instruction.

The dental environment also must appear clean and tidy. For example, leather and vinyl products should be cleaned regularly with an oil soap that will prevent drying and cracking. The crease where the chair back and seat meet should be cleaned by placing the back of the chair all the way down, and the chair base should be wiped daily to remove dust and debris. This attention to specific cleaning needs as well as general disinfection is important for long service and pleasant appearance.

The best check of a clean unit is to take the role of a patient yourself—enter the operatory, sit in the dental chair, and look around both from an upright and reclining position. This provides a patient's-eye view of the otherwise hidden spot of blood, the bespeckled light reflector, the cobweb in the corner, and the red disclosing solution under the lip of the infamous cuspidor.

The benefits of this attention to detail include positive patient responses to the general environment; more dependable, functional equipment; improved safety for the patient, clinician, and assistant; and longer-lasting, newer-looking equipment.

• • •

This chapter has addressed some general points concerning cleanliness and prevention of cross-contamination. Chapter 3 focuses on aseptic techniques and control of microorganisms in the dental operatory.

ACTIVITIES

1. In groups of three, use a search-and-discovery technique to explore a dental operatory in the dental hygiene clinic and elsewhere. (Students should rotate from clinician to patient to assistant roles.) Locate and operate the following items:
   a. Dental chair
      (1) Raise and lower
      (2) Tilt chair back
      (3) Lower back of chair
      (4) Adjust headrest
      (5) Rotate
   b. Dental unit
      (1) Master switch(es)
      (2) Air-water syringe
         (a) Air
         (b) Water
         (c) Air-water spray
      (3) Handpiece
         (a) Mount to hose
         (b) Operate forward and reverse
         (c) Clean, lubricate, and prepare for sterilization
         (d) Differentiate high and low speeds
      (4) Prophylaxis angle
         (a) Mount on handpiece
         (b) Attach cup and brush
         (c) Run forward and backward
         (d) Clean, lubricate, and prepare for sterilization
      (5) Suction
         (a) Insert high-speed suction tip and funnel
         (b) Attach saliva ejector tip
         (c) Activate
         (d) Clean surfaces and traps
   c. Adjust stool to proper height
      (1) Assistant's stool
      (2) Operator's stool
   d. Turn on overhead light
      (1) Change lamp in overhead light
      (2) Clean reflector and shield
   e. Identify presence of
      (1) Ultrasonic and/or sonic scaling equipment
      (2) Amalgamator
      (3) Radiographic equipment
   f. Clean the dental chair
   g. Clean the dental unit
   h. Operate sink and soap dispenser
2. Inspect dental equipment for proper function. Discuss how breakage or wear could be prevented.

3. Visit dental offices with modern equipment and offices with older equipment to determine how different models function and how they are maintained.
4. Attend a professional meeting at which equipment is displayed. Learn about and report the differences and similarities regarding function and recommended maintenance. Calculate what an operatory of equipment costs, itemizing each essential component.
5. Change a belt on a belt-driven engine.

REVIEW QUESTIONS

1. The overhead light (should/should not) be left on throughout a treatment sequence.
2. The proper sequence for adjusting the dental chair when seating a patient is (five steps).
3. The three functions of the air-water syringe are ___.
4. If a prophylaxis angle "freezes" or will not move, even though the handpiece itself is functional, the probable cause is _____.
5. The clinician's stool should be adjusted so that ___.
6. The assistant's stool should be adjusted so that ___.
7. Typical equipment used for cleaning and sterilizing instruments includes _____.

REFERENCES

ADA Councils on Dental Materials, Instruments and Equipment; Dental Practice and Dental Therapeutics: Infection control recommendations for the dental office and dental laboratory, *JADA* 116:241, 1988.

Carter LM, Yaman P: *Dental instruments,* St Louis, 1981, CV Mosby.

Centers for Disease Control: Recommended infection-control practices for dentistry, *MMWR* 35:237, 1986.

Centers for Disease Control: Recommendations for prevention of HIV transmission in health-care settings, *MMWR* 36:1, 1987.

Chasteen JE: *Essentials of clinical dental assisting,* ed 4, St Louis, 1989, CV Mosby.

Cottone JA, Terezhalmy GT, Molinari JA: *Practical infection control in dentistry,* Philadelphia, 1991, Lea & Febiger.

Gerwatowski LJ, McFall DB, Stach DJ: Carpal tunnel syndrome: risk factors and preventive strategies for the dental hygienist, *J Dent Hyg* 66:89, 1992.

Harris NO, Crabb, LJ: Ergonomics: reducing mental and physical fatigue in the dental operatory, *Dent Clin North Am* 22:331, 1978.

Miller CH: Sterilization and disinfection: what every dentist should know, *JADA* 123:46, 1992.

New dentist buying guide, Chicago, 1992, American Dental Association.

Richardson RE, Barton RE: *The dental assistant,* ed 5, New York, 1978, McGraw-Hill.

Snyder TL, Domer LR: Personalized guide to practice evaluation. In Snyder TL, Felmeister CJ, editors: *Mosby's dental practice series,* vol 1, St Louis, 1983, CV Mosby.

Sockwell CL: Dental handpieces and rotary cutting instruments, *Dent Clin North Am* 15:219, 1971.

Weinert AM: An evaluation of the dental lounge chair, *Dent Clin North Am* 15:129, 1971.

Williams KV, Williams FT: The maintenance of dental equipment. II. Chairs and lights, *Br Dent J* 153:71, 1982a.

Williams KV, Williams FT: The maintenance of dental equipment. III. Delivery and disposal systems, *Br Dent J* 153:113, 1982b.

Young JM: Dental equipment asepsis, *Dent Clin North Am* 35:391, 1991a.

Young JM: Maintaining dental equipment, *JADA* 122:83, 1991b.

3 DISEASE TRANSMISSION THEORY AND CONTROL OF CONTAMINATION AND BLOODBORNE PATHOGENS

Catherine Davis
Nancy Stutsman Young

Catherine Davis
Nancy Stutsman Young

LEARNING OUTCOMES

The dental hygienist will be able to

1. Explain the theory of disease transmission and the necessity for asepsis in dentistry.
2. Identify common pathogenic organisms that may be found in the oral cavity and the diseases they produce.
3. Define *direct* and *indirect* contamination and give examples that illustrate understanding of these terms.
4. Identify precautionary measures that must be taken by dental personnel to prevent disease transfer from patient to patient, patient to clinician, and clinician to patient.
5. Differentiate among the terms *sanitization, disinfection,* and *sterilization.*
6. Identify the major sources of contamination in the dental office and describe an effective method of controlling contamination or eliminating it from each source.
7. Discuss five accepted methods of instrument sterilization and identify the advantages and disadvantages of each.
8. Discuss the choice and use of chemical disinfectants.
9. Perform hand washing.
10. Prepare instruments for sterilization/disinfection.
11. Operate an autoclave and dry heat oven.
12. Discuss indications for the use of gloves, safety glasses, and face masks.
13. Follow infection control procedures for the laboratory.
14. Discuss the legal implications of following recommended infection control guidelines.
15. Follow the current Centers for Disease Control (CDC) recommendations for control of bloodborne pathogens.
16. Identify all current Occupational Safety and Health Administration (OSHA) standards regarding bloodborne pathogens.
17. Describe Hazard Communications laws.
18. Identify key components of Material Safety Data Sheets (MSDS).
19. Follow the rules and regulations regarding medical waste disposal.

With each educational component of professional preparation, the student hygienist gains a new dimension of respect for the oral environment. This respect should center on the nature of the relationship of the hygienist to the pathogenic (disease-producing) organisms of the oral cavity. Direct and indirect exposure to these organisms occurs practically every minute of the working day.

Dentists and hygienists are in constant contact with blood, saliva, mucous membranes, and other body fluids that may be infectious. It has been estimated that a single drop of saliva may contain up to 600,000 bacteria and a spoon excavator full of dental plaque may contain an average of 200 million bacteria (Palenik and Miller, 1984a). The potential exists for infection of the clinician and coworkers as well as patients. Managing disease transmission or, more positively, preserving the health of patients and dental care providers depends on rigid application of high standards of asepsis (freedom from pathogenic material). This chapter reviews oral as well as bloodborne pathogens and modes of microbial transfer as well as the current standards, at the date of publication of the book, established by the Occupational Safety and Health Administration (OSHA) for control of bloodborne pathogens. Controlling levels of contamination and procedures for maintaining asepsis are also discussed.

Some professionals may be skeptical about the need for strict standards of infection control for dental professionals and office environments. Dental treatment may seem benign compared with the aseptic and postinfection concerns of the medical-surgical arena. After all, patients are seen for relatively short periods of time, and the treatment in general seems superficial. For example, the risk of transmission of the human immunodeficiency virus (HIV) to a health care worker after percutaneous exposure to HIV-infected blood is 0.3%. This is considerably lower than the 30.0% risk of hepatitis B (HBV) transmission. However, exposure to HIV as well as HBV-contaminated blood can lead to lethal, untreatable infections (Gerberding et al, 1987; Henderson et al, 1990).

Because the oral cavity supports one of the most concentrated microbial populations of the body, length of time has little significance when procedures (periodontal instrumentation, injection, extraction, endodontics) that expose the underlying tissues to external agents are performed. These procedures cannot be classified as superficial. The main routes for disease transmission occur through contact with the bloodstream and through respiratory nasal/oral secretions. Except for the surgeon, few health professionals come in closer patient contact for longer periods of treatment than the dental team. Remember, the public is very aware of the transmission of the HIV virus from a dentist to five of his patients. Currently, this is the only report of HIV transmission from an infected health care worker to patients during invasive procedures. It has been documented that the dentist did not consistently adhere to the use of barrier protection or universal precautions (Centers for Disease Control [CDC], 1991).

It is important that the student develop an awareness of the infectious nature of oral organisms and their potential for transfer. Beyond this, maintaining aseptic practices is unquestionably the hygienist's professional responsibility.

MICROFLORA OF THE ORAL CAVITY

The oral cavity provides an excellent environment for supporting a variety of organisms, including many types of bacteria, yeasts, certain fungi, mycoplasmas, protozoa, and viruses. The indigenous flora of the oral cavity are listed in Table 3-1. The nature of the oral structures—the mucosa, tongue, and gingival crevice—and the variation in dental anatomy promote the adherence and growth of diverse microbial populations. Salivary components, exudates, and epithelial cells are an abundant intrinsic nutritional source for oral flora. In addition, the foods we ingest are extrinsic nutritional sources. These nutritional sources, the variety of epithelial surfaces for attachment, temperature, and moisture create the perfect environment for an active microbial community. In fact, the concentration about the gingival sulcus and in plaque is about 200 billion cells per gram of sample (Burnett and Schuster, 1978).

The normal resident flora and the host generally have a cooperative relationship. Innate bacterial antagonism, salivary lysozyme and peroxidase, and immunoglobulins act to regulate the oral flora and protect the host against potential pathogens. It is important that you understand the body's protective mechanisms before potential pathogens are described. Intact skin and mucous membranes offer a physical barrier against microbial invasion of the bloodstream and deeper tissues. It is interesting to note that the secretions of sweat glands maintain an average dermal pH of 5.2 to 5.8, which is bactericidal and fungicidal (Burnett and Schuster, 1978). To a large extent, once foreign particles enter the oral cavity, are trapped in the mucus or saliva, and are swallowed; they will be destroyed by gastric acid in the stomach. In a similar fashion, the respiratory tract has a mucous coat to trap large particles (10 to 50 mg) and a specialized ciliated epithelium that constantly moves the mucus down from the nasopharynx or away from the bronchi of the lungs in order to be swallowed. Smaller particles (0.5 to 5.0 mg) have the greatest potential for penetration and retention in the lung (Miller and Micik, 1978). Therefore a number of important factors, including the individual's innate or acquired immunity and the protective physical and chemical factors work in cooperation to protect against an overt infection.

Tables 3-2 and 3-3 summarize the bacterial and viral pathogens that may be active in the oral cavity or are significant in providing a means for transmission by way of the respiratory tract. Hep-

Table 3-1. Microorganisms indigenous to man

Microorganisms	Sites
Pathogenic staphylococci	Skin, human milk, nasal passages, vagina (during pregnancy), throat, gastrointestinal tract, oral cavity, feces
Micrococci and nonpathogenic staphylococci	Skin, mucous membranes, nose, throat, vagina, postpartum uterus, oral cavity
Anaerobic micrococci	Tonsils, uterus, vagina, respiratory tract
Streptococci	Mucous surfaces, mouth, pharynx, lower intestine, genital tract, vagina
Anaerobic streptococi	Mucous surfaces, vagina, postpartum uterus, oral cavity, human feces
Enterococci	Lower intestine, feces genitourinary tract, oral cavity, tonsils
Common neisseriae	Oral cavity, nasopharynx, nasal cavity, urethra, vagina
Veillonellae	Oral cavity
Lactobacilli	Oral cavity, gastrointestinal tract, vagina
Actinomyces	Oral cavity, throat
Corynebacteria	Mucous membranes, vagina, skin, conjunctiva, oral cavity, feces
Mycobacteria	Preputial and clitoral secretions, feces, tonsils
Clostridia	Gastrointestinal tract, feces
Enterobacteria	Feces, gastrointestinal tract, vagina, oral cavity, throat
Moraxella, Mima (Herellea) species	Conjunctiva, nose, genitourinary mucous membranes, respiratory tract
Pseudomonas species	Feces, skin, hands, external ear, axilla, perineum
Alcaligenes faecalis	Feces
Haemophilus	Conjunctiva, nose, pharynx, oral cavity, vagina
Bacteroides	Predominant in feces, lower intestine, oral cavity
Fusobacteria	Oral cavity, intestine, throat, genitalia
Anaerobic spirilla and vibrios	Oral cavity
Spirochetes	Oral cavity, genitalia, throat, tonsils, feces, GI tract, genitourinary tract
Candida species	Oral cavity, body surfaces, throat, feces, vagina
Pityrosporum ovale	Skin
Torulopsis glabrata	Skin, mucous membranes
Dermatophytes	Skin
Trichomonads	Oral cavity, intestine, genitourinary tract
Amebas	Oral cavity, intestinal tract, vagina, genitourinary tract
Pleuropneumonia-like organisms, L forms, spheroplasts, protoplasts	Vagina, male urethra, oral cavity, throat

Modified from Burnett GW, Schuster GS: *Pathogenic microbiology,* St Louis, 1978, CV Mosby.

atitis, tuberculosis, syphilis, herpes simplex infections, and acquired immune deficiency syndrome (AIDS) are discussed in this chapter as contagious diseases that can be transmitted during dental procedures.

PATHWAYS OF DISEASE TRANSMISSION

Diseases are transmitted by inanimate or human sources in a variety of ways.

Direct transmission occurs when organisms are transferred from one host to another, usually by way of the bloodstream, saliva, or respiratory secretions. Entrance to the bloodstream usually occurs when the skin or mucosa is penetrated by a contaminated instrument or needle or when organisms introduced into an open wound, such as a cut or torn cuticle on the clinician's hand.

The proximity of the patient and clinician makes respiratory sources important. As Tables 3-2 and 3-3 indicate the majority of potential pathogens inhabit the nasopharynx area (Nolte, 1982). During breathing, conversation, coughing, or sneezing, organisms are sprayed into the environment, producing an aerosol (Johnson & Johnson, 1969; Miller and Micik, 1978). This collection of articles suspended in the air is capable of transmitting pathogens. The organisms may stay suspended for a period of time or may fall rapidly to contaminate the environment and the people in the operatory. Aerosol production is more significant when one considers the equipment and procedures performed by dental clinicians. Handpieces, trisyringes (air-water syringes), ultrasonic scalers, instrumentation, and even instruction of a patient in toothbrushing are responsible for creating serious aerosols (Williams et al, 1970). One investigator collected and cultured a sample of air from a carrier that yielded 41 viable colonies of

Table 3-2. Summary of bacterial pathogens that may be transmitted by way of the oral cavity during dental treatment

Organism	Bacterial disease	Mode of transmission	Other
Mycobacterium tuberculosis	Tuberculosis of lungs, lymph nodes, meninges, kidneys, bone, skin, oronasopharynseal tissues	Organism found in sputum; transmitted by respiratory droplet or contact with contaminated inanimate objects	Microorganisms resist chemicals and survive well on dry surfaces for weeks
Treponema pallidum	Syphilis Primary: chancre of skin, lips, tongue, oral mucosa Secondary: recurrent patch of mucosa Tertiary: gummas of oral cavity, larynx, vocal cords	Contact with oral lesions harboring organism; transmitted by contact with contaminated blood or by penetration of epithelium	Disease is highly contagious in primary and secondary stages; because of nature of symptoms women may be unaware of the disease in early stages; lesions of secondary syphilis may persist or recur for 2 to 3 years
Staphylococcus aureus	Wound infection, abscesses, cellulitis, meningitis, osteomyelitis, toxic shock syndrome	Organism found in nose, mouth, skin; transmitted by contact with contaminated blood or inanimate objects	Organism survives well on dry surfaces; 30% of population are asymptomatic nasopharyngeal carriers
Streptococcus pyogenes, viridans, and *pneumoniae*	"Strep" throat, peritonsillar abscesses, pharyngitis, scarlet fever, rheumatic fever, glomerulonephritis, subacute bacterial endocarditis, pneumonia with secondary septicemia, empyema, pericarditis, and meningitis	Found in saliva, nasopharynx; transmitted by contact with contaminated blood or inanimate objects	Organism survives well on dry surfaces; approximately 10% of general population are asymptomatic nasopharyngeal carriers
Pseudomonas aeruginosa	May cause infection in almost all organs, especially in patients with lowered resistance	Lives in water supplies; transmitted through bloodstream by contaminated water supplies	Regular monitoring of water filtering system and maintenance of germ-free lines necessary to prevent transmission of organism
Candida albicans	Adult: candidiasis Child: thrush infection of skin or mucous membrane	Mouth, nails, lungs, skin, gastrointestina tract, vagina; transmitted by contact with contaminated source	Lesion of the labial commissures similar to that of riboflavin deficiency
Actinomyces israelii	Actinomycosis of oral cavity, face, neck, abdominal cavity, lungs	Organism inhabits tonsils, carious teeth, calculus, open wounds, extraction sites, pulp exposures; transmitted through bloodstream and tissue inoculation	Tissue infection usually occurs after repeated exposure to organism following surgery, injury, or chronic irritation
Chlamydia trachomatis	Lymphogranuloma venereum	Oral lesion (primarily tongue) can infect hands of dental personnel	Type of venereal disease seen most often in tropics
Haemophilus influenzae	Pharyngitis, sinusitis, respiratory tract infection, meningitis	Inhabitant of nasopharynx, mucus, sputum; transmitted by respiratory droplet and by contaminated objects	Organism incapsulated and may resist chemicals; organism survives longer on inanimate objects than do other organisms; 33% to 66% of normal adults are nasopharyngeal carriers

Continued.

Table 3-2. Summary of bacterial pathogens that may be transmitted by way of the oral cavity during dental treatment—cont'd

Organism	Bacterial disease	Mode of transmission	Other
Bordetella pertussis	Whooping cough	Transmitted by respiratory droplet	Affects 90% of nonimmunized population; vaccine greatly reduces morbidity; incubation 1 to 2 weeks; course of disease runs to 6 weeks
Clostridium tetani	Tetanus	Inhabits soil and intestinal tract; dust-borne spore transmission by spores entering wound site	Spores are highly resistant to physical/chemical agents. Protection: DPT vaccine

Table 3-3. Summary of viral pathogens that may be transmitted by way of the oral cavity during dental treatment

Organism	Viral disease	Mode of transmission	Other characteristics
Respiratory virus: adenovirus, coxsackievirus A, echovirus, respiratory syncytial virus, rhinovirus, polio virus	Upper respiratory tract infection (sore throat, cough, nasal discharge, fever, chills, muscle aches, fatigue); lower respiratory tract infection; conjunctiva; lesions of oral cavity; meningitis	Organism inhabits nose, mouth, eye; transmitted by respiratory droplet, aerosols, contaminated surfaces	Viruses occur worldwide; peak incidence in fall and winter; asymptomatic carriers and variety of strains make control difficult; all factors of transmission may not be identified as yet
Herpes virus	Simplex: "cold sores," dermatitis, keratitis (eye infection), whitlow (lesion of fingers); varicella-zoster: chicken pox (child), shingles (adult)	Saliva, direct contact with lesions, respiratory tract transmission	Repeated active phases of herpes simplex may result in chronic problem; chickenpox immunity after childhood episode; only 0.5% to 2% of population may acquire zoster varicellosus
Epstein-Barr (EB) virus	Infectious mononucleosis	Throat-oral respiratory transmission	Incubation period 4 to 49 days; possibility of treating patient in early stages
Hepatitis viruses: A B Other, as yet unidentified viruses Delta virus	Infectious hepatitis Serum hepatitis Non-A, non-B hepatitis Delta hepatitis	Saliva, feces, blood, tears, semen, sweat; transmitted by means of respiratory droplet or contact with contaminated blood	Disease on rise in general population; patient may be a carrier with or without acute episode; incubation period makes treating patient in undiagnosed or carrier state possible
Papillomavirus	Warts	Direct contact or contact with contaminated surface	Patient protection necessary if dental personnel are affected
Mumps virus Rubeola virus Rubella virus	Mumps Measles German measles	Respiratory secretions, saliva, blood, urine, contaminated surfaces	Transfer may occur during incubation phase (18 to 21 days). Vaccine available. Rubella is of special concern for pregnant women, since disease may cause congenital defects or death of fetus

Mycobacterium tuberculosis. The highest concentration of microorganisms was found within 2 feet in front of the patient, where the clinician is usually positioned (Johnson & Johnson, 1969).

Aerosols and organisms carried in dust make up airborne sources of disease transfer. Patients and clinicians moving in and out of the treatment area are carriers of pathogens and constantly stir up the airborne dust, contaminating the environment. Some organisms (see Tables 3-2 and 3-3) are able to survive on inanimate objects—countertops, sinks, operatory equipment—for extended periods and provide a source of cross-infection. When a pathogen is transferred from one person to another by way of an intermediate source or a source other than the original carrier, indirect transmission has occurred.

As well as being the primary contact between the environment and the patient or between one patient and another, the clinician can be the source of disease. A clinician with an upper respiratory tract infection or, more seriously, a blood-borne pathogen can infect patients. Wearing a mask and gloves protects both the clinician and the patient. Methods for maintaining asepsis and applying the theory of universal precautions during patient treatment are discussed later in the chapter.

Also, a patient may harbor organisms naturally in the oral cavity that can produce disease if they enter his or her own bloodstream. The resultant condition is referred to as an autogenous infection, meaning that the patient is the source of the pathogen. Some of the most prevalent organisms in the oral cavity capable of producing autogenous infection are the various types of streptococci. If organisms are carried into deep tissues during an injection, or if a bacteremia (bacteria circulating in the normally sterile bloodstream) of viable organisms into the bloodstream occurs as a result of instrumentation, these organisms may cause soft tissue or bone infection. In some patients a serious disease called bacterial endocarditis may result (see Chapter 6). If the bacteria are not cleared by the reticuloendothelial system, this could lead to death.

An awareness of the variety of pathways by which microorganisms, particularly pathogenic ones, may be transmitted in the course of dental treatment is important. All human beings have the potential to contaminate themselves, each other, and the environment by direct or indirect trans-mission. In most cases it is difficult to identify the exact source of an infection. This only emphasizes the need for clinics and offices to establish and follow a strict program of infection control.

Hepatitis

The viral illnesses known as hepatitis are of special concern to the dental clinician because they can be transmitted in operatory conditions and because infected carriers are often unaware of their condition. At least twenty different viruses may cause human hepatitis (Cottone, et al, 1991). There are at least four different types of viral hepatitis, called A; B; non-A, non-B; and delta. Common signs and symptoms include malaise, fever, loss of appetite, nausea, abdominal discomfort, and vomiting. Jaundice may or may not occur.

Hepatitis A has a short incubation period (2 to 6 weeks) after being transmitted predominantly by the oral-fecal route. Children and young people are most often infected. It appears to be acute (having a rapid onset), but there are no residual effects after recovery. There are no carriers of this disease. A vaccine for hepatitis A is under development.

In contrast, hepatitis B is transmitted by contact with body secretions (Table 3-4). This virus is found most commonly in the blood, but can also be present in saliva, sputum, crevicular fluid, and other body fluids. Only minute quantities of contaminated blood or saliva are required to cause infection. Intraorally, the greatest concentration of HBV is at the gingival sulcus, a location of prime concern to the hygienist as well as the dentist (Sampson, 1982). In the dental operatory, hepatitis B may be transmitted percutaneously through wounds from sharp instruments or contaminated needles. A second mode of transmission can occur nonpercutaneously from the transfer of infected saliva or blood into breaks in the skin or mucous membranes. Transmission can also occur from contact with surfaces, such as equipment or clothing, that have been contaminated by dental aerosols.

Hepatitis B has a long incubation period (2 to 6 months). Symptoms are often mild. They may mimic other common conditions such as influenza or stress-related illnesses and may include fatigue, loss of appetite, nausea, and abdominal and joint pain. Jaundice does not always occur. Hepatitis B may result in chronic hepatitis, cirrhosis, liver

Table 3-4. Comparison of the traditional two types of viral hepatitis

	Infectious hepatitis (A)	*Serum hepatitis (B)*
Virus transmission	Fecal-oral route; also parenteral	From blood and blood products; primarily parenteral; can be by means of oral route and contact with carrier
Incubation period	About 30 days (15 to 50)	30 to 180 days
Age preference	Children, young adults	All ages
Duration of infectious period	Virus in feces and blood 1 to 2 weeks before disease; remains 3 to 4 weeks longer	Virus in blood 3 months before disease; occasional asymptomatic carrier for as long as 5 years
Virus present	Saliva, feces, blood	Blood, feces, saliva
Clinical features*		
Onset	Acute	Slow, usually insidious
Fever	Common before jaundice	Less common
Jaundice	Rare in children, more frequent in adults	Rare in children, more frequent in adults
Severity of disease	Less severe	More severe
Prognosis	Good	Less favorable
Laboratory evaluation†		
Thymol turbidity†	Increased	Normal
Abnormal SGOT‡	Transient, 1 to 3 weeks	Prolonged, 1 to 8 months
HAA (Australia antigen) in blood	Not present	Present during incubation period and acute phase; occasionally persists
Prevention and control		
Prophylactic effect of gamma globulin	Good	Possibly beneficial
Dental precautions and control	1. Emergency care during acute phase 2. Mask, gloves, and safety glasses worn 3. Sterilization of contaminated items 4. Disposables used if sterilization is impossible 5. Care with anesthetics (amides) metabolized by liver	1. Emergency care during initial phase 2. Mask, gloves, and safety glasses worn 3. Sterilization of contaminated items 4. Disposables used if sterilization is impossible 5. Care with anesthetics (amides) metabolized by liver 6. Update history at every recall visit for carrier status

Modified from Smith AL: *Principles of microbiology,* ed 9, St Louis, 1982, CV Mosby.
*Many clinical features are the same.
†Test of liver function.
‡The enzyme serum glutamic-oxaloacetic transaminase level is elevated with liver disease.

cancer, and even death. There is no known cure or effective treatment for hepatitis B. Treatment with interferon is currently being evaluated (Mandell et al, 1990).

A number of population groups have been cited as being at high risk for contact with HBV (Cottone, 1985). These include persons who receive frequent large-volume transfusions (hemophiliacs); persons in renal dialysis unit; persons in institutions for the mentally handicapped; persons who are immunosuppressed or immunodeficient; persons with a recent history of jaundice; military personnel; intravenous drug abusers; promiscuous homosexual males; female prostitutes; and immigrants from developing countries (particularly Haiti and Indochina). This list is extensive, yet it only identifies those with a high risk of hepatitis B infection. Obviously, the safest recommendation is that of the National Centers for Disease Control (CDC), which states that an effective infection control program must operate under the assumption that *all* dental patients have the potential for transmitting this disease (that is, requires universal precautions).

Hepatitis B is a major occupational hazard for dental care providers. The general practitioner and hygienist may have a three times higher risk of hepatitis B infection than the general population, and specialists such a oral surgeons and periodontists may have an even higher risk (Cottone, 1985). The gingival sulcus is the primary site of periodontal instrumentation and is frequently treated by the dental hygienist. For this reason, the hygienist has been demonstrated to be at as much risk as the dentist (Schiff et al, 1986).

In an estimated 80% of cases of hepatitis B, the infected individual is asymptomatic or suffers only subclinical symptoms and is therefore unaware of the infection. Approximately 10% of those infected with the disease will become chronic carriers who are capable of infecting others, perhaps for years. Therefore medical histories and examinations cannot be relied on to identify patients who are capable of transmitting the disease in the dental environment. Dental practitioners may be lulled into a false sense of security if they gauge their potential for contracting this disease solely on medical history information. An office that treats 20 patients per day might expect to encounter an active carrier of hepatitis B once in every 7 working days (Crawford, 1985). Although a few reports have documented the transmission of hepatitis from dental professionals to patients, it is far more likely that the flow of transmission is from patient to dental professional. Therefore if universal precautions are not observed, dental professionals may not only find themselves infected, but also may unwittingly infect their family members or others with whom they have intimate contact.

The best prevention against HBV is for all dental personnel to be vaccinated with one of the hepatitis vaccines (Engerix-B [Smith Kline] or Recombivax-HB [Merck, Sharp & Dohme]). These vaccines have been proven to be safe and effective methods for prevention of hepatitis B. The plasma-derived vaccine (Heptavax B) is no longer available in the United States. The vaccination schedule most often used for adults and children has been three intramuscular (IM) injections. The second and third injections are given 1 and 6 months, respectively, after the first. This vaccination route and schedule has been reported to produce antibodies in 80% to 95% of recipients (Francis et al, 1982; Steven et al, 1987; Szmuness et al, 1980). It has been noted that some organizations have given $1/10$ of the dose intradermally (ID); however, hepatitis B vaccine is not licensed by the Food and Drug Administration (FDA) for ID administration, and use of this method has led to inadequate immune response (CDC, 1991). Booster doses of the vaccine have not been rec-

ommended because the protective efficacy persists 9 years after vaccination (Wainwright et al, 1989). Postvaccination testing should be done on health care workers who are at risk of injury from contaminated sharp instruments. This posttesting should be completed 1 to 6 months after completion of the vaccine series. Revaccination with one or more additional doses should be considered for those who do not seroconvert. The OSHA has mandated that its new bloodborne pathogen standard must contain several components, one of which is a postexposure evaluation (OSHA, Dec. 1991) (Table 3-5).

The second part of this chapter discusses infection control measures that should be incorporated into dental practice to further protect against transmission of HBV and other infectious agents. These recommendations should be instituted for all dental patients and not just those who are known to be infectious or from high-risk population groups.

The less common so-called non-A, non-B (NANB) hepatitis has been diagnosed. In general, this form appears similar to hepatitis B and follows a similar clinical course after an incubation period of approximately 7 weeks (Smith, 1982). There are two forms of transmission; parenteral and enteric. Fifty percent of patients with parenterally transmitted NANB hepatitis develop chronic carrier state. There is a low incidence of carrier state following infection with enterically transmitted NANB hepatitis (Kuo et al, 1989).

Delta hepatitis is a newly recognized form of viral hepatitis that has been shown to be a coinfection with hepatitis B (Cottone, 1986). It contains limited genetic material and requires HBV to act as a helper in its replication. Infection with the delta hepatitis virus may occur concurrently with HBV infection, in which case the symptoms and course of the infection are similar to those of hepatitis B. Infection of delta hepatitis can also occur in an individual who is already a chronic HBV carrier. These persons are more likely to have a serious and acute fulminant form of hepatitis that can progress rapidly, resulting in severe liver damage and ultimately death. Delta hepatitis, like hepatitis B, is usually transmitted by percutaneous or permucosal exposure and can be controlled by the infection control measures recommended for hepatitis B. Fortunately, the HBV vaccine will also protect against delta hepatitis virus, which is dependent on the former for survival.

Table 3-5. Recommendations for hepatitis B prophylaxis following percutaneous exposure

Exposed person	Treatment when source is found to be		
	HBsAg positive	*HBsAg negative*	*Unknown or not tested*
Unvaccinated	Administer HBIG × 1* and initiate hepatitis B vaccine	Initiate hepatitis B vaccine	Initiate hepatitis B vaccine
Previously vaccinated			
Known responder	Test exposed person for anti-HBs 1. If adequate, no treatment 2. If inadequate, hepatitis B vaccine booster dose	No treatment	No treatment
Known nonresponder	HBIG × 2 or HBIG × 1, plus 1 dose of hepatitis B vaccine	No treatment	If known high-risk source may treat as if source were HBsAg positive
Response unknown	Test exposed person for anti-HB† 1. If inadequate, HBIG × 1, plus hepatitis B vaccine booster dose 2. If adequate, no treatment	No treatment	Test exposed person for anti-HBs† 1. If inadequate, hepatitis B vaccine booster dose 2. If adequate, no treatment

Modified from *MMWR* 40:22, 1991.
HBsAg, hepatitis B surface antigen; *HBIG,* hepatitis B immune globulin; *anti-HBs,* antibody to HBsAg.
*Dose 0.06 mL/kg intramusculary.
†Adequate anti-HBs is 10 milli-International Units.

Acquired immune deficiency syndrome

Since its official recognition by the CDC in 1981, acquired immune deficiency syndrome (AIDS), for which there is no cure, has become a worldwide epidemic of frightening proportions. It has achieved unprecedented publicity, sometimes leading to panic, and is challenging established social, ethical, moral, legal, and medical beliefs and principles. The dental clinician is inevitably involved in these developments because of the deadly syndrome's tendency towards transmission through the exchange of body fluids.

It has been established that AIDS is caused by infection from the human immunodeficiency virus (HIV), which is transmitted through exposure to blood or other body fluids of an infected individual. The retrovirus enters the bloodstream and replicates in cells of the immune system. This replication is lytic in nature and therefore destroys many cells that are essential to the proper functioning of the immune system. This makes the victim vulnerable to opportunistic bacteria, viruses, fungi, and protozoans that would normally be harmless. The HIV incubation period varies widely among individuals, with the result that many carriers who can transmit HIV are unaware of their own infection. Clinical signs of HIV infection begin with mononucleosis-like illness symptoms and progress as opportunistic infections, such as pneumonia, tuberculosis, viral infections, meningitis, and cancers, invade the body, eventually resulting in death. Individuals at highest risk for AIDS are sexually active homosexual and bisexual males and intravenous drug abusers. AIDS is also transmitted through the use of contaminated needles, from mothers to unborn and nursing children, as well as through heterosexual behavior, with the result that its spread into the community at large is well under way.

The number of AIDS cases increases each year. It was predicted that by 1991 there will be 270,000 cases of AIDS in the United States. The cumulative number of AIDS-related deaths is estimated to reach 179,000 by the end of 1991 (U.S. Public Health Service, 1986 [USPHS]). Approximately 1.5 to 2.0 million persons are carriers of HIV who may be infectious, and the number of carriers is constantly increasing. Time from the initial infection to the appearance of overt symptoms and diagnosis may be as long as 7 years in some individuals (CDC, 1986b; Landesman et al, 1985; USPHS, 1986).

The HIV infection occurs in three stages. The first is an asymptomatic carrier phase in which the person may be infectious without exhibiting symptoms. An estimated 80% of infected individuals may be infectious to others. The second stage of infecton is known as AIDS-related complex (ARC) and occurs in an estimated 25% of those infected with HIV. Clinical signs include long-term fever, weight loss, lymphadenopathy, chronic diarrhea, fatigue, and night sweats. Oral findings may include candidiasis, hairy leukoplakia, herpes simplex, xerostomia, acute gingival infections resembling acute necrotizing ulcerative gingivitis (ANUG), and accelerated periodontal destruction. The third stage of infection is AIDS. Patients live an average of 56 weeks after the diagnosis of this stage. These patients frequently manifest a malignant skin cancer known as Kaposi's sarcoma. This tumor may appear intraorally, especially on the hard palate, as single or multiple painless, reddish blue, flat or elevated areas that are highly vascular. Other clinical findings are similar to those described for ARC (Neupert, 1987).

The primary means of transmission of HIV is through contact with contaminated body fluids. The blood-borne route is the primary route for transmission of the virus to health care workers. Although HIV has been found in saliva, no specific cases have proven transmission from saliva (Gotto, 1991).

The best means of protection for dental professionals against HIV infection are barrier protective techniques and compliance with the infection control procedures recommended by the CDC and the American Dental Association (ADA),which are discussed later in this chapter. These guidelines agree that transmission control is best achieved through the constant use of gloves, masks, and eye protection; the effective sterilization of dental instruments; cleanup of instruments and surfaces in the operatory; and proper disposal of contaminated materials. Special care should always be taken when handling sharp instruments. Clothes exposed to HIV can be safely used after a normal laundry cycle or dry cleaning. The clinician must remember that it is impossible to recognize someone who has HIV infection without clinical manifestations, and that the only method

of protection is to assume that every patient has HIV and use barrier mechanisms accordingly.

The dental professional has a responsibility to treat AIDS patients just as those suffering from other diseases. Although the right of a dentist to refuse or refer treatment of a prospective new patient who has AIDS has not yet been tested in the courts, refusal to treat a suspected or known AIDS carrier may be considered illegal on the grounds that it constitutes discrimination against a handicapped individual (Logan, 1987). The Colorado State Board of Dental Examiners recently adopted a rule that states "Colorado dentists and dental hygienists may not refuse to treat an individual solely because of an individual's HIV serotype status. Failure to treat these patients can be grounds for revocation of the professional license" (Department of Regulatory Agencies, 1992). When appropriate barrier precautions are implemented, dental professionals can safely treat these individuals. Dental clinicians are especially important because oral findings of certain infections play a significant role in the diagnosis and treatment of symptoms. The dental professional is also responsible for keeping informed about AIDS through the rapidly proliferating literature so that he or she can implement the latest breakthroughs in diagnosis and treatment.

Tuberculosis

More than 20,000 cases of tuberculosis are reported annually in the United States. Groups at high risk are the elderly, minorities, and HIV-infected and foreign-born individuals (Fox, 1990). Tuberculosis is of special concern for dental personnel, because the oral cavity is one of the chief pathways of transmission. Sputum laden with tubercle bacilli presents the greatest danger for persons in contact with the patient. *Mycobacterium tuberculosis* is resistant to many chemical disinfectants and survives well on dry surfaces, making it a matter of concern in maintaining asepsis in the dental environment.

Tuberculosis can be spread by a variety of modes. In the past it was frequently spread by contaminated milk; however, the pasteurization process has controlled this mode of transmission. There have even been reports of contamination of skin abrasions of laboratory personnel (prosector's warts). The most common mode of transmission is inhalation of droplet nuclei (Riley, 1982). Tuberculosis most often affects the lungs, but other sites of the disease include the mouth (especially a lesion of the tongue), skin, gastrointestinal tract, bone, and salivary glands (Burnett and Schuster, 1978; Rowe and Brooks, 1978).

Urban areas characterized by poor socioeconomic conditions have higher rates of tuberculosis than do areas with high incomes and low population densities (Nolte, 1982).

Effective therapy with medication has significantly reduced the number of deaths caused by tuberculosis. Treatment consists of excision of the tubercular lesion and a regimen of medications in various combinations. Choice of medication is dependent on the antimicrobial sensitivities of the particular strain of organisms involved. Common medications include isoniazid, rifampin, ethambutol, streptomycin and pyrazinamide. For those frequently exposed to tuberculosis, such as family members of a tubercular patient or medical personnel working in urban areas or developing countries, a vaccine of attenuated strain is available. Protection may be only temporary with the Bacille Calmette Guérin (BCG) vaccine. Most evidence indicates that the BCG vaccine will decrease the incidence of tuberculosis by 60% to 80% (Luelmo, 1982). However, this is only applicable to tuberculin-negative people. The vaccine does not prevent infection but limits its proliferation (Sutherland and Lindgren, 1979).

Because of the increased risk of dental personnel for contracting tuberculosis, periodic skin testing is recommended (Rowe and Brooks, 1978).

Once tuberculosis patients have been treated and cleared, they are generally followed for a yearly sputum culture and chest x-ray examination to determine any recurrence. A patient who reports a history of tuberculosis but has current medical clearance may be treated as a routine patient.

Syphilis

The organism that causes syphilis is *Treponema pallidum*, a spirochete that enters the body through a break—which need not be obvious—in the skin. It can be transmitted by sexual contact, congenitally, orally, though blood transfusions or by accidental direct inoculation (Kampmeier, 1943).

Syphilis has three stages. Each may be characterized by oral manifestations. From 10 days to 3 months after initial contact, a primary stage lesion may occur. The classic primary chancre begins at the sight of inoculation as a single, painless papule. This chancre most often occurs on the genitalia, but between 5% and 12% of patients develop extragenital lesions. Multiple chancres do occur, especially in patients infected with HIV (Chapel, 1978). Greater than 50% of these extragenital chancres occur on the lips, with the tongue and tonsils being other common oral sites. Dental personnel who contract syphilis may develop a chancre of the finger(s). Transmission may occur through mishandling of contaminated dental instruments or inanimate objects such as drinking cups.

The secondary stage can appear before or after the primary stage and can affect virtually any organ. The oral manifestation of this phase is termed a *mucous patch* and appear as silver-gray patches with a red periphery. These lesions are teeming with organisms and are highly infectious. The secondary stage may last as long as 6 weeks and is followed by a nonspecific latent period. Only about one third of persons with untreated syphilis develop destructive lesions of the tertiary stage (Nolte, 1982). Although tertiary lesions are rarely seen, tumors of granulomatous tissue, called gummas, may appear in the oral cavity. The most common site is the palate.

Treatment with antibiotics, usually penicillin, is indicated for syphilis. If possible, treatment should begin before the primary lesion occurs.

The dental professional should approach the examination and treatment of each patient carefully. The health history may be helpful in revealing a past episode of syphilis; as always, universal precautions should be followed. For example, some patients may be unaware of having syphilis. Primary stage lesions of the genitalia may go unnoticed, especially in women, and oral lesions may not occur at all. The primary and secondary stages pose the greatest risk for transmitting infection. At any stage, misdiagnosis of oral lesions may occur unless serologic studies are performed. For the added protection of dental personnel, some large clinics, such as those in dental schools, require a blood test as part of the admissions/screening procedure.

Herpes simplex virus infections

Infections caused by the herpes simplex virus are among the most common viral infections affecting humans and are of particular concern to the dental professional. Transmission of these infections can occur via direct contact with oral herpetic lesions or oral secretions containing the virus, via aerosols, or via fomites such as dental instruments, handpieces, or impressions (Merchant, 1982). It has been shown that these viruses, as well as bacteria, can be transmitted by dental charts touched by contaminated gloves (Thomas et al, 1985). Four diseases caused by herpes simplex viruses are presented here. These are acute gingivostomatitis, recurrent herpes labialis, ocular keratitis, and herpetic whitlow.

Primary herpetic gingivostomatitis is commonly acquired in small children (2 to 3 years of age). Initial symptoms may mimic many acute infections, with generalized malaise, fever, regional lymphadenopathy, headache, pain on swallowing, fretfulness, sleeplessness, and refusal to eat. Within a few days the mouth and gingiva become intensely painful and inflamed. The lips, tongue, buccal mucosa, palate, pharynx, and tonsils may become involved. Scattered aphthous-like lesions appear as crops of small ulcers that coalesce to produce large, shallow, irregular ulcers with surrounding inflammation (Gross, 1981). Merchant (1982) reports that only about 10% of oral infections are clinically apparent, indicating that some children especially may be infectious without usual symptoms or complaints. Within 7 to 14 days the vesicles and ulcers heal spontaneously with no scar formation.

Primary infections are usually asymptomatic but may present as gingivostomatitis. The hallmark of the secondary infection is usually a prodromal itching, tingling, or tenderness that may be present in the area 6 to 28 hours before the lesion occurs. The vesicles (the lay term for which is *cold sores*) on the lip or at the mucocutaneous junction generally progress to a crusted stage within 2 to 4 days. Discomfort is most severe during the first 24 hours, with the course of the disease running 7 to 10 days. Generally, no scar formation occurs.

The herpes virus may remain latent at the site in the regional nerve ganglia for years. The virus may be activated by trauma, febrile illness, exposure to sunlight, fatigue, menstruation, pregnancy, allergies, or emotional stress with shedding of the virus as the result. The virus shedding may or may not produce a lesion but may put at risk susceptible individuals who are in contact.

The proof of an antibody titer to herpes simplex virus does not necessarily protect against reinfection (Merchant, 1982).

The typical features of ocular keratitis include a foreign body sensation in the affected eye, followed several hours later by redness, tearing, light sensitivity, and pain. Dendritic ulcers of the cornea can occur. Only one eye is usually involved. Complete recovery occurs within about 3 weeks (Rowe et al, 1982). Ulcers may develop on the cornea, producing ocular damage. The possible debilitation and its effect on employment make recurrent ocular keratitis a serious condition for the clinician.

Herpetic whitlow is a herpes simplex virus infection of the fingers. It usually follows a puncture wound or passage of the virus through broken skin around fingernails. The site presents with extreme pain and itching within 3 to 5 days. The digit frequently swells, and one or more vesicles containing clear to turbid, but never purulent, fluid develop. Typically these lesions occur in the areas around the fingernail, although other areas of the finger can be involved as well. The lesion usually resolves within 14 to 21 days, but the clinical course may be prolonged (Merchant, 1982). Rowe and others (1982) state that the risk of contracting herpes simplex virus infection of the finger or hand for the practicing dental clinician is approximately twice what it would be if he or she were employed in some other field. There is no effective drug cure for herpetic whitlow, and because any clinician with this problem is a risk to patients and associates, a 10- to 14-day leave from practice may be indicated (Palenik and Miller, 1982).

Unlike hepatitis B, no vaccine is available to prevent herpes simplex virus infections. As stated previously, the proof of an herpes simplex virus antibody titer does not protect against reinfection. Treatment of herpes simplex infection is basically supportive in nature, with an emphasis on the prevention of secondary infection.

Topical anesthetics and compounds placed on the lesion to maintain moisture and prevent discomfort have been tried. Gross (1981) reports that topical applications of steroids have been used but have been shown to attenuate the attack and disperse the infection over a larger area. Therefore topical applications of corticosteroid creams should not be used. Compounds such as lysine (Tankersley, 1964) and bioflavonoid ascorbic acid (Terezhalmy et al 1978) have been reported to accelerate healing time. Currently, acycloguanosine (Acyclovir) has shown promise as a therapeutic agent, and research continues to find other agents to prevent, treat, and diminish recurrences of herpes simplex infections. The use of acyclovir in oral-labial herpes simplex virus infection has not been extensively studied. Anecdotal reports suggest its use in primary attacks, but it is not generally recommended for recurrent herpes labialis (Mandell et al, 1990).

Protection and prevention are best obtained by taking a history to identify patients with frequent episodes of herpes. Patients with active oral lesions should not be treated when elective care can be postponed. Standard infection control measures, including barrier protection, will reduce the risk of exposure to virus-containing aerosols and saliva.

CONTROL OF MICROORGANISMS

We live in an environment that is filled with microorganisms, including the air we breathe and every surface we touch. In addition, we carry immense communities of bacteria, viruses, and other microorganisms in our own bodies. The richest reservoir of these is the mouth. Many of these microorganisms are harmless to our health, and some are necessary to assist normal functioning of the human body. Others, such as the bacteria and viruses already discussed, cause serious communicable diseases. Many pathogens, including the tubercle bacillus, hepatitis viruses, and other durable viruses and infectious bacteria, can survive for a week or more in dried body fluids on surfaces and clothing, where they can be transmitted to dental personnel, other patients, and family members.

All health professionals are concerned about preventing disease transmission and maintaining an environment in which patients can be treated without the risk of contracting infection or debilitating disease. Total asepsis of the dental office is both impractical and impossible, but all attempts towards asepsis improve the chances of preventing cross-contamination of pathogens from objects in the dental environment to a person or from one person to another. An absolutely sterile office is impossible, but a safe environment is achievable. It is crucial that dental professionals be aware of the presence of pathogenic microorganisms and their potential for causing and transmitting disease. Clinicians must exercise all possible measures to reduce the numbers of pathogens and thus minimize the threat to patients and themselves.

The CDC has warned dental practitioners that medical histories and examinations cannot be relied on to identify all patients who are infected with the viruses that cause hepatitis, AIDS, and other bloodborne infections. Therefore, "universal" precautions designed to prevent transmission of these diseases should be followed for all patients (CDC, 1987). The recommendations in this chapter describe the standards of care currently accepted by the CDC and the ADA. It is the responsibility of every dental professional and student to seek all current information regarding future additions and changes in these guidelines to protect the health of themselves, their families, their coworkers, and those whom they serve. All members of the dental hygiene profession need to be aware of the OSHA Bloodborne Pathogens Standard (OSHA, 1991) which imposes a number of requirements regarding employees who could be occupationally exposed to infectious materials. The rule went into effect on March 6, 1992. Various timelines were established to help implementation. By May 5, 1992, all dental offices were required to have a written exposure control plan and as of June 4, 1992, record keeping requirements and training regarding rules must be provided to employees. All employees had to be offered the hepatitis B vaccination. Chemical containers must be labeled, and copies of applicable Material Safety Data Sheets (MSDS) must be on record. Personal protective equipment must be provided to employees, procedures for handling contaminated sharps and regulated waste must be developed, and a protocol for postexposure evaluation must be implemented. In order to understand these requirements, it is necessary to understand some of the theory behind them.

This chapter will discuss six important steps necessary to prevent disease transmission within the dental environment: (1) identification of contaminated surfaces; (2) sanitization of the dental environment; (3) disinfection procedures; (4) sterilization procedures; (5) use of effective barriers; and (6) personal hygiene and vaccinations.

The following definitions may be helpful in understanding contamination control terminology and recommendations:

antiseptic. Substance that inhibits the growth and reproduction of microorganisms; usually applied to living tissues as opposed to inanimate objects.

asepsis/aseptic. Absence of infection or infectious materials or pathogens.

-cidal. Suffix meaning "to kill" (e.g., virucidal, bactericidal, fungicidal, sporicidal, germicidal, tuberculocidal).

cross-contamination. Transmission of a pathogen from one person to another or from a surface to an individual.

disinfectant. Liquid chemical agent that destroys most but not all microorganisms.

disinfection. Process that destroys most but not all microorganisms.

HBV. Hepatitis B virus.

HIV. Human immunodeficiency virus.

sanitization. Process of mechanical removal or reduction of the number of microorganisms, dirt, or debris (e.g., cleaning.

-static. Suffix meaning "to restrain the development of" (e.g., bacteriostatic).

sterilant. Agent capable of resulting in sterilization.

sterilization. A process that results in the complete destruction of all microorganisms.

Identification of contaminated surfaces

Surfaces in the dental environment can be contaminated by direct contact with blood, saliva, mucous membranes, or other body fluids; aerosols; splatter droplets generated during dental treatment; or by contact with other contaminated surfaces or hands. Contamination control of environmental surfaces involves covering them with disposable drapes or wraps, avoiding unnecessary contact with surfaces during dental treatment, and treating them with recommended disinfection and sterilization procedures. In order to select the appropriate level of contamination control for each surface in the dental environment, one must first consider the level of contamination to which it is exposed and its potential as a source of cross-contamination. When considering the level and type of contamination, the prudent dental professional will remember that the recommended standards for infection control are based on the assumption that all patients are potential carriers of infectious diseases, including HBV and HIV. Although complete contamination control is the ideal goal, some items cannot be sterilized because of their size or their inability to withstand sterilization procedures. All surfaces and items in the dental environment may be classified in one of three ways:

1. Critical surfaces are those which actually enter the mouth and have direct contact with blood, saliva, mucous membranes, or other body fluids (e.g., all dental instruments, dental handpiece and prophy angle, air-water syringe tip, saliva ejector or high-speed evacuation tip, x-ray film holders) These instruments must either be sterilized before reuse or disposed.

2. Semicritical surfaces are those which may have frequent contact with aerosols generated during dental treatment or are touched by the patient or the contaminated hands of the clinician or assistant during patient treatment. These items may touch mucous membranes but do not enter sterile body areas. (e.g., chair and unit controls, lamp handle and switch, bases of the air-water syringe, saliva ejector, high-speed suction and handpiece, chair armrests, drawer pulls, supply container lids, bracket table rims or handles, countertops, x-ray head and controls, water faucet handles, and examining mirrors). These items should be treated with high-level disinfectants or be covered with barrier protection.

3. Noncritical surfaces are those which are present in the dental environment but unlikely to be contaminated by oral pathogens or touched during patient treatment (e.g., floors, walls, furniture, chairs, blinds, surfaces outside the dental operatory). Intermediate-level disinfectants can be used on these items.

All critical surfaces must be sterilized before reuse or discarded after one use (if disposable). Most of the items listed in the semicritical category cannot be moved or are too large for or incompatible with accepted sterilization methods. Therefore they must be kept covered and/or treated with accepted chemical solutions after each patient contact. Most noncritical surfaces require routine cleaning and disinfection.

Contamination control procedures are most effective if all office staff agree to follow predetermined written guidelines specifying what surfaces can and cannot be touched during patient treatment, as well as which disinfectants to use and how to use them properly. This disciplined behavior will ensure that prescribed contamination control procedures are consistently used to treat all contaminated areas in the most effective manner and that time will not be wasted trying to clean and disinfect surfaces that should never have been contaminated. Restricting the number of surfaces that fall within the semicritical category and following recommended guidelines that specify optimal treatment of all surfaces according to their categories can ensure maximal infection control. Following identification and categorization of contaminated surfaces in the operatory, sanitization—the first step in the infection control process—can be instituted.

Sanitization

Sanitization (cleaning) involves the physical removal of germ-laden dust and dirt from floors, walls, furniture, equipment, and surfaces. The elimination of visible soil is the first step in creating a safe environment and must precede all recommended disinfection and sterilization procedures. Sanitization reduces the numbers of microorganisms on surfaces and equipment, thus increasing the effectiveness of disinfection or sterilization procedures that follow. The presence of excessive numbers of microorganisms, soil, and organic matter (such as blood or saliva) can inhibit or even prevent methods of disinfection or sterilization from destroying the target pathogens. For this reason, routine cleaning and scrubbing of all surfaces in the dental office, especially those surfaces in the dental operatory which come into contact with patients, clinicians, or dental aerosols, is mandatory as the first step in the process to prevent disease transmission.

The general working environment of the dental office should be kept meticulously clean and free of dust. This includes walls, floors, furniture, curtains, cabinets, and countertops. Daily sanitization of all horizontal surfaces is necessary to remove bacteria-laden soil and dust that has entered from the outside environment. Other surfaces, including walls, furniture, drapes, and blinds, should be cleaned whenever they become visibly soiled. Cleaning and dusting is best accomplished with a vacuum system that removes the particles rather than a method that pushes them around the room and back into the air. Vacuum cleaning should be followed by use of a detergent solution. The detergents or soaps used for cleaning not only enhance the ability of water to remove surface dirt and films but also have mild destructive capabilities against some less resistant pathogens. In addition, a chemical disinfectant that has been registered by the Environmental Protection Agency (EPA) as a "hospital" disinfectant should be used on contaminated surfaces to destroy pathogenic bacteria and viruses that remain after mechanical cleaning. The directions on the label should be followed closely. This disinfectant should kill *M. tuberculosis*.

An especially critical area for contamination control is the lavatory, where pathogens that are spread by means of the oral-fecal route are frequently encountered. Sanitization of lavatories should include not only daily cleaning of all surfaces but also the use of strong and effective hospital disinfectants to destroy the large numbers of bacteria found there. In addition, all bathroom supplies such as towels or cups should be disposable.

Sanitization of the dental operatory is especially important because its surfaces are constantly exposed to oral pathogens during patient treatment. Operatory sinks should be kept clean, and any standing water should be removed from sink counters after hand washing. Foot-operated faucets are the best way to reduce contamination during washing. Hand faucets should be kept cleaned and disinfected. Because these surfaces may be difficult to disinfect thoroughly, contamination can be reduced by covering them with disposable plastic film, which is replaced after each patient, or by handling them with disposable paper towels rather than with contaminated hands. All disposable refuse should be kept out of sight in trash receptacles that have been lined with disposable bags. Appropriate puncture-resistant containers should be available for disposal of contaminated needles or other sharp items. Trash containers should be emptied promptly when full. Methods of disposal for all contaminated waste materials should comply with local and state ordinances. Items that pose a health hazard to others, such as disposable needles, syringes, blood-soaked materials, or hazardous chemicals, require special handling and disposal.

All surfaces in the dental operatory that would be at or above the eye level of the supine patient should be kept especially clean. Not only will these surfaces be contaminated by aerosols produced during dental procedures, but they will also be frequenty touched during treatment and within the viewing range of the patient. All surfaces on the semicritical list must be routinely cleaned before being disinfected and/or covered. To check the effectiveness of operatory sanitization, it is a good idea to recline in the dental chair and take a close look at the dental operatory from where the patient sits. Cobwebs near the ceiling, a spot of blood on the dental unit, or fingerprints on the light shield that went undetected from the clinician's vantage point may now be visible. These areas not only indicate inconsistencies or omissions in the cleaning routine but also affect the patient's opinion of office cleanliness. Patients may view these lapses in sanitization as a reflection of a general lack of concern not only for asepsis but also for their own health and well-being. Areas that need special spot cleaning and dusting should be attended to whenever necessary so that visible soil and dust accumulations on surfaces are promptly removed. Remember, cleaning is an essential step in disinfection and sterilization. It reduces the biologic burden and prevents the development of fomites by allowing effective disinfection and sterilization.

Disinfection

Methods of disinfection include the use of chemicals or heat to destroy microorganisms or to suppress the growth of organisms remaining after sanitization procedures. Disinfection methods that employ heat as the destructive agent include boiling water and hot oils. These methods are used to treat instruments or other items that are both heat resistant and small enough to be immersed in containers of the hot liquid. Because almost all instruments used in dentistry are categorized as critical surfaces, they need to be treated by sterilization methods; thus disinfection by boiling water or hot oil is not an acceptable substitute. Disinfection should be used only to control contamination on surfaces or items within the dental environment that cannot be sterilized; that is, those too large or too fragile to undergo accepted methods of sterilization.

Chemical disinfection. Chemical disinfectants may be used for immersion of small items or for disinfection of surfaces within the dental environment. Disinfectants should be chosen according to the range of bacteriostatic or bactericidal activity that is needed. Although some agents can effectively destroy microorganisms, others can only suppress their growth and multiplication. Agents that are lethal for bacteria are called bactericides. Others, called virucides, are effective against viruses. Corresponding results are obtained by fungicides and sporicides. The term *germicide* is used to describe an agent that is effective against vegetative bacterial cells but not the more resistant microbes such as *M. tuberculosis* or HBV. Even less effective are disinfectants described as bacteriostatic, which inhibit or suppress future bacterial growth but do not actually destroy all bacteria present on the affected surface.

Various chemical agents have been recommended for use in dentistry as disinfectants. Only those disinfectants that are registered by the EPA as hospital disinfectants and are tuberculocidal and virucidal for both lipid and hydrophilic viruses have been accepted for use in dentistry (Council on Dental Materials, Instruments, and Equipment [CDMIE], 1988, 1990). Table 3-6 provides a list of specific disinfectants that are accepted by the ADA for immersion and surface disinfection (CDMIE, 1988). Chemical disinfectants may be classified as high-, intermediate-, or low-level disinfectants depending on their range of effectiveness against pathogenic microorganisms. Table 3-7 shows the microbes that are destroyed by each level and identifies examples of disinfectants in each category.

Chemical disinfectants are effective only if the following critical factors are controlled: (1) all surfaces or items to be disinfected must first be precleaned; (2) optimal concentration of the chemical must be maintained; (3) surfaces to be treated must be in contact with the chemical for the recommended exposure time; (4) chemicals must not be used beyond their expected shelf life or period of stability; (5) solutions must be used at the recommended temperature; and (6) solutions must be used only during activated use and/or reuse periods. Specific manufacturer's recommendations must be followed carefully for each type of chemical disinfectant to maximize control of each of these factors.

Even under ideal conditions, however, chemical solutions cannot guarantee complete and consistent decontamination of all surfaces or instruments. Chemical solutions cannot penetrate into small recesses and destroy pathogens that may lie protected in jointed, hinged, or serrated instruments. Even after recommended exposure to chemical solution, these surfaces may remain contaminated and serve as sources of cross-contamination. Chemicals are most effective on smooth nonporous surfaces that can be adequately precleaned and can provide intimate contact between the pathogen and the solution. Any semicritical surface in the dental office that cannot be effectively cleaned and/or disinfected between patients must be kept covered to prevent contamination. An additional limitation of chemical disinfectants is the lack of standard, reliable methods for monitoring their effectiveness; thus there can be no guarantee that safe levels of protection have actually been achieved. This problem alone should make dental professionals wary of depend-

Table 3-6. Guide to chemical agents for disinfection and/or sterilization

Chemical classification* accepted products	Dilution	Disinfectant†, time (minutes)‡	Temperature (20° C = 68° F) (25° C = 77° F)	Sterilant‡
Surface/immersion				
Chlorine compounds				
Alcide LD	10:1:1	3	20° C	NA§
Exspor	4:1:1	3	20° C	4:1:1, 6 hours, 20° C
Bleach[a] (5.25% sodium hypochlorite)	1:10	10	20° C	NA
Iodophors				
Biocide and Surf-A-Cide	1:213	10	20° C	NA
ProMedyne-D	1:213	25	25° C	NA
Combination phenolics				
Multicide, Omni II, Vitaphene	1:32	10	20° C	NA
Phenolic-alcohol combinations—Lysol[b]	Full strength	10	20° C	NA
Immersion				
Phenolic-alcohol combinations—Decident[c]	Full strength	10	20° C	NA
Glutaraldehyde-phenolic combinations	1:16	10	20° C	Full strength, 6¾ hours
Sporicidin¶	1:16	10	20° C	Full strength, 6¾ hours, 20° C
ColdCide	1:4	10	20° C	Full strength, 6 hours, 20° C
2% Glutaraldehyde acidic	1:40	30	20° C	1:10, 10 hours, 25° C
Banicide concentrate	1:40	30	20° C	1:10, 10 hours, 25° C
Banicide, Sterall, and Wavicide-01	1:4	30	20° C	Full strength, 10 hours, 15° C
2% Glutaraldehyde neutral				
Glutarex	Full strength	—	—#	Full strength, 10 hours 20° C
2% Glutaraldehyde alkaline				
Cidex activated alkaline	Full strength	45	25° C	Full strength, 10 hours, 25° C
Cidex 7	Full strength	90	25° C	Full strength, 10 hours, 25° C
Germ-X	Full strength	—	—#	Full strength, 10 hours, 20° C
Asepti-Steryl 28, Dentacide, Glutall, Omnicide, Orthicide, Sporex, Vitacide	Full strength	45	20° C	Full strength, 10 hours
Steril-Ize	Full strength	45	25° C	Full strength, 10 hours, 20° C
CoeCide XL, K-Cide, Maxicide, Metricide 28, Procide 14	Full strength	20	20° C	Full strength, 6 hours, 20° C
Procide 30, Protec-top, Veratex	Full strength	10	25° C	Full strength, 6 hours, 20° C
3.2% Glutaraldehyde alkaline—Cidex Plus	Full strength	20	25° C	Full strength, 10 hours, 20° C

*ADA-accepted products as of March 1, 1990; a list of currently accepted products may be obtained by contacting the Council on Dental Therapeutics. [a]Bleach is not an accepted product. [b]For use on surfaces only. [c]For use on handpieces.

†Always use disinfectant/sterilant products according to the instructions specified on the product label.

‡The conditions listed reflect the time required for tuberculocidal activity for reused solution, if such use is possible, at the minimum temperature and maximal dilution specified on the EPA-approved product label. Tuberculocidal test methods may vary. Consult label or manufacturer for specifics.

§Not approved for use as a sterilant.

‖Alternate conditions, such as increased temperature or fresh solutions as opposed to reused solution, may decrease disinfection time. Consult label instructions for alternate uses.

¶Sporicidin was withdrawn from the market December, 1991.

#Data not available at time of publication; *NA,* Not applicable.

Table 3-7. Level of activity of chemical disinfectants and sterilants

Level of disinfection	Vegetative bacteria	Tubercle bacillus	Spores	Fungi	Lipid virus	Nonlipid virus	Disinfectants or sterilants
			Organisms destroyed				
High	Yes	Yes	Yes	Yes	Yes	Yes	2% glutaraldehyde-phenate 2% glutaraldehydes
Intermediate	Yes	Yes	No	Yes	Yes	Yes	Iodophors Sodium hypochlorite Phenolic compounds
Low	Yes	No	No	Yes	Yes	No	Quaternary ammonium compounds*

Modified from Terezhalmy GT et al: *Compend Contin Educ Dent* 9:114, 1987.
*Quaternary ammonium compounds are not acceptable for use as disinfectants of critical or semicritical surfaces in dentistry according to CDC and ADA guidelines.

ing on chemical solutions for treatment of instruments or other critical items that could undergo accepted methods of sterilization. Remember to consult MSDS sheets for each product used regarding its potential for effects on health, flammability, reactivity and any protective equipment that is needed to use it.

Surface disinfection. All surfaces or items that are contaminated during patient treatment by either direct or indirect contact with oral pathogens are sources for cross-contamination for patients and dental personnel. After identifying the critical, semicritical, and noncritical items or surfaces in the dental office, one can determine which disinfectant(s) will provide effective and safe levels of contamination control.

All critical items, especially dental instruments, handpieces, and air-water syringe tips, must be sterilized after each use. Any critical item that cannot undergo sterilization must be treated by a high-level disinfectant under recommended conditions. High-level disinfectants are those that are effective against all vegetative bacteria and viruses, including the tubercle bacillus, bacterial spores, and viruses such as the hepatitis B virus.

Many semicritical surfaces in the dental operatory can be protected from contamination by covering them with plastic-backed paper, plastic film, aluminum foil, or custom-designed disposable materials. Barrier covers are especially useful for surfaces that are difficult to clean and disinfect adequately in the time available between patient appointments. These disposable covers are replaced after each patient and discarded. Gloves

should always be worn when removing contaminated covers. Clean gloves should be used when replacing clean barrier covers. All surfaces in the semicritical category should be treated by an intermediate-level disinfectant. Intermediate-level disinfectants are effective against all microorganisms except for bacterial spores. Both the ADA and the CDC recommend the use of iodophors for surface disinfection. Iodophors are highly recommended because of their many advantages (Table 3-8). However, if you use an iodophor, be aware that it stains hard surfaces and linens (Block, 1991). Items that cannot be sterilized, disposed of, or covered must be precleaned and treated with an effective disinfecting solution for the prescribed length of time after each patient contact. Noncritical items or surfaces can be safely treated with low-level disinfectants, which are only effective against vegetative bacteria and some viruses.

The importance of adequate precleaning of all contaminated surfaces should not be underestimated. The process of physically removing microorganisms from surfaces by cleaning is as effective as directly killing them by chemical or other methods. The term *scrubbing*, rather than *wiping*, is appropriate to describe the cleaning process. This emphasizes the need to use pressure and repeated strokes over the contaminated surface while applying enough disinfectant solution to wet the surface thoroughly. Large surfaces such as chairs or countertops should be sprayed with disinfectant, scrubbed and sprayed again. They should be allowed to soak for the proper time and then scrubbed thoroughly (Fig. 3-1). Smaller

Table 3-8. Advantages and disadvantages of accepted chemical agents

Clinical agent	Advantages	Disadvantages
Chlorine compounds	Fast acting Effective against a wide variety of microbes, including HBV and tubercle bacillus Economical Recommended for hard surface disinfection	Unstable; prepare fresh solution daily Effectiveness reduced by presence of organic matter or altered pH Unpleasant odor Can corrode metals Irritates skin, eyes Can damage plastic and rubber materials Bleaching effect on clothing and other materials
Iodophors (high recommended as a hard surface disinfectant)	EPA-licensed surface disinfectant; broad spectrum effectiveness Economical Few physical side effects Color change from amber to clear indicates loss of effectiveness Residual activity on hard surfaces continues after solution has dried 3- to 30-minute contact time required for effective disinfection	Not classified as a sterilant Somewhat unstable with age at high temperature May stain light-colored surfaces after prolonged use Corrosive to some metals Inactivated by hard water Solution loses effectiveness with age Must be prepared fresh daily
Phenolic compounds	Active in presence of detergents Broad-spectrum effectiveness; some are tuberculocidal Primary use for floors, walls, etc.	Not recommended for disinfection of critical or semicritical surfaces Not sporicidal Irregular viricidal activity; ineffective against hydrophilic viruses (e.g., HBV) Inactivated by organic matter and hard water Can damage plastics and vinyl Potentially irritating to hands
Glutaraldehydes	Used primarily for immersion of heat and/or pressure-sensitive instruments that require high-level disinfection or sterilization	Irritating to skin, mucous membrane, eyes; wearing gloves and eyeglasses recommended Odor and fumes may be offensive; use in well-ventilated room Thorough rinsing of all treated materials is required Overnight immersion can corrode some metals

items such as handles and cords for air-water syringes and saliva ejectors should be wrapped in protective barriers.

Clinicians should be aware that the term *cold sterilization* is a misnomer when it is used to describe a chemical method of treating instruments. Cold sterilization has been traditionally used to describe the immersion of instruments in a disinfectant between patients. Because sterilization is the only accepted means of treating instruments and all chemical sterilants require immersion of instruments for at least 6¾ to 10 hours, it is clear that the use of chemical disinfecting solutions to treat contaminated dental instruments is not an acceptable procedure. Many of the chemicals still being used in dental offices do not provide an acceptable level of safety against resistant bacteria, bacterial spores, or HBV. Knowing this, dental professionals must consider their legal and ethical responsibilities to the patient before using chemical disinfecting solutions for treatment of instruments and other critical items when more effective and proven methods of sterilization are readily available.

Boiling water and hot oils. Both boiling water and hot oil solutions use heat as the destructive agent. Most vegetative cells are destroyed after immersion in vigorously boiling water (100° C, 212° F) for 10 minutes. However, because many spores and certain viruses may survive this

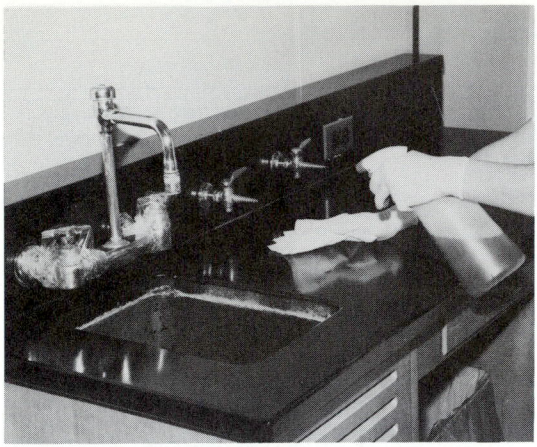

Fig. 3-1. Cleaning and disinfection of large surfaces can be accomplished efficiently with a spray bottle of disinfectant solution and a paper towel or large gauze sponges.

treatment, boiling cannot be considered a sterilization process. An additional problem with boiling is the corrosive effect of the water on metal. The addition of trisodium phosphate or sodium carbonate to the water will help reduce the corrosion as well as aid in removing debris from the instruments. These additives should not be used for aluminum instruments which can be corroded by the chemicals (Council on Dental Therapeutics [CDT], 1984).

Immersion of instruments in hot oils or silicone fluids will produce the following effects:

Disinfection: 150° C (300° F) for 15 minutes
125° C (260° F) for 20 to 30 minutes

Sterilization: 160° C (320° F) for 60 minutes minimum

Almost any instrument that can withstand such heat may be treated by this method. A special word of caution: hypodermic needles and syringes are never to be treated with hot oil because of the danger of retained oil being injected into the bloodstream and causing an embolus. Other disadvantages of the immersion method include the need to clean excess oil off items after sterilization or disinfection, difficulty in safely handling the hot oil solutions, and the possibility of unpleasant vapors and fumes from some heated solutions (CDT, 1984).

Antiseptics. Antiseptics are used in dentistry to reduce the number of microorganisms on living tissues, such as in the mouth or on the clinician's hands. Antiseptics are usually chemical disinfecting solutions that have been diluted so that they will not have a toxic or irritating effect when applied to human tissues. As a result of this dilution, antiseptics have a more limited ability to destroy bacterial cells than do disinfectants used on inanimate objects. Nonetheless, antiseptics can significantly reduce the chances of introducing pathogenic bacteria into the bloodstream during certain procedures. Antiseptics are commonly used before dental injections to cleanse the area so that the needle will not carry a large number of microorganisms deep into the tissue and blood supply. Antiseptics may also be used to clean an area of the mouth before a surgical procedure. The use of antiseptic mouthwashes can reduce the numbers of bacteria in the mouth before dental treatment. Many clinicians also use an antiseptic hand scrub to enhance the degerming effect of hand washing. The antiseptic may be contained in the soap or detergent that is used to cleanse the hands, or it may be a separate solution that is applied to the hands after scrubbing. Hand washing is discussed in more detail on page 56.

Sterilization

The highest level of contamination control is sterilization. Sterilization results in the total destruction of all forms of microbial life. Several methods of sterilization are approved for use by the ADA: steam under pressure (autoclaving), dry heat, ethylene oxide gas, chemical vapor sterilizers, and chemical solutions (Table 3-9). Of these methods, the first two, involving heat as the destructive agent, are preferred. Moist heat under pressure is considered the most efficient and reliable of all methods (CDT, 1984). Current recommendations regarding the preferred method(s) for sterilization of critical items in dentistry are listed in Table 3-10.

Autoclaving. Sterilization is accomplished by the action of steam under pressure in a metal chamber called an autoclave (Fig. 3-2). The pressure enables the temperature to reach a level high enough to ensure destruction of even bacteria that have endospores. Water at normal atmospheric pressures cannot be heated to a temperature higher than boiling (100° C, 212° F), which is not high enough to ensure complete microbial destruction. When water is heated under pressurized conditions, however, its temperature can be elevated beyond the boiling point to produce a

Text continued on p. 46.

Table 3-9. Methods of sterilization

Method	Standard conditions*	Uses	Advantages	Disadvantages	Packaging materials
Steam under pressure (autoclave)	Temperature: 121° C (250° F) Pressure: 15 psi Time: 20 minutes	All materials except oils, greases, powders, and items that cannot withstand the required temperatures and pressure	Most reliable method Quick and efficient Wide variety of materials can be sterilized	Cannot be used for oils, greases, powders, and heat-sensitive materials May dull cutting edges of carbon steel instruments May corrode metal instruments if precautions not taken Metal and glass containers must be open to penetration by steam	(Steam permeable) Paper Muslin Nylon Open containers
Dry heat (dry heat oven)	Temperature: 160° to 170° C (320° to 340° F) Time: 60 min. (170° C) or 120 min. (160° C)	Metal and glass equipment Oils, waxes, greases, powders Needles and other small instruments enclosed in glass or metal	Large capacity Low cost of equipment Does not dull cutting edges of carbon steel Only method for oils, greases, powders Does not erode ground glass surfaces Does not corrode metals Simple to operate Can penetrate closed glass and metal containers Items are dry after cycle	Requires longer time to sterilize than moist heat or chemical vapor Cannot be used on some heat-sensitive materials; temperatures above 170°C (340°F) will disjoin soldered instruments Instruments must be dry before sterilization to prevent rusting Cannot be used on liquids	(Heat permeable) Aluminum Paper Some cloth Open or closed containers
Ethylene oxide gas	Temperature: 49° C (120° F) Time: 2 to 3 hours or Temperature: room temperature Time: 12 hours	Sterilization of commercial products and items in hospital environments Most dental supplies and instruments	Useful for sterilization of handpieces that cannot be autoclaved Useful for heat-sensitive items	Causes irritation to eyes and nose Inhalation must be avoided; adequate ventilation required Toxic odor may be absorbed by some plastic or rubber items; requires aeration for 1 day or more before use Impractical for routine sterilization between patients Equipment may be more expensive than other methods	(Gas permeable) Paper Nylon Open containers

Continued.

Table 3-9. Methods of sterilization—cont'd

Method	Standard conditions*	Uses	Advantages	Disadvantages	Packaging materials
Chemical vapor	Temperature: 132° C (270° F) Pressure: 20 to 40 psi Time: 20 minutes	Any item tested for vapor penetration	Does not require high temperatures of dry heat Relatively short cycle useful for handpieces Will not corrode metals (metal instruments should be predried) Items are dry after cycle	Cannot be used for materials that are sensitive to the necessary temperature or pressure Vapor must penetrate through all materials Some materials may be incompatible with the chemicals used Exposure to fumes requires ventilation	(Gas permeable) Paper Open containers
Chemical solutions (glutaraldehyde)	Temperature: room temperature Time: 6¾ to 10 hours Requires optimal concentration of chemical solution	Plastics and other heat-sensitive materials that cannot withstand heat sterilization	Does not require heat to achieve sterilization Plastics, rubber, and other heat-sensitive materials can be sterilized Good for instruments containing bonded parts (e.g., lenses, mirrors, handpieces) Chemical not affected by soaps and detergents	Requires immersion of objects for minimum of 6¾ to 10 hours to achieve sterilization Destruction of hepatitis virus is probable but not proven Irritates skin and mucous membranes; should be rinsed off instruments before their use May corrode carbon steel after 24 hours of immersion	

*Recommended conditions may vary depending on model, wrapping, size of load. Follow manufacturer's instructions and monitor with spore tests.

Table 3-10. Sterilization and disinfection of dental instruments, materials, and some commonly used items*

	Steam autoclave	Dry heat oven	Chemical vapor	Ethylene oxide	Chemical disinfection/ sterilization	Other methods/comments
Angle attachments*	+	+	+	++	+	
Burs						
Carbon steel	−	++	++	++	−	
Steel	+	++	++	++	+	
Tungsten-carbide	+	++	+	++	+	
Condensers	++	++	++	++	+	
Dappen dishes	++	+	+	++	+	
Endodontic instruments (broaches, files, reamers)						Hot salt/glass bead sterilizer 10 to 15 seconds, 218° C (425° F)
Stainless steel handles	+	++	++	++	+	
Stainless with plastic handles	++	++	−	++	−	
Fluoride gel trays						
Heat-resistant plastic	++	− −	−	++	−	
Nonheat-resistant plastic	− −	− −	−	++	−	Discard (++)
Glass slabs	++	++	++	++	+	
Hand instruments						
Carbon steel	−	++	++	++	−	
	[Steam autoclave with chemical protection (1% sodium nitrite)]					
Stainless steel	++	++	++	++	+	
Handpieces*						Sterilizable preferably
Sterilizable*	(++)*	−	(+)*	++	− −	
Contra-angles*	−	−	−	++	+	Combination synthetic phenolics or iodophors (−)
Nonsterilizable*	−	−	−	++	+	
Prophylaxis angles*	+	+	+	+	+	
Impression materials						Table 2
Impression trays						
Aluminum metal	++	+	++	++	−	
Chrome-plated	++	++	++	++	+	
Custom acrylic resin	− −	− −	− −	++	+	
Plastic	− −	− −	− −	++	+	Discard (++); preferred
Instruments in packs	++	+ Small packs	++	++ Small packs	− −	
Instrument tray setups						
Restorative or surgical	+ Size limit	+	+ Size limit	++ Size limit	− −	
Mirrors	−	++	++	++	+	
Needles Disposable	− −	− −	− −	− −	− −	Discard (++) Do not reuse
Nitrous oxide						
Nose piece	(++)*	− −	(++)*	++	(+)*	
Hoses	(++)*	− −	(++)*	++	(+)*	
Orthodontic pliers						
High-quality stainless	++	++	++	++	+	
Low-quality stainless	−	++	++	++	−	
With plastic parts	− −	− −	− −	++	+	
Pluggers	++	++	++	++	+	
Polishing wheels and disks						
Garnet and cuttle	− −	−	−	++	− −	
Rag	++	−	+	++	− −	
Rubber	+	−	−	++	+	
Prostheses, removable	−	−	−	+	+	

Continued.

Table 3-10. Sterilization and disinfection of dental instruments, materials, and some commonly used items*—cont'd

	Steam autoclave	Dry heat oven	Chemical vapor	Ethylene oxide	Chemical disinfection/ sterilization	Other methods/comments
Rubber dam equipment						
Carbon steel clamps	−	+ +	+ +	+ +	−	
Metal frames	+ +	+ +	+ +	+ +	+	
Plastic frames	−	−	−	+ +	+	
Punches	−	+ +	+ +	+ +	+	
Stainless steel clamps	+ +	+ +	+ +	+ +	+	
Rubber items						
Prophylaxis cups	−	−	−	+ +	−	Discard (+ +)
Saliva evacuators, ejectors						
Low-melting plastic	−	−	−	+ +	+	Discard (+ +)
High-melting plastic	+ +	+	+	+ +	+	
Stones						
Diamond	+	+ +	+ +	+ +	+	
Polishing	+ +	+	+ +	+ +	−	
Sharpening	+ +	+ +	+ +	−		
Surgical instruments						
Stainless steel	+ +	+ +	+ +	+ +	+	
Ultrasonic scaling tips	+	− −	− −	+ +	+	
Water-air syringe tips	+ +	+ +	+ +	+ +	+	
X-ray equipment						
Plastic film holders	(+ +)*	− −	(+)*	+ +	+	
Collimating devices	−	− −	− −	+ +	+	

From Council on Dental Materials, Instruments, and Equipment; Council on Dental Practice; and Council on Dental Therapeutics: *JADA* 116:241, 1988.
The table is adapted from *Accepted Dental Therapeutics and Dentists' Desk Reference: Materials, Instruments, and Equipment.*
*As manufacturers use a variety of alloys and materials in these products, confirmation with the equipment manufacturers is recommended, especially for handpieces and the attachments.
+ +Effective and preferred method.
+Effective and acceptable method.
−Effective method, but risk of damage to materials.
− −Ineffective method with risk of damage to materials.

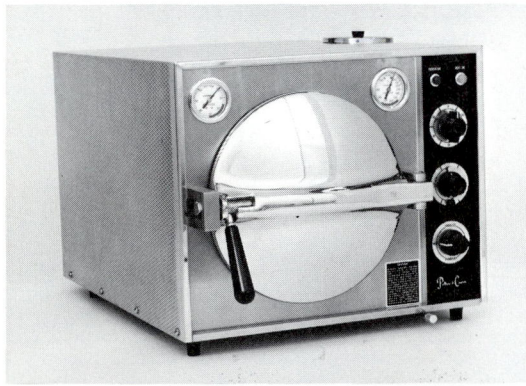

Fig. 3-2. Autoclave unit.
(Courtesy of Pelton and Crane, Charlotte, North Carolina).

superheated effect that is capable of sterilization. No living thing can survive 10 minutes of direct exposure to saturated steam at 121° C (250° F), a temperature that is attained under ideal conditions with 15 pounds of pressure per square inch (psi) in an autoclave. However, an additional 5 to 10 minutes is usually added as a safety factor because it takes a while to reach critical temperature.

Operation of the autoclave. Preparation of the autoclave should begin by checking the water supply in the unit. Steam for sterilization is provided by distilled or deionized water. The water level may be viewed by lifting the cover at the top of the chamber. During the operating cycle, there must be enough water available to produce sufficient steam to fill the entire chamber. Therefore the tank always should be kept filled to the indicator line.

Any package, instrument, or container to be autoclaved is loaded onto a metal tray that will be inserted into the chamber. Materials to be sterilized in the autoclave should be wrapped in muslin, paper, or steam-permeable plastic bags or be held in open glass or metal containers. Do not package materials to be autoclaved in sealed or closed jars or in aluminum foil. When loading trays, place wrapped packages uniformly on edge, with no more than two layers on each tray; place open jars or containers on their sides. Packages or containers should not touch the chamber walls. The success of the sterilization procedure depends on the ability of the superheated steam to come in contact with all items; thus, they should be packed loosely on the tray to permit an easy flow of steam in and around all materials (Fig. 3-3). If the completely sealed bags are jammed tightly against each other, it will be much more difficult for the steam to penetrate through to the innermost layers (Fig. 3-4). When trays are improperly loaded, microorganisms that are insulated or protected from the effects of the moist heat may not be killed during the usual sterilization cycle.

After the trays are placed in the sterilization chamber, the control knob should be turned to the "fill" position, allowing the water that will later be converted to steam to enter the chamber. To ensure a sufficient amount of water, the metal cover plate at the front of the chamber floor must be completely covered before the knob is turned to the "sterilize" position. At this time, the chamber door should be closed and locked into place. All packages should be completely sealed inside the chamber and should not be caught in the chamber door, which would prevent a complete seal within the chamber. In such a case, the temperature inside the chamber would not rise high enough to achieve sterilization.

When the knob is turned to the "sterilize" position, water will stop entering the chamber, and the inside temperature of the autoclave will begin to rise. The thermostatic controls on the front of the unit should be set so that when the desired temperature is reached, along with its corresponding pressure, the heat will be maintained at that level for the remainder of the sterilization cycle. Every autoclave should be equipped with a safety valve to prevent the inner chamber from reaching

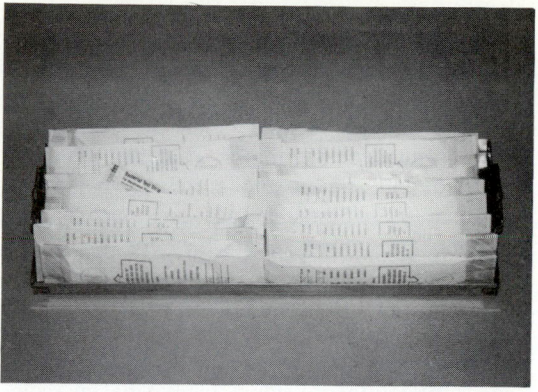

Fig. 3-3. Properly loaded trays will allow flow of steam through and around all surfaces.

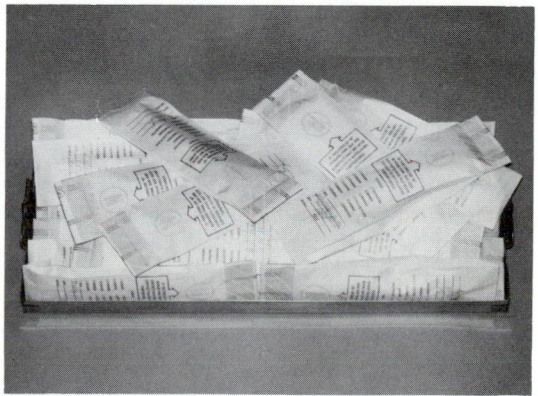

Fig. 3-4. Improperly loaded tray. Instruments are packed tightly together and tray is overloaded.

an unnecessarily high temperature or pressure. Once the chamber has reached the appropriate conditions for sterilization (usually 121° C at 15 psi), the timer on the unit should be set for the desired length of time. In most instances this will be 15 to 20 minutes. Timing of the sterilization cycle should not begin until the recommended conditions have been reached and the temperature of the contents has reached 121° C. These conditions must then be maintained for the entire length of the cycle. At the end of this period, as indicated by the timer, the control knob can be turned to the "vent" position. The steam will escape from the chamber to release pressure, and the chamber will begin to cool. These changes should be indicated by the temperature and pressure gauges, which move slowly toward zero. When both levels have been reduced to zero, the chamber door can be opened. No attempt to open the door should be made until the pressure has been eliminated within the chamber. The door should be left ajar for several minutes before trays are removed so that the bags and other materials have a chance to dry before they are stored. Even after a few minutes of cooling, however, the metal trays and their contents will still be hot and should be handled with care.

Monitoring sterilization. The effectiveness of any sterilization procedure cannot be guaranteed unless it is certain that the desired conditions such as temperature, pressure, time, and/or chemical exposure are consistently met. Even the best gauges are not foolproof, and periodic maintenance and tests should be performed to ensure the effectiveness of all equipment. Studies of the effectiveness of dental office sterilizers have indicated that up to one third may fail testing procedures (Hastreiter, 1991; Palenik et al, 1986; Simonsen et al, 1979; Skaug, 1983; Palenik and Miller, 1986a). Any number of factors can contribute to sterilization failure including: improper packaging or wrapping, overloading, disregard for manufacturer's instructions, or mechanical malfunction. Proper maintenance of the sterilization equipment, observation of units as they are operating, and the use of external and internal chemical monitors and biologic monitors are all important steps in ensuring that sterilization occurs.

Biologic spore tests (Fig. 3-5) are the most reliable way of ensuring the effectiveness of sterilization procedures. Biologic monitoring methods are available for testing the effectiveness of autoclaves, dry heat ovens, chemical vapor sterilizers, and ethylene oxide gas sterilizers. There are currently no standard procedures for biologic monitoring of chemical sterilant solutions used for immersion of instruments. Biologic monitoring uses special bacterial spore test strips or vials that are placed at the center of a normal load in the sterilization unit and then submitted to the usual sterilization cycle. Spore strips consist of filter paper that has been impregnated with spores and enclosed in an envelope. After sterilization, the spores are placed in a sterile growth medium and incubated for 7 days. If spores grow they turn the solution cloudy, indicating that sterilization has

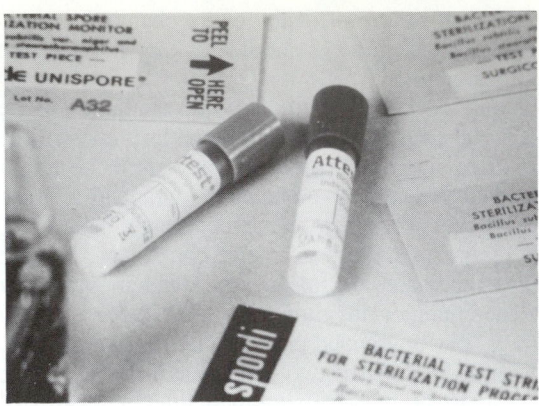

Fig. 3-5. Spore strips and test ampules are placed inside packages or containers during sterilization procedures to test whether or not sterilization has occurred. (Courtesy of 3M Co, Minnesota.)

failed. Spore test vials may contain a spore strip and an ampule of growth medium. After processing, the vial is squeezed to crush the ampule and then incubated for 24 to 48 hours. Another type of vial contains spores in a test medium that changes colors if spore germination occurs. An inexpensive incubator can be purchased to perform this test in the dental office, or test materials can be mailed to one of a number of sterilization monitoring services (Farah and Powers, 1986).

Autoclaves and chemical vapor sterilizers are tested using the organism *Bacillus stearothermophilus*, a bacterial spore that can withstand all but the most stringent sterilization conditions and is used for monitoring chemiclaves and autoclaves. The organism *Bacillus subtilis* var. *niger* is used to test dry heat ovens and ethylene oxide sterilizing equipment. Evidence of bacterial growth following incubation indicates that some of the bacterial spores survived the sterilization process and that equipment malfunction or other errors have occurred during the sterilization procedure. Sterilization equipment must be tested weekly by this method and documented in a log book (CDMIE, 1988; CDC, 1986, 1991).

A second step toward ensuring sterilization is the use of chemical indicators (Fig. 3-6) that change color when subjected to sterilization conditions. External chemical indicators include labels on autoclave bags and special heat-sensitive tape used to seal bags. The color change occurs when the indicator has been exposed to steriliza-

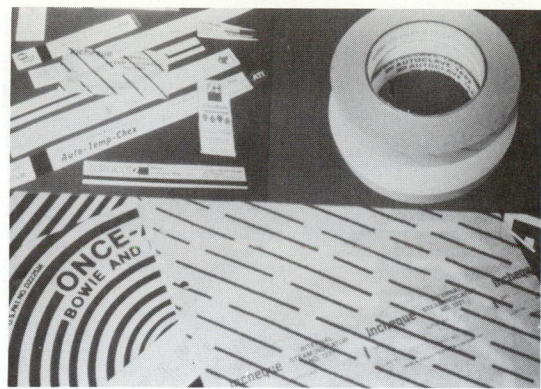

Fig. 3-6. Examples of internal *(top left)* and external chemical indicators.
(Courtesy of 3M Co, Minnesota.)

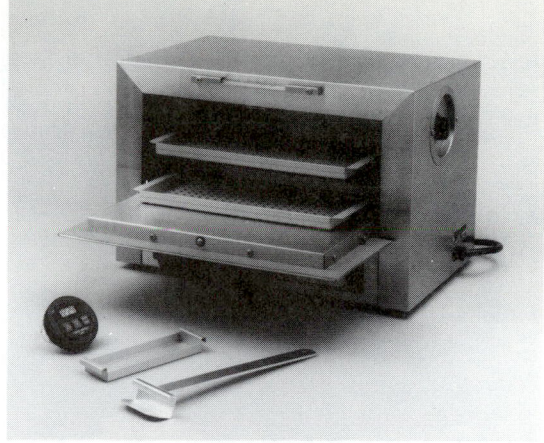

Fig. 3-7. Dry heat oven (Dri-Clave).
(Courtesy of Columbus Dental, St Louis, Missouri.)

tion temperatures, but this does not document that the instruments have been sterilized for the proper amount of time. Chemical indicators provide an easy way of discriminating between processed and nonprocessed items. Internal chemical indicators are placed inside wrapped packages to ensure that the contents of the packages were exposed to appropriate conditions. All bagged items for sterilization must be sealed and have a heat-sensitive indicator placed on them. Although chemical indicators provide a quick means of identifying a failure in sterilization procedures, they cannot be relied on to guarantee that sterilization has actually occurred. They indicate that the materials were exposed to the appropriate temperature or chemicals, but they do not prove that the exact conditions and time required for sterilization have been met. The only method that provides conclusive evidence that sterilization has occurred is biologic monitoring with spore tests.

Maintenance of the autoclave should follow manufacturer's instructions and include daily checking of the temperature, pressure, and timer gauges. The door gasket should be checked regularly for signs of wear or damage. The inner surface of the chamber should be washed periodically with a mild detergent and rinsed well. Dental offices should keep written records to document sterilization monitoring procedures. Runnells (1985) recommended that these records be kept and stored for at least 3 years. Records should include the type of monitoring performed, sterilization conditions, dates on which tests were

performed, results of biologic monitoring tests, and maintenance procedures (Miller, 1987).

Dry heat. Dry heat may be used for materials that cannot withstand steam under pressure, such as oils, powders, greases, and some dental instruments and handpieces. Dry heat is the method of choice for fine endodontic instruments. The dry heat oven is much like a regular oven (Fig. 3-7). The same conditions for loading the oven apply as for loading the autoclave to ensure that all contents reach sterilization temperatures within the prescribed length of time. Instruments should be packaged in a manner that will allow the heated air to circulate freely around them. Appropriate wrapping materials include foil or closed glass or metal containers or trays. Cloth and paper materials may char or scorch because of the high temperatures, and some plastics may produce toxic fumes when heated.

Because some microorganisms are extremely resistant to dry heat, it is necessary to maintain high temperatures for a prolonged period until all spores have been killed. An internal temperature of 160° C for 2 hours or 170° C for 1 hour (320° F to 340° F) must be achieved and maintained for the required time. More specific instructions as to the recommended temperatures and time required for certain materials are given in Tables 3-6 and 3-9. The length of time required to achieve the proper internal temperature depends on the size of the load, the materials being heated, and the wrapping materials used. For example, a few unwrapped metal instruments could be heated to

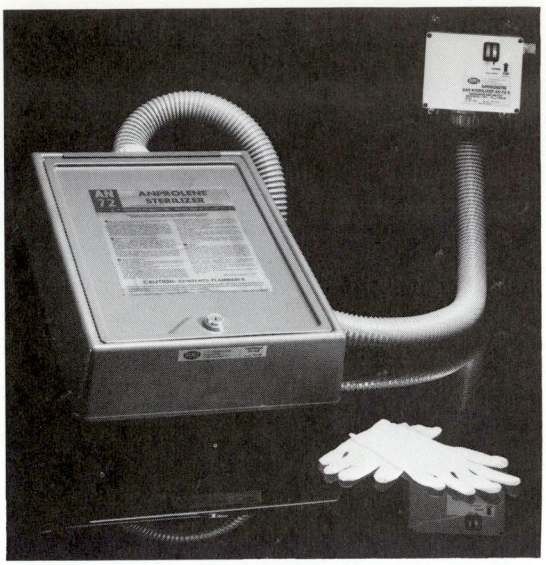

Fig. 3-8. Ethylene oxide sterilizer (Anprolene model). (Courtesy of HW Anderson Products, Inc, Chapel Hill, North Carolina.)

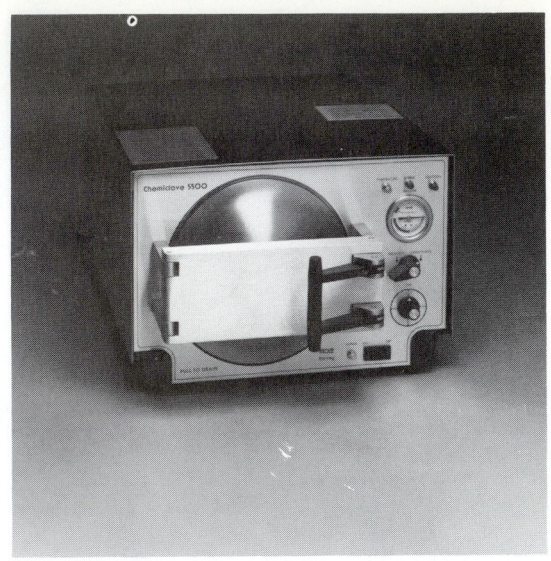

Fig. 3-9. Chemical vapor sterilizer (Chem-Clave). (Courtesy of MDT Corp, Torrance, California.)

sterilization temperatures much faster than a large number of heavily wrapped bundles. Since a certain amount of time is required to heat the entire contents of the oven to this temperature, a total sterilization period of 2 hours is often recommended. Avoid overloading the oven. Separate items by at least ½ inch and load packages no more than two layers deep, with the top layer at right angles to the bottom layer. Check the temperature with a thermometer that indicates the internal temperature of the oven. Bacterial spore tests are recommended to monitor the effectiveness of this equipment in achieving sterilization. Dental offices using this method of sterilization should use a unit that has been tested and approved by the FDA as a commercial sterilizer.

Ethylene oxide gas. A third method of sterilization is ethylene oxide gas. This method is used mainly by hospitals, where large quantities of materials and instruments must be sterilized. It is also used for sterilization of some commercial products. Recently, smaller sterilizing units that are more suitable in size and expense for the dental office have been made available (Fig. 3-8). The main advantage of ethylene oxide gas sterilization is that it does not require the high temperatures of the autoclave or the dry heat oven, which means that heat-sensitive materials, including plastic items and all handpieces, can be safely

sterilized. Some units operate with cycles that require no additional moisture or pressure, and sharp items and fragile pressure-sensitive items can be safely sterilized by this method. A major disadvantage of the ethylene oxide method is its long sterilization cycle (10 to 16 hours) and the additional time required for aeration of some items; these render it impractical for routine sterilization of all dental instruments or supplies. In addition, ethylene oxide gas does have some toxic properties that make it irritating to the eyes and nose. These toxic fumes can be retained by plastics or rubber materials. Rubber and plastic materials that can absorb the gas should be aerated for 24 hours or longer before being used. Prolonged inhalation of the gas in even low concentrations should be avoided, and the sterilizing unit should be used only in properly ventilated areas (CDT, 1984).

Chemical vapor. Chemical vapor sterilization is another method available for use in dental practices. The chemical vapor sterilizer is an autoclave-like device (Fig. 3-9) that uses a mixture of chemical vapors, including alcohol, ketone, acetone, and formaldehyde, which are heated together with water to a temperature of 270° F, under 20 psi of pressure, for 30 minutes. It is effective for materials that are heat sensitive and cannot withstand autoclaving or dry heat temperatures. The risk of damage by rust or corrosion is aso diminished because of the low water content. The chemical vapor sterilizer should not be used for any material that cannot withstand the necessary temperatures or is incompatible with the chemical agents. An additional disadvantage of this method is the production of chemical fumes that can destroy heat-sensitive plastics. Therefore these units should be operated only in well-ventilated areas. Fumes can be minimized by opening the chamber door slightly at the end of the cycle so that vapor condenses on the inside of the chamber or by venting the unit to the outside.

Wrapping materials or containers must be permeable to the chemical vapors to ensure effective exposure of chemicals to all surfaces. Do not use sealed glass jars, closed containers, or aluminum foil to hold or wrap items that will be sterilized using this method, as these materials do not permit penetration of the chemical vapor. Packages should be wrapped so as to prevent air pockets but not so tightly that airflow is obstructed. Chemical vapor sterilization should be monitored with spore test organisms to ascertain that all conditions for sterilization are being met. Maintenance should follow manufacturer's instructions and should include regular checking of all fittings and seals and weekly cleaning.

Chemical solutions. Table 3-6 lists chemical solutions that are approved for use in dentistry as sterilants (ADA, 1990). The only chemical solution that has been shown to achieve true sterilization is 2% glutaraldehyde. It should be noted that Sporicidin (Ash Dentsply, York, Pa.) was recalled from the market by the FDA in December, 1991 (Ingersoll, 1991). Glutaraldehyde has been shown to destroy fungi, viruses, and bacteria, including *M. tuberculosis*, after immersion for 10 minutes (disinfection). It is also capable of killing bacterial spores after immersion for 6 ¾ to 10 hours (sterilization). Exposure times vary depending on the product used and the amount of biocidal activity desired (CDMIE, 1988). The manufacturer's directions for use of these chemicals should be followed carefully to ensure optimal results.

Glutaraldehyde can probably destroy HBV under recommended conditions, but this cannot be guaranteed as the etiologic agent for HBV cannot be cultured. Bond and others (1983) tested the effectiveness of a number of intermediate- and high-level disinfectants, including iodophors, sodium hypochlorite, and two types of 2% glutaraldehyde, against the HBV by treating HBV-infected human plasma for 10 minutes with each disinfectant and then injecting the neutralized plasma into chimpanzees. After 9-month observation period, none of the animals had developed hepatitis B. Although these preliminary tests indicate that glutaraldehyde and certain intermediate-level disinfectants may destroy HBV, further studies are needed before it can be considered safe to treat critical surfaces that have been exposed to the hepatitis B virus by anything other than approved sterilization methods.

Chemical sterilant solutions should not be depended on as a substitute for other approved measures such as the autoclave, dry heat oven, or chemical vapor sterilizer because the effectiveness of solutions is difficult to verify. Although individual manufacturers provide tests for monitoring the concentration of active glutaraldehyde remaining in solution for reuse, there is no accepted standard for biologic monitoring of this method as there is for the other accepted methods. In addition, the 6 ¾ to 10 hours required for sterilization by 2% glutaraldehyde preparations makes them impractical for routine treatment of instruments and other critical items between patients. Glutaraldehyde solutions should be considered, however, for obtaining a high degree of disinfection or sterilization for any immersible items that cannot be sterilized by heat, such as plastics or rubber items. If this method is used, the items must be rinsed with sterile water and then properly bagged.

Gloves and goggles or a face shield should be worn when using chemical sterilants, as they are irritating to the skin and eyes. Holding containers should be kept closed and the solutions should be used in well-ventilated areas. Instruments treated in these solutions should be rinsed thoroughly with sterile water. Because some rubber and plastic materials can retain the chemical after repeated exposure, rinsing of these items must be particularly thorough so that the glutaraldehyde is not carried to the patient's skin, mouth, or bloodstream (Palenik and Miller, 1984a).

Several other methods of sterilization including ultraviolet light, microwaves, and other forms of radiation, have been used as methods of sterilization. At the present time, none of these methods is a practical alternative for use in dental offices (Runnells, 1985).

Disposable supplies and instruments

The ADA states that the proper handling and preparation of instruments in the dental office should provide the practitioner with instruments that are completely free of viable bacteria, viruses, and spores while maintaining their usefulness (ADA CDT/CDMIE, 1990). This can be accomplished by sterilizing reusable instruments by one of the methods discussed or by using disposable items that are discarded after one use. Many dental supplies, such as tongue blades, cotton-tipped applicators, aspirator tips, saliva ejectors, radiograph holders, rubber polishing cups, fluoride trays, syringes, and needles are available in disposable form. Disposable prophylaxis angles are also available. All disposable supplies are intended to be used only once and then discarded; they are not meant to be cleaned and reused under any circumstances. Disposable supplies should be stored in sterile, dry containers. Transfer of supplies into storage containers or from containers to the operating area should be accomplished using clean, gloved hands and/or sterile forceps or cotton-pliers.

There are a number of advantages to using disposable supplies. The most important advantage is prevention of cross-contamination, because these items are used only once and then discarded. The use of disposable needles is especially valuable in the prevention of hepatitis B and AIDS, because contaminated needles are known to be one of the chief causes of transmission of these serious diseases. The use of disposable supplies saves considerable time and money that would otherwise be expended in cleaning and sterilization. Disposable tray covers, patients' napkins, and headrest covers not only protect the patient and the working environment from contamination by bacterial aerosols and splatter, but also reduce the time and effort needed to disinfect surfaces between patients. Use of disposable hand towels is a necessity in the dental office. Cloth towels become contaminated after only one use and cannot be safely reused until they have been cleaned and sterilized. The advantages of using disposable supplies should be weighed against the cost of purchasing them. Whenever possible, dental professionals should consider the use of disposable items for purposes of convenience and as a means of preventing cross-contamination

Preparing instruments for sterilization

Cleaning instruments. Any instrument or other item that is to be sterilized or disinfected must be prepared by thorough cleaning, rinsing, and drying before it undergoes sterilization. The presence of blood saliva, soap films, and other organic debris not only increases the numbers of microorganisms that must be killed but also protects them against the destructive agent. The more a microorganism is protected by insulating debris, soap residue, or other microorganisms, the longer it will take for it to be destroyed. Recommended sterilization and disinfection conditions (time, concentration, temperature) depend on the intimate contact of the chemical or heating agent with the microorganism. Therefore thorough washing, rinsing, and drying of all instruments must precede the disinfecting or sterilization process.

Instruments should be cleaned as soon as possible after they have been used to expedite removal of blood and debris before they dry. If immediate cleaning is not possible, instruments should be soaked in a cool detergent or disinfectant solution. Ultrasonic cleaning is preferred for instrument preparation over hand scrubbing because the ultrasonic cleaner can dislodge contaminated material from grooves, hinges, and other surfaces that are not easily reached with a brush. Ultrasonic cleaning is also safer because it reduces the need to handle contaminated instruments. Protective rubber gloves should always be worn when handling contaminated instruments to prevent accidental injury and infection. Scrubbing spatters contamination and creates unnecessary aerosol.

Use of the ultrasonic cleaner. Gross debris may be rinsed from contaminated instruments before cleaning. They are then placed into the cleaning solution, which can be either a nonfoaming commercial detergent (see manufacturer's instructions) or a solution of 1 part iodine surgical scrub solution to 19 parts detergent (Crawford, 1986). Do not use a chemical sterilant—it can be volatilized and accidentally inhaled. The instruments should be treated for 5 minutes in the ultrasonic bath with the cover in place to avoid splattering of the solution onto adjacent surfaces. After cleaning, the instruments should be removed with forceps or heavily gloved hands, rinsed, inspected for debris, and then either rinsed in alcohol to enhance drying or dried with paper towels. Carbon steel instruments or low-quality stainless steel instruments that are likely to rust as a result of autoclaving should be dipped in protective solutions such as 1% sodium nitrite (Crawford, 1986) or amine compounds to prevent corrosion. The cleaned instruments can then be wrapped or placed in trays for sterilization. At the end of the day, the solution in the ultrasonic cleaner should be discarded and the reservoir and tray disinfected with 0.5% sodium hypochlorite (Crawford, 1986). Monitoring can be done by placing a small piece of tin foil in the bath during operation. Generalized pitting should be noted on the foil if the machine is operating properly.

Wrapping instruments. Unless an instrument or item will be used immediately after it is sterilized, it should be wrapped or contained in a material compatible with the sterilization method to be used (see Table 3-9). Follow the recommendations of sterilizer manufacturers regarding the best types of packaging materials to use for each method. Sterilization bags are constructed so that, once they are sealed, they maintain the sterility of their contents unless the bag is torn or punctured. Damage to the sterilization bag can be prevented by wrapping sharp instruments in a paper towel or shielding sharp edges with cotton rolls or gauze sponges before inserting them into the bag. Instruments that can be damaged by contact with other instruments, such as the head of the mouth mirror, should be wrapped separately so that they are protected from damage. The most common type of sterilization bag is made of paper and is disposable. These bags come in a variety of shapes and sizes, depending on the number and type of instruments to be sterilized. To increase practice efficiency, it is advisable to wrap instruments together as a "tray" specific to a designated procedure. By wrapping instruments according to their intended use, only one or two sterile packages need to be opened to furnish the entire tray set-up. This is important because whenever a bag is opened, its entire contents are exposed to environmental contaminants and can no longer be considered sterile. When instruments are wrapped with this in mind, bags need not be opened unless all instruments are to be used. Infrequently used instruments should be packaged individually. Each bag should be labeled so that instruments for any given tray setup can be identified easily. As an added convenience, some sterilization bags

are made of transparent materials so that the contents can be identified without the need for labelling or opening the bag. These bags are especially useful for singly wrapped instruments. Following are examples of instruments that may be packaged together:

Treatment procedure	Tray setup (package together)
Initial examination	Mirror, explorer, probe, gauze sponge, tongue blade
Scaling	Assorted scalers and/or curettes
Periodontal debridement	Gracey curettes, explorer, mirror

Once the wrapped instruments and supplies are inserted into the labeled bag, the open end of the bag should be closed with a double fold and sealed with a piece of specially designed sterilization tape. The tape should be long enough to seal the entire fold and to lap around to the opposite side on both ends. Sealing and taping in this way will help ensure that the bag is properly sealed against recontamination during storage. Plastic bags may also be heat sealed. Muslin or paper-wrapped packs should be resterilized if not used within 30 days. Tape-sealed paper and plastic packs should be resterilized after 4 months, and heat-sealed plastic packs can last up to 6 months before requiring resterilization (Crawford, 1986).

Instrument transfer. Clean gloves should always be worn when handling clean or sterile supplies in preparation for the next patient or when transferring supplies from one location to another. Sterile supplies should be transferred by means of sterile forceps rather than with the fingers. This precaution will help ensure that pathogens transmitted by the hands are not introduced into an otherwise aseptic environment. Sterile cotton pliers may be included on each tray setup for this purpose. When supplies are being transferred from a covered container, it is best to hold the lid top up with one hand while removing the supplies with the forceps in the other hand (see Fig. 3-5). This prevents airborne bacteria from settling onto the inside of the lid, which is then replaced on the sterile container. If it is necessary to lay the lid down, however, it should be put down with the inside surface up so that its rims are not contaminated by the countertop.

Aseptic technique should be used when removing sterile instruments from an autoclave bag for positioning on the tray. Because the bag has contacted the storage drawer and has been handled since it left the autoclave, the outside is no longer sterile. Therefore placing the bag on the tray contaminates that surface. Instead, tear off the end of the bag and slide the wrapped instruments onto the tray without permitting contact of the bag with the contents of the tray. The contents of the tray should be kept covered until they are needed.

Reducing airborne contamination

Dental aerosols and splatter. Dental aerosols are tiny, invisible particles of contaminated water, blood, and saliva generated from the patient's mouth during dental procedures. Large numbers of aerosols are produced during use of the high-speed handpiece, the air-water syringe, the ultrasonic scaler, and the air polishing unit, as well as during engine polishing and tooth brushing. The small size of these particles permits them to enter the body through the nose, mouth, and eyes. After they have entered the respiratory tract, they can penetrate deeply into its linings. Aerosols can remain suspended in the air for as long as 24 hours (Micik et al, 1969), where they continue to be sources of contamination long after the patient has left.

In addition to aerosols, the air can be contaminated by larger droplets of saliva-borne microorganisms and debris known as splatter. Splatter droplets are usually large enough to be visible. Their larger diameter and weight cause these particles to fall out of the air more quickly than aerosols so that they are most likely to accumulate on surfaces in the immediate treatment area, contaminating them with microorganisms from the patient's oral flora as well as other pathogens.

Miller and others (1971) compared the aerosol and splatter production of specific dental procedures with those of common nasal-oral activities. They found that using the high-speed handpiece or washing the teeth with a combined air-water spray produced contamination equal to sneezing, hissing, or tooth brushing. A prophylaxis procedure produced the same amount of aerosol contamination as gargling, and using the ultrasonic scaler produced the same amount of contamination as a cough. Certainly, anyone would dislike having another person sneeze, hiss, gargle, or cough directly at him or her within a distance of only 8 to 12 inches, and yet most dental clinicians have to contend with these same levels of aerosol and splatter contamination continuously.

Both aerosols and splatter can contaminate the mucous membranes of the oral cavity, nose, or eyes and lead to disease in a susceptible host. Aerosols can be the source of transmission for serious diseases, including hepatitis, tuberculosis, herpes simplex, other viral infections, and respiratory tract infections. Treatment of patients known to be infectious should be postponed until they are no longer contagious. Clinicians should avoid procedures that produce high amounts of aerosols on patients in high risk categories, such as carriers of HBV, HIV, or tuberculosis.

Reducing aerosol production. There are a number of ways in which the dental professional can control and reduce the amount of dental aerosols and splatter generated during treatment. The use of the rubber dam during operative procedures or at other times when this type of isolation is practical reduces aerosol production. High-speed evacuation during procedures involving the ultrasonic scaler or high-speed handpiece or when rinsing the mouth is essential. When the air-water syringe is used, the clinician should apply water to the area, followed by air, rather than dispensing both at the same time to produce a forced spray of water. Because bristle brushes generate more splatter during polishing procedures than do rubber cups or polishing points, use of brushes should be limited.

The number of microorganisms within the patient's mouth can be significantly reduced through the use of an antiseptic mouthwash before dental treatment (Litsky et al, 1976). Wyler and others (1971) demonstrated that the use of a pretreatment rinse with a commercially available antiseptic mouthwash reduced bacterial counts by 10 to 100 times. Although the main effect of mouth rinsing is mechanical removal, the antiseptic properties of some mouthwashes could enhance the overall reduction of microorganisms.

The direction of airflow within the dental operatory will also affect aerosols. Installation of a ceiling-to-floor laminar airflow system to direct the circulation of air in the operatory has been shown to reduce aerosols. The use of laminar airflow will also reduce the amount of surface contamination from airborne particles (Pollock et al, 1970).

Cross-contamination from aerosols and splatter should be controlled by using disposable paper covers on all countertops; keeping all clean and sterile supplies in closed containers, drawers, or cabinets; and disinfecting all contaminated surfaces thoroughly between patients. Touching of various surfaces should be controlled. Use overgloves for answering the phone, if you must, during patient procedures or if you need to reach into a drawer while treating a patient. See Fig. 3-10 for another suggestion on reducing cross- contamination. Dental personnel should protect themselves from aerosols and splatter through the use of barrier techniques including masks; safety glasses or face shields; gloves, and full-coverage uniforms, laboratory coats or gowns. Disposable paper or plastic aprons, jackets, and bibs provide additional protection in decreasing the amount of contamination to which uniforms are exposed, thereby reducing the potential of soiled uniforms to serve as cross-contaminants to the wearer and to other patients (Fig. 3-11). Disposable head covers and gowns provide effective barriers for dental personnel involved in the treatment of high-risk patients. Dental practitioners also can reduce their exposure to aerosols and splatter by observing proper patient-operator positioning and through effective tissue retraction. Maintaining a safe operating distance from the patient's mouth, retracting soft tissues in ways that reflect liquid aerosols and splatter away from the operator, and operating from behind the patient rather than in front will all reduce exposure to airborne contaminants.

Personal hygiene and protection

Personal hygiene of all dental staff is an important step in the control of transmissible diseases. Important considerations include choice and care of uniforms or disposable coverings; hand washing and care of nails; avoiding direct contact with infected persons or lesions; wearing disposable masks, gloves, and glasses; and other practices to prevent transmission of pathogens from the office environment to the home environment.

All operating personnel—the dentist, the hygienist, and the assistant—participate in patient treatment and are potential sources of contamination. Dental personnel, by means of their occupation, are exposed to more disease-producing microorganisms than are most other people. If a member of the dental team contracts any sort of contagious disease, all efforts should be made to avoid transmission to other people in the office and to patients. A responsible health care provider

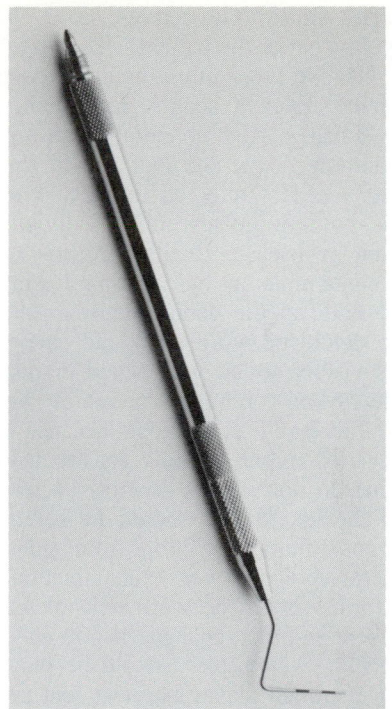

Fig. 3-10. This instrument could prevent cross-contamination of surfaces. Why?
(Courtesy of Hu-Friedy, Chicago, Illinois.)

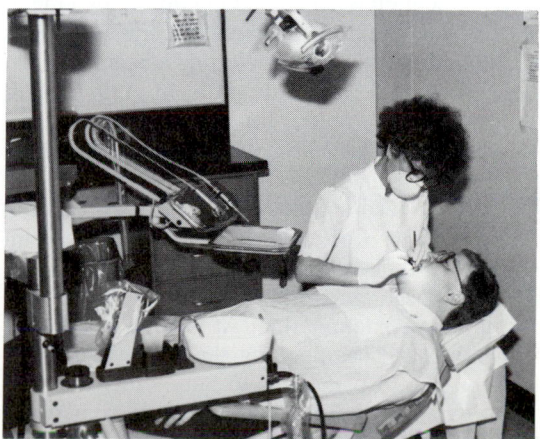

Fig. 3-11. Note the number of barrier techniques shown in this photo. How many do you see? What would you add?
(Courtesy of Hu-Friedy, Chicago, Illinois).

will not risk transmitting active disease. When either the clinician or the patient is known to have a disease, elective procedures should be postponed.

Uniforms. Even a healthy individual, patient or professional, carries potentially harmful bacteria on clothing, skin, and hair and in the mouth and nose. Carriers may be unaffected by these microbes, but in more susceptible individuals they may result in disease. Health care providers can control contamination by wearing freshly laundered clothing in the dental environment. Clean clothing should be worn daily and changed if it becomes visibly soiled with blood or other contaminants. Many clinicians prefer to wear uniforms or full-length clinic coats because they are easily cleaned and are usually constructed of materials that do not readily give off bacteria-laden lint and threads. Styles should be selected that provide maximum protection from splatter and dental aerosols. To prevent contamination of others, uniforms should be worn only in the dental environment and then changed before leaving that environment. Soiled garb should be placed in a properly identified plastic bag and sent to a commercial launderer by the employer.

Personal hygiene is mandatory for all health care workers. Because bacteria are known to shed along with skin cells, dandruff, and dust from the hair and body, all exposed skin and hair must be as clean as possible. In addition, the longer the hair, the more likely it is to shed dandruff and bacteria because of its movement and contact with the shoulders and face. The clinician's head and face are kept close to the patient during treatment, and cross-contamination between oral pathogens and the clinician's hair (including a beard or mustache) can pose a health problem. Longer hair may also be a problem for the clinician in terms of maintaining a clear field of vision. For these reasons hair should be kept short, pinned, or tied close to the head and out of the field of operation. Individuals who provide dental treatment for infectious or high-risk patients may consider wearing a disposable covering over their hair to protect it from contamination. At the end of the day, showering and shampooing the hair will prevent transmission of pathogens to family members.

Jewelry may be another source of contamination and should be kept to a minimum, if worn at all. Because the hands and wrists cannot be adequately cleaned unless they are bare, no jewelry—including all rings, bracelets, and watches—should be worn on the hands while treating patients. All exposed jewelry, including earrings and necklaces, can trap and hold contaminants that are difficult, if not impossible, to remove, becoming potential reservoirs of contamination to the wearer and to other surfaces they contact.

Care of nails and hand washing. Ideally, any object that enters the patient's mouth should be sterilized or disposable to minimize the potential for cross-contamination. The most obvious and unavoidable failure of this rule is the clinician's hands. There is no acceptable way to sterilize human hands. For the protection of both the clinician and the patient, all direct-care providers should wear disposable gloves during all intraoral dental procedures. As an additional measure of protection it is imperative that dental care providers give close attention to the washing and care of the hands both before putting on a new pair of gloves and after removing them. For the clinician's own protection, hands should be closely inspected to ensure that there are no potential portals of entry for bacteria. Hangnails, or small cuts, or irritated areas are potential gates for infectious bacteria to enter the bloodstream. Clinicians with oozing dermatitis or exudative lesions should avoid direct patient contact until the condition has subsided (CDMIE, 1988). All breaks in the skin should be protected by keeping them covered during patient treatment procedures.

Hands and nails should be thoroughly cleaned before donning gloves and after gloves are removed. Nails should be kept short so that they will not interfere with patient comfort and effective instrument handling during intraoral procedures, and because long nails may cause tears in disposable gloves (Parker and Williams, 1987). The protected area beneath the nail has been found to harbor residual blood and bacteria for up to 5 days in clinicians who do not routinely wear gloves (Allen and Organ, 1982). These same studies demonstrated that the area under the nails is a potential source of cross-contamination for other patients, for the clinician, and for family members. Therefore, the hand washing procedure should begin with a thorough cleaning around and under the nails with an orangewood stick, combined with lathering with a liquid soap or hand detergent and copious rinsing with cool water.

Two levels of bacteria reside on the hands. A superficial layer of microorganisms, or transient bacteria, is found on the outer layers of the skin, under the fingernails, and around the nails. These bacteria include all the microorganisms that are picked up in the environment. A deeper level, called resident bacteria, forms part of the normal flora of the skin and lies deep in the crevices and folds of the skin. A quick, superficial washing will not dislodge these bacteria. This fact is significant, as many of these organisms are potential pathogens. Any technique of washing must be thorough enough to remove most transient bacteria and as many of the resident microorganisms as possible.

The goals of hand washing are to remove all surface dirt and contamination and to remove as much of the deeper (resident) bacteria as possible. An effective hand washing procedure should start with an initial scrub that includes a thorough lathering and scrubbing of all surfaces of the nails, fingers, hands, and lower arms. This is possible only if the hands and arms are bared of all jewelry and clothing at least to the elbow. The most important aspect of hand washing is mechanical rubbing of all surfaces to remove soil and microorganisms, which are then rinsed away by the running water. This initial scrub should consist of three latherings, each followed by a thorough rinsing with cool to lukewarm water, and may last for 2 to 3 minutes (Crawford, 1986; Palenik and Miller, 1984b). The initial scrub can be performed by repeated rubbing of one hand with another or with the aid of a soft, sterile brush or disposable sponge. Overzealous use of a stiff bristle brush, however, can abrade and lacerate the skin, increasing the risk of infection by oral pathogens. Scrubbing should include all surfaces of the hands and fingers and should emphasize the dominant hand, which is likely to be the more contaminated and less scrubbed hand (Maloney and Kohut, 1987.

Soap or detergent helps loosen dirt, oils, and bacteria from the skin. The use of a liquid soap dispenser containing an antimicrobial soap rather than a bar of soap reduces cross-contamination during hand washing; a cake or bar of soap can serve as a nutrient source and reservoir for bacteria growth after it has been used. Use of antiseptic handscrubs enhances the destruction of bacteria in the deeper recesses of the skin. The professional should be aware of the claims of different manufacturers regarding the bactericidal and bacteriostatic effects of antiseptic handscrubs. Whatever product is chosen should be nonirritating and gentle to the skin. Select one that has chlorhexidine gluconate, parachlorometaxylenol, or an iodophor and use it throughout the day to enhance its residual effects. The constant use of a harsh product can lead to excessive drying and skin irritation, reducing the ability of the skin to form an effective barrier against infection. A listing of accepted antimicrobial hand cleaners is available from the ADA Council on Dental Therapeutics (1986).

When the hands are being rinsed, the water should flow from the fingertips down towards the elbow. The water should not be allowed to run back over an area that has been previously rinsed, and contaminated rinse water should not come into contact with an already clean area. The hands should be dried with a paper towel, moving from the fingers to the hands and finally to the arms. A separate paper towel should be used for each hand. The faucet should be turned off either with foot controls or with a paper towel if hand controls are used. The paper towels should then be discarded. Care should be taken not to touch the sink, paper towel dispenser, or waste receptacle after the hands have been washed.

In addition to the initial scrubbing procedures, individuals involved in direct patient contact must wash their hands thoroughly between patients, immediately after removing gloves, and before donning clean gloves. This routine of hand washing should include two or three latherings followed by cool water rinses. Hands should be dried thoroughly before gloves are donned. Use of hand creams should be restricted to after-work hours since these preparations can become microbially contaminated (Palenik and Miller, 1987).

Wearing disposable gloves. The use of sterile gloves by dental clinicians affords the highest degree of hand hygiene and protection against cross-contamination. Disposable gloves can achieve and maintain a safer level of contamination control than is possible with bare hands alone. Most important, they provide an effective barrier against the entry of serious pathogens, including those responsible for syphilis, hepatitis, and other diseases transmitted by the blood or saliva of infected patients. Because it is not always possible to detect which patients carry infectious diseases, the dental professional must wear gloves for all intraoral procedures, especially those in which bleeding is likely to occur. The CDC and the ADA recommend that gloves be worn for all procedures involving contact with blood, saliva, mucous membranes, or surfaces contaminated with body fluids or secretions. This includes all intraoral procedures and examination of oral lesions (CDC, 1986a; CDMIE, 1988. Nitrile gloves should also be worn when handling soiled or contaminated instruments, surfaces, or supplies and when handling contaminated materials such as impressions or prostheses in the laboratory (Palenik and Miller, 1987).

Four types of gloves may be used in dental practice (Fig. 3-12). Sterile surgical gloves are the highest quality, most expensive, and best-fitting disposable gloves. They are used most commonly for surgical or invasive procedures in which maximum protection against infection must be provided for the patient and the clinician. Nonsterile, latex examination gloves are the most commonly used for routine dental procedures. They are available in a variety of sizes and may come with or without a cornstarch lubricant for ease in getting them on and off. Because there is a wide variation in sizing (palm width, finger width and length) among different manufacturers, clinicians should sample several different brands and choose the one that fits best. Some individuals may develop hypersensitivity reactions either to the latex material or to the cornstarch lubricant in disposable gloves. This problem is usually alleviated through the use of nonpowdered surgical gloves or latex-free (neoprene or vinyl) examination gloves. Heavy-duty, puncture-resistant utility gloves should be worn when handling and cleaning contaminated instruments or supplies, when using chemical sterilant solutions, and for general operatory cleaning. These gloves can be washed, disinfected or sterilized, powdered with cornstarch, and reused (Palenik and Miller, 1987).

All disposable gloves should be considered as single-use items because their present composition does not permit them to be safely washed and reused with other patients (CDC, 1986a; CDMIE, 1988). Contact with hot water, soaps, detergents, and other chemicals can negatively affect glove materials by making them "tacky" and more prone to tearing. Clinicians should always inspect gloves carefully before putting them on and during treatment for signs of tears, punctures, or tackiness and should replace damaged gloves im-

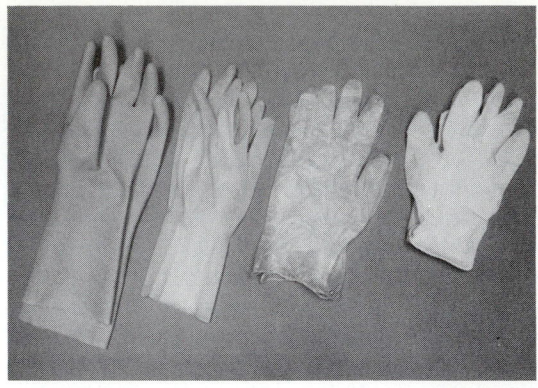

Fig. 3-12. Types of gloves. *From left to right:* puncture-resistant nitrile utility gloves, regular surgical gloves, vinyl examination gloves, latex examination gloves.

mediately before proceeding. Rings and watches and long fingernails should not be worn under gloves because of their potential for causing holes. Even new gloves may already have minute holes or tears and should be carefully inspected (Clinical Research Associates, 1985; Skaug, 1976). A good test is to inflate gloves with air and then hold them closed to see if there is significant leakage indicating the presence of a defect in the material. Gloves should not be worn for more than 1 hour on a single patient procedure. Dental personnel must be careful during patient treatment not to touch any part of their clothing or bodies or any other surfaces that are not protected by barrier covers, disinfection, or sterilization. If they must leave the operatory or touch surfaces that are not routinely treated or covered between patients, they should remove their gloves and wash their hands before touching other surfaces. Hands must then be rewashed and new gloves put on before returning to patient treatment.

Inexpensive vinyl gloves, such as those used by food handlers or cafeteria workers, may also be placed over examination or surgical gloves that have been rinsed in cool water and dried when it is necessary to touch radiographs, chart, and the phone. The second pair of gloves should then be removed before returning to the patient (CDMIE, 1988).

Use of face masks. Current CDC and ADA guidelines recommend that surgical masks or chin-length plastic shields be worn for all dental procedures in which splashing or spattering of blood or other body fluids is likely (CDC, 1986a, 1987, 1991; CDMIE, 1988). A well-fitting face mask is an effective means of protection in two ways. First, it protects the patient from contamination by a clinician who has a cold or other condition that is transmittable by respiratory droplets. Because the clinician's face is so close to the patient, this kind of transfer could easily occur. Second, it may also protect the clinician from bacteria- or virus-containing aerosols generated during dental treatment.

An effective mask not only mechanically blocks larger particles of blood, saliva, and oral debris, but also filters out aerosols. Face masks should also be comfortable, fit well, and have minimal marginal leakage. Face masks are available in a wide variety of styles and materials, including paper, cloth, foam, fiberglass, and other synthetic materials. Of these, the paper, cloth, and foam masks have proven least effective and those made of fiberglass or synthetic fiber most effective in filtering aerosols. Thus fiberglass or synthetic masks are the best for dental procedures (Micik et al, 1971; Underhill et al, 1986) (Fig. 3-13).

Most face masks available to dental personnel are disposable and should be discarded after each patient or when they become visibly contaminated or wetted (Christensen et al, 1991; Craig and Quayle, 1985). Although disposable face masks have been shown to be effective in reducing contamination, they do not totally prevent the passage of potentially dangerous microorganisms. Additional measures for controlling airborne contaminants are discussed later in this chapter.

Use of protective eyeglasses. Protective eyeglasses with side shields or a face shield must be worn by all dental personnel involved in chairside treatment (CDC, 1986A, 1991; CDMIE, 1988). This important safety measure can prevent damage from bacteria-laden aerosols, accidental trauma, or flying debris. The use of ultrasonic scalers and high-speed handpieces increases the presence of aerosols containing large numbers of infectious bacteria, which pose a risk to clinician and patient alike. The herpes virus is one example of a pathogen that could be transmitted from saliva or an active lesion into the eye by means of aerosols or splatter droplets. The resulting infection, recurrent herpetic keratitis, leads to impaired vision and, in some cases, blindness (Brooks et al, 1981). Safety glasses prevent eye damage that

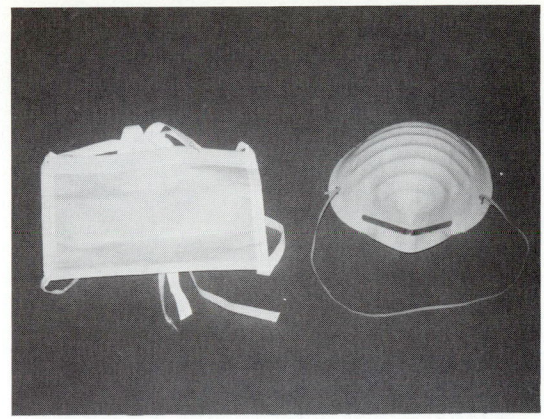

Fig. 3-13. Two popular styles of masks used in dentistry.

could result from a particle of calculus being snapped from the tooth and propelled out of the mouth or from a slurry of abrasive and saliva that might splatter against the clinician's face during polishing procedures. Clinicians who wear glasses can see the evidence of splatter and debris on the lenses after patient treatment. As the eyes of both the patient and the dental team are so close to the working area, the risk of eye injury is high. In a survey of dental hygienists, 44% had suffered the following foreign bodies in their eyes as a result of treatment procedures: pumice/prophylaxis paste, calculus, dental materials, and contaminated water spray (Gravois and Stringer, 1980).

Clinicians who already wear glasses should be advised that they must have a separate pair that meet OSHA requirements and that are worn during working situations *only*.

Some practitioners prefer plastic face shields because they protect the eyes, nose, and mouth and do not interfere with communication (Fig. 3-14). Disadvantages of these shields are that they still require use of a mask because they are not closely adapted to the face and must be completely disinfected after each patient.

Most eyeglasses fitted by prescription are now made of shatter-resistant materials, and lenses can be coated to make them scratch and fog-resistant. Side shields can also be added. The clinician's glasses can be treated with commercially available antifogging cloths or cleaners to prevent the problem of fogging. Plastic safety glasses can be safely treated by immersion in 2% glutaraldehyde

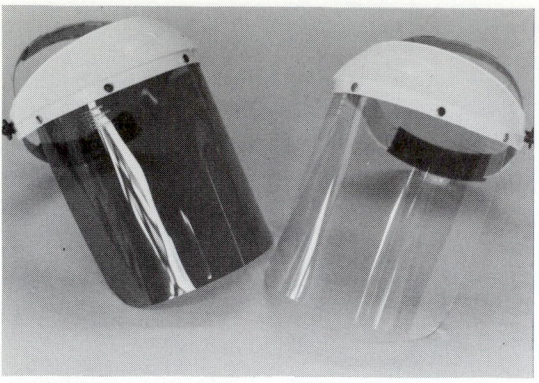

Fig. 3-14. Examples of protective shields
(Courtesy of American Shield Co, Orlando, Florida.)

between patients (Gleason and Molinari, 1987).

The patient's eyes are extremely vulnerable to damage from oral debris and aerosols and from falling or mishandled instruments and dental materials. This is especially true for patients in the supine position (Cooley et al, 1978). Incorrect transfer of instruments or supplies over the patient's face could result in trauma to the eye or impaction of a foreign body. Safety glasses should be provided for patients who do not normally wear glasses. They may be either disposable or sterilized or disinfected between patients. Most patients will appreciate this precaution if the dental professional explains that it is recommended out of concern for their health and safety. Tinted lenses in the glasses provided for patient use will also provide shielding from overhead lighting.

ESTABLISHING AN EFFECTIVE ROUTINE FOR CONTAMINATION CONTROL BETWEEN PATIENTS

Now that methods of contamination control for dental personnel and the dental environment have been discussed in general, here are some of the important factors to be considered in establishing an effective and efficient routine for treating contaminated surfaces between patient appointments. Because time is limited, the person responsible for performing these tasks should already have identified the critical, semicritical, and noncritical items in the dental environment and should know which methods of treatment are appropriate for each item. In addition, care must be taken during treatment of patients not to enlarge the list of critical surfaces by touching and contaminating additional surfaces. After they have been contaminated by the patient's oral flora and saliva, the dental professional's hands should not touch any surface that is not routinely sterilized or disinfected until the hands have been washed.

Following is a discussion of specific surfaces or items that require infection control measures both before and after patient treatment, along with recommendations for specific measures.

Before cleaning and disinfecting the dental operatory at the beginning of the day, wash hands and put on nitrile gloves. Clean and disinfect all semicritical surfaces with an intermediate-level surface disinfectant. Whenever possible, cover semicritical surfaces with clean, disposable barrier covers to prevent them from becoming recontaminated during treatment. In most cases it takes far less time to cover these items than it does to clean and disinfect them between patients. Use of barrier coverings is especially important for surfaces or items that cannot be easily cleaned. Surfaces that may be covered include the dental chair (especially headrest and armrests), chair and unit control buttons, lamp handles and switch, bracket table and handles, equipment cords, counter and cart surfaces, sink faucets, and any equipment or supply containers that are exposed to dental aerosols (e.g., ultrasonic and air polishing units, storage containers, and patient education materials) (Figs. 3-15 to 3-18). In general, all clean or sterile supplies should be kept in covered containers

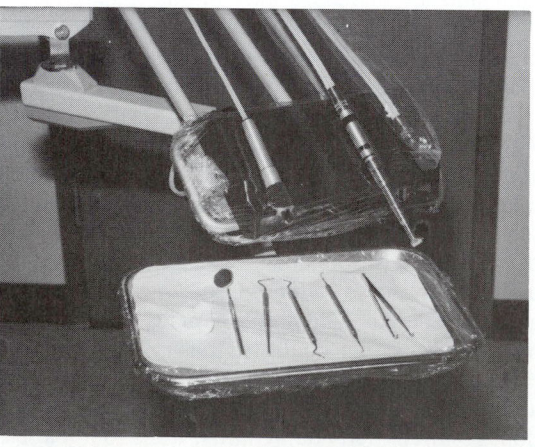

Fig. 3-15. Surface on units and bracket table, including hoses, can be covered with clear plastic film.

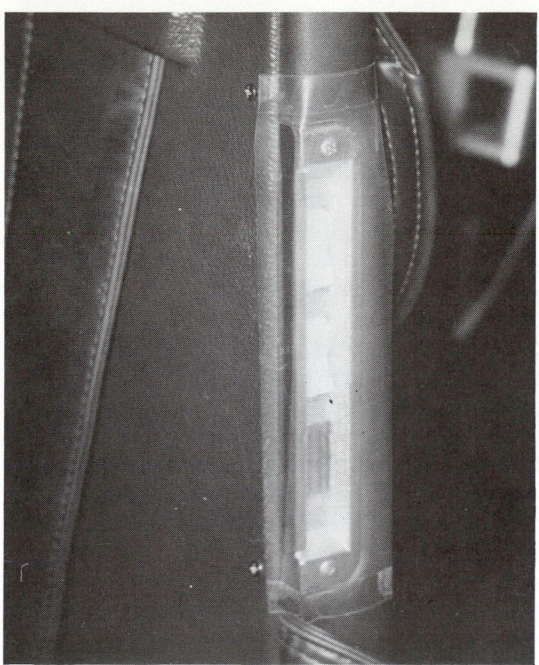

Fig. 3-16. Chair controls are easily contaminated and difficult to disinfect. Plastic covers with self-adhesive ends are a convenient way to protect these surfaces.

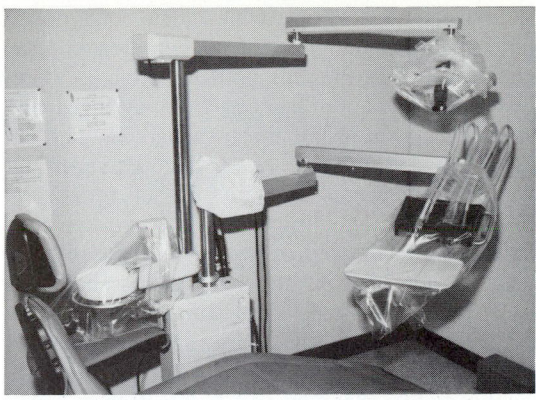

Fig. 3-18. At the end of the day, cleaned and disinfected surfaces can be kept covered overnight to protect them from aerosol particles and dust that settle out of the air.

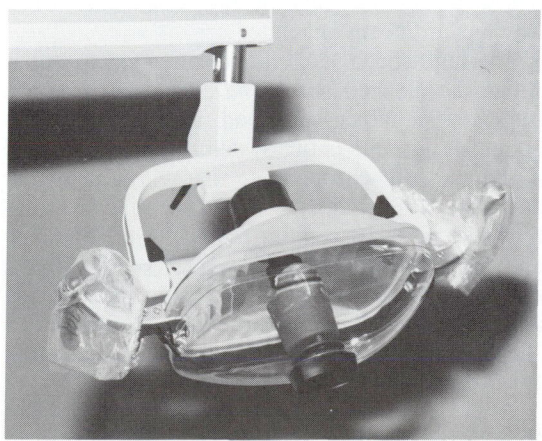

Fig. 3-17. Light handles are frequently touched during treatment. Covering them with plastic covers or film is an effective way to prevent cross-contamination.

or in drawers where they are protected from dental aerosols and should be brought into the dental environment in quantities sufficient for each patient. Surfaces should be disinfected as needed, and clean barrier coverings replaced after hands have been washed and clean gloves put on.

All semicritical surfaces that cannot be covered, including bases for the saliva ejector, high-speed suction, hand-held cuspidor, and handpiece, must be scrubbed and disinfected between patients. Disinfection should be done only with approved chemical solutions and should follow manufacturers' recommendations for use.

In many instances the water supplies in dental units can become contaminated with bacterial concentrations higher than those considered acceptable for public consumption. When water supplies are allowed to sit for long periods without being used, the effectiveness of chlorine in controlling bacterial growth begins to decrease. The subsequent growth of microorganisms provides a source of contamination when the water lines are again used and delivered directly into the patient's mouth by way of the drinking cup, air-water syringe, ultrasonic scaler, air polisher, and water-cooled handpiece. In addition, many modern handpieces and syringes are equipped with retraction devices that are designed to prevent water from dripping out of them after use. When this excess water is retracted back into the handpiece or syringe, it is often accompanied by contaminated water and saliva, which then contaminate the water line and the next patient treated. The best way to prevent this contamination is to remove the retraction devices from syringes and handpieces or to install check valves (Bagga et al, 1984). In addition, all hoses that deliver water from the dental unit should be flushed for several minutes at the beginning of the day, between each patient and at the end of the day. Disposable air/water syringe tips or autoclavable tips should be used. After use, water-cooled handpieces, ultrasonic and air polishing units, and air-water syringes should be flushed with water for 20 to 30 seconds before cleaning and disinfection or sterilization (CDC, 1986a and 1991; CDMIE, 1988).

Equipment used for delivering nitrous oxide analgesia should be disinfected after each use. The nitrous oxide nosepiece should be disinfected after each use to prevent transmission of viral and upper respiratory tract infections from one patient to another. This equipment cannot be routinely sterilized because it is composed of rubber or plastic materials that cannot withstand the high temperatures of the autoclave or dry heat oven. Yagiela and others (1979) compared the effectiveness of a number of different methods for disinfecting this equipment and concluded that the most effective procedure was to wash the nosepiece thoroughly after each use with soap and water, immerse it in a 2% alkaline glutaraldehyde solution for 10 minutes to achieve disinfection, and then rinse it thoroughly in tap water. This equipment should be sterilized nightly, when immersion for a full 6 ¾ to 10 hours and a 1-hour rinse can be accomplished.

The x-ray supplies and equipment, including the cone, head, and controls, should be protected from contamination with disposable barrier covers. If this is not done, these items must be scrubbed and disinfected after each use. Because the clinician is constantly going back and forth between the intraoral placement of radiographic films and the x-ray equipment, they are prime sources of cross-contamination. Whenever possible, disposable paper towels should be used to handle the head and cone. Contaminated film packets should be placed on disposable paper towels or a disposable cup until film is removed. Film should be ejected from packets without being touched and contaminated by the fingers (CDMIE, 1982). Intraoral radiographic film holders are critical surfaces and should be made of materials that are disposable or can be sterilized between patients. X-ray viewboxes should be left on and should not be touched unless hands are clean.

The pens and pencils used for recording patient data, patients' charts, and patient education materials are often overlooked as sources of contamination. Pens and pencils should be wiped thoroughly with a high-level disinfectant after each patient appointment. Look at Fig. 3-10 again to see how the pen-probe combination can help. Another safeguard is to delegate all recording and chart handling to an assistant, so that the clinician's contaminated hands never touch them. If an assistant is not available, the clinician's hands must be washed before handling these items and then washed again before resuming intraoral procedures. An alternative is to use a computerized chart with voice activation or a sterilizable or disposable data entry surface. Chart folders and contents should be handled only with clean hands. Pens and pencils that are used in the treatment room should remain there and not be carried to other areas, where they could transfer pathogens to other patients or family members. Mirrors, demonstration models, and instructional booklets that are used during patient education should never be handled when the hands are contaminated after patient treatment. Mirrors and models should be cleaned and disinfected after being handled by patients. Instructional materials (i.e., posters, flip charts) should be laminated to withstand disinfection. Materials should not be left exposed on countertops during treatment, when aerosols are being generated.

The high-speed suction and saliva ejector tubes should be cleaned out at the end of each day to remove residual saliva, blood, and debris. To accomplish this, the entire system should be flushed at the end of each operating day with a detergent and water followed by use of a disinfectant solution such as 1:10 sodium hypochlorite (Maloney and Kohut, 1987). Disposable suction traps should be used and switches should be scrubbed and disinfected. Exact instructions as to how this should be accomplished should be obtained from the manufacturer of the equipment.

After all surfaces have been cleaned, disinfected, and sterilized, sterile supplies and instruments should be placed on the bracket tray aseptically, using sterile forceps and clean, gloved hands. These items should then be kept covered until they are needed.

Laboratory asepsis

Principles of contamination control apply to all areas in the dental office, not just the dental operatory. Another area in which stringent infection control guidelines must be applied is the dental laboratory. All laboratory materials, impressions, and intraoral appliances should be cleaned and disinfected before being handled, adjusted, or sent to a commercial dental laboratory (CDC, 1986a; CDT, 1985).

Handling of intraoral prosthetic appliances. Dentures should be rinsed thoroughly to remove blood, saliva, and oral debris. They should then be placed in a disposable plastic cup or a disposable zip-lock plastic bag. If dentures are to be cleaned, the appropriate solution should be added to the bag, which is then sealed and placed in the ultrasonic cleaner for the prescribed length of time. After cleaning, the denture should be removed from solution and rinsed thoroughly. The bag should be emptied and rinsed thoroughly and the denture replaced in the bag and returned to the dental operatory.

When adjustments or polishing of dentures using laboratory equipment is required or when dentures are to be returned to a commercial laboratory, they should be disinfected before being handled and treated. Dentures can be disinfected by immersion in 1:10 sodium hypochlorite solution for 10 to 30 minutes (CDT, 1985). Prolonged immersion of dentures with metal parts can lead to corrosion and should be done cautiously. Another method for disinfection of dentures has been described by Henderson and others (1987), in which dentures are scrubbed with a denture brush for 1 minute with 4% chlorhexidine gluconate (Hibiclens), placed in a zip-lock bag with either undiluted or diluted (1:16) buffered, alkaline glutaraldehyde, and ultrasonically treated for 10 minutes. The denture and bag are then rinsed thoroughly and the denture again ultrasonically treated for 3 minutes in sterile water.

Impression materials should be handled with gloves, rinsed gently under water to remove blood and saliva, and disinfected before pouring stone casts. Manufacturer's recommendations should be followed regarding appropriate choice of disinfectants that will not distort impression material (CDMIE 1991; Merchant, 1990). Alginate and reversible hydrocolloid impressions may be distorted by prolonged submersion in disinfectant. At the very least, these impressions should be sprayed with an iodophor (1:213 solution) or be soaked in iodophor disinfectant for 10 minutes (Crawford, 1986). Herrera and Merchant (1986) reported that short-term (30-minute) immersion of impression materials in 1% sodium hypochlorite did not significantly affect the dimensional accuracy of the resulting casts and that glutaraldehyde, povidone-iodine solution, and halogenated phenol disinfectants had no apparent effect on the dimensional stability of rubber impression materials. Minag and others (1986, 1987) recommended immersion of silicone rubber impression materials in sodium hypochlorite solution for 60 minutes and immersion of irreversible colloid and hydrophilic impression material in 2% glutaraldehyde for 60 minutes as a means of preventing cross- contamination of viral diseases. An alternative to disinfecting impression materials is to handle the impression with gloves, pour the stone model, discard the contaminated impression and gloves, wrap the stone cast, and sterilize it using ethylene oxide gas.

If impressions are sent to a commercial laboratory, both parties should understand the disinfection procedures that have been used. If impressions are disinfected at the dental office before transfer to the laboratory there is no need for additional disinfection at the laboratory, which might distort or harm the materials. All materials from high-risk patients must be clearly marked on the outside of the delivery package for the protection of dental laboratory personnel. Dentures returned from a commercial laboratory should be disinfected and rinsed thoroughly before being handled and returned to the patient. Packaging materials in which appliances are received from dental laboratories should be discarded and not reused.

Aerosols and flying debris generated by machine grinding and rag wheel polishing is another potential problem. Safety glasses must be worn. Pumice should be replaced daily and mixed with a 1:20 sodium hypochlorite solution to which 3 parts of green soap has been added to keep the pumice suspended (CDT, 1985). Pumice pans can be easily cleaned if they are covered with a large disposable plastic bag at the beginning of the day. At the end of the day the bag can be turned inside out, and carefully removed so that the contaminated pumice is neatly discarded. Rag wheels should be sterilized. In offices in which wheel polishing is done infrequently, a sterilized rag wheel can be held ready for use with only a small amount of pumice dispensed into a covered or disposable pan as needed. Pumice pans should be cleaned out daily or after use with an iodophor disinfectant. Preferred methods of disinfection and sterilization for other items used in the laboratory are listed in Table 3-9.

Barrier covers are recommended for laboratory equipment whenever possible. All contaminated surfaces should be cleaned and disinfected after each use with a spray bottle of an approved surface disinfectant and absorbent disposable towels or gauze sponges. For obvious reasons, dental employees should be discouraged from eating or smoking in the dental laboratory.

LEGAL ASPECTS OF INFECTION CONTROL

The alarming spread of lethal diseases such as hepatitis B and AIDS in recent years has not only led to major changes in standards for infection control in dentistry but has also caused dental professionals to reassess the legal implications of potential infection transfer in their practices. Failure to act in accordance with the current standard of care may be viewed by the courts as a breach of required duty and result in liability for negligence (Baker and Hawkins, 1985). Employer dentists who do not implement current infection control guidelines as set forth by the CDC and ADA may be held liable by employees or patients who contract infectious diseases as a result of dental treatment (Logan, 1987). Dental hygienists must assume a similar legal responsibility for all recommended precautions in the treatment of patients.

OSHA has issued standards to ensure a safe and healthy dental workplace. These require that all dentist employers provide appropriate infection control barriers to all employees in quantities that allow for gloves, masks, and glasses to be changed with each new patient or in accordance with current infection control principles (e.g., CDC and ADA guidelines). OSHA also requires that employees use these infection control barriers. Employers must inform their employees about OSHA regulations and keep them updated regarding changes in health and safety requirements. Employees must also be informed that failure to comply with these regulations is grounds for dismissal.

OSHA's existing and new standards will apply to 316,237 employees in 100,174 dental offices nationwide (ADA, 1992). Offices should have copies of the December 6, 1991 *Federal Register* as well as OSHA's publication, *Compliance Assistance Guideline for the February 27, 1990 OSHA Instruction CPL 2-2.44B Enforcement Procedures for Occupational Exposure to Hepatitis B Virus and Human Immunodeficiency Virus* (US Department of Labor, 1991). The following are some guidelines to help you come into compliance with the guidelines. Make sure that you know the *current* guidelines.

First, the following general workplace safety regulations must be in place. The Job Safety and Health Protection poster (#2203, revised 1989) must be displayed in a prominent place. Injuries in offices with eleven or more employees must be reported using Forms #200 and #101. The office must have a written fire safety policy, and employees must be given training in this area. All exits must be marked. If gases are used (i.e., oxygen or nitrous oxide), they must be maintained in a safe condition. Eyewash stations must also be available for employee use.

Any employer who has one or more employees must follow OSHA's guidelines for prevention of bloodborne pathogens. Each employee must have an exposure determination prepared. For example:

Category 1—potential exists for contact with blood or body fluids during routine work.

Category 2—normal work routine does not involve contact with blood or body fluids, however, a potential exists if asked to help.

Category 3—normal work conditions NEVER involve contact with fluids.

It should be noted that saliva is often mixed with blood, and OSHA has therefore concluded that saliva should be treated as potentially infectious. Saliva itself carries pathogenic microorganisms and should be treated with the same respect given to blood.

A written exposure control plan must have been implemented by May 5, 1992. This must include exposure classification, barrier techniques, hepatitis B vaccination, education and documentation, housekeeping, protocol for disinfection of contaminated work surfaces and equipment, handling of regulated waste, postexposure evaluation and follow-up, communication of bloodborne pathogen hazards to employees, and record keeping. All employees must have access to the plan, which must be updated to reflect any changes and updated annually.

Exposure control precautions

Barrier techniques must be used for exposure control. For example, gloves are required whenever hand contact with infectious material is probable. Utility gloves must be worn when disinfecting instruments, work surfaces or pouring hazardous chemicals. Gloves must be changed when they become contaminated (at least after every patient) and may not be rewashed. If the gloves are punctured during a procedure, they must be replaced immediately. The employer must provide gowns and other protective equipment. The selection of gown style is based on the quantity and type of exposure anticipated. Gowns must be changed if penetrated by body fluids. Soiled clothes must be placed in a red biohazard bag, and personal protective equipment must be worn when soiled clothes are handled by the commercial launderers.

Masks and eyewear are required when any blood/and or saliva aerosolizes, or splatter could occur, or when eye, nose, or mouth contamination is anticipated. Protective equipment and clothing must be used by employees at all times unless there is a sudden change in patient status that puts the patient's life in jeopardy. Providing pediatric dental care is not an exception. Handwashing facilities must be provided by employers and used by employees immediately before and after use of gloves.

Contaminated sharps (needles, slides, wires) must be placed in a closable, puncture-resistant container that is leakproof on the sides and bottom. The container must be marked with the universal biohazard symbol and be red or labeled BIOHAZARD. A sharps container should be located at each site at which contaminated disposable sharps are generated. Containers should be disposed of in accordance with any applicable state medical waste law. Needles may not be recapped with two hands or broken. The one-handed scoop technique or a mechanical recapping device may be used.

All employees must be offered the HBV vaccine at no charge. Training regarding HBV needs to be provided 10 days before the vaccine is offered. Any FDA-approved HBV vaccine given at the recommended doses and time schedule is acceptable. An employee may refuse the vaccine, but this must be documented.

Post exposure evaluation and follow-up

The postexposure evaluation and follow-up procedure is designed to evaluate an employee's health following an occupational exposure of the eye, mouth, mucous membrane, or broken skin or after parenteral contact with potentially infectious body fluid. The employer will provide, at no cost to the employee, a confidential medical evaluation. Items that need documentation are:

1. Route of exposure
2. Source—try to obtain a test of the source individual's blood
3. Collection and testing of consenting employees's blood
4. Medical prophylaxis as recommended by the U.S. Public Health Service
5. Counseling
6. Evaluation of illness after the incident

Record keeping

Documentation of the exposure incident and its management must be kept by the employer and include the employee's name and social security number, copy of the hepatitis B vaccination status, any medical opinions with test results, and details of exposure incidents.

Housekeeping

Employers must make sure that the worksite is clean. There must be a written schedule in each location as to tasks performed in that area and the type of surface to be cleaned.

Training

Training is considered the key to OSHA compliance. The education must be provided during the workday at no charge to the employee and presented at an appropriate educational level. Each employee should be given the following:

1. Explanation of the epidemiology and transmission of bloodborne pathogens, specifically HBV and HIV
2. Copy of the office's exposure control plan and standard for bloodborne pathogens—OSHA form 29 CFR 1910.1030
3. Protocol for using personal protective barriers (i.e., gloves and masks)
4. Methods to identify tasks involving occupational exposure
5. Information on HBV vaccine (safety and efficacy) and that it will be provided at no charge
6. Information on what actions to take and who to contact if an occupational exposure occurs
7. Explanation of biohazard labels

8. Explanation of actions to take in an emergency.

This training must be done annually and any time procedures that affect an employee's occupational exposure are changed. Records of the training need to be kept.

Waste

OSHA does not regulate disposal of contaminated waste. Contact your state agency for information regarding this aspect of infection control. However, OSHA does regulate handling of contaminated waste in the office. Blood-caked or saliva or blood-soaked items and contaminated sharps must be disposed of in accordance with this law. Orange biohazard warning labels need to be affixed to these items, or they may be placed in red biohazard containers.

Hazards communications

All hazardous chemical containers must be labeled. Labels must include the chemical's generic name, an appropriate hazards warning sign, dilution factor if applicable, and name and address of manufacturer. Material Safety Data Sheets (MSDS) for all hazardous products in the office must be cataloged, employees must be trained in dealing with hazardous materials, and records of this training must be maintained. Training is to be offered at:

1. The start of a program
2. Within 90 days for new employees
3. When introducing new hazardous materials into the office
4. When modifying handling procedures
5. At least annually for employees.

If the employer dentist does not comply with these regulations, the employee should first discuss the problem with the employer to make sure that he or she is aware of the regulations. If compliance is still not implemented, the employee has the right to file a complaint with the local branch of OSHA. When filing a written and signed complaint, the employee may request that his or her name be withheld from the employer and that he or she desires notification of OSHA actions regarding the complaint. Enforcement of regulations will be implemented through inspections of dental offices as necessary and the imposition of fines against dentist employers who are in violation of the rules (ADA, 1987a, 1987b; American Dental Hygienists Association, 1987; Yokom, 1988).

In light of these new legal implications concerning safety in the dental practice, several recommendations could prevent clinicians from encountering legal problems (Palenik and Miller, 1986b). These include (1) be aware of state-of-the-art infection control techniques as well as those used by other clinicians; (2) be sure all office staff are educated as to procedures for minimizing cross-infection; (3) if you have any indication of an infection, cease patient contact immediately and seek medical advice; and (4) consult an attorney if the issues become too complex.

CONCLUSION

It should be apparent that control of contamination when preparing the site for the patient is a very important step in patient care. Such control makes possible a comfortable, efficient, and safe environment for the patient and for dental personnel.

Although the time needed for this preparatory phase may diminish with experience, its importance in providing quality care should remain a primary consideration in all phases of care.

ACTIVITIES

1. Purchase or prepare Petri dishes containing 5% sheep red blood cells in trypticase soy agar, which should support the growth of several types of organisms. Using sterile cotton swabs, collect microbial samples from different parts of the clinic (such as countertops, sink, trisyringes, dental chair) or from yourself (such as skin, clothing, shoes). Wipe the contaminated swab over the agar medium and incubate for 24 to 48 hours at 37° C. Observe the growth on the plates for a visual representation of the organisms present in the clinical area. As an extension of this activity, compare culture samples from before and after sterilization and disinfection procedures. Evaluate the success of contamination control practices in the clinic.
2. Obtain a copy of "Enforcement Procedures for the Occupational Exposure to Bloodborne Pathogens Standard, 29 CFR 1910. 1030." Perform an audit on your clinics' operating procedures for management of exposure to bloodborne pathogens. Does your clinic meet the standards?
3. With a laboratory partner, role play performing an intraoral procedure. Identify the possible sources of contamination in the area, and demonstrate how direct and indirect transmission occur.
4. Observe and report on aseptic practices in other parts of the school or other clinics.
5. Observe asepsis control in a hospital operating room.
6. Review the literature for statistics relating to the

incidence of hepatitis and HIV seropositivity among dental professionals and patients.

7. Discuss the implications of contracting serum hepatitis or HIV for the career of a dental professional.

8. Discuss the legal ramifications of compromising safety of practice through ineffective contamination control. Determine if malpractice suits related to this issue have been brought against health professionals in your state or others. Consult a lawyer about the legalities of this issue.

9. Make a specific list of each item in the student's instrument kit and determine how it would best be sterilized/disinfected.

10. Ask students to inspect their safety glasses after a patient appointment for signs of splatter droplets of blood and saliva or other debris.

11. Compare the germicidal effects of all disinfectants, soaps, and antiseptics available in the clinic from manufacturers' descriptions and descriptions in *Accepted Dental Therapeutics*.

12. Wipe red tempera paint on a surface normally contaminated during dental treatment to simulate saliva contamination. Have students attempt to remove it with disinfectant-soaked gauze squares. Discuss how much scrubbing was necessary to remove all traces of the paint, and compare this with the amount of wiping students may normally use.

13. Trace the recall of Sporicidin. See the *ADA News* 23:28, January 6, 1992 and Ingersoll B: *Wall Street Journal*, p. B4, Dec. 16, 1991.

14. View the videotape *"What if Saliva Were Red"* by I. Crawford, University of North Carolina.

15. Inspect your clinic using the current OSHA standards. Does anything need attention? Make a list.

16. Discuss how OSHA addresses protection from tuberculosis transmission.

REVIEW QUESTIONS

1. Discuss the susceptibility of the dental clinician to sources of infection.

2. State the bacterial or viral disease caused by the following organisms (give the mode of transmission for each):
   a. *Mycobacterium tuberculosis*
   b. *Treponema pallidum*
   c. *Clostridium tetani*
   d. Respiratory virus (e.g., adenovirus)
   e. Hepatitis B virus
   f. Rubeola virus
   g. HIV

3. True or false:
   a. Hepatitis A usually has no residual effects after recovery.
   b. Jaundice occurs in all cases of hepatitis.
   c. Hepatitis B virus may be transmitted by means of the saliva.

   d. *Mycobacterium tuberculosis* is routinely destroyed by surface disinfection.
   e. Because of an increased opportunity for contracting tuberculosis, dental personnel should have periodic skin testing.
   f. When the patient's saliva enters the clinician's blood by way of a break in the skin, direct transmission has occurred.
   g. When the hygienist punctures his or her hand while cleaning instruments, indirect transmission has occurred.
   h. Aerosol production is responsible for contaminating a major portion of the dental operatory.
   i. Syphilis is only contagious in the primary stage.
   j. A chancre is a primary-stage syphilitic lesion.

4. Define the terms *sanitization*, *disinfection*, and *sterilization*.

5. Describe an effective hand washing procedure.

6. List five accepted methods for instrument sterilization.

7. Describe the conditions required for sterilization when using each of the methods listed in question 6.

8. Describe the recommended procedure for decontaminating the trisyringe and the handpiece between patients.

REFERENCES

Allen AL, Organ RJ: Occult blood accumulation under fingernails: a mechanism for the spread of blood-borne infections, *JADA* 105:455, 1982.

American Dental Association: What the new standards require, *JADA* 123:32, 1992.

American Dental Association News 18(3):1, 1987a.

American Dental Association News 18(16):1, 1987b.

American Dental Hygienists Association: OSHA mandates protective wear, *Access*, p 1, November 1987.

American Health Consultants: Companies, hospitals, scientists debate safety of disposable gloves, *AIDS Alert* 2:207, 1987a.

American Health Consultants: Latex vinyl gloves offer same protection against HIV, *AIDS Alert* 2:210, 1987b.

Bagga BS et al: Contamination of dental units cooling water with oral microorganisms and its prevention, *JADA* 109:712, 1984.

Baker CH, Hawkins VI: Law in the dental workplace: legal implications of hepatitis B for the dental profession, *JADA* 110:637, 1985.

Block S: *Disinfection, sterilization and preservation*, ed 4, Philadelphia, 1991, Lea & Febiger.

Bond WW et al: Inactivation of hepatitis B virus by intermediate-to-high level disinfectant chemicals, *J Clin Microbiol* 18:535, 1983.

Brooks SL et al: Prevalence of herpes simplex virus disease in a professional population, *JADA* 102:31, 1981.

Burnett GW, Schuster GS: *Oral microbiology and infectious disease*, Baltimore, 1978, Williams & Wilkins.

Centers for Disease Control: Recommendations for protection against viral hepatitis, *MMWR* 34:313, 1985.

Centers for Disease Control: Recommended infection control practice for dentistry, *MMWR* 35:237, 1986a.

Centers for Disease Control: Update: acquired immunodeficiency syndrome—United States, *MMWR* 35:141, 1986b.

Centers for Disease Control: Update on hepatitis B prevention, *MMWR* 36:353, 1987.

Centers for Disease Control: Inadequate response among public safety workers receiving intradermal vaccination against hepatitis B—United States, 1990- 1991, *MMWR* 40:659, 1991a.

Centers for Disease Control: Update: Transmission of HIV infection during invasive dental procedures—Florida, *MMWR* 40:377, 1991b.

Chapel TA: The variability of syphilitic chancres, *Sex Transm Dis* 5:68, 1978.

Christensen RP et al: Efficiency of 42 brands of face masks and 2 face shields in preventing inhalation of airborne debris, *Gen Dent P* 414, Nov-Dec 1991.

Clinical Research Associates: Subject: gloves, disposable operating, *Clin Res Assoc Newsletter* 9(9):2, 1985.

Cottone JA: Hepatitis B virus infection in the dental profession, *JADA* 110:617, 1985.

Cottone JA: Delta hepatitis: another concern for dentistry, *JADA* 112:47, 1986.

Cottone JA, Baker BR: Hepatitis B: recent advances and 1986 preview, *Can Dent Assoc J* 13:36, 1985.

Cottone JA et al: *Practical infection control in dentistry*, Philadelphia, 1991, Lea & Febiger.

Council on Dental Materials, Instruments, and Equipment, *JADA* 122:110, 1991.

Council on Dental Materials, Instruments, and Equipment: Recommendations for radiographic darkroom practices, *JADA* 104:886, 1982.

Council on Dental Materials, Instruments, and Equipment; Council on Dental Practice; and Council on Dental Therapeutics: Infection control recommendations for the dental office and the dental laboratory, *JADA* 116:241, 1988.

Council on Dental Therapeutics: *Accepted dental therapeutics*, ed 40, Chicago, 1984, American Dental Association.

Council on Dental Therapeutics: Accepted therapeutic products, *JADA* 113:1018, 1986.

Council on Dental Therapeutics and Council on Prosthetic Services and Dental Laboratory Relations: Guidelines for infection control in the dental office and the commercial dental laboratory, *JADA* 110:969, 1985.

Council on Dental Therapeutics and Council on Dental Materials, Instruments, and Equipment, *Monograph on safety and infection control*, ed 1, Chicago, ADA, 1990.

Craig DC, Quayle AA: The efficiency of face masks, *Br Dent J* 158:87, 1985.

Crawford JJ: *Clinical asepsis in dentistry*, ed 3, Mesquite, Texas, 1986, RA Kolstad.

Crawford JJ: State of the art practical infection control in dentistry, *JADA* 110:629, 1985.

Department of Regulatory Agencies, Colorado State Board of Dental Examiners: *Newsletter* 1:3, 1992.

Farah JW, Powers JM, editors: Infection control, *Dental Advisor, Materials, Instruments and Equipment Quarterly* 3(3):4, 1986.

Fox JL: TB: a grim disease of numbers, *ASM* 56: 363, 1990.

Francis DP et al: Prevention of hepatitis B with vaccine: report from the Centers for Disease Control multi-center efficacy trial among homosexual men, *Ann Intern Med* 97:363, 1982.

Gerberding JL et al: Risk of transmitting the human immunodeficiency virus, cytomegalovirus and hepatitis B virus to health-care workers exposed to patients with AIDS and AIDS-related conditions, *J Infect Dis* 157:1, 1987.

Gleason MJ, Molinari JA: Stability of safety glasses during sterilization and disinfection, *JADA* 115:60, 1987.

Gobette JP, et al: Hand asepsis: the efficacy of different soaps in the removal of bacteria from sterile, gloved hands, *JADA* 113:291, 1986.

Goto Y et al: Detection of proviral sequences in saliva of patients infected with human immunodeficiency virus type I, *AIDS Res Hum Retroviruses*, 7:343, 1991

Gravois SL, Stringer RB: Survey of occupational health hazards in dental hygiene, *Dent Hyg* 54:518, 1980.

Gross ML: Herpes: an overview on diagnosis and treatment, *J Ky Dent Assoc* 33(3):26, 1981.

Hastreiter RJ et al: Effectiveness of dental office sterilization procedures, *JADA* 122:51, 1991.

Henderson CW et al: Evaluation of the barrier system, an infection control system for the dental laboratory, *J Prosthet Dent* 58:517, 1987.

Henderson DK et al: Risk for occupational transmission of human immunodeficiency virus type 1 (HIV-1) associated with clinical exposures; a prospective evaluation, *Ann Intern Med* 113:740, 1990.

Herrera SP, Merchant VA: Dimensional stability of dental impressions after immersion disinfection, *JADA* 113:419, 1986.

Ingersoll B: US takes steps against product from Sporicidin, *Wall Street Journal* B4 p. ?, Dec 16, 1991.

Johnson & Johnson: *Handbook of Dental Practice Asepsis*, East Windsor, NJ, 1969, Dental Products Co.

Kampmeier, RH: *Essentials of Syphilology*, ed 3, Philadelphia, 1943, JB Lippincott.

Kane MA, Lettau LA: Transmission of HBV from dental personnel to patients, *JADA* 110:634, 1985.

Kuo G et al: An assay for circulating antibodies to a major etiologic virus of human non-A non-B hepatitis, *Science* 244:362, 1989.

Landesman S et al: The AIDS epidemic, *N Engl J Med* 312:521, 1985.

Litsky BY et al: Use of antimicrobial mouthwash to minimize the bacterial aerosol contamination generated by a high speed drill, *Oral Surg* 29:25, 1976.

Logan MK: Legal implications of infectious disease in the dental office, *JADA* 115:850, 1987.

Luelmo F: BCG vaccination, *Am Rev Respir Dis* 125:70, 1982.

Maloney JM, Kohut RD: Infection control: barrier protection and the treatment environment, *Dent Hyg* 61:310, 1987.

Mandell R et al: *Principles and practices of infectious diseases*, ed 3, New York, 1990, Churchill Livingston.

Manzella JP et al: An outbreak of herpes simplex virus type I gingivostomatitis in a dental hygiene practice, *JAMA* 252:2019, 1984.

Merchant VA: Herpes simplex virus infection: an occupational hazard in dental practice, *J Mich Dent Assoc* 64:199, 1982.

Merchant VA: Disinfection of dental impressions, *Dent Teamwork* 3:13, 1990.

Micik RE et al: Studies on dental aerobiology. I. Bacterial aerosols generated during dental procedures, *J Dent Res* 48:51, 1969.

Micik RE et al: Studies on dental aerobiology. III. Efficiency of surgical masks in protecting dental personnel from airborne bacterial particles, *J Dent Res* 50:626, 1971.

Miller CH: Heat sterilization assures microbe-free instruments, *Dentist* Nov- Dec 1987.

Miller RL et al: Studies on dental aerobiology. II. Microbial splatter discharges from the oral cavity of dental patients, *J Dent Res* 50:621, 1971.

Miller RL, and Micik RE: Air pollution and its control in the dental office, *Dent Clin North Am* 22:453, 1978.

Minagi S et al: Disinfection method for impression materials: freedom from fear of hepatitis B and acquired immunodeficiency syndrome, *J Prosthet Dent* 57:451, 1986.

Minagi S et al: Prevention of acquired immunodeficiency syndrome and hepatitis B. II: Disinfection method for hydrophilic impression materials, *J Prosthet Dent* 58:462, 1987.

Molinari JA et al: Comparison of dental surface disinfectants, *Gen Dent* 35:171, 1987.

Neupert AH: AIDS and the dental team, *Dent Hyg* 61:314, 1987.

Nolte WA: *Oral microbiology*, ed 4, St Louis, 1982, CV Mosby.

OSHA: Bloodborne pathogens standard, *Federal Register* 56:64175, 1991.

Palenik CJ, Miller CH: Occupational herpetic whitlow, *J Indiana Dent Assoc* 61:25, 1982.

Palenik CJ, Miller CH: Approaches to preventing disease transmission in the dental office. Part I, *Dent Asepsis Rev* 5(9), 1984a.

Palenik CJ, and Miller CH: Handwashing review, *Dent Asepsis Rev* 5(7), 1984b.

Palenik CJ, Miller CH: The need to properly monitor the office sterilizer, *Dent Asepsis Rev* 7(11), 1986a.

Palenik CJ, and Miller CH: Infection control telecast. Part II. Procedures and legalities, *Dent Asepsis Rev* 7(4), 1986b.

Palenik CJ, Miller CH: Use of gloves in the dental operatory, *Dent Asepsis Rev* 8(6):1, 1987.

Palenik, CJ et al: A survey of sterilization practices in selected endodontic offices, *J Endodontics* 12:206, 1986.

Parker ME, Williams H: Cross-infection and cross-contamination: the relationship between subgingival bacteria and fingernail length, *Dent Hyg* 61:68, 1987.

Pollock NL et al: Laminar air purge of microorganisms in dental aerosols, *JADA* 81:1131, 1970.

Price PB: Bacteriology of normal skin: a new quantitative test applied to a study of the bacterial flora and the disinfectant action of mechanical cleansing, *J Infect Dis* 63:301, 1983.

Riley RL: Disease transmission and contagion control, *Am Rev Respir Dis* 125:16, 1982.

Rowe NH et al: Herpetic whitlow: an occupational disease of practicing dentists, *JADA* 105:471, 1982.

Rowe NH, Brooks SL: Contagion in the dental office, *Dent Clin North Am* 22:491, 1978.

Runnells RR: Heat and heat/pressure sterilization, *Can Dent Assoc J* 13:46, 1985.

Sampson E: Hepatitis B-protection of patient, dentist, and staff. In *Proceedings of a symposium on hepatitis B: risk, prevention and the vaccine*, One hundred twenty-third annual session of the American Dental Association, Las Vegas, 1982.

Schaefer ME: Infection control in dental laboratory procedures, *CDA J* 13:81, 1985.

Schiff ER et al: Veterans Administration cooperative study on hepatitis and dentistry, *JADA* 113:390, 1986.

Simonsen RJ et al: An evaluation of sterilization by autoclaving in dental offices, *J Dent Res* 58:400, 1979 (abstract).

Skaug N: Micropunctures of rubber gloves used in oral surgery, *Int J Oral Surg* 5:220, 1976.

Skaug N: Proper monitoring of sterilization procedures used in oral surgery, *Int J Oral Surg* 12:153, 1983.

Smith AL: *Principles of microbiology*, ed 9, St Louis, 1982, CV Mosby.

Steven CE et al: Yeast-recombinant hepatitis B vaccine: efficacy with hepatitis B immune globulin in prevention of perinatal hepatitis B virus transmission, *JAMA*, 257:2612, 1987.

Sutherland I, Lindgren I: The protective effect of BCG vaccination as indicated by autopsy studies, *Tubercle* 60:225, 1979.

Szmuness W et al: Hepatitis B vaccine: demonstration of efficacy in a controlled clinical trial in a high-risk population in the United States, *N Engl J Med* 303:833, 1980.

Tankersley RW: Amino acid requirements of herpes simplex virus in human cell, *J Bacteriol* 87:609, 1964.

Terezhalmy GP et al: The use of water-soluble bioflavonoid-ascorbic acid complex in the treatment of recurrent herpes labialis, *Oral Surg* 45:56, 1978.

Thomas LE et al: Survival of herpes simplex virus and other selected microorganisms on patient charts: potential source of infection, *JADA* 111:461, 1985.

Underhill TE et al: Prevention of cross-infections in the dental environment, *Compend Contin Educ Dent* 7:260, 1986.

US Public Health Service: Coolfont report: a PHS plan for prevention and control of AIDS and the AIDS virus, *Public Health Rep* 101:341, 1986.

US Department of Labor, Occupational Safety and Health Administration: *Compliance assistance guidline for the February 27, 1990 OSHA instruction CPL 2-2.44B enforcement procedures for occupational exposure to hepatitis B virus and human immunodeficiency virus*, 1991.

Wainwright RB et al: Duration of immunogenicity and efficacy of hepatitis B vaccine in a Yupik Eskimo population, *JAMA* 261:2362, 1989.

Williams GH et al: Laminar air purge of microorganisms in dental aerosols: prophylactic procedures with the ultrasonic scaler, *J Dent Res* 49:1498, 1970.

Wyler D et al: Efficacy of self-administered preoperative oral hygiene procedures in reducing the concentration of bacteria in aerosols generated during dental procedures, *J Dent Res* 50:509, 1971.

Yagiela JA et al: Disinfection of nitrous oxide inhalation equipment, *JADA* 98:191, 1979.

Yokom NG: Infection control, the government, and you, *IDHA Newsletter*, January 1988.

4 THE COMPLETE DENTAL RECORD

Donna J. Stach

LEARNING OUTCOMES

The dental hygienist will be able to

1. Explain the purposes of a complete dental record and its component parts.
2. Apply the guidelines for making chart entries, especially progress notes.
3. Evaluate dental charts using a chart audit format.
4. Discuss the advantages of the electronic dental record.

In all likelihood, you have at one time or another been treated by a physician, nurse practitioner, nurse, dentist, or dental hygienist. Think about your treatment and the treatment records that the health care providers used to assist them. What would you expect to see in the record? What would you want excluded from the record? Have you ever read (or peeked at) the record? If so, what was your impression of its contents and of the health care providers who had written in the record?

Undoubtedly, you have come to expect that the health care provider will have an accurate, legible recording of each of your conditions or problems, visits, treatments, tests, and test results, as well as the progress of your condition. In a nutshell, you expect the provider to be able to glean from the record all the pertinent information needed to treat your present condition knowledgeably and adequately. In addition, you probably expect that entries will be written objectively and that the entire record will be treated with respect and confidentiality. Patients will rightfully have these expectations of *you*, as a dental health care provider, regarding *their* dental record.

Good record keeping is increasingly important in today's dental practice. Patients have more sophisticated expectations, government agencies have more regulations, third-party payers have an interest in treatment, and litigation is increasingly common.

The purpose of this chapter is to familiarize you with the functions of the dental record, its inclusions, and the approaches to maintaining a complete dental record. In addition, confidential-

ity, legal responsibility, chart audits, and the use of computers are discussed.

A MEDICOLEGAL DOCUMENT

A complete dental record should include all of the information necessary to treat a patient safely and knowledgeably. The record must contain a data base that includes the patient's past and present medical and dental histories, present dental status, diagnosis of present conditions, consultation reports, treatment plan, patient consent, treatment rendered, outcomes, referrals, and conversations with patients. The complete dental record and associated materials, such as study models, radiographs, laboratory test results, and photographs, are medicolegal documents. The records are medical documents because they concern the general health of a patient and the ensuing treatment. They are legal documents because they are admissible in a court of law as evidence either for or against the health care provider or the patient (Miller, 1970, Pollack, 1987). As a legal document, the chart protects both the patient and the clinician, so the chart should be complete, thorough, accurate, and legible.

Miller (1970) states, "A cautious dentist (dental hygienist) will never rely on memory. He [she] will record *all* facts pertinent to a patient's history, examination, diagnosis, visits, treatments, fees, and observations, and will identify each fact by specific date. . . . Everything pertinent to a dentist's [dental hygienist's] treatment should be included in the record file...."Any treatment, diagnostic aid, or diagnosis performed with the patient must be noted in the permanent record. It is important to document every interaction and treatment to ensure continuity of care for the patient and legal protection for the patient and dental personnel.

The dental record is important not only for the provision of quality care for the patient, but also as legal protection. The dental health care provider is legally responsible for protecting and respecting the personal and property rights of the patient, for providing only necessary and agreed-on care, for completing care within a reasonable amount of time, for achieving reasonably satisfactory results, for exercising "reasonable care" in performing services, and for charging reasonable fees (Miller, 1970; Morris, 1976; Woodall, 1989). In turn, the patient is responsible for paying the fee and cooperating in treatment (Miller, 1970; Morris, 1976; Woodall, 1989). If either the health care provider or the patient does not fulfill any of these responsibilities, the other party can take legal action. In most such legal cases the dental record would be used as evidence; therefore it is crucial that the record be accurate and legible. Legal action may take place years later when memory may not accurately recall details. The dental record should provide sufficient information to recreate the event. For a further discussion of patient and health care provider responsibilities, as well as malpractice, consult Woodall (1987).

Two elements of the health care provider's responsibility for protecting and respecting the personal and property rights of the patient—confidentiality and informed consent—must be emphasized. Protecting the patient's confidentiality involves respecting communications among the health care providers and the patient. It does not mean that everything between the patient and the health care provider is secret; if that were so, continuity of care would be impossible. Rather, protecting a patient's confidentiality involves ensuring that the records are not visible to other patients and that the patient's name or identifying information is removed from records being used in a professional presentation. Another example of protecting this confidentiality is not releasing a patient's records without his or her permission. Perhaps the most important way to respect a patient's confidentiality is by writing objective, truthful, and respectful chart entries. Such chart entries are discussed later in the chapter.

Informed consent, discussed in Chapter 18, means that the patient has enough information about his or her condition and treatment options available to be able to accept or reject the recommended treatment knowledgeably. The patient's informed consent should be recorded in the dental record.

NECESSARY INCLUSIONS AND RECORD ORGANIZATION

Considering the importance of the dental record, medically and legally, it becomes apparent that a health care provider should know what must be included in a complete dental record. The necessary inclusions for a dental record are the patient's name on all pages; the patient's residence and employment addresses and phone numbers; the patient's date of birth, sex, and occupation; the physician's name, address, and phone number; the name of the person to contact in an emergency; medical and dental histories; examination findings and diagnosis; treatment goals; the treatment plan; the treatment provided, with dates and signatures; results of treatment, especially unexpected results; radiographs; fees charged and paid; and copies of all correspondence (Miller, 1970). Although financial information is part of the patient's record, it should be kept on separate forms and not on the same sheets as treatment progress records (Pollack, 1987).

The chart should be logically organized so that it is easily read and understood. Records can be organized in many different ways. The most common format is to have a folder or envelope that contains all the forms and radiographs. It is helpful if chart folders have an envelope or pocket attached to hold the radiographs and intraoral photographs. Forms should be fastened in the sequence in which they will be prepared or reviewed at the time of the appointment.

The usual sequence of forms is basic demographic data, the patient's past and present medical and dental histories, examination findings and diagnosis, treatment goals or problem list, the treatment plan, patient's agreement to treatment, the treatment provided with dates and signatures, and results of treatment. Radiographs, intraoral photographs, copies of correspondence, and records of fees charged and paid follow or are stored in the folder pocket.

Some charts have a symbol, colored tape, or the words "medical alert" in a prominent position on the front of the chart to alert the clinician to a medical condition that must be considered *before* treatment is begun. On seeing such an alert, the health care provider can then open the chart, refer to the medical history, and become familiar with the patient's condition. The use of symbols, tape, or "medical alert" is preferable to writing the condition (e.g., hepatitis) on the front of the chart, because it is more respectful of the patient's right to confidentiality.

The chart should also have an area for notation of special needs of the patient. Such needs may include provisions to accommodate a wheelchair or referral to a specialist.

Some charts provide an area for notation of nicknames, hobbies, or special interests of the patient (Kilpatrick, 1974); these may provide the dental professional with information to put the patient at ease. It is also helpful to note emotional traumas that a patient may mention to the provider, such as the death of a spouse or a recent separation; these emotional traumas may affect the patient's overall and dental health. The health care provider should remember to write these statements objectively and descriptively without violating the patient's privacy.

GUIDELINES FOR CHART ENTRIES

Considering the importance of the complete dental record, some general guidelines to complete a chart may be helpful. The following should be considered whenever making an entry in a patient's record.

All entries should be *complete, accurate, legible, with the author easily identified, and in ink or some other permanent form* (Pollack, 1987). To be admissible as evidence in court, the data must be discernible, and it must be obvious that entries were made during the course of treatment and not after a suit was filed. Ink and computer entries can be evaluated for the length of time since they were made; thus they are valid as evidence if they reflect legitimate records of the progress of care. Pencil entries are easily changed and the time of entry is difficult to evaluate; therefore pencil records in some instances may not be admissible as evidence. It should be obvious from these facts that entries should be made at each visit and that, in the face of a suit, *no attempt should be made to alter records* to try to prove a point. Such an attempt is foolish and an obstruction of justice (Stetler, 1962; Woodall, 1987). If errors are made in the record entry, a single line should be drawn through it, the word *error* written above it, and the correction made on the next available line (Pollack, 1987).

Records should be retained for at least 10 years past the time a file becomes inactive (Miller, 1970) and perhaps forever (Pollack, 1987). Depending on the state, a patient may file suit against a health care provider up to 6 to 10 years *after* the encounter that triggered the dissatisfaction (Stetler, 1962). The record may be the only evidence in support of the health care provider. Therefore, even if the only treatment rendered for that patient was an extraction, the record must be kept for the duration of the state's statute of limitations.

Documentation of all services rendered, data collection, and procedures performed should be entered in the record when they are done. The progress notes should reflect the patient's needs identified during data collection, the diagnosis, and treatment planning. For example, a progress note stating that an amalgam was placed in tooth No. 30 should only be present if a carious lesion was charted for tooth No. 30 during data collection and subsequently included in the treatment plan.

The progress note should contain descriptive, objective statements dated and signed by the health care provider. It is always wise to compose the progress notes in a specific order so that the necessary information is always present. One such order is to report the patient's subjective findings, if any; the clinician's objective findings; any medication administered, such as a local anesthetic; the procedure performed; complications and/or results observed; the patient's reactions; whether the treatment is complete or incomplete; the treatment to be performed at the next appointment; and the amount of time required before the next appointment. Following is a sample progress note:

3/5/92: Patient reports that her gums are tender and bleed when brushing. Gingiva is marginally red, edematous, and bleeds on probing. Calculus generalized, moderate to heavy subgingivally. Bleeding index 35%, plaque index 50%. Reviewed periodontal chart, no significant changes. Discussed importance of plaque and bleeding in periodontal disease. Demonstrated Bass brushing—patient performed it well and agreed to brush twice daily. Reviewed and corrected flossing technique—patient not carrying floss subgingivally. Gave left posterior superior alveolar, middle superior alveolar, anterior superior alveolar, greater palatine and nasopalatine injections using 2.7 ml of 2% lidocaine with epinephrine 1:100,000, used benzocaine topical. Debrided maxillary left quadrant with ultrasonic and hand instruments. Advised patient of possible root sensitivity post-operatively. No adverse reactions to local anesthesia or to treatment observed or reported. Plan: reevaluate maxillary left and debride mandibular left with anesthesia. Next appointment: 1 week.

DJS

Chart entries can be shortened by using commonly accepted abbreviations. It is still important to include information transmitted and clinical impressions as well as procedures performed. The chart entry above could be shortened as follows:

3/5/92. Patient reports gums tender and bl. on TB. Ging. marg. red, edem., BOP. Calc. gen. mod.-heavy sub. BI 35%, PI 50%. Review perio ch. No sig. changes. Discussed role of pl. and bl. in perio. Demo. & return Bass brushing. Pt. did well and agreed to do 2x/day.Review & correct floss tech.—not taking floss sub. Gave lf. PSA, MSA, ASA, GP, NP w/2.7 ml 2% lido w/epi 1:100,000. Benzo topical. Debride max. lf. w/ultrason. & hand inst. Advis. pt. of possible rt. sensitivity post. op. No adverse reaction obs. or report. Plan: reeval max. lf. debride w/LA mand. lf. N/A: 1 week.

DJS

It is important to enter progress notes using accepted dental terminology or abbreviations and descriptive, objective sentences for two reasons. First, other health care providers must be able to understand the terminology used in the entry to continue care; second, the patient can gain access to the record, so no derogatory or subjective comment should be entered in the record (Howard, 1975, Pollack, 1987). For example, it is highly inappropriate to enter, "Ms. Jones is a real complainer—ignore her for her own good." The following sample entry may be more appropriate: "Ms. Jones said that she hates the scraping noise of the instruments on her teeth and that she does not want me to make that noise. I explained why the noise was necessary and reassured her that the scaling was being done properly. At the end of the appointment, Ms. Jones said that she still didn't like that sound, but her teeth feel smooth." The second entry describes the situation more completely, and if the patient ever read the entry, it is not likely that she would be offended or feel discredited. Abbreviations could be used to shorten the length of this entry.

An entry should be supported with data whenever possible so that the next health care provider can better understand the situation. If an entry stated, "Patient has poor home care procedures," the next health care provider would not have much concrete information to evaluate. However, the entry "Patient has consistently high plaque and bleeding indices; patient reports that she brushes once a day when she remembers to brush" gives the next health care provider more information about the patient's dental status without subjective judgments.

APPROACHES TO RECORD STYLE

The system for record keeping should be easy to use, organized, and allow quick retrieval of needed information. So far the necessary inclusions in a dental record have been discussed, but the styles of record keeping have not. Currently two approaches are commonly used. The traditional style is the *treatment-oriented record*. It has three major components: data base, treatment plan, and progress notes. The other style, which is increasingly the standard of care, is the *problem-oriented* record. It has four major components: data base, problem list, treatment plan, and progress notes (Barsh, 1981; Weed, 1969).

The addition of the problem list allows the development of a more organized and comprehensive treatment plan. It should address systemic as well as specific dental needs and is especially helpful if the patient has multiple or complex problems. It is an analytical tool used to interpret the data collected in the examination and patient interview. Each sign or symptom is identified as a problem, and each problem has an individual treatment plan with a priority number so that the most threatening problems are treated first (Weed, 1969). Just as the treatment plan flows from the problem list, the progress notes will also follow the same sequence and address identified needs. This helps to meet the requirements that a good dental record show the sequence and progress of treatment in a clear and concise manner (Barsh, 1981).

In the problem-oriented approach, there is a specific step, formulating the problem list, for analysis of the data and then logical assignment of priorities. In the treatment-oriented approach, this step is not present; rather, the clinician analyzes the data directly in preparing the treatment plan (Fig. 4-1).

Comparison of Record Approaches

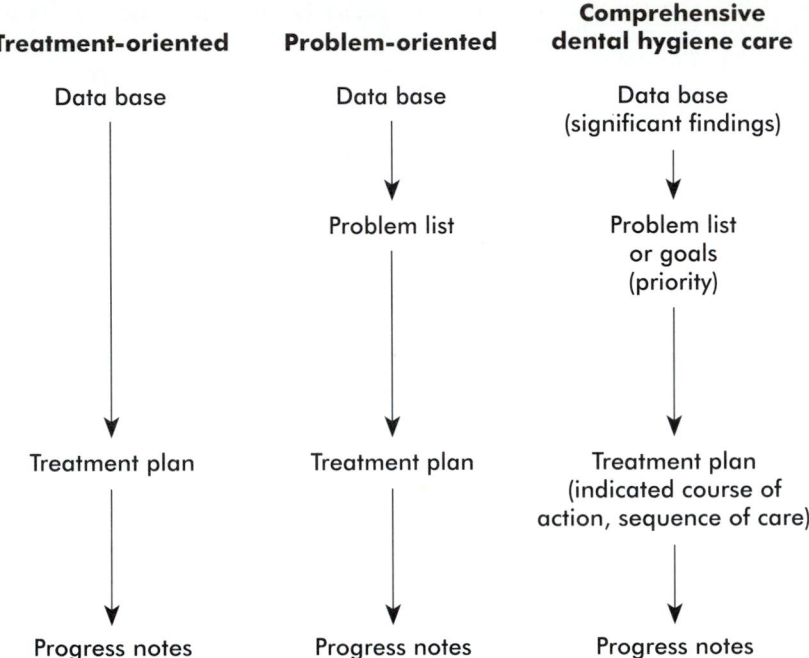

Treatment-oriented   **Problem-oriented**   **Comprehensive dental hygiene care**

Treatment-oriented	Problem-oriented	Comprehensive dental hygiene care
Data base	Data base	Data base (significant findings)
	Problem list	Problem list or goals (priority)
Treatment plan	Treatment plan	Treatment plan (indicated course of action, sequence of care)
Progress notes	Progress notes	Progress notes

Fig. 4-1. Treatment-oriented and problem-oriented approaches are compared in the first and second columns. Note that the treatment-oriented approach does not include a problem list. The approach presented in this book, a problem-oriented approach, is in the third column. Consult Chapter 18 for further explanation of terms in parentheses.

The approach to records and treatment planning presented in this book is a problem-oriented one. This approach is described more fully in Chapter 18.

ELECTRONIC DENTAL RECORD

The computer is essentially a sophisticated electronic filing system that can store all necessary patient data (Forest, 1986). Any information that can be stored in written form can be kept in a computer file. A tremendous advantage of the computer is its ability to sort and reference all available data across all patient records with minimal time and effort from the office staff. The second major advantage of a computer record system is the completion of several functions from one or two entries.

The computer can integrate aspects of record keeping, financial management, patient management, clinical functions, and some miscellaneous functions. For a new patient, data-base information, such as patient identification, insurance and billing, and medical/dental status, is entered into the computer. Medical alerts can be programmed to appear not only in the patient's record but also each time he or she has an appointment scheduled.

After the clinical examination, the treatment plan is entered so that the computer can monitor status and progress whenever it is requested. Given the desired appointment length and the task to be performed, the computer can seek and schedule appropriate appointments. A series of specific instructions can customize the scheduling function; for example, extensive debridement may only be scheduled at 8:00, 11:00, and 1:00, or no more than two initial patient visits may be scheduled in a row.

The computer is excellent for financial management. It can complete insurance forms and generate monthly billings automatically. The computer can generate correspondence through its word-processing function. This can be a customized version of a form letter or a short note such as

THE COMPLETE DENTAL RECORD

DENTAL RECORD AUDIT

Patient _____ Date _____

Chart number _____ Reviewer _____

Note in each box whether the item is Satisfactory (S), Unsatisfactory (U), or Not Applicable (NA). Note the reason of each NA on the back of this form. Place your initials and the date of the review in the appropriate boxes.

Auditor's Initials

Date   Date

1. Medical history complete, updated, signed
2. Medical consult present, if needed
3. Oral exam complete, updated, signed
4. Chartings complete, updated, signed
5. Satisfactory radiographs taken/present
6. Satisfactory study models present, if taken
7. Satisfactory photographs present, if taken
8. Additional records present, if taken
9. Home care procedures assessed
10. Problem list completed and prioritized
11. Treatment plan recorded
12. Patient informed of needs, treatment, and
    consent signed
13. Home care planned, implemented, evaluated
14. Treatment plan followed/revised
15. Progress notes complete, dated, signed
16. Recall date recorded
17. Financial records complete
18. Demographic data complete

Additional comments:

Fig. 4-2. Sample dental record audit form. See text for explanation of how to use this form.

"Happy Holidays" on a monthly statement. The patient recall interval can also be monitored by the computer and reminder postcards printed and addressed automatically. This list of the uses of a computer in dental practice is not exhaustive but touches only on the dental record aspects.

Computer terminals are becoming part of the dental operatory equipment. Advances in graphics packages are making computers more useful for clinical data gathering and recording. Computer-generated dental charts that use multiple colors and anatomically accurate restorations and abnormalities are now possible. Automated data entry can greatly increase the ease and speed of this phase of record management. Some systems also offer significant advantages in the maintenance of an aseptic chain by allowing direct data entry through voice activation, touch screen (Suddick, 1986), and periodontal probes with electronic sensors that can feed data about pocket depth directly to the computer. It is possible to generate a periodontal chart that shows the level of the gingival margin and epithelial attachment; the difference between the two—the pocket—is shaded (Agudio, 1985). The resulting printout is more diagrammatic and understandable to the patient in its portrayal of gingival status. Future projections for electronic probe and computer systems include sulcular fluid volume readings and tissue antibody measurements. The combination of this information in the computer format will make the computer an integral tool in diagnosis.

Computers are not problem solvers; necessary information must be entered and appropriate questions asked. Computers are data management systems, which makes them valuable tools in today's dental practice.

RECORD AUDITS

With the increasing emphasis on thorough, complete, and accurate records and the increasing interest of third-party carriers, such as insurance companies, in the prevention of fraud in filing claims, many health care practices have instituted record audits to ensure that the charts are being completed accurately and that the necessary inclusions are present (Woodall, 1987). Fig. 4-2 is a sample chart audit form that has been used in a health care practice to audit dental records.

The audit form is completed at the conclusion of a patient's course of treatment by a clinician other than the one responsible for the patient's treatment. When performing an audit, the clinician checks the record for each of the items listed in the left column. If the item is present and satisfactory, an "S" is placed in the appropriate space; if the item is missing or unacceptable, a "U" is written in the space. Once the audit is completed, the auditor initials and dates the form at the top of the column. If any items are missing or unsatisfactory, the clinician responsible for the patient's care is asked to rectify the situation. Because there are several columns, the same audit form can be used after each course of a patient's treatment.

It is a wise practice to review all patient records regularly using an audit form to identify missing or inaccurate entries and to be certain that the care being delivered is appropriate for the patient's needs. By maintaining thorough, complete, and accurate charts, the health care provider will be better able to provide continuous high-quality care and provide protection for both the dental personnel and the patient.

ACTIVITIES

1. Secure sample charts from several dental care practices and:
   a. Review the charts for organization.
   b. Review the charts for the necessary inclusions.
   c. Review the progress notes for thoroughness and completeness.
   d. Rewrite some of the progress notes in a format that meets the criteria described in this chapter.
2. Invite a speaker from one of the companies that print dental records or market computer software packages for dental records and have him or her explain the company's record form.
3. Take a hypothetical patient, Mrs. Smith, from first contact with office through data gathering, treatment planning, appointment scheduling, multiple appointment scaling and root planing, insurance and billing, and 3-month recall maintenance using a pen and paper record system.
4. Repeat activity 3 using a computer record system.
5. Develop a chart audit system that could be used in a dental practice.

REVIEW QUESTIONS

1. Explain the purposes of dental records.
2. List the inclusions that should be part of a dental record and justify each item.
3. Name one major difference between the treatment-oriented and the problem-oriented approaches to record keeping.
4. What is the purpose of a chart audit?
5. Describe a format for writing progress notes.

REFERENCES

Agudio G, Prato GP, Bartolucci EG: Computerized charting of probing depths, *J Periodontal* 56:766, 1985.

Barsh L: *Dental treatment planning for the adult patient*. Philadelphia, 1981, WB Saunders.

Forrest JL, Williams C, Gurenlian JR: Improved communication through computer technology, *Dent Hyg* 60:558, 1986.

Howard WW: *Dental practice planning*, St Louis, 1975, CV Mosby.

Miller SL: *Legal aspects of dentistry*, New York, 1970, GP Putnam's Sons.

Morris WO: Some thoughts on dental malpractice, *Int Dent J* 26:175, 1976.

Pollack BR: *Handbook of dental jurisprudence and risk management*. Littleton, Mass, 1987, PSG Publishing.

Stetler CJ, Moritz AR: *Doctor and patient and the law*, St Louis, 1962, CV Mosby.

Weed LL: *Medical records, medical education, and patient care*, Cleveland, 1969, Case Western Reserve University, Year Book Medical.

Woodall IR: *Legal, ethical, and management aspects of the dental care system*, ed 3, St Louis, 1987, Mosby-Year Book.

SUGGESTED READINGS

Boyce JS: Risk management: an introduction for the dental practice, *Dental Hyg* 61:504, 1987.

Conger SX: The law and dental hygiene practice, *Dent Hyg* 57:14, 1983.

Council on Insurance: Informed consent: a risk management view, *JADA* 115:630, 1987.

Kilpatrick HC: *Work simplification in dental practice: applied time and motion studies*, Philadelphia, 1974, WB Saunders.

Kiser A: Informatics futures in dental practice: professionals viewpoint #1, the ADA, *J Dent Educ* 55:267, 1991.

Murrell C: Recordkeeping: its role in dental hygiene malpractice avoidance and defense, *Dent Hyg* 60:324, 1986.

Murrell C: Recordkeeping: patient responses to treatment, *Dent Hyg* 60:420, 1986.

Nerburger EJ, Diehl MC: The past and future of the electronic dental record from the practioner's view, *J Dent Educ* 55:269, 1991.

Rozovsky FA: *Consent to treatment: practical guide*, Boston, 1990, Little, Brown.

Suddick RP, Collins EM: Computerized charting of the electronic dental record: dentistry's entre' to the computer age, *Dental School Quarterly (UTH SCSA)* 1986.

Valenza JA, Berg JH: *Computers in the dental office*, Chicago, American Dental Association (in press).

Wood NK editor: *Treatment planning: a pragmatic approach*, St. Louis, 1978, CV Mosby.

PART THREE

ASSESSMENT

In the development of any program or project, it is wise to take time to *assess* the situation. Moving directly to implementation without taking time to determine the reasons for the project or the unique needs of the persons for whom the project is being developed can cause considerable difficulty, delay progress, or lead to the ultimate failure of the project. Even the best efforts in implementation can be fraught with difficulty if they are aimed at nonexistent needs or at needs that the subjects of the project do not wish to have modified. A more scientific approach to project development is to set aside assumptions and personal beliefs about the needs and reasons for a project and investigate objective data from which reasons can be inferred.

Assessment includes not only objective data but also the more subjective responses and feelings of the people for whom or with whom the project will be carried out. Even though objective signs are clear indicators of the need for change, subjective responses may override those indicators. People may not want change, or they may want change to be gradual.

In providing clinical care for patients, the principle of assessment is particularly important. Assessment data provide the baseline information for determining the general and oral health status of each patient and provide the dental professional with the opportunity to evaluate the patient's perceptions of the need or desire for change. Assessment can prevent, or help the provider anticipate, emergency situations; it can allow for the individualization of care; it provides baseline data for comparing progress and outcomes with the patient's initial status; and it allows for rational planning.

This section will provide you with the information and skill to work with patients to determine their needs. You will learn the basics of interpersonal interaction with patients, the components of a comprehensive health history, what to do in the event of a medical emergency, and how to perform a general physical and oral examination. You also will learn how to use dental instruments to conduct an examination and to sit at the dental chair with comfort and good vision. Further, you will learn how to interpret a radiographic survey and conduct dental chartings, including a comprehensive periodontal examination. Plaque and gingival indices, occlusion, preparation of study models, and intraoral photography will round out the procedures you will learn in anticipation of your first patient.

5 THE PATIENT'S PERCEPTIONS

Irene Woodall

LEARNING OUTCOMES

The dental hygienist will be able to

1. Adopt language patterns that reinforce that the patient is a partner in care.
2. Given case descriptions of two views of proposed treatment (the patient's and the hygienist's), identify discrepancies in wants, needs, and expectations.
3. Identify the probable impact of discrepancies in wants, needs, and expectations on the success of treatment.
4. Given case presentations, identify ways in which the dental hygienist can gather information regarding the patient's perspectives (wants, needs, and expectations).
5. Describe and develop a helping relationship with patients.
6. Differentiate a helping relationship and a dependency relationship.
7. Differentiate professional closeness and excessive familiarity.
8. Identify ways to blend responsiveness to patients' needs with professional responsibility to provide the "best" care.
9. Explain preliminary plans for assessment phases of care to a series of hypothetical patients who have a variety of wants, needs, and expectations regarding dental hygiene care.

A person may decide to become a dental hygienist for many reasons. Motivations related to self-esteem, a flexible working schedule, and a comfortable income and working environment are related mostly to "self" needs. A second group of motivations is based largely on the desire to perform technical procedures with one's hands and to work with fascinating equipment and instruments that can improve the function and appearance of teeth and their surrounding tissues. Although this second group of reasons is "other"-oriented, it focuses largely on the procedural aspects of practice. A third kind of motivation is that of helping persons achieve positive health changes or maintain their health. Most health care providers have traces of all three motivations that, in balance, can provide satisfaction with the profession as well as favorable outcomes for patients.

According to communications theory regarding the building of interpersonal relationships, the person with a major interest in helping people maintain and achieve health is most likely to encourage and develop the patient's role as a cotherapist or a partner in care. If the health care provider's major interests are self-oriented or proce-

dure-oriented, the patient is more likely to be viewed as an object of care or as a means to an end.

THE PATIENT AS A PARTNER IN CARE

The health care provider who views the patient as a partner in care is more likely to be interested in the patient's wants, needs, and expectations rather than in creating an independent set of needs based solely on clinical data. The partner-in-care concept includes opportunities for the patient to self-assess personal needs, as well as oral conditions, under the guidance of the dental hygienist. Partners in care arrive at mutually satisfying treatment plans and appointment sequences to maximize the partners' ability to complete preventive and therapeutic phases of care (Clark and Morton, 1977).

Basic communications theory explains that people are more likely to feel a commitment to a project or a goal if they share in its development and if its development clearly meets their individual needs (Collins, 1977; Keltner, 1973). While sharing in the design of the plan, participants learn about needs they did not know they had and begin to feel some ownership of the entire proposal. Thus, in a partnership between the dental hygienist and the patient, the dental hygienist learns about the patient's specific needs and limitations, and the patient learns about those of the hygienist (Cohen, 1975; Dworkin, Ference, and Giddon, 1978). Mutual respect for each other's wants and needs can emerge and a clear set of reasonable expectations can be defined, which both people will be more likely to fulfill. Unshared expectations are difficult to meet. Unilateral treatment planning is often unrealistic, because it focuses on issues of low priority to the patient (Dworkin, Ference, and Giddon, 1978). The classic example is the treatment plan that is based on carefully gathered clinical, radiographic, and laboratory findings; prepared by the brightest, most incisive diagnostician; scheduled into logical, perfectly spaced appointments; and presented to the patient with beautiful slides and a well-ordered outline of objective findings and related plans, but for which the patient never appears. Regardless of how well prepared the health care provider's procedures are, if the patient does not believe his or her needs are addressed and being met, the likelihood of compliance is remote. The patient has the final say in whether care will be delivered. If it is not in the form of a "no" at the time of the case presentation, it may be a canceled or "forgotten" appointment.

The patient can usually detect whether he or she is an object or a partner in care. The language that health care providers use is an indicator. Do health care providers perform a procedure *for* or *with* someone, or do they do it *to* someone? Which expression connotes partnership and which connotes object? Is the person scheduled for an appointment at 3:00 PM referred to as the "Class III prophylaxis" or as the "Class II amalgam," or is that person referred to by name, with a diagnosis or planned treatment described as his or her condition? Compare the following two statements: "The upper denture case is in operatory 3." "Ms. Wolfe is in operatory 3, waiting for a try-in of the upper denture." Though the second phrasing may be a few words longer, it connotes a different image of just what is residing in operatory 3. Patients often hear our descriptions of them; if they are viewed as partners in care, they are likely to be referred to as people and not as conditions (Collins, 1977).

Davis (1989) describes how our own needs, values, and prejudices can complement or compli-

cate our interactions with patients. Even though we may want to provide ethical, high-quality care for every patient, individual encounters with patients create reactions that do not fit well with our expectations and thus compromise our ability to be objective and to deliver the highest standard of care. For instance, you may find yourself working with patients who are in poor health because of a long history of self-neglect (those who have avoided dental care for years; tobacco smokers or chewers; or bulimic patients) or because of "foolish" impulsive choices (removing a bottle cap with the teeth) that affect their health. In such cases it may be difficult to avoid being judgmental; yet making the judgment even mentally is often transmitted to the patient, setting up negative barriers to the helping relationship.

To maximize effective communication, you should be aware of when you are feeling angry, resentful, or condemning about a patient's behavior or state of health and recognize where those feelings are coming from. Davis (1989) gives these examples, among others:

1. Paying more attention to some patients and acting cool and aloof with others can mean an underlying prejudice or indifference.
2. Continuing criticism of the patient so that he or she feels nothing is right can also originate from prejudice, as well as from values of perfectionism or rigidity.
3. Treating the patient as an object rather than as a person with feelings of pain, worry, and insecurity can come from a bias of depersonalization.
4. Treating the patient as a child incapable of understanding or making wise choices is patronizing and condescending, reflecting egocentrism.
5. Refusing to let the patient work independently and giving constant supervision and instruction fosters dependence and can arise from a personal need to be needed.
6. Always "fitting the patient in" rather than focusing on his or her individual needs implies that other values (the schedule, your treatment preferences) are more important and that your selfish interest is more important than the patient's.
7. Refusing to listen to or acknowledge the patient's stories of pain and difficulties reflects a need to defend yourself against personal feelings of fear and insecurity.

Though we may each think we would never adopt any of these negative behaviors, it is quite likely that we will, even in subtle ways, find ourselves reacting with control or defensiveness to some of our patients. The key is to pay attention to our feelings and what we are conveying to the patient, and how that behavior will affect the patient's ability to acquire and keep health.

PATIENT INVOLVEMENT IN PLANNING CARE

Involving the patient in the preparation of a treatment plan and in the design of appointment sequences is a difficult concept for many health care providers to accept. The most frequent response to this idea is that the patient does not really know what he or she needs. That is why the patient has come to the health care provider—to find out what is wrong and to have it fixed. Although it is certainly true that the health care provider has far greater knowledge of the patient's objective, observable needs, most patients have important information or notions about their health status or particular needs that can greatly influence the outcome of care. Such information may not emerge except during a discussion of wants, needs, and expectations. Even if the patient has little to contribute to modify suggested care, inclusion in the decision-making process may improve the likelihood that he or she feels a sense of commitment to the process and help ensure that the disease state is avoided in the future (Clark and Morton, 1977; Collins, 1977; Keltner, 1973; Purtilo, 1990).

Evaluate the following two case presentations for the extent to which they include the patient in the decision-making process:

Presentation 1: Well, Mr. Brennan, I've taken a careful look at your examination findings and have decided that you need three appointments for complete periodontal debridement. You have some problems with your gums, and the dentist and I concur that the best way to reverse that problem is to remove all the hard calculus from your teeth and to debride the areas subgingivally in the pockets between your teeth and gums. Now, I know you are interested in having those front teeth turned so they are better looking, but I think your highest priority should lie with getting these gum problems under control. So, we have decided to delay discussing orthodontic treatment until these appointments are complete. If you'll see the receptionist, you can schedule those appointments some time in the next 2 weeks.

Presentation 2: As I remember our initial conversation, Mr. Brennan, your primary interest in dental care was to have those front teeth straightened. Is that still a primary concern for you? (Discuss with patient.) You may recall that during the guided self-assessment we did of your teeth and gums, we found a lot of red, swollen tissue and quite a bit of hard accumulations of calculus on your teeth. Well, the x-ray films confirm that you do have gum or periodontal problems. Take a look at these films; I think if you compare the bone around the molars with the bone around your lower front teeth, you will see a difference in appearance and in height around the teeth. The bone around the molars appears to be in an active state of destruction. I consulted the dentist, and we agree that you may want to postpone the movement of the teeth until we modify the state of the supporting tissues for all your teeth. The bone and the gingiva should be made healthy before we put any additional stress on them. And even after their health has improved, we will have to decide whether tooth movement is advisable. The dentist has agreed that an orthodontist should completely review your case after the initial preparation is complete. We are suggesting that the efforts to move your teeth now might cause harm to the rest of your teeth if we don't attend to these other problems first. Is this set of priorities acceptable to you? Would you agree that we should proceed with the removal of these hard deposits? (Discuss with patient.) Once we have the irritants off your teeth, we'll show you a way to prevent their recurrence, since these gingival and bone problems will recur if plaque builds up on your teeth and if hard deposits form again. (Pause for response; check nonverbal response.) And, after the plaque is under control, we'll assess the tissues to see if further treatment is needed. This will require three appointments, spaced over the next few weeks to allow time between each appointment for healing. Then, when all this is accomplished, we'll reevaluate orthodontic care. Does this sound reasonable to you? Do you have suggestions that could make it easier for us to accomplish our goal together? Are you as interested in having your supporting tissues heal and remain solid as you are in having those front teeth moved? (Discuss after each sample question.)

Which case presentation is more patient centered? Pick out the phrases that tell you the clinician views the patient as a partner rather than a person expected to agree. In which case can you imagine the hygienist making eye contact frequently with the patient? What other differences in nonverbal behavior can you imagine would be evident between these two case descriptions? The differences intended between the two styles of case presentation are in the patient's degree of opportunity to react to the suggested treatment plan and the extent to which the patient's need (tooth movement for esthetics) is kept in mind as a serious priority. Patients may not necessarily value certain elements of dental health (or general health, for that matter) as much as health care providers do (Collins, 1977; Purtilo, 1990). Certainly, explanation of the rationale for altering the treatment plan and for including more in the plan than the patient expected is essential and valid. In patient-centered care, this explanation is given with the underlying premise that the patient's wants and needs are equally important in designing the total plan and that the patient has the right to be involved in the discussion and decision making (Collins, 1977; Dworkin, Ference, and Giddon, 1978). The patient should always be asked if he or she is satisfied with the proposed treatment plan (Clark and Morton, 1977).

Though this chapter focuses on the interpersonal responsibility and wisdom of keeping a patient fully informed and of seeking the patient's verbal consent, this responsibility is also a legal one. It is not enough to be right about what a patient needs. The attitude of engaging a patient as a partner in decision making is supported by the law as well as by the need for harmony and cooperation (American Dental Association Council, 1987; Broonten and Chapman, 1987; Rosoff, 1981; Rozovsky, 1984).

An obvious outcome of sharing plans, discussing priorities, and asking opinions is that the patient may disagree with what the provider believes is right. There are times when the patient may not wish to compromise desires for care, despite the careful discussion of rationales for including other phases of care or delaying or eliminating the phases of care the patient believes are needed to improve appearance or health. A case in point would be the person who appears with perfectly healthy teeth and periodontium but insists that he or she will have all the teeth extracted and dentures made. A patient who is convinced that this course of treatment is best certainly deserves discussion of some alternatives and a careful analysis of why and how he or she came to this conclusion. In some cases it may not be possible to convince the patient that other approaches should be followed. The health care provider then has to decide whether to provide the procedures the patient wants or to refuse care. Generally speaking, if a patient requests care that, in the opinion of the

dentist or hygienist, is totally inappropriate or dangerous, the health care provider should refuse care. The alternative is to write out all the adverse possible outcomes of such care and have the patient sign the statement. Such a statement should relieve the health care providers from responsibility for the negative outcomes of such treatment and place full responsibility on the patient. Because of the critical nature of such a disclaimer, it is absolutely essential that an attorney draw up this document.

The patient who demands unreasonable care is certainly a challenge to health care providers, because the only realistic decision may be to refuse care. The professional must then allow the patient to leave with untended real problems to seek another professional to solve the imagined problems. For the patient, however, the labels for those problems are just the opposite, and efforts to solve what the patient sees as imaginary problems and what the health professional sees as real ones will probably result in further patient dissatisfaction.

Another challenge is the patient who says he or she is satisfied but does not act that way. The patient may act resentful or miss appointments. If there is a discrepancy between what the patient says and does, he or she should be asked about it (Purtilo, 1990).

LISTENING

The first step in developing an attitude that will "let the patient in" as a partner is to practice good listening skills. Many new clinicians are concerned about what to say to a patient. Your first priority is to *listen* to what the patient says and to let the patient know you understand. This is *not* accomplished by saying, "I understand." Even though these words of assurance are spoken, the patient is left wondering what it is you think you understand.

Listening involves rephrasing (1) the *content* of the message the patient has sent and (2) the patient's *affect* or emotion behind it. Listening requires "immediate, genuine, concrete, and empathic reaction to verbal and nonverbal messages" (Okun, 1987). Usually what people say—the actual words they speak—conveys an apparent message, but the way they say it and their subtle choice of words often provide an underlying message that should not be ignored (Okun, 1987). Reading those messages, reflecting them back accurately, and using those new insights is a highly refined, but essential, skill that helpers develop as they work with people (Gottschalk, Lolas, and Viney, 1986).

For instance, a new patient arriving for dental hygiene care says, "I sure hate coming to a dental office." Listening would involve reflecting back the content and effect by saying, "It sounds like you don't enjoy these visits very much and you'd rather be elsewhere right now." The patient responds to correct an inaccuracy, such as:

Well, no. I don't look forward to being here. But I know I should have this done. So here's the place to be.

Or the patient may confirm the hygienist's reflection and elaborate:

You bet. My mouth must be very sensitive, because I feel *everything*. Having my teeth cleaned really hurts.

Further listening would be:

So you've had your teeth cleaned many times before, and it always hurts.

The patient:

Yes, it does. Every time an instrument touches my teeth, I feel like a needle is touching the nerve.

The hygienist:

So what hurts is a metal instrument touching the tooth rather than your gums feeling sore.

The patient:

Yes. My gums don't bother me at all. It's the teeth. I just have to hang on for fear of crying. I wish someone could do something so I wouldn't feel the pain.

The hygienist:

Having your teeth cleaned must be awful for you— like you're "white knuckling" it through the appointment. Anesthesia hasn't worked for you.

The patient:

Well, no one has given me anesthesia. I just put up with it and keep quiet.

After all that *listening* it may now be time for the hygienist to begin *talking*. It appears that the patient could benefit from anesthesia, and the hygieniest could suggest it. But imagine that the hygienist had not used active listening. Typical responses to a patient's complaint about being in a dental office could be:
• Don't worry. I'll be gentle.

• Everyone hates to be in a dental chair—even I don't like it.
• Dentistry is an evil necessity, isn't it?
• Do you come to the dentist regularly?
• You should try relaxation exercises.
• Well, we're just cleaning your teeth today. It won't be bad.

Any one of those typical comments shuts off the communication. The patient either gives up and suffers again or has to start up with another entry to get the hygienist to listen. Even the question responses shut off communication because they redirect the patient to talk about what the hygienist suspects is behind the problem. The patient's message is lost, and thus a critical insight to his or her needs and expectations is missed.

Poor communication with patients results in two important roadblocks. First, the patients will not understand what you are saying and cannot act appropriately on what you say even if they want to. Second, the patients become convinced that you do not care whether they understand or not—that you do not value their feelings and needs (Purtilo, 1990). Nonverbal behavior can close out communication as well. One example is the smile that conveys no warmth, acceptance, or respect. These negative "smiles" include those which say:

1. *I know something you don't know*. The hygienist smiles this way when thinking, "You think your teeth are in good shape, but they're really not."
2. *Poor, poor you*. This smile accompanies the hygienist's intervention to change a person's flossing technique after smugly watching him or her try for 5 minutes.
3. *Don't tell me*. The hygienist asks how the patient is and smiles a "how wonderful" even before he or she speaks.
4. *I'm smarter than you*. This smile is a nonverbal reprimand, perhaps because a hygienist's recommendations were not followed, resulting in expensive treatment.
5. *I don't like you either*. This smile is given when the patient's beliefs are backed up by the dentist or some other authority, contrary to what the hygienist has said. The patient looks at the hygienist to note the "victory"; the hygienist smiles through his or her teeth.

These are destructive, nonverbal messages that hurt more than words, and are difficult to combat verbally (Purtilo, 1990).

Nonverbal messages reveal a great deal about what the communicator really means. "Negative smiles," a touch that carries anger or disinterest, failure to make eye contact, and other distancing behaviors can undo all the carefully selected phrasing. A person will see right through a beautifully prepared speech about warmth and caring and see the true feelings. Accepting people for who they are and learning to enjoy their foibles and to see the bright side of each encounter can help the hygienist learn how to feel warmth and caring and then communicate it naturally.

Compassion "is a value that is fueled with imagination and the ability to envision what is possible from the other person's perspective" (Davis, 1989). It occurs when we (1) value each patient as an individual human being, (2) we take action and speak from moral values that enhance healing, (3) we treat patients as adults who are in charge of their own lives and can make appropriate choices, (4) we respect what patients say and its confidentiality, (5) we attend to them with interest, and (6) we obtain their informed consent for therapy (Davis, 1989). When compassion is present, you can discover the other person and determine with him or her how you can be of help.

THE HELPING RELATIONSHIP

The first basic element of the helping relationship in which the patient is a partner in care is the patient *wanting* to be helped (Purtilo, 1990). Patients must have the freedom to refuse help (even if help is *good* for them). If help is requested as a result of discussions with the patient, the relationship can grow.

Second, the function of the helper is to meet the needs of the "helpee," not those of the helper. A true helper should not be working to change other people to fit an image of something better. The helper and helpee work together to seek the best solution and determine how to implement it. Helping is a mutual learning process (Okun, 1987).

Third, the helping relationship should build toward patient self-reliance (Purtilo, 1990). A sound helping relationship enables the patient to accept responsibility for self-care, for preventing disease, and for seeking professional help to maintain health. The alternative is a dependency relationship in which the patient sees the health care provider as the one responsible for his or her dental health.

The helper must be able to work with people in the affective domain (feelings and emotions), the cognitive domain (thinking), and the behavioral domain (actions) (Okun, 1986). This is important in dentistry, because people arrive for care with a basketful of emotions about what they expect will happen, previous experiences, and the appearance and health of their teeth. People arrive with misinformation, and they often have unhelpful health habits or omit practices that are necessary for their oral health.

In the practice of dental hygiene, it is common to encounter patients who believe that as long as they have their teeth checked and cleaned every 6 months, their responsibility toward good dental health is fulfilled; the rest is up to the dentist and hygienist. Having clean teeth 2 days out of the year (every 6 months) and having restorations placed year after year result in detrimental long-term effects. Periodontists who treat patients who have "graduated" to their care from years of this kind of care refer to it as supervised neglect. The patient has become dependent on the professionals for something they cannot possibly provide. Daily self-care in removing plaque and debris and in monitoring diet are critical components of dental health that cannot be assigned to the dental hygienist or dentist.

Certainly, there is a degree of dependence on the health care provider in some early stages of care, when considerable therapeutic time and skill are required to correct disease status. The goal throughout these early stages, however, should be to shift primary responsibility from the health care provider to the patient (Purtilo, 1990), beginning with (1) involving the patient in the diagnostic phases of care by means of a guided self-assessment of oral conditions; (2) including the patient in making decisions about treatment; and (3) facilitating the shift of responsibility for maintaining health through dental health education, nutritional guidance, and mechanisms for self-evaluation of oral status between appointments. Thus "constructive dependence" grows towards the interdependence of a partnership (Purtilo, 1990).

This relationship may be difficult to achieve for professionals whose major motives are self-oriented or technically oriented. Likewise, this may be a difficult relationship for the patient who would rather not be bothered with responsibility for health, saying, "You're the doctor! Do what you need to." Usually the partnership relationship develops at different rates, depending on the perceptions and needs of the health care provider and the patient. Usually the health care provider leads the way in developing the partnership; in this era of heightened consumer awareness, however, the patient may lead by seeking information, input, and shared responsibility. Adopting these fundamental assumptions from Okun (1987) can help clinicians work more effectively with people:

1. People are responsible for and capable of making their own decisions.
2. People are controlled to a certain extent by their environment, but they do have control of their lives—often more than they realize. Even in the face of restricted options, they have the freedom to choose.
3. What people do is goal directed and purposive—even if the purposes seem unclear and vague.
4. People want to feel good about themselves; they want others to see them as worthwhile.
5. People are capable of learning new behavior if there are visible reinforcements for those changes that fit their own values and beliefs.
6. People's problems may arise from unfinished business (conflicts from the past) or from a perception that does not match others' views of reality.
7. Problems can result from environmental or societal conditions; those conditions can be managed or altered through personal choice and action (Okun, 1987).

Patients' values are changing in tandem with the growing emphasis on consumer rights over the last 25 years. These values include a greater sense of independence (less reliance on a health care provider's words), self-determination, and egalitarianism. Patients look past the status-claiming medical or dental degree and seek second opinions, inquire about alternatives, and question the conclusions presented (Gallagher, 1976). Thus the patients you encounter may expect to be involved more than you expect they will be.

PROFESSIONAL CLOSENESS

Relationships with dental patients in particular may last many years and involve families as well as individuals. Thus there is considerable opportunity for developing trust and refining ways to move in and out of a dependency relationship with each person, depending on the patient's social and economic needs, growth, and overall

health status (Purtilo, 1990). This is among the most satisfying aspects of the practice of dental hygiene.

This high degree of trust with a patient is professional closeness. During a series of appointments, and especially over a period of years, the patient and you may be able to share personal ideas and judgments and perhaps feelings and emotions. You may be able to share laughter, grief, solutions to the world's problems, a new recipe, or an easy method for adjusting the carburetor. In any case, you will have passed the stage of cliche conversation about the weather and facts about plaque levels and gingival conditions.

You can gauge your closeness with others by assessing the "level" of content you discuss.

1. Cliche conversation involves no genuine human sharing. It is superficial and usually involves standard questions and replies: "How are you today?" "Fine."
2. Reporting facts at least includes a sharing of information, but typically on "safe," impersonal topics: "How about those Mets?"
3. When personal ideas and judgments are shared, information about oneself is shared. You express an idea, a judgment, or decision. It is usually guarded and is modified by the listener's response. If the response is negative, little else will be shared.
4. People who share a deep trust express their feelings and emotions: "I'm really hurting today. I've lost a dear friend and all I can think about is how much I will miss her." If that statement is judged ("You should just get over it and go on with your life."), no further sharing is likely to occur. It is important that the sharing of feelings be understood as deep and that the person sharing is vulnerable in sharing them.
5. Peak communication occurs when there is sufficient mutual trust and honesty; the deepest secrets, hurts, desires, and needs are expressed and understood. The fact that the person feels them makes them accepted; there is no judgment. All five levels of communication occur, but this one is rarest. It is usually reserved for closest friends and those patients with whom an extraordinary trust is developed (Purtilo, 1990).

There is a critical balance between aloofness and excessive familiarity—this is professional closeness (Purtilo, 1990). Both verbal and nonverbal expressions declare which side of the balance the hygienist has found. Aloofness is cold, factual, precise, and uncomplicated by human feeling.

Excessive familiarity is inappropriately casual or chummy, filled with expressions or feelings that are seen as overreactions, but still uncomplicated by much true understanding of human feelings. Such familiarity shows lack of awareness of the other person's boundaries. The patient has the freedom to move toward an open relationship or to reserve such a response for somewhere other than the dental environment. Professional closeness, in contrast to these two extremes, is largely in response to the patient's expressed needs and is, above all, a genuine expression of caring for a fellow human being (Collins, 1977). It includes an interest in the patient as a person with values, needs, and beliefs that deserve respect (Collins, 1977; Goldberg, Plume, and Nacman, 1973; Murray and Weise, 1975; Purtilo, 1990), and it recognizes that efficiency and formality can express caring when they do not impose rigid limits on interaction. Issues regarding the use of first names or last names with patients require individual judgment of outcomes based on the patients' *expressed* preferences and a careful analysis of the hygienist's personal preferences (Purtilo, 1990).

One useful guideline in developing a professional relationship with a patient is to ask what the patient prefers: "What would you prefer I call you?" or "Do you prefer to have me talk to you during the appointment, or do you like it better if I work quietly?" After a while, experience seems to help you know when to talk, when to remain silent, when to work efficiently with minimal conversation, and when to set aside instruments and discuss an issue. In some ways, developing a professional relationship is much like establishing a friendship, with the complicating factors of specifying wants and needs, which may be considered appropriate by the patient for inclusion in a plan of care.

The patient-professional relationship is a unique combination of closeness and distance. For all its genuine emotional content, closeness, and honesty of communication, the therapeutic relationship is peculiarly distanced, circumscribed, and asymmetrical. Most of the time, one person talks and the other listens. The client almost always talks about himself and the therapist almost never does. There is money exchanged. There are tight procedural, businesslike rules that limit the monetary exchange, the time spent, the scheduling of encounters, and sexual behavior or conventions of friendship. The therapist is not a moralist, but helps people make their own judgments. Still, the therapist is a model of behavior to the client (Bellah, et al, 1985).

INTRODUCING THE PATIENT TO INITIAL PHASES OF CARE

Often the dental hygienist's initial encounters with the patient center on the critical issue of what shall or shall not be included in care. This issue can be a major one if the patient thinks that one or two specific procedures will be completed to meet his or her needs. For instance, if the patient has been accustomed to having his or her teeth cleaned on request, the patient may not expect to have a complete medical history, a complete series of radiographs, and plaque and gingival indices recorded. The patient may be even more aghast at having a facial massage (actually an extraoral examination) and blood pressure taken.

For this reason, it is wise to describe for the patient exactly what is routinely included in the first visit, how long it will take, and how much it will cost. The "laundry list" of procedures should be prefaced by a few introductory comments regarding the need at the first appointment to gather some baseline information, which forms the basis for decisions regarding treatment. As each procedure is begun, the patient should be told what the procedure is, why it is important to perform the procedure, how it is done, and how the patient can cooperate in the effort. A simple request to proceed should be made before the procedure is begun.

Some patients may be put at ease if the health care provider describes aloud what he or she is doing as each phase is performed. The patient may wish to observe in a hand mirror. Significant findings can be shared with the patient. For instance, the hygienist may say, "I can feel the muscles in the floor of your mouth, and I see the normal structures that carry saliva to your mouth and that attach your tongue to the floor of the mouth. There is some normal tonsillar tissue on the side of your tongue."

Use assessment data to make a dental hygiene diagnosis and a preliminary, dental diagnosis which will be confirmed by the dentist. You may discuss the significance of the findings with the patient in greater detail. Most patients would like to know more about themselves, including their oral health, as long as the technical language is kept to a minimum and the descriptions are clear and relevant.

At the conclusion of the first appointment, the dental hygienist should tell the patient what will occur at the next appointment and approximately how long it will take (Clark and Morton, 1977). If an additional charge will be made, an estimate of cost should be provided. Usually all subsequent needs are addressed in a treatment plan as discussed in Chapter 18.

What if the patient refuses a phase of care? As mentioned earlier, the patient does have this right. For preliminary procedures, it may be helpful to explain how the missing data will affect the accuracy of the diagnosis. If the patient still elects to refuse a specific phase of care, the health care provider can elect to terminate care, have an attorney draw up a disclaimer similar to that suggested for patients who request care that is not in their best interests, or postpone care until other aspects not reliant on the rejected procedure can be completed. Sometimes, after a few appointments and some low-pressure discussion, the patient will reconsider and decide to include the procedure, especially if the undesirable result of its exclusion becomes increasingly apparent.

If the patient can see the health care provider as a trustworthy person who views him or her as an individual with unique needs rather than as an object for demonstrating technical prowess or as a means to a lucrative end—he or she may see the professional as a partner in care rather than as a necessary evil. The patient may then ask to have the omitted procedure performed.

In some instances this relationship depends on an initial lowering of apparent control over the environment. Sharing a bit of the control may eventually yield more freedom to suggest and implement care. Insisting on immediate, total control may send many patients away or may unintentionally foster a dependency relationship in which the patient hears the message, "Doctor knows best. Hygienist heals all."

ACTIVITIES

1. Tape record interactions between a health care provider and a patient and listen to the recording to determine signs of:
   a. Listening
   b. Dependence/partnership
   c. Aloofness, closeness, and familiarity
   d. Conflicts of wants, needs, and expectations
2. Role-play vignettes to demonstrate:
   a. A helping relationship
   b. A dependency relationship
3. Role-play the explanation of preliminary assessment procedures to a patient who is:
   a. Interested only in restorative care
   b. Concerned about excess exposure to radiation from x-rays
   c. Convinced he or she will need dentures in another 10 years
   d. Accustomed to *no* preliminary procedures in a dental office other than two x-ray films and a caries charting
   e. Afraid he or she has oral cancer
4. Watch carefully for "negative smiles" during day-to-day interaction. Record the circumstances resulting in the negative smile, and share those observations in a small group.

REVIEW QUESTIONS

1. The patient wants her front teeth polished so she will look nice for her son's wedding. The hygienist wants to do something about her inflamed gingivae and the heavy calculus on her molars. How might this discrepancy affect the outcome of care?
2. The patient wants his cavities filled. He does not want to hear the hygienist's eighteenth rendition of how to floss and the need to eat fewer sweets. The hygienist wants to end the string of recurrent caries that is evident from the patient's record. How might this discrepancy affect the outcome of care?
3. A hygienist's patient looks up and says contentedly, "I know that as long as you take care of me, I'll never lose my teeth." What might that statement imply?
4. Identify whether each of the following vignettes reflects professional aloofness, professional closeness, or excessive familiarity:
   a. The hygienist slaps a new patient on the back and says, "Well, Joe, how's tricks?"
   b. The hygienist decides she prefers to wear a clinic coat over her street clothes. To verify this decision, she asks several patients what they think of the new garb.
   c. A long-term patient complains that she has been under considerable tension lately and knows she has not taken proper care of her teeth. The hygienist elects not to discuss the unusually bad state of the gingivae other than to show the plaque index and a few selected papillae (by means of a mirror) to the patient. Later during the appointment, the hygienist gently asks

whether the patient has been able to get some help for her tension.

    d. The dental hygienist checks a plaque index and sees that it is actually worse than at the previous visit. The hygienist launches into her "plan B" speech on the merits of brushing and flossing and states that care will fail if the patient does not comply with these directives.

5. What measures can a health care provider take if a patient refuses a phase of care that is essential for diagnostic or therapeutic purposes?

6. Give a listening response to each of these patient comments:
    a. "I don't think you are going to like the way my teeth look!"
    b. "I never have liked these dental chairs where I have to lie flat."
    c. "You really dig a lot deeper than other hygienists I've had."
    d. "I want the dentist and not some girl to clean my teeth."
    e. "I've always had my teeth polished all the way around, and I expect you'll do that today, or I won't pay."

7. How does each of these nonlistening replies to the statements in question 6 cut off further communication and understanding?
    a. "Don't worry. I *always* like the way your teeth look!"
    b. "Well, these new ones are much better for posture than those old clunkers."
    c. "I could give you some anesthesia."
    d. "I'm not 'some girl.' I'm a licensed hygienist who is highly skilled at cleaning teeth and many other procedures."
    e. "Fine. I'll polish your teeth, but it is a waste of time and energy."

REFERENCES

American Dental Association Council on Insurance: Informed consent: a risk management view, *JADA* **115:**630, 1987.

Bellah RN et al: *Habits of the heart: individualism and commitment in American life*, Berkeley, 1985, University of California.

Broonten KE, Chapman S: *Malpractice: a guide to avoidance and treatment*, Orlando, 1987, Grune & Stratton.

Clark JD, Morton JC: Behavioral assessment: an appraisal of beliefs and behaviors relating to treatment, *Dent Clin North Am* 21:515, 1977.

Cohen DW: Preventive periodontics, *J Indian Dent Assoc* (special issue), p. 273, 1975.

Collins M: *Communication in health care: understanding and implementing effective human relationships*, St Louis, 1977, CV Mosby.

Davis C: *Patient practitioner interaction*, Thorofare, NJ, 1989, Slack.

Dworkin SF, Ference TP, Giddon DB: *Behavioral science and dental practice*, St Louis, 1978, CV Mosby.

Gallagher EB: *The doctor-patient relationship in the changing health scene*, Washington, DC, 1976, US Department of Health, Education, and Welfare.

Goldberg HJ, Plume M, Nacman M: The importance of attitude in the delivery of health services, *J Public Health Dent* 33:35, 1973.

Gottschalk LA, Lolas F, Viney LL: *Content analysis of verbal behavior: significance in clinical medicine and psychiatry*, New York, 1986, Springer-Verlag.

Keltner JW: *Elements of interpersonal communication*, Belmont, Calif, 1973, Wadsworth.

Murray BP, Weise HJ: Satisfaction with care and the utilization of dental services at a neighborhood health center, *J Public Health Dent* 35:170, 1975.

Okun B: *Effective helping: interviewing and counseling techniques*, ed 3, Monterey, Calif, 1987, Brooks/Cole.

Purtilo R: *Health professional and patient interaction*, ed 4, Philadelphia, 1990, WB Saunders.

Rosoff AJ: *Informed consent*, Rockville, Md, 1981, Aspen Systems.

Rozovsky FA: *Consent to treatment: a practical guide*, Boston, 1984, Little, Brown.

SUGGESTED READINGS

Cohen LC et al: Caring and controlling dimensions in patient relations: the dental student perspective, *J Am Coll Dent* 47:180, 1980.

Faden RR, Beauchamp TL: *A history and theory of informed consent*, New York, 1986, Oxford University Press.

Weinstein P et al: Oral self-care: a promising alternative behavior model, *JADA* 107:67, 1983.

6 COMPREHENSIVE HEALTH HISTORY

Catherine Davis
Bonnie Dafoe

LEARNING OUTCOMES

The dental hygienist will be able to

1. Explain the reasons for a comprehensive health history to a skeptical patient.
2. State the rationale for combining questionnaire and interview techniques to obtain the necessary patient information.
3. Identify and use the communication skills that help ensure a thorough health history.
4. List the components of a comprehensive health history and explain the relevance of each.
5. Identify responses that necessitate consultation with the dentist and/or physician.
6. Identify specific conditions and/or responses that indicate the need for antibiotic premedication, sedation, change in medication, special appointment planning, additional laboratory studies, and special precautions to prevent disease transmission and allergic reactions.
7. List history update questions to be asked at recall appointments.
8. Given various responses to questions, identify appropriate follow-up questions or procedures to ensure gathering of complete data.
9. Given a patient with a variety of medical problems, conduct a complete health history and prepare a review of systems.
10. Explain the rationale for a medical classification system.
11. Explain the rationale for a medical release letter.
12. Use the *Physicians' Desk Reference*.
13. List the types of patients who would need premedication with antibiotics recommended by the American Heart Association.
14. List the standard and alternative antibiotic dosing regimens as recommended by the 1990 American Heart Association committee on prevention of bacterial endocarditis.

Observing necessary precautions that may relate to specific medical problems or medications is a professional responsibility. Before dental services are offered to any patient, an assessment of the overall health status is necessary. Providing safe treatment is the prime objective in planning dental care consistent with a patient's health status. Advances in medical diagnosis and therapeutic agents enable many people with serious medical conditions to function at a near-normal level of activity. For this reason, completing a comprehensive health history is essential to familiarize the health care provider with each patient's unique health profile.

RATIONALE FOR COMPLETING A HEALTH HISTORY

There are a number of reasons for completing a health history. First, the information provides *continuity between medical and dental care*. Establishing communication and cooperation between the physician and the dental professional ensures that all aspects of the patient's health needs can be addressed. Oral conditions and other physical conditions are often closely related. Measles, for instance, may be diagnosed by the recognition of Koplik's spots (white or bluish spots surrounded by an inflamed red zone) found on the buccal mucosa 24 hours before the general skin rash appears (Kerr and Ash, 1978). Conditions such as a red, swollen tongue and cracking skin at the corners of the mouth may be observed, which may indicate a nutritional deficiency in riboflavin. In chronic medical conditions such as diabetes mellitus, the patient's resistance to infection may be lowered, making him or her prone to periodontal disease.

Explaining to the patient how medicine and dentistry are related is important in providing total patient care. For example, medications prescribed by the physician may affect oral conditions. Phenytoin (Dilantin) is an anticonvulsant medication often prescribed for the treatment of epilepsy. This medication has the potential to increase the gingiva's response to irritation (plaque, calculus) (Angelopoulous, 1975; Braham, 1977; Israel, 1974). For many patients the result of taking this medication is gingival enlargement, or hyperplasia.

A number of patients still find routine visits to the dentist anxiety producing. Patients with medical conditions such as angina pectoris or hypertension may be adversely affected by stress. Patients with medical or emotional conditions may be aggravated by the stress of dental care.

A complete health history may help the dental care provider *avoid medical emergencies* and *identify precautions* the clinician and patient should observe. It is not difficult to imagine what could happen if a medically compromised patient were treated without proper assessment of health status. Administering a local anesthetic agent to a patient who is sensitized or allergic to one of its constituents could produce a severe and possibly fatal anaphylactic reaction. Another reason for completing a health history is *to identify patients for whom a bacteremia can have serious health consequences*. This will be discussed later in the chapter.

Information gained through the comprehensive health history aids in *identifying the need for antiinfective precautionary measures*. As mentioned in Chapter 3, disease transmission from patient to patient or patient to clinician can occur with some medical conditions. Hepatitis, sexually transmitted diseases, and the common cold are examples. To prevent the transmission of such diseases the clinician should try to reschedule a patient to a time when he or she is not infectious. However, some patients may not have overt signs of infection, especially during incubation stages. Therefore it is very important to adhere to the universal precautions as recommended in Chapter 3.

Undiagnosed conditions can also be detected as a result of the complete health history. A dental problem may be the one reason why an apparently healthy person seeks any professional care over a period of years. A complete health history provides a unique opportunity to review the general health status of such a person. The patient will discuss a symptom, unaware of its significance, that could necessitate a medical consultation. Taking the blood pressure at each recall visit may reveal a jump in blood pressure levels or indicate a pattern worthy of medical advice. Additionally, taking the pulse and noting the ease and rate of respiration may help in assessing the patient's need to consult a physician. A discussion of vital signs, hypertension, and the role of the dental team in screening these patients is contained in Chapter 8.

The *overall physical and psychologic state of the patient can be assessed* in general through the health history. The opportunity to talk candidly with the patient in discussing personal physical health allows the clinician to appreciate how the patient feels about himself or herself. Is the patient generally optimistic or pessimistic? Is the patient relaxed or anxious? The sensitive interviewer may be able to identify other significant tendencies. Is the patient cooperative or defensive? Compulsive or indifferent? In addition, the patient's ability and comfort in expressing himself or herself can be noted. The patient's attitudes about dentistry are usually revealed during the interview. Evaluation of both the physical and psychologic factors will be helpful in providing individualized care.

Gathering the health history data is often the *first opportunity to establish professional trust*. Each patient desires to feel valued as an individual with special needs that the dental team will address. With an understanding of the patient's past and current health status and an appreciation of the patient's wants and needs, the dental care provider has guidelines on which to establish rapport and build a professional helping relationship. In the framework of such a relationship, dental treatment issues become easier to address, and trust increases.

The health history *aids in diagnosis and treatment planning*. Questions related to dental status reveal the nature of the patient's chief complaint. For example, the patient may be aware of carious lesions in the posterior teeth but be most concerned about the appearance of a discolored front tooth. A patient may report sensitivity to hot or cold liquids in a particular area but be unable to locate the exact tooth that seems to be affected. Such information is helpful in guiding the dental team in performing diagnostic services (e.g., radiographs and vitality testing) and in directing care to satisfy patient concerns.

Collecting detailed health information and updating the history at regular intervals *provide a legal record* as well as an important source of information about the patient when treatment is planned and delivered. The patient signs the health history to indicate that the information is accurate to the best of his or her knowledge. This record becomes an important reference when treating the patient over time.

Occasionally a patient may feel skeptical about the need for a comprehensive health history. Often this stems from feelings of invaded privacy, defensiveness about medical problems, or a desire to simply get the dental visit over with as quickly as possible. The patient should be informed of the dental professional's responsibility to keep information confidential. The patient should be assured that the information is necessary to provide safe treatment. Examples may be given of the way health information can affect dental treatment. One can agree that gathering information is time consuming, but explain that this time is well spent. On occasion, some practitioners may choose not to provide elective treatment if the patient refuses to cooperate with the health history. Generally, most patients are agreeable and extremely helpful once the professional's sincere desire to provide the best possible care has been demonstrated.

COMMUNICATION: THE QUESTIONNAIRE AND INTERVIEW

For gathering information, a questionnaire provides a thorough and time-saving tool. Fig. 6-1 is an example of one of the health questionnaires, copyrighted by the American Dental Association. An interview provides a flexible and personal approach to obtaining and clarifying information. The combined questionnaire and interview technique is a practical and sensitive method for assessing the patient's health (Froelich and Bishop, 1977).

The most important aspect of this portion of needs assessment and planning patient care is that the written history must be verbally reviewed with the patient for clarification and accuracy. In a 1991 study de Jong and others tested the validity of a patient-administered risk-related medical questionnaire for dental patients. The gold standard was the verbal history taken by a physician. There was good correlation between the two assessment methods; however, several patients failed to answer questions because they did not understand them. The authors noted that false positives could be identified by short verification of all affirmative replies and false negatives prevented by carefully checking all answers and linking replies to different questions (de Jong et al, 1991).

The outcome of the comprehensive health history, using a questionnaire and interview technique, is determined to a great extent by the professional's ability to communicate. Conducting an interview demands a high level of communication skill. The interviewer must respond to both the attitudes and behaviors of the patient. A good interviewer is nurturant, supportive, and helpful (Froelich and Bishop, 1977). It is not always easy for the patient to share highly private information about his or her personal or family history. The interviewer must listen and accept the patient's attitudes and perceptions without judging. As the interviewer responds to the patient by listening and clarifying statements, the patient begins to have a feeling that the problem is well understood. At this point information may be shared with the patient to allay fears or anxiety. In this way the good interviewer may be able to convey to the patient a conceptual model by which the patient can better understand his or her problem or disease (Froelich and Bishop, 1977). When acquiring the comprehensive health history using a questionnaire and interview format, the health professional not only gathers information and builds rapport but creates the environment and opportunity to educate and counsel the patient.

Interviewing skills

Awareness of and sensitivity to the kinds of messages communicated are important to counseling and interviewing (see Chapter 5). Communication involves words, facial expressions, gestures, body movements, tone of voice, rate of speech, and silence. The interviewer must become an active listener by being aware of the patient's total communication effort and being able to respond in a way that the patient will interpret as attentive and concerned (Froelich and Bishop, 1977).

Body communication signifies to the patient

Text continued on p. 96.

Medical History

Date _____

Name _____ Address _____

    Last   First   Middle   Number, Street

City _____ State _____ Zip _____ Home _____ Business _____
                            Code   Phone   Phone

Date of Birth _____ Sex __ Height _____ Weight _____ Occupation _____

Social Security No. _____ Single _____ Married _____ Name of Spouse _____

Closest Relative _____ Phone _____

If you are completing this form for another person, what is your relationship to that

person? _____

Referred by _____

In the following questions, circle yes or no, whichever applies. Your answers are for our records only and will be considered confidential.

1. Are you in good health?. . . . . Yes   No

2. Has there been any change in your general health within the past year? . . Yes   No

3. My last physical examination was on _____

4. Are you now under the care of a physician? . . . . Yes   No
   If so, what is the condition being treated? _____

5. The name and address of my physician is _____
   _____
   _____

6. Have you had any serious illness or operation? . . . . Yes   No
   If so, what was the illness or operation? _____

7. Have you been hospitalized or had a serious illness within the past five (5)
   years? . . . . Yes   No
   If so, what was the problem? _____

8. Do you have or have you had any of the following diseases or problems?
   a. Damaged heart valves or aritifical heart valves, including heart murmur . Yes   No
   b. Congenital heart lesions . . . . Yes   No
   c. Cardiovascular disease (heart trouble, heart attack, coronary insufficiency, coronary occlusion, high blood pressure, arteiosclerosis, stroke). Yes   No
      1. Do you have pain in chest upon exertion?. . . . . Yes   No
      2. Are you ever short of breath after mild exercise?. . . . . Yes   No
      3. Do your ankles swell?. Yes   No
      4. Do you get short of breath when you lie down, or do you require extra
         pillows when you sleep?. . . . . Yes   No
      5. Do you have a cardiac pacemaker?. . . . . Yes   No
   d. Allergy . . . . Yes   No
   e. Sinus trouble . . . . Yes   No
   f. Asthma or hay fever . . . . Yes   No
   g. Hives or a skin rash . . . . Yes   No
   h. Fainting spells or seizures. . . . . Yes   No
   i. Diabetes . . . . Yes   No
      1. Do you have to urinate (pass water) more than six times a day?. . . Yes   No
      2. Are you thirsty much of the time?. . . . . Yes   No
      3. Does your mouth frequently become dry?. . . . . Yes   No

Fig. 6-1. American Dental Association health questionnaire.
(Copyright by the American Dental Association. Reprinted by permission.)

Continued.

Medical History—cont'd

j. Hepatitis, jaundice or liver disease	Yes	No
k. Arthritis	Yes	No
l. Inflammatory rheumatism (painful swollen joints)	Yes	No
m. Stomach ulcers	Yes	No
n. Kidney trouble	Yes	No
o. Tuberculosis	Yes	No
p. Do you have a persistent cough or cough up blood?	Yes	No
q. Low blood pressure	Yes	No
r. Venereal disease	Yes	No
s. Epilepsy	Yes	No
t. Psychiatric problems	Yes	No
u. Cancer	Yes	No
v. AIDS or other immunosuppressive disorders	Yes	No
w. Other _____		

9. Have you had abnormal bleeding associated with previous extractions, surgery, or trauma? . . . .   Yes   No

    a. Do you bruise easily? . . . .   Yes   No

    b. Have you ever required a blood transfusion? . . . .   Yes   No
       If so, explain the circumstances _____
       _____

10. Do you have any blood disorder such as anemia? . . . .   Yes   No

11. Have you had surgery, x-ray or drug treatment for a tumor, growth, or other condition of your head or neck? . . . .   Yes   No

12. Are you taking any drug or medicine? . . . .   Yes   No
   If so, what? _____

13. Are you taking any of the following:

a. Antibiotics or sulfa drugs	Yes	No
b. Anticoagulants (blood thinners)	Yes	No
c. Medicine for high blood pressure	Yes	No
d. Cortisone (steroids)	Yes	No
e. Tranquilizers	Yes	No
f. Antihistamines	Yes	No
g. Aspirin	Yes	No
h. Insulin, tolbutamide (Orinase) or similar drug	Yes	No
i. Digitalis or drugs for heart trouble	Yes	No
j. Nitroglycerin	Yes	No
k. Oral contraceptive or other hormonal therapy	Yes	No
l. Other _____		

14. Are you allergic or have you reacted adversely to:

a. Local anesthetics	Yes	No
b. Penicillin or other antibiotics	Yes	No
c. Sulfa drugs	Yes	No
d. Barbiturates, sedatives, or sleeping pills	Yes	No
e. Aspirin	Yes	No
f. Iodine	Yes	No
g. Codeine or other narcotics	Yes	No
h. Other _____		

Fig. 6-1—cont'd. American Dental Association health questionaire.

Continued.

Medical History — cont'd

15. Have you had any serious trouble associated with any previous dental treatment? . . . .   Yes   No
If so, explain _____
_____

16. Do you have any disease, condition, or problem not listed above that you think I should know about? . . . .   Yes   No
If so, explain _____
_____

17. Are you employed in any situation which exposes you regularly to x-rays or other ionizing radiation?. . . . .   Yes   No

18. Are you wearing contact lenses? . . . .   Yes   No

19. Have you had anything to eat or drink in the last 4 hours?. . . . .   Yes   No

20. Are you wearing removable dental appliances? . . . .   Yes   No

Women

21. Are you pregnant? . . . .   Yes   No

22. Do you have any problems associated with your menstrual period? . . . .   Yes   No

23. Are you nursing? . . . .   Yes   No

Chief Dental Complaint

I certify that I have read and understand the above. I acknowledge that my questions, if any, about the inquiries set forth above have been answered to my satisfaction. I will not hold my dentist, or any other member of his/her staff, responsible for any errors or omissions that I may have made in the completion of this form.

_____
Signature of Patient

_____
Signature of Dentist

Fig. 6-1—cont'd. American Dental Association health questionaire.

that the interviewer is listening. The interviewer should find a comfortable and relaxed position. The interviewer and patient should be at approximately the same eye level. Eye contact should be made with the patient when he or she is talking. Affirmative head nods also are used to indicate listening. Facial expressions should agree with the feelings being expressed by the patient.

The verbal communication and attitude of the interviewer can strongly influence the atmosphere of the interview. Techniques for verbal communi-cation include using a vocal tone that reassures the patient, helping the patient develop and pursue a topic through affirmative words that indicate understanding, not interrupting the patient if possible, fitting comments into the context of the topic, and using silence to aid the interview communication. For most inexperienced interviewers, silence is uncomfortable. Often a question is hastily asked and may not be helpful. Interviewer-initiated silence can be used to communicate the desire for the patient to continue to provide information or to choose the topic. Silence allows the patient time to think about the response to the questions. Silence can be supportive and signify interest. Patient-initiated silence may mean that the patient needs time to think, is examining himself or herself, or wishes to avoid the topic. Each function of silence is important to the communication effort.

The following are interviewing suggestions from Froelich and Bishop (1977):

1. Introduce yourself. Ask a direct, open question, such as "What situation brings you here today?"
2. Have a plan or order for obtaining information.
3. Guide the interview; do not dominate it.
4. Respond by showing support and empathy.
5. Restate or reflect a patient's response to clarify meaning.
6. Avoid questions that can be answered "yes" or "no." Such questions permit the patient to avoid discussing a topic or allow the patient to give a response that he or she thinks the interviewer is looking for. An appropriately phrased question is, "When does this pain bother you?" as opposed to "Does it hurt when you eat something cold?"
7. Avoid antagonistic "why" questions that make the patient account for behavior, such as "Why didn't you seek care sooner?"
8. Stay with a topic until it is fully discussed.
9. Use verbal and nonverbal signals to encourage the patient to say more.
10. Complete the interview with a summary to clarify what has occurred and affirm mutual understanding.

COMPONENTS OF THE COMPREHENSIVE HEALTH HISTORY

Three areas of information are explored in the comprehensive health history: the patient profile, the patient's current health status, and the patient's historical health data.

The patient profile includes the patient's name, address, telephone number, date of birth, and physician's name and office telephone number. Each practitioner may develop his or her own version of the patient profile section of the chart. Items that may be included are the patient's occupation, business telephone number, marital status, number of children, and dental insurance or preferred billing plan; the name of the person who referred the patient; days and times preferred for appointments, and the names and telephone numbers of the patient's physician and who to contact in case of an emergency. The patient completes this information on the questionnaire. The interviewer should be familiar with this basic information before greeting the patient. Follow-up on this information is usually indicated only when a response needs clarification.

The patient's current health status and historical health data require more attention. The interviewer should take a few minutes to review the patient's questionnaire responses and note the questions to which an affirmative response has been indicated. These areas need specific follow-up during the patient interview. The following format with the accompanying descriptions is designed as a guide for directing the interview and organizing patient data.

Current health status

Chief complaint (CC). This usually is stated in the patient's own words and refers to the symptoms for which the patient is seeking treatment.

History of present illness (HPI). Signs and symptoms of the current problem should be described in this section, along with the location, onset, intensity, and duration of the problem. Additional probing questions may be needed to define and clarify the nature of the patient's needs, such as, "When did this problem first occur?" "Describe the discomfort for me." "When does it bother you the most?"

Medications (Meds). It is important to note clearly the medications that the patient is currently taking. This includes over-the-counter remedies or preparations such as vitamins, aspirin, and weight control pills in addition to prescribed medications. Record the reason for taking the medication and the dosage of the product. *The Physicians' Desk Reference* (described later in the chapter) gives additional information. Note medication allergy or intolerance **in bold letters.** Inquiring into the patient's social habits, such as frequency of consumption of alcoholic beverages and coffee and tobacco use, is appropriate at this time. If the patient is currently taking Antabuse, do not recommend an oral rinse product that contains alcohol. Antabuse can trigger a violent reaction if the patient is exposed to alcohol.

Review of systems (ROS). This allows information from the questionnaire and interview to be organized into physical systems. At this point the professional is interested in the current (within 6 months) status of each system. The past medical and dental history will be summarized later.

Body symptoms should be reviewed noting any signs and/or symptoms that could indicate disease. The patient should be asked if he or she is bothered by any of these.

General constitution (Gen). Recent significant weight gain or loss, weakness, fatigue, fever, chills, insomnia, irritability, and change in general vigor. If the patient has experienced any of these signs and symptoms, additional probing questions should be asked. The interviewer should summarize the patient's response. It is advisable to repeat the summary so that the patient can verify its content. Otherwise the interviewer may record "patient denies" the specific symptoms.

Head, ears, eyes, nose, and throat (HEENT). Reports of headache, trauma, dizziness, disturbance of vision, loss of hearing acuity, ringing in ears, loss of balance, disturbances of smell, discharge, symptoms of obstruction, hoarseness, and difficulty in swallowing.

Respiratory (Resp). Difficulty in breathing, chest pain, coughing blood or sputum, wheezing, and effect of exercise.

Cardiovascular (CV). Chest pain, palpitation, difficulty in breathing when lying flat, murmurs, and blood pressure.

Gastrointestinal (GI). Abdominal pain, nausea, vomiting, indigestion, food intolerance, hernia, and change in bowel habits.

Genitourinary (GU). Painful urination, blood in urine, frequency of urination, flank pain, and change in menstrual cycle.

Muscles, bones, and joints (MBJ). Pain, stiffness, swelling, limitation of movement, arthritis, and back problem.

Central nervous system (CNS). Fainting, seizure, stroke, paralysis, spasm, tremor, and loss of feeling.

Endocrine (Endo). Change in growth or development; thyroid function; change in appetite or tolerance to temperature; diabetes; and excessive urination, thirst, or hunger.

Hemopoietic (Hemo). Tendency to bruise or bleed excessively after injury, recent blood transfusion, and exposure to radiation.

Medical and dental history
Past medical history (PMH). Summarize the medical status previous to current history. Include general health and vigor, childhood diseases, past infectious diseases, chronic diseases, injuries, accidents, hospitalizations (include name of hospital and dates), history of immunizations, allergies and type of allergic reactions, and service-related disability.

Family history (FH). Summarize data on the state of immediate family members, past hereditary diseases, and the presence of infectious or chronic disease in the family.

Past dental history (PDH). Summarize the nature of dental care the patient has had in the past. Include type of clinic, treatment by specialist, experience with local and general anesthetics, degree of preventive education, and satisfaction with past treatment.

BACTEREMIA: CONSEQUENCES AND PREMEDICATION

Bacteremia refers to the presence of viable bacteria in the circulating blood. Surgical instrumentation involving a variety of mucosal surfaces can cause bacteremias that are transient (i.e., that rarely persist more than 15 minutes).

Baltch and others (1982) studied 56 patients with moderate to severe periodontal disease. Twenty-eight with valvular heart disease received intravenous penicillin before an oral prophylaxis was performed, and 28 without known disease did not receive the drug. None of the subjects had bacteremia before the prophylaxis, but 5 minutes after the procedure, 61% of the group that had not received penicillin were bacteremic compared with 11% of the treated group. From these patients 71 different microorganisms were isolated, including 53 anaerobes and 18 aerobes. Only 11 of the isolates were found in the patients receiving prophylaxis with the antibiotic.

As bacterial endocarditis is of particular concern in dental care, the disease process is described in some detail here. Such bacteria may attach to the susceptible person's affected cardiac valve endothelium or artificial prosthesis. Members of the viridans streptococci or alpha-hemolytic streptococci are the bacteria most commonly found as the cause of bacterial endocarditis, although other bacteria, including *Staphylococcus aureus,* have been implicated as the cause of the infection (Durack, Kaplan, and Bisno, 1983; Kaye, 1983). The organisms proliferate, forming bacterial masses and clumps. With the growth of these bacteria and the consequent infection and destruction of the cardiac tissue, the valve is unable to maintain its function. In other patients the surgical graft becomes infected and incompetent. Clinically the patient exhibits a low-grade fever, slowly developing anemia, loss of appetite, and fatigue. With undiagnosed and untreated bacterial endocarditis, the patient's life expectancy seldom exceeds 3 to 6 months. Sudden death may occur when a bacterial clump breaks off and causes a fatal embolism. The most common cause of death results from congestive heart failure attributed to valve destruction or myocardial damage (Weinstein and Schlesinger, 1974; Kaye, 1983). The heart fails when the infected valve becomes incompetent, preventing the proper emptying of the heart chamber. The blood literally backs up because the valve is no longer able to close and permit the proper blood flow out of the heart to the rest of the body.

Some patients are susceptible to developing bacterial endocarditis after the inevitable bacteremia that occurs during procedures such as prophylaxis, currettage, endodontic therapy, tooth extraction, or more extensive periodontal surgery (Kaye, 1983; Weinstein and Schlesinger, 1974; Prevention, 1985). Antibiotic protection is recommended with all dental procedures that are likely to cause trauma to the tissue and allow oral bacteria to enter the bloodstream in individuals with these conditions (Dejami et al, 1990).

These include:
1. Prosthetic cardiac valves, including bioprosthetic and homograph valves,
2. Previous bacterial endocarditis, even in the absence of heart disease,
3. Surgically constructed systemic-pulmonary shunts
4. Most congenital cardiac malformations
5. Rheumatic and other acquired valvular dysfunction even after valve surgery
6. Hypertrophic cardiomyopathy, and
7. Mitral valve prolapse with valvular regurgitation.

Patients with a history of systemic lupus erythematosus and Down syndrome may be at risk of infective endocarditis, which is not always identifiable by ausculatory cardiologic examinations (Zysset et al, 1987; Barnett et al, 1988). The American Heart Association (AHA) also notes several specific situations and circumstances that need special attention.
1. Concurrent rheumatic fever treatment. Antibiotic regimens used to prevent recurrence of acute rheumatic fever are inadequate for preventing bacterial endocarditis in a patient with active disease. This treatment may have been selected for bacteria that are resistant to penicillin, amoxicillin, and/or ampicillin. Another AHA-recommended antibiotic should be substituted in its place for premedication.
2. Anticoagulant therapy. Patients who report the use of heparin and warfarin sodium should not be given intramuscular (IM) injections for endocarditis prevention.
3. Renal dysfunction. It may be necessary to modify or omit the second dose of gentamicin because aminoglycosides are associated with adverse renal effects. This is also necessary with vancomycin hydrochloride use. The patient's physician should be consulted before the patient is premedicated.
4. History of cardiac surgery. The risk of developing endocarditis appears to continue even after the placement of prosthetic heart valves. There is no evidence that coronary artery bypass graft surgery introduces a risk for patients developing endocarditis.
5. Patients with prosthetic joints. Currently no national dental or medical organization has produced official guidelines supporting the use of prophylactic antibiotics for the prevention of infection of prosthetic joints in patients receiving dental treatment. However, most orthopedic surgeons still recommend antibiotic coverage. Therefore the decision to premedicate or not should be made by the dentist in consultation with the patient's physician (ADA Council on Dental Therapeutics, 1990).

Antibacterial prophylaxis

With early diagnosis and appropriate antibiotic treatment, 90% of patients survive bacterial endocarditis (Durack, Kaplan, and Bisno, 1983). The clinician's role is to prevent the disease from occurring by screening susceptible patients with the comprehensive health history and providing the proper antibiotic protection before treatment.

In a recent study, 52 cases of endocarditis prophylaxis failure were reported to a national registry established by the AHA (Durack, Kaplan, and Bisno, 1983). Forty-eight cases (92%) occurred after dental treatment. Only six patients (12%) had received the antibiotic treatment currently recommended by the AHA. These data indicate that endocarditis prophylaxis failures may be more common than was previously believed, and most regimens used in patients with prophylaxis failure did not conform to current recommendations.

The 1990 AHA recommended prophylactic regimen (antibiotic premedication) for dental procedures is:

1. Standard regimen—Amoxicillin, 3 g, orally 1 hour before procedure, then 1.5 g after initial dose
2. Standard regime for patients allergic to penicillin or amoxicillin—Erythromycin ethylsuccinate, 800 mg, or erythromycin stearate, 1 g, to be taken orally 2 hours before procedure, then half of the dose 6 hours after initial dose

   For adults: Erythromycin, 1 g, 1 hour before the procedure, and then 500 mg 6 hours later.

   For children: Erythromycin, 20 mg/kg 1 hour before the procedure, then 10 mg/kg 6 hours later (1 kg=2.2 lbs).
3. For amoxicillin or penicillin-allergic patients—300 mg Clindamycin, to be taken orally 1 hour before procedure and 150 mg 6 hours after initial dose
4. For patients allergic to amoxicillin, ampicillin, and penicillin who are considered to be at high risk—Intravenous administration of vancomycin, 1 g over 1 hour, starting one hour before procedure; no repeat dose necessary

Initial pediatric doses are amoxicillin, 50 mg/kg; clindamycin, 10 mg/kg; and vancomycin, 20 mg/kg. Follow-up doses should be one half the initial dose. Total pediatric doses should not exceed total adult doses.

Pollock (1991) noted that the 1990 AHA guidelines contained an error regarding the amount of erythromycin to be taken. He states that 1600 mg of erythromycin ethylsuccinate (EES) should be taken 2 hours before the appointment rather than 800 mg, as 400 mg of EES is equivalent to 250 mg of erythromycin stearate (Pollock, 1991).

The following are recommended for patients unable to take oral medications:

1. Ampicillin—IV or IM administration of 2 g 30 minutes before procedure; then IV or IM administration of 1 g or oral administration of amoxicillin, 1.5 g, 6 hours after initial dose
2. Clindamycin (for patients allergic to ampicillin, amoxicillin, and penicillin)—IV administration of 300 mg 30 minutes before procedure, then IV or oral administration of 150 mg 6 hours after initial dose; alternatively, the parenteral regimen may be repeated 8 hours after initial dose
3. Vancomycin (for patients allergic to ampicillin, amoxicillin, and penicillin) who are considered at high risk—IV administration of 1 g over 1 hour, starting 1 hour before procedure; no repeat dose necessary
4. Ampicillin, gentamicin, and amoxicillin (for patients considered at high risk and who are not candidates for standard regimen)—IV or IM administration of ampicillin, 2 g, plus gentamicin, 1.5 mg/kg (not to exceed 80 mg) 30 minutes before procedure; followed by amoxicillin, 1.5 g, orally 6 hours after initial dose; alternatively, the parenteral regimen may be repeated 8 hours after initial dose

Initial pediatric doses are ampicillin, 50 mg/kg; clindamycin, 10 mg/kg; gentamicin, 2 mg/kg; and vancomycin, 20 mg/kg. Follow-up doses should be one half the initial dose. Total pediatric doses should not exceed the total adult doses.

The choice of penicillin V rather than amoxicillin for prophylaxis against alpha-hemolytic streptococci is considered rational and acceptable. However, amoxicillin provides higher serum levels and is absorbed from the stomach better. *Tetracycline and sulfonamides are not recommended for endocarditits prophylaxis.*

The 1990 AHA guidelines also recommend that "dental professionals should attempt to decrease gingival inflammation in at-risk patients through the use of brushing, flossing, fluoride rinse and chlorhexidine gluconate (CHXG). CHXG that is painted on isolated and dried gingiva 3 to 5 minutes prior to tooth extraction has been shown to reduce postoperative bacteremia" (Dejani et al, 1990; ADA-CDT, 1991). These statements could be interpreted to endorse the prolonged use of CHXG or to primarily advocate its use before dental treatment (Pallasch and Slots, 1991). There is concern that CHXG allows a greater predominance of other bacteremic microorganisms, such as pseudomonads and enterococci, in the human mouth (Rams et al, 1990; Spijkervet et al, 1989). Pallasch and Slots (1991) recommend that "the rules of antibiotic endocarditis prophylaxis are the same whether the antimicrobials are used systemically or topically." They caution against prolonged use of an antimicrobial.

Patients with a history of rheumatic fever without a residual organic heart murmur need not be premedicated. Patients classified as having "functional" heart murmurs or heart sounds not associated with structural defects do not need antibiotic protection. However, consulting the patient's physician for the exact nature of a cardiac condition is advisable. This can be accomplished by using a form of the medical release letter described later in this chapter. It should also be recognized that patients with localized juvenile periodontitis harbor some members of the "HACEK" group of bacteria (i.e., genera *Haemophilus, Actinobacillus, Cardiobacterium, Eikenella,* and *Kingella* species) (Barco, 1991). Both *Capnocytophaga* and *Actinobacillus species* are usually resistant or of intermediate sensitivity to penicillin (Grace et al, 1988). Since 1988, 13 cases of endocarditis caused by *Actinobacillus* have been reported (Grace et al, 1988). Ampicillin *plus* an aminoglycoside given parenterally have been suggested for these patients (Kaye, 1986). Such patients should *not* be given tetracyclines immediately before or after premedication with ampicillin, because tetracyclines inhibit protein biosynthesis and therefore interfere with cell wall biosynthesis (target of ampicillin).

MEDICALLY COMPROMISED PATIENTS

The following section provides the dental hygienist with information on common medical conditions that should be identified by the health history. A basic definition of the problem is presented, along with common signs or symptoms the patient may report. In some cases examples of medications the patient may be taking are given by generic name. The significance of the disease is presented followed by precautions recommended for dental treatment.

Heart disorders

Rheumatic heart disease. Rheumatic heart disease results from rheumatic fever and causes rigidity or deformity of the heart valves.

Patient reports: History of rheumatic fever or heart murmur. Patient may be taking antibiotics (e.g., penicillin) on a regular basis.
Significance: Patient is susceptible to bacterial endocarditis.

Precautions:
1. Obtain consultation letter from physician on the nature of heart involvement.
2. Antibiotic premedication is necessary (Kaye, 1983; Prevention, 1985; ADA- CDT, 1991).
3. Be sure patient has taken antibiotic as prescribed before dental treatment.
4. Avoid unnecessary trauma to tissues during instrumentation.

Congenital heart defect. This term refers to structural defects of the heart (e.g., a hole in the common wall between heart chambers) that is present at birth.

Patient reports: History of heart murmur, "hole in heart," or other heart abnormality, corrective heart surgery, or valve replacement.
Significance: Patient is susceptible to developing bacterial endocarditis.
Precautions:
1. Obtain letter from physician on the nature of defect and correction.
2. Antibiotic premedication may be necessary (Kaye, 1983; Prevention, 1985; ADA-CDT, 1991).

Surgical valve replacement. A diseased heart valve caused by rheumatic heart disease or congenital heart defect is replaced with an artificial prosthesis.

Patient reports: History of heart surgery. Patient may be taking anticoagulant.
Significance: Patient is susceptible to developing bacterial endocarditis.
Precautions:
1. Obtain letter from physician as to heart status and surgical correction.
2. Antibiotic premedication is necessary (Kaye, 1983; Prevention, 1985; ADA- CDT, 1991).
3. Patient may be taking anticoagulant (e.g., warfarin or coumarin). Consult physician. Testing for bleeding time may be necessary before treatment, or patient may be advised to stop medication for a few days before appointment. Antibiotic premedication should not be given IM (Dejani et al, 1990).

Coronary artery disease. Coronary circulation is inadequate for metabolic demands on the heart. This disease results from hardening of arteries (arteriosclerosis), which causes blockage or narrowing of the vessels.

Patient reports: Episodes of substernal pain (angina pectoris), typically radiating to left arm and jaw. Pain is precipitated by activity and anxiety and is relieved by rest and certain medications. Patient may be taking vasodilators, nitroglycerin, or propranolol.

Significance: Patient may have angina attack in dental office.

Precautions:
1. Obtain letter from physician to clarify medical status.
2. Have patient's vasodilator medication accessible.
3. Use local anesthetic without vasoconstrictor, or keep vasoconstrictor use to minimum—less than 0.04 mg (Bennett, 1984).
4. Keep appointments to reasonable length, avoiding unnecessary stress and anxiety.

Coronary thrombosis (myocardial infarction). The blood supply through the coronary arteries is insufficient to meet the metabolic demands of the heart. This differs from angina pectoris in that the damage is irreversible (i.e., a portion of the heart muscle dies).

Patient reports: History of angina pectoris, previous heart attack, taking vasodilators.

Significance: Patient may have angina attack or myocardial infarction.

Precautions:
1. Obtain letter from physician as to severity of disease.
2. Do not treat patient if heart attack occurred within 6 months.
3. Have vasodilator medication ready.
4. Avoid vasoconstrictors in local anesthetic or keep to minimum.
5. Keep appointments short.
6. Be prepared to resuscitate patient. Should cardiac arrest occur, call emergency rescue team.

Congestive heart failure. Blood backs up behind a failing chamber, causing congestion of circulation and pooling of blood in organs. For example, if the left ventricle fails, blood backs up in the pulmonary circulation and lungs. Forward flow from the failing chamber is also diminished.

Patient reports: Shortness of breath, swollen ankles, sleeping on two or more pillows. Patient may be taking diuretics and/or digitalis.

Significance: Patient may have difficulty in breathing when supine in dental chair. If inhalation anesthetics are used, oxygenation of blood may be poor because of fluid in lungs.

Precautions:
1. Obtain letter from physician as to severity of disease.

2. Keep patient in semiupright position.
3. Keep appointments short.
4. Supplemental oxygen may be needed.

Cardiac arrhythmias. This is a disturbance of the heart's electrical conduction system. The heart beats at too rapid or too slow a pace or at an irregular pace (either continuously or with occasional odd beats).

Patient reports: Fast or irregular heart beat, palpitations (awareness of rapid heart beats), recurrent fainting, surgical implant of pacemaker. He or she may be taking digitalis or other antiarrhyhmic medication.

Significance: Patient may faint. Also, a pacemaker device may be affected by electromagnetic interference. Dental office equipment such as ultrasonic scaling devices, pulp testers, electrodesensitizing equipment, electrosurgical instruments, microwave ovens, and motorized dental chairs may adversely affect some devices. Patient may exhibit gingival overgrowth if taking nifedipine or other calcium channel blocker.

Precautions:
1. Obtain letter from physician as to severity of disease and surgical history. Ask about the need for antibiotic premedication and type of pacemaker device implanted.
2. Avoid use of equipment or proximity to such equipment being used on other patients if patient's pacemaker will be affected.

Hypertension

Hypertension is high arterial blood pressure (see Chapter 8).

Patient reports: History of elevated blood pressure, frequent dizziness, headaches, nosebleeds. Patient may be taking antihypertensive or diuretic drugs.

Significance: Patient may have a stroke (cerebrovascular accident). Disease can cause cardiac enlargement, impair kidney function, and accelerate arteriosclerosis.

Precautions:
1. Take blood pressure at each appointment.
2. Obtain letter from physician for patients whose diastolic reading exceeds 95 mm Hg or systolic reading exceeds 160 mm Hg.
3. Do not provide dental treatment if diastolic blood pressure is greater than 115 mm Hg or systolic blood pressure is greater than 160 mm Hg.
4. Determine if antihypertensive medication has been taken as prescribed.
5. Use local anesthetic without vasoconstrictor, or do not exceed 0.1 mg epinephrine (Bennett, 1984).
6. Avoid sitting patient up rapidly. This may cause

fainting (orthostatic or postural hypotension), an effect of some antihypertensive drugs.

7. Have patient remain sitting upright for several minutes before he or she leaves the dental chair.

Diabetes mellitus

Diabetes mellitus is a disorder of glucose intolerance manifested by hyperglycemia (increased blood glucose) (Kaye, 1983). In general there are two types of diabetes mellitus. Insulin-dependent (type 1) diabetes has its onset in youth. Hyperglycemia is due to a lack of insulin normally produced by the pancreas. Adult-onset (type 2) diabetes occurs in older patients and is often associated with obesity. Although the amount of insulin produced by the pancreas is adequate, this type of diabetes is characterized by insulin insensitivity of the tissues.

Patient reports: Personal or family history of disease; excessive thirst, hunger, urination; high birth weight children. Patient may be taking injectable insulin or oral hypoglycemics.

Significance: Patient has low resistance to infection, is prone to periodontal disease and poor healing, and may have episode of insulin shock, especially if he or she missed a meal before the appointment.

Precautions:

1. Determine if disease is under control (frequency of urine testing, medication taken as prescribed, recent incidents of diabetic coma, insulin shock, or diabetes-related hospitalizations). Obtain letter from physician to determine status of other diabetes-related conditions. Patient with severe diabetes may have compromised vascular system, renal impairment, or loss of vision.

2. Determine if patient has eaten. Schedule appointments around eating schedule.

3. Have sugar source available in case of impending shock, which patient can usually anticipate.

Epilepsy

Epilepsy is a disorder characterized by convulsions (seizures) or disturbances of consciousness (e.g., momentary inattentive staring), usually associated with a disturbance of electrical activity of the brain (Braham, 1977; Kaye, 1983).

Patient reports: History of seizures. Seizures can be petit mal (trancelike state, fixed posture, blinking) or grand mal (twitching, seizing, loss of consciousness, incontinence). Patient may report a peculiar sensation that heralds a seizure (aura), such as a specific odor or visual sensation; he or she may be taking phenobarbital, phenytoin, or another anticonvulsant.

Significance: Patient may have a seizure. Phenytoin (Dilantin) may cause gingival hyperplasia or orofacial changes (Angelopoulous, 1975; Israel, 1974).

Precautions:

1. Determine if anticonvulsant medication has been taken.

2. Make appointments when patient is rested; keep them short.

3. If seizure occurs, do not try to restrict patient. Remove equipment from striking distance, and keep patient from injuring self. After seizure, keep airway open by tilting head back or turning patient on his or her side. Saliva, and/or blood (from biting tongue), may require suction or manual removal.

Allergies

Allergies are localized or systemic reactions caused by a variety of substances (allergens). The reaction may be mild, causing itching or a rash. A severe reaction may cause a rapid fall in blood pressure, airway obstruction from swelling of oral mucosa, and/or cardiac arrest (anaphylaxis).

Patient reports: Reaction to a known substance (e.g., penicillin).

Significance: Reaction may occur to substances used in dental treatment.

Precautions:

1. Determine exact cause and severity of previous reaction.

2. Avoid allergen or related substance.

3. Use caution administering anesthetics and antibiotics.

4. If patient is unsure of specific anesthetic agent that caused previous allergic reaction, request physician to perform skin patch test. (See Chapter 32 on local anesthesia.)

5. If anaphylaxis should occur, be prepared to support patient with cardiopulmonary resuscitation and to call emergency rescue team.

Kidney disease

Patients with kidney disease have impairment of renal function with accumulation of waste products and fluid, resulting from congenital abnormalities, infection, diabetes, or other disease processes. The patient may be maintained on an artificial kidney machine (hemodialysis) or have a kidney transplant.

Patient reports: History of renal failure, hemodialysis, headache, swelling of extremities, fever, flank pain, nausea, mental dullness, excessive fatigue, easy bruising; or if kidney transplant, will be taking immunosuppressant medication.

Significance: Patient is prone to infection and poor healing, and bleeds easily. Medications metabolized by kidney (e.g., local anesthetics of amide type) will remain in circulation longer.

Precautions:

1. Obtain letter from physician on the extent of disease. If patient is immunosuppressed, obtain recommendations for precautions during dental treatment. These patients are susceptible to bacterial endocarditis at site of hemodialysis shunt or transplanted kidney graft, making prophylactic antibiotic coverage necessary (Dejani et al, 1991).
2. If medication is to be administered, check with physician, *Physicians' Desk Reference,* or pharmacist about renal metabolism.
3. Exercise care in instrumentation.
4. If the patient requires antibiotic premedication with ampicillin OR gentamicin, check with the patient's physician. Gentamicin may be contraindicated.

Infectious or contagious diseases
Hepatitis. Hepatitis is an inflammation of the liver caused by several different viruses (see Chapter 3).

Patient reports: History of disease, fatigue, loss of appetite, nausea, fever, dark urine, tender liver, sore joints. Patient may appear jaundiced (yellow).

Significance: Patient may bleed excessively and have impaired metabolism of drugs broken down in liver (e.g., local anesthetics of the ester type). There is a high risk for transfer of disease to dental professional or other patients.

Precautions:

1. Do not treat patient with active, overt disease.
2. Follow universal precautions. Wear gloves, face mask, and glasses. Maintain strict sterilization and asepsis of all objects in contact with patient.
3. If medication is administered, consult physician, *Physicians' Desk Reference,* or pharmacist about possible liver metabolism.
4. Follow Occupational Safety and Health Administration's recommendation for hepatitis B prevention through proper vaccination in advance of any patient treatment.

Tuberculosis (TB). Tuberculosis most commonly affects the lungs. It is caused by the organism *Mycobacterium tuberculosis.* AIDS patients are also susceptible to *Mycobacterium avium intercellarae.*

Patient reports: History of disease, positive TB test, fever, weight loss, night sweats, cough, blood in sputum and tender lymph nodes. The patient may be taking streptomycin, ethambutol, isoniazid, or other antituberculosis medication.

Significance: Patient may transmit disease to others. Documented TB patients are generally followed up yearly with a sputum culture and chest x-ray examination. If medical clearance is given for noncontagious patient no special precautions are required for treatment.

Precautions:

1. Obtain letter from physician determining if disease is active. Additional TB tests may be necessary.
2. Follow universal precautions. Wear gloves, face mask, and glasses. Maintain strict sterilization and asepsis of all objects in contact with patient.

Sexually transmitted diseases. STDs are acute or chronic infectious diseases, such as syphilis, gonorrhea, or chlamydia, typically acquired through sexual intercourse or other close physical contact.

Patient reports: History of disease, painful urination, urethral or vaginal discharge, sore throat, skin eruptions, painless ulcer with firm rolled edges involving oropharyngeal mucosa or genitalia (chancre), mucous patch in oral cavity (gumma).

Significance: Patient may transmit disease to others.

Precautions:

1. Follow universal precautions. Wear gloves, face mask, and glasses. Maintain strict sterilization and asepsis of all objects in contact with patient.

Blood diseases
Anemia. Anemia is a deficiency of red blood cells (erythrocytes) in the circulating blood. Anemia may result from a vitamin or iron deficiency, bone marrow problems, excessive loss of blood, or red cell destruction.

Patient reports: Fatigue, weakness. The patient appears pale and may be taking iron and vitamin supplements.

Significance: Patient has lowered resistance to infection and possibly delayed healing.

Precautions:

1. Exercise care in instrumentation.
2. Advise patient to consult physician for further investigation of problem.

Leukemia. Patients with leukemia have an excessive number of immature white blood cells (leukocytes), which do not function normally. This disease is a type of blood cancer. Cells may overpopulate bone marrow and crowd out normal blood cells and other components such as red blood cells and platelets.

Patient reports: History of multiple infections, fatigue, and fever. The patient bruises easily and may be taking medications (chemotherapeutic agents) directed at controlling proliferation of these abnormal leukocytes.

Significance: Patient is extremely prone to infection. Patient may also have may have lesions of oral mucosa, xerostomia, more acidic saliva, and aggravated periodontal conditions as a result of chemotherapy. These conditions necessitate modifications in oral hygiene. Excessive bleeding caused by marrow depression and decreased platelets may affect healing time. Before periodontal treatment or extractions, consultation with the patient's physician is indicated.

Precautions: Obtain letter from physician on disease status and recommended procedures for dental intervention.

Hemorrhagic disorders (hemophilia, other). Hemophilia is a hereditary disorder characterized by excessive bleeding due to lack or deficiency of a coagulation factor (Grossman, 1975; Kaye, 1983). Types include classical hemophilia (factor VIII, hemophilia A), Christmas disease (factor IX, hemophilia B), and von Willebrand's disease. Other hemorrhagic disorders include clotting factor deficiency (e.g., vitamin K deficiency can cause depression in certain clotting factors, as do certain drugs such as warfarin and heparin) and platelet dysfunction (platelets are crucial to clotting); aspirin and certain drugs, including dipyridamole, interfere with platelet aggregation).

Patient reports: Family history of hemophilia, spontaneous or excessive bleeding, tendency to bruise easily.

Significance: When blood fails to clot, the patient is in danger of aspirating blood or even bleeding to death (exsanguination) if bleeding is not arrested. Medical measures are necessary when a large quantity of blood is lost. Patient may have received blood plasma factor replacement therapy and may carry hepatitis B antigen or have history of hepatitis and/or HIV infection (Evans, 1977).

Precautions:
1. Obtain letter from physician as to severity of disease. Medication before treatment (e.g., transfusion of deficient factor) may be needed.

2. Limit treatment to a specific area per appointment. If factor replacement therapy has been necessary before dental treatment, allow sufficient time for procedure to be completed in one visit on one day to reduce risks and expense of multiple transfusions (Evans, 1977).

3. Do not prescribe aspirin or aspirin-related products for pain control. Substitute acetaminophen, codeine, propoxyphene hydrochloride, or other analgesic.

4. Follow universal precautions. Wear gloves, face mask, and glasses. Maintain strict sterilization because of risk of exposure to bloodborne pathogens.

MEDICAL CLASSIFICATION

A medical classification system, as described in Table 6-1, is useful for identifying a patient's

Table 6-1. Sample format for medical classification system

Classification	Description
1	*Minimal risk.* Patient in good health. All dental procedures may be carried out with no special precautions.
2	*Some precautions must be observed* (e.g., patients with drug allergies, rheumatic heart disease without decompensation, controlled diabetes, or controlled hypertension).
3	*Deferred classification.* Patients have questionable health status but have given insufficient information regarding their ailment, abnormality, or treatment status. Consultation with local physician is usually required (e.g., patients taking unknown medications, patients with possible blood dyscrasias or with heart murmurs of unknown nature, and patients taking anticoagulants).
4	*Unable to withstand prolonged, difficult, or stressful dental procedures because of overall health status.* Degree of decompensation must be ascertained on an individual basis.
5	*Should be hospitalized for treatment or referred for care by more qualified health care providers.* Experienced health care providers should exercise high-level precautions during treatment, preferably under hospital conditions (e.g., patients with uncontrolled hypertension, uncontrolled diabetes, severe congestive heart failure, or hemophilia).

medical status. A standardized system of marking the medical classification in bold numbers on the chart provides a simple mechanism for conveying information quickly while preserving patient privacy.

UPDATING THE RECORD

A person's health is dynamic. Performing the comprehensive health history and classifying the medical status at the initial visit are only the first steps in providing safe treatment for the patient. Reviewing the chart at every visit is imperative. Should an emergency arise, precious time can be lost fumbling for information on medical problems or medications that would have been noted by a minute's review of the health history before beginning the day's treatment. Updating the chart at recall intervals is recommended. The dental professional should make a sincere inquiry about the patient's general health at every dental visit and note additional information.

Following are appropriate questions to ask the patient for updating the health history:

1. How has your health been lately?
2. What medications are you currently taking?
3. Have you been hospitalized for any reason since your last visit?
4. How has your (state specific medical condition) been since the last appointment?
5. How did you get along with the dental care you received last time?

These questions are direct but open to allow the patient to respond with as much information as possible.

The dental professional should measure the patient's blood pressure the day of the visit and compare it to previous entries. The health history form should have a specific update summary area, as important information can be easily missed when one is looking through a long series of treatment notes.

THE MEDICAL RELEASE LETTER

A medical release form is used for the patient to give consent for health professionals to exchange otherwise confidential information. This is necessary for acquiring pertinent medical details that the patient may be unable to provide about an illness or medication. This is also useful in obtaining dental-related information when a patient transfers from one office or clinic to another.

A standard three-carbon copy format is practi-

cal (Fig. 6-2). A form such as this saves the staff from having to write individual letters. It allows the office to retain an original copy and the physician or dentist to mail back the reply copy and keep a copy for his or her own records.

PHYSICIANS' DESK REFERENCE

The *Physicians' Desk Reference (PDR)* is published annually and is used as a reference by health professionals when seeking information about medications. The *PDR* is used to check such information as drug dosage, composition, contraindications, and the interactions of one drug with another. Today, with the huge number of medications available, a drug dictionary of this nature is essential for providing information about current and newly released medicaments.

It is important for dental professionals to use the *PDR* to investigate the medications their patients take. In this way the dental professional will be familiar with the reason why the patient is taking the medication and will be aware of possible contraindications or interactions between medication and dental treatment. For example, warfarin (Coumadin) is a blood anticoagulant, often prescribed for patients with phlebitis. Before a scaling procedure is performed, a consultation with the patient's physician may be necessary to change the patient's dosage to prevent prolonged bleeding during treatment.

Acetyl sulfisoxazole (Gantrisin) is an antibiotic used for the treatment of urinary tract infections. Procaine, once used as a primary dental local anesthetic, and sulfonamides (such as Gantrisin) are chemically related. Taken together, an antagonistic response occurs, rendering both medications ineffective.

Pharmacologic terms to be familiar with include brand name, generic name, and drug classification. The *brand name* is the name given to a particular medication or product by its manufacturer. Many manufacturers make the same product but market it under their own brand name. The *generic name* is the chemical name of the product. The use of generic names is advised because these always remain the same, give more chemical information, and do not limit prescription to one commercial preparation. For example, the product ibuprofen (generic name) is made by several manufacturers and marketed with the brand names Motrin, Advil, Heprin, and Rofen.

Drug classification refers to the broad category

```
Dentist_____    Patient_____

Address_____     Address_____

Phone_____      Phone _____




REQUEST  Date_____

Dear Dr._____,


The patient named above was recently seen in our office as a new patient.
Before dental therapy is initiated, I would appreciate information
regarding the patient's health status in the following areas.  Thank you.













                                       _____



I, _____ , hereby consent to the release of my medical/
dental records to t'.e office of_____.
                                       (Patient signature)

REPLY  Date_____










                                       (Consultant signature)
```

Fig. 6-2. Sample medical release letter.

to define drugs sharing similar actions. For example, analgesics are products that alleviate pain, diuretics promote urination, and sedatives induce a quiet, calm state.

The *PDR* consists of cross-referenced indices of products arranged alphabetically by manufacturer, brand name, generic name, and drug classification. If a sample medication is available, a picture identification section is included. The largest portion of the book is the product information section. Descriptions of each product include its chemical composition, the form in which it is supplied, its action and suggested use, administration, recommended dosage, contraindications, precautions, and side effects. Other sections include information on diagnostic products and management of drug overdose. Between the yearly publication dates, quarterly supplements are issued to update product information or describe new products.

Procedure for using the *PDR*

The dental hygienist should obtain as much information as possible from the patient about the drug he or she is taking. Perhaps the patient has brought the medication. The hygienist should read the prescription, look at the product, and ask the following questions:

1. For what condition are you taking this medication?
2. How often do you take it?
3. How long ago was it prescribed for you?
4. Do you take the medication exactly as prescribed?
5. When did you last take the medication?
6. Besides the manner in which this medication helps you specifically, does it change the way you feel in general?

Generally, patients are aware of the name and nature of the medication and the prescribed regimen for administration. Knowing the dosage is not as common. Dental hygienists should follow-up by checking the prescription or the *PDR*.

The patient should be asked whether he or she is taking the medication as directed by the physician. One may discover that the patient is altering the dosage in some way. This often happens when the patient "feels good" regardless of the state of the illness. Patient noncompliance in taking medications is a common problem. In a professional manner, one should reinforce the prescribed routine and suggest that the patient check with the physician for approval of the change. The hygienist should explain that not taking a medication as prescribed alters the control of the medical condition, which may create a risk to the patient and may affect reactions during dental treatment.

Often medications have minor effects that patients cope with readily. For example, antihistamines can make people sleepy, antibiotics can cause nausea, and asthma medications can make people agitated or tremulous. The conditions may or may not affect dental therapy, but the clinician's understanding of these states may help put the patient at ease, making treatment more comfortable.

After asking the above questions, the hygienist should note the name of the medication, the reason for its prescription, and the patient's dosage in the appropriate history or update section. The *PDR* is checked for drug action and any complication that might affect dental treatment. It is also advisable to have copies of the following articles on the effects of drugs and the oral cavity for reference:

Seymour RA, Hearsman PA: Drugs and the periodontium, *J Clin Periodontol* 15:1-16, 1988.

Matthews TG: Medication side effects of dental interest, *J Prosthet Dent* 64:219-226, 1990.

SUMMARY

This chapter has discussed one part of the dental appointment: obtaining a comprehensive health history. It has been an introduction to some ways in which medicine and dentistry are interrelated. Other courses, such as anatomy/physiology and oral medicine/pathology, will enrich the student's understanding of normal conditions and specific diseases in relation to dental care. The important points of this chapter are recognizing the need for a thorough review of health conditions before dental treatment and detailing the contents of such a review to identify medical conditions that may necessitate changes in dental care. In addition, the history-taking experience provides an opportunity for the clinician and patient to interact in a way that can lay the foundation of the professional relationship.

ACTIVITIES

1. Provide sample health history information for small groups to discuss. Practice completing the patient write-up using this information.
2. Role play the medical interview. Discuss communication skills and hygienist-patient interactions observed.
3. Practice using the *Physicians' Desk Reference* by identifying medications, contraindications, side effects, and so on.
4. Observe and critique health histories (interviews or written documentation) completed by students during their final year of clinical education. Discuss the observations in small groups.
5. Complete a comprehensive health history for a student partner. Preserve the complete data for use in treatment planning (discussed in Chapter 18). Stu-

dents should note that recording such data also ensures safe practice of intraoral procedures for a student partner.

6. Prepare a report summarizing the most recent research on viral hepatitis, acquired immunodefiiency syndrome (AIDS), or heart disease.

REVIEW QUESTIONS

1. Respond to this situation: Mrs. Jones is a new patient. Part-way through the health history interview she states, "This is just wasting time. I want my teeth checked."
2. Which of the following conditions should be followed up by a physician's consultation and why?
   a. Rheumatic heart disease
   b. History of myocardial infarction
   c. Blood pressure reading of 160/100
   d. Hemophilia
   e. All of the above
3. List the medical conditions that require antibiotic premedication before dental treatment to prevent bacterial endocarditis.
4. List several communication principles that help ensure a thorough medical history and a helping relationship with the patient.
5. How is the *Physicians' Desk Reference* useful to the dental hygienist?

REFERENCES

ADA Council on Dental Therapeutics: Preventing bacterial endocarditis: a statement for the dental professional, *JADA* 122:87, 1991.

ADA Council on Dental Therapeutics; Management of dental patients with prosthetic joints, *JADA* 121:537, 1990.

ADA Council on Dental Therapeutics: *Accepted dental therapeutics*, ed 40, Chicago, 1984, American Dental Association.

Angelopoulous AP: Diphenylhydantoin gingival hyperplasia: a clinicopathological review, *J Can Dent Assoc* 41:103, 1975.

Baltch AL et al: Bacteremia following dental cleaning in patients with and without penicillin prophylaxis, *Am Heart J* 104:1335, 1982.

Barco CT: Prevention of infective endocarditis: a review of the medical and dental literature, *J Periodontol* 62:510, 1991.

Barnett ML et al: The prevalence of mitral valve prolapse in patients with Down's syndrome: implications for dental management, *Oral Surg Oral Med Oral Path* 66: 445, 1988.

Bennett CR: *Monheim's local anesthesia and pain control in dental practice,* ed 7, St Louis, 1984, CV Mosby.

Braham L, editor: *The dental implications of epilepsy: report to the Commission for the Control of its Consequences, by the ad hoc committee of the Academy of Dentistry for the Handicapped,* ASA Pub. No. 1, 78-5217, Washington, DC, 1977, Department of Health, Education and Welfare.

Dajani AS et al: Prevention of bacterial endocarditis: recommendation by the American Heart Association, *JAMA* 264:2919, 1990.

deJong KJM et al: Validity of risk-related patient-administered medical questionnaire for dental patients, *Oral Surg Oral Med Oral Pathol* 72:527, 1991.

Durack DT, Kaplan EL, Bisno AL: Apparent failure of endocarditis prophylaxis: analysis of 52 cases submitted to a national registry, *JAMA* 250:2318, 1983.

Evans BE: *Dental care in hemophilia*, New York, 1977, Cutter Laboratories and the National Hemophilia Foundation.

Froelich RE, Bishop FM: *Clinical interviewing skills: a programmed manual for data gathering, evaluation, and patient management,* ed 3, St Louis, 1977, CV Mosby.

Grace CJ et al: *Actinobacillus actinomycetemcomitans* prosthetic valve endocarditis, *Rev Infect Dis* 10:922, 1988.

Grossman R: Orthodontics and dentistry for the hemophilic patient, *Am J Orthod* 68:391, 1975.

Israel H: Abnormalities of bone and orofacial changes from anticonvulsant drugs, *J Public Health Dent* 34:104, 1974.

Kaye D: Prophylaxis for infective endocarditis: an update, *Am Intern Med* 104:419, 1986.

Kaye D et al: *Internal medicine for dentistry*, St Louis, 1983, CV Mosby.

Kerr D, Ash M Jr: *Oral pathology: an introduction to general and oral pathology for hygienists,* ed 5, Philadelphia, 1986, Lea & Febiger.

Pallasch TJ, Slots J: Letters to the editor: author's response, *J Periodontol* 62:227, 1991.

Physician's Desk Reference, ed 41, Oradell, NJ, 1987, Medical Economics.

Pollack SM: Letters to editor re: antibiotic prophylaxis for medical risk patients, *J Periodontol* 62:227, 1991.

Prevention of bacterial endocarditis: a committee report of the American Heart Association, *JADA* 110:98,1985.

Rams TE, et al: Subgingival occurrence of enteric rods, yeasts and staphylococci after systemic doxycycline therapy, Oral Microbiol Immunol 5:166, 1990.

Spijkervet FKL et al: Effect of chlorhexidine rinsing on the oropharyngeal ecology in patients with head and neck cancer who have irradiation mucositis, *Oral Surg Oral Med Oral Pathol* 67:154, 1989.

Sullivan BV et al: The cardiac patient: chemoprophylaxis considerations, *Dent Hyg* 60(10):462, 1986.

Weinstein L, Schlesinger J: Pathoanatomic, pathophysiologic, and clinical correlations in endocarditis, I and II, *N Engl J Med* 291:832, 1122, 1974.

Zyssett MK et al: Systemic lupus erythematosus: a consideration for antimicrobial prophylaxis, *Oral Surg Oral Med Oral Pathol* 64:30, 1987.

SUGGESTED READINGS

ADA Council on Dental Therapeutics: *Accepted dental therapeutics*, ed 40, Chicago, 1984, American Dental Association.

Bodak-Gyovai LZ: *Diagnostic center manual*, Philadelphia, 1978, Department of Oral Medicine, University of Pennsylvania School of Dental Medicine.

Butler RT et al: Drug-induced gingival hyperplasia: phenytoin, cyclosporine, and nifedipine, *JADA* 114:56, 1987.

Mohammad AR et al: Assessment of dental patients' comprehension of health questionnaire, *J Oral Med* 38:74, 1983.

Small I: *Introduction to the clinical history,* ed 2, Flushing, NY, 1971, Medical Examination Publishing.

Tzukert AA et al: Prevention of infective endocarditis: not by antibiotics alone, *Oral Surg Oral Med Oral Pathol* 62:385, 1986.

Woodall IR, editor: *Curriculum guidelines,* ed 3, Chicago, 1975, American Dental Hygienist's Association.

7 BASIC EMERGENCY PROCEDURES

Donna Karras

Donna Karras

LEARNING OUTCOMES

The dental hygienist will be able to

1. Explain briefly why a dental hygienist should:
   a. Identify promptly the early signs and symptoms of medical emergencies.
   b. Follow an established emergency protocol system when managing a medical emergency.
   c. Successfully complete a comprehensive course in medical emergency management, basic life support, and cardiopulmonary resuscitation (CPR) at level C.*
2. Select drugs and equipment that would constitute a basic emergency kit for a dental clinic.
3. Identify and know the appropriate use of advanced emergency drug therapy.
4. Operate an oxygen tank and know the appropriate uses for the various delivery systems demanded by various emergency situations.
5. Use a complete, reviewed medical history and preoperative vital signs to help prevent, predict, and identify medical emergencies.
6. Explain the importance of stress management in preventing medical emergencies.
7. Use "universal precautions" as a necessary protective mechanism for emergency preparedness.
8. Appropriately manage specific medical emergencies in response to given signs and symptoms.
9. Develop an emergency protocol for a given clinical setting and explain how it will be implemented in a variety of emergency situations.
10. Identify and follow proper emergency preparedness measures when working with homebound and nursing home patients.
11. Identify and follow basic fire, accident, and personal injury prevention guidelines for a clinical setting.

Before beginning clinical practice, a dental hygiene student must be able to identify and respond to basic emergency signs that may occur during patient care. It is also important for the student to recall significant patient assessment data that may indicate the likelihood and nature of an emergency situation. To this end, the student's approach to emergency treatment should emphasize prevention with the goal of averting a medical emergency. This can best be accomplished through thorough patient assessment before treatment. McCarthy (1989) advises a four-step approach known as *RAM-E: R* recognition of disease; *A* assessment of the risk; *M* management for safety and comfort; and *E* emergency care. Where a regular course of comprehensive therapy is followed, the need for emergency treatment should be minimized and uncommon. This chapter will strive to alert the student to the rudiments of responsible attention to safety in practice. *A complete course in first aid and basic life support, in-*

*The American Heart Association recommends level C certification for health care providers. Level C certification includes one- and two-man CPR on the infant, child, and adult, as well as management of the obstructed airway for the infant, child and adult.

cluding cardiopulmonary resuscitation (CPR) and techniques for clearing the airway, is also essential.

THE HYGIENIST'S ROLE

A dental hygienist is often the first to recognize a potential medical emergency, as he or she may be the one to perform the medical history and record vital signs. Likewise, working with a patient in a private or semiprivate operatory frequently makes the hygienist the sole observer of the patient's condition and responses to various phases of care. It is the competent hygienist's responsibility to monitor the patient's responses throughout care, remaining constantly aware of changes in expression, skin tone, muscle tonus, respirations, and verbal expression. As intraoral procedures are performed, the clinician should, through peripheral vision, watch for signs of distress, relaxation, puzzlement, and other indications of the patient's state.

An additional responsibility is to be able to classify the kinds of responses and know when an emergency situation seems imminent. Prompt, appropriate reaction to signs of distress may avert an emergency and even save a life. The hygienist's ability to provide complete descriptions of signs of distress to the dentist or attending medical team can hasten the provision of appropriate care.

A further responsibility that may be assumed following a comprehensive first aid and life-support course is that of administering care to reverse an emergency or to sustain life until help can be secured. This role is essential for hygienists who function in their own practice or under general supervision, when a dentist or physician may or may not be present. All members of the dental team should be qualified to administer oxygen, record vital signs, perform basic life support procedures to open an airway, and perform CPR. As a primary provider of care, the dental hygienist certainly has this responsibility.

Once the signs of distress are noted, the clinician should be able to respond with a logical, rehearsed pattern of behavior— the emergency protocol. The response may be simply to move instruments and other pieces of potentially harmful equipment away from the patient, to raise the back of the chair, to lower the back for a full supine position, to go for help calmly, to push the emergency signal button, or to let the patient rest quietly for a moment. It may include preparing a syringe for an intramuscular (IM), intravenous (IV), or subcutaneous injection; performing CPR; or directing an emergency squad to the right location. For each possible situation, the clinician should be prepared to respond in a predetermined fashion, as there may be little time for contemplation or consulting references.

BEING PREPARED TO ACT

Responding to a medical emergency involves many steps that can and should be divided among dental team members according to their skill levels and their abilities to react quickly and appropriately under stress. All team members should be aware of the possible problems and proper responses to ensure that everyone participates knowledgeably and according to a well-rehearsed plan. Though procedures should be divided and delegated to individual team members, the division should be flexible enough to ensure that all steps are taken even when a team member is missing or is the subject of the emergency care.

A rehearsal of one of the possible emergencies should be held monthly, according to a carefully delineated script. For instance, in the event of aspiration of a foreign object into the lung, the clinician would follow predetermined steps to assist the patient and alert another team member to notify the dentist and the emergency squad.

Emergency phone numbers must be readily accessible; ideally, they should be attached to the phone itself. Procedures for alerting other team members of the occurrence of an emergency should be unmistakable, but a calm atmosphere should be preserved as much as possible.

Many tasks to be performed must be assigned and rehearsed. Eleven generic functions described by Kinne (1982) as part of any emergency are as follows:

1. Evaluate the vital signs.
2. Diagnose the nature of the emergency.
3. Decide on the appropriate treatment.
4. Instruct others what to do.
5. Phone for help.
6. Prepare for treatment administration.
7. Administer treatment.
8. Monitor vital signs.
9. Reassure the patient.
10. Record events that occur.
11. Ensure privacy and/or manage other patients.

Once the entire dental team has completed life-support and emergency management courses, they should write out specific protocols for action in the event of medical emergencies. Specific assignments should be made to individuals to ensure that all designated procedures are completed. The protocols should be posted, reviewed monthly, and rehearsed.

MEDICAL EMERGENCIES IN THE DENTAL ENVIRONMENT

Any medical emergency can occur in the dental office. Patients with a predisposition to a medical emergency (such as those with high blood pressure, cardiac insufficiency, asthma, or angina) may be more likely to experience an emergency in a dental office, as anxiety levels may be high in the anticipation or experience of dental care. The combination of a medical problem and anxiety may trigger a physical response that can be classified as an emergency (Trieger, 1982). Accordingly, patient anxiety levels are of prime concern to the practitioner, even in the "healthy" patient. Preventive procedures must include assessment of the patient's ability to cope mentally with the dental procedure. In other words, the "total" patient must be considered before therapy begins. An effective means of assessing patient anxiety (see box) was developed by Corah (1969). Using this Dental Anxiety Scale as part of the total patient evaluation will allow the practitioner to recognize patient anxiety, modify dental therapy, and prevent an emergency.

Table 7-1 summarizes the signs, symptoms, and treatments for the medical emergencies presented in this section. The emergency situations are presented by disease or emergency (for example, syncope, cardiac arrest, angina pectoris). However, when a medical emergency occurs, the clinician will be faced with specific signs and symptoms, such as unconsciousness or convulsions. It is strongly suggested that you complete activities 8 and 9 on p. 126 to prepare for responding to a medical emergency.

Emergency supplies and equipment

An integral part of any emergency protocol system is a strategically and conveniently located emergency kit. Even more important are the contents of the kit. What should the kit contain? At this time the experts cannot agree. The increasing numbers of medically compromised people seeking dental care, the frequently changing methods of managing emergencies, and the varied levels of

---

Dental Anxiety Scale

1. If you had to go to the dentist tomorrow, how would you feel about it?
   a) I would look forward to it as a reasonably enjoyable experience.
   b) I would not care one way or the other.
   c) I would be very uneasy about it.
   d) I would be afraid that it would be unpleasant and painful.
   e) I would be very frightened of what the dentist might do.
2. When you are waiting in the dentist's office for your turn in the chair, how to you feel?
   a) Relaxed.
   b) A little uneasy.
   c) Tense.
   d) Anxious.
   e) So anxious that I sometimes break out in a sweat or almost feel physically sick.
3. When you are in the dentist's chair waiting for him or her to get the drill ready and begin working on your teeth, how do you feel? (Same choices as question 2.)
4. You are in the dentist's chair to have your teeth cleaned. While you are waiting and the dentist is getting out the instruments with which to scrape your teeth around the gums, how do you feel? (Same choices as question 2.)
5. In general, do you feel uncomfortable or nervous about receiving dental treatment?
   a) Yes
   b) No

From Corah N: *J Dent Res* 48:596, 1969.

---

skill and training in emergency management techniques make it difficult to develop prepackaged emergency kits to meet all needs. Indeed, the American Dental Association Council on Dental Therapeutics (1986) has refrained from endorsing any commercial kit, suggesting instead that emergency kits be "individualized to meet the special needs and capabilities of each practitioner."

Accordingly, where prepackaged kits are considered, practitioners should commit sufficient time to developing their knowledge of and familiarity and skill with the contents of kits. Otherwise they may develop a false sense of confidence in their emergency management skills because of the mere presence of the kit. In certain cases, this could lay the groundwork for malpractice claims.

Table 7-1. Emergencies: signs, symptoms, and treatments

Emergency	Signs and symptoms	Treatment
Acute adrenal insufficiency (Adrenal crisis)	Confusion Weakness Nausea, vomiting Hypotension Severe pain in abdomen, lower back, legs Syncopal episodes Coma	*CONSCIOUS PATIENT* Terminate therapy Monitor vital signs Place in supine position Administer oxygen (5-10 liters per minute) Summon medical assistance *UNCONSCIOUS PATIENT* Recognize unconsciousness Place in supine position Provide basic life support* Emergency kit O₂ Summon medical assistance Transfer to hospital
Vasodepressor syncope	**Presyncope** EARLY Feeling of warmeth Loss of color Heavy perspiration Complaints of feeling bad Nausea Blood pressure approximately baseline Rapid heart rate LATE Pupillary dilation Hyperpnea Coldness in hands and feet Hypotension Bradycardia Dizziness **Syncope** Loss of consciousness	EARLY Recognize signs and symptoms Terminate therapy Place in supine position, feet slightly elevated Reassure patient Waft ammonia vaporole under patient's nose Administer oxygen; patient may hold mask Attempt to determine cause of presyncopal signs LATE Terminate therapy Place patient in supine position, feet slightly elevated Establish patient airway using head tilt, chin lift method Check breathing Artificial ventilation (if necessary) Check circulation Monitor vital signs Support patient Waft ammonia vaporole under patient's nose Cold towels to forehead Blankets if cold and shivering Attempt to determine cause of syncope Arrange for transportation Modify future therapy
Insulin shock Insulin reaction (hypoglycemia)	RAPID ONSET Moist and pale skin Full and bounding pulse Respirations, normal to shallow Blood pressure baseline to normal Bizarre behavior; may appear intoxicated but with no odor of alcohol Loss of consciousness (sometimes) Tremors Convulsions (in late stages)	Terminate therapy Recognize hypoglycemic symptoms *CONSCIOUS PATIENT* Assess ABCs† Administer oral carbohydrates *UNCONSCIOUS PATIENT* Provide basic life support* Summon medical assistance Carbohydrate IV or IM

*American Heart Association Guidelines
†Advanced training is required for safe and effective use of these devices.

Continued.

Table 7-1. Emergencies: signs, symptoms, and treatments—cont'd

Emergency	Signs and symptoms	Treatment
Diabetic coma (hyperglycemia)	**GRADUAL ONSET** Dry, flushed skin Dry mouth Intense thirst Vomiting Abdominal pain Rapid respiration (Kussmaul) Acetone odor to breath Low BP Weak, rapid pulse Loss of consciousness (sometimes)	Terminate therapy Recognize symptoms of hyperglycemia Summon medical assistance Provide basic life support* Transport to hospital (This patient needs insulin; however, due to complications associated with injectable insulin, it should *never* be a part of the emergency kit)
Respiratory problems		

Choking (aspiration)*	**Upper airway obstruction**
	Partial obstruction
	   Good air exchange
	   Coughing
		Terminate therapy
		Do not interfere
		Allow patient to cough

	PARTIAL OBSTRUCTION Poor air exchange High-pitched, crowing sound Cyanotic Ineffective cough Panic	Terminate therapy Treat as totally obstructed airway Transport to hospital
	TOTAL OBSTRUCTION *CONSCIOUS PATIENT* Ominous quiet Patient clutches throat (universal choking symbol Cyanotic Panic UNCONSCIOUS PATIENT	Perform Heimlich maneuver until obstruction is relieved‡ Reassure patient Transport to hopsital Summon medical assistance Heimlich maneuver (6-8 times) Finger sweep to remove obstruction (adults only) Attempt to ventilate Continue sequence until obstruction is relieved †Cricothyrotomy if obstruction cannot be relieved Monitor vital signs Artificial ventilation (if necessary) CPR (if necessary) Transport to hospital
	Lower airway obstruction Not as immediately life-threatening Object usually goes to right main bronchi and into right lung Patient may be unaware or may cough	Terminate therapy *Unless object is retrieved,* patient must be transported to hospital to locate and retrieve object
Hyperventilation	Acute anxiety Rapid breathing Shortness of breath Tingling in extremities and perioral area Dryness of mouth Chest pain Palpitations Muscle cramps and pain	Terminate therapy Position patient comfortably (this patient usually does not want to recline) Have patient place a paper bag, full face mask, or cupped hands over mouth and nose to breath CO_2-enriched air Drug management—Diazepam (only when the above therapy is ineffective) Attempt to determine cause of anxiety

Table 7-1. Emergencies: signs, symptoms, and treatments—cont'd

Emergency	Signs and symptoms	Treatment
Acute asthmatic attack	Intense coughing Intense wheezing Perspiration Cyanosis of nail beds and mucous membranes Flushing Fatigue Mental confusion	Terminate therapy Position patient comfortably (sitting or standing) Administer bronchodilator (use patient's prescription whenever possible) or subcutaneous epinephrine Administer O_2 Summon medical assistance
Chest pain		
Acute congestive heart failure and acute pulmonary edema	Weakness and undue fatigue Dyspnea on exertion Cyanotic Skin cold and clammy Wheezing (moist rales) Frothy sputum Pulsus alternans	Terminate therapy Place patient in an upright position Administer O_2 Monitor and record vital signs Attempt to alleviate apprehension Summon medical assistance
Angina pectoris	Pain usually substernal, but may radiate Brought on by exertion or stress Patient may hold clenched fist over chest (Levine's sign) Elevated BP and heart rate Dyspnea Feeling of faintness	Terminate therapy Place patient in upright position Administer nitroglycerin (patient's prescription whenever possible) Administer O_2 If pain persists, administer nitroglycerin again Monitor vital signs Summon medical assistance Modify therapy at future appointments
Myocardial infarction	Severe, prolonged substernal pain (30 minutes or more); pain may radiate (nitroglycerin provides no relief) Dyspnea Weakness Nausea and vomiting Severe distress Heart rate bradycardia to tachycardia BP baseline to low (may drop precipitously in first few hours)	Terminate therapy Record vital signs Administer nitroglycerin Initiate basic life support* as needed Summon medical assistance Administer O_2 Reassure patient Administer an analgesic for pain Transport to hospital
Cardiac arrest	Ashen gray appearance Skin cold and clammy Absence of adequate pulse Absence of respiration Most common cause is cardiovascular disease May occur as a result of complications to other emergency situations (such as airway obstruction, overdose, anaphylaxis, asthma, seizure disorders)	Terminate therapy Provide basic life support* Summon medical assistance
Altered consciousness		
Hypoglycemia Hyperglycemia Hypothyroidism	See insulin shock See diabetic coma Dry skin Coarse hair Lethargy Slow speech Edema of eyelids Gain in weight	 No special management Prior medical consultation Judicious use of drugs

Table 7-1. Emergencies: signs, symptoms, and treatments—cont'd

Emergency	Signs and symptoms	Treatment
Hyperthyroidism (thyroid storm; life-threatening; extremely rare)	Hyperpyrexia Profuse sweating Nausea, vomiting Abdominal pain Tachycardia Disorientation Agitation Coma	Terminate therapy Supine position Provide basic life support* O₂ Summon medical assistance
Seizure disorders		
Epilepsy (tonic-clonic seizures)	PRODROMAL STAGE Increase in anxiety or depression Aura Loss of consciousness ICTAL STAGE Cyanosis Tonic and clonic movements Frothing Occasionally urinary and fecal incontinence POSTICTAL STAGE Deep sleep to comatose Disoriented Headache Muscle soreness	Terminate therapy Place in supine position Protect from injury Provide basic life support* Monitor vital signs Allow patient to recover If duration is longer than 5 minutes, summon medical assistance Continue to monitor vital signs
Cerebral vascular accident		
(Sudden onset)	Flushed Bounding pulse Paralysis Headache Dizziness Drowsiness Nausea, vomiting Loss of consciousness	Terminate therapy Provide basic life support* Manage signs and symptoms Monitor vital signs Summon medical assistance
Allergic reaction	One or more body systems must be affected Reaction may be mild or severe Itching Urticaria Wheezing Nausea, vomiting Abdominal cramps Urinary, fecal incontinence Cardiac dysrhythmias Obstructed airway	Terminate therapy For mild reaction (slow onset—longer than 1 hour), administer antihistamine and arrange for medical consultation For severe reaction (anaphylaxis) administer epinephrine, provide basic life support,* summon medical assistance, and arrange medical consultation for future therapy
Toxic (overdose)		
Reaction to local anesthetic or vasoconstrictor	MILD TO MODERATE OD Confusion Excitedness	Terminate therapy Reassure patient

*Basic life support (BLS) does two things: (1) prevents circulatory or respiratory arrest or insufficiency through prompt recognition and intervention, and (2) externally supports circulation and respiration of a victim of cardiac or respiratory arrest through CPR.

†ABCs refers to airway, breathing, and circulation.

‡The Heimleich maneuver is performed differently in infants, children, and adults. A course in BLS provides information and practice for this procedure.

Data from American Heart Association (1985), Malamed (1987), Rose (1981), McCarthy (1982), and Braun (1979).

Continued.

Table 7-1. Emergencies: signs, symptoms, and treatments—cont'd

Emergency	Signs and symptoms	Treatment
	Slurred speech	Administer O_2 and instruct patient to
	Headache	hyperventilate
	Blurred vision	Provide basic life support*
	Numbness in perioral area	Monitor vital signs
		Recovery
		Medical consultation for further therapy
	MODERATE TO HIGH OD	
	Tonic-clonic seizures	Terminate therapy
	CNS depression	Supine position
	Depressed BP, heart rate, and respiratory rate	Manage seizure
	May lose consciousness	Provide basic life support*
		Monitor vital signs
		Summon medical assistance
		Transport to hospital
		Medical consultation for future therapy

Ideally, the practitioner should select emergency kit items after an exhaustive research of current literature, a consultation with referral physicians, a review of pharmacologic texts, and an examination of community emergency medical systems. This allows the informed practitioner to select only drugs and equipment that are effective, economical, and suited for the job. All clinicians should recognize their limitations in this area, however, and endeavor to enhance needed emergency skills.

In any medical emergency, time is of the essence. Seconds lost fumbling with unfamiliar drugs or equipment can compromise the outcome of most critical medical situations. Accordingly, actual medical emergencies are not the time for "trying out" or "practicing" emergency techniques for the first time.

When an emergency kit is developed, the anticipated arrival time of backup advanced life support should be considered. A clinician must be able to manage a critical situation for at least as long as it takes for expert help to arrive. Thus the emergency kit for a practice located in a large medical building or an emergency medical clinic is likely to differ in content from the kit for a rural practice that depends on a volunteer ambulance department whose arrival time may be more than an hour.

Most emergency situations can be managed using basic life support (without use of drugs) until advanced life support can arrive. Therefore the emergency kit must remain simple and, whenever doubt exists, no medication should be given (Malamed, 1987). (An important exception is treatment for acute anaphylaxis, where epinephrine is the drug of choice.)

A basic emergency kit should normally include aromatic ammonia capsules, portable oxygen (O_2) with delivery system (separate from the nitrous oxygen unit), nitroglycerin, and epinephrine. Aromatic ammonia capsules are one of the most commonly used drugs in emergency management. They should be readily available in each operatory and in the emergency kit itself. An ammonia capsule taped to the back of the patient's chair can provide practitioners with quick and easy access to the medication in case of a syncopal episode (Malamed, 1987).

Oxygen is also used to manage many emergency situations, from minor to very serious. Portable equipment is essential, as emergencies do not occur exclusively in the operatory. Patients may require oxygen in waiting rooms, hallways, restrooms, and other parts of the practice setting. Practitioners should acquire an "E"-size portable cylinder, providing at least 30 minutes of oxygen, and an additional backup cylinder, so that 1 full hour of total emergency oxygen is available for use in patient treatment and transport. Every staff member should know how to replace oxygen tanks in an emergency. In addition, a written record of oxygen use should be plainly presented on all tanks to ensure a verifiable and adequate supply.

A reliable method of delivering oxygen is also important. If a patient is not breathing (that is, in respiratory arrest), the practitioner must have access to a mechanism capable of forcing air into the victim's lungs. One such device is the positive pressure mask (Robertshaw). When attached to the oxygen tank, this mask will deliver 100% oxygen to the patient. Another device, the portable self-inflating resuscitation bag (Ambu bag), can be attached to the O_2 tank to deliver 100% O_2, or may be used alone to deliver 20% atmospheric O_2. During a cardiac emergency, the patient will benefit most from 100% oxygen.

Masks for either of these devices should be clean and transparent, allowing the operator optimal visibility to monitor vomitus, blood, or other substances that may be expelled. Ensuring an airtight seal is also critical. Masks come in adult, pediatric, and infant sizes to facilitate proper fit and seal. Accordingly, a complete kit should contain a full range of mask sizes. Basic competence with any delivery system is, of course, realizable only through diligent and conscientious practice. In addition, strategic location of resuscitation equipment will minimize the need for mouth-to-mouth resuscitation. Should mouth-to-mouth resuscitation be necessary, however, a CPR microshield must be available (OSHA, 1991).

Nitroglycerin is a vasodilator used for the treatment of chest pain, such as angina pectoris and myocardial infarction. Nitroglycerin is available in spray or tablet form; spray is recommended because of its longer shelf life. Whenever possible, a patient's own prescription should be used.

Epinephrine is used in the treatment of acute anaphylaxis. Because time is critical in this type of emergency, preloaded syringes are recommended. Hollister-Stier Laboratories offers a preloaded, metered syringe that allows only a preset or recommended dosage of epinephrine to be administered, thereby minimizing the risk of overdose. To administer an additional dose, the syringe plunger must be rotated. The importance of this built-in safety device cannot be overstated (Malamed, 1987).

Many other types of drugs and equipment could be included in any functional emergency kit. Primary drugs and equipment—those necessary for prompt, successful management of a crisis—should receive priority consideration. Secondary drugs and equipment, although important, are less critical for crisis management and often require advanced training for use. A third group of drugs and equipment, designed for practitioners with advanced cardiac life support (ACLS) training, would not be included in the normal emergency kit unless an operator has received such training (Malamed, 1987).

A suggested list of primary drugs and equipment is as follows (see Table 7-2 for additional information):

1. Primary injectable drugs
   a. Epinephrine
   b. Antihistamine
   c. Anticonvulsant
   d. Narcotic antagonist
2. Primary noninjectable drugs
   a. Oxygen
   b. Vasodilator
3. Primary emergency equipment
   a. O_2 with delivery system
   b. Suction and suction tips
   c. Tourniquets (for practitioners skilled in venipuncture)
   d. Syringes for drug administration (Malamed, 1987)

Finally, a complete and plainly visible log of drugs should always be affixed to any emergency kit. This log should list and identify drugs by both generic and proprietary name and include the expiration date of each to minimize confusion in a crisis and to prevent the use of outdated drugs.

Care of emergency equipment

"The term 'universal precautions' refers to a system of infectious disease control which assumes that every direct contact with body fluids is infectious" (OSHA, 1990). Accordingly, practitioners must use comprehensive office infection control procedures for contamination and cross contamination during emergency treatment and for care of emergency equipment (including stethoscopes and blood pressure cuffs that come in contact with blood and/or body fluids).

Disposable emergency equipment is the ideal, and new items are continually being developed; therefore, the clinician should be alert for new products. Reusable equipment will require standard sterilization and disinfection procedures to prevent hepatitis B (OSHA, 1990). Each practitioner should know what method of asepsis is necessary for the equipment in the office. For example, some Ambu bags require disinfection, while others are autoclavable or disposable.

Table 7-2. Emergency drugs and equipment

Category	Drug of choice	
	Generic	Proprietary
I. Injectable drugs		
PRIMARY DRUGS		
Allergy	Epinephrine	Adrenalin
Antihistamine	Chlorpheniramine	Chlor-Trimeton Maleate
Anticonvulsant*	Diazepam	Valium
Narcotic antagonist†	Naloxone	Narcan
SECONDARY DRUGS		
Analgesic	Morphine sulfate	
Vasopressor	Methoxamine HCl	Vasoxyl
Corticosteroid	Hydrocortisone succinate	Solu-Cortef
Antihypoglycemic	50% Dextrose	—
	Glucagon	Glucagon
ADVANCED CARDIAC LIFE SUPPORT INJECTABLES		
	Sodium bicarbonate	
	Atropine sulfate	
	Lidocaine	Xylocaine
	Calcium chloride	

*Anticonvulsant is a primary drug only when the practitioner is able to administer the drug intravenously.
†Narcotic antagonist is primary drug if any narcotic is employed in patient management. It need not be present if narcotics are never used.

Category	Generic	Proprietary
II. Noninjectable drugs		
PRIMARY DRUGS		
Oxygen	Oxygen	—
Vasodilator	Nitroglycerin	Nitrolingual spray
SECONDARY DRUGS		
Respiratory stimulant	Aromatic ammonia	—
Antihypoglycemic agent	Carbohydrate	Many available, plus juice, icing tubes
Bronchodilator	Metaproterenol	Alupent

III. Emergency equipment	
Equipment	Description
PRIMARY EMERGENCY EQUIPMENT	
Oxygen delivery system*	Positive pressure/demand valve or self-inflating bag-valve-mask *and* clear full face masks
Suction and suction tips	Large-diameter, round-ended suction tips or tonsil suction tips (high-volume suction)
Syringes for drug administration	Disposable syringes
Tourniquets	Rubber tourniquet or latex tubing or sphygmomanometer
SECONDARY EMERGENCY EQUIPMENT	
Scalpel or cricothyrotomy device†	
Artificial airways†	Oropharyngeal airways
	Nasopharyngeal airways
Airway adjuncts†	Laryngoscope and endotracheal tubes

*Advanced training is required for safe and effective use of these devices. All dental personnel should be trained in their use.
†Advanced training is required for safe and effective use of these devices. *Do not* include in emergency kit if personnel are not trained to use properly.
Adapted from Malamed SF: *Handbook of medical emergencies in the dental office*, ed 3, St Louis, 1987, CV Mosby.

Care in specific situations

Altered consciousness. *Syncope,* or simple fainting, can occur if the patient's brain fails to receive adequate oxygen and glucose as the result of vasodilation or loss of vasomotor tone. The signs of simple syncope are loss of color from the skin (pallor), perspiration, slight confusion, complaints of nausea or dizziness, and sometimes loss of consciousness from which the patient can be roused. In coma, by comparison, the patient cannot be roused (Miller, 1982). Because most dental procedures are performed with the patient in the supine position, which facilitates adequate blood flow to the brain, syncope is probably a less likely occurrence now than in the era of the upright position (Miller, 1982). Sitting up rapidly after being in a supine or recumbent position can, however, bring on syncope.

If a patient does exhibit signs of syncope and complains of discomfort, instruments should be moved away, the chair should be adjusted to the full supine position, and another team member should be alerted. Oxygen should be readied for administration, a cool cloth may be applied to the patient's forehead, and an ammonia ampule should be ready for wafting under the patient's nose.

Many times, prompt action can avert loss of consciousness. If the patient does retain consciousness, he or she should be allowed to rest comfortably. Essential procedures such as suturing an area should be completed, and the patient should be allowed to leave when fully recovered.

If the patient does lose consciousness, an ammonia ampule can be broken and wafted under his or her nose (Dunn and Booth, 1975; Malamed, 1987; Miller, 1982). A quick whiff will usually restore consciousness. Oxygen can then be administered along with comforting words. When fully recovered, the patient should be allowed to leave. It may be necessary to escort the patient home.

If a woman in the late stages of pregnancy loses consciousness, the back of the chair should be lowered and the patient should be turned onto her side (Malamed, 1987). Placing a woman in the third trimester of pregnancy on her back, especially on a hard surface, can cut off circulation in the venous system; the weight of the uterus impinging on the vena cava can encourage loss of consciousness.

A patient recovering from syncope (or another emergency) may be frightened or even embarrassed. During the recovery stages, the patient may appreciate care and comfort without undue solicitousness.

Syncope is only one of the possible reasons for a patient to lapse into unconsciousness. In the beginning stages of syncope, the patient has a lowered blood pressure and increased pulse. Recovery is usually rapid if the actions previously described are taken. If recovery is not immediate, the clinician should check for respirations. The mouth mirror can be placed close to the mouth or nose to check for fogging, or the clinician can listen for sounds of respiration by placing his or her ear close to the patient's mouth. The pulse can be checked by placing the fingers in the area of the carotid artery between the larynx and the anterior border of the sternocleidomastoid muscle. If either sign is absent, help should be summoned immediately. Someone should be directed to call a rescue team, after which basic life support procedures are begun. The clinician clears and maintains an airway, forcing oxygen into the lungs, and performs external cardiac massage if there is no pulse (Dunn and Booth, 1975; Malamed, 1987; McCarthy, 1982).

Acute adrenal insufficiency, wherein the adrenal gland does not produce sufficient amounts of cortisol, rendering the body incapable of coping with stress, is another possible cause of loss of consciousness. Patients likely to experience acute adrenal insufficiency fall into three groups: persons in the late stages of Addison's disease (adrenocortical insufficiency) who have not yet been diagnosed and are not yet taking medication; persons who are suddenly withdrawn from steroid hormones; and persons experiencing stress, particularly those with compromised function of the adrenal or pituitary glands (patients receiving corticosteroids) (Malamed, 1987). Many diseases (Addison's disease, asthma, herpes zoster, ulcerative colitis, rheumatoid arthritis, and lichen planus, to name only a few) are treated with steroid hormones. Athletes and body-builders often use self-prescribed steroids indiscriminately. A thorough dialogue review of the patient's medical history (Brady, 1980), including medications being taken or recently stopped, is imperative to uncover factors that may predispose a patient to acute adrenal insufficiency. A patient experiencing acute adrenal insufficiency is in danger of death from shock and cardiac arrest. The hygienist should summon assistance, initiate CPR, and relate the symptoms to the dentist or physician, who may administer cortisone to counteract the crisis.

A person with diabetes mellitus may lose consciousness as a result of low blood sugar levels (hypoglycemia) secondary to a relative excess of insulin. This can happen if the patient omits a meal, exercises heavily and uses available blood glucose, or takes an overdose of insulin (insulin shock). For the conscious patient, orange juice or any carbohydrate can reverse the condition. For the unconscious patient, IV or IM glucose is indicated, accompanied by basic life support.

Hypoglycemia can also occur in patients who do not have diabetes. Patients who skip meals before dental treatment and are anxious about the dental visit may experience a drop in the blood glucose level. Alcoholics suffer from hypoglycemia because of a lack of stored glycogen in the liver and poor nutrition.

Hyperglycemia is a possible cause of loss of consciousness in patients with diabetes. In this case insulin levels are insufficient; the blood sugar rises above safe levels. Insulin is necessary to reverse this situation. If the patient has a history of insulin shock, this should be included in the medical history. The patient may carry a supply of insulin for injection, of which the clinician should be aware. Coma associated with hyperglycemia occurs most frequently in juvenile diabetics, usually when the condition is first diagnosed. In most cases a comatose patient is hypoglycemic and needs glucose. The response to glucose should be immediate. The hyperglycemic patient will not improve with glucose.

In addition to patients in early stages of hypoglycemia or hyperglycemia, *altered consciousness* can be observed in patients who are intoxicated; patients with hypothyroidism or hyperthyroidism, or patients entering a convulsive state, such as epilepsy. These patients should be monitored to ensure they do not lose vital signs and should be escorted home (in the case of excess alcohol) or taken for physical evaluation by a physician. In severe cases, hospitalization may be indicated. In the case of epilepsy, it is important to ensure that a patent airway be maintained during tonic-clonic seizures. Removable dental appliances or objects forced between the victim's teeth often result in obstruction. Placement of any object in the oral cavity usually is *not* indicated during tonic-clonic seizures (Malamed, 1987).

An additional cause of altered consciousness is a *cerebral vascular accident* in which a blood vessel in the brain breaks or is occluded, preventing adequate blood supply to the brain. Accompanying signs are intense headache, weakness or paralysis of speech and extremities, dizziness, and nausea. The patient should be positioned in a semierect position. The symptoms should be managed until assistance can be summoned.

Respiratory difficulty. Patients may experience respiratory difficulty in a number of ways. A patient may be *choking* on excess water, *vomitus*, or a foreign object, or may need to cough for some other reason. If the patient is able to cough, the clinician should not interfere. Coughing will help remove the object and indicates good air exchange (American Heart Association, 1985).

If choking is caused by a foreign object, such as a prophy cup in the oropharyngeal area, the patient must not be allowed to sit up. Instead, the chair is placed in a head-down (Trendenlenberg) position, allowing gravity to return the object to the oral cavity where it can be retrieved by coughing or forceps. The clinician must not allow the patient to sit up if the object has progressed into the trachea. The patient is placed in the head-down position, lying on the right side, and encouraged to cough, if coughing does not occur spontaneously (Malamed, 1987). If the patient cannot cough and begins to express panic, assistance may be necessary to free the air passage. The recommended procedure is the Heimlich maneuver, in which the air in the lungs is forced out by upward compression on the diaphragm. This technique should be learned under supervision as part of a life-support course.

If the patient vomits while in a supine position, the emesis maneuver is performed to prevent aspiration (McCarthy, 1989). The patient is rolled onto his or her side, the head and shoulders directed toward the floor. The patient's head, neck, and chest should thereafter be in a dependent position, making aspiration virtually impossible.

A second form of respiratory difficulty is *hyperventilation* (Dunn and Booth, 1975; Malamed, 1987), usually resulting from anxiety, in which insufficient carbon dioxide is present in the bloodstream because of prolonged rapid breathing. It is characterized by tingling fingers and toes, lightheadedness, acute anxiety, and rapid breathing. Perioral tingling or numbness is also characteristic of hyperventilation. Usually, having the patient breathe in and out of a bag (a headrest cover, perhaps) will permit inhalation of sufficient amounts of carbon dioxide to reverse the problem. The patient should be calmed. A tranquilizer may be necessary in severe cases.

There are two kinds of *asthmatic attacks*. The mild form is more typical and is characterized by a feeling of thickness in the chest, coughing, wheezing, slow and labored breathing, heightened anxiety, a slightly elevated blood pressure, and an elevated heart rate. Treatment for a mild attack includes steps 1 to 3 and 8 below, which will usually be effective; steps 4 and onward can be taken in the case of a severe attack or if relief is incomplete (Malamed, 1987).

1. Terminate the dental therapy.
2. Position the patient comfortably (usually either sitting up or standing).
3. Administer an aerosol spray of epinephrine or similar drug. (Most patients who suffer from these attacks carry a bronchodilator for such emergencies.)
4. Administer oxygen.
5. Give an IM or subcutaneous injection of aqueous epinephrine if necessary.
6. Summon medical assistance if steps 1 to 5 are ineffective.
7. Give IV medication if necessary.
8. After recuperation, reevaluate for recovery, continued therapy, and eventual dismissal.

Cardiovascular problems. *Chest pain* associated with cardiovascular problems can result from heart failure, angina pectoris, or myocardial infarction. These diseases are discussed further in Chapter 6.

Heart failure will cause respiratory difficulty (Malamed, 1987). The signs of onset include chest pain and palpitation, a feeling of suffocation, coughing including bloody sputum, and sometimes cyanosis. The difficulty in breathing results from the filling of the interstitial tissues of the lungs with serous fluid. As long as the patient is conscious, he or she should be positioned in an upright position, which allows the excess lung fluid to settle in the lower lung areas to permit some air exchange in the tissues. Oxygen should be administered; use of a mask should be avoided, if possible, to minimize the patient's sensation of suffocation. Emergency assistance and hospital transport must be summoned. Diuretics to reduce the fluid and digitalis to improve heart contractility may be administered by ACLF personnel as a part of medical treatment.

Angina pectoris is a temporary lack of oxygen in the heart muscle resulting from (1) narrowed coronary arteries; (2) exertion, excitement, or eating a heavy meal; or (3) an increased work load. The pain ranges from mild to severe and often radiates to the left shoulder or arm. It usually is not as intense as the pain caused by a myocardial infarction, wherein the blood supply is cut off to a portion of muscle, causing tissue death. Vasodilators, such as nitroglycerin, are used to treat angina. The vasodilator allows the circulatory capacity of the heart muscle to dilate, improving flow and reducing the work load and thus the pain. Currently, nitroglycerin spray (developed in 1986) is most commonly used for the treatment of an anginal episode. At the onset of pain, one dose of nitroglycerin spray is administered sublingually. If the pain persists beyond 10 minutes and three doses of nitroglycerin, emergency medical help should be summoned (American Heart Association, 1985; Malamed, 1987; McCarthy, 1982).

Myocardial infarction, also called *coronary occlusion*, results when the coronary artery flow to some portion of the heart muscle is stopped. The affected muscle dies from lack of oxygen. About 75% of cases are caused by a thrombus (blood clot). Symptoms are similar to those of angina pectoris, but the pain is more crushing and is not relieved by nitroglycerin. The patient is often in a cold sweat, weak, and restless. In contrast, the patient with angina stays still, knowing that movement heightens the pain. An infarction often is accompanied by nausea, light-headedness, coughing, wheezing, and abdominal bloating (which may cause the patient to mistake the problem for indigestion) (McCarthy, 1982).

The first step in treating an infarction is to administer nitroglycerin and watch for pain relief. If the pain continues or increases, emergency assistance should be summoned, oxygen administered, and vital signs monitored. Drugs for relief of pain can be administered. The emergency medical team should manage complications such as arrhythmia. In the event of cardiac arrest, CPR must be begun to prevent death (Blair, 1982a; Malamed, 1987; McCarthy, 1982).

Cardiac arrest occurs when the heart has stopped beating or "circulation of blood is absent or inadequate to maintain life" (Malamed, 1987). Myocardial infarction is only one cause of cardiac arrest. Others include airway obstruction, drug overdose, anaphylaxis, seizure disorders, and acute adrenal insufficiency. The treatment is to restore circulation. In a dental office, the method of choice is CPR, in which a heartbeat and respiration are created for the patient through external cardiac compression and ventilation.

All dental health care providers must complete a course in CPR. The American Heart Association recommends level C certification for health care providers and annual recertification (American Heart Association, 1985).*

Reactions to a local anesthetic

Patients can have reactions to local anesthetics, ranging from syncope (psychogenic reaction) to a toxic reaction (overdose) to an allergic reaction (Malamed, 1987). It is extremely important that a member of the dental team who is capable of recognizing an emergency situation remains with the patient after he or she has received an injection, because a minor or severe immediate reaction can occur in 3 to 5 minutes. Most patients are anxious before and during an injection. Syncope is the most common reaction to a local anesthetic injection; its signs and symptoms and the methods for treating it have been described. Another stress-related reaction that can occur is hyperventilation, which also has been described.

A *toxic reaction* results from an absolute or relative overdose of a local anesthetic agent or vasoconstrictor. It is caused by injection of more solution than the patient's body can metabolize and excrete. This reaction can be prevented by aspirating before injecting, by injecting the solution slowly, by injecting only the recommended amount according to the patient's body weight, and by checking the patient's history for the presence of disease or previous reaction to local anesthetic. During a mild toxic reaction the patient will appear restless, talkative, and agitated. The clinician should stop administering the agent, instruct the patient to hyperventilate O_2 from the O_2 mask (Malamed, 1987), and allow the patient's system to remove some of the anesthetic; a mild toxic reaction can reverse itself. A severe toxic reaction is characterized by an excitatory stage (agitation or possibly convulsions), followed by a corresponding depression. A patient suffering from such an attack needs immediate medical at-

tention. The clinician should begin life-support measures, alert the supervising dentist immediately, and have someone notify a rescue squad.

Another possible reaction is an *allergic reaction,* which can be a delayed mild reaction or an immediate severe reaction. The immediate and severe reaction, called *anaphylaxis*, often begins with itching and urticaria but rapidly progresses to a life-threatening stage including muscle spasms, fluid accumulation, swelling in the throat causing inability to breathe, and cardiovascular collapse and death (Stroh and Johnson, 1982). Anaphylaxis requires immediate attention, including epinephrine IM or IV, an antihistaminic IM or IV, and a corticosteroid IM or IV. Further assistance from a medical team should be sought.

At the first signs of itching or urticaria, the clinician should stop dental treatment and retrieve the preloaded syringe of epinephrine (0.3 ml of 1:1000 aqueous) for subcutaneous injection (Malamed, 1987). Do basic life support as indicated. If the reaction progresses, summon emergency assistance and administer the epinephrine immediately. If the patient is already in shock, the quickest route for distribution of the drug is IV. Because peripheral veins may be collapsed at this stage, injection is best accomplished into the highly vascular underside of the tongue. Such injections have been shown to assist resuscitation (Shaber and Smith, 1982; Stroh and Johnson, 1982).

A mild allergic reaction is characterized by a skin rash and itching; often this will be a delayed reaction. The patient may call the office several hours after the injection, complaining of a rash and itching. A mild allergic reaction is treated by administering an antihistaminic; the patient should be referred for further medical care.

It is extremely important to record accurately *any* untoward reaction of a patient during treatment. Many of the medical emergencies described could recur or may indicate a severe physical condition that needs prompt medical attention. The supervising dentist should refer a patient for a medical evaluation if a previously indicated medical condition seems apparent.

In addition to helping to ensure the patient's safety, accurate records are necessary in case of later legal proceedings. Thorough, objective, accurate progress notes about a medical emergency are part of the dental personnel's best defense.

*The American Heart Association recommends level C certification for health care providers. Level C certification includes one- and two-man CPR on the infant, child, and adult, as well as management of the obstructed airway for the infant, child, and adult.

Accident, personal injury, and fire prevention

Although many emergencies in the dental office relate to the disposition of patient medical emergencies, other kinds of emergencies can be precipitated by negligence, carelessness, or unforeseeable circumstances.

To prevent accidents, it is important to ensure that all equipment is safe and functioning properly. A loose hinge, a missing bolt, or a short circuit can lead to unfortunate accidents that can harm the patient and the dental professional. It is the clinician's responsibility to protect the patient from harm caused by faulty equipment and to eliminate hazards that could cause harm, such as a tangle of cords in the patient's pathway or a wet, slippery floor.

Personal injury can result from criminal acts of intruders as well as from physical hazards in the office. It is always wise to have a co-worker available to summon assistance in case of a medical emergency and to dissuade persons (including perhaps, a patient) from assaulting the dental professional. Working alone in a quiet office in proximity with a patient may stimulate a patient or provoke erratic behavior in an emotionally disturbed patient.

Drugs and cash or checks should be locked away in an unnoticeable place to reduce the likelihood of robbery during or after office hours.

The department of education and safety of local police forces provides many individualized programs, such as self-protection, personal safety for women at work, safety for women when alone, and crime prevention, to ensure the safety of the dental staff and office. The programs are free and of invaluable service.

Fire prevention is an additional factor in preventing emergencies. Flammable substances should be kept clear from Bunsen burners and radiators. The laboratory, in particular, is a hazardous area, because the open flame of a Bunsen burner may ignite hair, electrical wiring, papers, or other materials. A fire extinguisher should be kept in the laboratory for prompt response to such occurrences. The natural gas supplied to operatories and the laboratory is a potential hazard if there is a leak or if a gas jet is left open. If such a leak goes undetected and fills the room, the spark or static electricity produced by simply turning on a light switch can cause a sudden explosion.

Fire departments routinely inspect public buildings; however, they will provide additional educational courses on request to help ensure the safety of office personnel and patients. These courses are free.

Routes for fire escape, procedures for extinguishing fires that are contained, and procedures for summoning assistance should be drafted by the team, reviewed, and rehearsed. Smoke detectors should be installed. A main valve for natural gas should be installed and closed at the end of each working day. Again, procedures to follow in the event of a police or fire emergency should be rehearsed. This preparation could save a person's life.

EMERGENCIES IN NONTRADITIONAL SETTINGS

As the role of the dental hygienist expands into nontraditional settings, so must the hygienist's emergency management skill. The nursing home hygienist should inform the head nurse of his or her presence before beginning therapy. It is important to be familiar with the emergency protocol of each facility and to review it thoroughly before entering. This procedure should also be followed by hygienists in industry, schools, elder care centers, and other nontraditional practice settings. The hygienist working with homebound patients should invest in an emergency kit and create an emergency protocol for each home visited. It is important to know the location of phones and emergency numbers and to be familiar with the local emergency medical services before beginning dental therapy.

ACTIVITIES

1. Identify the location of the emergency kit in the clinic. Note the contents of the kit and the purposes of each item. Also note the expiration date of each drug. Discuss the security system for guarding against theft of drugs while ensuring ready access to drugs by the dental staff during an emergency.
2. Locate and operate the oxygen mask and supply for the conscious and unconscious patient.
3. Role-play various emergency situations, such as the following:
   a. Cardiac arrest
   b. Syncope
   c. Hypoglycemia
   d. Respiratory difficulty
4. Design an emergency protocol for several different clinical settings. Consider office personnel, office design, emergency equipment, and location. Your plan must consider contingencies in the event that

a staff member is the victim or is out of the office.

5. Review a variety of medical histories of medically compromised patients. In groups of three or four, plan for potential medical emergencies and simulate the proper emergency responses for the entire class.

6. Refer to Absi EG: *Br Dental J* 163:199, 1987, for a case history of cardiac arrest in the dental chair. As a group, discuss the protocol followed before, during, and after the incident.

7. Simulate a fire emergency evacuation from the clinical setting.

8. Refer to the "Appendix/Quick-reference Section to Life-threatening Situations," in Malamed SF: *Handbook of medical emergencies in the dental office,* St Louis, 1987, CV Mosby, pp. 392-397. Have your emergency team discuss each of the emergency situations contained in this appendix.

9. Refer to Blair DM: *Dent Clin North Am* 26:163; 1982 and have your emergency team discuss each of the errors shown and described.

10. Locate your own carotid pulse by palpating with your fingers between your larynx and the anterior border of the sternocleidomastoid muscle. Check for respirations by using a stethoscope on a partner's larynx and by placing a dental mirror under the nose.

11. Refer to Fast TB: *JADA* 112(4):1986. Have a group discussion on the report of emergency preparedness among dental practitioners.

12. Arrange for a local law enforcement body to provide a personal safety and crime prevention course for the class.

13. Obtain a copy of the Center for Disease Control's (CDC) "Guidelines for hospital environmental control: cleaning disinfection and sterilization of hospital equipment" (CDC Building #1, Room 2209, D-14, 1600 Clifton Road Northeast, Atlanta, GA 30333).

REVIEW QUESTIONS

1. Why is it essential for a dental hygienist to have completed a comprehensive course in first aid and basic life support?

2. List the suggested primary drugs and equipment for an emergency kit and their use.

3. How can the dental team prepare for an emergency?

4. What do you do if:
   a. Your patient becomes ashen and agitated and complains of nausea and dizziness?
   b. Your patient complains of severe chest pain?
   c. Your patient suddenly loses consciousness?

5. Explain how oxygen delivery to the conscious victim will differ from oxygen delivery to the unconscious victim.

6. What type of disinfection/sterilization is necessary for the Ambu bag in your clinic?

REFERENCES

American Dental Association Council on Dental Therapeutics: Office emergencies and emergency kit, *Council Report,* 101:305, 1980, Chicago, The Association.

American Heart Association: *Instructor's manual for basic life support,* Dallas, 1985, The Association.

Blair DM: Cardiac emergencies, *Dent Clin North Am* 26:49, 1982a.

Blair DM: Common errors in handling medical emergencies, *Dent Clin North Am* 26:163, 1982b.

Blitz P: Personal communication, 1979.

Brady W et al: Validity of health history data collected from dental patients and patient perception of health status, *JADA* 101:642, 1980.

Corah N et al: Assessment of a dental anxiety scale, *JADA* 97:816, 1978.

Dunn MJ, Booth DF: *Dental auxiliary practice: internal medicine and systemic emergencies,* Baltimore, 1975, Williams & Wilkins.

Kinne RD: Training for the effective management of medical emergencies, *Dent Clin North Am* 26:147, 1982.

Malamed, SF: *Handbook of medical emergencies in the dental office,* ed 3, St Louis, 1987, CV Mosby.

McCarthy F: *Essentials of safe dentistry for the medically compromised patient,* Philadelphia, 1989, WB Saunders.

McCarthy, FM: *Medical emergencies in dentistry,* ed 8, Philadelphia, 1982, WB Saunders.

Miller AG Jr: Syncope, *Dent Clin North Am* 26:119, 1982.

OSHA Instruction CPL 2-2.44B, February 27, 1990.

OSHA. Occupational exposure to bloodborne pathogens: final rule, 29 CFR, Part 1910. 1030, Part II, Dec 6, 1991.

Shaber EP, Smith RA: Techniques of drug administration, *Dent Clin North Am* 26:35, 1982.

Stroh JE Jr, Johnson RL: Allergy-related emergencies in dental practice, *Dent Clin North Am* 26:87, 1982.

Trieger N: Special care of the medically compromised patient, *NY State Dent J* 48:451, 1982.

SUGGESTED READINGS

American Dental Association Council on Dental Materials, Instruments, and Equipment: *Dentist's desk reference: materials, instruments and equipment,* Chicago, 1981, The Association.

Bodak-Gyovai LZ: *Oral medicine: patient evaluation and management,* Baltimore, 1980, Williams & Wilkins.

Braun R: *Dentists' manual of emergency medical treatment,* Reston, Va, 1979, Reston.

Capello J et al: Medical emergencies: the dental team approach, *Dent Surv* 53:24, Aug 1977.

Emergency Medical Services—Equipment Supplement, 1991.

Emergency Medical Services, Sept, 1991.

Freeman NS et al: Office emergencies: causes, symptoms, treatment, *Oral Health* 67:60, Oct 1977.

Howell RB: *Office emergency procedures: a self-study course,* Chicago, 1979, American Dental Hygienists' Association.

Jaffe M: Teaching medical emergencies in a dental hygiene program, *NY State Dent J* 48:456, 1982.

Lown B: Lidocaine to prevent ventricular fibrillation, *N Engl J Med* 313:1154, 1985.

Maitland RI: Patient assessment in the dental office emergency, *NY State Dent J* 48:442, 1978.

Malamed SF: *Handbook of medical emergencies in the dental office,* ed 3, St Louis, 1987, CV Mosby.

Martin M et al: Skills in cardiopulmonary resuscitation: a survey of dental practitioners, *JADA* 112:501, 1986.

McCarthy F: A new-patient administered medical history developed for dentistry, *JADA* 111:595, 1985.

McCarthy F: Vital signs—the six minute warnings, *JADA* 100:682, 1980.

McCarthy F, Malamed S: Physical evaluation system to determine medical risk and indicated dental therapy modifications, *JADA* 99:181, 1979.

Morrow GT: Designing a drug kit, *Dent Clin North Am* 26:21, 1982.

Perks ER: The diagnosis and management of sudden collapse in dental practice, I, *Br Dent J* 143:196, 1977.

Proy HG et al: Minicomputer simulation of medical emergencies and advanced life support, *J Dent Educ* 46:657, 1982.

Rose L: Diagnosis and management of medical emergencies in the dental office, *Cont Dent Educ* (self-instruction series) 1:3, 1977.

Rose LF, Hendler BH: *Medical emergencies in dental practice,* Chicago, 1981, Quintessence.

Ryan DE, Bronstein SL: Dentistry and the diabetic patient, *Dent Clin North Am* 26:105, 1982.

Safar P: *Cardiopulmonary cerebral resuscitation,* Stavenger, Norway, 1981, Asmund S Laerdal.

Sanger RG et al: Training program in emergency medical service for the dental profession, *JADA* 98:695, 1979.

Shannon ME: Strokes, *Dent Clin North Am* 26:99, 1982.

Shijatshky M: *Life threatening emergencies in the dental practice,* Chicago, 1975, Quintessence (Translated by HM Koehler).

Solomon AL: Emergency treatment: local and general anesthesia, *NY State Dent J* 48:447, 1982.

Tillis T, Karras D: A preclinical medical emergencies exercise, *Education Update* 5:3, Mar 1987.

Trieger N: Special care of medically compromised patient, *NY State Dent J,* 48:451, 1982.

Trieger N et al: The art of history taking, *J Oral Surg* 36, Feb 1978.

Turner R: First aid in acute myocardial infarction, *Br Med J* 1:356, 1976.

West K: The TB comeback, *Emerg Med Serv,* 1991, pp 63-5.

Woodworth JV, Woodworth CE: Emergency! The dentist's role in prevention and treatment. I, *Gen Dent* 26:35, May-June 1978.

Woodworth JV, Woodworth CE: Emergency! The dentist's role in prevention and treatment. II, *Gen Dent* 26:46, July-Aug 1978.

Woodworth JV, Woodworth CE: Emergency! The dentist's role in prevention and treatment. III, *Gen Dent* 26:56, Sept-Oct 1978.

Zinman EJ: Emergency care: some legal implications, *Dent Surg* 55:46, 1979.

8 GENERAL PHYSICAL EVALUATION AND THE EXTRAORAL AND INTRAORAL EXAMINATION

Catherine Davis
Bonnie Dafoe
Nancy Stutsman Young

LEARNING OUTCOMES

The dental hygienist will be able to

1. State the purposes and advantages of performing a complete general and oral examination for each patient.
2. Identify the characteristics to observe in assessing a patient's general appearance and state why they may be significant to treatment.
3. Use the proper techniques for obtaining a patient's vital signs.
4. Discuss the role dentistry plays in identifying and monitoring hypertension.
5. Describe and use the extraoral and intraoral examination, including:
   a. The names of all structures to be visually inspected and palpated.
   b. Normal landmarks associated with these structures.
   c. The prescribed method of palpation for each structure.
   d. Common abnormalities that may be detected.
6. Given an illustration of an abnormal lesion, describe its location in the mouth, size, and clinical characteristics using medical descriptions of the type of lesion represented.
7. Use the four different methods of examination—inspection, palpation, auscultation, and percussion.

A complete head and neck examination is a vital component of comprehensive health services. The total procedure combines a subjective and objective appraisal of the patient's health and an examination of extraoral structures of the head and neck and intraoral structures. In the appointment sequence, the clinical examination procedures described in this chapter should follow the gathering of all pertinent data in a comprehensive health history. Information recorded in the patient's health history provides not only a summary of his or her health background, but also valuable insight into potential health problems or clinical manifestations that might be detected during the head and neck examination.

The treatment plan designed for the patient must be based on a *thorough identification and description of all observed and suspected health problems*. At this point in treatment, the health history has already provided information regard-

ing past health experiences and insight into current problems of which the patient is aware. The clinical examination will *supplement and update this history by identifying and/or describing the patient's current health status*. The information gathered in the examination will also help the clinician *determine what preventive methods and education* are most appropriate for each patient's needs.

Potential *need for further consultations* with dental or medical specialists is also identified through information gathered in the head and neck examination. Cooperative efforts among health professionals are necessary to provide comprehensive care. The clinical examination will provide clues as to whether the services of specialists such as pathologists, periodontists, endodontists, oral surgeons, or the patient's physician are needed.

Total patient care involves a responsibility for

more than just the patient's teeth and gingiva. It includes an awareness of other health problems that may be manifested during the head and neck examination. Often, *systemic disorders can be identified* through extraoral or intraoral signs and symptoms. The complete examination may reveal signs of nutritional deficiencies or imbalances that have dental implications.

Early detection of diseases that are progressive and irreversibly destructive in nature is a critical factor in determining their extent of destruction. This is especially true of oral cancer. A thorough head and neck examination performed at regular intervals could greatly reduce the incidence of deaths from oral cancer. It is estimated that in 1987 there were 29,800 new cases of oral cancer, 12,100 cases of cancer of the larynx, and 25,800 cases of skin cancer (some of them in the head and neck area). The number of deaths each year from oral cancer alone is estimated at 9,400 (American Cancer Society, 1987). An estimated 30,000 new cases of oral cancer (buccal cavity and pharynx) were expected to occur during 1992 (Boring et al, 1992). Early detection and diagnosis of these malignancies are critical to reduce deaths caused by oral and other cancers.

It is every dental hygienist's responsibility to apply the necessary skills and knowledge to ensure that all patients are not only examined thoroughly, but educated to perform frequent and effective self-examination and thus increase the chances of early detection of cancer. The self-examination procedure is discussed in greater detail later in this chapter. As each patient will be seen at regular recall intervals, you will likely be able to detect health or tissue changes from one appointment to another and thus identify the need for prompt and early treatment of disease or malignancies. You can also use recall appointments to revise or reinforce patient education and self-care methods based on new information gathered at each updated clinical examination. Frequent examinations enable you to become familiar with a patient's normal oral manifestations and to identify deviations.

Throughout the clinical examination, you should *identify contraindications to dental treatment* that would affect the health of the patient, the clinician, or both. Clinical signs of transmissible diseases (such as hepatitis B, acquired immunodeficiency syndrome, (AIDS), syphilis, or severe sore throat) or of other potentially dangerous conditions (such as uncontrolled hypertension) may be apparent at the time of the examination, even if they were not discussed in the health history. Because some oral lesions may be pathognomonic of a human immune deficiency virus (HIV) infection or AIDS, early diagnosis and treatment may prolong and improve the quality of life of people with AIDS (Greenspan et al, 1987; Murray et al, 1985; Silverman et al, 1986). Referring these patients back to their physicians for care protects the health both of the patient and the dental team.

The information gathered from the initial head and neck examination serves as *valuable baseline data* on the patient's health status at the time of the initial appointment. These data form a standard by which to measure progress through treatment and preventive procedures. They are the primary starting point from which the dental professional can measure effectiveness in treatment. If those problems identified in the clinical examination are not resolved through treatment and home care, the professional must reevaluate the current treatment plan to determine what factors may be causing the lack of success and whether or not those factors can be alleviated. Clinical examinations at recall appointments will provide additional data to be added to the patient's overall health profile and ensure a constant reevaluation of present oral conditions.

It is important that the patient's general health and oral conditions be described as completely as possible in the patient's chart to facilitate its use as a *legal record*, if that should become necessary. Documentation needs to be comprehensive and concise. All entries should be in ink and dated (Zarkowski, 1991). Evaluation of the information recorded in patient records is also becoming more and more prevalent in situations involving third-party insurance carriers or when peer review is used to evaluate treatment.

CLINICAL HEAD AND NECK EXAMINATION

The clinical head and neck examination is divided into four basic components: (1) general appraisal, (2) vital signs, (3) extraoral examination, and (4) intraoral examination.

In the following descriptions of each component, the tissues, structures, or functions to be examined are given, along with the suggested examination technique and sequence and possible significant findings. In most cases one of the following four methods of examination will be used to gather clinical information:

inspection. Systematic visual assessment of body tissues, structures, or systems to identify normal and abnormal appearances and/or functioning.

palpation. Use of the fingers or hands to examine the texture, form, and function of soft and hard tissue structures.

auscultation. Listening for sounds produced within the body (such as clicking of the temporomandibular joint [TMJ], abnormal breathing sounds, or vocal fremitus).

percussion. Striking tissues with the fingers or an instrument to hear the resulting sounds and patient response.

Objective information (signs) gained from one or more of these methods, combined with the patient's subjective responses (symptoms), provides a complete description of clinical findings.

General appraisal

Many aspects of the patient's health and general disposition may be detected from simple observation of overall appearance, movements, and responses. The examination methods used are inspection and auscultation. As the patient enters the office or operatory, observe his or her general body weight, height, posture, and gait for abnormal signs. For example, obesity or excessive height deviations may not only provide clues to possible nutritional or endocrine disorders but also indicate necessary alterations in patient positioning. The patient's posture and gait may signal back problems or other conditions that would also affect positioning in the chair. Does the patient limp or seem uncoordinated? Deficiencies of motor or sensory functions, including hand or arm movement, affect the type of home care the patient is capable of performing. Are there additional signs of paralysis, tremors, or other dysfunctions that will affect the patient's needs or treatment? What do the rate and character of the gait or gestures indicate about the patient's level of anxiety? While looking at the extremities, glance at the patient's legs and ankles for signs of swelling or other indications of poor circulation.

Observe the patient's face. Is the skin color normal, pale, or flushed? Does it appear dry or moist? What might the patient's facial expression indicate about his or her general attitude? Are there any signs of facial paralysis, tremors, asymmetry, or other abnormalities?

Monitor the patient's respiration rate. Is it shallow or deep? Is it fast or slow? Is it regular or punctuated with gasps, puffs, or wheezes? Are there signs that the patient has difficulty breathing through either the nose or mouth? Does the chest cavity appear particularly shallow (caved in), or is the patient barrel-chested? Any deviation from normal breathing may be an indication of respiratory or cardiac problems or of an anxiety response to the dental appointment.

Once the patient is seated and engaged in conversation, the clinician can take a closer look at the appearance of the skin, hair, eyes, and nose for signs of abnormalities. Also evaluate the speech for hoarseness, rate, pitch, and general quality. This information may assist in recognizing problems of the larynx (vocal cords) and, again, the patient's anxiety level. A nervous patient may speak at a pitch and rate higher than normal.

Observe the patient's hands to acquire valuable information about his or her general health and attitude. Does the patient bite or chew the nails? Are the palms dry or moist? Are the hands fidgeting and gesturing nervously? Look between the first and second fingers for signs of tobacco stain from cigarettes. A constant tremor or paralysis of the hands or fingers may indicate nerve damage. The hands may also manifest signs of systemic or local diseases. For instance, a patient with anemia may exhibit spoon-shaped nails. Clubbing of the fingers may be associated with cardiac or pulmonary disorders. Swollen, painful finger joints are observed in the arthritic patient. Any of these specific signs would likely have an effect on the overall treatment plan and should be noted.

Because this general appraisal is your first clinical introduction to the patient, it is important to retain the impressions and information you accumulate and use them to guide later discussion with the patient concerning the health history and reactions to dental treatment. As subjective observations are confirmed through the health questionnaire or discussion with the patient, record the final objective findings in the patient's chart.

After reviewing the health history with the patient, if there is no obvious contraindication to proceeding (such as a current contagious disease), the hygienist should explain the content and purpose of the clinical examination. Hopefully, the patient and hygienist will have developed a feeling of mutual trust and confidence and the patient will feel free to ask questions about the procedures and will share responsibility by reporting any symptoms that occur as the examination progresses. When all examination procedures have been explained and agreed to by the patient, assuming there are no contraindications to treatment at this point, the hygienist is ready to proceed with the next portion of the examination—taking the vital signs.

Vital signs

Pulse rate, respiration rate, temperature, and arterial blood pressure constitute the patient's vital signs. Usually this part of the physical examination is performed as one of the initial procedures in the appointment. For some patients, however, apprehension about the dental appointment or rushing to be on time may increase vital sign readings. An attempt should be made to relax the patient through conversation or a calm atmosphere to ensure accuracy of the findings. Repeating the pulse and blood pressure measurements near the end of the appointment may be helpful to ensure accuracy.

Pulse rate. An arterial pulse that reflects the count of heartbeats may be palpated at the following locations that are accessible to the clinician:

radial. Located on the thumb side of the patient's wrist over the radial bone.
brachial. Located in the antecubital fossa before the brachial artery branches into the radial and ulnar arteries in the lower arm.
carotid. Located on the lateral aspect of the neck on either side of the trachea.
temporal. Located slightly above and in front of the ear.
facial. Located at the border of the mandible in the mandibular notch.

Because of its accessibility, the radial pulse in the wrist area is most commonly used for determining the pulse rate during the physical examination. The pulse rate may be affected by age, exercise, and emotional status. Generally, a rate of 60 to 80 beats per minute is considered normal for most adults. Patients accustomed to regular exercise may have lower pulse rates because of the strength and efficiency of the heart muscle's pumping ability. The normal pulse rate for children is 90 to 120 beats per minute.

Technique. (Klimaszewski and Grim, 1985; Malasanos et al, 1986). Seat the patient with the arm supported comfortably at his or her side. Place the first three fingers on the patient's radial

artery. (The clinician's thumb is not used to determine the pulse because it contains a pulse, which may create confusion when determining the patient's pulse rate.) Gently compress the artery against the underlying bone. Count the pulse for 1 minute while noting the rate, rhythm, and character of the beat (Fig. 8-1). If a pulse rate is abnormally fast, slow, irregular, or inconsistent in character, note this in the chart. Repeat the procedure a few minutes later to confirm the previous measurement. Be alert to unusual findings, and discuss the situation with the patient. A physician's consultation may be suggested.

Respiration rate. The hygienist should also note the quality and rate of respirations, especially for patients reporting a health history of respiratory symptoms such as asthma, congestive heart failure, or allergic reactions or for apprehensive patients prone to hyperventilation. Count the inspiration and expiration of air as one breath. Note the rate, rhythm (regular, irregular), type (strong, labored, weak), and depth (shallow, deep) of the patient's quiet breathing. Listen for wheezing sounds, and observe whether breathing occurs primarily through the nose or the mouth.

Record the findings on the chart. Notify the dentist of unusual or abnormal recordings.

Temperature. The average temperature of the body is 98.6° F (37.0° C) for most individuals. There is a certain amount of variation from one individual to another; the normal temperature may range from 97.0° to 99.6° F (36.1° C to 37.6° C) (Malasanos et al, 1986). The temperature also

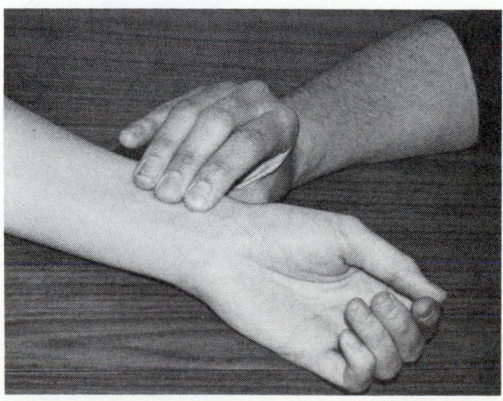

Fig. 8-1. Technique for pulse determination. Place fingers on radial artery. Gently compress artery against bone and count pulse for 1 minute.

fluctuates slightly depending on the time of day, the influence of hormones or drugs, and recent exercise, but for the most part it remains quite stable. When the temperature rises a full degree or more above normal, the patient is said to have a fever. This usually indicates infection or tissue injury. Temperatures below normal may occur with shock or when the patient has been overly exposed to cold. The accepted normal temperature has been established by the oral method, but body temperature can be taken rectally or externally in the axillary or groin areas if the oral method is contraindicated (Kerr, Ash, and Millard, 1983). Standard normal temperature by the rectal method is 99.6° F and by the external methods 97.6° F. The oral temperature method is contraindicated for infants, unconscious patients, those unable to breathe through the nose, or patients unable to hold the thermometer or understand the procedure.

Technique. Using an oral thermometer, shake the mercury indicator to below 96° F or, if digital, clear the reading. Insert the thermometer under the patient's tongue. Ask the patient to hold the thermometer with the lips. Avoid taking the temperature immediately after the mouth has been rinsed with hot or cold liquids. Do not engage the patient in conversation when determining the temperature. Remove the thermometer after 3 min-

utes. Read the thermometer, and repeat the procedure if the accuracy of the reading is in doubt. Record the temperature in the chart. Use a disposable barrier to cover the thermometer.

As an efficiency measure, the pulse and respiration rate may be recorded while the thermometer is in the patient's mouth.

Arterial blood pressure. Blood pressure is the measurement of the force of the blood pushing against the walls of the blood vessels. This pressure is influenced by the physical condition of the heart, the volume of blood being pumped, and the resistance of the arteries to the flow of blood (peripheral resistance). The blood vessel most commonly used for blood pressure determination is the brachial artery in the arm. The normal adult blood pressure is 120/80 mm Hg. The top number refers to systolic pressure, the pressure in the blood vessel at the point of ventricular contraction of the heart. The systolic pressure is the maximal pressure that the arteries undergo when the heart is working. The bottom number refers to diastolic pressure, the pressure in the blood vessel during ventricular relaxation (Fig. 8-2). The diastolic pressure is measured when the heart is at rest and reflects the minimal pressure that is constantly sustained by the arteries. A diagnosis of hypertension is confirmed in adults when the average of two or more diastolic measurements on at least

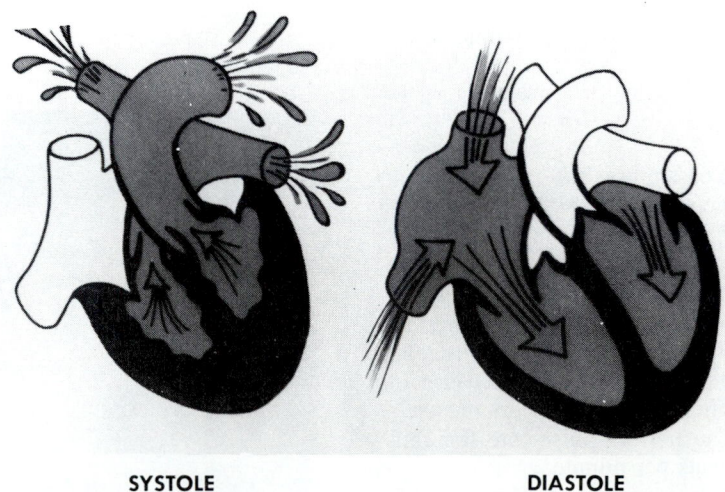

SYSTOLE   DIASTOLE

Fig. 8-2. Heart chamber during ventricular contraction (systole) and during ventricular relaxation (diastole). (From Anderson J, Geistfeld NC: *Hypertension . . . the silent killer,* Minneapolis, University of Minnesota.)

two subsequent visits is 90 mm Hg or higher or when the average systolic measurement on two or more visits is greater than 140 mm Hg (Joint Council, 1984a).

Dental professionals can provide a valuable service for dental care consumers by detecting elevated blood pressure levels of which patients are unaware. It is also important to detect uncontrolled hypertension before dental treatment because of the potential risk to the patient when the stress of dental treatment is added to an already stressed cardiovascular system. Detection of hypertension, patient education, and appropriate referrals and consultations with the patient's physician are all important aspects of the patient assessment procedures. The following information regarding hypertension will help the dental professional understand the nature of hypertension and its significance to dentistry.

Hypertension. Hypertension (high blood pressure) is a common disease, found in approximately 20% of white and 30% of black Americans. Dental professionals can estimate that about 10% to 20% of their patients will suffer from hypertension and that about one-third of these will be unaware of the problem (Cutler, 1986). Hypertension is the second most common cardiovascular disease in the United States. It is the principal risk factor in congestive heart failure, stroke, and kidney failure and a predisposing factor in the acceleration of arteriosclerosis. Undiagnosed or untreated hypertension can shorten a life by 10 to 30 years (Silverberg, 1976). The prevalence of this disease increases with age. Certain population groups are at a higher risk for developing hypertension, including African-Americans, obese individuals, and people with a family history of high blood pressure. Blood pressure screening is an important part of the clinical examination of all dental patients. Many patients visit their dentists more frequently than their physicians, making the dental office a prime location for detecting patients who may require medical consultation and treatment. The American Dental Association has stated that blood pressure measurement for screening purposes is appropriate for all new patients, including children, and for recall patients once a year. The procedure should be part of the office routine for taking or updating the health history (American Dental Association, 1985).

Singer and others (1983) reported that during dental hygiene treatment, diastolic pressure fluctuates an average of 2.1 mm Hg for patients with normal blood pressure, 1.0 mm Hg for nonmedicated hypertensive patients, and 0.1 mm Hg for medicated hypertensive patients. These findings indicate that the stress of anticipated dental treatment does not significantly increase blood pressure and that blood pressure readings taken in the dental office are quite reliable.

Referral. Classification of blood pressure measurements and suggestions for appropriate referral and follow-up are listed in Table 8-1.

Because an increase in diastolic pressure generally results from a narrowing of the arterioles throughout the body, this figure is considered more significant. A diastolic blood pressure of 90 to 104 mm Hg is considered mild hypertension, a diastolic pressure of 105 to 114 mm Hg is considered moderate hypertension, and a diastolic pressure greater than 115 mm Hg is considered severe hypertension (Joint Council, 1984). External influences on blood pressure include exercise, emotional status, and ingestion of stimulants (such as caffeine and nicotine) or depressants (such as alcohol). Systolic pressure tends to be more influenced by external factors than diastolic pressure. Systolic pressure may also be influenced by the age of the patient. Diastolic pressure tends to rise 0.5 to 1.0 mm Hg per year until the seventh decade of life. Therefore slightly elevated systolic readings may be within normal limits for an elderly adult (Cutler, 1986).

Patients whose diastolic blood pressure is between 85 and 89 mm Hg should be informed that their blood pressure reading is higher than normal and that it should be checked annually. These individuals may have a higher risk for developing diagnosed hypertension. If the diastolic blood pressure is between 90 and 104 mm Hg or the systolic measurement is 140 to 199, the patient should be informed that the blood pressure should be checked by a physician. If the diastolic blood pressure is between105 and 114 mm Hg, the patient should be referred for medical confirmation. A telephone consultation with the patient's family physician is appropriate to determine whether dental treatment should be continued for the day and to establishcommunication for following the patient's medical status. If the diastolic blood pressure is greater than 115 mm Hg or the systolic blood pressure is greater than 200 mm Hg, the patient should be allowed to remain quiet for at least 5 minutes and the reading should be con-

Table 8-1. Classification of blood pressure readings and recommendations for individuals aged 18 years or over

Blood pressure	Classification	Recommended follow-up
Diastolic (mm Hg)		
<85	Normal blood pressure	Recheck at each appointment
85 to 89	High normal blood pressure	Inform patient that blood pressure reading was high and recommend medical evaluation
90 to 104	Mild hypertension	Refer patient for evaluation by physician within 2 months; request medical consultation; use routine dental management and stress reduction protocol
105 to 114	Moderate hypertension	Refer patient for evaluation within 2 weeks; request medical consult before dental therapy; use stress reduction protocol
≥115	Severe hypertension	Refer patient for medical evaluation immediately; postpone all elective dental procedures until blood pressure is controlled; request medical consultation
Systolic (mm Hg)		
(When DBP is <90 mm Hg)		
<140	Normal blood pressure	Recheck at each recall appointment; use routine dental management
140 to 159	Borderline isolated systolic hypertension	Refer patient for medical evaluation within 2 months; request medical consultation; use routine dental management and stress reduction protocol
≥160	Isolated systolic hypertension	Refer promptly for medical evaluation; request medical consultation before beginning dental therapy
≥200		Refer promptly for medical evaluation (within 2 weeks); postpone elective dental procedures until blood pressure is controlled; request medical consultation before beginning dental treatment

firmed. If the blood pressure is still elevated after two or more measurements, dental treatment should be delayed and *immediate* medical referral and confirmation obtained.

In most cases hypertension is an asymptomatic disease. Some patients with hypertension may complain of symptoms including severe headaches, dizziness, blurred vision, or signs of renal disease. Blood pressure readings should be correlated with findings such as these in the medical history.

When a medical referral is made, the patient should understand that: (1) his or her blood pressure exceeds normal limits; (2) hypertension is often asymptomatic, (3) uncontrolled high blood pressure has serious consequences; (4) long-term follow-up and therapy are necessary, and (5) therapy will control but not cure high blood pressure (Joint Council, 1984a).

In addition to the role of screening patients for untreated or uncontrolled hypertension, the dental professional must consider the implications of this disease for dental treatment. Recommendations

for dental management of hypertensive patients and the need for medical consultation should be followed. Patients with uncontrolled high blood pressure may have a higher risk of suffering a medical emergency as a result of the stresses of dental treatment. The dental professional must assess whether these patients can safely tolerate the physical and psychologic stresses of the planned dental procedures.

In addition to referring the patient for prompt diagnosis and treatment and obtaining a medical consultation, certain modifications of the dental appointment can help to reduce the potential medical risks of dental treatment for hypertensive patients. Dental professionals should recognize signs of anxiety in these patients and work to eliminate their causes by taking time to explain all procedures and providing reassurance and moral support during the procedures. The dentist may prescribe premedication for anxious patients before the dental appointment. Nitrous oxide analgesia and adequate pain control measures also help to reduce anxiety and discomfort during the dental visit. Appointments should be scheduled early in the day when patients are well rested and should be kept as short as possible (Shapiro and Avery, 1984). Postoperative pain and anxiety control should also be implemented as needed.

Dental professionals should record the names and dosages of all medications prescribed for treatment of hypertension. Dentists and hygienists should be aware of the side effects of these drugs and of potential contraindications or interactions with anesthetic solutions or other drugs used in dental treatment. The degree of patient compliance with the prescribed antihypertensive therapy should also be determined before dental treatment. Patients diagnosed as hypertensive must understand the importance of complying with prescribed drug therapy to control their condition.

In a case tried by the New Jersey Supreme Court, a dentist administered a local anesthetic with an epinephrine vasoconstrictor to a patient for a routine restoration. The patient collapsed with a stroke and died a few days later. Negligence was alleged in this case because the dentist failed to make a physical evaluation or to complete a medical history before administering anesthesia. Because of these omissions the clinician was unaware of the patient's cardiovascular status. The court upheld the ruling of negligence. This is probably the most specific case dealing with a dentist's failure to conduct a physical examination that may have detected hypertension and altered the series of events (Conway, 1980).

Treatment. In mild cases of hypertension, weight reduction and control of sodium intake may bring the blood pressure into normal range. When drug therapy is necessary, a "stepped-care" program is advisable. This approach entails initiating therapy with a small dose of antihypertensive medication, increasing the dosage of that drug, and adding one medication after another gradually as needed until the goal blood pressure is achieved, side effects become intolerable, or the maximum dose is reached (Joint National Committee, 1984a). Depending on the patient, several medications may be necessary, making medical follow-up an important part of ongoing care. Generally, the need for treatment continues for life (Silverberg, 1976).

Diuretics are the first drug of choice for treating mild hypertension. These medications promote the renal excretion of water and sodium ions. Positive results occur in about 50% of mildly hypertensive patients (Gaynor, 1983). Common diuretics include hydrochlorothiazide, furosemide, and spironolactone. The second step after diuretics is adrenergic inhibiting agents, such as reserpine, methyldopa, clonidine, and propranolol hydrochloride. These agents deplete or inhibit norepinephrine. A vasodilator such as hydralazine may be added as the third step in medical therapy. For severe hypertension, the fourth step would include an additional adrenergic inhibiting agent such as guanethidine sulfate.

Implications for dental treatment. Antihypertensive medications often cause postural hypotension (positional low blood pressure); this necessitates raising the patient slowly from the supine position to prevent dizziness or syncope. Antihypertensive medications may affect the fluid balance in the oral cavity, causing a dry mouth with resultant dental complications. A saliva substitute and concomitant fluoride therapy may need to be recommended for patient use. Analgesic agents (cyclopropane, halothane) may produce a decrease in oxygen in the blood and may cause a rapid increase in blood pressure for these patients. Local and general anesthetics and vasopressors may potentiate the hypotensive effects of the antihypertensive medication, possibly causing cardiovascular collapse and shock. Epinephrine in the form of a gingival retraction cord or in a local anesthetic is contraindicated in patients taking guanethidine, reserpine, or methyldopa. It may potentiate the pressure effects of catecholamine, possibly causing a rapid increase in blood pressure. In a well-controlled hypertensive patient, 0.1 mg of epinephrine is allowed if necessary.

The dental team and physician need to cooperate in detecting, treating, and following the hypertensive patient. Noting the blood pressure at each dental visit is a preventive health service that cannot be overlooked. For the patient with a history of hypertension, the medical history should be updated at recall intervals by inquiring about current medications and recent visits to the physician, in addition to recording the blood pressure for the day.

Technique. Obtain a stethoscope and a sphygmomanometer (blood pressure apparatus). This usually includes an inflatable bladder enclosed in an unyielding cuff, which will be wrapped around the patient's arm. The cuff must be the correct width for the diameter of the patient's arm. The width of the bladder should be slightly less than half the circumference of the arm, and the length of the bladder should be at least 80% of the arm circumference. Approximately two-thirds of the upper arm should be covered by the cuff when it is in place. If the cuff is too narrow, the blood pressure reading will be erroneously high; if it is too wide, the reading may be too low. Several sizes of cuffs are available to fit small to obese patients. The circumference of the arm, not the age of the patient, is the determining factor in selecting the proper sphygmomanometer. Attached to the cuff is a rubber bulb to pump air into the bladder and a gauge (aneroid dial or mercury column) that reflects the pressure in the blood vessel as the air in the bladder is deflated by regulation of the air-release valve.

Also available is equipment that inflates and deflates the cuff automatically and displays a computerized digital readout of the blood pressure. Units that provide electronic digital readouts of blood pressure measurement are easy to use because a stethoscope is not needed. They are especially useful for individuals who are hearing impaired. Disadvantages of these units are (1) they are more expensive than standard manual equipment and (2) they are more likely to result in erroneous measurements, because their readings are sometimes inaccurate and because they are battery-dependent.

The following steps should be followed when taking a blood pressure measurement using a standard sphygmomanometer and stethoscope:

1. Allow the patient to relax in the chair for at least 5 minutes before taking the blood pressure to allow the blood pressure to stabilize. Seat the patient in a comfortable position in which the arm can be easily supported at heart level. Ask the patient to roll up a sleeve or to slip the arm out of the clothing to permit access to the brachial artery. Rest the arm in a slightly flexed position with the hand open and relaxed.

2. Wrap the cuff around the patient's arm with the arrows centered over the brachial artery. The lower border of the cuff should be 1 inch (or about the width of 2 fingers) above the bend in the arm. Place the manometer gauge (either a mercury gauge or an aneroid gauge) in a position where it can be viewed easily (Fig. 8-3). With a mercury manometer, the gauge should be viewed so that the meniscus is at eye level.

3. Find the radial pulse just above the thumb at the wrist joint. Close the valve of the pressure bulb (rotate clockwise until tightened) and inflate the cuff until the pulse is no longer felt. Note the pressure registering on the gauge. Open the air-release clamp until the cuff is

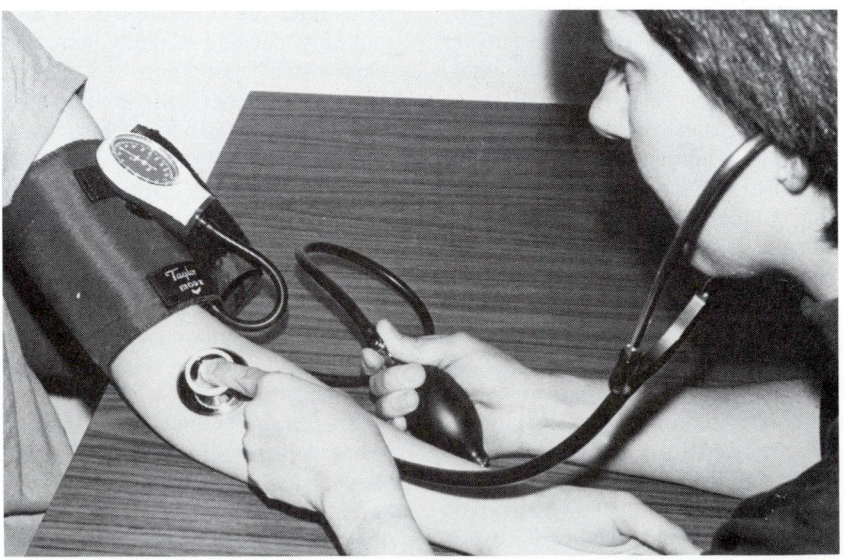

Fig. 8-3. Place cuff 1 inch above bend in arm with gauge in position for easy viewing.

completely deflated. Wait 30 to 60 seconds before reinflating.

4. Place the stethoscope comfortably in the ears with the earpieces directed forward. Place the diaphragm of the stethoscope over the brachial artery approximately 1 inch from the bend in the arm, towards the hand, and close to the inner aspect of the forearm (Fig. 8-4). The diaphragm should be in total contact with the skin and positioned just below (but not touching) the cuff or tubing.

5. Inflate the cuff 20 to 30 mm Hg higher than the pressure at which the radial pulse disappeared, as noted in step 3.

6. Using the air-release valve, slowly deflate the cuff at a rate of about 2 to 3 mm Hg per heartbeat. Note the pressure at which the first pulse beat is heard. This is the systolic pressure. Continue to release the air in the cuff. The pulse sound will increase in intensity, then become muffled and disappear. Note the pressure at which the last sound occurs. This is the diastolic pressure. Continue listening during the entire range of deflation and at least 22 mm below the diastolic reading. On occasion there will be what is known as an "auscultatory gap" in which the sounds disappear for 10 to 15 mm Hg and then return. Errors in measurement caused by the "auscultatory gap" can be prevented if the clinician inflates the cuff beyond the point where the pulse is lost and listens to the entire range of sounds, continuing past the last sound. If the sounds are too faint to allow an accurate reading, ask the patient to open and close the fist 8 to 10 times after the blood pressure cuff is inflated above the systolic level; then take the readings as usual. Or elevate the patient's arm for several seconds before inflating the cuff; then inflate the cuff with the arm still elevated. Lower the arm and deflate the cuff in the normal manner while taking the measurement readings.

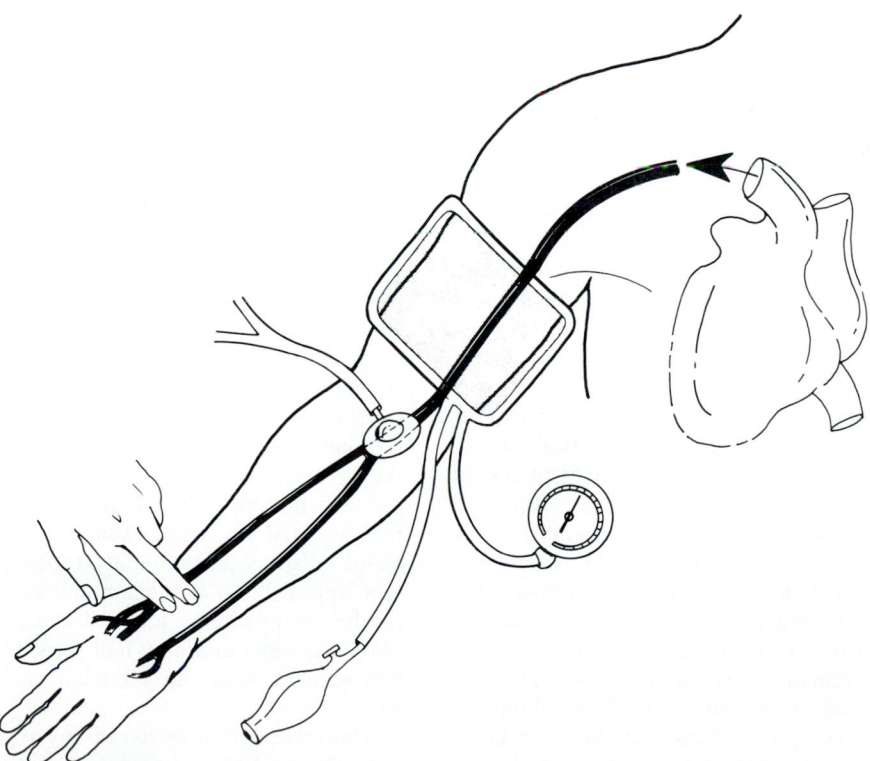

Fig. 8-4. Place diaphragm of stethoscope over branch of brachial artery. This is approximately 1 inch from bend in arm towards hand and close to inner aspect of forearm.
(From Boundy SS, Reynolds, NJ: *Current concepts in dental hygiene*, vol 2, St Louis, 1979, CV Mosby.)

7. Record the blood pressure measurements as a fraction, as follows:

Systolic pressure/diastolic pressure: $\frac{120}{80}$

This number is spoken as "120 over 80." Also make a note of the arm position of the patient (e.g., $\frac{120}{80}$ RAS reg [right arm sitting, regular adult cuff]).

8. Let the patient relax the arm once again before repeating the procedure to confirm the reading. Avoid repeating the procedure several times in a row without allowing the patient's circulation to return to normal. This may arouse anxiety in the patient, affect the reading, and make the arm quite uncomfortable.

9. Compare the current reading with past blood pressure readings (if available). Consult the dentist and physician when the systolic pressure is greater than 160 mm Hg or the diastolic pressure is greater than 95 mm Hg. Note any unusual findings or changes in the pattern of blood pressure recordings as compared with past visits.

Table 8-2 shows the upper limits of blood pressure for children. When recording blood pressure readings for children, three numbers should be recorded (as in 110/80/70), compared with two numbers for an adult (as in 110/70). The first number (110) is the systolic reading recorded when the first two regular beats are heard. The second number (80) is recorded when the tapping sounds become muffled and lower in pitch. This point is the accepted diastolic reading for children. The third number (70) is the cessation or disappearance of all sound.

Extraoral examination

Once vital signs are recorded, the hygienist begins the extraoral examination. For this part of the head and neck examination, the patient should be seated in an upright or semisupine position. It is difficult to examine the deeper structures of the neck and submandibular area with the patient in a full supine position because many of the soft tissue structures tend to fall back into the deeper structures of the head and neck and are less accessible for examination and palpation. The clinician will be working either in front of or behind the patient, depending on which structures are being examined. At all times, the patient should be positioned for maximum visibility. All supplies that are needed for the examination procedure should be assembled and accessible to the clinician.

Table 8-2. Upper limits of normal blood pressure in children

Age (in years)	Arterial pressure (mm Hg) systolic/diastolic
14-18	<135/90
10-14	<125/85
6-10	<120/80
<6	<110/75

Modified from Joint National Committee on Detection, Evaluation and Treatment of High Blood Pressure, *Arch Intern Med* 144:1045, 1984.

The following guidelines should be considered while the examination is being performed:

1. The clinician should be able to locate each structure in the head and neck region that will be examined.
2. All structures being examined should be accessible for observation or palpation.
3. The clinician should use a thorough technique to examine each structure.
4. The clinician should use a sequence of examination that is systematic and efficient in time and motion.

Patient considerations. The patient's needs for privacy and comfort should be carefully considered during the head and neck examination. Patients appreciate a clinical attitude that demonstrates professional interest in their feelings and concerns. Before beginning the clinical examination, the clinician should explain the procedure and why it is an important part of dental health care. The clinician should speak in a quiet and friendly voice so that the conversation will not be overheard by other patients or personnel outside the operatory. Patients deserve to have all procedures explained to them and to be considered as partners in care rather than objects of care. During the head and neck examination, the clinician should display a confident attitude and a competent approach to the examination. Patients may not be used to being touched and examined in so close a manner and may feel some shyness or embarrassment until the clinician can put them at ease.

Many patients may avoid any type of physical examination because they fear the results of the procedure. The clinician can ease this apprehension by explaining the importance of regular professional examinations and self-examinations and by reinforcing this behavior in the patient. The patient's fears may be heightened if the clinician discusses the clinical findings in technical jargon that the patient cannot understand. The clinician can accomplish a great deal of patient education on self-assessment of oral conditions by using language that is easily understood and by thoroughly discussing the significance of diagnoses with the patient in lay terms. For instance, while examining the extraoral and intraoral structures, the clinician can describe what is being examined and why. This eliminates any guesswork and potential misunderstanding by the patient. An excerpt from such a conversation might sound like this:

Mrs. Willis, the next thing I will be examining is your tongue. Have you ever looked closely at your tongue? If you will watch me in the mirror you're holding, I'll show you how it can be examined and what to look for. First, I'd like you to place the tip of your tongue on this gauze square so that I can move it easily. Good! Now, as I look at the top of the tongue, I can see that it has a slight coating. This can be easily removed by brushing the tongue with a toothbrush. Otherwise, your tongue looks very pink and healthy. These bumps back here are normal papillae. Now I'm going to check the sides of the tongue for any areas that look like sores or for any white or red patches. The sides of the tongue and the floor of the mouth are two areas where oral cancer may sometimes occur, so you will want to take the opportunity to inspect these surfaces yourself at home. After seeing them here and at home, you'll have a good idea of what they normally look like and it will be easier for you to recognize any changes that might occur. These structures in the back of your tongue are also normal. They are the lingual tonsils. Now I'm going to feel your tongue for lumps or hard areas. Everything looks and feels fine, Mrs. Willis. Do you have any questions about what I've shown you?

In this way the patient will gain an understanding of the normal structures of the mouth while observing the clinician's examination and listening to the clinician's explanations. In addition, patients should be given the following instructions regarding their own oral self-assessments: (1) they should look for unusual lumps or bumps in the mouth; (2) they should check for unusual color changes that may appear as white, red, or bluish patches, or areas that appear to be speckled with both white and red areas; (3) they should establish a sequence for examining all parts of the mouth; (4) they should perform their own oral examina-

tion on a monthly basis; and (5) they should observe any unusual lesion for 2 weeks to make sure it heals; if not, they should report it to a dentist or physician promptly (Glass et al, 1975).

Not only will patients benefit from the health information you provide but they will also appreciate your interest in taking the time to answer their questions and discuss their concerns. This process will help make each patient a more educated and prevention-oriented health consumer. A more detailed explanation of self-assessment techniques for dental patients is given later in this chapter.

Visual inspection. The extraoral examination includes two components. The first is a visual inspection of each structure, which is followed by palpation and auscultation.

For the visual inspection the patient should be seated in an upright or semisupine position, with the clinician seated facing him or her. Glasses should be removed, and clothing that restricts access to the neck (such as tight-fitting collars and tie) should be loosened. Starting from the top of the head and neck area and moving downward, examine the hair for texture, amount, and distribution. Note any apparent scalp lesions, such as scars, sores, or growths. Examine for the presence of lice or other transmittable conditions within the hair.

Next examine the face for symmetry, form, and profile. Observe the skin of the face for abnormal pigmentation, hair, texture, scars, or lesions. Facial asymmetry may be indicative of inflammatory conditions such as dental abscesses or mumps. Stroke victims or others who suffer from unilateral paralysis of facial muscles (Bell's palsy) are unable to produce normal facial expressions on the affected side. The muscles and soft tissues of the affected side may have a drooping or flaccid appearance.

Note the general color of the skin. An abnormal redness may indicate the presence of inflammation, fever, sunburn, or increased vascularity resulting from excitement or exertion. Abnormal paleness could indicate anemia, systemic illness, or shock. Patients with a history of heart or pulmonary disorders may exhibit a slightly bluish cast to the skin. Jaundice or yellow skin may be indicative of liver disease (hepatitis), red blood cell disorders, or drug toxicity.

Question the patient about the presence of any raised lesions, such as moles, to determine how long they have been present and whether they have undergone any changes in size, texture, color, or tendency to bleed. Malignant melanoma is a deadly type of skin cancer that can appear as lesions similar to common skin moles. More than 32,000 new cases of melanoma were predicted to occur in 1992 (Boring et al, 1992).

The clinician should be aware of the risk factors and clinical characteristics of melanoma to aid in its detection during the head and neck examination. Factors that may increase the risk of this cancer include light-colored complexion or eyes; history of severe sunburn during childhood, teenage, and early adult years; extensive sun exposure as a result of occupation or recreational habits; presence of xeroderma pigmentosum or increased number of pigmented nevi in childhood; and family history of malignant melanoma.

Malignant melanoma can result from an abnormal change in a preexisting pigmented nevus or can develop as a totally new lesion, particularly in individuals 40 years or older. Because its appearance can be similar to that of other common, benign skin lesions, the clinician should be familiar with the characteristics that distinguish a benign lesion from a potentially malignant lesion. Most benign pigmented lesions (common moles) have round and symmetric shapes, regular margins, and uniform color and are less than 6 mm in diameter. In contrast, early malignant melanomas have asymmetric shapes with irregular borders, variegated color (multiple shades), and diameters greater than 6 mm.

The following changes in a raised skin lesion should be considered danger signs (Friedman et al, 1985):

Change in color to variegated shades of dark brown, black, red, white, or blue or a spread of color from lesion into surrounding skin

Change in size that is sudden or continuous

Change in shape resulting in irregular margins

Change in elevation

Change in surface, including scaliness, erosion, oozing, crusting, ulceration, or bleeding

Change in the surrounding skin, including redness or swelling

Change in sensation, including itching, tenderness, or pain

Change in consistency, including softening or friability

If the clinical head and neck examination and the patient's report of relevant signs or symptoms indicate that skin lesions may be abnormal, the patient should be promptly referred to his or her physician for a definitive diagnosis. Early detection and treatment of malignant melanoma significantly increase the chances for survival.

Scars are indications of past trauma to the head or face. Discuss the cause of the trauma to determine its relevance to the patient's medical and dental history.

While examining the eyes, observe the following structures:

sclerae. Note color and signs of irritation.
pupils. Note size and reactivity to stimuli such as light.
eyelids. Note texture, form, color, and habits (blinking).
conjunctivae. Note color, degree of moisture, and presence of foreign bodies; examine by retracting the lower lid in a downward direction with the tip of the index finger.

Examine the nose for form, symmetry, and obstructions. The airflow can be examined by placing the dental mirror underneath the patient's nostrils during normal respiration.

Examine the lips for symmetry, form, texture, color, and habits. Note signs of irritation, chapping, or breaks in the skin, especially at the corners of the mouth. Chapped lips should be protected with a coating of petroleum jelly or other lubricant to prevent the dried tissues from breaking open during the examination. Mouth ulcers or intact and healing vesicles on the lips should never be touched with unprotected hands. Always follow universal precautions as described in Chapter 3. A recurrent viral infection, herpetic whitlow, can be established in the fingers of the clinician in this manner. Examine the function of the lips by asking the patient to open and close the mouth. Note lack of closure or mouth-breathing tendencies.

Examine the ears for form, texture, hair, symmetry, and color. Be sure to look behind the ears for possible lesions that would normally be shielded from view.

Check the neck area for symmetry of the structures in the neck. Examine the skin of the neck for pigmentation, texture, scars, obvious swellings, or lesions.

Description of significant findings. It is important to describe all abnormal or unusual findings in the patient's chart in terminology that is clear, concise, and descriptive and provides the dentist and/or oral pathologist with sufficient data on which to base a diagnosis. The color, morphology, surface texture, size in millimeters or centimeters, and symptoms of all lesions should be described. The patient should be questioned about the history of each lesion. Determine whether or not the patient has been aware of the lesion, how long it has been present, and what symptoms it has caused. The following descriptive categories and terminology may help the dental hygienist to describe the clinical findings accurately (McCann and Wesley, 1987):

1. Morphology. Note whether the lesion is localized or generalized, single or multiple, and whether multiple lesions are separate or coalescing.
   a. Raised lesions.
      Are lesions filled with clear fluid or pus (vesicles, pustules, bullae) or solid (papule, nodule, tumor, plaque)?
      Do lesions have a sessile or a pedunculated base?
   b. Depressed lesions (ulcers).
      Is there a regular or irregular border or outline?
      Is the margin raised or smooth?
      Is it superficial or deep?
   c. Flat lesions.
      Are borders regular or irregular?
2. Surface texture. Describe the texture of the lesion as verrucous, papillomatous, fissured, corrugated, crusted, or smooth.
3. Consistency. Do raised or palpable lesions feel hard, firm, or soft?
4. Size. Measure the dimensions of visible lesions in millimeters with a probe; estimate the size of palpable lesions that lie beneath the surface of the skin or mucous membrane.
5. Color. Does the lesion display a single, uniform color or multiple colors or shades?
6. Symptoms. Is the lesion associated with pain, tenderness, itching, swelling, or other discomfort?

Lesions detected during the examination should be described using the following descriptive terms:

petechiae. Red-purple discoloration less than 0.5 cm in diameter.
purpura. Red-purple discoloration greater than 0.5 cm in diameter.
ecchymoses. Red-purple discoloration of variable size.
macule. Flat, nonpalpable circumscribed lesion less than 1 cm in diameter (such as freckles, flat moles, rubeola, and rubella).
patch. Flat, nonpalpable, irregularly shaped lesion larger than 1 cm.
papule. Elevated, palpable, firm, circumscribed lesion less than 1 cm in diameter (such as warts or pigmented nevi).
plaque. Elevated, flat-topped, firm, tough, superficial lesion greater than 1 cm in diameter.
nodule. Elevated, firm, circumscribed, palpable lesion, 1 to 2 cm in diameter (such as lipomas, traumatic fibromas, and lesions associated with rheumatoid arthritis, leprosy, and syphilis).
tumor. Elevated, solid mass greater than 2 cm in diameter (such as tori, polyps, papillomas, and neoplasms).
vesicle. Elevated, circumscribed, superficial, lesion that is filled with clear fluid and less than 1 cm in diameter (blister).
bulla. Vesicle greater than 1 cm in diameter.
pustule. Similar to vesicle but filled with pus (as in acne).
cyst. Elevated, circumscribed, palpable, lesion that is encapsulated and filled with liquid or semisolid material.
fissure. Linear crack or break (such as angular cheilosis).
erosion. Depressed, moist, glistening lesion that follows rupture of vesicle or bulla; larger than a fissure.
ulcer. Defect in the skin or mucosa that extends beyond the surface epithelium and into the underlying tissues. Reddened border may be ragged or punched out; depressed bases may appear soft or indurated with a floor that is smooth, granular, glazed, pus-covered, or hemorrhagic; may be painless or extremely sensitive (as in acute necrotizing ulcerative gingivitis, traumatic injuries, certain types of oral cancer).
hyperplasia. Increased number of cells resulting in an overgrowth of tissue.
keratosis. Abnormal thickening of the outer layers of skin or mucosa that may appear as white, gray, or brown lesions; may occur as localized or diffuse areas (as in linea alba, cheek biting, nicotine stomatitis, certain lesions of lichen planus, and leukoplakia).

Lesions may be further delineated through the use of the following descriptors:

confluent. Blending or occurring together; originally separate but subsequently combined.
corrugated. A rippled surface.
crusted. A hard, scablike surface.
discrete. Separate, not blending or occurring together.
induration. Hardened area of tissue.
pedunculated. Elevated papillary-type lesion attached to underlying tissue by a stem or narrow connector.
papillomatous. Nipplelike growths.

sessile. Attachment of a lesion by a broad base.
verrucose. A wartlike surface.

Extraoral palpation. The clinician is now ready to continue the extraoral examination by palpating all extraoral structures. One of the following methods of palpation will be indicated for each structure, or several techniques may be combined.

digital palpation. Use of a finger to examine tissues.
bidigital palpation. Use of one or more fingers and the thumb to examine tissues by grasping the tissue between thumb and fingers.
manual palpation. Use of all the fingers of one hand to examine tissues.
bimanual palpation. Use of both hands by grasping tissues between them for examination.
bilateral palpation. Examination of structures on both sides of the face or neck simultaneously to detect differences between the two sides.
circular compression. Moving the fingertips in a circular pattern over a structure while simultaneously applying pressure to the tissue.

It is important for the clinician to palpate soft tissue structures against a harder structure such as underlying bone, other fingers, or hands. If the soft tissues are not supported by some means, there is greater possibility that abnormal masses might be displaced away from the examining fingers and not detected. Firm yet gentle pressure should be applied to the soft tissues to feel through all layers of skin and muscle. A hesitant examination technique that evaluates only the surface of the skin will not accomplish this goal.

Sequencing the palpation. The following sequence of the palpation procedure is designed to examine all structures in a logical and systematic order that avoids "hopping" from one area of the head to another. Following a set pattern of examination guarantees that the clinician always knows which structures have or have not been examined in case the procedure is interrupted, and provides for efficient time and motion management. As you begin the examination, ask the patient to report any feelings of discomfort or tenderness in the areas being palpated.

The first structure to be palpated is the mentalis muscle. This muscle attaches to the lower lip and inserts into the symphysis of the mandible. Palpate it with digital compression, rolling the tissue over the mandible. Have the patient swallow and observe the function of this muscle in swallowing. Patients with abnormal swallowing habits often grimace and wrinkle the chin when using this muscle to assist in swallowing. (A glass of water may help the patient in swallowing at various points during the examination.)

Examine the anterior border of the mandible next. From a position behind the patient, use bidigital and circular compression of the soft tissues, starting at the symphysis of the mandible and moving posteriorly along the borders of the mandible (Fig. 8-5). Through palpation, examine the soft tissues and underlying bone to locate normal bony landmarks, deviations in symmetry, tenderness, and crepitus (cracking sounds). Continue this method of palpation bilaterally until the angle of the mandible is reached.

The occipital lymph nodes are located at the base of the skull at the back of the head. Ask the patient to lean his or her head forward, and apply digital circular compression bilaterally with your fingertips. Palpation should begin at the back of the neck and extend horizontally to the sternocleidomastoid muscle (Fig. 8-6). The occipital lymph nodes drain the posterior scalp region. Therefore any deviations in lymph nodes in that region may indicate an infection or other alteration in the scalp region.

The auricular and parotid lymph nodes are located behind, beneath, and in front of the ears. Begin by applying the fingertips in digital compression and circular movement to the area of the posterior auricular nodes. These nodes drain the ear and parotid area. If you notice any deviations (e.g., pain, fixation, or hardness) evaluate the sites that the nodes drain to locate the sources of a potential lesion. The palpation should be done bilaterally to identify deviations from one side to another. Continue this palpation, moving around the base of the ear and anterior to the ear, examining the parotid nodes and the anterior auricular nodes, which are located anterior to the tragus of the ear. Note enlargements, tenderness, degree of mobility, and firmness of nodes (Fig. 8-7).

Palpate the temporomandibular joint bilaterally by placing the index fingers of each hand just anterior to the outer meatus of the ear and asking the patient to open and close the mouth slowly several times. As the patient opens and closes, observe the face for deviations in mandibular function. Feel for abnormal function of the joints and differences in function between the right and left sides (Figs. 8-8 and 8-9). Question the patient about any painful symptoms associated with these

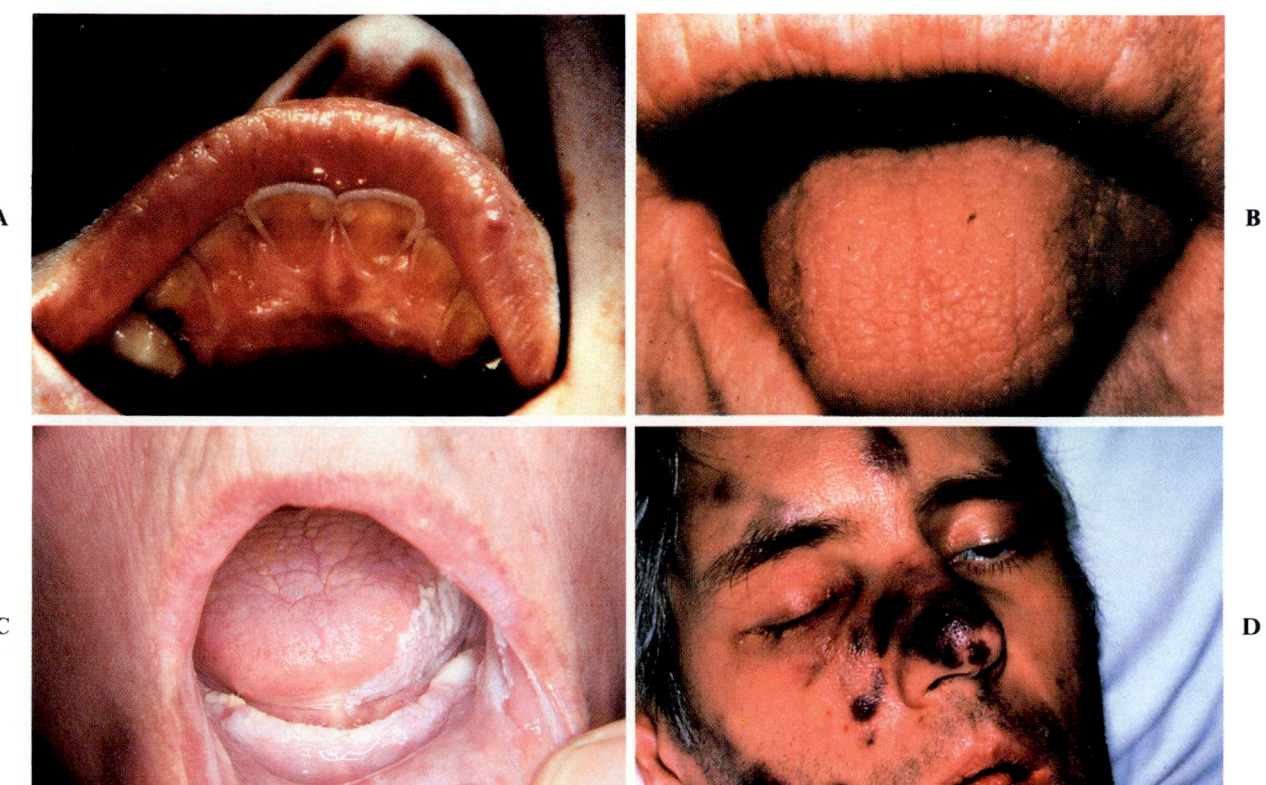

Plate 1. A, Maxillary lingual view of a bulimic patient who had self-induced vomiting for 5 years. **B,** Postradiation therapy patient exhibiting severe xerostomia and cobblestone appearance of tongue (scrotal tongue). **C,** Tobacco lesion in a denture wearer. Tobacco was placed beneath denture, inducing a large leukoplakia lesion on ventral and lateral surfaces of tongue and on alveolar ridge. **D,** Extraoral multiple purple lesions consistent with Kaposi's sarcoma in AIDS patient.

(*C* from Smith-Turner-Robbins: *Atlas of oral pathology*, St Louis, 1991, Mosby–Year Book. *D* courtesy Dr. Michael Finkelstein, Iowa City, Iowa.)

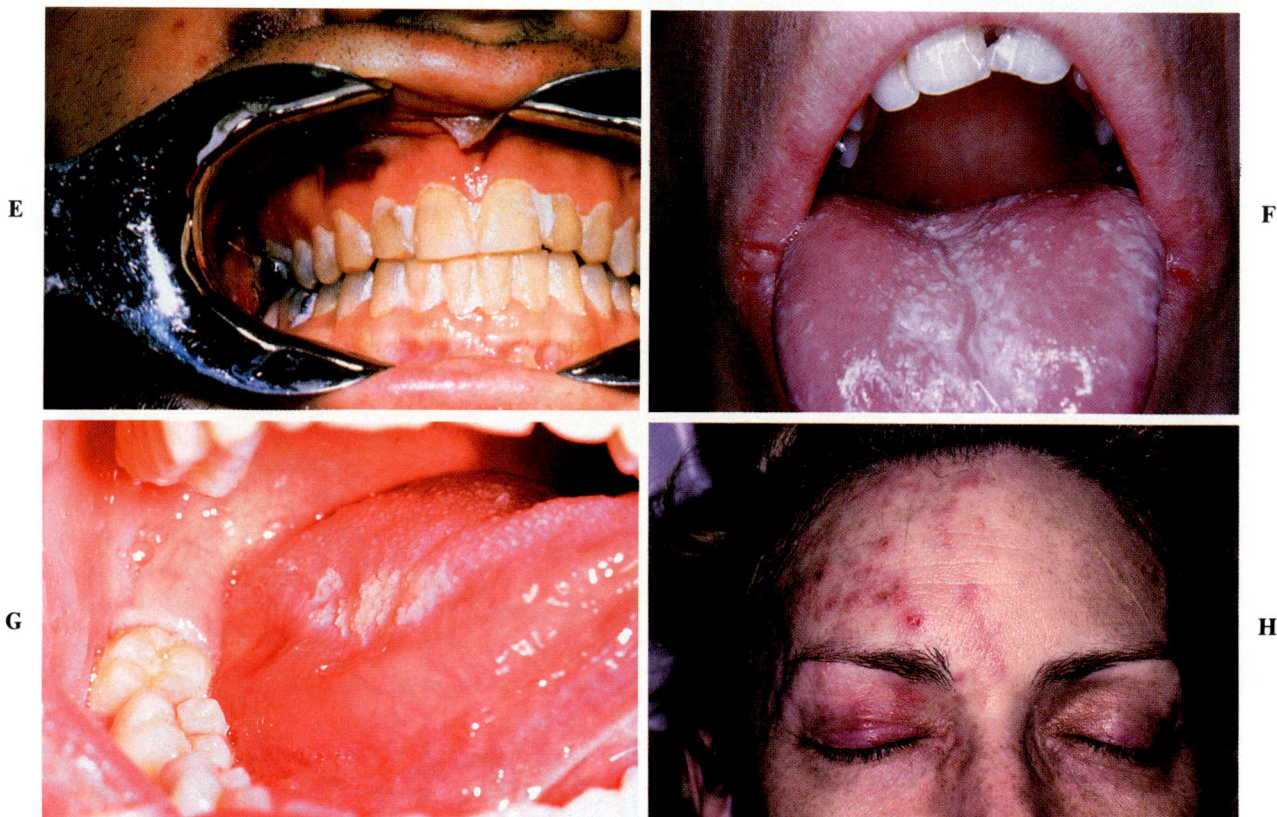

Plate 1, *cont'd*. **E,** Intraoral view of same patient as in **D. F,** Candidiasis of tongue. **G,** Hairy leukoplakia on lateral border of tongue in an HIV-positive patient. **H,** Note unilateral distribution of painful vesicles along V-1 in patient suffering from herpes zoster (i.e., shingles).
(*E* and *G* courtesy of Dr. Michael Finkelstein, Iowa City, Iowa. *F* and *H* from Smith-Turner-Robbins: *Atlas of oral pathology,* St Louis, 1991, Mosby – Year Book.)

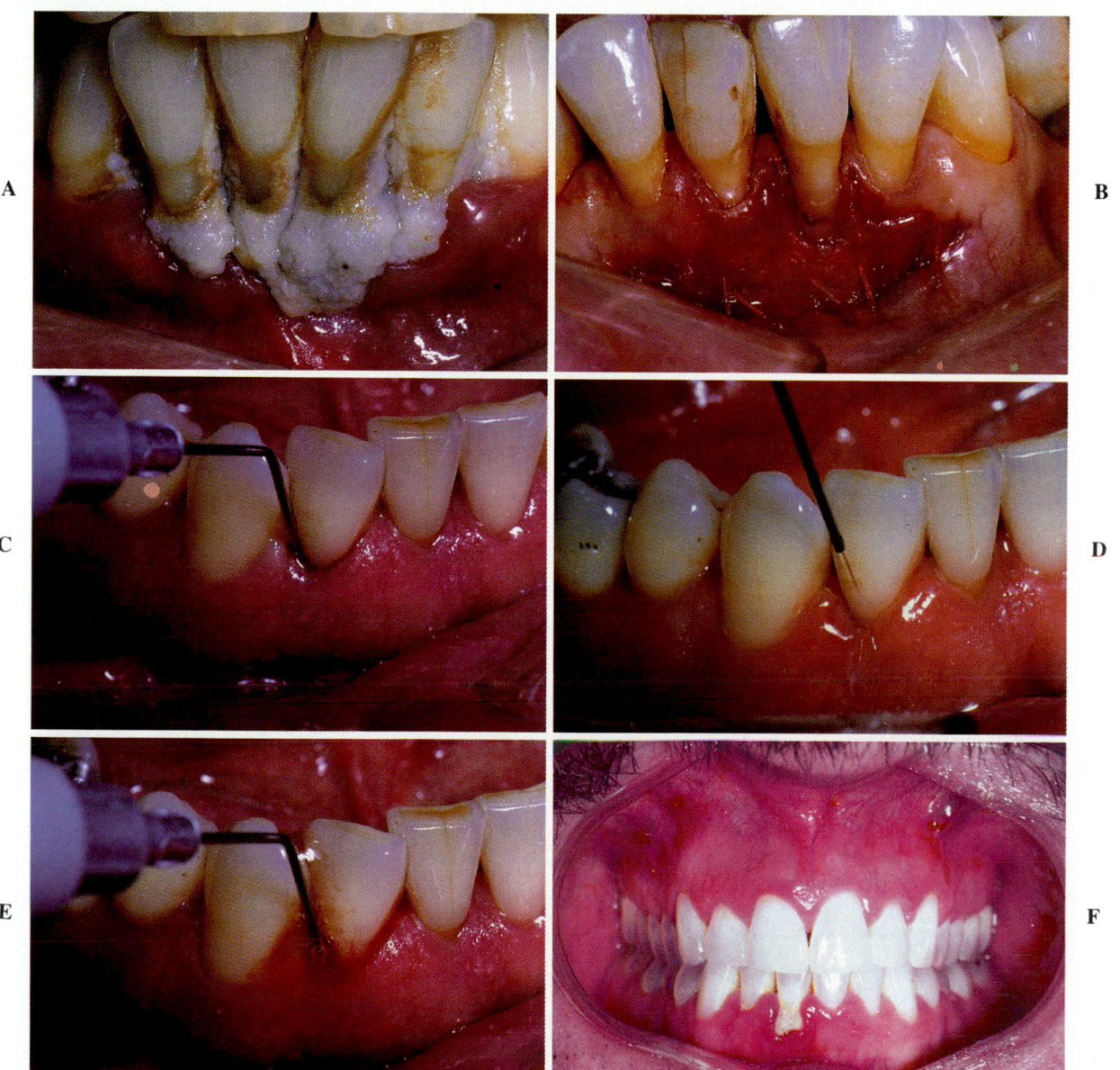

Plate 2. **A,** Continuous bridge of calculus covers anterior teeth facially (and lingually) and is covered with materia alba. **B,** Teeth in **A** were scaled and tissue resected; note residual ledge on mesiofacial of No. 24 despite careful instrumentation. **C,** Subgingival cannula placed in the periodontal pocket to deliver antimicrobial solution following scaling. **D,** Gentle stream of liquid emerging from end-port cannula. **E,** Liquid emerges from the pocket as the tip is activated subgingivally. **F,** Obvious pathology on No. 25 but remainder of tissue shows minimal inflammation.

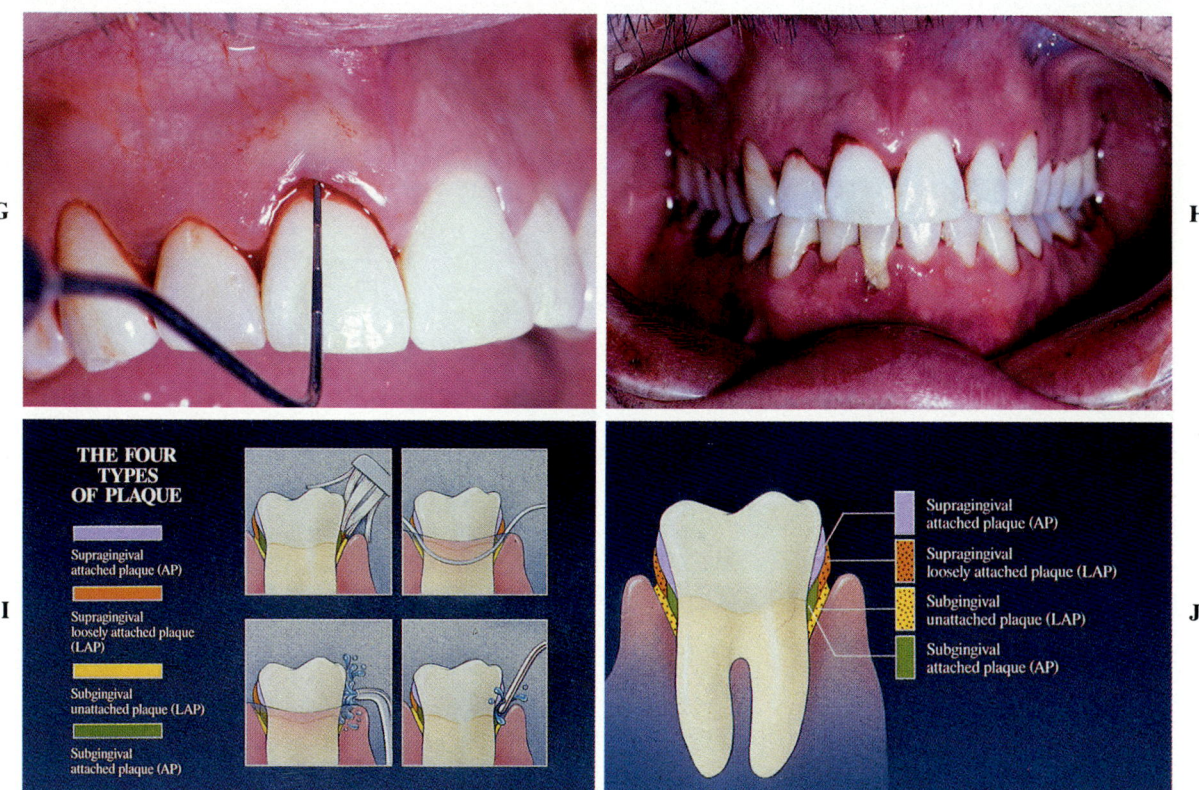

Plate 2, *cont'd.* **G,** Probing prompts sulcular and papillary bleeding, indicating ulcerated lining of pockets. **H,** Probing reveals generalized soft tissue bleeding. **I,** Four types of plaque. **J,** Relationship of the four types of plaque to the periodontal pocket.

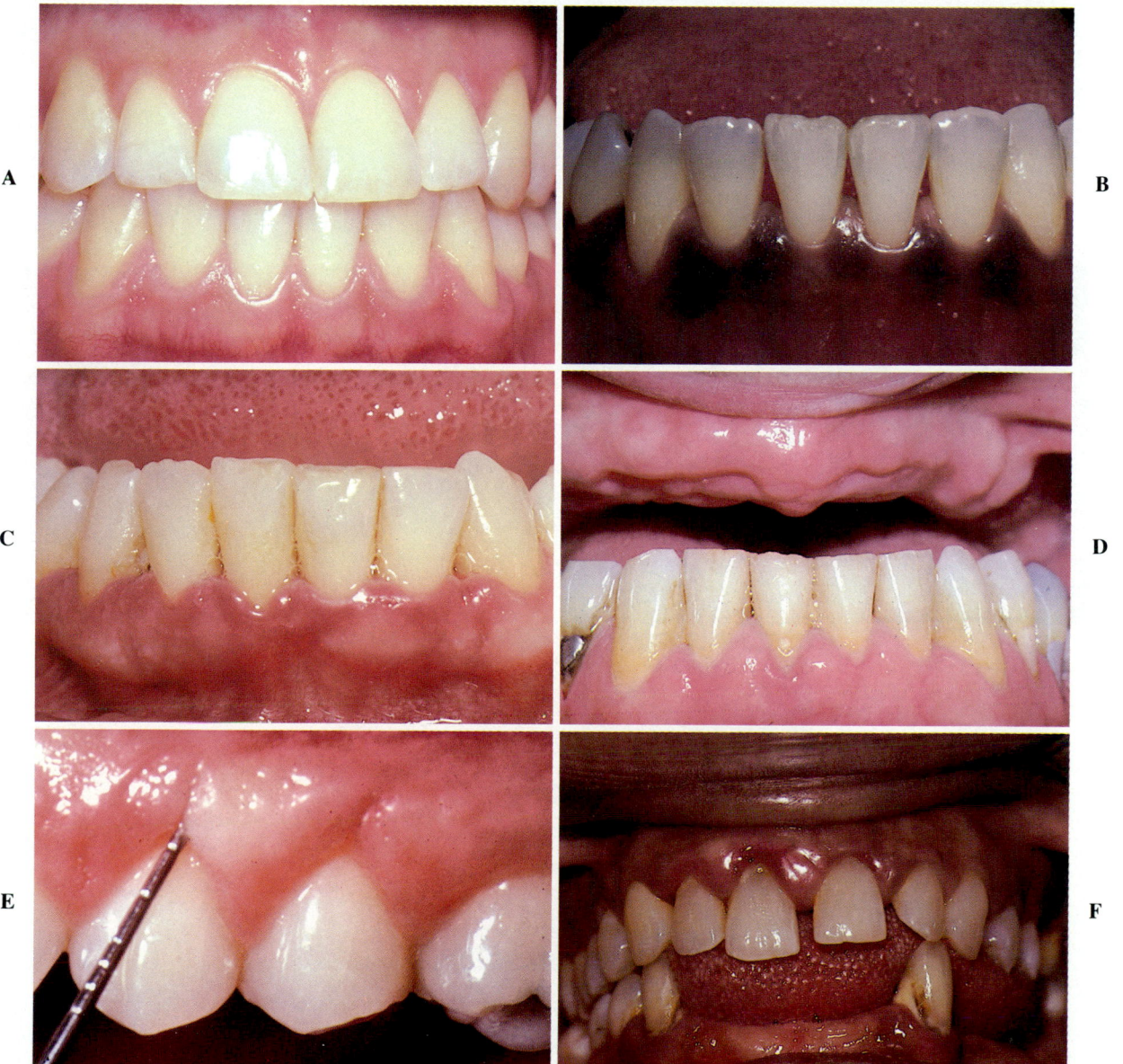

Plate 3. **A,** Clinically healthy gingiva. **B,** Normal melanin pigmentation is visible on free and attached gingiva of this patient. **C,** Signs of marginal inflammation are visible, including redness, rolled margins, and loss of contour. Papillae appear blunted and swollen. Note differences in appearance between attached gingiva and alveolar mucosa. **D,** Fibrotic (hyperplastic) tissue, as seen in mandibular arch of this patient, may appear normal or near normal in color and has a very firm, hard consistency. **E,** Gingival clefting is evident on facial surfaces on premolars. **F,** Marginal gingivitis and periodontitis. Clinical signs of inflammation are visible, especially around Nos. 6 to 10. Note open contacts between teeth and extrusion of maxillary right central incisor, indicating loss of periodontal support. Melanin pigmentation can also be seen in patient's gingiva.

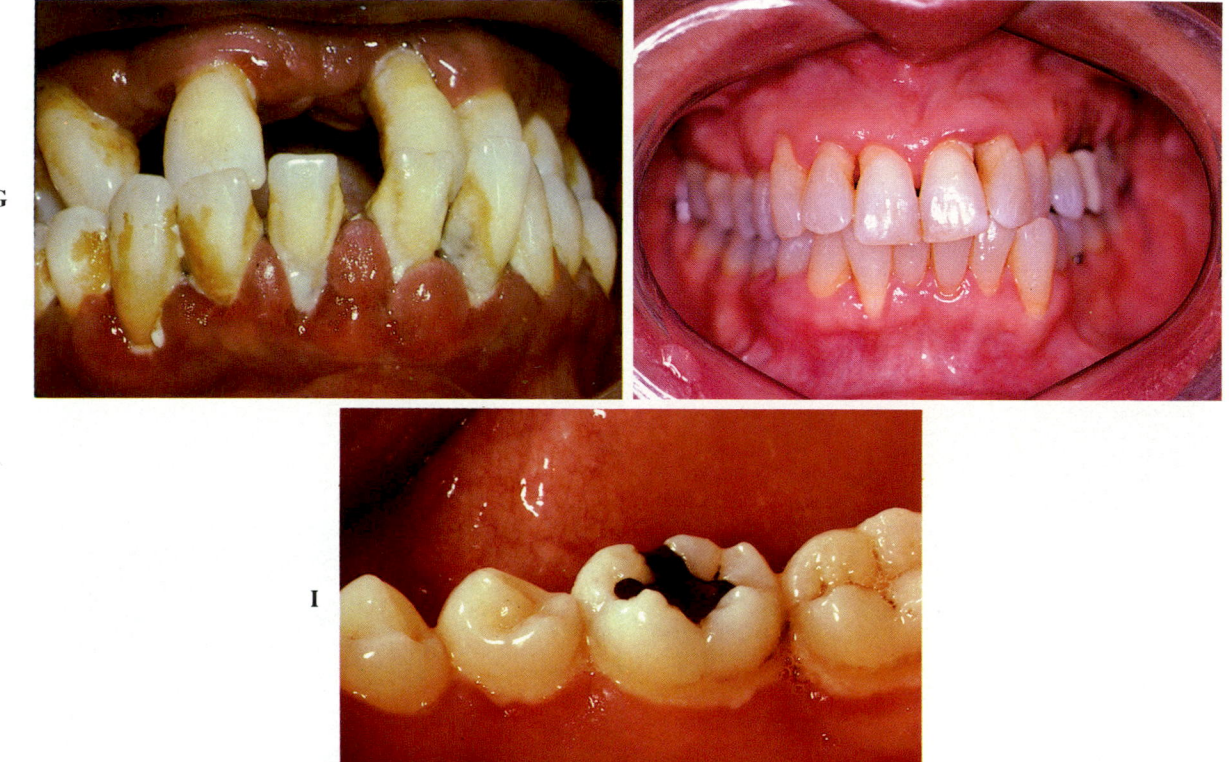

Plate 3, cont'd. **G**, Severe periodontal disease. Presence of heavy hard and soft deposits can be seen. Gingiva exhibits signs of both acute (redness, edema) and chronic inflammation (hyperplasia). Note presence of extruded and shifted teeth and recession as a result of periodontal destruction. Anterior teeth are clinically mobile. **H**, Generalized recession of maxillary gingivae resulting from periodontal disease. **I**, Clinical signs of acute necrotizing ulcerative gingivitis can be seen. Tissues are red, swollen, and extremely painful. Necrotic ulceration, which began in interdental papillae, now includes marginal gingiva in this patient. Yellowish "pseudomembrane" is actually a collected mass of bacteria, dead inflammatory cells, and necrotic tissue.

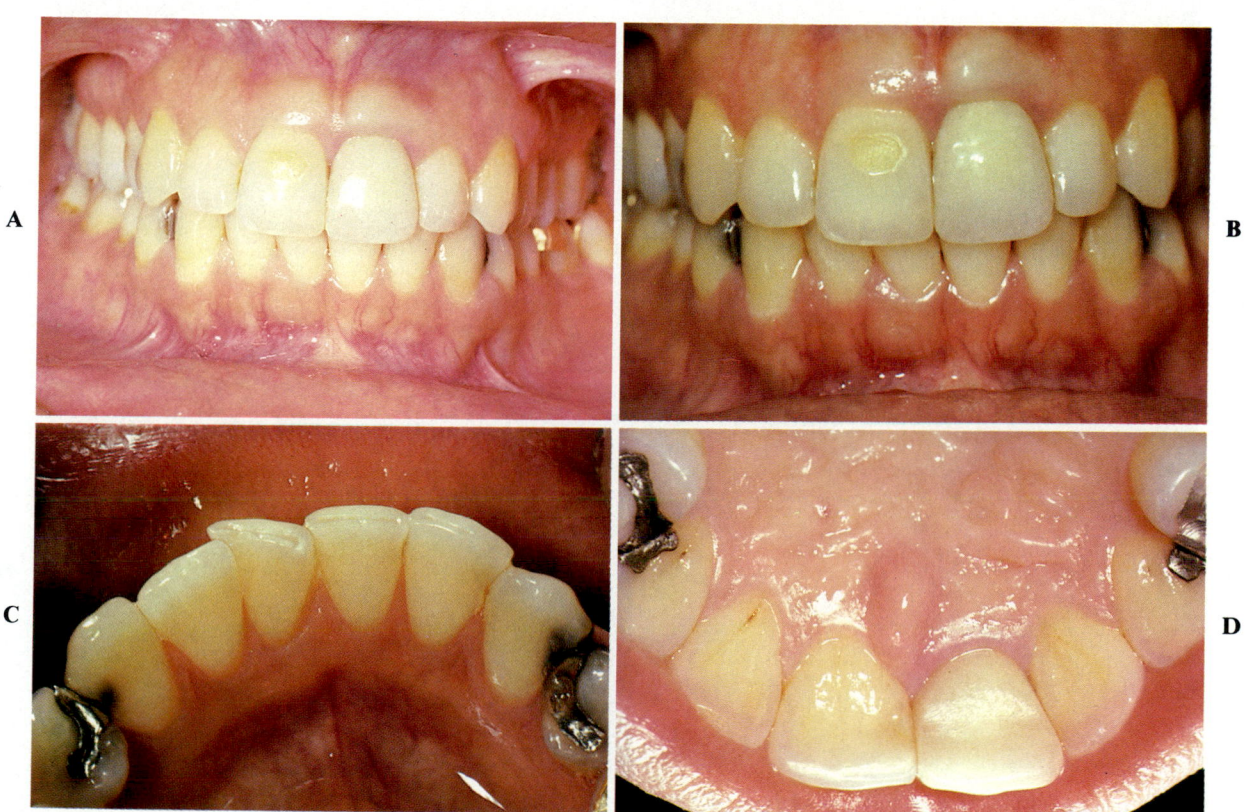

Plate 4. Complete intraoral series. **A,** Full direct view. **B,** Anterior direct view. **C,** Mandibular anterior lingual view. **D,** Anterior palatal view.

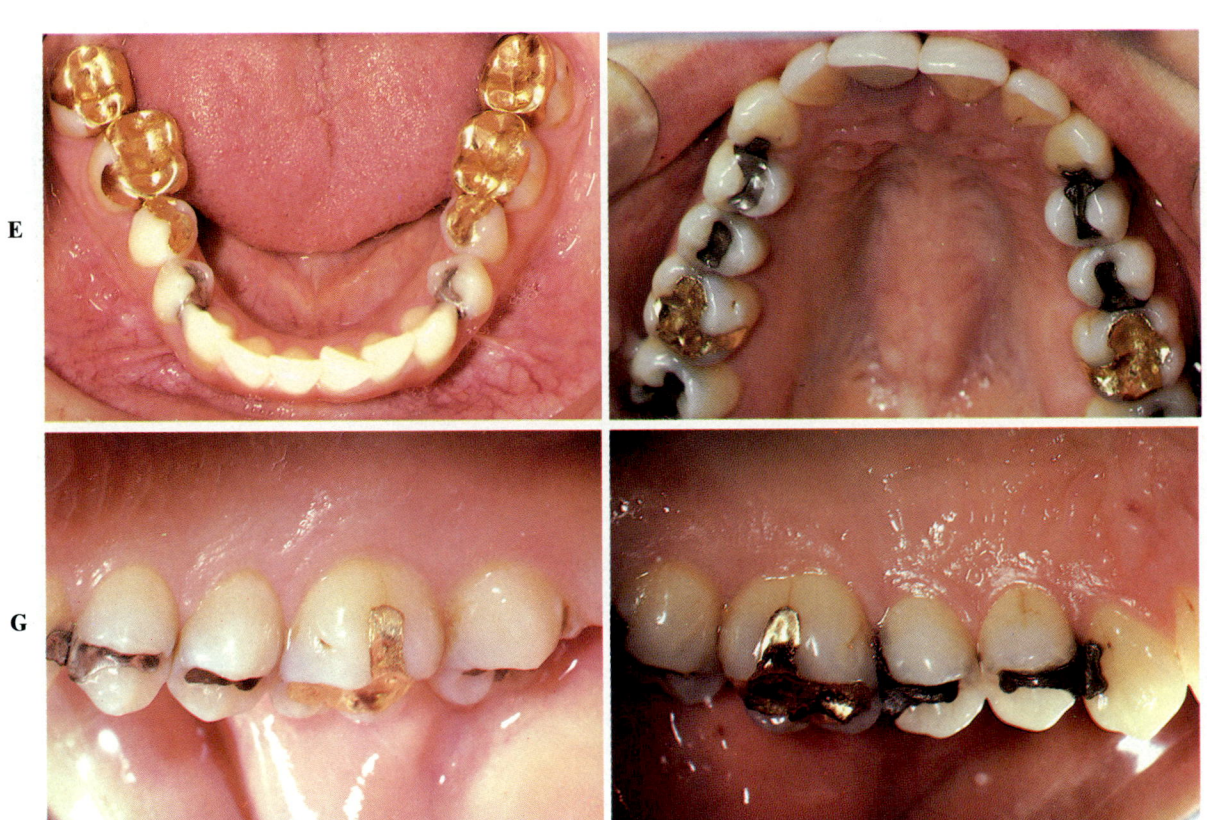

***Plate 4**, cont'd*. **E**, Mandibular occlusal view. **F**, Maxillary occlusal view. **G**, Right posterior palatal view. **H**, Left posterior palatal view.

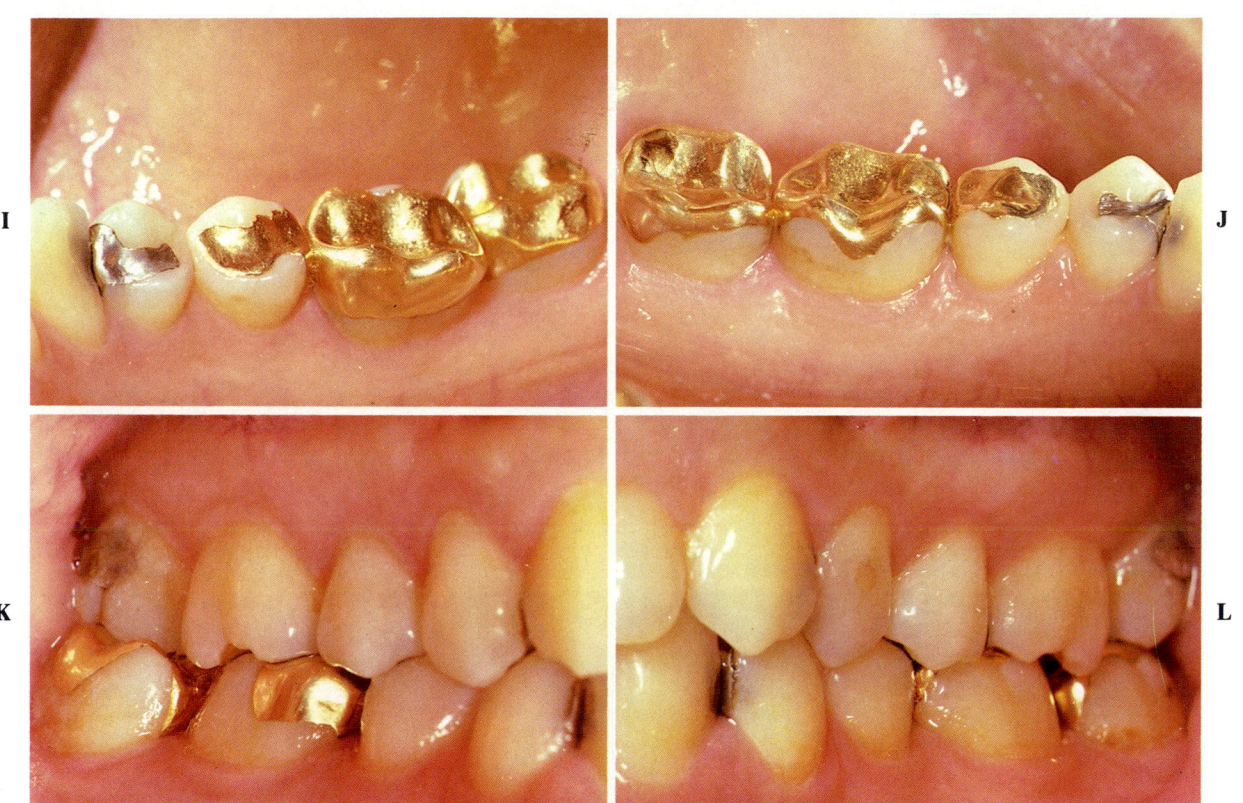

Plate 4, *cont'd*. **I**, Right posterior lingual view. **J**, Left posterior lingual view. **K**, Right buccal view. **L**, Left buccal view.

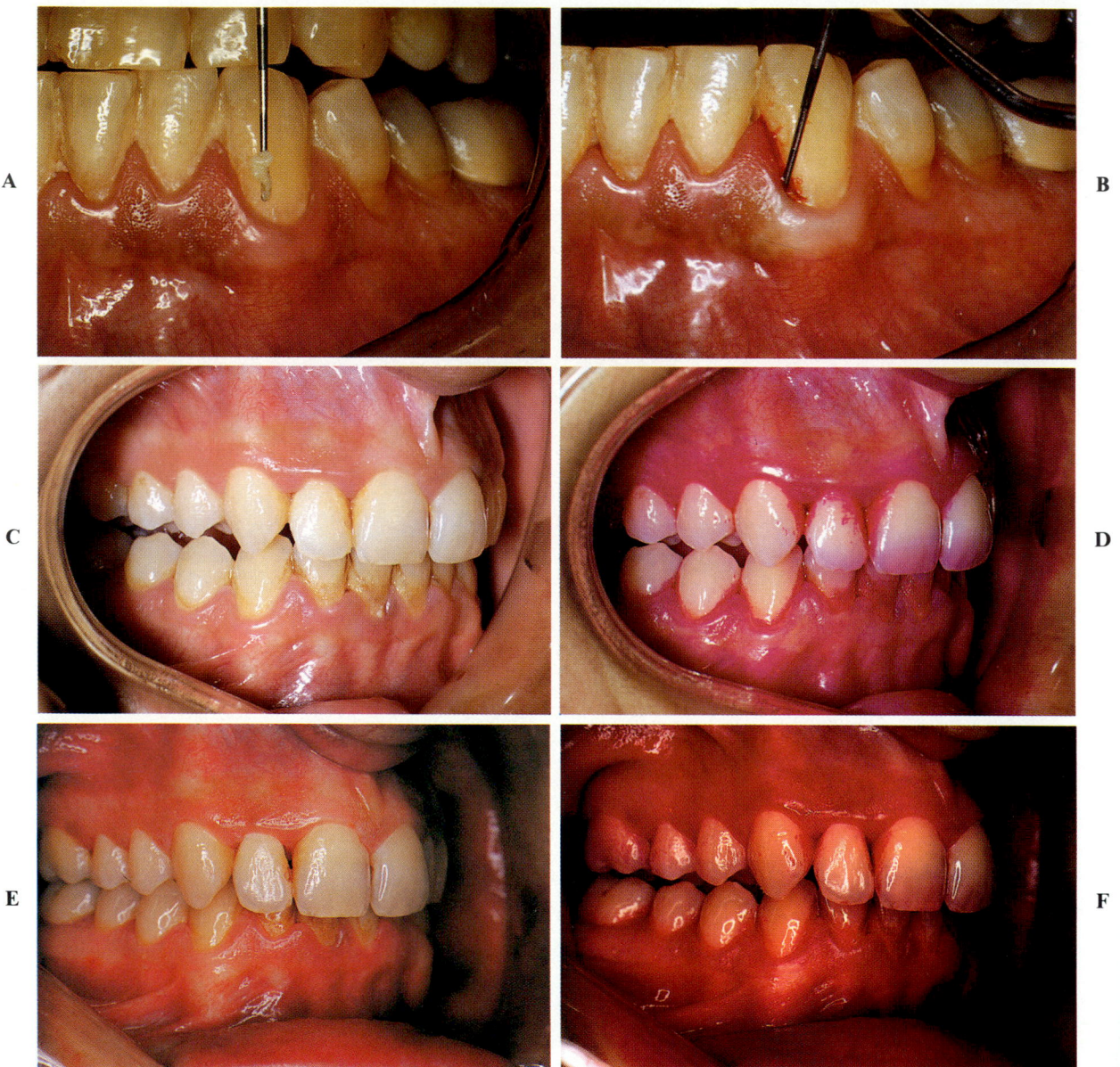

Plate 5. **A,** Plaque accumulated on periodontal probe before disclosant is applied. **B,** Probe stimulates bleeding of inflamed adjacent gingiva. **C,** Subject #1; marginal gingivitis and anterior calculus. **D,** Subject #1. Erythrocine dye shows plaque interdentally and at gingival margin; calculus is stained red. **E,** Subject #1, 14 days after being instructed to use a toothbrush to remove plaque. **F,** Subject #1, 14-day results with disclosant; note minimal improvement.

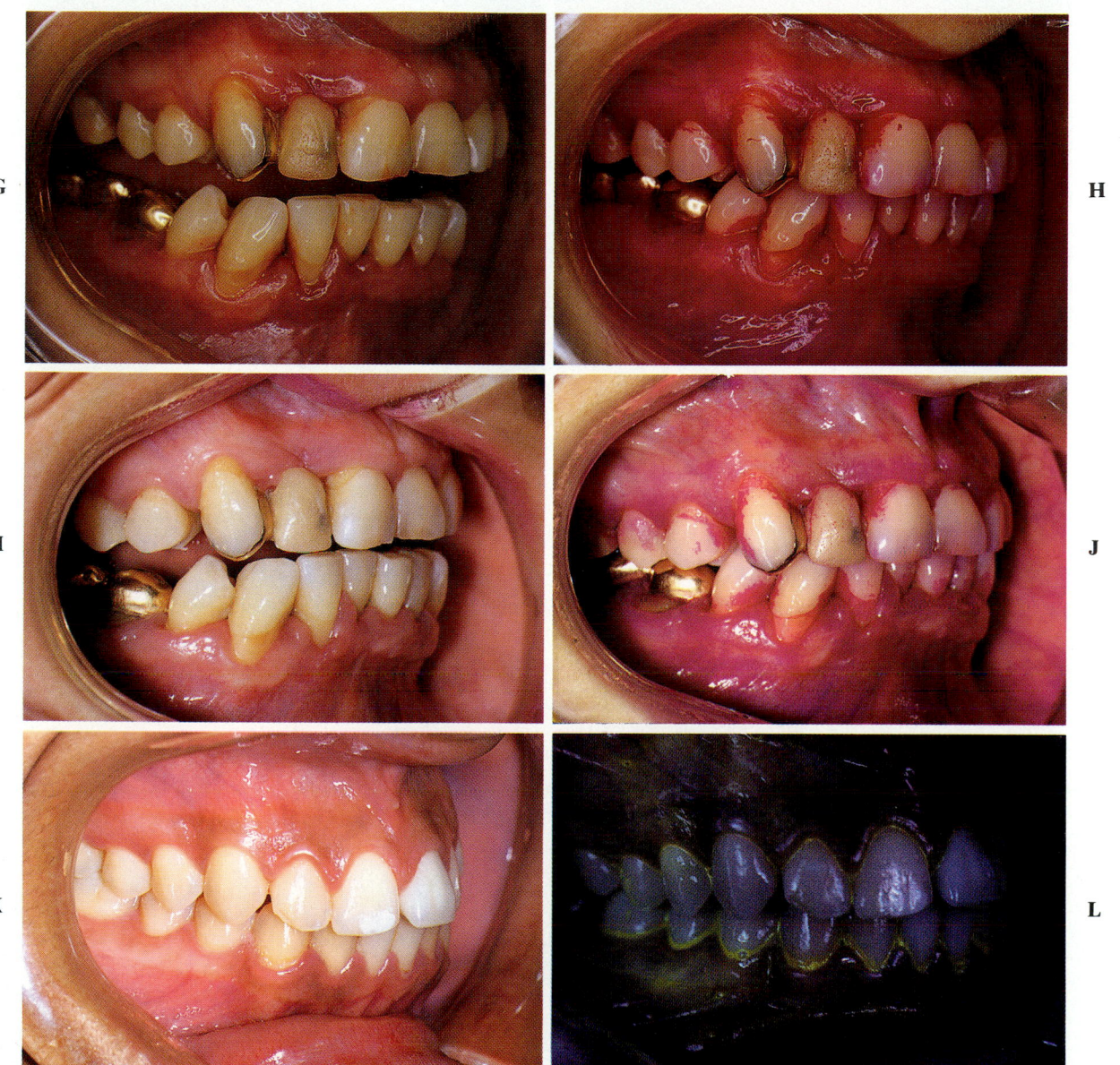

Plate 5, cont'd. **G,** Subject #2; marginal gingivitis complicated by extensive restorations. **H,** Subject #2. Erythrocine dye shows plaque interdentally and at gingival margin; note accumulations near malposed teeth and restorations. **I,** Subject #2, 14 days after instruction to use disclosant as a normal part of oral hygiene and to use a brush to remove visible plaque. **J,** Subject #2, 14-day results with disclosant; note minimal improvement. **K,** Subject #3; marginal gingivitis. **L,** Subject #3. Fluorescein dye (under blue light) shows heavy plaque at gingival margins and interdentally.

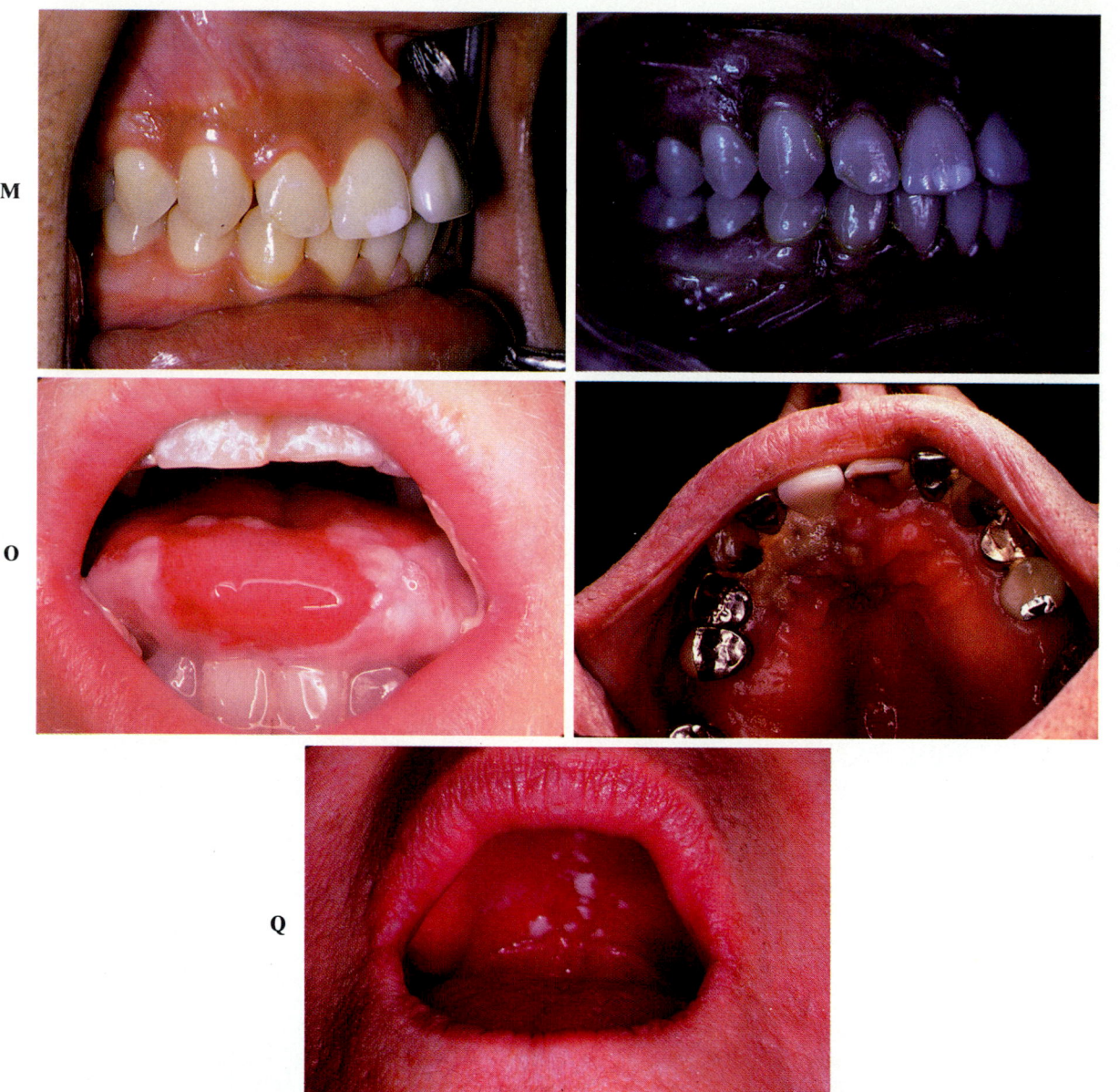

Plate 5, *cont'd*. **M,** Subject #3, 14 days after instruction to use disclosant as a normal part of oral hygiene and to use a brush to remove visible plaque. **N,** Subject #3, 14-day results with disclosant; reduction of plaque is representative of results obtained in controlled clinical trial. **O,** Severe oral mucositis in a patient with colon cancer resulting from direct stomatotoxic effect of antineoplastic chemotherapy. **P,** Herpes simplex virus involving hard palate and adjacent gingival tissue in a patient with acute myelogenous leukemia therapy. Lesion occurred 14 days after initiation of antileukemic therapy. **Q,** Candidiasis of the hard palate in an edentulous patient. Treatment includes removal of prosthesis and treating both soft tissues and dental appliances with antifungal medication.

(A and B courtesy Dr. Dennis Thompson, Denver, Colorado; C to N actual data from a clinical trial [Squillaro et al, 1975] courtesy of Dr. Norman Stoller, University of Colorado, who recorded the results of the trial while at the University of Pennsylvania.)

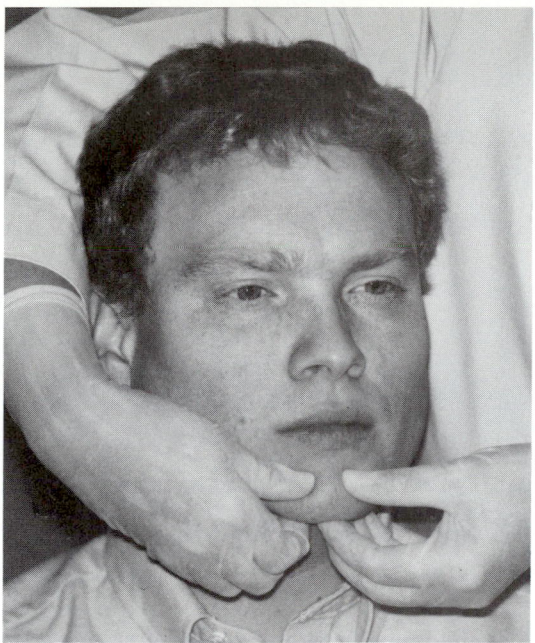

Fig. 8-5. Anterior border of mandible as it is palpated using bidigital compression and circular motion of soft tissues against bone.

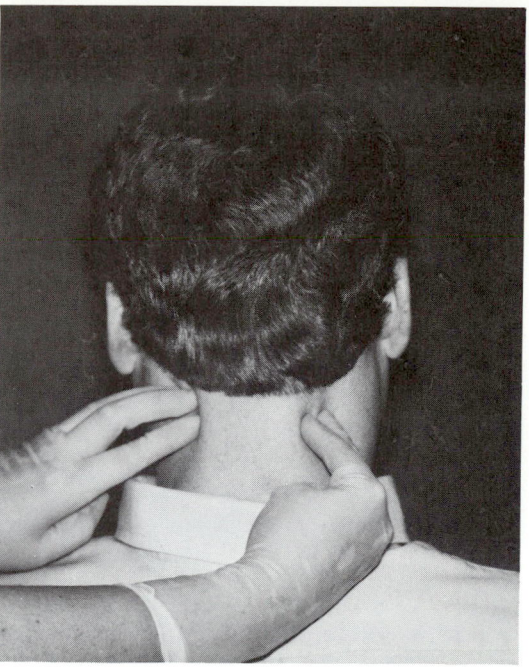

Fig. 8-6. Occipital nodes are being examined. Circular compression is applied at base of skull.

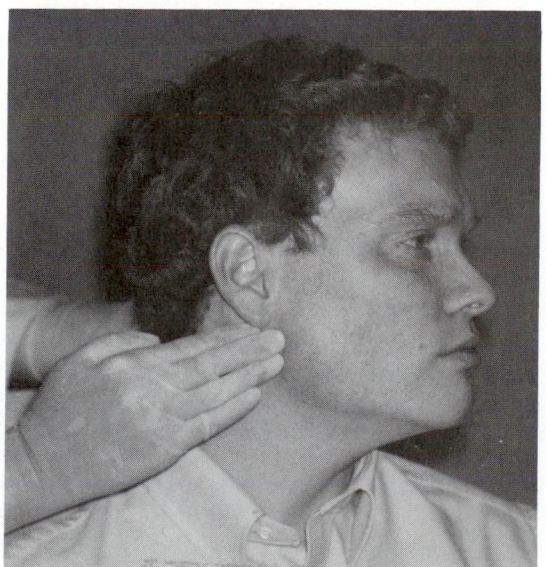

Fig. 8-7. Inferior auricular nodes are being examined by circular compression against tissues. Both anterior and posterior auricular nodes are examined in this manner.

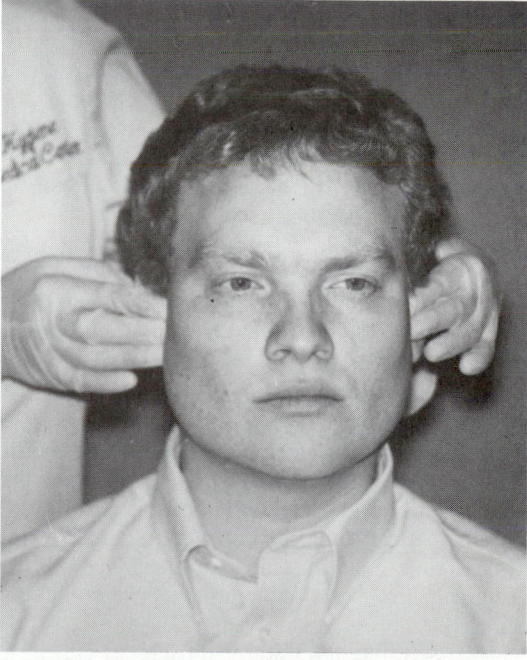

Fig. 8-8. Palpation of temporomandibular joint; fingertips are placed bilaterally just anterior to outer opening of ear.

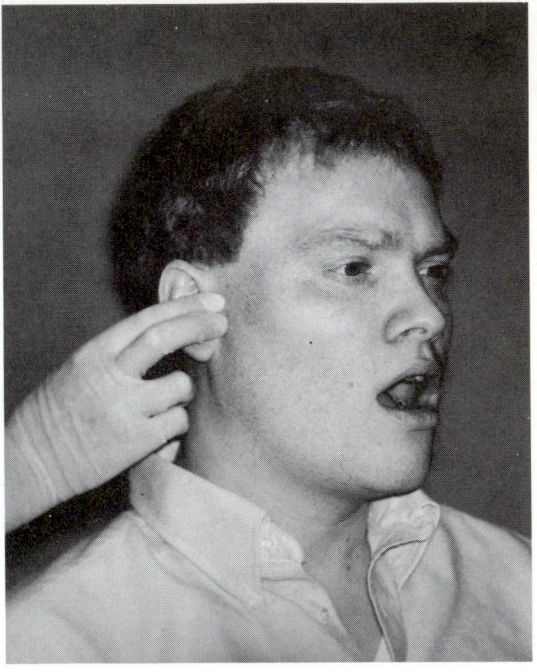

Fig. 8-9. Patient is asked to perform a variety of jaw movements as temporomandibular joint is palpated. Here patient is slowly opening his mouth as far as is comfortable while clinician feels for abnormal movement or clicking in joint.

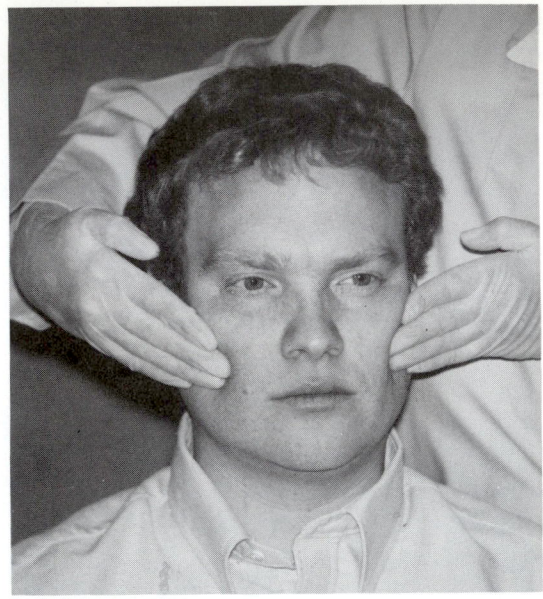

Fig. 8-10. Area of parotid gland is palpated with circular compressions over entire area of gland. This is a large gland that extends from in front of ear to cheek area and down to angle of mandible.

jaw movememts. The joint is auscultated during movement to detect the presence of clicking, popping, or grating sounds. Also ask the patient to perform right and left lateral movements with the teeth apart and to make protrusive movements with the teeth together and then apart.

Palpate the area of the parotid gland (including the parotid nodes) bilaterally using digital compression and circular movement. Begin anterior to the tragus of the ear and extend the palpation inferiorly to the angle of the mandible. Note any deviations in form, density, or size or tenderness in the area (Fig. 8-10).

Palpate the masseter muscle by placing the fingers of each hand over the angle of the mandible and extending the hand up onto the cheek. Then ask the patient to clench the teeth together several times, and examine the muscle bilaterally for size, function, and deviations between the two sides.

Examine the temporalis muscle in much the same way as the masseter muscle. Place the hands bilaterally across the muscle on the patient's tem-

ples, and ask the patient to clench the teeth together several times. Check for muscle function and tenderness.

Examine the submental region (including the lymph nodes) using digital compression and circular motion behind and beneath the symphysis of the mandible. Examine for swelling, enlargements, tenderness, firmness, and mobility of lymph nodes. For locations of lymph nodes of the head and neck see Figs. 8-11 and 8-12.

Palpate the submandibular region (including the glands and nodes) using bidigital compression and circular movements. Ask the patient to lower the head so that the skin and muscles beneath the chin are not taut. This adjustment will make it easier to gain access to the deeper soft tissues of the submandibular area. Starting at the anterior border of the mandible, push the tissue from the left submandibular area over to the right and grasp it with the fingertips of the right hand. The examining fingers should be cupped slightly to grasp the tissues effectively. Then use the fingertips to roll the soft tissue over the right border of

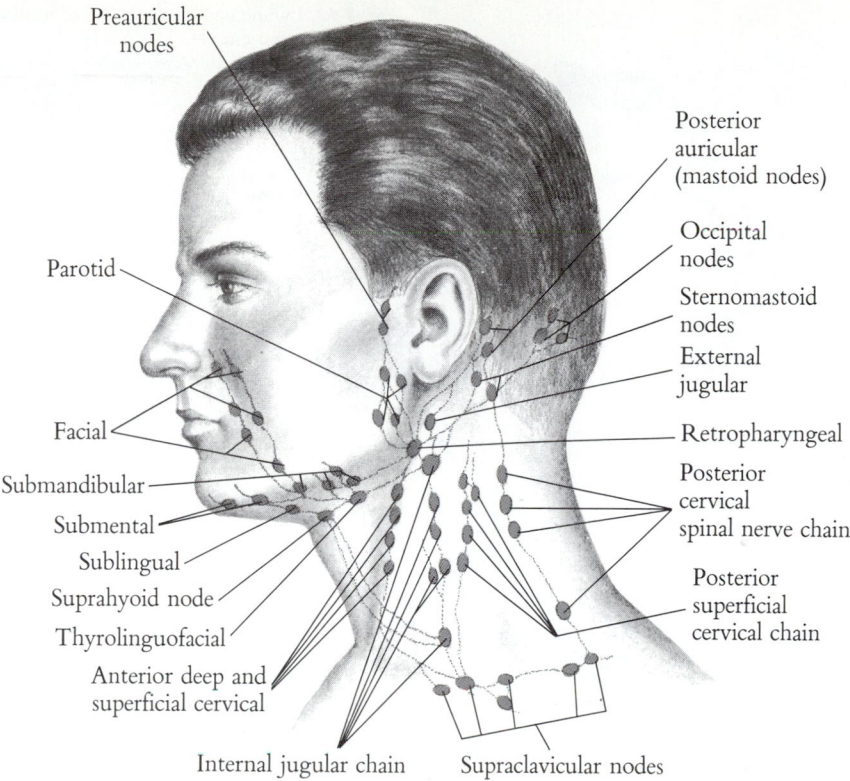

Fig. 8-11. Lymphatic drainage system of head and neck. If the group of nodes is often referred to by another name, the second name appears in parentheses.
(From Seidel HM et al: *Mosby's guide to physical examination,* St Louis, 1987, CV Mosby.)

the mandible, feeling for swelling or enlargements, tenderness, mobility, and firmness of lymph nodes. Reverse this procedure for the left submandibular area. Finally, use the fingertips to compress the soft tissues of the submandibular region bilaterally. Start this palpation at the midline of the submandibular area, and proceed outward to the borders of the mandible and posteriorly to the angle (Fig. 8-13).

To examine the structures of the neck, start with the sternocleidomastoid muscle. Ask the patient to turn the head to the left and lower the chin. This will cause the muscle on the right side of the neck to be more prominent, increasing its accessibility for the examination. The left hand of the clinician should support the patient's head at the chin, and the right hand should grasp the muscle between the thumb and fingers.

Begin bidigital palpation, starting from behind the ear and continuing all the way down the mus-

cle until you reach the clavicle. Remember that for thorough examination of the structures of the neck, tight collars or ties should be loosened to expose the neck area. Repeat the examination on the left side of the neck. Examine the muscle for rigidity, tenderness, induration, presence of masses, and difference in function from one side to the other (Fig. 8-14).

The superficial cervical lymph nodes are located anterior and posterior to the sternocleidomastoid muscle. Apply digital compression and circular movement to this area, extending from the angle of the mandible in a downward direction along the anterior and posterior aspects of the muscle (Fig. 8-15). The patient's head should be in an upright and forward position. Palpate the area bilaterally to examine for deviations from normal. Look for enlarged lymph nodes, and note their tenderness, degree of mobility, and firmness. *Text continued on p. 148.*

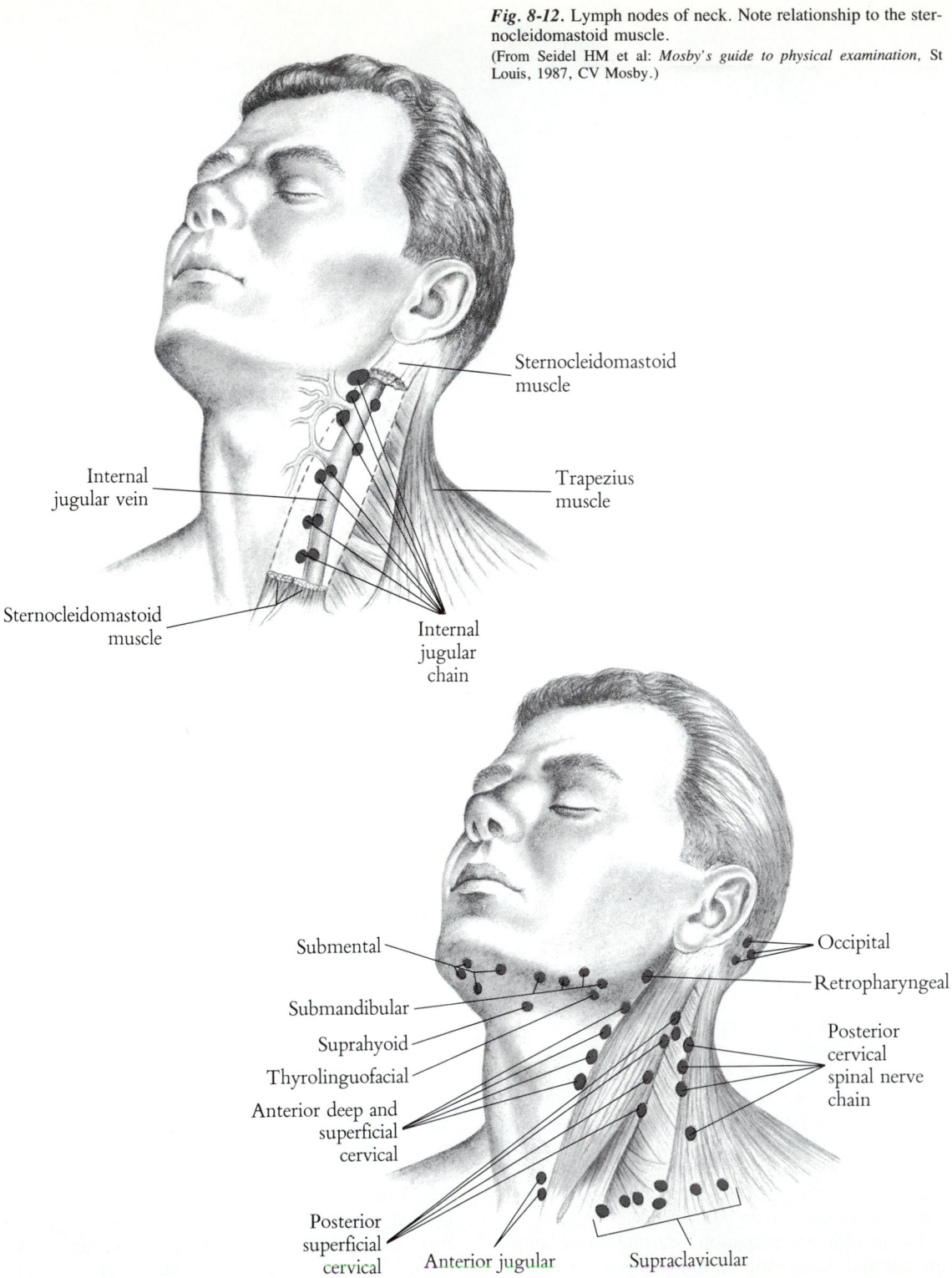

Fig. 8-12. Lymph nodes of neck. Note relationship to the sternocleidomastoid muscle.
(From Seidel HM et al: *Mosby's guide to physical examination*, St Louis, 1987, CV Mosby.)

Sternocleidomastoid muscle

Internal jugular vein

Trapezius muscle

Sternocleidomastoid muscle

Internal jugular chain

Submental

Occipital

Retropharyngeal

Submandibular

Suprahyoid

Thyrolinguofacial

Posterior cervical spinal nerve chain

Anterior deep and superficial cervical

Posterior superficial cervical

Anterior jugular

Supraclavicular

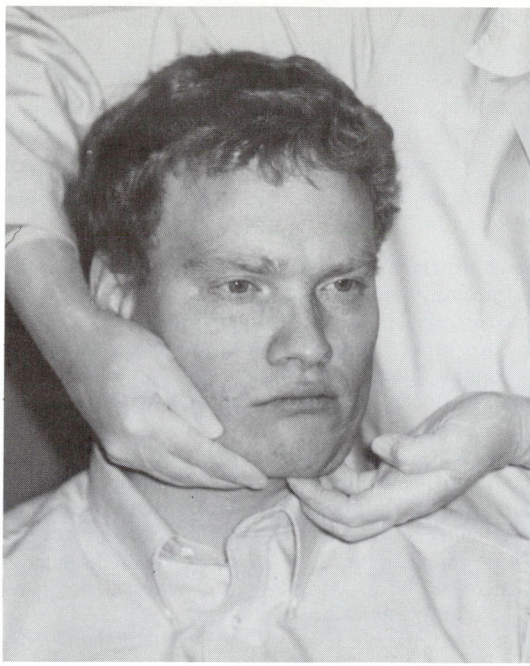

Fig. 8-13. Palpation of submandibular area. Note that clinician has pushed tissue from patient's left side over to opposite side where it is being grasped and rolled over angle of mandible. Opposite side will be examined in same way.

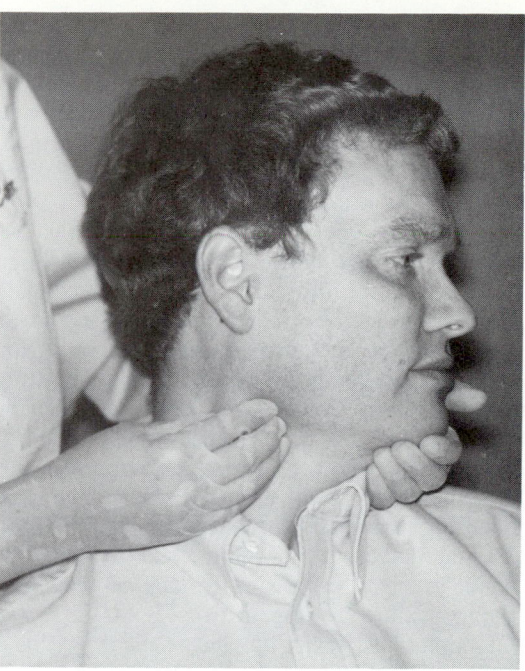

Fig. 8-14. Note patient positioning for palpation of sternocleidomastoid muscle. His head is turned to side and slightly down while chin rests in clinician's free hand. This causes muscle to protrude so that it is easily seen. Palpation is by bidigital compression starting from below ear and continuing whole length of muscle to clavicle.

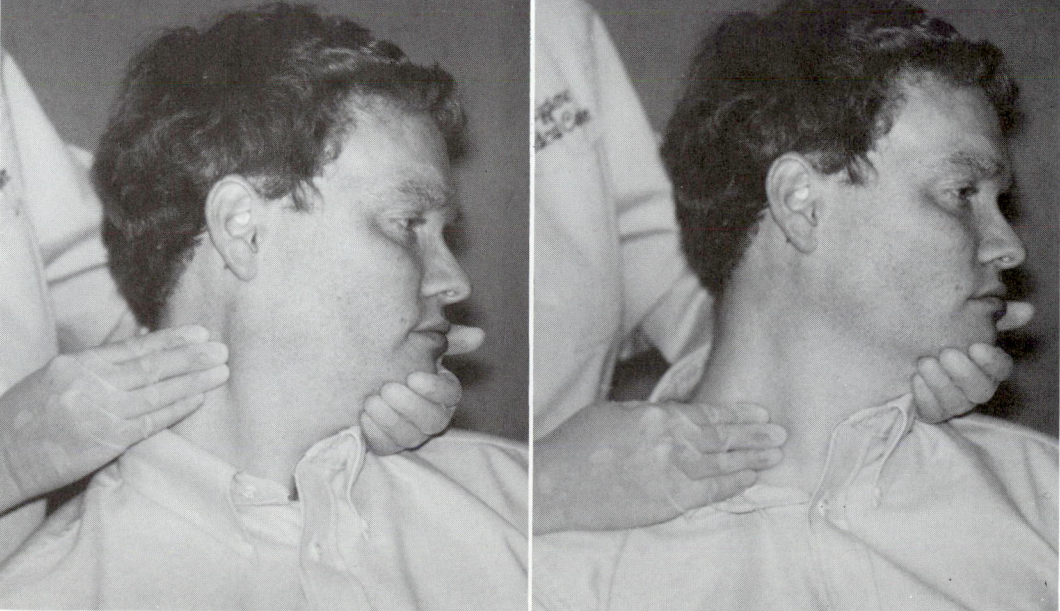

Fig. 8-15. Circular, digital compression is used to examine cervical chain of lymph nodes anteriorly and posteriorly to sternocleidomastoid muscle.

The deep cervical lymph nodes are located along and behind the sternocleidomastoid muscle. The technique of palpation is the same as for the anterior cervical lymph nodes, but an increased effort is made to place the thumb and fingers behind the muscle to locate nodes in the deeper, less accessible tissues.

The thyroid gland normally is not visible. It is located vertically between the cricothyroid ligament and the fourth tracheal ring and horizontally between the sternocleidomastoid muscle and the trachea. It can be palpated from behind or in front of the patient. With one hand place the fingers on one side of the trachea and gently displace the thyroid tissue over to the other side of the neck. With the opposite hand apply gentle circular digital compression to the tissues. Palpate the thyroid gland for enlargements, tenderness, and mobility. Ask the patient to swallow, and examine the gland for signs of masses or lack of movement during swallowing (Fig. 8-16).

Examine the larynx by placing the fingertips of one hand bilaterally over the structure and applying alternate pressure in a medial direction against it. A normal larynx should be freely movable and should ascend and descend during the process of swallowing. A slight fremitus (palpable vibration or movement) may be noted when the normal larynx is displaced during palpation (Fig. 8-17).

This completes the extraoral examination. All significant findings should be described and recorded in the patient's chart to aid in diagnosis and treatment planning. Significant palpation findings to include in the chart may be summarized as follows:

bony structures. Record abnormal anatomy, growths, fractures, crepitus, and pain.

muscles. Record hyperfunction or hypofunction, deviations between the two sides, swellings, masses, indurations, and tenderness.

glands. Record abnormal swellings, tenderness, and hard masses.

lymph nodes. Record palpable nodes and describe their size (estimate diameter), firmness (hard or soft), mobility (fixed or freely movable), tenderness (sensitive or painless), and how long they have been present. Determine if the presence of lymph node enlargement can be traced to current manifestations of disease or recent history of disease.

skin. Describe all lesions using the terminology discussed earlier.

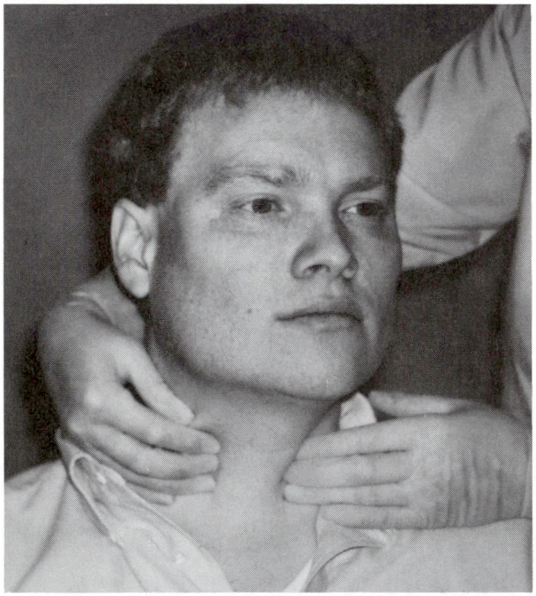

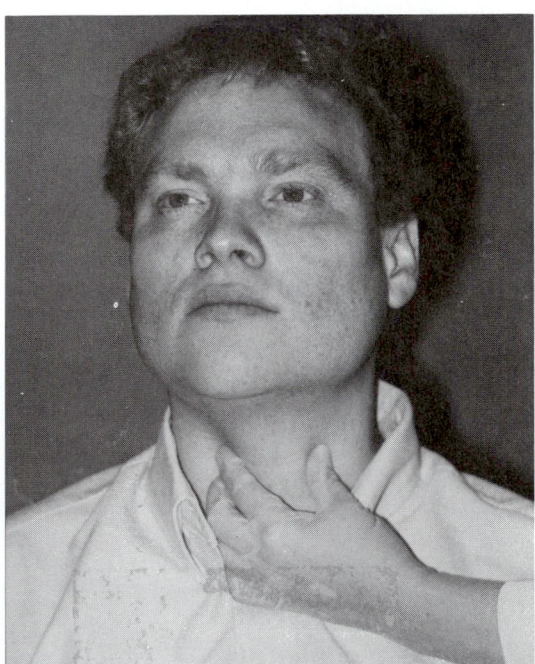

Fig. 8-16. Thyroid is being palpated from rear of patient. One hand gently displaces tissue to one side while fingers of other hand carefully feel for enlargements or abnormal masses.

Fig. 8-17. Gentle medial pressure is used in area of larynx to check for mobility of larynx and trachea. Inability to move this structure slightly might indicate problems.

Significance of lymph node examination

Normal lymph nodes are not visible or palpable during the head and neck examination. When the presence of swollen lymph nodes can be detected by either of these methods, the clinician should continue evaluating the patient to determine what the cause of the abnormality might be. Lymph nodes of the head and neck area can become swollen and tender from infections that originate in the areas that they drain. The clinician must have a clear understanding of human anatomy and the lymph node system to trace a detectable lymph node back to its associated cause. Enlargement of lymph nodes as a result of acute or chronic infections is known as lymphadenitis. Lymph nodes may become temporarily enlarged because of localized infections such as a dental abscess, regional infections such as tonsillitis, or systemic infections such as tuberculosis or syphilis. In most cases of acute inflammation, resolution of the infection allows the lymph nodes to return to their normal state. In some cases chronic infections cause enlargement of affected lymph nodes because of the presence of scar tissue; in this case nodes remain palpable as nontender firm or fibrotic single masses even after the source of the infection has been removed. Because many of these same characteristics might be found in nodes associated with malignant or metastatic diseases, the patient's medical history should be explored and he or she should be interviewed to determine possible explanations for the presence of these nodes. In general, nodes arising from acute inflammatory conditions are tender, soft, enlarged, and freely movable.

Lymph node involvement resulting from malignant diseases may display different characteristics. Detection and examination of these nodes reveals that they are often hard, nontender, and fixed to underlying tissues. Multiple nodes that are matted together may be involved. The patient may indicate no recent history of local or systemic infection to explain the presence of the detectable nodes. Bilaterally enlarged nodes may indicate the presence of systemic infection or an advanced malignancy. The presence of unilateral node enlargement may indicate either localized infection or possibly early metastatic disease. The alert clinician combines information from the patient's medical and dental history, the oral examination, the lymph node examination, and an up-to-date knowledge of the demographics of patients who are at high risk for malignant diseases to evaluate the potential significance of detectable lymph nodes. When lymph node involvement suggests malignant changes, the clinician should examine the areas served by those nodes for signs of abnormal tissues. Although many detectable nodes may be easily explained by the presence of local, regional, or systemic infections, the dental professional should refer all questionable findings to the patient's physician or a specialist for a definitive diagnosis (Kerr, Ash, and Millard, 1983; Kutcher et al, 1981).

Intraoral examination

The supplies and instruments needed for the intraoral examination include a mirror, explorer, probe, gauze squares, and a tongue depressor. For this and all other intraoral procedures, the clinician should follow universal precautions (see Chapter 3).

The following factors help ensure optimal examination technique: (1) lighting, (2) positioning, (3) tissue retraction, and (4) sequence. A complete and thorough examination cannot be performed without optimal consideration of all of these factors.

Direct lighting is provided by directing the central beam of the overhead light onto the area being examined. Care should be taken not to direct the light into the patient's eyes. The light beam must be readjusted as different areas of the mouth are examined. This responsibility should be assumed by the chairside assistant if one is present. Supplementary indirect lighting is also provided by the mouth mirror. This is especially useful for the posterior parts of the mouth where it is difficult to use the direct beam of the overhead light.

The patient and clinician should be positioned such that both are comfortable and all areas are accessible for complete examination. When necessary, the patient must be instructed as to where to turn the head to place the tongue so that all areas are visible. The clinician should follow the principles of good positioning, discussed in previous chapters. Whenever possible, the clinician should seek a direct view of the structure to be examined. If a direct view cannot be obtained without violating the principles of effective positioning, such as in the maxillary tuberosity area, the dental mirror should be used to examine that area thoroughly.

The third factor for good examination technique is thorough, but gentle, retraction of soft tissues so that the entire area can be observed. There is no guarantee that lesions will not occur behind folds of tissue or at the hidden corners of the mouth. Failure to examine all tissues completely regardless of their accessibility can only be considered negligent.

The establishment of an efficient sequence is also an important factor. Optimal time and motion management, use of a logical order, and asepsis should all be considered in determining the sequence of examination. Because the examination of some intraoral structures, such as the labial and buccal mucosa and the floor of the mouth, requires external retraction or palpation technique, these structures should be done consecutively as a group.

Thus the sequence presented in this chapter will be as logical and efficient as possible.

The clinician must be fully acquainted with the hard and soft tissue anatomy of the head and neck and especially of the oral cavity. To perform a comprehensive examination, the clinician must be able to discriminate normal from abnormal appearances. For records to be universally understandable, the clinician must be well acquainted with the specific names and terminology associated with the structures to be examined and record all findings accurately.

To begin the intraoral examination procedure, lower the back of the dental chair to a semisupine position. Seat yourself at the 9 o'clock (3 o'clock for left-handed clinician) position, where you can obtain a direct view of the oral cavity and structures. Ask the patient to remove all dental appliances that are not permanent, and place them in appropriate containers until they can be examined. Radiographs should have been reviewed before the appointment, if they were available. Information from the radiographs will be correlated with the head and neck examination to aid in the detection of clinical findings. Assemble all necessary forms and supplies and place them within easy reach. Because this is the first intraoral procedure that you are likely to perform, wash your hands thoroughly and put on gloves before the examination.

Before beginning a detailed examination of each structure, it is wise to perform a cursory screening of the intraoral tissues with a mouth mirror or tongue blade. This screening is done to determine whether contagious lesions are present that should not be contacted because of the risk of disease transmission (as with herpes simplex or syphilis) or patient discomfort (as with mouth ulcers or other traumatic lesions). Briefly inspect the following structures: lips, labial mucosa, buccal mucosa, hard palate, soft palate, tongue, floor of mouth, and alveolar ridges (Figs. 8-18 and 8-19). The clinician should also check the throat for signs of severe sore throat or other manifestations that would suggest that the patient should be seen or treated by a physician before any intraoral procedures are performed. A serious consequence of examining the oral tissues in the presence of a severe sore throat could be the introduction of multitudes of streptococci into the bloodstream. If the patient has a history of heart disease, bacterial endocarditis could result. Postpone additional treatment until any acute infections have subsided or until infective lesions have healed. This will protect not only the patient but also dental personnel and other patients who could encounter the disease pathogens indirectly from contaminated surfaces or supplies.

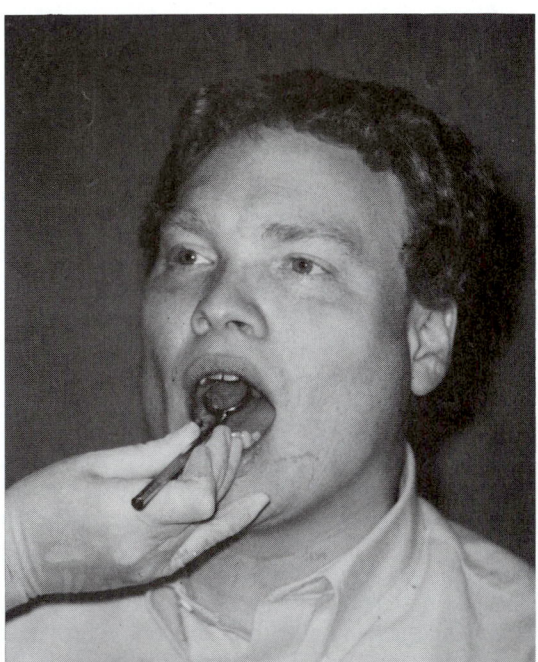

Fig. 8-18. A quick but thorough inspection of all areas of the mouth should be made before clinician begins more comprehensive examination of intraoral structures. In this view, a mirror is being used to examine palate and back of mouth.

When the initial screening is complete and no contraindications to continued treatment have been detected, start the inspection and palpation of all intraoral structures using the following sequence:

1. *Lips*. Inspect the clinical appearance of the lips before retracting them. The skin should be intact and have a semimoist, firm texture. They should be free of all lesions, discolorations, growths, or swellings. Common abnormalities that might be detected include chapped lips, cracks at the corners of the mouth, traumatic lesions such as from lip biting, blisters, ulcers, and cold sores. Protect dry and cracked areas from further trauma by applying petroleum jelly to lubricate the area during retraction. Avoid touching ulcers or blisters.

2. *Labial mucosa*. Retract the mandibular labial mucosa down and away from the teeth. Grasp the tissues so that the thumb is placed intraorally and the fingers are kept extraorally. Try always to use this same arrangement so that the fingers used extraorally do not go back inside the mouth at any time unless the hands have been washed again;

this helps reduce contamination during the examination. On the labial mucosa, check for a moist red surface with no abnormal lesions, masses, or color deviation. You might notice small white or yellowish bumps just below the mucosal lining. These are probably the labial sebaceous glands (Fordyce's granules) and are normal for this tissue. Examine the labial frenum for any tissue tags or lesions. Check also to make sure that this muscle attachment is not pulling on the gingival tissues and causing recession. Continue inspecting and retracting around the corners of the mouth and up onto the maxillary labial mucosa. Palpate this tissue using bilateral, bidigital compression, feeling the tissues between the thumb and fingers. Note any swelling, hard masses, or tenderness (Figs. 8-20 to 8-22).

3. *Buccal mucosa*. Retract the buccal mucosa out and slightly away from the teeth so that its surface can be inspected from the labial mucosa back to the retromolar area. Alternately extend and examine the vestibular areas. As with the labial mucosa, the tissue should be moist and red. The soft tissue structure visible opposite the max-

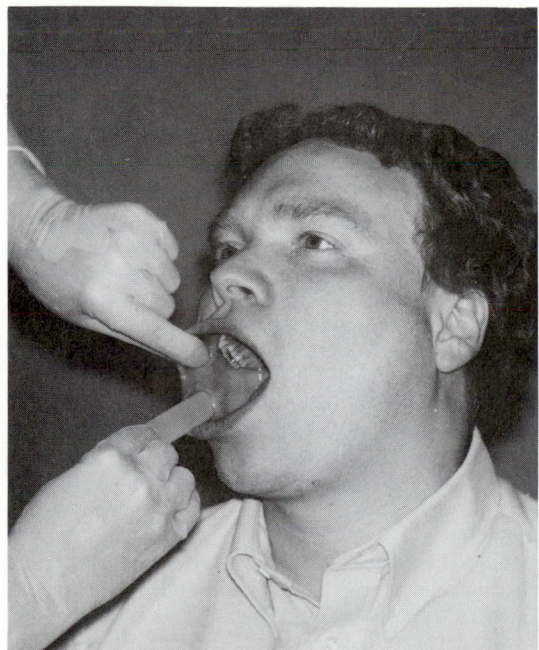

Fig. 8-19. A tongue blade may also be used to assist in tissue retraction during intraoral inspection.

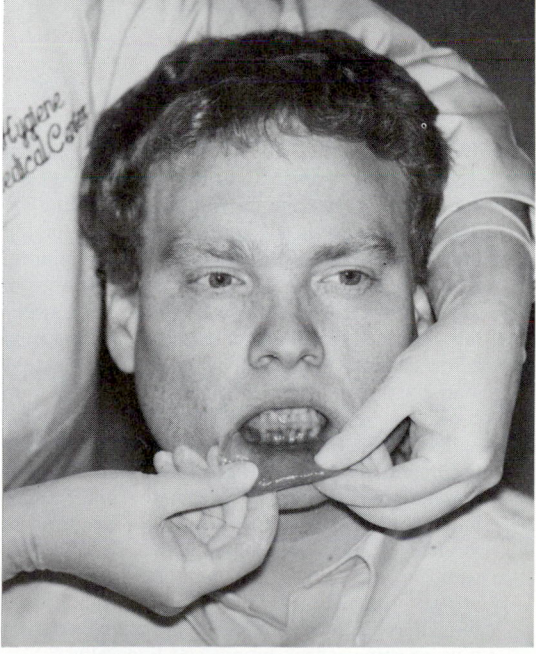

Fig. 8-20. Mandibular labial mucosa is retracted and examined. General appearance of gingiva and frenum attachments is also assessed.

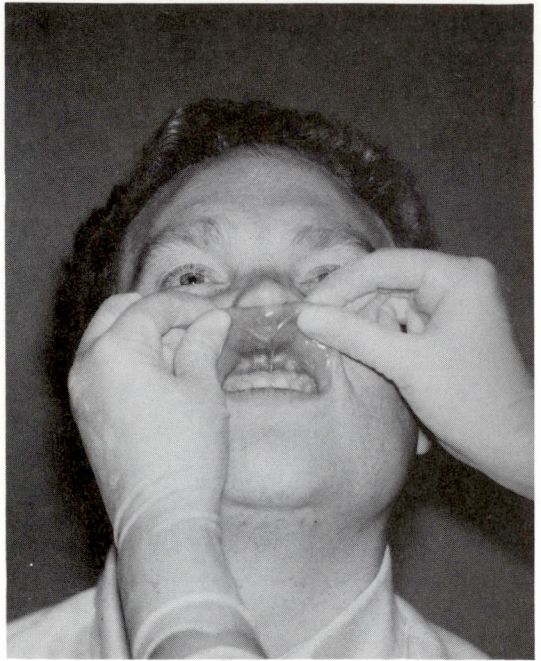

Fig. 8-21. Maxillary labial mucosa is retracted.

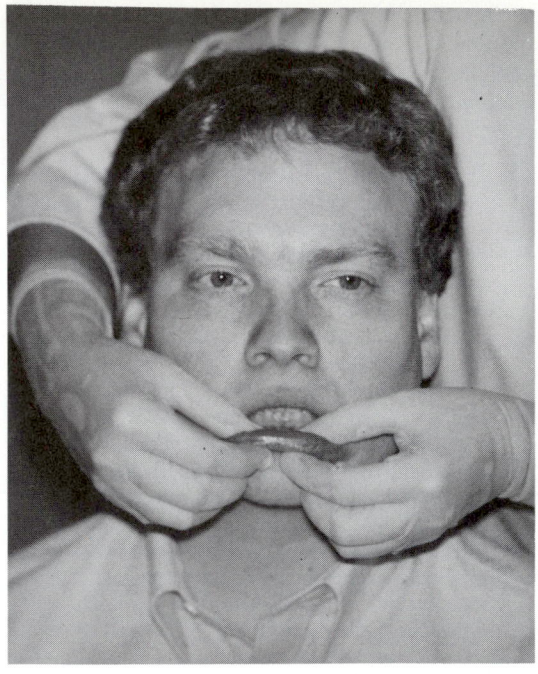

Fig. 8-22. Labial mucosa is palpated with bilateral bidigital compression, moving from midline to corners of mouth.

illary molar area is the parotid papilla. It houses the opening of Stensen's duct of the parotid salivary gland. Check the salivary flow by drying the duct opening with a gauze square and applying light, intermittent external pressure to the parotid gland. Watch for evidence of salivary flow from the duct opening. Examine the tissues for swelling, lesions, breaks in the mucosa, or abnormal color changes, including white or red patches. Variable amounts of brown melanin pigmentation could be present, depending on the race of the patient. Palpate this area bimanually by placing the fingers of one hand intraorally while supporting the tissues extraorally with the other hand. Palpate the tissue between the two hands from the front of the mouth all the way back to the retromolar area. Note all abnormal swellings, masses, or tenderness (Fig. 8-23). Common findings may include Fordyce's granules, xerostomia, scarring, cheek biting, and linea alba.

4. *Floor of the mouth.* Examine the floor of the mouth. Ask the patient to lift the tongue to the roof of the mouth. This area should appear moist and extremely vascular. Examine the following structures of the floor of the mouth:

lingual vein. This vein courses up either side of the ventral surface of the tongue. Varicosities may be seen in the older patient.

plica fibriata. These are small hairlike projections of tissue that lie along the lingual vein.

lingual frenum. This is the muscle attachment between the tongue and the floor of the mouth. An extremely short lingual frenum will restrict the movement of the tongue (ankyloglossia or "tongue-tie"). This is often detected when the tongue cannot touch the palate. It may also be manifested in abnormal speech patterns.

sublingual caruncle. This is located at the base of the frenum and appears as a small rounded projection. It houses the opening of Wharton's duct for the submandibular salivary gland. Test the action of this duct by drying the floor of the mouth with a gauze square and then applying intermittent compression to the submandibular tissue between the ducts. Observe

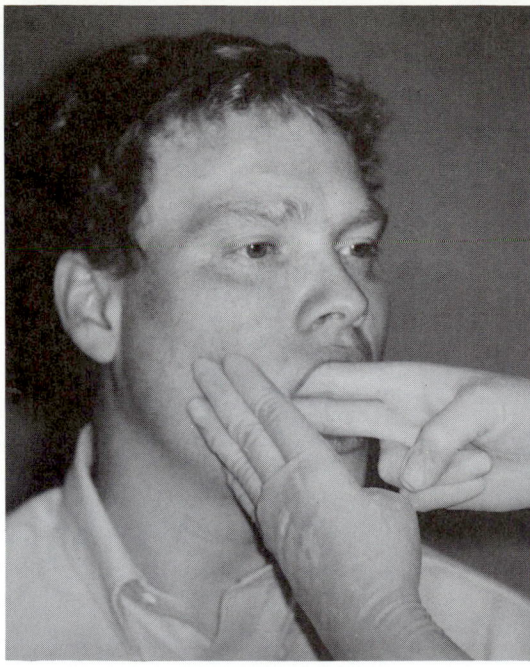

Fig. 8-23. Buccal mucosa is palpated bimanually with fingers of one hand inside mouth and fingers of other hand supporting tissues extraorally.

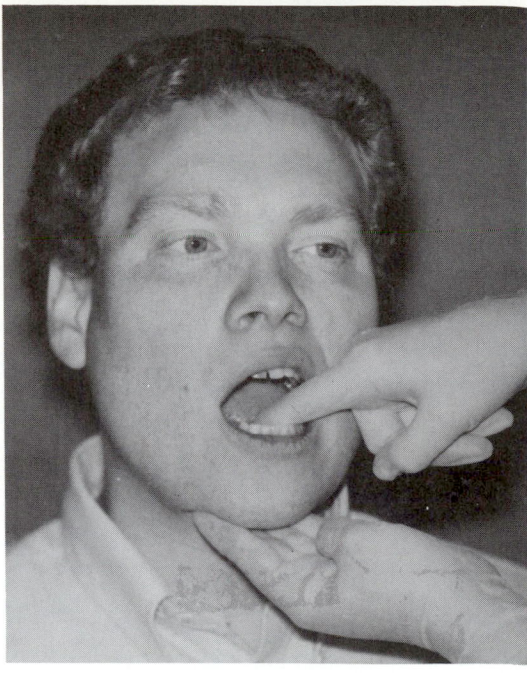

Fig. 8-24. Floor of mouth is palpated bimanually by placing one hand intraorally and supporting tissues against extraoral hand. Entire floor of mouth should be examined in this way.

the floor of the mouth for the rate and amount of saliva flow entering the area.

sublingual folds. These appear as two elevations or ridges running along the floor of the mouth on either side of the tongue. These tissues house the ducts of Rivinus that service the minor sublingual salivary gland in the floor of the mouth.

plica lingualis. These are small hairlike projections of tissue that lie along the crest of the sublingual folds.

While inspecting these structures, inspect the floor of the mouth for lesions or abnormal color changes. Palpate the area by placing the right hand intraorally and the left hand extraorally and feeling the tissues between the two hands (bimanual palpation) (Fig. 8-24). Note any swellings, masses, white or red patches, the comparative size of glands, and any tenderness described by the patient.

The next area to be examined is the hard palate. With the light source directed up onto the palate, inspect the surface for lesions, swellings, and color deviations. A normal palatal surface will appear light pink and will have the following anatomic structures:

incisive papilla. A protuberance of soft, firm tissue located between the two central incisors. It covers the incisive foramen, which is the opening for the blood and nerve supply to this area of the palate. This papilla is normally slightly redder than the surrounding palatal tissue because of its increased blood supply.

medial palatal raphe. A white line extending from the incisive papilla to the soft palate.

palatal rugae. Irregular ridges of tissue radiating from either side of the raphe.

palatine foveae. Two small depressions, one on either side of the midline, at the junction of the hard and soft palate.

Inspection of these structures may reveal abnormalities such as nicotine stomatitis, inflamed incisive papilla, ulcerations, palatal tori, or redness and irritation caused by dentures.

Palpate the palate using digital compression of one or two fingers against the palatal surface (Fig. 8-25). Take care not to extend this technique onto the soft palate, as this could initiate gagging in

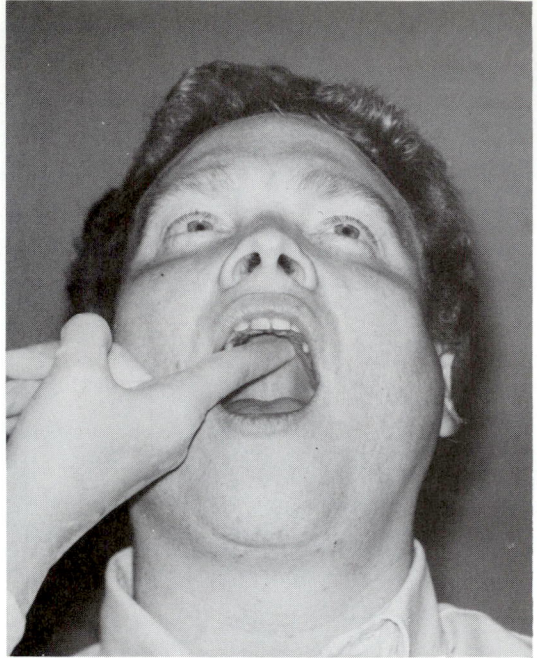

Fig. 8-25. Hard palate is palpated using firm digital pressure against hard tissues.

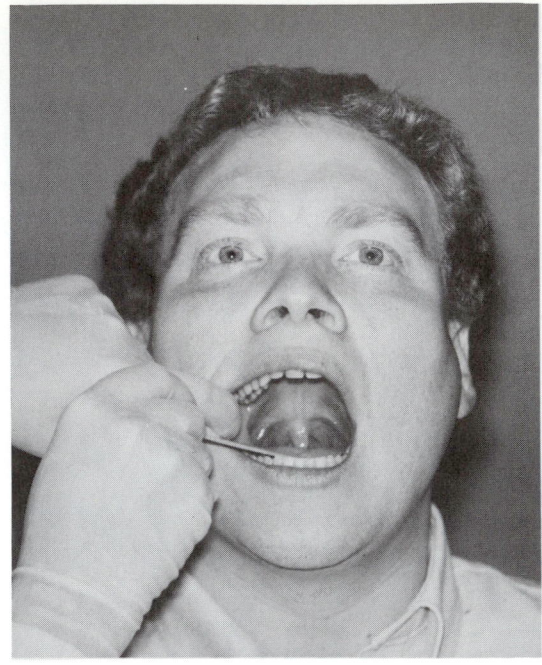

Fig. 8-26. Because the tongue normally shields the oral pharynx from view, this area is examined by placing a mirror or tongue blade on anterior third of tongue and asking patient to say "ah."

some patients. Firm on-and-off pressure against the tissue is more comfortable than light circular pressure, which tends to "tickle" the palate. Palpate for swellings or hard masses (e.g., palatal tori), tenderness, and continuity of the underlying bone.

Next inspect the back of the mouth and examine the soft palate for color and lesions (Fig. 8-26). Observe the palatine uvula for deviations in form or color. To examine the oral pharynx, place a tongue depressor on the middle third of the dorsum of the tongue and ask the patient to say "ah." As the patient does this, the posterior third of the tongue should lower, providing a full view of the entire area. Observe also the movement of the uvula as the patient is saying "ah." Note any deviation of movement to either the right or the left. With the pharynx clearly visible, locate the following structures and examine them for color and signs of abnormal lesions or form: posterior wall of the pharynx, posterior pillars, palatine tonsils, and anterior pillars. Note any redness, signs of exudation, lesions, or tenderness.

The examination of the tongue is specific for each of four surfaces: the dorsal (top), ventral (bottom), and the two lateral borders. Examine the dorsal surface first for color, lesions, symmetry, and form. The normal structures of this surface of the tongue include:

filiform papillae. Plentiful hairlike papillae covering the dorsal surface of the tongue. These generally have a whitish color, although they often are stained extrinsically by food, tobacco, or medication.

fungiform papillae. Flat, broad papillae that appear as red, mushroom-shaped elevations and are scattered among the filiform papillae. They house taste buds for sweet, sour, or salty stimuli.

circumvallate papille. A series of large papillae located in a V-shaped formation on the posterior dorsal surface. They contain taste buds that respond to bitter stimuli only.

Retract the tongue by wrapping a gauze square around the anterior third to obtain a firm grasp and pulling it anteriorly as far as it will extend comfortably. Palpate the dorsal surface using digital compression over the entire surface (Figs.

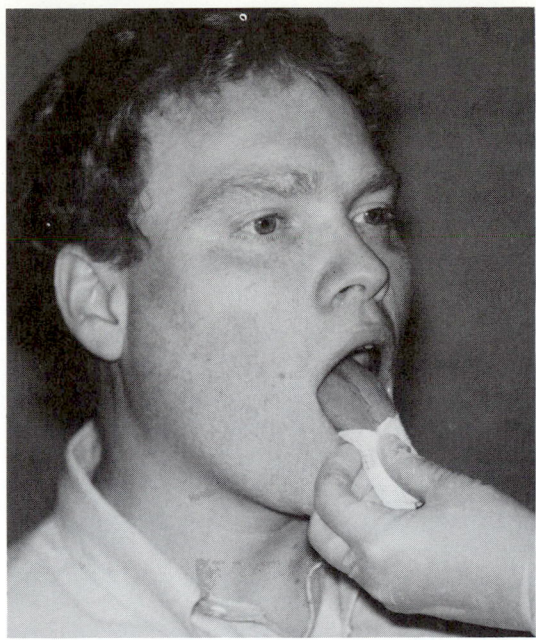

Fig. 8-27. Tongue is grasped by holding it with a folded gauze square and retracting it so that entire dorsal surface can be examined.

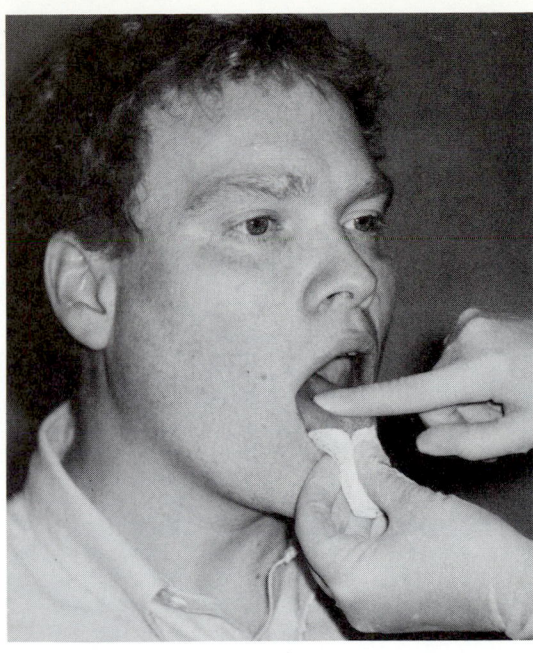

Fig. 8-28. Palpation of dorsal surface of tongue is done with digital compression over entire surface.

8-27 and 8-28). Feel for abnormal masses, indurations, or swellings. Common abnormalities that may be detected on the dorsal surface of the tongue include a coated tongue, black hairy tongue, geographic tongue, and fissured tongue.

While still retracting the tongue out from the mouth, inspect the lateral borders by turning the tongue slightly over on its side to obtain a full view of the border (Fig. 8-29). Examine this area carefully for abnormal redness, red or white patches, swellings, ulcerations, or masses, because it is a common site for oral cancer. The normal structures found on the lateral borders of the tongue are the foliate papillae, which appear as a series of vertical ridges on the posterior borders. These papillae house taste buds for sour and acidic stimuli. Inspect the other side of the tongue in the same way. Palpate the lateral borders using bidigital compression of the tissue between the thumb and fingers, beginning at the posterior borders and moving to the anterior borders after removing the gauze (Fig. 8-30).

Ask the patient to move his or her tongue superiorly (Fig. 8-31). Inspect and palpate the entire

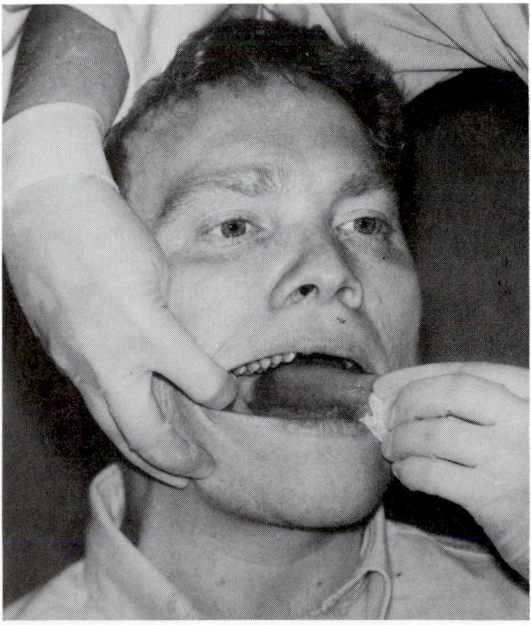

Fig. 8-29. An inspection of lateral borders of tongue involves retracting tongue out using a gauze square and turning it slightly over on its side so that entire lateral border can be closely examined. This is a common site for oral cancer.

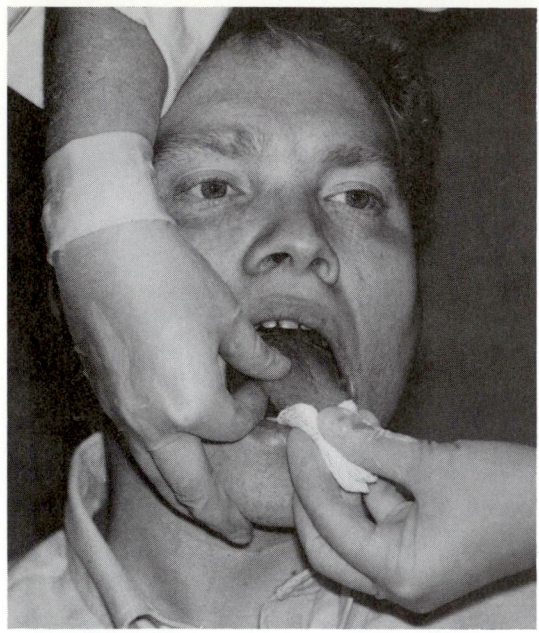

Fig. 8-30. Lateral borders of tongue are palpated with bidigital compression. While one hand stabilizes tongue, the other palpates. This procedure is repeated for other side.

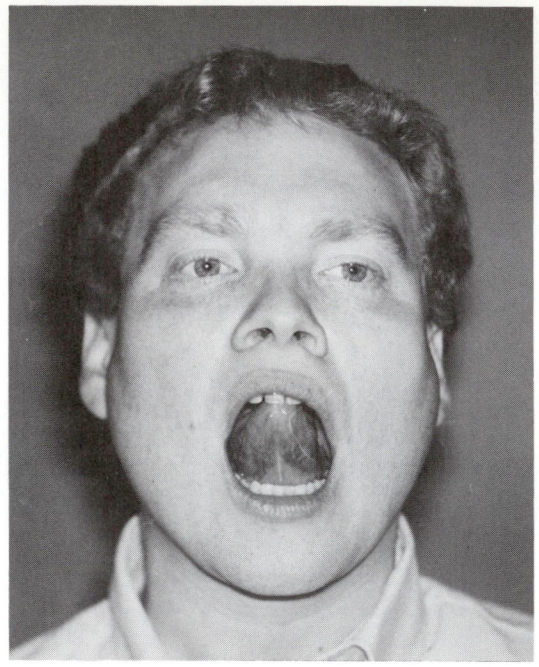

Fig. 8-31. Ventral surface is inspected by asking patient to lift tip of tongue to roof of mouth. With use of a mirror or tongue blade, the floor of the mouth can be examined simultaneously. Palpate the surface.

ventral surface of the tongue using digital compression.

Use the mirror to aid in the inspection of the maxillary tuberosity and retromolar area. Note any deviations in form, color, or size; presence of abnormal growths of tissue; or lesions. Palpate the retromolar areas and maxillary tuberosities using digital compression. Common findings may include scarring from third molar extractions, overgrowth of tissue, inflammation, or tenderness caused by erupting third molars.

Examine the alveolar ridges thoroughly for signs of redness, color deviations, swellings, or lesions. Retraction of the buccal mucosa and tongue is necessary for good visibility of these structures. Palpate the ridges using bidigital compression with the thumb and index finger opposing each other. Examine the ridges for hard masses (tori), swellings, or crepitus, and note any tenderness experienced by the patient (Fig. 8-32).

The general and oral examination of the patient is now complete. After recording all significant findings, the clinician can continue the examination and assessment with more specific evalua-

tions of the dental and periodontal structures. Use of other diagnostic tools, combined with the information obtained from the general and oral portion of the examination, will be used to construct a total picture of the patient's needs.

IDENTIFICATION OF PATIENTS WITH SPECIAL NEEDS

During patient examination, the dental professional may encounter signs and symptoms of conditions that demand the attention of medical and other professionals. As health professionals, the dentist, hygienist, and dental assistant should be alert to the presence of conditions that require referral. Specific situations discussed in this chapter include nutritional disorders, anorexia nervosa, child neglect or abuse, xerostomia, smokeless tobacco use, and AIDS.

Nutritional disorders

A number of conditions observed during the physical evaluation may indicate nutritional disorders. For example, the hair may lack luster and be thin and sparse; the fingernails may appear spoon

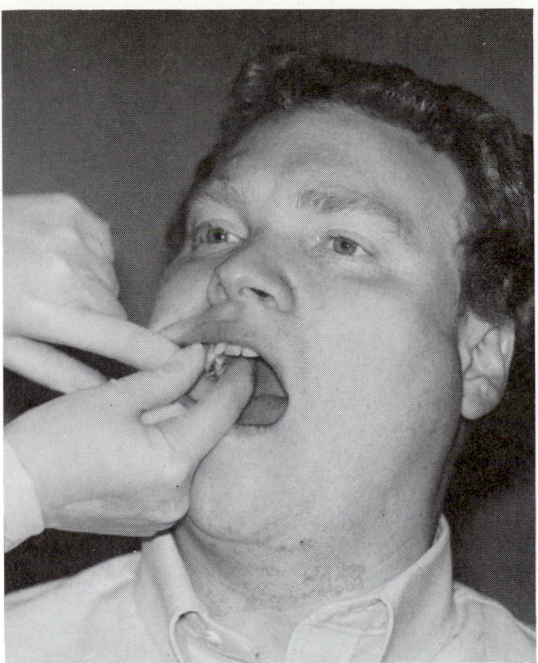

Fig. 8-32. Alveolar ridges are shown being palpated with bidigital compression. Any signs of abnormal masses or lack of continuity in the bone should be noted. Patient should also be requested to report any symptoms experienced during palpation.

shaped, dry, and brittle; the skin may lack color and appear dry and flaky; bruised areas may be visible under the skin because of subdermal bleeding; there may be an abnormal lack of body fat; the face may appear red and swollen; areas under the eyes may appear dark and shadowed; the eyes may appear dull or bloodshot; and the corners of the eyes and lips may be dry, red, and fissured.

Intraoral signs that may indicate nutritional deficiencies include gingivae that bleed easily and a tongue that appears deep red and raw, abnormally smooth, and glossy. The tongue may also exhibit sores or hypertrophy of papillae on the dorsal surface. The teeth may show evidence of decay or abnormal eruption patterns.

Other signs of nutritional deficiency may include an increased heart rate, hypertension, enlargement of the abdominal cavity caused by liver or spleen enlargement, mental irritability, loss of normal reflexes in the knees and ankles, and muscle weakness. This list of signs and symptoms is by no means specific to nutritional disorders, as other medical conditions could produce similar effects. The clinician should combine these findings with information gathered during the patient interview, however, to assess the need for including a nutritional survey in the preventive treatment plan. Additional data from that survey may provide sufficient information to allow you to ascertain the contribution of nutrition to these conditions.

Anorexia nervosa/bulimia nervosa. Individuals suffering from anorexia or bulimia nervosa may be seen in the dental practice. Dental care providers may be the first to suspect these conditions because of the presence of certain oral complications. In general, these patients do not recognize their condition as a health hazard, and they need support and understanding to encourage them to seek professional help. Patients most likely to display signs of anorexia and bulimia nervosa are teenage or young adult women who have poor self-images and a preoccupation with weight control.

Anorexia nervosa causes avoidance of eating, leading to significant weight loss and signs of malnutrition. Anorexics may exhibit electrolyte imbalance, insomnia, constipation, skin disorders, brittle or thin hair and nails, hypotension and/or a low pulse rate (Rollins and Piassa, 1978). Untreated cases have been known to result in death, usually from cardiac failure or suicide.

Patients with bulimia alternate between eating "binges" and "purges" (induced vomiting). Reports indicate that known bulimics may binge and purge an average of 12 times a week. These episodes are often precipitated by emotional stress. In addition to inducing vomiting, these individuals may use laxatives, diuretics, and cathartics to effect weight loss. The resulting physical complications may include acute stomach dilation, electrolyte imbalance, alkalosis, hypochloremia, edema, kidney disorders, and cardiac arrhythmias. Oral symptoms and signs include dental caries, gingivitis, parotid gland enlargement, erosion of enamel (Plate 1, *A*), and dental hypersensitivity brought on by the presence of gastric acids in the mouth (Roberts and Li, 1987).

Patients suffering from these problems usually deny that the problems exist and deny vomiting. They do not respond positively to criticism, so an empathetic yet direct approach to the problem is needed. The treatment of this condition is not within the dental professional's area of training, so referral is necessary. The dental professional can be instrumental, however, in providing information and encouragement to convince the patient of the need to seek professional help. The dentist or hygienist can also help by telling the patient how to minimize the oral complications of frequent vomiting until the condition is brought under control. Patients should be advised to use a sodium bicarbonate or magnesium hydroxide rinse after vomiting to neutralize the effects of excess acids. In addition, the use of daily fluoride rinses or fluoride gels may be indicated to prevent the occurrence of decay and to minimize enamel erosion and related hypersensitivity. Patients should also be advised not to brush immediately after vomiting, because doing so might increase the eroding effect of the acids. Usual approaches to plaque control should be encouraged, although these individuals do not seem more susceptible than the general population to periodontal destruction (Roberts and Li, 1987).

Child neglect or abuse

The general appraisal and head and neck examination of children may lead to suspicions regarding the presence of child neglect or abuse. Dental professionals are especially likely to detect the signs and symptoms of maltreatment during their examinations because an estimated 50% of these injuries occur to the head, face, and intraoral areas (Becker et al, 1978; Kittle et al, 1981).

There is a difference in the meaning of the terms *child neglect* and *child abuse*. Child neglect refers to physical or emotional negligence of a child and usually represents a case of omission (failure to provide health, food, and medical and dental care). Child neglect in terms of dental care might include such findings as untreated rampant caries, untreated dental pain or infection, or a lack of continuity of dental care in the presence of known disease (Davis et al, 1979).

Child abuse includes any physical, sexual, or emotional act directed against a child. During the general appraisal of the patient, the dental professional might notice that the child appears fearful, withdrawn, or watchful and provides no eye contact or spontaneous smiles. There may be signs of malnutrition, uncleanliness, limping, or a slumped or withdrawn posture. During the extraoral examination, signs of bruises, slap marks, bite marks, black eyes, cigarette burns, or abrasions and lacerations in unusual places should be noted. The ears should be examined for signs of trauma caused by twisting, pulling, or pinching. Marks on the neck that might have been caused by strangling may also be detected (Davis et al, 1979).

Intraorally, signs of child abuse may include teeth that have been fractured or displaced; scars on the lips, mucosa, or tongue; binding marks at the corners of the mouth where the child has been gagged; darkened or nonvital teeth; or laceration to the maxillary frenum. Jaw fractures also might result from abuse.

More than 1 million cases of child abuse or neglect are reported each year in the United States; at least 2,000 children die from these causes annually (Kittle et al, 1981; Winters, 1985). Those numbers translate into six deaths a day or one every 4 hours (Stimson, 1984). The true incidence of child maltreatment is probably much higher than these figures indicate, as only about half of all child abuse cases are reported to authorities (Sopher, 1977).

Surveys of child abuse have shown that there are no reliable predictors for its occurrence. The age distribution varies from birth to 17 years. Children from all socioeconomic groups are affected (Davis et al, 1979; Kittle et al, 1981). Schwartz and others (1977) found little difference in the incidence of the problem based on racial, religious, economic, or educational grounds. Obviously, this problem is a serious one that deserves the attention and action of the dental community to assist in its detection and solution.

Dental professionals as well as others in the community are mandated by law to report suspected cases of child abuse or neglect to the appropriate local authorities. It is not the responsibility of dental professionals to prove that maltreatment has occurred, only to report that they suspect it. Other health and welfare authorities must then investigate.

The dentist or dental hygienist should follow several steps before reporting suspected child maltreatment. First, the presence of unexplained or unusual injuries must be recognized and documented in the dental record. Color photos of suspicious injuries may also be taken to document their appearance. The child and/or parents should be asked how injuries occurred, and the explanations should be correlated with the appearance of the wounds. Parents should be approached not in an accusatory or critical manner but in a way that demonstrates genuine concern for the child (Stanley, 1981). The dentist or hygienist should explain to the parents the legal responsibility of health professionals to ask about unusual injuries. If the explanations seem unsatisfactory to account for the nature of the injuries, the dental professional may seek assistance through consultation with the family's physician or with special agencies set up to deal with these problems.

Information regarding procedures for reporting suspected child abuse usually can be obtained from state or local welfare or health departments. Laws in most states require dental professionals to report suspected cases of child abuse or neglect to the appropriate state agency for investigation. Failure to do so can result in a fine, imprisonment, or both. In addition, all states and the District of Columbia protect dental professionals and others from civil and criminal lawsuits when the reports of child abuse or neglect are made in good faith (Schwartz et al, 1977).

Xerostomia

Xerostomia (dry mouth) is a common oral sign of postradiation therapy treatment. Ionizing radiation can destroy salivary gland architecture so that the serous component of saliva is lost; function of the gland rarely returns (Marks et al, 1981). Patients may complain of difficulty in swallowing, difficulty retaining a maxillary denture, burning mouth, cracked lips, and/or difficulty in swallowing (Plate 1, *B*). Other factors that can induce xerostomia include AIDS, bulimia, and drugs such as antihypertensives, diuretics, antidepressants, and antihistamines (Matthews, 1990). Appropriate care should be designed for these patients. An over-the-counter saliva substitute could be recommended especially for patients with afunctional glands. Some groups advocate the use of topical pilocarpine to stimulate saliva; this should be used only by patients with functional salivary glands. Postradiation therapy patients cannot use pilocarpine. Frequent recalls and home fluoride therapy should be recommended for dentulous patients. An air humidifier and petroleum jelly for the lips could be recommended for patient use during sleep.

Smokeless tobacco

Smokeless tobacco has been associated with oral leukoplakia in a variety of locations in the oral cavity (National Institute of Dental Research [NIDR], 1990). In the NIDR report, snuff users were reported to have a much higher prevalence of oral leukoplakia than tobacco chewers (Plate 1, *C*). Snuff users are more likely to have loss of attachment and root caries at sites where they held the tobacco. Although leukoplakia can be a precursor to oral cancer, biopsies of lesions in the NIDR study showed that they were not cancerous. The investigators suggested that this may have been because the subjects in the study had not been using snuff long enough.

AIDS

In 1981, the Centers for Disease Control announced several unusual cases of *Pneumocystis* pneumonia in homosexuals. Those early reports were the first glimpses of what is now known to be AIDS. This syndrome has several intraoral manifestations that may be prognostic of the disease. Plate 1, *D* is a facial view of an AIDS patient who initially presented to the clinician with multiple purple nodules on the face. These same types of nodules were present in the mouth (Plate 1, *E*). On biopsy, the lesions were found to be consistent with Kaposi's sarcoma, one of the first lesions to appear in an AIDS patient's mouth (Silverman et al, 1986; Wescott, 1990). After diagnosis of this malignant lesion, death occurs within 3 years (Keenly et al, 1987).

Candidiasis is also noted to occur in AIDS patients (Plate 1, *F*). This disease is caused by the dimorphic fungus *Candida albicans*. Infections may appear as white curdlike plaques on a variety of mucous membranes. This intraoral lesion has been identified in 88% of heterosexual as well as homosexual HIV-positive patients (Silverman et al, 1986). Dental professionals should be aware of the implications of discovering oral candidiasis in an otherwise healthy person.

Hairy leukoplakia of the tongue (Plate 1, *G*) was first described in patients with human T-lymphotrophic virus III (also known as HIV) disease (Greenspan et al, 1987). It appears to result from a proliferation of Epstein-Barr virus, possibly in association with the papilloma virus, within the superficial layers of the squamous epithelium of the tongue. In AIDS-related complex, this leukoplakia is usually associated with a poor prognosis. It is seldom symptomatic.

Herpes zoster is also very common, occurring in 25% of patients with AIDS and AIDS-related complex. The unique unilateral distribution of painful pustules along V-1 of cranial nerve V is noted in Plate 1, *H*. Clinically, its course does not appear to be more severe and dissemination is rare.

The abilities of dentists, dental hygienists, and dental assistants to recognize HIV/AIDS-associated intraoral lesions was recently investigated (Tilliss and Stach, 1991). Recognition scores for all groups indicated that the dental health team may not be recognizing these important oral manifestations of a deadly disease.

SELF-EXAMINATION FOR ORAL CANCER
Oral cancer self-examination: teaching approach

The first time the patient performs the self-examination for oral cancer, guide him or her through the steps of the examination and confirm the findings. Ideally, the patient should sit in front of a large mirror and you should stand behind or sit at the patient's side; from either of these positions, both can see into the patient's mouth. At the beginning of the examination, it may be helpful to remind the patient that he or she is examining the face, neck, and mouth to become familiar with the normal forms and structures so that any changes can be noticed during subsequent examinations. Also, you will be helping the patient identify the normal structures within the mouth. The patient should follow the outline or pamphlet that he or she will be using at home and should perform as much of the examination on his or her own as possible. This is a difficult balance to strike, because you are playing the dual role of teaching the procedure and fostering some independence in the patient. Ultimately, at the end of the session, the patient will have learned the examination and will be confident enough to perform it at home at regular intervals. In addition, you have the challenge of motivating the patient to want to perform the examination regularly. The approaches for motivating a patient to perform the oral cancer self-examination are the same as those for motivating a patient to perform home care procedures. In this situation, however, the potential benefits to the patient are even greater—his or her life.

The oral cancer self-examination is composed of several steps in which the face, neck, and mouth are examined (Atterbury, 1979; Burzynski, Moore, and DeJean, 1970; Carl et al, 1982; Engelman and Schackner, 1966; Glass et al, 1975;

Olsqewski, 1976). A pamphlet such as *Early Detection of Oral Cancer May Save Your Life,* published by the American Cancer Society (Eastern Great Lakes, 1976), can be given to the patient. Many dental and dental auxiliary schools also have pamphlets outlining the steps of the oral cancer self-examination for use by the patient.

While the patient is learning to perform the examination, the clinician should point out the normal structures in each area and review with the patient the kinds of changes that should be noted.

At the completion of the examination, it should be emphasized to the patient that the earlier any changes are brought to the attention of the dentist the better. Any change or lesion that is present for 2 weeks should be checked by the dentist; waiting even until the next 6-month checkup may be too risky. It may be helpful to reassure the patient that the dentist would rather be asked to check a thousand changes in the patient's mouth that turn out to be normal rather than not asked to check the one change that may lead to cancer.

The following outline for the lay person describes one way a dental hygienist can teach oral cancer self-examination (Eastern Great Lakes, 1976; Glass et al, 1975).

Oral cancer self-examination: guidelines for the lay person

This outline is to be used as a guide when you perform the oral cancer self-examination. It lists each of the areas to be examined and the kinds of changes that may be significant and should be brought to the dentist's attention. In general, you are looking for any of the following changes:

1. Any sores on the face, neck, or mouth that do not heal within 2 weeks
2. Any white, red, or dark patches in the mouth
3. Any swelling, lump, bump, or growth
4. Repeated bleeding for no apparent reason
5. Pain or loss of feeling in any area of the face, neck, or mouth

A mirror and good lighting are needed for the examination. Following are the steps of the oral cancer self-examination.

1. *Facial symmetry*. Look at yourself in the mirror. Both sides of your face and neck should be the same size, shape, and form. No person's face is absolutely symmetric, but the two sides are basically the same. Any swellings, lumps,

bumps, or growths appearing on one side of your face should be noted; if they appear on both sides of your face, they are probably normal (Fig. 8-33).

2. *Face*. Look at the skin on your face and neck. You are looking for any changes in skin color, moles that have changed, lumps, or sores. If you wear glasses, take them off and examine the areas covered by them—the bridge of the nose. Finally, palpate your face by gently pressing fingers of each hand against all areas of your face. By palpating both sides of your face at the same time, you will notice any differences between one side of your face and the other side (Fig. 8-34).

3. *Side of neck*. With the fingers of both hands, palpate both sides of your neck at the same time. As with your face, you are feeling for any lumps, bumps, or swellings that appear on one side of your neck but not on the other (Fig. 8-35).

4. *Center of neck*. Gently place your fingers against your "Adam's apple" and swallow; it should move when you swallow. Then grasp your Adam's apple and gently move it from side to side (Fig. 8-36). Once again, check for any lumps or bumps, and note any hoarseness that does not clear up within 2 weeks.

Any dentures or partial dentures should be removed at this point.

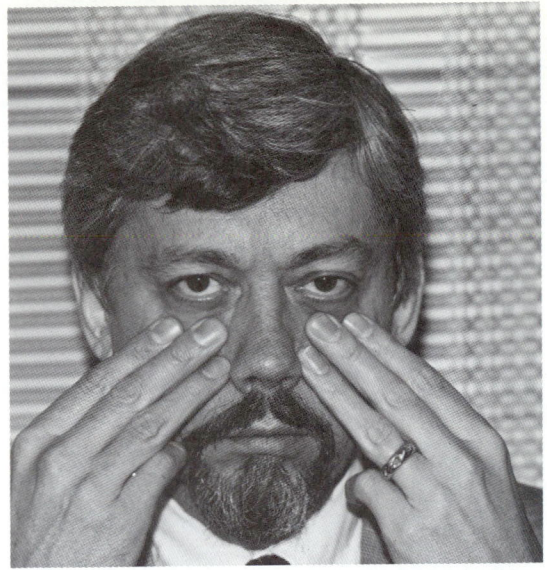

Fig. 8-34. Palpating face with both hands.

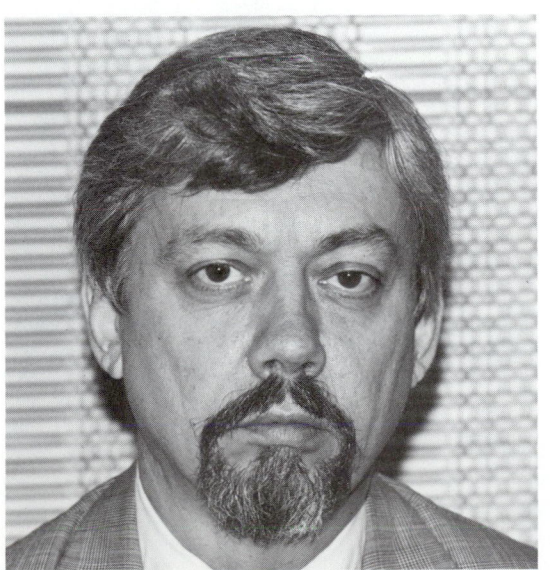

Fig. 8-33. Examining facial symmetry visually.

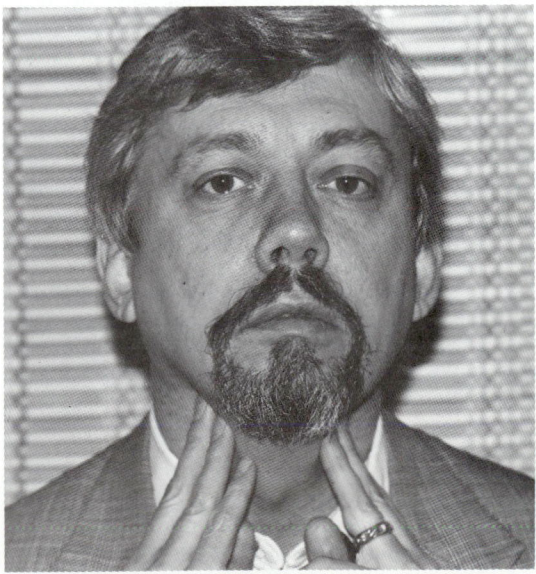

Fig. 8-35. Palpating neck with both hands.

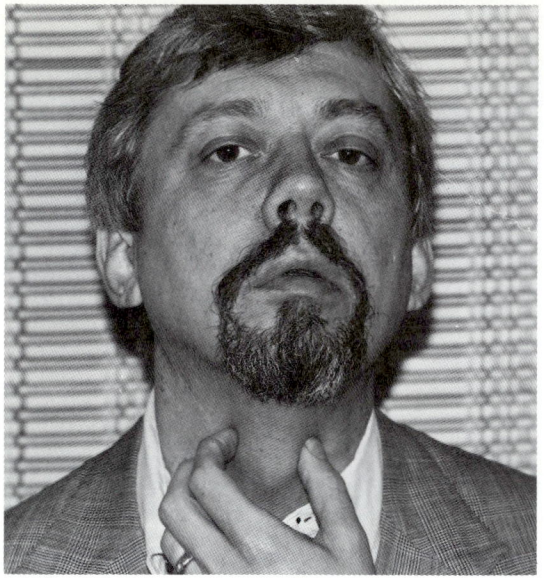

Fig. 8-36. Palpating center of neck ("Adam's apple").

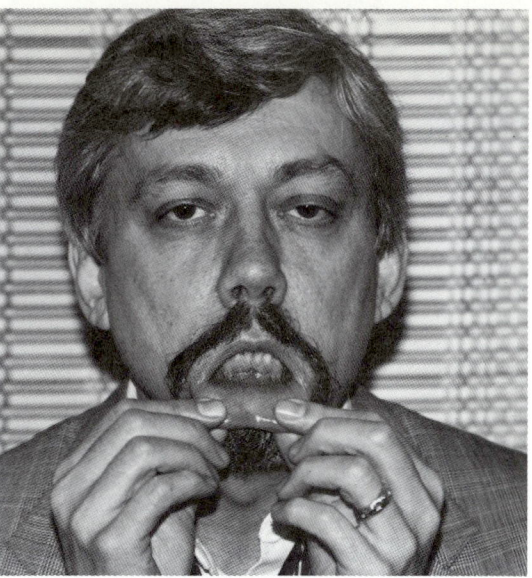

Fig. 8-37. Examining inner surface of lips.

5. *Lips*. Pull your lower lip down and look for any sores or color changes. Gently squeeze your lip with your fingers to feel for any swellings, lumps, bumps, or tenderness. Repeat this procedure for your upper lip (Fig. 8-37).

6. *Cheek*. Pull back your cheek with your fingers so you can see the tissue inside your cheek. Look for any color changes—red, white, or dark areas. Place your thumb on the outside of your cheek and your index finger inside and gently squeeze your cheek. Note any swellings, lumps, or bumps. Repeat this procedure for your other cheek (Fig. 8-38).

7. *Roof of mouth*. Tilt your head back and look at the roof of your mouth. Note any color changes—white, red, or dark areas—or any lumps. With your index finger gently press against the roof of your mouth to feel any lumps, bumps, or swellings (Fig. 8-39).

8. *Gingivae*. Look at your gingivae for any color changes—red, white or dark areas—lumps, bumps, or growths. Are there any sores that have not healed for longer than 14 days or any areas that bleed without cause (Fig. 8-40)?

9. *Tongue and floor of mouth*. Place the tip of your tongue to the roof of your mouth. Look at the un-

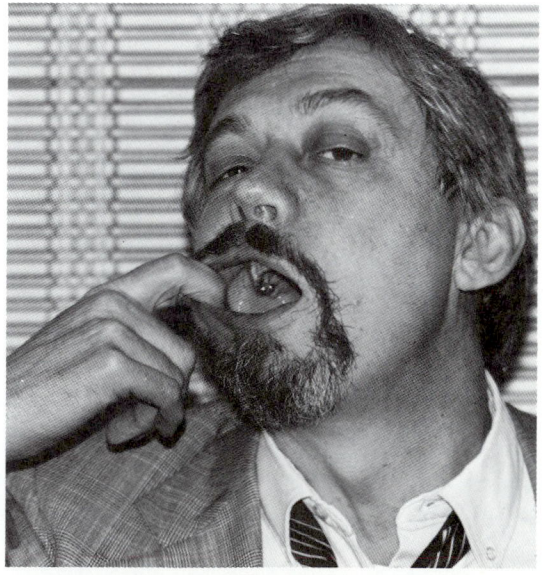

Fig. 8-38. Examining inner surface of cheek.

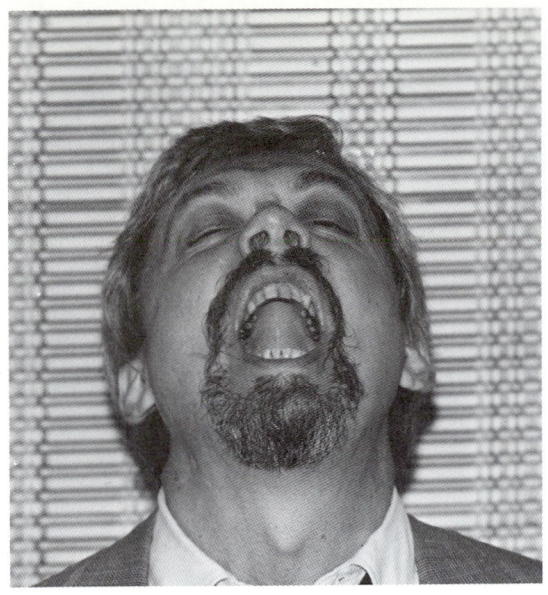

Fig. 8-39. Examining roof of mouth.

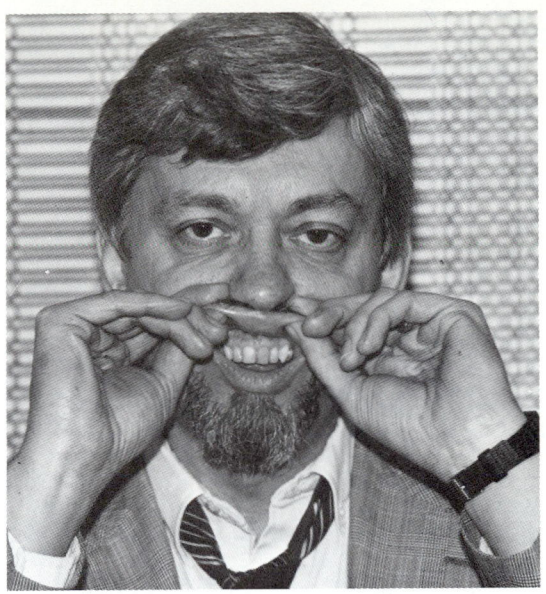

Fig. 8-40. Lifting lip to examine gums.

derside of your tongue and the floor of your mouth for any color changes, lumps, bumps, or growths. Palpate the floor of your mouth by gently pressing your finger against it to feel any lumps, bumps, or growths. Extend your tongue and look at its top side. Using a gauze square, grasp the tip of your tongue and gently pull it to one side. Look at the side of your tongue and palpate it. Note any color changes, lumps, bumps, or sores that have not healed. Repeat this procedure on the other side of your tongue (Figs. 8-41 to 8-44).

SUMMARY

At the completion of the examination, the clinician can ask if the patient has any questions about the procedure. This is also a good time to ask patients if they have any concerns or hesitations about performing the examination. The clinician should be sensitive to patients' responses; some patients may express their concerns about actually finding oral cancer. Perhaps the patients' fears can be acknowledged and discussed as appropriate. The patients should be encouraged to perform

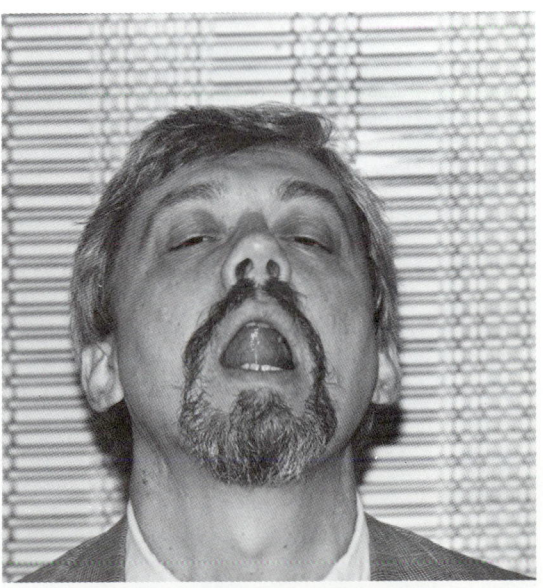

Fig. 8-41. Raising tongue to examine its undersurface and floor of mouth.

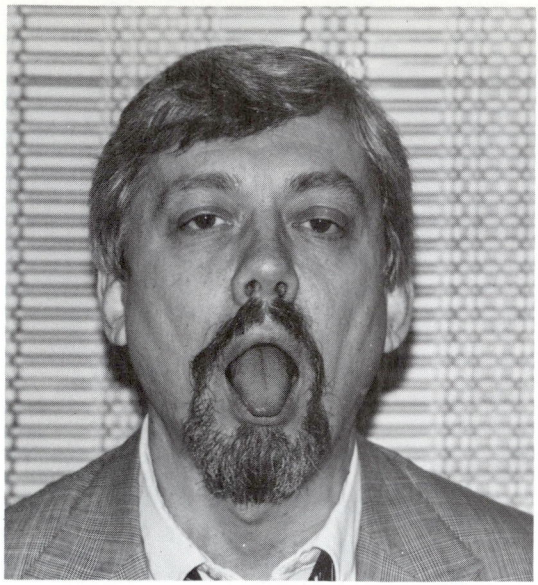

Fig. 8-42. Examining upper surface of tongue.

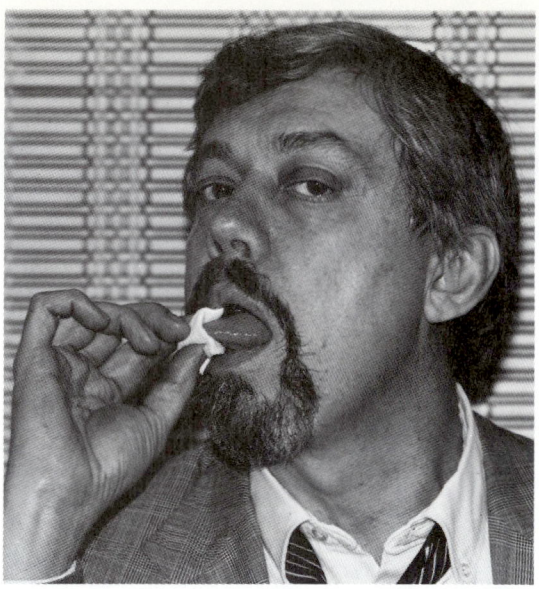

Fig. 8-43. Grasping tip of tongue with gauze and examining side of tongue.

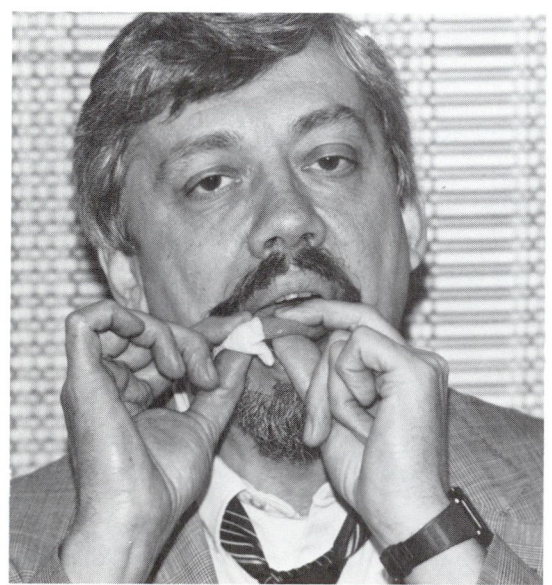

Fig. 8-44. Palpating tongue.

the examination routinely and to call the office as needed.

CONCLUSION

Teaching the guided self-assessment and oral cancer self-examination are important preventive adjuncts in dental hygiene treatment. The procedures and findings of the examination will need to be reviewed with patients at subsequent visits to ensure proper completion of the examinations. These examinations benefit both the patient and the dental health professional. The patients become knowledgeable about their oral conditions and able to detect oral cancer in its early stages. The professional is able to work with patients who are truly partners in care.

ACTIVITIES

1. Obtain a presentation designed to teach the concepts of blood pressure screening and hypertension, such as *Hypertension . . . The Silent Killer: Screening* (14:41) B-1460 and *Practice in Blood Pressure Reading* (13:40) B-315.*

*Written by Jane Anderson and Nancy Champlin Geistfeld. Produced by Health Sciences Learning Resources, Dental Audio-Visual, Biomedical Graphic Communications, University of Minnesota, Minneapolis.

2. Practice the procedures for determining each of the four vital signs on a laboratory partner or clinic patient.

3. Practice the procedures for intraoral and extraoral examination with a laboratory partner or clinic patient. To sharpen tactile perceptions during the palpation of hard and soft tissues, work in pairs and practice palpating individual structures on a laboratory partner with your eyes closed. Concentrate on the different anatomic structures and textures that you feel and describe them to your partner.

4. Arrange for a guest speaker from the oncologic department of a nearby hospital to speak on the incidence of oral cancer in your area; check with the local American Cancer Society to get the latest pamphlets, statistics, and public information on oral cancer.

5. Have a group discussion about students' feelings regarding touching another person's body as in the head and neck examination. Some students react at first with embarrassment at having to perform this procedure for strangers. Discuss ways of dealing with these feelings. Role-play explaining the purpose and use of the oral examination to a patient. Include in the role-playing a situation in which a suspicious lesion that might be cancerous is detected. What would you say to the patient in that situation? When discussing the role-playing, ask the "patient" what feelings or reactions he or she had to a thorough examination.

6. Contact the state or local child welfare department to find out the exact procedures required for reporting child neglect or abuse in your state.

7. Show slides of a variety of intraoral and extraoral lesions and have students write a clinical description of each lesion.

8. List some of the classic signs and symptoms of AIDS and AIDS-related complex involving the oral cavity as well as other sites.

REVIEW QUESTIONS

1. Give five reasons for performing a complete general and oral examination.
2. List the four vital signs.
3. State the normal range for each of the following:
   a. Adult pulse.
   b. Adult respiration rate.
   c. Adult temperature.
   d. Adult blood pressure.
   e. Borderline temperature for fever.
   f. Borderline blood pressure for hypertension.

4. Describe the procedure for obtaining the following from a patient:
   a. Pulse rate.
   b. Blood pressure
5. State the four methods of examination described in the text and give an example of how each is used.
6. Describe the palpation technique recommended for the following structures:
   a. Submandibular lymph nodes.
   b. Floor of the mouth.
   c. Buccal mucosa.
7. Why must the initial inspection of the mouth be done before the clinician's hands enter the mouth?
8. What chain of lymph nodes is located near each of the following structures?
   a. Ear.
   b. Sternocleidomastoid muscle.
   c. Base of the skull.
   d. Floor of the mouth.

REFERENCES

American Cancer Society: Cancer statistics, 1987, *CA* 37:13, 1987.

American Dental Association Council on Dental Health and Health Planning and Bureau of Health Education and Audiovisual Services: Breaking the silence on hypertension: a dental perspective, *JADA* 110:781, 1985.

Atterbury RA: Self-examination of paraoral tissues for detection of early oral cancer, *Dent Surv* 55:18, 1979.

Becker DB et al: Child abuse and dentistry: orofacial trauma and its recognition by dentists, *JADA* 97:24, 1978.

Boring C et al: Cancer statistics, 1992, *CA* 42:19, 1992.

Burzynski NJ, Moore C, DeJean E: Basic steps in mouth-throat examination for cancer detection, *JADA* 81:932, 1970.

Carl W et al: Early detection of oral cancer: another aspect of preventive dentistry, *Quintessence Int* 13:1179, 1982.

Conway BJ: High blood pressure screening and referral by dentists: legal implications of blood pressure measurement in the dental practice, *RI Dent J* 13:16, Dec 1980.

Cutler LS: Evaluation and management of the dental patient with cardiovascular disease. II. Hypertension, *J Conn Dent Assoc* 60(4):230, 1986.

Davis GR et al: The dentist's role in child abuse and neglect, *J Dent Child* 46:185, 1979.

Eastern Great Lakes Head and Neck Cancer Control Network and Department of Oral Medicine: *Early detection of oral cancer may save your life*, New York, 1976, American Cancer Society.

Engelman MA, Schackner JS: *Oral cancer examination procedure*, Poughkeepsie, NY, 1966, St Francis Hospital.

Friedman RJ et al: Early detection of malignant melanoma: the role of physician examination and self-examination of the skin, *CA* 35:130, 1985.

Gaynor AM: Commonly used drugs in dentistry and the hypertensive patient, *W Va Dent J* 57(1):18, 1983.

Glass RT et al: Teaching self-examination of the head and neck: another aspect of preventive dentistry, *JADA* 90:1265, 1975.

Greenspan D et al: Relationship of oral hairy leukoplakia with HIV and the risk of developing AIDS, *J Infect Dis* 155:475, 1987.

Joint National Committee on Detection, Evaluation and Treatment of High Blood Pressure: *1984 report,* Washington, DC, 1984a, US Department of Health and Human Services, Public Health Service, National Institutes of Health, pub no 84-1088.

Joint National Committee on Detection, Evaluation and Treatment of High Blood Pressure: *Arch Intern Med* 144:1045, 1984b.

Kerr DA, Ash MM, Millard HD: *Oral diagnosis,* ed 6, St Louis, 1983, CV Mosby.

Keeney K et al: Oral Kaposi's sarcoma in acquired immune deficiency syndrome, *J Oral Maxillofac Surg* 45:815, 1987.

Kittle PE et al: Two child abuse/child neglect examinations for the dentist, *J Dent Child* 48:175, 1981.

Klimaszewski DL, Grim CM: *Blood pressure measurement: standardization and certification program manual,* Indianapolis, 1985, Indiana University Hospitals.

Kutcher MJ et al: Oral medicine in general dental practice. I. physical evaluation of the dental patient, *Compend Contin Educ Dent* 2:79, 1981.

Malasanos L et al: *Health assessment,* ed 3, St Louis, 1986, CV Mosby.

Marks J et al: Selective measurements of parotid salivary function after electron beam therapy, *Int J Radiat Oncol Biol Phys* 7:1013, 1981.

Matthews TG: Medication side effects of dental interest, *J Prosthet Dent* 64:219, 1990.

McCann AL, Wesley RK: A method for describing soft tissue lesions of the oral cavity, *Dent Hyg* 62:219, 1987.

Murray HW et al: Patients at risk for AIDS-related opportunistic infections, *N Engl J Med* 313:1504, 1985.

National Institute of Dental Research: Dental researchers link smokeless tobacco to oral lesions, *NIDR Res Dig* Sept. p. 2, 1990.

Olsqewski V: The role of the dental hygienist in oral cancer detection, *Dent Hyg* 50:169, 1976.

Roberts MW, Li H: Oral findings in anorexia nervosa and bulimia nervosa: a study of 47 cases, *JADA* 115:407, 1987.

Rollins N, Piazza E: Diagnosis of anorexia nervosa: a critical reappraisal, *J Am Acad Child Psychiatry,* 17:126, 1978.

Schwartz S et al: Oral manifestations and legal aspects of child abuse, *JADA* 95:586, 1977.

Shapiro S, Avery K: An office protocol for treating patients with hypertensive disease, *Ark Dent J* 55(4):15, 1984.

Silverberg DS: The dentist's role in hypertension detection, *J Can Dent Assoc* 42:549, 1976.

Silverman S et al: Oral findings in people with or at high risk for AIDS: a study of 375 homosexual males, *JADA* 112:187, 1986.

Singer J et al: Blood pressure fluctuations during dental hygiene treatment, *Dent Hyg* 57:24, Aug 1983.

Sopher I: The dentist and the battered child syndrome, *Dent Clin North Am* 21:113, 1977.

Stanley RT: Child abuse—what's a dentist to do? *Ohio Dent J* 55(9):16, 1981.

Stimson PG: Battered child syndrome, *Tex Dent J* 101(9):10, 1984.

Tilliss T, Stach DJ: Recognition of HIV/AIDS-associated oral lesions by the dental team, *Clin Prev Dent* 13:5, 1991.

Wescott W: *Malignant neoplasms and lesions of unknown etiology in the impact of HIV infection on dentistry,* taped broadcast, Regional Learning Resources Center, St Louis VAMC, 1990.

Winters R: *Child abuse digest,* Tampa, Fla, 1985, Winters Communications.

Zarkowski P: Legal considerations in periodontal therapy, *Dent Hyg News* 4:3, 1991.

SUGGESTED READINGS

Abbey LM et al: A resurvey of hypertensive patients detected in a dental office screening program, *J Public Health Dent* 36:244, 1976.

Abbey LM et al: Hypertension screening among dental patients, *JADA* 93:996, 1976.

Baden E: Prevention of cancer of the oral cavity and pharynx, *CAS* 37:49, 1987.

Barkmeier WW et al: Anorexia nervosa: recognition and management, *J Oral Med* 37:134, 1982.

Malamed SF: Blood pressure evaluation and the prevention of medical emergencies in dental practice, *J Prev Dent* 6:183, 1980.

Rawson RD: Child abuse identification, *J Can Dent Assoc* 14:21, 1986.

PRINCIPLES OF INSTRUMENTATION AND POSITIONING

Irene Woodall
Laura Mueller-Joseph

The dental hygienist will be able to

1. Determine the basic purposes of the following instruments in the assessment phase of dental hygiene care:
   Mouth mirror
   Explorer
   Periodontal probe
2. Identify the specific parts of an instrument; handle, working end(s), shank, and terminal shank.
3. Identify single-ended, double-ended, and paired instruments.
4. Identify instruments by their shapes and recognize variations in shape and design.
5. Determine the appropriate positioning of the dental chair, clinician, patient, and chairside assistant to enhance instrumentation procedures.
6. Adjust the positions of the clinician, patient, and chairside assistant to provide maximum access and visibility of any area in the dentition.
7. Given any tooth surface, adjust himself or herself to the proper position; adjust the patient's head position and the over head light; use the mouth mirror to maximize access and vision; and establish a modified pen grasp, finger rest, and wrist motion to generate vertical, overlapping strokes on a tooth.
8. Establish proper positioning, access, vision, grasp, finger rest, wrist motion, and stroke for each area in the recommended sequence of positions.
9. Use proper positioning, grasp, wrist motion, instrument adaptation, and stroke for the following instruments:
   Periodontal probe
   Paired explorer (cowhorn, pigtail)
   Straight-shanked explorer (No. 17 or 20)
10. Explore for caries using the shepherd's hook (No. 23) explorer.

Instrumentation is a term used to describe the use of hand-held instruments in the practice of dental hygiene. The principal skills necessary to perform instrumentation procedures include grasp, finger rest, and wrist motion, in addition to proper patient/operator positioning.

INSTRUMENT DESIGN

Most instruments are designed with four specific parts; the handle, shank, terminal shank, and working end. (Fig. 9-1 demonstrates the parts of the instrument.) Knowledge of instrument parts and designs enhances instrument selection and facilitates discussion of variations.

The *handle* is the part grasped by the clinician or assistant. Handles come in various shapes and sizes, including variations of hexagonal, round, and tapered. They can be smooth or have knurls or a grooved pattern to prevent them from slipping in the user's hand (Pattison and Behrens, 1973; Pattison and Pattison, 1992; Ward and Simring, 1978;). New handles designed by Hu-Friedy

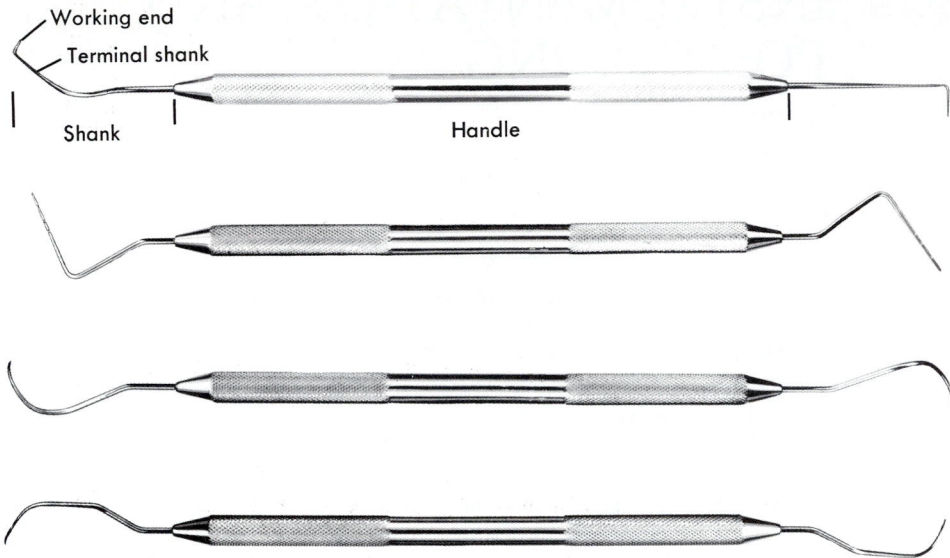

Fig. 9-1. Handle of instrument is connected to a thinner shank angled to permit access to various areas of the dentition. Working end is at tip of instrument. Part of shank closest to working end is called the terminal shank. All instruments shown are double ended. Bottom two instruments are paired. (Courtesy of Hu-Friedy Co., Chicago, Illinois.)

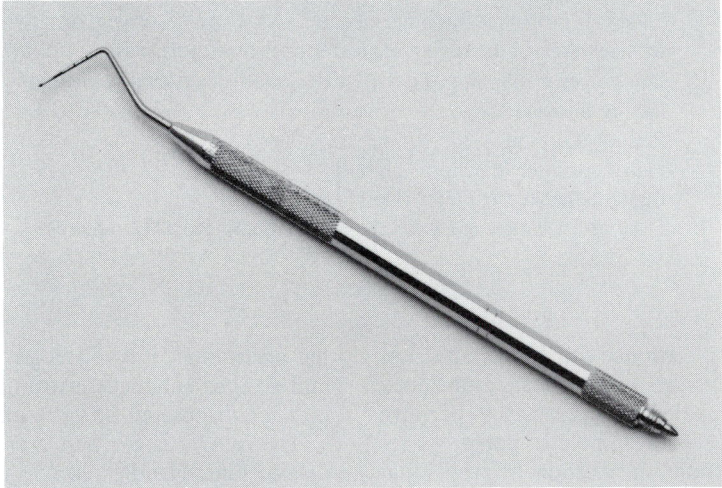

Fig. 9-2. Entire instrument is autoclavable to reduce cross-contamination during charting. Pen Probe. (Courtesy Hu-Friedy Co., Chicago, Illinois.)

(Chicago, Ill.) incorporate a pen at one end (Fig. 9-2). These handles can only be used with single-ended instruments and are most commonly found on explorers and probes to limit cross-contamination during charting.

The *working end* of the instrument refers to the end of the instrument that comes into contact with the tooth and performs the intended task. The working end can have a point, blade, blunt nib, pincers for grasping an object, or some other useful configuration (Pattison and Behrens, 1973; Pattison and Pattison, 1992; Ward and Simring, 1978).

Joining the working end and the handle is the *shank*, which determines the accessibility of the instrument to various places in the mouth and the flex and strength of the instrument. The angles and convolutions in the shank permit access to posterior areas and proximal surfaces while allowing the clinician's hand to enter from the front of the mouth. The thickness and tensile strength of the shank dictate the amount of stress that it can endure in intraoral procedures requiring considerable pressure. Shank shape and strength are therefore particularly important considerations when selecting instruments for removing heavy, tenacious deposits from the teeth (Pattison and Behrens, 1973; Pattison and Pattison, 1992; Ward and Simring, 1978).

The *terminal shank* is the part of the shank that is closest to the working end. It is important to be able to locate the terminal shank on instruments with simple and complex shanks, because the terminal shank is one important cue in adapting the instrument to the tooth. This term is used frequently in this chapter to describe the procedure for selecting the correct end of the instrument and for ensuring that it is being used safely and correctly.

Some instruments have two working ends, one at each end of the handle. These are referred to as *double-ended* instruments. Using double-ended instruments necessitates fewer instrument changes and minimizes the number of individual instruments on the tray, reducing clutter. However, when changing ends of an instrument, one must take care to prevent touching the patient with the instrument. Instrument changes should occur away from the patient's face, usually over the patient's chest, as is the practice in four-handed dentistry. All of the instruments shown in Fig. 9-1 are double ended.

Two of the double-ended instruments in Fig. 9-1 are also examples of *paired instruments*. The ends of a paired instrument are mirror images of each other. One end is intended for use on the proximal surface of a tooth from the facial aspect. Its pair is intended for entry from the lingual aspect. Thus the bends in the shank allow access to a given proximal surface from both aspects.

A more complete discussion of where instruments may be used and how pairs are identified is presented in later chapters. At this point in developing an awareness of instruments and their use, it is helpful to remember that many instruments are used in pairs, permitting universal access to tooth surfaces.

Fig. 9-2 shows and innovative pen-probe instrument that enables one end to assess periodontal conditions while the other is used to record findings. The pen is autoclavable when reversed inside the handle (Hu-Friedy, Chicago, Illinois).

As each instrument is introduced and used in assessing patient needs and implementing care, it may be helpful to identify the parts of the instrument and to project what function it might serve and where it could be adapted. This approach to instrument selection will enable the clinician to identify instruments on the basis of their shapes and sizes rather than by the numbers engraved in the handle. It also will help the clinician develop a working familiarity with instruments, permitting experimentation with a variety of designs as skill and experience grow.

Another important reason for knowing and analyzing instrument design is that the original shape must be preserved as instruments are sharpened. Strokes with a sharpening stone are more likely to sharpen without damaging the working end if the clinician has a clear concept of the proper shape.

BASIC INSTRUMENT SKILLS: GRASP, FINGER REST, AND WRIST MOTION

The hand instruments used in dental hygiene care serve a variety of functions in the assessment, implementation, and evaluation phases of care. However, before learning and performing any additional assessment procedures, it is important to develop basic skills in handling instruments and working at chairside.

Holding an instrument is different from the way most people hold writing implements. Fig. 9-3 shows a typical pen grasp with the thumb and first finger grasping the handle, supported by the mid-

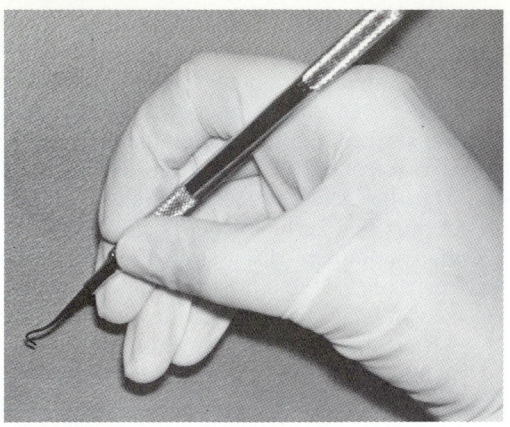

9-3. Typical pen grasp, with thumb and first finger grasping handle. Middle finger supports instruments from underneath.

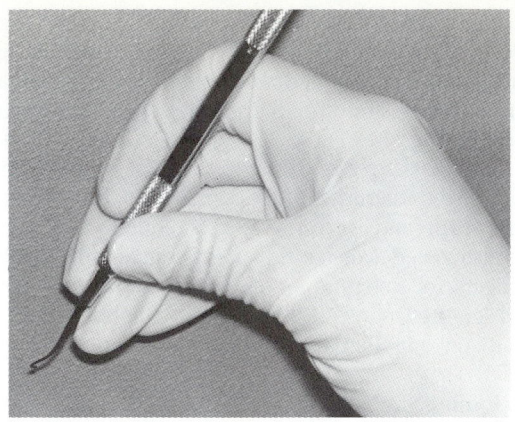

Fig. 9-4. Modified pen grasp with both first and second fingers holding handle, opposed by thumb. Third finger is in position to rest on tooth structure to create stability and to act as a finger rest for moving the instrument.

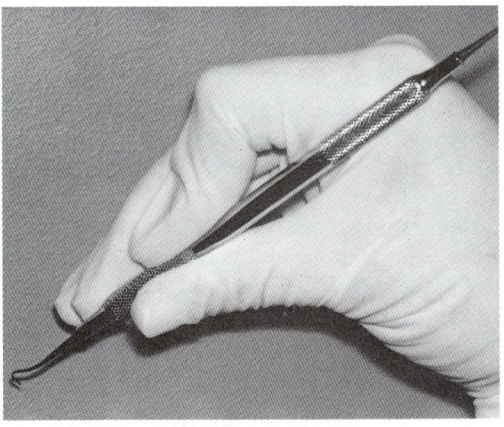

Fig. 9-5. Incorrect modified pen grasp because knuckle of first finger is buckled. Handle should lie flat against first two sections of first finger, as shown in Fig. 9-4.

dle finger under the handle. Fig. 9-4 shows the *modified pen grasp*, in which the first and second fingers are placed on the instrument, opposed by the thumb. This grasp is commonly used in holding dental instruments. Fig. 9-5 shows a common error made in grasping a dental instrument. The first two knuckles of the first finger should be flat on the instrument to improve stability and to ensure tactile sense. The third finger should serve as a *finger rest*, or pivot point, often called a *fulcum.* With this grasp and finger rest, it should be possible to see the palm of the hand when looking past the instrument from the thumb, as evident in Fig. 9-4. The *wrist motion*, or wrist rock, begins in this position and moves on the finger rest point as a unified movement of the arm, wrist, and hand in a side-to-side, rock-and-return oscillation (Fig. 9-6). When using wrist motion, the instrument should move up and down on the tooth surface without changing the angle of the instrument shank to the tooth. A heavily accentuated wrist rock that starts with the palm cupped downward can cause the shank to move in and out from the tooth surface, thereby changing the established angle.

Another motion that can be useful in areas where lateral rocking is difficult is the vertical, or

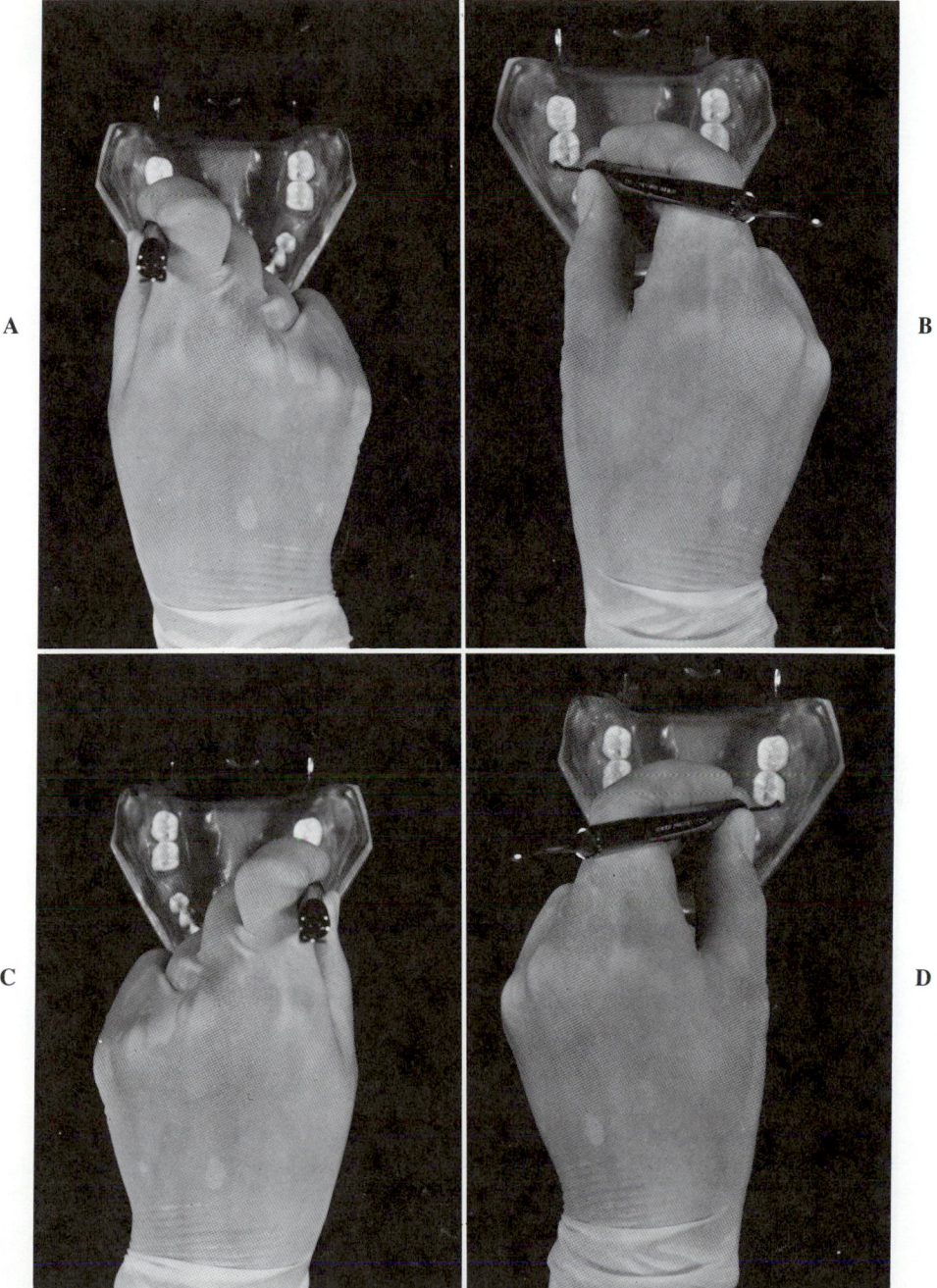

Fig. 9-6. **A,** Beginning position for lateral wrist motion, with modified pen grasp and solid finger rest. **B,** Hand rocks laterally to the right, moving working end of instrument in coronal direction. Rocking back to position in **A** moves working end of instrument apically. Thus instrument strokes are accomplished by rocking the hand back and forth. **C,** Beginning position for left-handed clinician. **D,** Hand rocked laterally to the left.

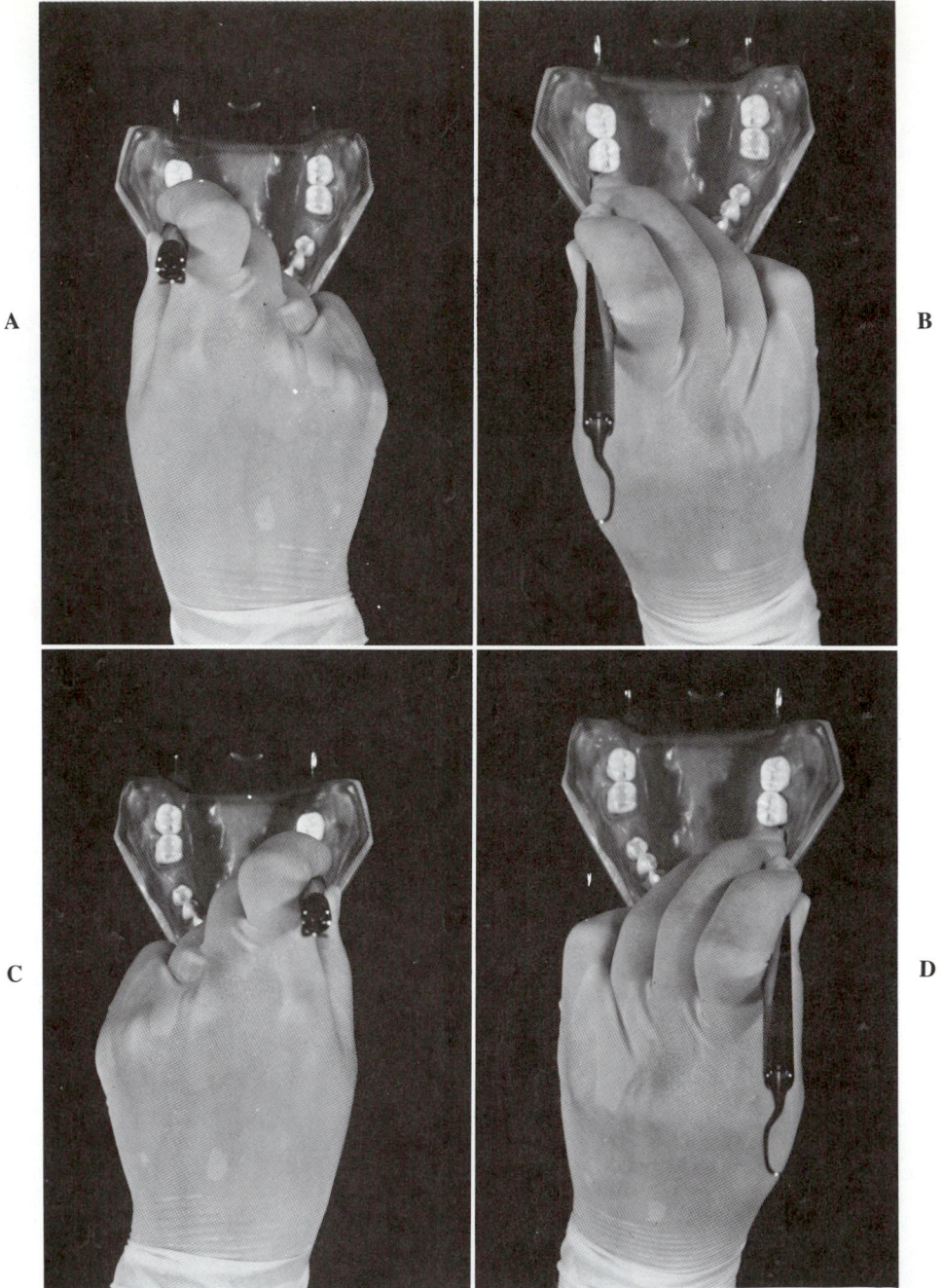

Fig. 9-7. **A,** Beginning position for vertical wrist motion. **B,** Hand moves in vertical plane by bending the wrist. Bending the wrist moves instrument tip coronally, and returning to position in **A,** moves instrument tip apically. **C,** Beginning position for left-handed clinician. **D,** Hand moved by lowering the wrist while maintaining a finger rest.

forward-and-back, wrist rock motion (Fig. 9-7). The instrument is moved up and down the tooth in the same stroking pattern, but the hand movement is performed by lowering the wrist while maintaining a finger rest.

EFFICIENCY AND MOTION ECONOMY IN INSTRUMENTATION

When any instrument is used in performing intraoral procedures, effectiveness is improved and fatigue reduced if a few simple guidelines are followed. Proper positioning of the clinician, patient, and dental assistant during the very first efforts at instrumentation can help you develop safe practice habits that will enhance efficiency and aid in mastery of instrumentation skills.

Proper positioning at the chair makes it easier to see the operative site, to maintain a stable finger rest, and to adapt the instrument. Additionally, good positioning reduces muscle strain and fatigue for the entire dental team.

Therefore as the basic principles of instrumentation are introduced and practiced, principles of motion economy, including proper positioning, will be implemented as well. The basic premises underlying this approach are that good instrumentation learned from detrimental or impossible positions does not transfer readily to a useful pattern of clinical practice, while instrumentation learned from ideal positions makes mastery of basic manipulation much easier. This mastery is enhanced by good vision, finger rest placement, and access.

BASIC POSITIONS OF THE DENTAL TEAM

Instrumentation procedures are performed with the clinician in a sitting position: for this to be possible the patient needs to be placed in a supine position. As described in Chapter 2, this is best accomplished by tilting the entire chair back to ensure that the patient's hips are seated in the angle of the chair. The back of the chair is then lowered to just above the lap of the seated clinician or even with the clinicians' elbows when at rest. The headrest should be adjusted and a protective drape and napkin placed on the patient. The patient's feet should be at approximately the same height as his or her head.

The clinician should be seated with the thighs parallel to the floor and the feet flat on the floor. If the clinician's stool has an abdominal rest, it should be located just below the ribs to provide

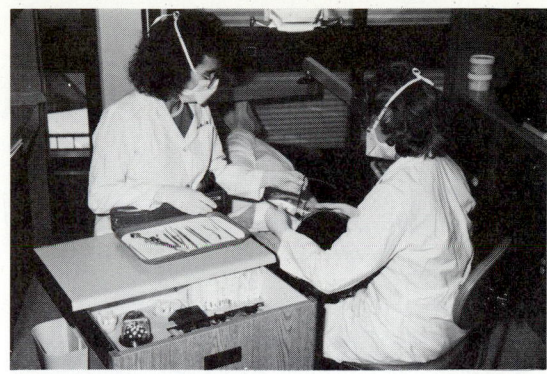

Fig. 9-8. Properly positioned patient; right-handed clinician and assistant.

support as he or she inclines the upper body forward from the waist.

The chairside assistant should be seated so that his or her eye level is 4 to 6 inches above the clinician's eye level. Depending on the assistant's height, a foot support on the stool may be needed to enable the thighs to be parallel to the floor.

With the three members of the team in this basic seating arrangement, the clinician may move from a front to a rear position at the chair, with the assistant making appropriate minor adjustments to ensure proper instrument transfers and visibility. The right-handed clinician's position at the chair is approximately 8:30 to 10 o'clock at the chair for the front position and 10:30 to 12 o'clock for the rear position. Left-handed clinicians occupy the 3:30 to 2 o'clock and 2:30 to 12 o'clock positions for front and rear positions, respectively (Figs. 9-8 and 9-9). Some areas of the mouth may also be reached from the 1:00 position for right-handed clinicians and the 11:00 position for left-handed clinicians.

Additional flexibility and access may be gained as the patient turns his or her head towards or away from the clinician. Additionally, the patient can raise or lower the chin. The back of the chair can be raised or lowered 1 to 2 inches for access to specific areas.

The combination of clinician position, patient head movement, and the wisely used mouth mirror eliminates the need for contorted positions to gain adequate vision. It is possible to gain access to all areas of the mouth while maintaining a healthful posture.

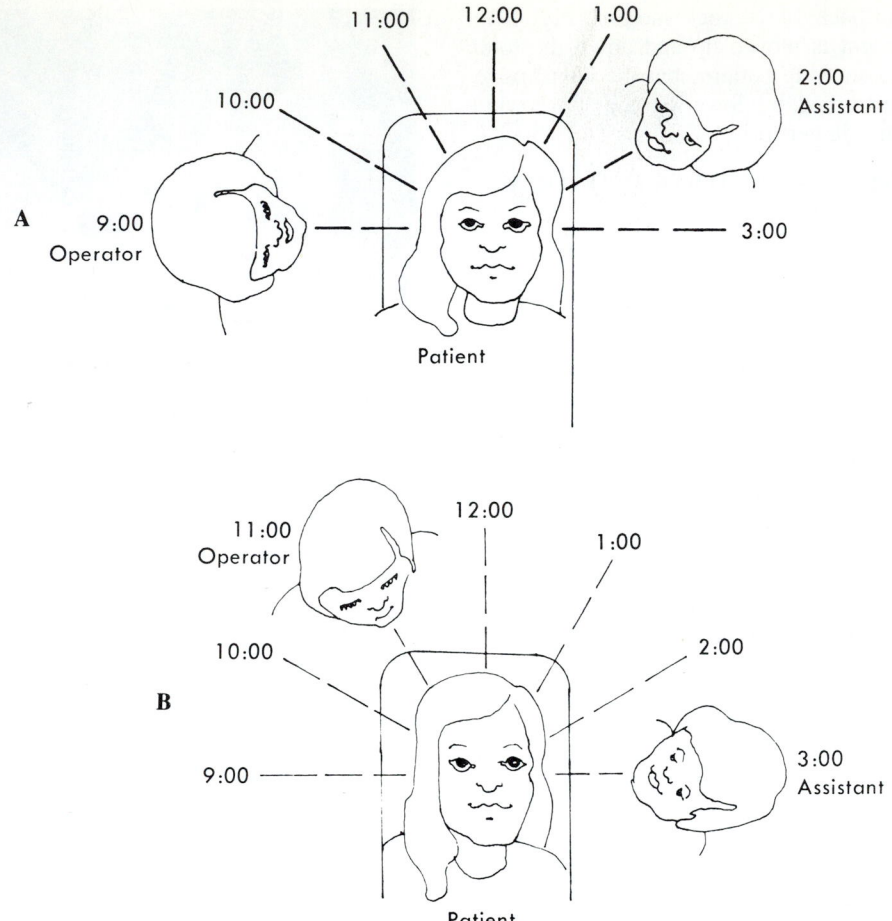

***Fig. 9-9.* A,** Right-handed clinician seated at approximately 9 o'clock with assistant at 2 o'clock position. **B,** Right-handed clinician seated at 11 o'clock position with assistant at 3 o'clock position. Left-handed clinician sits at 3 o'clock and 1 o'clock positions for front and rear positions, respectively.

TYPES OF HAND INSTRUMENTS

Hand instruments are classified according to their design, shape, and function. There are many hand instruments used in dental hygiene treatment classified under the general categories of mirrors, explores, probes, and scalers.

Mouth mirrors

One of the most important instruments in dental hygiene care is the mouth mirror. It is used to enhance vision in the recesses of the oral cavity. Mirrors are available in a variety of sizes and may

have a magnifying surface. The mouth mirror is used for *retracting* tissues such as the cheek and tongue, for *reflecting* light onto an area that otherwise would be in a shadow, for *indirect vision* of an area that cannot be seen directly (such as the distal aspect of the most posterior molar), and for *transillumination* (casting light through the teeth to determine the presence of caries or calculus by detecting variations in translucency).

An essential prerequisite skill in learning to use dental instruments is the effective use of the mouth mirror to ensure comfortable, adequate vi-

SINGLE END

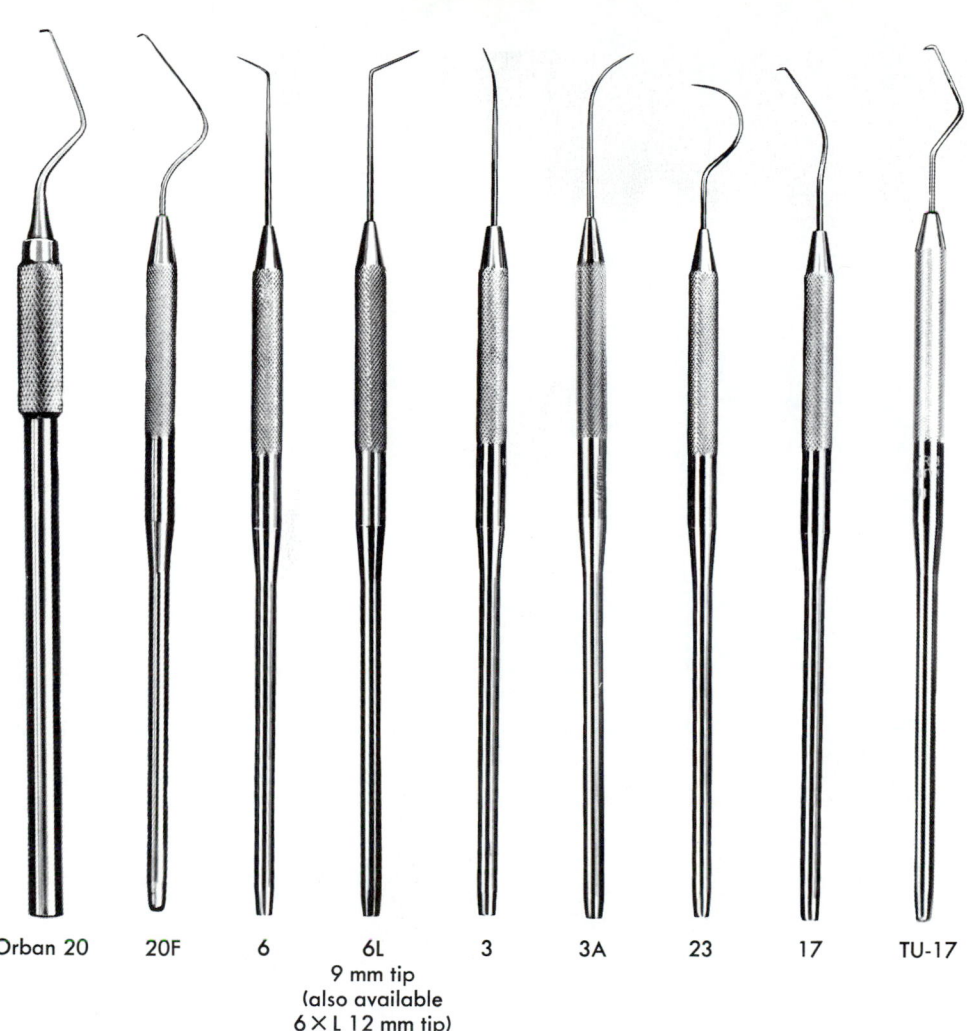

Orban 20   20F   6   6L   3   3A   23   17   TU-17

9 mm tip
(also available
6 × L 12 mm tip)

Fig. 9-10. Explorers used for detection of caries and for examining teeth for calculus and other irregularities are available in a variety of shapes and sizes.
(Courtesy of Hu-Friedy Co., Chicago, Illinois.)

sion of all areas of the mouth. An exercise at the end of this chapter outlines a method for developing this skill before the introduction of "working instruments." The goal should be careful, assertive placement of the mirror to obtain a clear view of the operative site and adequate space to locate a firm finger rest or finger rest for the working hand. This should be accomplished without clanking the mirror against the teeth, pinching the lip against the teeth, pressing the mirror head against the gingiva, or impinging soft tissue against bone.

Explorers

Other instruments are used to *examine* teeth and tissues by exploring the teeth and by measuring the size and location of tissue entities. Explorers are used primarily to examine the teeth for caries and for the presence of tooth irregularities such as calculus deposits, root roughness, anatomic defects, and margins of restorations. Explorers come in a variety of shapes and sizes—some best suited for exploring for caries and others for detecting fine subgingival irregularities. (Figs. 9-10

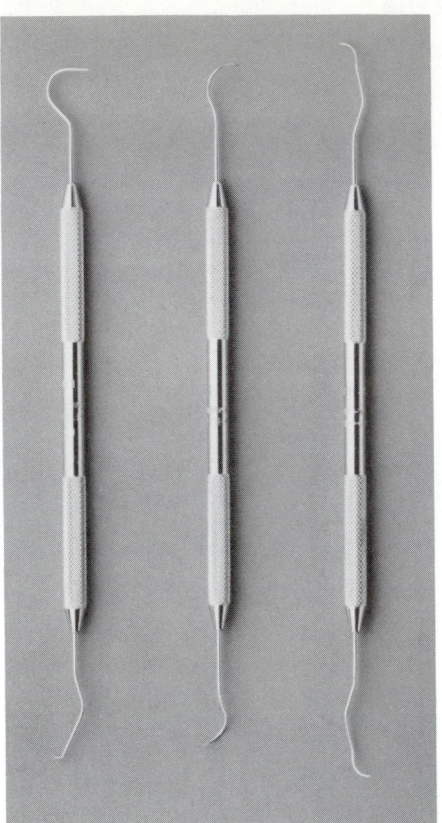

Fig. 9-11, left. Explorers are available in pairs, for instance, to gain access to a tooth from the facial aspect with one end and from the lingual aspect with the other end. Double-ended instruments may have two entirely different styles of working designs, such as TU17/23, on the left.
(Courtesy of Hu-Friedy Co., Chicago, Illinois).

Fig. 9-12, below. Periodontal probes, used primarily for examining sulcus and measuring its depths, are calibrated in millimeters. Some are color coded to improve readability. Shank length, angle, and working tip shape vary. *Left-to-right* CP-11, CP-12, CP-15 UNC, CP-NT2, and Williams.
(Courtesy of Hu-Friedy Co., Chicago, Illinois.)

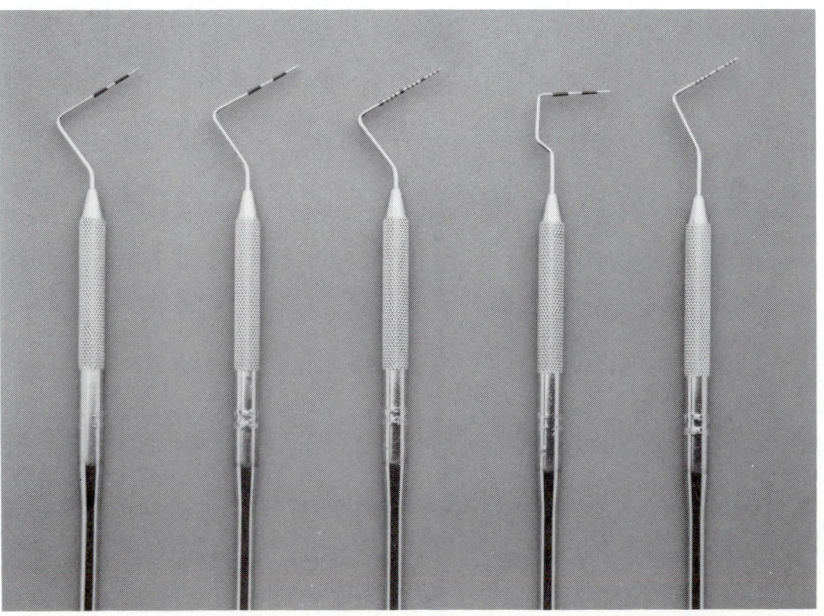

and 9-11 show several common types of explorers.) Because the dental hygienist's role includes identifying tooth characteristics and monitoring a patient's oral health, it is important to master the use of explorers early in clinical practice.

Probes

The periodontal probe also is used for examining oral tissues. However, it is not used for caries detection, because it does not have a sharp point for retention in carious areas. Probes are noted for their delicate design and are often used to detect root irregularities and hard deposits. Although the probe has other functions, its primary purpose is to measure the depth of the gingival sulcus or periodontal pocket (Pattison and Behrens, 1973; Ward and Simring, 1978). The periodontal probe's unique characteristic is its calibrations, marked in millimeters. How far the probe slides into the sulcus or a pocket indicates the level of the attachment of the gingiva to the tooth. The probe can trace the topography of the attachment around the tooth, providing the clinician with an idea of the extent of disease and the health status of the periodontium.

The calibrated probe also can be used to measure recession of the free gingiva, the amount of attached masticatory mucosa, or the size of a lesion. It is critical to know how the probe is calibrated, as some are marked in 3 mm increments and others are marked at 1, 2, 3, 5, and 7 mm; other variations are also seen (Fig. 9-12).

A probe recommended for general dentists by the American Academy of Periodontology and American Dental Association (AAP/ADA) has color-coded markings at 3.5, 5.5, 9, and 12 mm and a ball tip to help in detecting subgingival calculus and to provide comfort for the patient (see Fig. 9-2). Novatech probes manufactured by Hu-Friedy offer periodontal pocket probes with a right angle parallel tip design. This unique design provides more accurate and smooth placement of the tip into the interproximal and lingual aspects of posterior teeth (see Fig. 9-12).

Exercises described in this chapter provide opportunities for the clinician to use the mouth mirror for vision and the periodontal probe for exploring and measuring subgingival areas. A subsequent exercise advances the student to the use of a cowhorn explorer and a No. 17 explorer.

Once he or she can use the mouth mirror, probe, and explorers competently, the clinician is

prepared to assess the intraoral dental findings for a patient.

Other instruments

Instruments are used to *remove deposits* from teeth, such as scalers and curettes, and to *recontour or excise tissue*. Other working instruments, particularly in restorative dentistry, may be used to *place materials on or in the teeth and the surrounding tissues* and to shape those materials. In later chapters, as each phase of implementation of dental hygiene care is addressed, the design and use of each instrument are also discussed.

EXERCISES
Positioning exercises

To develop skill in gaining access to all areas of the mouth, students should divide into groups of three to practice the basic positions, each student serving once as patient, clinician, and assistant. The student who serves as chairside assistant should prepare the dental unit by disinfecting the equipment and placing sterile instruments on the tray (including a mouth mirror and a cotton-tipped applicator), seating the patient in a supine position, and placing the drape. The assistant should adjust his or her stool to the proper height in relation to the clinician and ensure an adequate view of each operative site by making minor adjustments in position.

The dental assistant should ensure proper adjustment of the overhead light. This is done by observing the target of the primary beam of light and adjusting the overall position and angle of the lamp so that the beam is on the operative site and is not blocked by a hand, the clinician's head, or some other obstacle. A general rule is to bring the lamp up over the patient's face and angle it downward (nearly perpendicular to the floor) for mandibular sites and to bring the lamp back over the patient's lap and angle it toward the mouth (so that the primary beam is nearly parallel to the floor) for maxillary sites (Fig. 9-13). From these two basic positions the lamp can be angled from one side or the other to eliminate shadows created by the hands.

The clinician should adjust his or her stool to the proper height and use the mouth mirror for retraction, indirect vision, and/or light reflection as appropriate for each area of the mouth. The mouth mirror should be held in the nonworking hand. The cotton-tipped applicator should be held

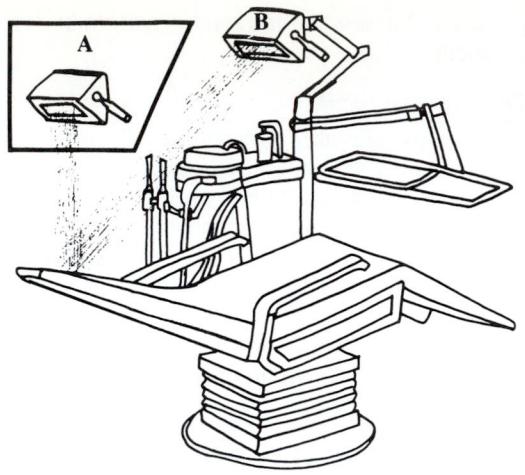

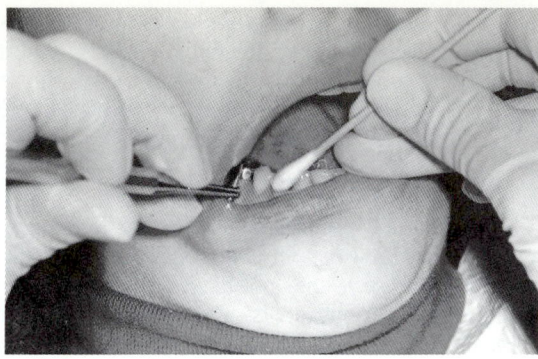

Fig. 9-14. Modified pen grasp for right-handed clinician, showing cheek retraction and stable third-finger fulcrum on teeth for access to mandibular right buccal area.

Fig. 9-13. A general rule in obtaining optimal intraoral illumination is to angle beam of overhead lamp nearly perpendicular to floor for mandible *(A)* and more parallel to floor. For maxilla *(B)* range of angulation is usually between 45 and 10 degrees to floor.

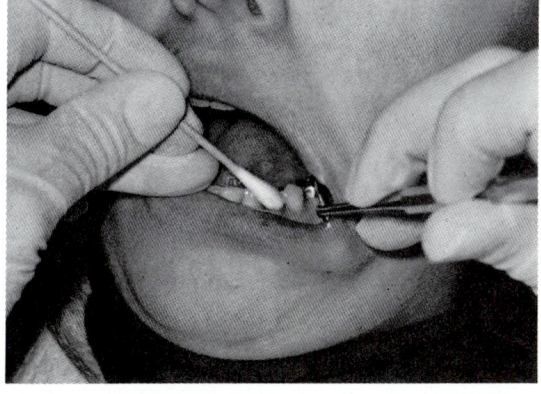

Fig. 9-15. Modified pen grasp for left-handed clinician, showing cheek retraction and stable third-finger fulcrum on teeth for access to mandibular left buccal area.

in the working hand. (Right-handed people use the right hand and left-handed people the left hand.) Moving sequentially from area to area of the dentition, the clinician should use the mouth mirror as indicated in Table 9-1 or 9-2. The clinician should establish a solid modified pen grasp with the working hand as shown in Figs. 9-14 and 9-15 for right- and left-handed clinicians, respectively; establish a finger rest on the teeth; and use wrist motion so that the cotton tip rides up and down the tooth in a vertical pattern of overlapping strokes. Two or three teeth in each area should be traced to provide practice in maintaining retraction and in using a stable grasp, finger rest, and wrist motion.

Figs. 9-16 to 9-27 show sample hand positions for right-handed clinicians; left-handed clinicians should follow Figs. 9-28 to 9-39. These hand positions should be referred to for this exercise. The student may progress to the probe and then to the cowhorn (as shown in the illustrations) after achieving basic skill with the cotton-tipped applicator.

The student playing the role of patient should comply with requests to turn the head to the right or left or to tilt the head up or down to facilitate access. It is also appropriate for this student to provide feedback about the careful use of the mouth mirror (reporting pain or discomfort) and to comment on the sense of confidence inspired

Table 9-1. Positioning for right-handed clinicians

Area of operation	Patient's head position*	Clinician position	Finger rest	Vision	Use of mirror
Mandible					
Right buccal	Left	9 o'clock	Bicuspid/cuspid	Direct	Retract cheek
Left lingual	Left	9 o'clock	Bicuspid/cuspid	Direct	Retract tongue
Right lingual	Right	9 o'clock	Bicuspid/cuspid	Indirect	Retract cheek; indirect vision and illumination
Left buccal	Right	11 o'clock	Bicuspid/cuspid	Direct	Retract cheek
Anterior lingual	Straight†	11 o'clock	Cuspid	Direct	Reflect light; retract tongue
Anterior labial	Straight†	11 o'clock	Cuspid	Direct or indirect	Indirect vision; retract lip
Maxilla					
Right buccal	Left	9 o'clock	Occlusal surface of tooth posterior to area of operation	Direct	Retract cheek
Left lingual	Left	9 o'clock		Direct	Reflect light
Right lingual	Right	11 o'clock		Indirect	Indirect vision; reflect light
Left buccal	Right	11 o'clock	Incisal edge	Direct	Retract cheek
Anterior lingual	Straight†	11 o'clock	Incisal edge	Indirect	Indirect vision; reflect light
Anterior labial	Straight†	11 o'clock		Direct	None

*Patient is in the supine position.
†Patient is asked to turn his/her head slightly as clinician moves from cuspid to cuspid in the anterior areas.

Table 9-2. Positioning for left-handed clinicians

Area of operation	Patient's head position*	Clinician position	Finger rest	Vision	Use of mirror
Mandible					
Left buccal	Right	3 o'clock	Bicuspid/cuspid	Direct	Retract cheek
Right lingual	Right	3 o'clock	Bicuspid/cuspid	Direct	Retract tongue
Left lingual	Left	3 o'clock	Bicuspid/cuspid	Indirect	Retract cheek; indirect vision and illumination
Right buccal	Left	1 o'clock	Bicuspid/cuspid	Direct	Retract cheek
Anterior lingual	Straight†	1 o'clock	Cuspid	Direct	Reflect light; retract tongue
Anterior labial	Straight†	1 o'clock	Cuspid	Direct or indirect	Indirect vision; retract lip
Maxilla					
Left buccal	Right	3 o'clock	Occlusal surface of tooth posterior to area of operation	Direct	Retract cheek
Right lingual	Right	3 o'clock		Direct	Reflect light
Left lingual	Left	1 o'clock		Indirect	Indirect vision; reflect light
Right buccal	Left	1 o'clock		Direct	Retract cheek
Anterior lingual	Straight†	1 o'clock	Incisal edge	Indirect	Indirect vision; reflect light
Anterior labial	Straight†	1 o'clock	Incisal edge	Direct	None

*Patient is in the supine position.
†Patient is asked to turn his/her head slightly as clinician moves from cuspid to cuspid in the anterior areas.

by the stability of the finger rest and the clinician's caring approach. From the beginning, the clinician should treat the patient as a person rather than as a mannequin or "object of care." The student playing the role of the patient may also hold the table of positions, areas, and approaches for the clinician's reference as the sequence is learned. As the sequence is mastered and approaches become more comfortable, the student-patient may wish to observe the student-clinician in a hand mirror.

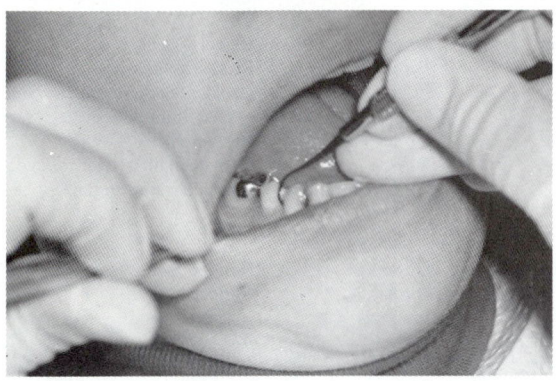

Fig. 9-16. Right-handed clinician. Hand position for instrumentation on mandibular right buccal aspect. Once cotton-tipped applicator has been used in each area, student may progress to periodontal probe to learn subgingival insertion and to explorer to learn adaptation. Mirror retracts cheek; finger rest is anterior to operative site, resting on occlusal surfaces.

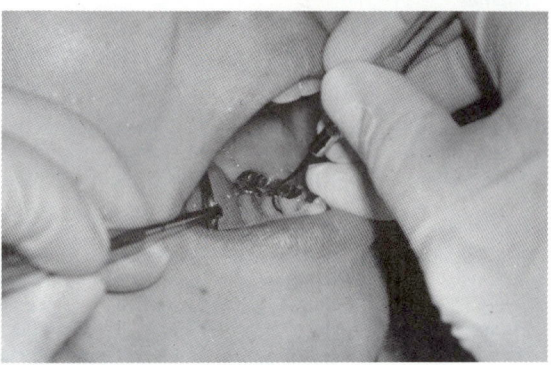

Fig. 9-17. Right-handed clinician: Hand position for instrumentation on mandibular left lingual aspect. Mirror retracts tongue. Finger rest is on facial-occlusal aspect of teeth in that sextant.

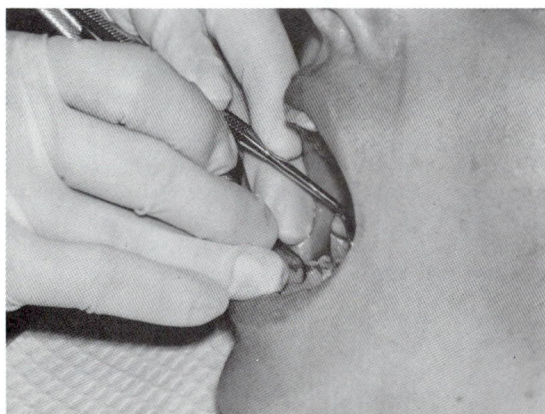

Fig. 9-18. Right-handed clinician: Hand position for instrumentation on mandibular right lingual aspect. Mirror retracts tongue but faces teeth, directing light onto area and providing indirect vision. Some clinicians prefer to approach this area from a rear position, with patient's head turned well towards clinician to enable direct vision.

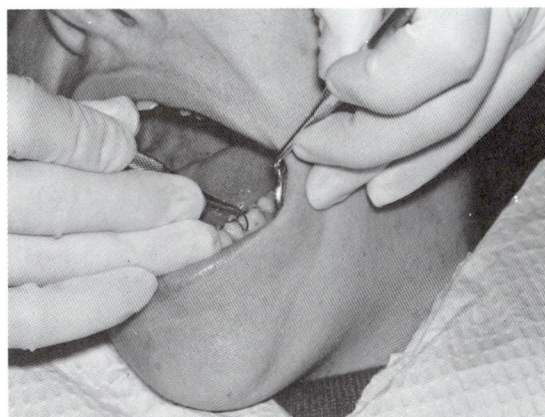

Fig. 9-19. Right-handed clinician: Hand position for instrumentation on mandibular left buccal aspect. With patient's head turned toward clinician, mirror retracts cheek, enabling direct vision. Clinician is seated in rear position.

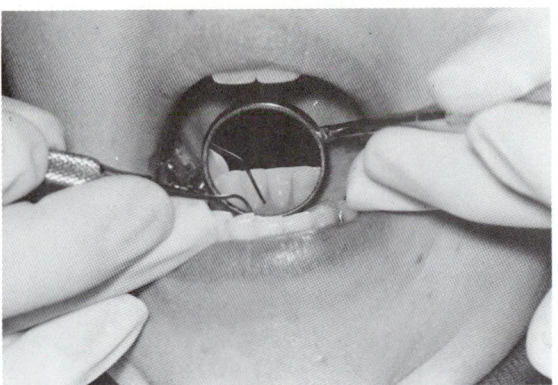

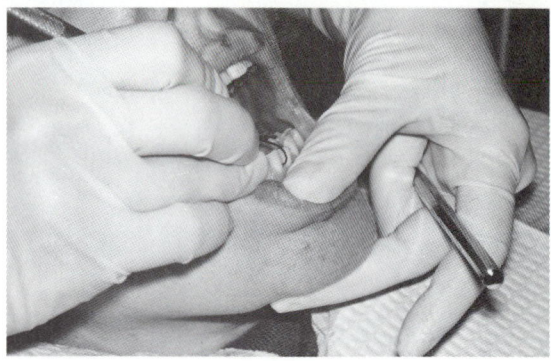

Fig. 9-20. Right-handed clinician: Hand position for instrumentation on mandibular anterior lingual aspect. Seated in rear position, clinician uses mirror to retract tongue and reflect light on area for direct vision.

Fig. 9-21. Right-handed clinician: Hand position for instrumentation on mandibular anterior facial aspect. Clinician is seated in rear position. Lower lip is retracted by thumb and finger, or mouth mirror. Direct vision is used. When indirect vision is difficult to achieve, mouth mirror can retract lip and provide indirect vision.

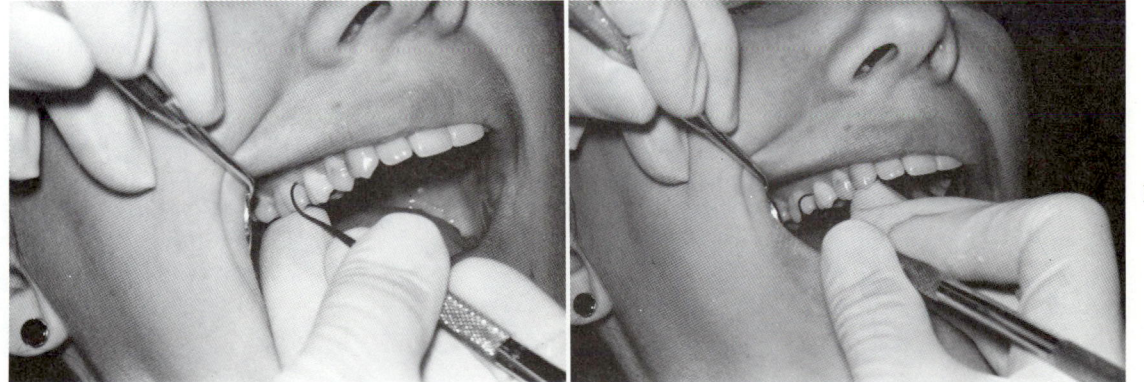

Fig. 9-22. Right-handed clinician: Two approaches to maxillary right buccal aspect. **A,** Palm up, finger rest on or posterior to operative site, giving stability and greater leverage for deposit removal during scaling. Clinician is seated at approximately 9:30 position. **B,** Palm down, finger rest anterior to area being explored. Clinician is seated in front position. Though this technique is easier to learn and is adequate for exploring, it provides less control and leverage during scaling. A vertical wrist motion (see Fig. 9-7) is used for this approach.

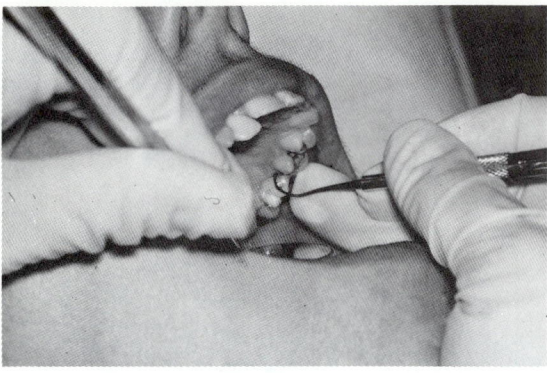

Fig. 9-23. *Right-handed clinician:* Hand position for instrumentation on maxillary left lingual aspect. Finger rest is placed on occlusal surface of tooth or slightly on buccal aspect. All fingers are kept together as a single unit to ensure a solid wrist motion and stroke. Mirror reflects light onto area. Direct vision is used with patient's head tilted away. Clinician is seated in front position.

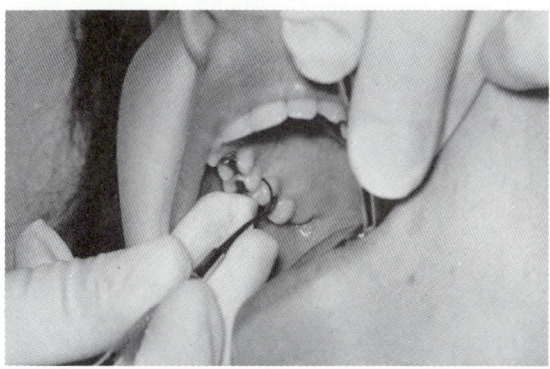

Fig. 9-24. *Right-handed clinician:* Hand position for instrumentation on maxillary right lingual aspect. Clinician is in rear position. Mirror reflects light and provides indirect vision. Finger rest is on occlusal aspect of sextant. Maintaining good posture, clinician holds mirror so it is visible, then angles mirror until light is cast on area to be explored and image is visible in mirror.

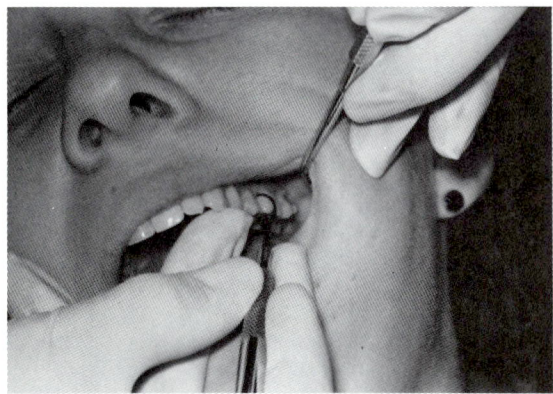

Fig. 9-25. *Right-handed clinician:* Hand position for instrumentation on maxillary left buccal aspect. Clinician is in rear position. Mirror retracts cheek, and finger rest is on occlusal aspect of teeth, with patient's head turned towards clinician for direct vision.

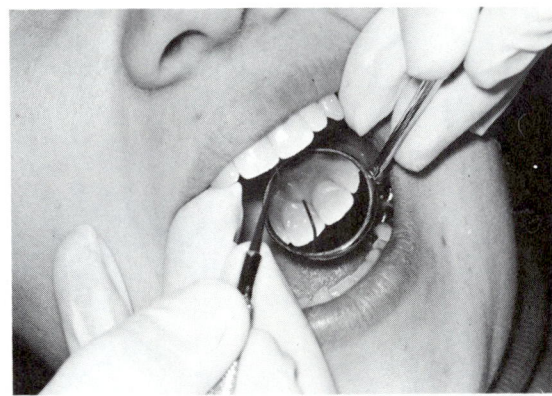

Fig. 9-26. *Right-handed clinician:* Hand position for instrumentation on maxillary anterior lingual aspect. Clinician remains in rear position and uses mirror to reflect light and provide indirect vision. Maintaining good posture, clinician holds mirror so it is visible, then angles mirror until area is illuminated and visible. Finger rest is on incisal edge with palm up for efficient wrist motion.

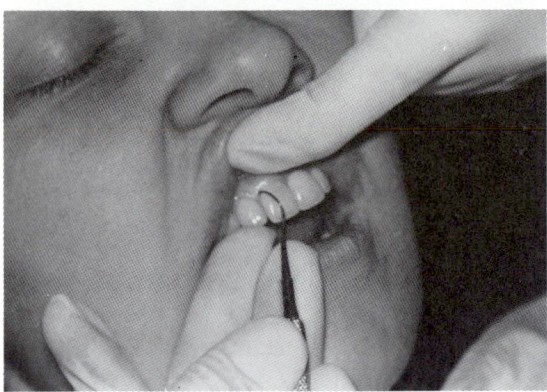

Fig. 9-28. Left-handed clinician: Hand position for instrumentation on mandibular left buccal aspect. Once cotton-tipped applicator has been used in each area, student may progress to the periodontal probe to learn subgingival insertion and to the explorer to learn adaptation. Mirror retracts cheek and finger rest is anterior to operative site, resting on occlusal surfaces.

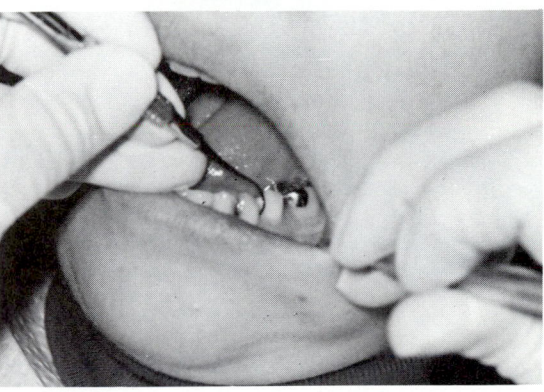

Fig. 9-29. Left-handed clinician: Hand position for instrumentation on mandibular right lingual aspect. Mirror retracts tongue. Finger rest is on facial-occlusal aspect of teeth in that sextant.

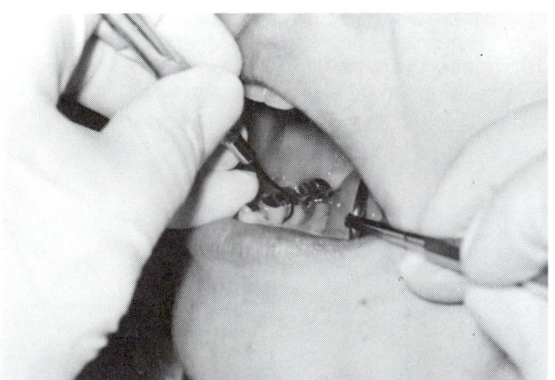

Fig. 9-27. Right handed clinician: Hand position for instrumentation on maxillary anterior labial aspect. To ensure a stable finger rest, rear position is preferred. Hand remains a solid unit, with all fingers resting on fulcrum, palm up. Direct vision is used, with forefinger retracting lip.

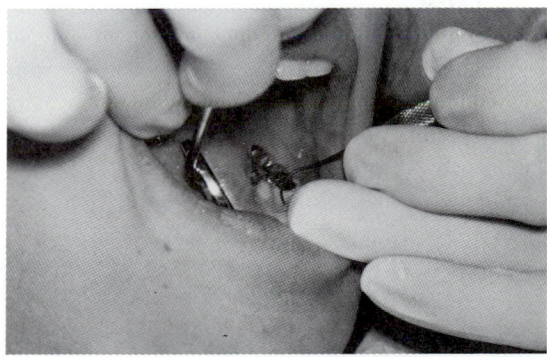

Fig. 9-30. Left-handed clinician: Hand position for instrumentation on mandibular left lingual aspect. Mirror retracts tongue but faces teeth, directing light onto area and providing indirect vision. Some clinicians prefer to approach this area from a rear position, with patient's head turned well toward clinician to enable direct vision.

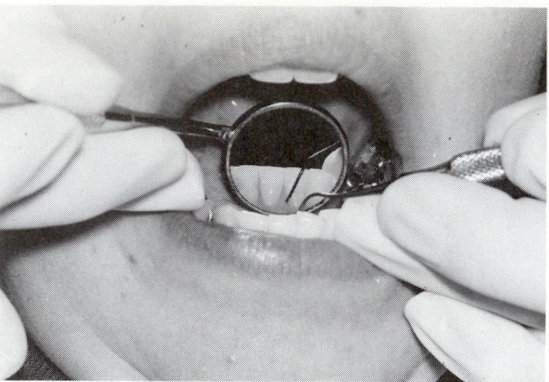

Fig. 9-31. *Left-handed clinician:* Hand position for instrumentation on mandibular right buccal aspect. With patient's head turned toward clinician, mirror retracts cheek, enabling direct vision. Clinician is seated in rear position.

Fig. 9-32. *Left handed clinician:* Hand position for instrumentation on mandibular anterior lingual aspect. Seated in rear position, clinician uses mirror to retract tongue and reflect light on area for direct vision.

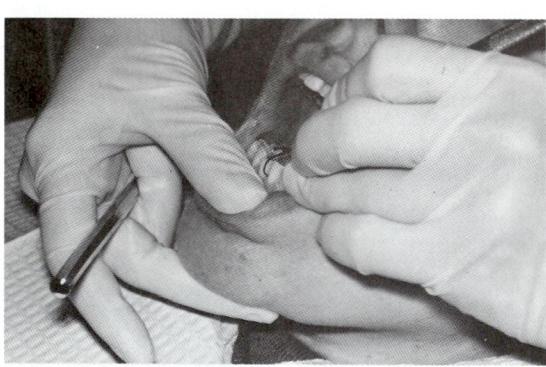

Fig. 9-33, left. *Left-handed clinician:* Hand position for instrumentation on mandibular anterior facial aspect. Clinician is seated in rear position. Lower lip is retracted by thumb and finger or mouth mirror. Direct vision is used. When direct vision is difficult to achieve, mouth mirror can retract the lip and provide indirect vision.

A 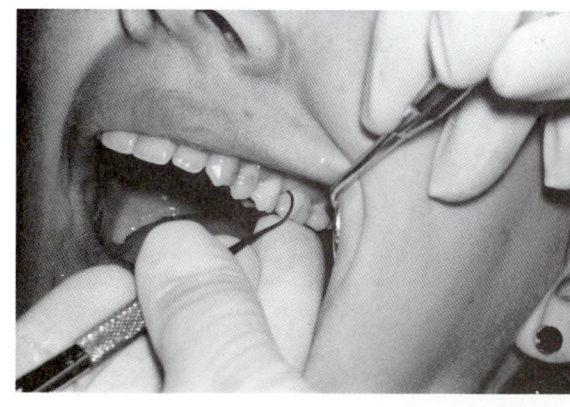 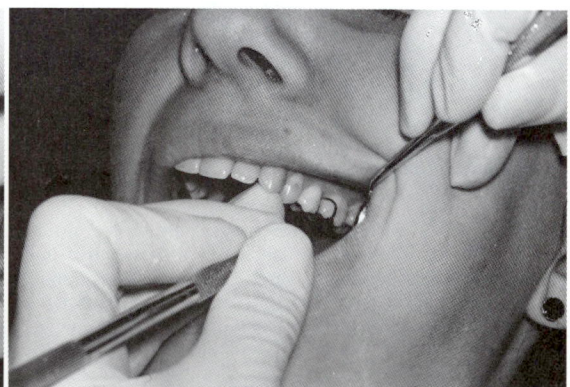 B

Fig. 9-34. *Left-handed clinician:* Two approaches to maxillary left buccal aspect. **A,** Palm up, finger rest is on or posterior to operative site, giving stability and greater leverage for deposit removal during scaling. Clinician is seated at approximately 2:30 position. **B,** Palm down, finger rest is anterior to area being explored. Clinician is seated in front position. Though this technique is easier to learn and is adequate for exploring, it provides less control and leverage during scaling. A vertical wrist motion (see Fig. 9-7) is used for this approach.

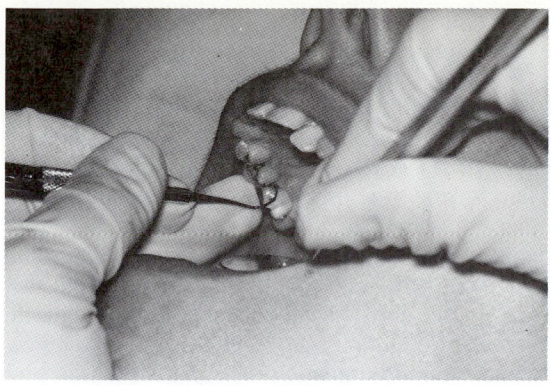

Fig. 9-35. *Left-handed clinician:* Hand position for instrumentation on maxillary right lingual aspect. Finger rest is placed on occlusal surface of tooth or slightly on buccal aspect. All fingers are kept together as single unit to ensure a solid wrist motion and stroke. Mirror reflects light onto area. Direct vision is used, with patient's head tilted away. Clinician is seated in front of patient.

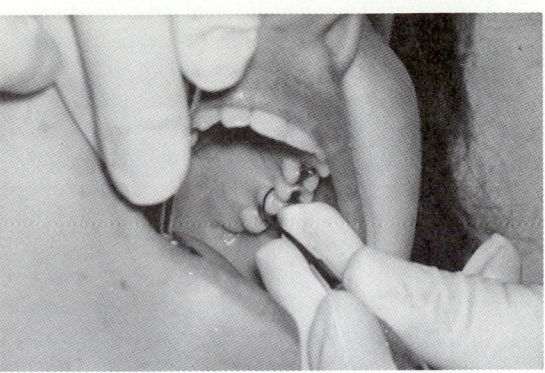

Fig. 9-36. *Left-handed clinician:* Hand position for instrumentation on maxillary left lingual aspect. Clinician is seated in a rear position. Mirror reflects light and provides indirect vision. Finger rest is on occlusal aspect of sextant. Maintaining good posture, clinician holds mirror so it is visible, then adjusts mirror until light is cast on area to be explored and image is visible in mirror.

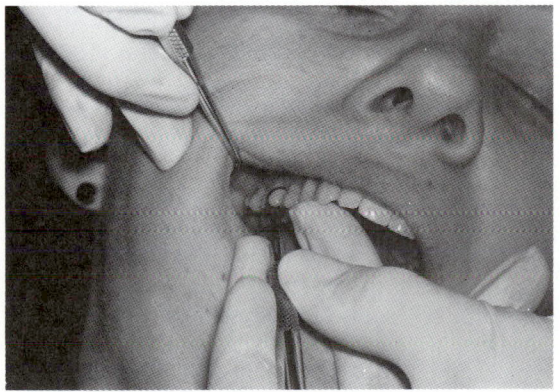

Fig. 9-37. *Left-handed clinician:* Hand position for instrumentation on maxillary right buccal aspect. Clinician is in rear position. Mirror retracts cheek, and finger rest is on occlusal aspect of teeth, with patient's head turned towards clinician for direct vision.

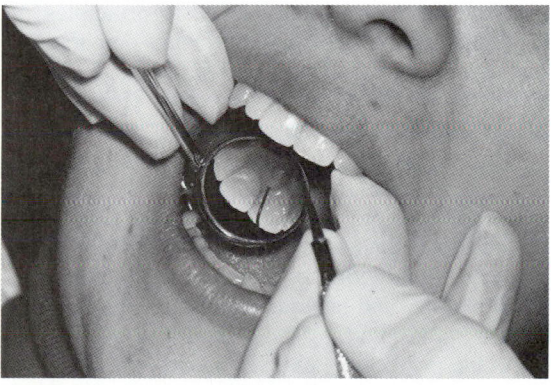

Fig. 9-38. *Left-handed clinician:* Hand position for instrumentation on maxillary anterior lingual aspect. Clinician remains in rear position and uses mirror to reflect light and provide indirect vision. Maintaining good posture, clinician holds mirror so it is visible, then angles mirror until area is illuminated and visible in mirror. Finger rest is on incisal edge, with palm up for efficient wrist motion.

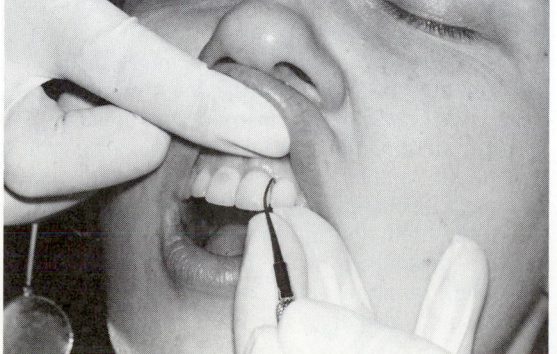

Fig. 9-39, left. *Left-handed clinician:* Hand position for instrumentation on maxillary anterior labial aspect. To ensure a stable finger rest, rear position is preferred. Hand remains a solid unit, with all fingers resting on finger rest, palm up. Direct vision is used, with forefinger retracting lip.

All three students should feel free to discuss comfortable ways of implementing each position. The instructor should circulate among the groups of students to check mirror use, pen grasp, finger rest placement, and wrist motion as well as basic positions and the location of the overhead lamp.

To see how the mirror can be used to reflect light through tissue (transillumination), the clinician should place the mirror behind the teeth and angle it until the teeth brighten from the light being reflected through them. The clinician should look at the teeth rather than the image in the mirror. The shadow of restorations should be visible, as should caries and interproximal or lingual calculus. Light is not as easily transmitted through substances other than healthy tooth structure. These substances or defects are thus usually visible as dark shadows.

As each clinician practices and completes the sequence of positions, the team should rotate to ensure each student an experience as clinician, assistant, and patient. All the basic principles of contamination control, including unit preparation, instrument sterilization, hand scrub, and aseptic chain should be practiced to reinforce previously learned skills.

After one or two practice sessions and study of the table of positions, students should be prepared to assume the proper position for any given area of the mouth and to assume each position in sequence. Skill with the mouth mirror should be considerable, and beginning skills for instruments used with the working hand should be apparent.

As the positioning exercise is implemented, the skills of the modified pen grasp, finger rest, and wrist motion should improve.

Following the arbitrary sequence of positions found in Tables 9-1 and 9-2 allows integration of time and motion economy with mastery of most dental hygiene instruments as each instrument is learned. The sequence is designed to minimize position and instrument changes and to provide a systematic approach to completing each arch or quadrant. Experienced clinicians may vary in their approach to specific areas, complementing or replacing some of the suggested positions and sequence.

Typically difficult areas to master are (1) the lingual surfaces of the mandibular quadrant closest to the clinician (Fig. 9-18 or 9-30), (2) the buccal surfaces of the maxillary quadrant closest to the clinician (Fig. 9-22 or 9-34), and (3) the

lingual surfaces of the maxillary quadrant closest to the clinician (Fig. 9-24 or 9-36).

Problems with the positions shown in Figs. 9-18 and 9-30 usually arise from the dual role of the mouth mirror in both retracting the tongue and cheek and serving as a source of indirect vision. Many times it is also used to reflect light on an otherwise dark area. Therefore the beginning clinician needs to acquire a high degree of control with the mirror. The shank retracts the cheek, the back of the mirror head retracts the tongue, and the face of the mirror serves as the primary source of vision and illumination. The patient's head position is critical in enabling all this to happen. Many clinicians prefer to approach this area from the rear, with the patient's head turned well toward them.

The maxillary right buccal (for right-handed clinicians) and maxillary left buccal (for left-handed clinicians) are controversial as well as difficult areas. Most people agree that the mirror retracts the cheek. The controversy centers around finger rest placement and hand position. The easiest approach to learn is to place the finger rest anterior to the area to be examined with the palm down. The wrist motion then becomes a back-and-forth vertical motion rather than a motion to the side (Figs. 9-22, *B,* and 9-34, *B).*

The more difficult position to learn is to place the finger rest finger on the occlusal surface of the tooth posterior to the tooth being examined, with the palm up. Although the clinician is in a front position, it usually is at 9:30 o'clock, (or 2:30 o'clock for left-handed clinicians) with the body turned towards the patient. The best way for beginners to practice this position is on the premolars, moving posteriorly tooth by tooth. As the clinician's hand moves back towards the last molar, the actual finger rest is less on the fingertip on the tooth and more on the side of the finger on the muscular resistance of the obicularis oris (Figs. 9-22, *A,* and 9-34, *A).*

This palm-up position may be more difficult to master but, according to the laws of physics, it increases control of the instruments, makes it possible to maintain proper terminal shank relation to the tooth, and allows for more efficient use of strength in engaging and removing hard deposits from the teeth and in root planing.

The difficulties with the lingual side of this problem quadrant are simpler to identify and overcome. Usually, the student has difficulty working with a mirror image at first. This area relies heavily on indirect vision by means of the mirror. Ways to overcome this problem are to bring the mirror to the front of the mouth and to maintain good posture. With the mirror in the anterior area, the seated clinician can clearly see the reflective surface. The mirror head is then angled until the area to be examined is visible in the mirror. Skill in moving the working hand in the intended direction while looking at a mirror image will develop with practice. This is one reason why rubbing the cotton-tipped applicator up and down the tooth structure is good practice. It is a safe instrument with which to learn indirect vision and instrument control.

Exercises with the periodontal probe

Once the student can move quickly and easily from area to area using the proper positioning, mirror function, grasp, finger rest, and wrist motion, he or she is ready to learn to use the periodontal probe.

Because the periodontal probe can be used on all surfaces (universally) and has no cutting edge or sharpened point, it is a relatively safe beginner's instrument. In addition, it is a key instrument in assessing oral health. Sliding it into the gingival sulcus reveals the depth of the sulcus and the presence of root irregularities and hard deposits. Gently bobbing the probe up and down in the sulcus (using an overlapping stroke pattern) as it travels around the tooth helps the clinician trace the topography of the attachment. Thus, even in the first phases of learning instrumentation, the clinician can learn about his or her partner's oral conditions.

Guidelines for using the probe include the following:

1. Using the same positioning, grasp, finger rest, and wrist motion as in the previous exercise
2. Sliding the probe into the sulcus until it meets the elastic resistance of the epithelial attachment
3. Using approximately 1 mm of the tip of the calibrated portion of the instrument to feel the side of the tooth as the probe slides in and out of the sulcus and around the tooth
4. Keeping the calibrated portion of the instrument parallel to the long axis of the tooth, except for modifications necessary to accommodate the flare of the crown of the tooth

5. Using wrist motion to move the instrument coronally for each stroke
6. Pivoting on the rest finger and rolling the instrument slightly in the fingers to move the bobbing instrument around the tooth

The probe should slide in gently so as to avoid causing pain, yet it must travel the full depth of the sulcus or pocket to yield valuable, accurate information. One frequent error is failure to "instrumentate" far enough across the proximal surfaces (Ward and Simring, 1978). If the probe is not placed to the base of the sulcus at the middle portion of the proximal surface, the most frequent site of early periodontal disease will remain unexamined. Examining this area, particularly below contact areas, may necessitate a *slightly* angled approach with the probe.

One way to begin probing a tooth is to *insert* the probe into the sulcus at the distofacial line angle and *bob* or *walk* it across the distal surface (at least slightly more than halfway); *retrace* the probing to the distofacial line angle and *across the facial* surface, past the facial line angle at least slightly more than halfway *across the mesial;* and *back out* to the mesial line angle. The probe should not emerge completely from the sulcus with each stroke. Rather, it should remain in a subgingival position as it travels around the tooth (Fig. 9-40).

The student serving as the assistant should record millimeter readings for the distal, facial, and mesial surfaces and then for the distal, lingual, and mesial surfaces for each tooth as it is probed in sequence. Otherwise, the clinician should record findings for at least two teeth in each sextant. The faculty member should circulate to help students improve their grasp, finger rest position, wrist motion, stroke (in and out of the sulcus), adaptation of the tip to the tooth, and pivot motion around the tooth.

At the completion of the exercise, the student should have probed all areas of the mouth and measured two teeth for sulcus depth in each sextant of teeth. The student should have acquired entry-level competence in at least six of the following skills:

Proper positioning
Grasp of instrument
Finger rest placement and use
Wrist motion
Adaptation of tip to tooth
Smooth sulcular bobbing and walking strokes
around tooth

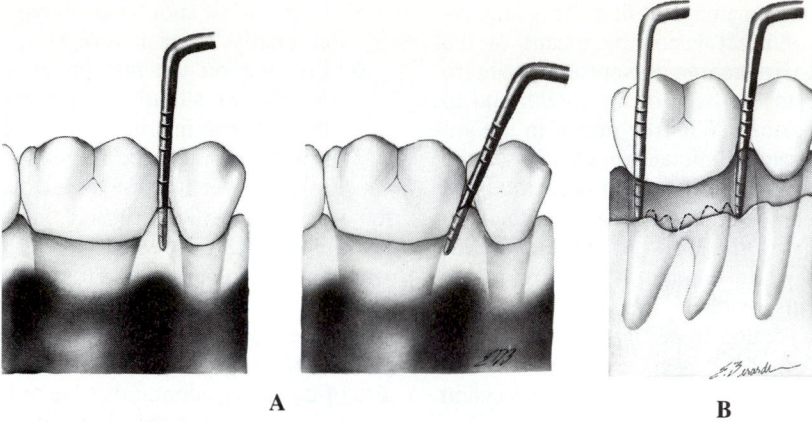

A   B

Fig. 9-40. Incorrect *(left)* and correct *(right)* adaptation of probe to tooth. Correct adaptation ensures that tip is adapted and is not free to engage soft tissue in sulcular wall. Walking, or bobbing, motion of probe in sulcus is shown in **B.** Note that probe follows topography of attachment.

Maintenance of calibrated position in parallel relation to long axis of tooth

Guidance of instrument at least slightly more than halfway across proximal surfaces

Measurements of sulcus accurate within 1 mm

Further practice sessions should allow students to concentrate on those areas in which they are not yet skilled.

Exercises with the paired explorer

Many of the basics of instrumentation given in the previous two exercises will prove helpful in learning to use the paired explorer (such as the cowhorn or pigtail). The student will learn to (1) select the appropriate end of the explorer for adaptation in each area of the dentition; (2) adapt the side of a sharp tip against the tooth to minimize discomfort; and (3) change (pivot) the direction of a tip moving out from the distal surface so as to guide it in an anterior direction across a facial or lingual surface, around the mesial line angle, and across the mesial surface.

For this exercise the same positioning, use of the mouth mirror, modified pen grasp, finger rest, and wrist motion are used. The stroke with the paired explorer is an overlapping pattern of vertical strokes around the tooth. The purpose for using this instrument subgingivally is to detect the presence of calculus, root irregularities, normal anatomic landmarks such as the cementoenamel junction (CEJ), and root furrows and contours. The thin shank and working end facilitate the transmission of vibrations to the clinician's fingers and thumb as they hold the shank and handle (tactile sensitivity). The paired explorer can be used supragingivally to examine the tooth for roughness and contours, confirming the visible findings.

In selecting which end to use, it is helpful to (1) select either end of the paired explorer, (2) assume the proper position for the first sextant (mandibular facial area closest to the clinician), (3) establish a proper modified pen grasp and finger rest, and (4) place the randomly selected end so that the tip is aimed across the mesial surface from the facial aspect in one of the teeth in the sextant. One of the two views in Fig. 9-41 should resemble this first effort.

The next step is to assess whether the instrument point is curling out towards the tissue as if ready to penetrate it if moved subgingivally. Depending on the selected end, the point will be directed toward either the soft tissue or the tooth. The latter, for obvious reasons, is preferable.

Another cue is whether the terminal shank (which is contiguous with the working tip) is horizontal or vertical. The point is curved towards the tooth when the terminal shank is vertical.

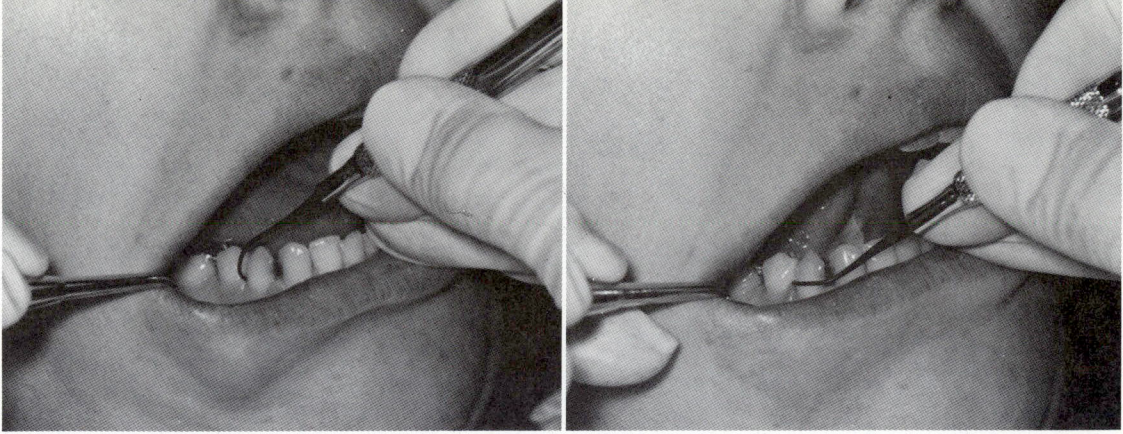

Fig. 9-41. **A,** Adaptation of one end of cowhorn explorer to mesial surface of tooth with point directed across mesial surface. Terminal shank is parallel to long axis of tooth; point is curved in towards tooth. **B,** Opposite end of explorer, which, although adapted in same area, has terminal shank in horizontal relationship with point curved toward gingiva. These cues help in selecting correct end of paired cowhorn explorer.

Thus a handy guide for determining which end to use is to look at the direction of the point and the terminal shank's relation to the long axis of the tooth. The end that aligns the terminal shank with the long axis of the tooth will provide correct adaptation for the distal, facial, and mesial surfaces of the first sextant of teeth. Fig. 9-41, *A,* meets these criteria.

Once the proper end is selected, the side of the tip (1 to 2 mm) should be placed on the distobuccal line angle. Wrist motion should be activated to move the instrument up and down. A pivot on the finger rest finger and a slight rolling of the instrument in the fingers should guide the tip around the line angle and across the distal surface at least slightly more than halfway (Pattison and Behrens, 1973). The clinician should concentrate on what can be felt with 1 mm of the side of the tip. He or she should explore for calculus, the CEJ, rough margins of restorations, and the root shape.

The side of the tip should then be bobbed back out to the distobuccal line angle. The tip should be pivoted so that it is aimed towards the anterior of the mouth, and the side of the tip should touch the facial aspect of the tooth. Again, a pivot of the hand on the finger rest finger and a slight rolling of the instrument in the fingers should allow the side of the tip to move past the mesiobuccal

line angle onto and across the mesial surface. The tip is then backed out to the mesiobuccal line angle and removed from the tooth (Figs. 9-42 to 9-47). It is critical to keep 1 to 2 mm of the tip in contact with the tooth. No more and no less should be used; otherwise (1) the tip may wander into the tissue, (2) it is less possible to determine exact locations of deposits, and/or (3) the point will merely scratch over the tooth, sending misleading vibrations to the clinician's hand (Pattison and Behrens, 1973).

It is also important to use overlapping strokes that cover the area. A few long, sweeping strokes do not thoroughly evaluate a tooth surface for the presence of miniscule deposits and root roughness (Pattison and Behrens, 1973).

As in probing, the explorer must drop to the attachment with each stroke to complete a thorough evaluation of subgingival areas (Pattison and Behrens, 1973). Gentle subgingival exploring does not allow the explorer to exit completely from the sulcus with each stroke. Reentry to the sulcus for each downward motion is unnecessary and may cause trauma to the margin of the gingiva.

A student exploring a partner's teeth should identify calculus, root irregularities, and margins of restorations while focusing on stroke and adaptation. The faculty member should circulate to help students improve their form and approach.

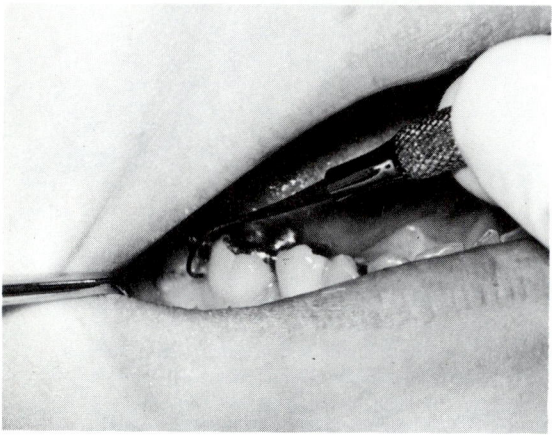

Fig. 9-42. Explorer is inserted on tooth's distobuccal line angle and is moved with vertical strokes around line angle into proximal area to fully explore distal surface.

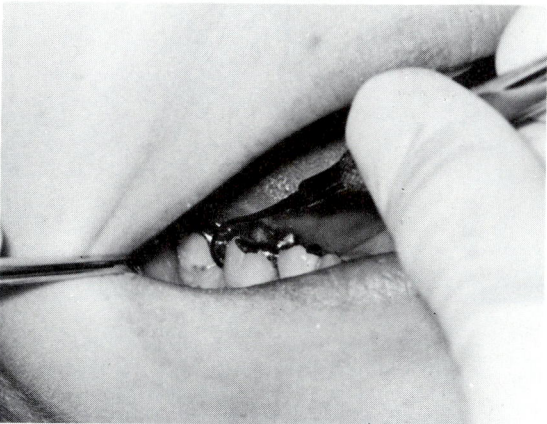

Fig. 9-43. Once explorer is more than halfway around the surface and has explored from attachment to margin of the gingiva, it should be backed out to distobuccal line angle with overlapping strokes.

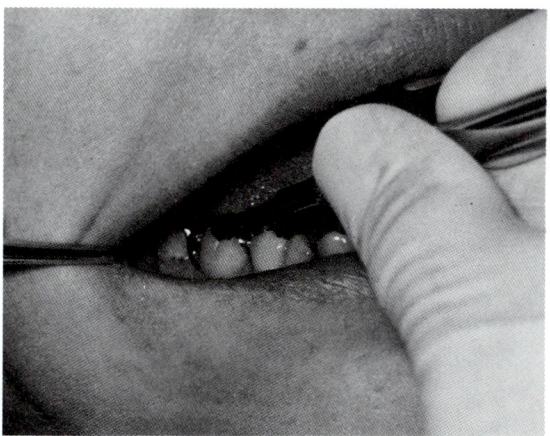

Fig. 9-44. At distolingual line angle, the point is pivoted so that it is directed toward mesial aspect of tooth and stroked in overlapping pattern across facial surface.

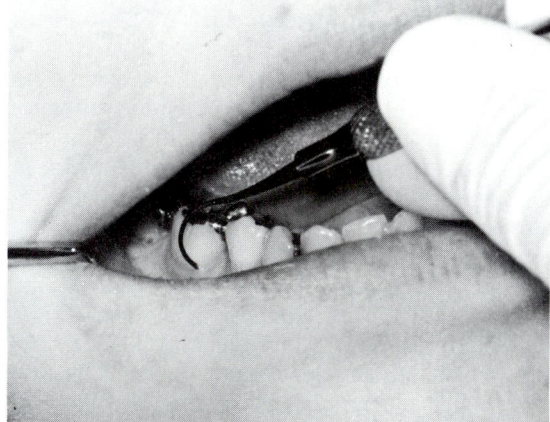

Fig. 9-45. When explorer reaches mesiobuccal line angle, tip is pivoted so that it stays in adaptation with tooth and does not wander into soft tissue. Stroking pattern continues around line angle and into mesial aspect to fully explore proximal surface.

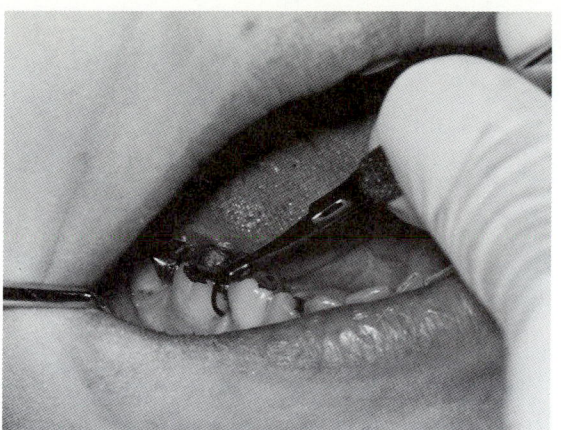

Fig. 9-46. Thorough exploration of mesial surface includes moving explorer in vertical and oblique pattern over all subgingival tooth surface, ensuring that area is fully explored to base of sulcus more than halfway across tooth.

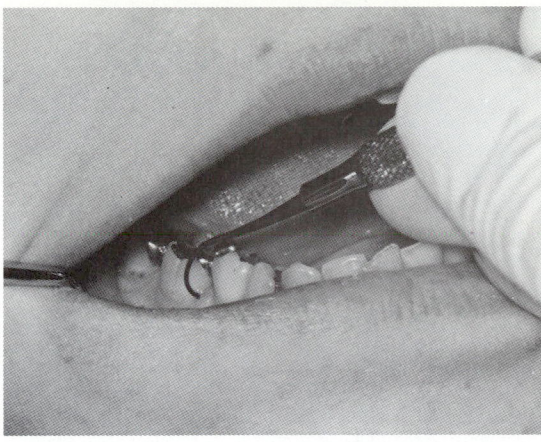

Fig. 9-47. After fully exploring mesial aspect of tooth, explorer is backed out to mesiobuccal line angle, where it is removed from sulcus. Tip of explorer should remain in subgingival position throughout its course around tooth to minimize trauma of reentering sulcus with each stroke.

Each student should be able to identify all areas in the dentition where each end of the explorer can be adapted simply by testing the direction of the point and the relationship of the terminal shank to the tooth's long axis. If one end can be adapted on the facial aspect of teeth No. 28 to 32, where else in the dentition can the *same end* be used?

At the completion of the exercise the student should have improved performance in the following basic skills:

Positioning and maintenance of vision

Grasp

Finger rest location and maintenance

Wrist motion

Exploratory stroke

The student should have learned how to select the correct end of a paired explorer for any sextant in the dentition and be able to adapt the tip safely and effectively. Safety and effectiveness should improve with practice.

Exercises with the "anterior" explorer

Once adaptation of the tip to the tooth has been added to the student's repertoire of entry-level skills, he or she can move from the paired contraangled explorer to the more simply designed "straight-shanked" explorer such as the No. 17 or No. 20. The shanks for these explorers do have bends and angles, but they do not have the contraangles that necessitate their use in pairs. The No. 20 explorer is shaped similarly to the No. 17; however, it is much finer and has a longer shank and thus more flex.

The No. 17 or No. 20 can be used almost universally; accessibility is limited by the relatively straight shank, which makes it difficult to obtain a solid finger rest and adaptation in posterior areas. For purposes of simplicity (and with the full acknowledgment that the instrument *can be* and *is* used in posterior areas), the instrument is referred to here as an *anterior* instrument. The maxim "the simpler the shank, the more anterior the intended use of the instrument," applies here for explorers and in later chapters that discuss scalers and curettes. Variations in areas of use can be added as the student gains experience and confidence.

One reason for calling the No. 17 or No. 20 explorer an anterior instrument is that it allows the student to learn some basic principles associated with adapting instruments into anterior teeth before learning about cutting edges.

When an anterior instrument is being used, the terminal shank is kept parallel to the long axis of the tooth. To do this, the finger rest must be on the same tooth or on the immediately adjacent one (Fig. 9-48). Allowing the finger rest to rest two or three teeth away causes the terminal shank to angle in the direction of the finger rest rather

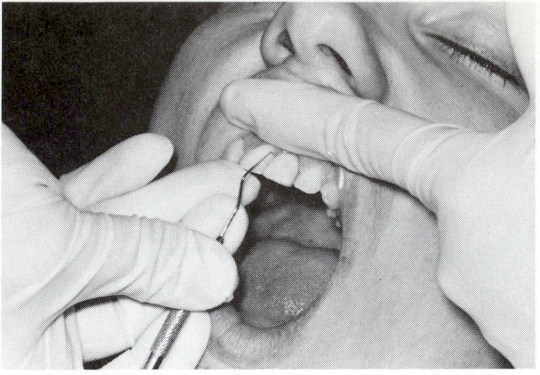

Fig. 9-48. When an "anterior" instrument is used, finger rest must be on same tooth or nearby tooth to ensure that shank is parallel to long axis of tooth.

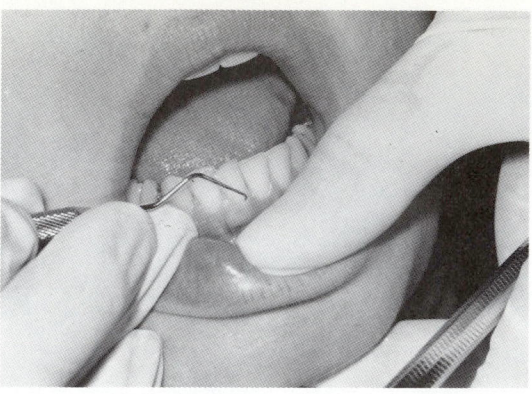

Fig. 9-49. Instruments may be used with a circumferential horizontal stroke around tooth. Tip is placed so that it is inclined apically and with terminal shank at 45-degree angle to the long axis of the teeth. Care must be taken to adapt carefully at line angles when using this stroke on facial and lingual aspects.

than remaining parallel to the tooth's long axis.

Many straight-shanked instruments can be used with a circumferential or horizontal stroke (as opposed to a vertical stroke) on the facial and lingual surfaces of teeth, including posterior teeth. The tip is angled more apically, the shank is *not* parallel to the long axis of the tooth, and the tip moves in short, overlapping oblique strokes from line angle to line angle (Fig. 9-49).

Another key factor is the need to accommodate the sharp line angles of the anterior teeth. If the tip is not carefully adapted to the tooth as the surface changes from facial to proximal, the sharp point will catch the gingiva, causing an iatrogenic hemorrhage point and accompanying discomfort.

Therefore practice in adapting the instrument is the focus in learning anterior instruments. The exercise also allows the student to improve skills in the following:

Positioning and maintenance of vision
Grasp
Finger rest location and maintenance
Wrist motion
Exploratory stroke
Detection of irregularities, landmarks, and calculus

After exploring the anterior teeth, the student should have achieved entry-level competence in all of the aforementioned skills and be able to explore anterior teeth and the direct facial and lingual surfaces of any tooth in the dentition without creating iatrogenic hemorrhage points or pain.

Shepherd's hook

Another straight-shanked explorer is the shepherd's hook (No. 23). It can be used for calculus detection but is frequently limited to caries detection because of the thickness of its tip and shank (Pattison and Behrens, 1973).

Fig. 9-50 shows the No. 23 explorer adapted for caries detection in the distal pit of tooth No. 28. The sharp point of the explorer is pressed into the pit to see if it sticks in soft tooth structure (caries). If resistance is felt as the explorer is removed from the tooth structure, the area is usually considered carious and worthy of further evaluation for restoration.

In addition to exploring pits for caries, the explorer can be used to check grooves, margins of restorations, and other caries-prone areas of the teeth, such as the gingival third of the facial and lingual surfaces and the proximal surfaces. Though it is usually necessary to examine a patient radiographically to rule out proximal caries, large lesions can often be found with an explorer.

The student should explore a partner's teeth for caries and for defective margins of restorations by placing the point into the pits and grooves, applying pressure, and detecting *retention* of the point in a *soft area*. Similarly, gently tracing the mar-

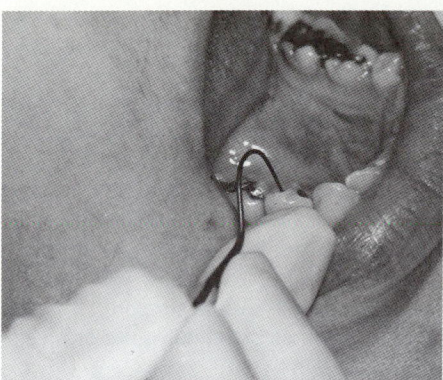

Fig. 9-50. Shepherd's hook (No. 23) explorer is usually reserved for caries detection because of its thick, resilient shank. Its sharp point is pressed into pits and grooves and suspicious margins of restorations to see if it sticks in soft tooth structure.

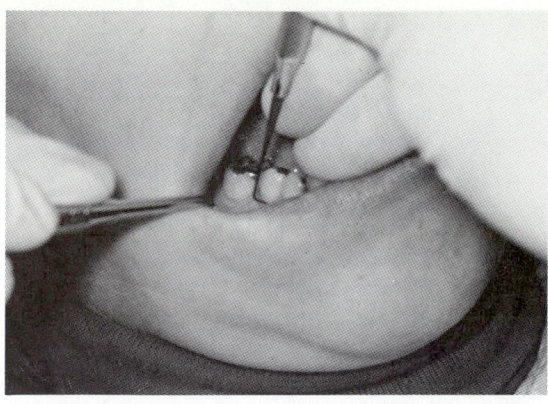

Fig. 9-51. Exploring for calculus with No. 6 explorer, a simply designed instrument with universal use.

gins allows the detection of caries and other defects around restorations.

Adjunct explorers

Refer again to Figs. 9-10 and 9-11 and note the variety of explorers available for calculus and caries detection. With greater experience a clinician can experiment with this range of available instruments.

Fig. 9-51 shows the No. 6 explorer being adapted in the posterior teeth. It has a simple design with only one angle in the shank. The terminal shank is the portion that is in the same plane as the handle, and it is maintained in a nearly parallel relationship to the long axis of the tooth. The tip is angled slightly downward into the sulcus, but not so that it points directly apically. This instrument can be used universally; its versatility makes it a popular choice.

Another explorer, O.D.U. 11/12, is designed as a highly sensitive instrument that combines the features of the curved pigtail-type explorer with the shank length of the straighter and longer #17 explorer. This instrument also can be used universally and is an excellent choice for exploring the mesial and distal surfaces.

SUMMARY

The principles of instrumentation discussed in this chapter will provide you with the skills necessary for instrument usage. Once you have mastered these principles you will be ready to advance to scaling procedures, which are discussed in subsequent chapters.

The instruments discussed in this chapter, as well as the exercises, are directed at the assessment phase of dental hygiene care. Mirrors, explorers and probes are used together to obtain pertainent diagnostic information relating to your patients present state of oral health.

ACTIVITIES

1. Compare a variety of instruments to determine the parts of the instruments, to distinguish between double-ended and paired instruments, and to examine shank shape and strength and the location of the terminal shank.
2. Ask a partner to grasp the handle of an instrument you are holding and try to move it while you are using each of the following grasps. Which grasp provides the most stability against movement? How would this grasp ensure best control of the instrument?
   a. A typical pen grasp used in holding a pencil
   b. The modified pen grasp, but with the knuckle buckled, as shown in Fig. 9-7, *B*
   c. The modified pen grasp, as shown in Fig. 9-7, *A*
3. *Exercises in positioning.* In groups of three, rotate from clinician to assistant to patient roles in completing the following procedures:

a. As chairside assistant
   (1) Disinfect unit
   (2) Place sterile mirror and cotton-tipped applicator on covered tray
   (3) Clear pathway for patient entry to chair
   (4) Position patient (supine position):
       (a) Tilt chair back
       (b) Lower back of chair
       (c) Adjust headrest
       (d) Place drape
   (5) Adjust assistant's stool to proper height and location
   (6) Adjust overhead light to ensure illumination of each area
b. As patient
   (1) Comment on seating comfort
   (2) Comment on comfortable use of mouth mirror and cotton-tipped applicator
   (3) Turn head as requested by clinician
   (4) Hold table of positions for clinician and assistant reference
c. As clinician
   (1) Adjust stool properly (thighs parallel to floor; feet flat on floor; abdominal rest below rib cage)
   (2) Seat self at chairside at 9 o'clock position (for right-handed clinician) or at 3 o'clock position (for left-handed clinician)
   (3) Use Table 9-1 or 9-2 to guide position, mouth mirror use, and finger rest placement for each of the following areas of the mouth:

Right-handed clinician	*Left handed clinician*
Mandibular	Mandibular
Right buccal	Left buccal
Left lingual	Right lingual
Right lingual	Left lingual
Left buccal	Right buccal
Anterior lingual	Anterior lingual
Anterior labial	Anterior labial
Maxillary	Maxillary
Right buccal	Left buccal
Left lingual	Right lingual
Right lingual	Left lingual
Left buccal	Right buccal
Anterior lingual	Anterior lingual
Anterior labial	Anterior labial

   (4) Use mouth mirror as indicated for each area
   (5) Use cotton-tipped applicator as dental instrument to explore two teeth in each area, using
       (a) Modified pen grasp
       (b) Finger rest
       (c) Wrist motion
       (d) Stroking pattern
   (6) Reflect light through anterior teeth with mirror and observe the presence of caries, restorations, or calculus
4. *Exercises with periodontal probe.* In dyads, serve as patient and as clinician in completing the following procedures:
   a. As patient
      (1) Comment on seating comfort
      (2) Comment on comfortable use of mouth mirror and probe
      (3) Monitor proper positioning of clinician
   b. As clinician
      (1) Use proper seating and positioning of self, patient's head, and mouth mirror for each area as described in Tables 9-1 or 9-2
      (2) With periodontal probe in working hand
          (a) Maintain modified pen grasp
          (b) Maintain firm finger rest
          (c) Gently insert probe in sulcus
          (d) Explore each area with probe
              From distobuccal line angle to direct distal
              From distal to distobuccal line angle and across facial aspect
              Past mesiobuccal line angle to direct mesial and back to mesiobuccal line angle
          (e) Explore with 1 mm of tip adapted to tooth
          (f) Maintain calibrated working end parallel to long axis
          (g) Bob or walk instrument from base of sulcus to free margin of gingiva while traveling around tooth
          (h) Measure depth of sulcus in millimeters
      (3) Record measurements of sulcus depth for at least two teeth in each sextant
5. *Exercise with paired explorer.* In dyads, serve as patient and as clinician in completing the following procedures:
   a. As patient
      (1) Comment on seating comfort
      (2) Comment on comfortable use of mouth mirror and paired explorer
      (3) Monitor proper positioning of operator
   b. As clinician
      (1) Use proper seating and positioning of self, patient's head, and mouth mirror for each area as described in Table 9-1 or 9-2

(2) With paired explorer in working hand
  (a) Maintain modified pen grasp
  (b) Maintain firm finger rest
  (c) Select proper end of explorer
  (d) Adapt side of point (1 mm) to tooth at distobuccal line angle in first area
  (e) Activate wrist motion to stroke instrument in overlapping vertical pattern around distal surface and back out to line angle
  (f) Pivot point at line angle so that it is aimed anteriorly, stroking vertically across facial surface
  (g) Continue stroking past mesiobuccal line angle and across mesial surface, using pivot on finger rest finger and rolling instrument slightly with fingers
  (h) Back instrument out of mesiobuccal line angle using vertical stroking pattern
  (i) Remove instrument from sulcus
(3) Explore root anatomy, margins of restorations, and calculus deposits
(4) Watch for iatrogenic hemorrhage points, and correct adaptation to ensure that side of point is in contact with tooth

6. *Exercises with anterior explorer*. In dyads, serve as patient and as clinician in completing the following procedures:
  a. As patient
    (1) Comment on seating comfort
    (2) Comment on comfortable use of mouth mirror and anterior explorer
    (3) Monitor proper positioning of clinician
  b. As clinician
    (1) Use proper seating and positioning of self, patient's head, and mouth mirror for each area as described in Table 9-1 or 9-2
    (2) With straight-shanked explorer in working hand
      (a) Maintain modified pen grasp
      (b) Establish finger rest close to site of operation in anterior teeth
      (c) Maintain terminal shank parallel to long axis of tooth
      (d) Adapt 1 mm of tip at line angles and activate vertical overlapping strokes with wrist motion to move instrument across proximal surfaces
      (e) Use horizontal or oblique stroke with terminal shank horizontal to long axis of tooth to explore direct facial and lingual surfaces of anterior and posterior teeth (tip toward base of sulcus)
      (f) Explore tooth for normal anatomy, margins of restorations, calculus, and irregularities
    (3) Using shepherd's hook explorer, explore for caries; direct point into pits, grooves, and around restorations with pressure to find areas of retention that feel soft

REVIEW QUESTIONS

1. What are four functions of a mouth mirror?
2. What are the functions (at least four) of a periodontal probe?
3. What are the functions (at least two) of explorers?
4. True or false:
  a. The terminal shank is that part of the shank closest to the working end.
  b. In exploring, the full length of the working end should contact the tooth.
  c. Generally, the simpler the shank, the more anterior the intended use of the instrument.
  d. In selecting one end of a paired instrument for a given area, one cue in selecting the right end is that the terminal shank is perpendicular to the long axis of the tooth.
5. Identify the proper clinician and patient's head positions for each of the following areas. For each area, designate whether the positions are for a right-handed or a left-handed clinician.
    a. Labial No. 8
    b. Lingual No. 18
    c. Buccal No. 3
    d. Buccal No. 12
    e. Lingual No. 5
    f. Lingual No. 14
    g. Buccal No. 31

REFERENCES

Carter LM, Yaman P: *Dental instruments,* St Louis, 1981, CV Mosby.

Nield JS, O'Connor GH: *Fundamentals of dental hygiene instrumentation,* Philadelphia, 1983, WB Saunders.

Pattison AM, Behrens J: *Dental hygiene: the detection and removal of calculus,* Reston, Va, 1973, Reston.

Pattison GL, Pattison AM: *Periodontal instrumentation,* Reston, Va, 1992, Reston.

Ward HL, Simring MR: *Manual of clinical periodontics,* ed 2, St Louis, 1978, CV Mosby.

10 RADIOGRAPHIC ASSESSMENT

Gail F. Williamson

LEARNING OUTCOMES

The dental hygienist will be able to

1. Use selection criteria to recommend radiographic surveys for new and recall patients.
2. View dental radiographs in a logical evaluation sequence under optimal viewing conditions.
3. Differentiate between the normal and abnormal appearance of tooth structure, supporting structures, and anatomic landmarks on dental radiographs.
4. Identify and record from radiographs restorations, caries, periodontal findings, periapical disease, and bony abnormalities.
5. Write a description of the radiographic features of a bony lesion observed on a patient's radiographs.
6. Discuss alternative imaging methods.

Radiographs are an essential component of patient assessment. Radiographs, in addition to the clinical findings, will provide a more complete picture of the patient's oral condition and assist you in determining appropriate treatment. Several questions come to mind when discussing the use of radiographs in patient assessment. When are radiographs indicated? In what circumstances will radiographs yield information that cannot be determined clinically? What is the recommended manner of viewing radiographs to obtain maximum information? What limitations are inherent in radiographs? What types of information can be gleaned from radiographs about caries, periodontal disease, periapical pathoses, and bony abnormalities? What technologic advances have taken place in dental radiography? The goal of this chapter is to address these questions and provide you with a broader knowledge base in radiographic assessment.

SELECTION CRITERIA

In the United States dental radiographic examinations are second only to chest film examinations in terms of numbers and cost (Health and Human Services, 1987). It has been a common practice for dental patients to have dental radiographs on a routine schedule without variation regardless of oral conditions. Despite the advances in radiographic film (E speed) and screens (rare earth phosphors) that reduce patient exposure, patients still receive ionizing radiation from dental radiographic procedures. Although radiation exposures are considered to be quite low, more research needs to be conducted to determine the actual risks of low-dose radiation exposures (White, 1990). Therefore you need to use discretion with ionizing radiation. In addition, you should provide appropriate lead shielding for all patients undergoing radiographic examinations regardless of age. This radiation safety precaution will assist in reducing exposure to the public.

In 1987 the U.S. Department of Health and Human Services published guidelines for selecting patients for dental radiographic examinations. Patient selection criteria were developed by the Food and Drug Administration and a panel of dental experts. These recommendations were designed to help dental practitioners determine when a radiographic examination should be performed and assist in the selection of patients for such examinations. Selection criteria include the age of the patient, type of patient visit, dental health status, and risk factors. These criteria can be used to design a radiographic survey appropriate for each patient considering the clinical presentation and medical/dental history. A summary of these guidelines appears in Table 10-1 (Health and Human Services, 1987). The recommendations contained in the chart are subject to the dentist's and your judgment and serve as a framework in decision making. Radiographic indicators are listed in Table 10-2. These guidelines suggest situations in which radiographs are likely to yield useful infor-

Table 10-1. Selection criteria guidelines

Patient category	Child (primary/transitional)	Adolescent (prior to third molar eruption)	Adult
New patient Assess dental disease, child/adolescent growth and development	**Primary:** Bitewings if proximals closed **Transitional:** Bitewings and selected periapicals/occlusals or bitewings and panoramic	Bitewings and selected periapicals or full mouth survey for generalized disease or history of extensive treatment	**Dentulous:** Bitewings/selected periapicals or full mouth for generalized disease or history of extensive treatment **Edentulous:** Full mouth or panoramic
Recall Clinical caries or high risk for caries	Bitewings at 6-month intervals until no caries	Bite wings at 6 to 12 month intervals until no caries	Bitewings at 12 to 18-month intervals
No clinical caries or low risk factors	12 to 24 month intervals	18 to 36-month intervals	24 to 36-month intervals
Periodontal disease Present clinically or history of disease	Selected bitewings and/or periapicals	Selected bitewings and/or periapicals	Selected bitewings and/or periapicals
Growth and development	**Transitional:** Selected periapical/occlusal, or panoramic survey	Periapical or panoramic survey to assess third molars	Not indicated

Adapted from *Dental Radiographic Examinations,* Health and Human Services Publication FDA 88-8273, 1987.

Table 10-2. Radiographic indicators

Positive historical findings

1. Previous periodontal or endodontic therapy
2. History of pain or trauma
3. Familial history of dental anomalies
4. Postoperative evaluation of healing
5. Presence of implants

Positive clinical signs and symptoms

1. Clinical presence of periodontal disease
2. Large or deep restorations
3. Deep carious lesions
4. Malposed or clinically impacted teeth
5. Swelling or evidence of facial trauma
6. Mobility of teeth.
7. Fistula or sinus tract infection
8. Clinically suspected sinus abnormality
9. Growth abnormalities or facial asymmetry
10. Oral involvement of systemic disease
11. Positive head and neck neurologic findings
12. Evidence of foreign bodies
13. Temporomandibular pain and/or dysfunction
14. Abutment teeth for fixed or removable prosthesis
15. Unexplained bleeding or tooth sensitivity
16. Unusual eruption, spacing, migration of teeth
17. Unusual tooth morphology, calcification, color
18. Missing teeth with unknown reason

High risk for caries

1. High level of caries experience
2. History of recurrent caries
3. Many multisurface or poor quality restorations
4. Poor oral hygiene
5. Inadequate fluoride exposure
6. Prolonged bottle or breast nursing
7. High sucrose diet
8. Poor family dental health
9. Developmental enamel defects
10. Developmental disability
11. Xerostomia
12. Genetic abnormality of teeth
13. Chemotherapy or radiation therapy

Adapted from *Dental Radiographic Examinations,* Health and Human Services Publication FDA 88-8273, 1987.

mation. Since it is common practice for the dental hygienist to take medical/dental histories and examine new and recall patients (Tilliss and Cross-Poline, 1989), the hygienist may participate in the selection of patients for radiographic examinations. The result of patient selection should be a radiographic examination tailored to the patient and not one of convenience for the clinician. The type and number of films to be taken should be adequate to provide the necessary information. Note that the only time-based radiographic procedure is the bitewing survey for caries evaluation. The time intervals vary based on the presence or absence of historical and clinical findings as well as risk factors (see Table 10-2).

VIEWING RADIOGRAPHS

Once radiographs have been taken and processed, the finished films should be mounted in an appropriate frame for viewing and for future reference. The most suitable film mount is one that is opaque to light, preferably black, which allows illumination of the film window only. Pocket film mounts are desirable, as they protect the mounted survey from fingerprints and contaminants (Block Drug Corp., Jersey City, New Jersey). The plastic cover design will allow for careful surface disinfection if the survey was handled or contaminated during a patient appointment.

Viewing conditions are an important aspect of examining radiographs for relevant information. Properly mounted radiographs should be examined on a viewbox with opaque glass and even light distribution. Subdued background lighting and elimination of extraneous viewbox light around the mount are recommended. The ideal viewbox allows changes in light intensity, so that the clinician can view films of different intensities by adjusting the level of viewbox light. Once the viewing conditions have been set, the eyes will adjust to the level of transillumination of the survey. In addition, a magnifying glass is a useful adjunct in viewing radiographs (Fig. 10-1). It enables the interpreter to more closely examine suspicious or questionable areas on the film survey.

When viewing radiographs for information, it is best to examine structures sequentially and focus on one aspect of evaluation at a time (Bodak-Gyovai and Manzione, 1980). A consistent and organized approach will ensure that all structures are viewed. A suggested format follows:

1. Examine film dot convexities for uniformity and proper film mounting.
2. Inspect the films for correct tooth and anatomic landmark location.
3. Examine the existing teeth. Note those that are missing, carious, or restored or that have changed in size, shape, or structure.
4. Examine the supporting bone structure. Note deviations in crestal bone height, overall density, trabecular pattern, and changes in the lamina dura and periodontal ligament spaces.
5. After examining the films for fine detail,

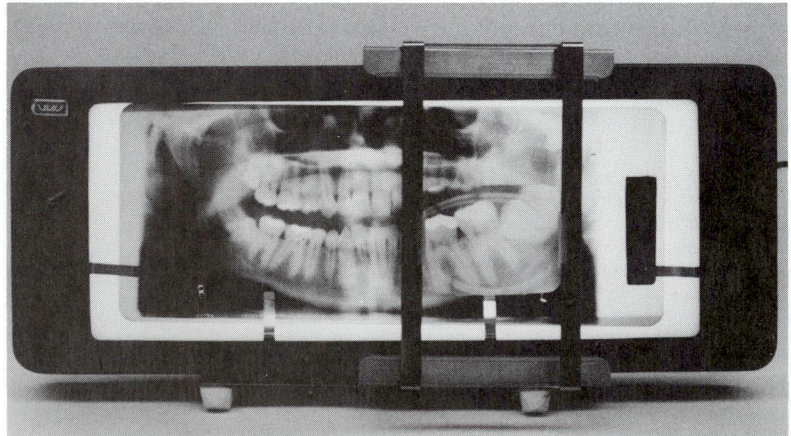

Fig. 10-1. Viewbox with magnifying lens. (Courtesy of Rinn Corporation, Elgin, Illinois.)

broaden your visual perspective. View the films as a composite and compare bilateral anatomic structures right to left for differences.

RECOGNITION OF NORMAL RADIOGRAPHIC ANATOMY

You must be familiar with the normal appearance of tooth structure and bony anatomy to observe abnormalities or disease. Each region of the arches displays characteristic features that identify its location and aid in differentiation between healthy structure and disease. Knowing tooth morphology is another key to area identification.

Radiographs are film records of structures with varying densities. Objects such as tooth enamel and bone attenuate the primary beam and are depicted as radiopacities. Objects such as the maxillary sinus and pulp chamber represent spaces in structures that allow free passage of x-rays and are recorded as radiolucencies. There are relative degrees of radiopacities, and radiolucencies depending on the size, density, and thickness of the structures. Other factors that influence the radiographic appearance are the projection technique used, the inherent layering effect of displaying three-dimensional objects in two dimensions, exposure factors, and processing techniques.

Tooth structure

The tooth is composed primarily of mineralized tissues: enamel, dentin, and cementum. The enamel is the densest and most radiopaque of these substances. It appears as a white cap overlying the coronal aspect of the tooth. A distinct margin—the dentinoenamel junction (DEJ)—separates the enamel from the underlying dentin. The dentin is less mineralized than enamel and appears gray or as a lesser radiopacity. Cementum and dentin have the same degree of opacity and cannot be distinguished from each other radiographically. In the body of the tooth is a space that houses the pulp tissues. The pulp of normal teeth is soft tissue and is shown as a radiolucency. In posterior teeth a broader horned configuration is seen with the pulp canals extending apically from the pulp chamber. In anterior teeth the pulp is a more uniform linear shape. The size of the pulp chamber and canals varies with age. Generally young individuals will display larger pulpal anatomy than older individuals. Developing teeth have large pulp chambers and canals and

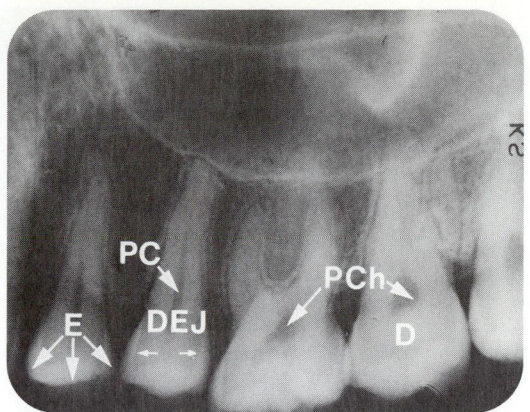

Fig. 10-2. Tooth is composed primarily of mineralized tissues such as enamel and dentin. *(E)* Enamel, the most dense and radiopaque of these structures, appears as a white cap overlying tooth crown. Dentinoenamal junction *(DEJ)* demarcates the interface between the dense enamel layer and the less calcified, less radiopaque *(D)* dentin, located beneath the enamel cap. Pulp canal *(PC)* and pulp chamber *(PCh)* are spaces inside tooth that house the nerve and vascular tissues. These structures appear radiolucent on dental radiographs.

incomplete apical development. Familiarity with tooth maturation stages is useful in differentiating between tooth development and possible periapical disease (see Fig. 10-2 to view these structures).

Supporting structures

The structures immediately adjacent to the tooth are the periodontal ligament space and the lamina dura (Fig. 10-3). The periodontal ligament is composed of flexible collagen fibers and therefore is seen as a thin radiolucent line surrounding the entire tooth root. The width of the periodontal ligament space of teeth in function is approximately 0.25 to 0.4 mm and may vary from tooth to tooth and from person to person (Shafer, Hine, and Levy, 1983). The lamina dura is the linear radiopaque bony lining of the tooth socket. In health the lamina dura will appear as a continuous opacity around the tooth root. Its thickness and degree of opacity vary with tooth function, being wider and more opaque with heavy occlusal stress, thinner and less opaque with loss of function (Goaz and White, 1987). The lamina dura also is continuous with the alveolar crest of bone. The alveolar crest is the bone that extends between the teeth near the gingival margin. This ra-

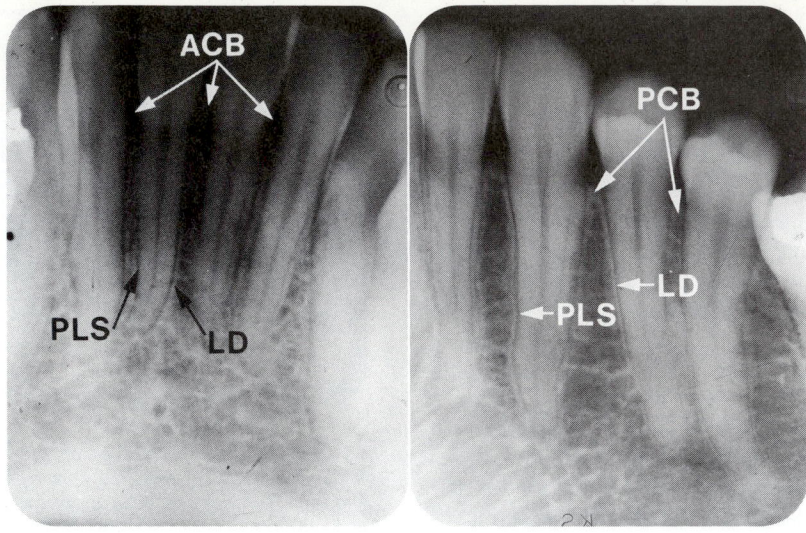

Fig. 10-3. Anterior crestal bone *(ACB)* has a narrow, pointed shape, whereas the posterior crestal bone *(PCB)* has a flat, angular configuration. Periodontal ligament space *(PLS)* appears as a thin radiolucent line surrounding entire tooth. Lamina dura *(LD)* is adjacent to ligament space and is seen as continuous radiopacity that outlines the tooth socket.

diopacity is located approximately 1.5 mm from the cementoenamel junction (CEJ) and should appear parallel to a line joining the CEJs of adjacent teeth. In the posterior regions the crestal bone has a flat, angular shape in contrast to the narrow, pointed shape of the anterior regions (see Fig. 10-3). The cancellous or trabecular bone is located between the outer cortical plates of the jaws. It has a spongy or honeycomb appearance radiographically. The trabecular pattern is seen as a mixture of radiopacities and radiolucencies representing the bone structure and marrow spaces. Its overall appearance is gray and may vary. In general the maxilla has a fine, compact trabecular pattern with small marrow spaces that become slightly larger in the posterior areas. In the mandible the trabecular pattern is not as fine, and the marrow spaces tend to be larger than the maxilla. As in the maxillary arch, the marrow spaces are often larger in the posterior regions.

Maxillary structures

The maxilla has many distinguishing anatomic landmarks that can be used to identify the area recorded whether or not teeth are present. The principal landmarks of the posterior maxilla are the coronoid process of the mandible, the pterygoid plates (lateral and medial), the tuberosity, the zygomatic process and bone, and the sinus cavity (Figs. 10-4 to 10-6). With the exception of the maxillary sinus, these landmarks are bony in origin and therefore radiopaque. The sinus is the predominant radiolucent landmark of the posterior maxilla. All of these structures appear bilaterally on radiographs. The primary landmarks of the anterior maxilla are the nasal fossae, the nasal septum, the anterior nasal spine, the inverted Y, the median palatal suture, and the incisive foramen (Figs. 10-5 to 10-8). The radiopaque structures include the septum, spine, and inverted Y, whereas the radiolucencies include the fossae, suture, and foramen. Only the nasal fossae and the inverted Y landmarks occur bilaterally. These landmarks are described more fully in the following text.

Coronoid process. The coronoid process of the mandible is frequently seen on maxillary molar periapical radiographs in the inferoposterior corner of the film. This radiopaque triangular or thumb-shaped structure represents the anterosuperior portion of the ramus. When the patient opens his or her mouth to allow for placement of the film in this area, the coronoid moves forward and is recorded. It is the only mandibular landmark

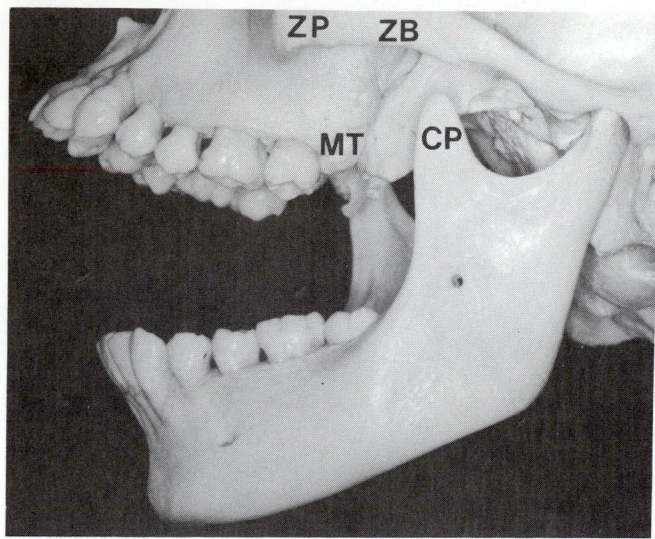

Fig. 10-4. Zygomatic process *(ZP)* and zygomatic bone *(ZB)* are structures that constitute the cheek bone. Maxillary tuberosity *(MT)* is the rounded, bony end of the maxillary alveolar ridge. Coronoid process *(CP)* of mandible is a triangular-shaped bony structure that provides insertion of the temporalis and masseter muscles.

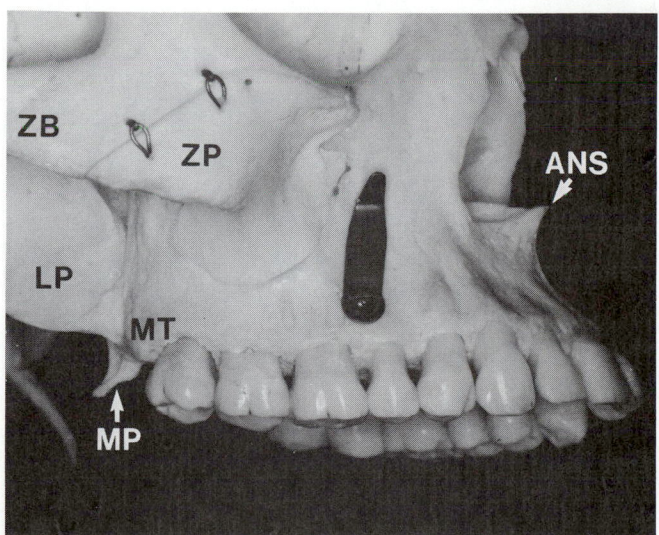

Fig. 10-5. Zygomatic bone *(ZB)* extends and broadens from curved prominence of zygomatic process *(ZP)* Anterior nasal spine *(ANS)* is a spike-shaped structure projecting from the central base of the nasal cavities. Lateral pterygoid *(LP)* plate is a thin wing of bone located behind the maxillary tuberosity *(MT)*. Medial pterygoid plate is a tiny finger of bone extending from the medial aspect of the pterygoid plate of the sphenoid bone.

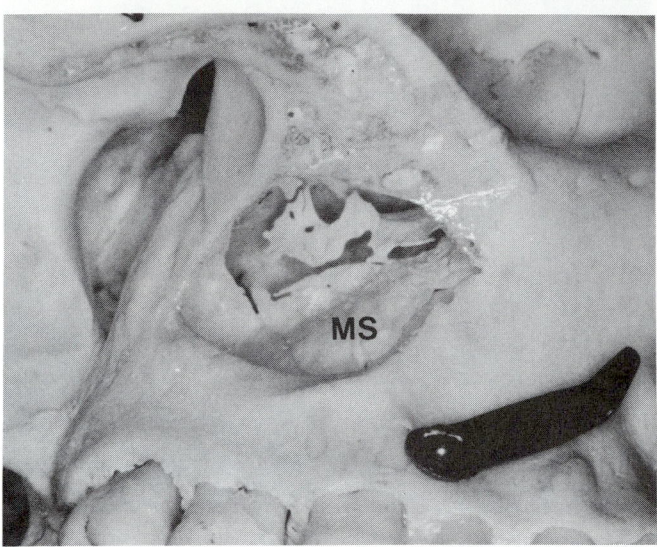

Fig. 10-6. Maxillary sinus *(MS)* is an air-filled cavity that extends from the distal part of the canine tooth to the tuberosity area. External wall of sinus has been removed to view this structure.

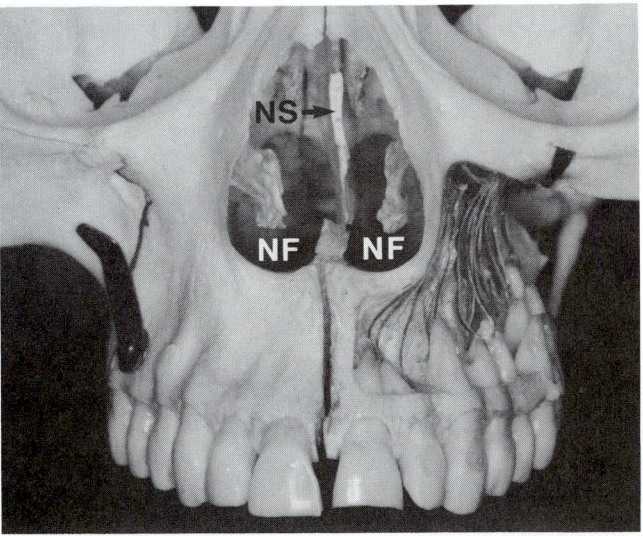

Fig. 10-7. Nasal septum *(NS)* is a bony and cartilaginous structure that separates the two nasal cavities in the midplane. Nasal fossae *(NF)* are the hollow air cavities of the nose.

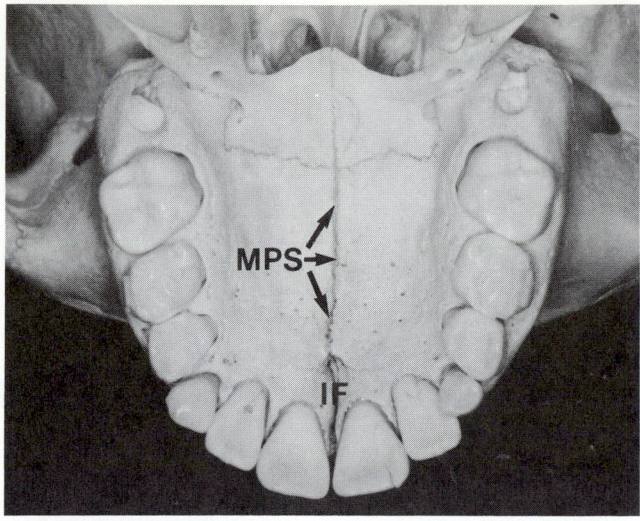

Fig. 10-8. Median palatal suture *(MPS)* is a thin linear space between the palatal processes of the maxilla. Incisive foramen *(IF)* is an oval-shaped, lingual opening in bone that serves as an orifice for the nasopalatine canal.

that appears on maxillary periapical radiographs (Fig. 10-9).

Pterygoid plates. The pterygoid plates appear superior to the coronoid process on the most posterior aspect of the molar film. These delicate bony plates are part of the sphenoid bone. The lateral pterygoid plate is a thin wing of bone extending toward the posterior aspect of the film. The medial pterygoid or hamulus is a fine, tiny finger of bone extending from the anteroinferior aspect of the medial plate (see Fig. 10-9).

Maxillary tuberosity. The maxillary tuberosity is the rounded posterior boundary of the alveolar ridge just distal to the third molar area. Beyond the tuberosity on each side is a small space called the hamular notch. Radiographically this space represents where the bony ridge ends and the pterygoid plates begin. The tuberosity may be recorded on molar bitewing views as well (Figs. 10-9 and 10-11).

Zygomatic process and bone. The zygomatic process of the maxilla is the prominent U-shaped radiopacity just apical to the first and second molars. The zygomatic bone or cheek bone extends posteriorly from the process and becomes a broader, less opaque structure. Both of these structures may superimpose over the regional

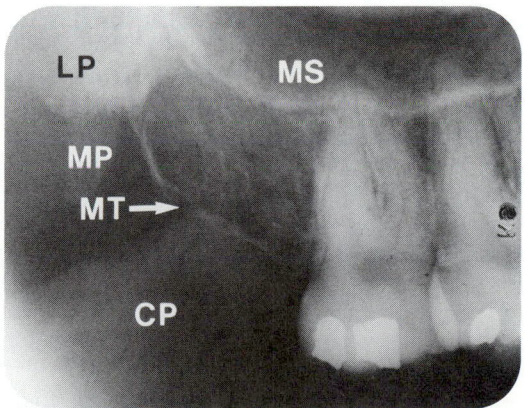

Fig. 10-9. Lateral pterygoid *(LP)* plate is the radiopaque wing of the sphenoid bone. Maxillary sinus *(MS)* is the radiolucent structure with a thin radiopaque border. Hamulus, or medial pterygoid plate *(MP)* is the radiopaque, fingerlike structure just posterior to the maxillary tuberosity *(MT)*, the rounded bony end of the maxillary ridge. The coronoid process *(CP)* of the mandible is the bony, thumblike structure extending upward toward the tuberosity.

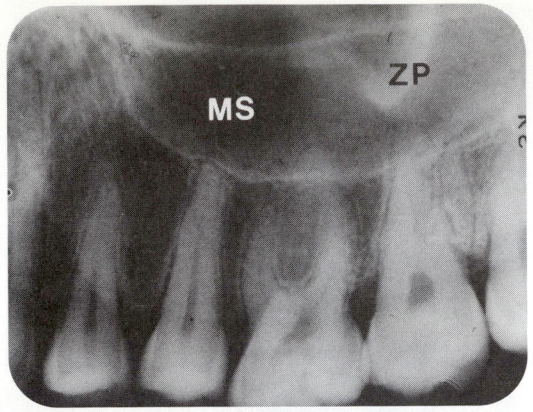

Fig. 10-10. Maxillary sinus *(MS)* is shown extending from first premolar to third molar tooth. It is bounded superiorly by the floor of the nasal fossa. Zygomatic process *(ZP)* is the radiopacity superior to the second molar and extending in a posterior direction.

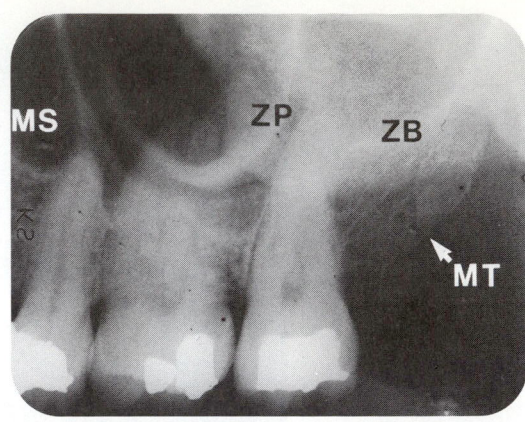

Fig. 10-11. Maxillary sinus *(MS)* is the radiolucent structure approximating the apices of the second premolar and first molar teeth. Note presence of a vertical septum within anterior body of the sinus. This is a variation in the anatomy of the sinus. U-shaped structure is zygomatic process *(ZP)*, and the broader radiopacity superimposed over the posterior sinus is the zygomatic bone *(ZB)*. Maxillary tuberosity *(MT)* is the rounded bony ridge distal to the second molar.

anatomy and the teeth, especially when a bisecting angle technique is used for periapical radiography (Figs. 10-10 and 10-11).

Maxillary sinus. The maxillary sinus is an air-filled cavity located just superior to the apices of premolar and molar teeth. The body of this structure is radiolucent, but its borders are thin linear radiopacities. The sinus extends from the distal of the canine tooth to the tuberosity area on each side of the maxilla. The inferior border or floor of the sinus may closely approximate the apices of the posterior teeth. The sinus can be viewed on most canine, premolar, and molar periapical radiographs (see Figs. 10-9 to 10-11).

Nasal fossae, septum, and spine. Radiographically the nasal cavities may be seen superior to the incisor teeth as two vertical oblong radiolucencies. These hollow chambers are divided by the nasal septum, a longitudinal band radiopacity. The nasal septum terminates at the central base of the fossae in a triangular point of bone, the anterior nasal spine. These anatomic landmarks are most frequently seen on central and lateral incisor periapical views (Fig. 10-12).

Inverted Y. The inverted Y is a radiographic landmark demarcating the bony borders of the anterior aspect of the maxillary sinus and the lateral aspect of the nasal floor. The shape of the borders looks like an inverted Y or, sometimes, an X. The inverted Y is bounded by two radiolucencies; the posterior one represents the sinus and the anterior one represents the nasal fossa. Typically this landmark is found just apical to each canine tooth. The inverted Y is especially useful in orienting and mounting edentulous radiographs (Fig. 10-13).

Median palatal suture. The median palatal suture is a thin radiolucent line found between the apices of the maxillary central incisor teeth. Anatomically it is located between the two palatal processes of the maxilla. Radiographically it may be seen to extend superiorly from the alveolar crest through the entire nasal midline (Fig. 10-14).

Incisive foramen. The incisive foramen or nasopalatine foramen is an oval-shaped radiolucency found between the apices of the maxillary central incisors. This opening in bone is located on the lingual aspect of the palate and is an orifice for the nasopalatine canal. The incisive foramen varies in size, shape, location, and definition (see Fig. 10-12).

Mandibular structures

The mandible has several anatomic features that aid in identifying specific regions in the mandible

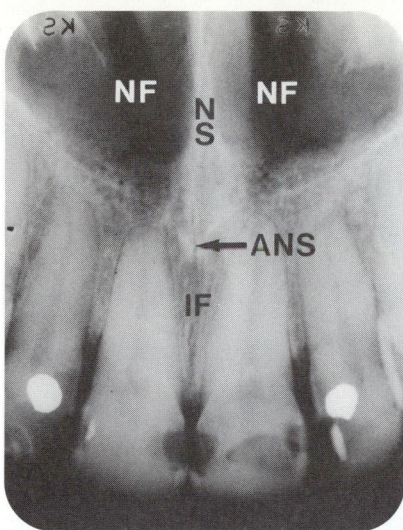

Fig. 10-12. Nasal fossae *(NF)* are the oblong radiolucencies divided by a vertical radiopacity, nasal septum *(NS)*. Anterior nasal spine *(ANS)* is the small, triangular radiopacity at the inferior base of the nasal septum. Incisive foramen *(IF)* is located between the apices of the maxillary central incisors and is seen here as a faint heart-shaped radiolucency.

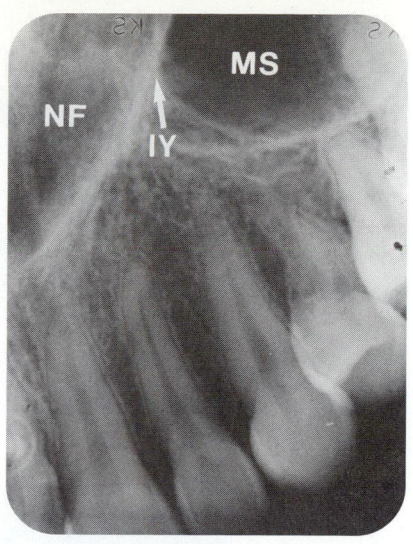

Fig. 10-13. Nasal fossa *(NF)* is located superior to the incisor teeth; its lateral border forms the anterior boundary of the inverted Y *(IY)*. Maxillary sinus *(MS)* is found superior to the premolar teeth; its anterior border forms the posterior boundary of the inverted Y.

and in differentiating it from the maxilla. The primary landmarks of the posterior mandible are the external oblique ridge, the internal oblique ridge, the mandibular canal, the inferior border of the mandible, and the mental foramen (Figs. 10-15 to 10-17). The oblique ridges and the inferior border of the mandible are bony in origin and appear as bilateral radiopaque structures on films. The mandibular canal and the mental foramen are the most common bilateral radiolucent landmarks seen in the posterior regions of the mandible. In the anterior portion of the mandible, the principal landmarks include the mental ridge, the genial tubercles, the lingual foramen, and the inferior border of the mandible (Figs. 10-18 and 10-19). With the exception of the lingual foramen, these landmarks are bony in origin and therefore radiopaque on radiographs.

External oblique ridge. The external oblique ridge is part of the anterior border of the ramus that extends downward from the coronoid process to the lateral aspect of the posterior alveolar process. The ridge serves as an attachment for the buccinator muscle. This diagonal radiopaque stripe is commonly seen distal to or superimposed

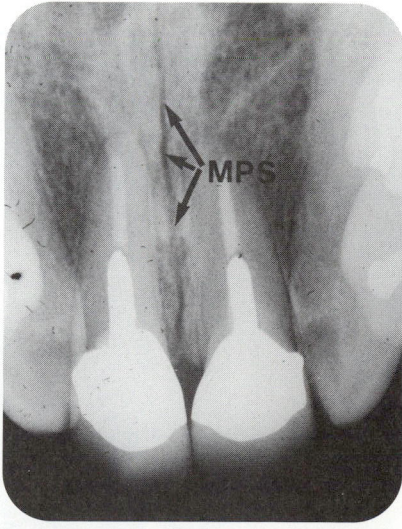

Fig. 10-14. Median palatal suture *(MPS)* divides the dental midline and is shown as a thin, radiolucent vertical line.

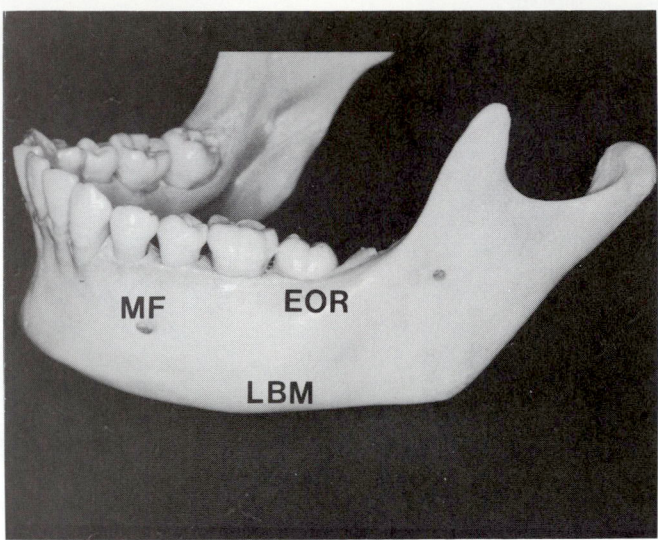

Fig. 10-15. Mental foramen *(MF)* is a circular bilateral opening in the premolar region of the mandible and serves as the anterior terminus of the mandibular canal. External oblique ridge *(EOR)* is a prominent ridge of bone on the external surface of the anterior ramus that provides attachment for the buccinator muscle. Lower border of the mandible *(LBM)* is found on the inferior aspect of the mandible and is composed of heavy cortical bone.

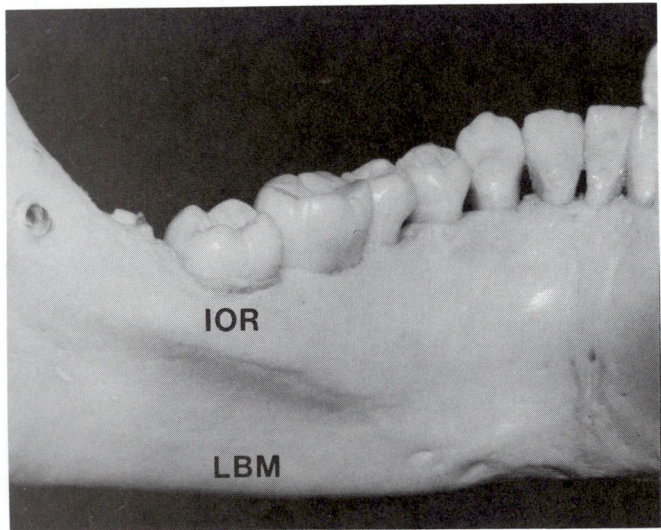

Fig. 10-16. Internal oblique ridge *(IOR)* is found bilaterally on the lingual surface of the mandible and serves as attachment for the mylohyoid muscle. Lower border of the mandible *(LBM)* is shown here from the lingual aspect.

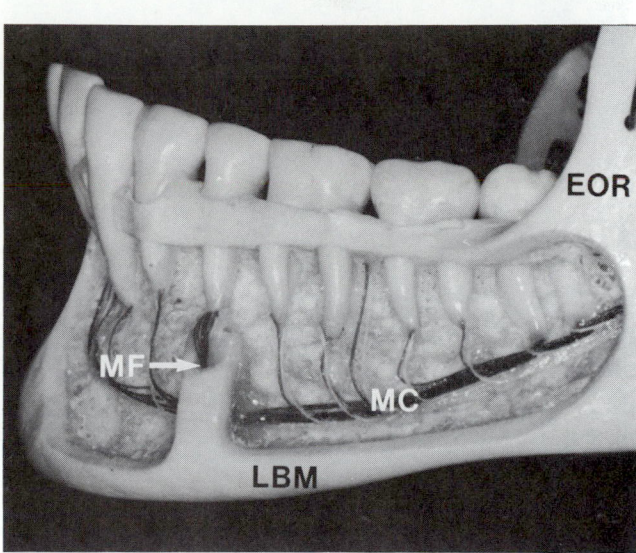

Fig. 10-17. External oblique ridge *(EOR)* extends downward from the anterior ramus, crossing the third molar crown in a diagonal fashion. Mental foramen *(MF)* is shown in relationship to the second premolar apex and mandibular canal *(MC)*. Note the inferior alveolar vessels and nerves that branch from the mandibular canal. Lower border of the mandible *(LBM)* is inferior to the mandibular canal.

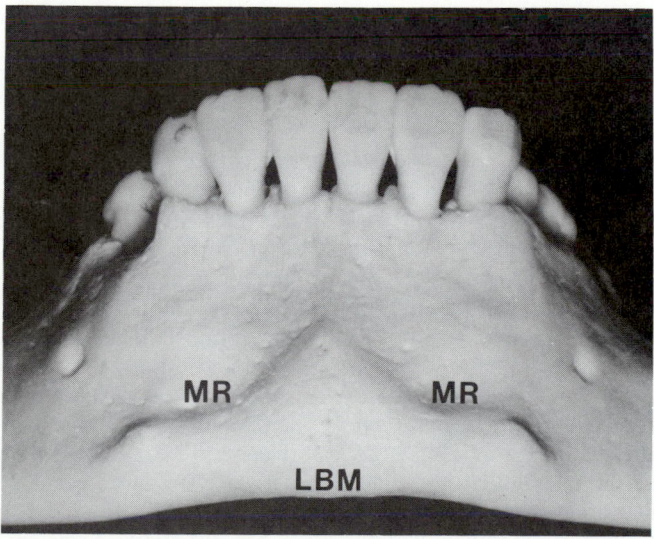

Fig. 10-18. Mental ridge *(MR)* is a prominence of bone on the facial surface of the mentum positioned just above the lower border of the mandible *(LBM)*.

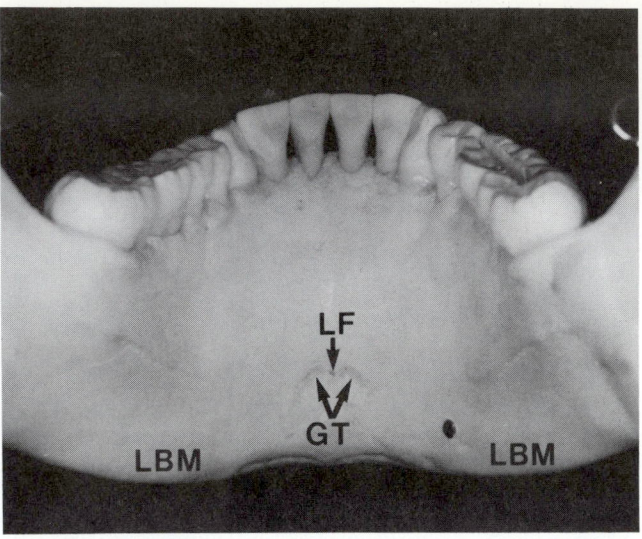

Fig. 10-19. Pinpoint opening of lingual foramen *(LF)* generally found in the center of the genial tubercles *(GT)*. These are small spines of bone on the lingual anterior mandible that provide attachment for the genioglossus and geniohyoid muscles. Lower border of the mandible *(LBM)* is located inferior to the tubercles.

over the third molar crown or ridge area. This landmark is typically found on the molar periapical and molar bitewing views (Figs. 10-20 and 10-21).

Internal oblique or mylohyoid ridge. The internal oblique or mylohyoid ridge is located on the lingual surface of the posterior mandible. It serves as an attachment for the mylohyoid muscle. Radiographically it appears as a diagonal radiopaque stripe superimposed over or inferior to the apices of the molar and sometimes the premolar teeth. The path of this bony line is parallel to the external oblique ridge. The internal oblique ridge is usually less defined than the external oblique ridge (see Fig. 10-20).

Mandibular canal. The mandibular canal is represented on radiographs as a diagonal radiolucent tube with thin radiopaque borders approximating the apices of the molar teeth. This structure is the pathway for the mandibular nerve and blood vessels. The canal originates at the mandibular foramen (lingual aspect of the ramus) and extends anteriorly into the premolar area, terminating at the mental foramen. Generally the course of this landmark runs parallel and inferior to the oblique ridges (see Fig. 10-21).

Inferior border of the mandible. The inferior border of the mandible may be seen on the inferior aspect of any mandibular periapical view. Radiographically this heavy layer of cortical bone is depicted as a prominent radiopaque band crossing the bottom of the film (Figs. 10-20 to 10-22).

Mental foramen. The mental foramen is a circular radiolucency located near the apices of the premolar teeth and may be viewed on premolar and canine periapical projections (Fig. 10-23). As previously discussed, this structure is the anterior terminus of the mandibular canal, allowing passage of the mental nerves and vessels. Its radiographic appearance is quite variable in size, location, and definition. Often the mental foramen is superimposed over the root of one of the premolar teeth and mimics an abnormality. Careful examination of the suspected tooth for a contiguous lamina dura should assist in differentiating between the two. Also, comparing the area to its appearance on an adjacent or an additional periapical film is useful.

Mental ridge. Occasionally the mental ridge is recorded on canine and incisor periapical films. This bilateral ridge of bone is located on the anterior surface of the mandible. Radiographically it forms a radiopaque inverted V or triangular shape and closely approximates the apices of the anterior teeth (see Fig. 10-22).

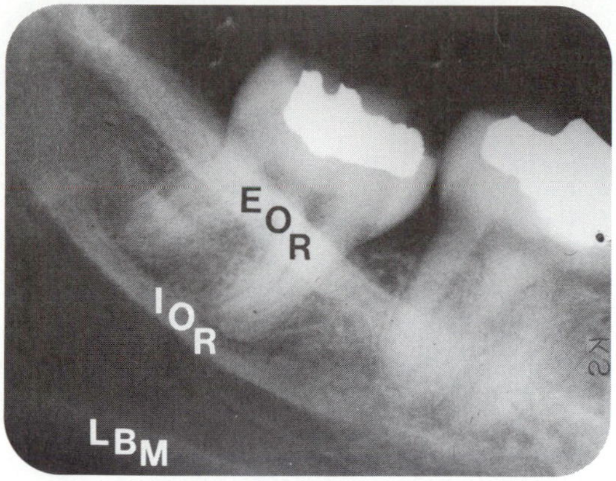

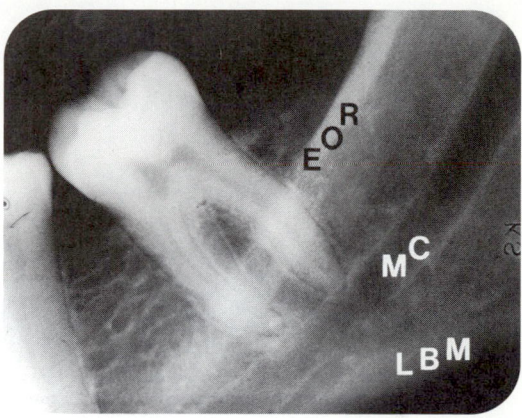

Fig. 10-20. External oblique ridge *(EOR)* is the heavy, diagonal radiopaque ridge of bone located above the internal oblique ridge *(IOR)*, which approximates the apices of the molar teeth and is generally less radiopaque than the external oblique ridge. Lower border of the mandible *(LBM)* is shown on the posteroinferior aspect of this radiograph as a horizontal radiopaque stripe of bone.

Fig. 10-21. External oblique ridge *(EOR)* is the prominent, diagonal radiopaque stripe crossing the molar tooth. Mandibular canal *(MC)* is the radiolucent tubelike structure with thin radiopaque superior and inferior borders. Lower border of the mandible *(LBM)* displays its typical radiopaque appearance on the posterioinferior aspect of this molar film.

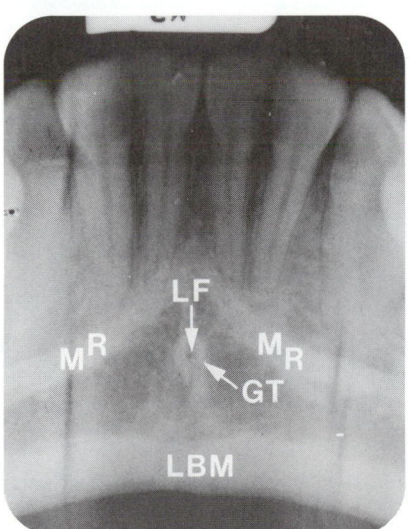

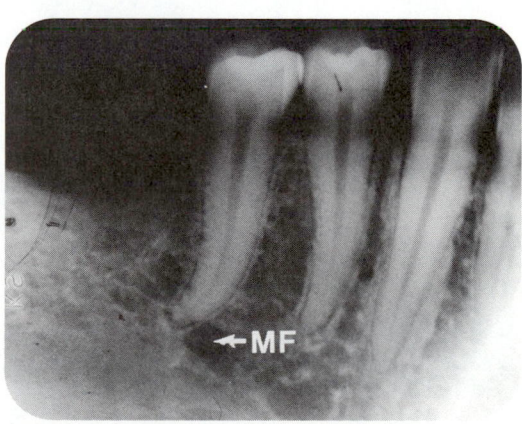

Fig. 10-22. Inverted v-shaped radiopaque structure is the mental ridge *(MR)*. Lingual foramen *(LF)* is shown here in the center of a ring of bony spines known as the genial tubercles *(GT)*. Lower border of the mandible *(LBM)* extends across the bottom of the anterior ridge.

Fig. 10-23. Mental foramen *(MF)* is located near the apex of the second premolar tooth. Its typical appearance is that of a circular radiolucency.

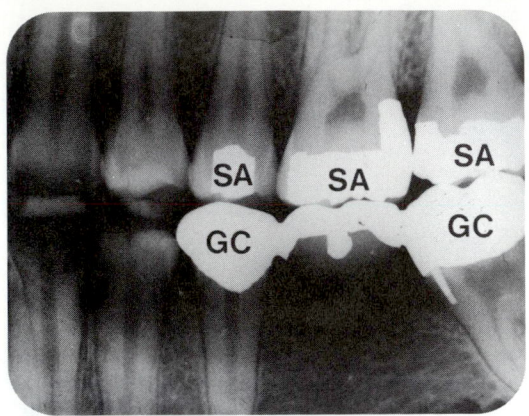

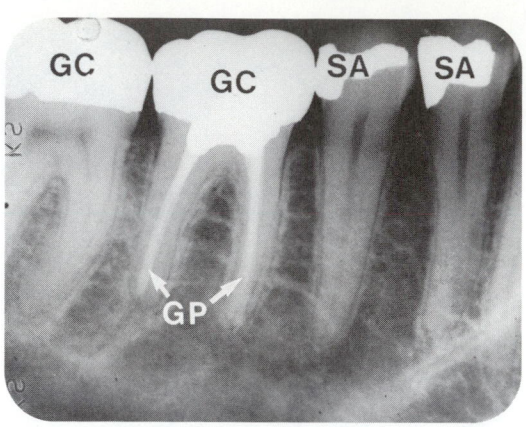

Fig. 10-24. Silver amalgam *(SA)* restorations are present in teeth Nos. 13, occlusal; 14, distalocclusal; 15, mesioocclusal. Gold crown *(GC)* abutments for a three-unit bridge are found on teeth Nos. 20 and 18, with a porcelain-metal pontic replacing tooth No. 19. Retention pin is present in tooth No. 18.

Fig. 10-25. Gold crowns *(GC)* are present on both molars, Nos. 30 and 31. No. 30 has post and core type of gold crown, which serves to better secure the crown on this endodontically treated molar. Gutta percha *(GP)* endodontic points fill the pulp canals of tooth No. 30. Silver amalgam *(SA)* restorations are present in teeth No. 28 and 29; both distal and occlusal surfaces are filled.

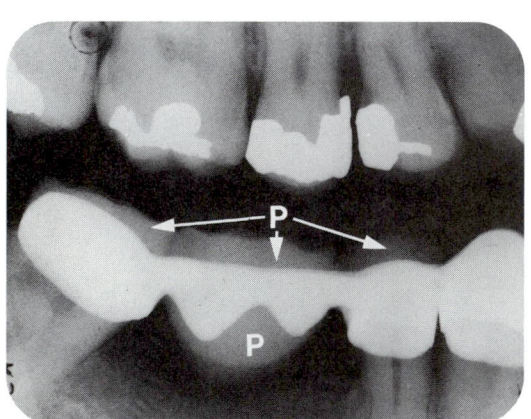

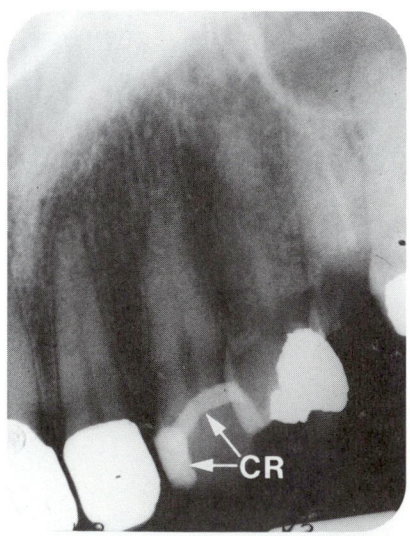

Fig. 10-26. Porcelain *(P)* fused to metal three-unit bridge extends from teeth Nos. 28 to 31, with No. 30 replaced by the pontic. The porcelain material is radiopaque, about the same density as dentin on dental radiographs. A single metal-ceramic crown covers tooth No. 27. In addition, silver amalgam restorations are found in the maxillary posterior teeth.

Fig. 10-27. Two radiopaque composite resin *(CR)* restorations are found in tooth No. 11, a mesial and a facial Class V.

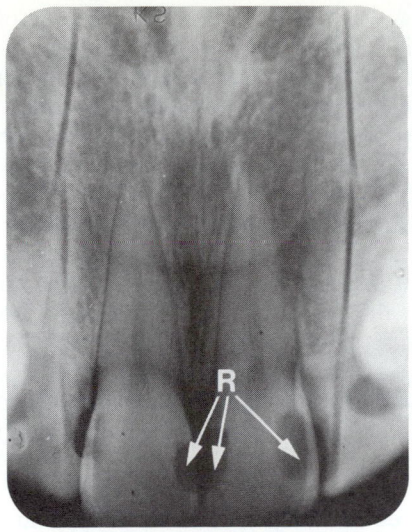

Fig. 10-28. Radiolucent interproximal R-resin *(R)* restorations are present in teeth No. 7, mesial; 8, mesial; 9, mesial and distal; and 10, mesial and distal. The distal interproximal radiolucencies on No. 8 are Class III carious lesions. Note the smooth, regular outlines of the restorations compared to the carious lesions.

Genial tubercles and lingual foramen. The genial tubercles are small spines of bone found on the lingual midline of the mandible and provide attachment for the genioglossus and geniohyoid muscles. Frequently seen on incisor projections, the genial tubercles form a radiopaque ring of bone around the lingual foramen. The lingual foramen is a pinpoint radiolucency on radiographs. This tiny opening in bone allows for passage for the terminal branches of the mandibular nerve. Often these landmarks appear together in the middle to inferior third of the film (see Fig. 10-22).

Dental materials

In addition to recognizing anatomic structures, the clinician needs to be familiar with the typical appearance of materials commonly used to restore the teeth. Metallic restorations such as gold; silver amalgam; endodontic silver points; orthodontic wire, bands, and brackets; implants; and stainless steel pins and crowns are prominent radiopacities appearing in the tooth structure. Examples of metallic restorations are seen in Figs. 10-24 and 10-25. Nonmetal materials such as porcelain, endodontic gutta percha points, base materials, and

some composite resins are radiopaque but not as distinctly radiopaque as metallic materials (Figs. 10-25 to 10-27). Silicates, resin, acrylic, and some composite resin anterior restorative materials appear radiolucent on radiographs (Fig. 10-28). Often the presence of these materials can be determined by observing the outline form of the cavity preparation or the presence of a base. Chapter 11 provides further examples of restored teeth and discusses the appropriate nomenclature for charting restored teeth.

RECOGNITION OF DENTAL DISEASE

Radiographs are an integral part of patient evaluation and disease assessment. Radiographs provide the practitioner with information that may not be apparent clinically. Often radiographs are used to verify conditions that are suspected clinically. Whatever the clinical circumstance, the radiographic findings must to be correlated with the patient's dental and medical histories as well as the data obtained from the oral examination for proper diagnosis and treatment. The clinician must realize that radiographs have limitations and serve as only one means of obtaining diagnostic information.

The first step in radiographic assessment of disease conditions is recognizing the normal appearance of the teeth, restorative treatments, and the supporting structures. From that baseline the teeth and supporting structures can be more critically examined for changes in configuration, density, size, and relative position. The second step in the radiographic assessment process is the systematic review by category for abnormal or disease condition. As previously discussed, this critical viewing should be conducted in an organized and sequential manner with consideration given to optimal viewing conditions. The disease categories to be discussed below are dental caries, periodontal disease, and periapical disease. In addition, a method for describing the radiographic features of pathologic lesions of the jaws is presented.

Dental caries

Dental caries is a pathologic process of demineralization and destruction of tooth structure by microorganisms. The incidence of caries is influenced by factors such as tooth composition, morphology, and position; salivary composition, pH, quantity, viscosity, and antibacterial properties; diet; and time (Shafer, Hine, and Levy, 1983).

The widespread use of fluoride in public water systems and the use of adjunctive fluoride products has reduced the incidence of caries in children (Goaz and White, 1987). Despite these reductions, dental decay is a recurring problem for many patients. The result of dental decay is loss of tooth structure and potentially the tooth itself.

Carious lesions are represented on dental radiographs as radiolucent areas at the site of the lesion. X-rays are able to pass through the area of undermined tooth structure and reach the film. However, approximately 40% demineralization is necessary for radiographic detection of a lesion (Goaz and White, 1987). Thus lesions may be somewhat larger in size than they appear on films. The clinician also must be aware that various dental anomalies, such as hypoplastic pits, cervical abrasion, erosion, and portions of teeth that have fractured off, may mimic caries. Therefore it is important to correlate radiographic findings with clinical findings.

Radiographs are especially valuable in detecting carious lesions on the surfaces of the teeth that are difficult to examine clinically. For example, occlusal, facial, and lingual decay are more readily found clinically, whereas interproximal and recurrent decay along the interproximal margins are more readily found radiographically. Bitewing radiographs provide the most undistorted view of tooth structure that aids in caries evaluation. Short-scale, low kilovoltage (70 kVp) exposure factors are recommended for sharp depiction of carious lesions. Periapicals taken with the paralleling technique are useful for comparison purposes and allow apical inspection of cariously involved teeth.

The nomenclature for classifying carious lesions by location was developed by G.V. Black (Sturdevant, 1985) and is as follows:

Class I: All pit and fissure cavities: occlusals of molars and premolars, occlusal two thirds of facial and lingual surfaces on molars, and lingual pits of maxillary molars.

Class II: Cavities on the proximal surfaces of molars and premolars

Class III: Cavities on the proximal surfaces of incisors and canines *not* involving the incisal angle

Class IV: Cavities on the proximal surfaces of incisors and canines *involving* the incisal angle

Class V: Cavities on the gingival one third of facial or lingual surfaces of all teeth

Class VI: Cavities on the incisal edge of anterior teeth or the cusp tips on posterior teeth

This system of classification does not include root or recurrent caries but provides basic terminology for reporting or discussing radiographic findings. (Refer to caries classification illustrations in Chapter 11.)

Interproximal caries. Radiographs are more efficient in revealing interproximal lesions than clinical inspection of the dentition. The bitewing film is the best radiographic means of recording the interproximal surfaces of the teeth. Interproximal caries occurs just below the contact point of the tooth. The susceptible zone extends from the contact point area to the free gingival margin, approximately 1 to 1.5 mm (Goaz and White, 1987). The typical lesion forms a classic V-shaped or triangular radiolucency with the tip of the V directed toward the DEJ. Other lesional shapes do occur and may be seen radiographically as a linear band, a diffuse notch, or a half moon. Once the decay has entered the dentin, the lesion will extend vertically along the DEJ and then spread out in a triangular fashion toward the pulp.

Interproximal lesions can be classified by degree of penetration into the tooth structure. Goaz and White (1987) describe the degree of carious involvement as incipient, moderate, advanced, or severe. Incipient lesions are those that are less than halfway through the enamel (Fig. 10-29). The moderate lesion category includes lesions that have penetrated more than halfway through the enamel layer but that do not involve the DEJ (see Fig. 10-29). Usually neither of these types of lesions requires restoration and may be charted as a "watch." Other risk factors, such as poor oral hygiene status, may influence the dentist's decision whether to restore moderate lesions. The dentist will determine when and in what manner teeth will be restored. The dental hygienist can participate by instituting preventive measures that may intervene in the caries process. Advanced lesions are those that have undermined the DEJ but have progressed less than halfway to the pulp (Figs. 10-29 to 10-31). The dentin will have a diffuse and often subtle radiolucent appearance. Finally, the severe lesion is one that has progressed more than halfway toward and may involve the pulp (Figs. 10-30 and 10-31). Sometimes interproximal lesions undermine so much of the dentin that the enamel will collapse from masticatory forces. Obviously the advanced and severe lesions require treatment by the dentist.

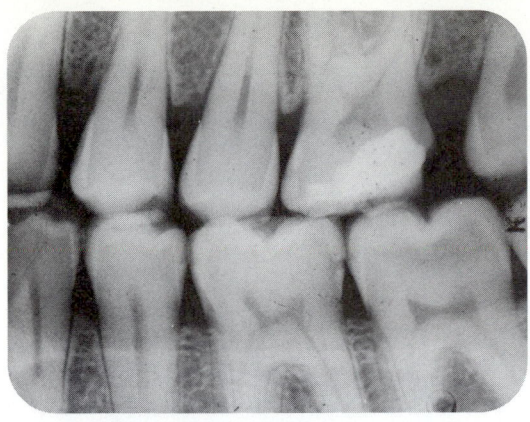

Fig. 10-29. Incipient interproximal caries: Teeth Nos. 12, mesiodistal; 18, mesiodistal; 19, mesial; 20, distal; and 21, distal. Moderate interproximal caries: Nos. 11, distal; 14, mesial. Advanced interproximal caries: Nos. 14, distal; 19, distal. Large occlusal caries in No. 18.

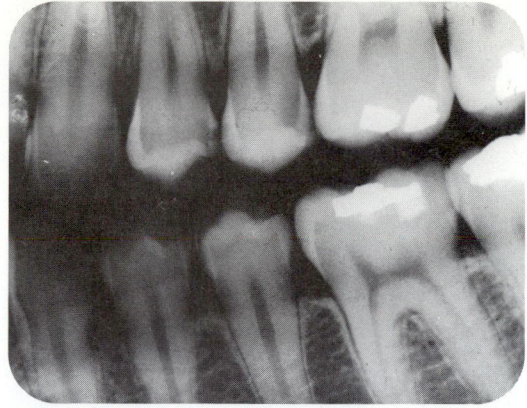

Fig. 10-30. Incipient interproximal caries: Teeth Nos. 14, distal; 19, mesial. Moderate interproximal caries: No. 19, distal. Advanced interproximal caries: No. 12, distal. Severe interproximal caries: No. 13, distal.

Occlusal caries. Occlusal lesions occur in the pits and fissures of posterior teeth and are more easily detected with an explorer during the clinical examination. Radiographs are not effective in demonstrating incipient lesions. However, once the lesion invades the dentin, the radiograph becomes a more useful assessment tool. The typical occlusal lesion is a triangular radiolucency beginning just below the enamel cap. Usually the occlusal point of entry is not demonstrated radiographically because of the thickness and anatomy of the enamel. In its early stages of penetration, the lesion may look like a radiolucent line under the enamel cap. The base of the lesion broadens as it penetrates into the dentin toward the pulp chamber. As the lesion enlarges, it becomes more obvious clinically as well as radiographically (Figs. 10-29 and 10-32).

Buccal and lingual caries. As with occlusal lesions, buccal and lingual caries can be determined better clinically than radiographically. Buccal and lingual lesions are difficult to distinguish from one another radiographically because of image superimposition. A radiolucent dot or circle is the typical appearance of these types of lesions (Fig. 10-31). The surrounding tooth structure will appear normal. Buccal or lingual caries may be confused with occlusal caries. Careful inspection of the radiographs and correlation with clinical findings will resolve the problem.

Buccal or lingual caries occurring in the cervi-

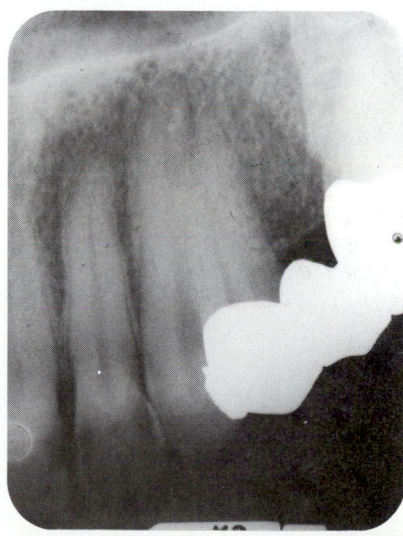

Fig. 10-31. Advanced interproximal caries: tooth No. 10, mesial. Severe interproximal caries: No. 10, distal. Lingual pit caries: No. 10.

cal portion of the tooth has a different appearance than described previously. Cervical lesions have a crescent-shaped radiolucent appearance and occur in the cervical third of the tooth crown (Fig. 10-33). A Class V radiolucent resin restoration often has the same radiographic appearance as a cervical carious lesion. Once again, these lesions or their restorative counterpart are recognized more readily during the clinical examination.

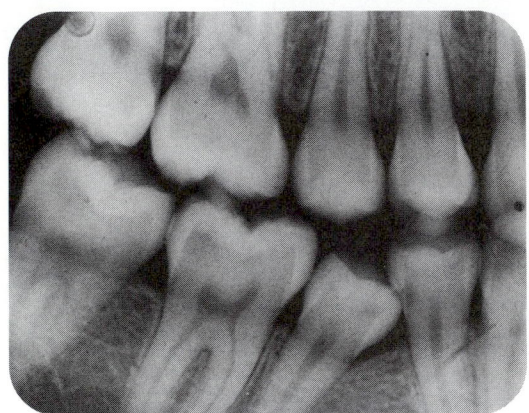

Fig. 10-32. Advanced interproximal caries: tooth No. 28, distal. Occlusal caries: Nos. 29, mesial pit; 30, distal pit; 31, distal pit.

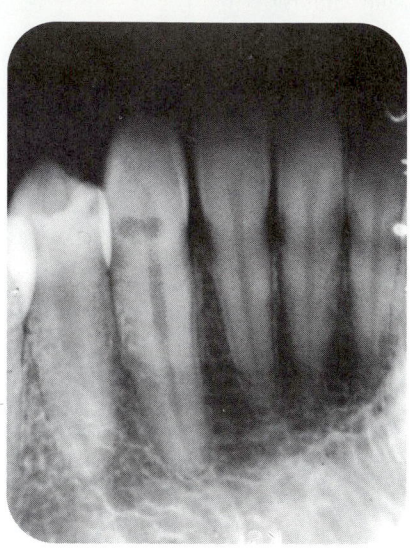

Fig. 10-33. Cervical caries: tooth No. 27. Class V radiolucent resin restorations have a similar appearance. Note areas of cervical burnout on Nos. 25 and 26.

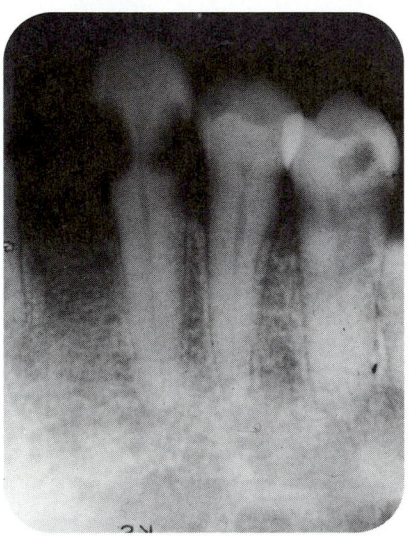

Fig. 10-34. Root caries: tooth No. 22, mesiodistal. Occlusal caries: No. 20, distal pit.

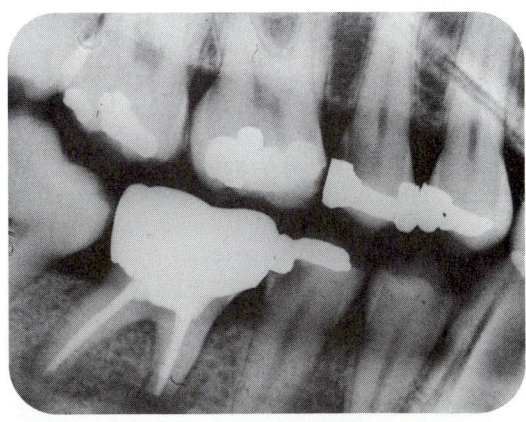

Fig. 10-35. Recurrent caries: Teeth Nos. 4, distal; 29, distal. Note areas of cervical burnout on Nos. 28 and 31.

Root caries. Root caries involves the cementum and dentin most typically on the buccal, lingual, and interproximal root surfaces (Katz, 1980). Root caries is more prevalent in older persons who have poor oral hygiene because of neuromuscular deficits, systemic disease that reduces salivary flow, or conditions requiring medications that induce xerostomia (Ettinger, 1989). Radiographically these lesions have an ill defined cupped-out or saucer-shaped radiolucent appearance just below the CEJ. They may become quite large and extend into the cervical enamel (Fig. 10-34). If enough tooth structure becomes involved, the tooth may break off at the gingival margin. Gingival recession is a necessary precondition for the development of root caries (Nyvad and Fejerskov, 1982).

At times the clinician may confuse root caries with cervical burnout. Cervical burnout is a phenomenon of x-ray penetration. The tissues at the neck of the tooth are thinner than the enamel above it and the alveolar bone below it. Consequently the x-rays are able to more completely penetrate this area and depict it as a radiolucent wedge adjacent to the CEJ (Figs. 10-33 and 10-35). The true root caries lesion will *not* show a root edge image as seen in cervical burnout. In addition, root caries has a diffuse, rounded inner border rather than a wedge configuration.

Recurrent caries. Recurrent caries is decay that occurs in close proximity to an existing restoration. The radiographic appearance is a radiolucent area underneath or adjacent to the restoration (see Fig. 10-35). It is most typically seen beneath the occlusal and interproximal margins. Incomplete caries removal, inadequate cavity preparation, and improper adaptation of the restorative material contribute to the incidence of recurrent decay (Langland et al, 1988). Evaluation of the margins of buccal and lingual restorations is better accomplished during the clinical examination.

Periodontal disease

By definition, periodontal disease is any pathologic process that affects the periodontium. The most typical form of periodontal disease is plaque associated. Chronic infection and inflammation produced by bacterial enzymes and endotoxins cause deterioration of the periodontium (Fedi, 1985). The progression of periodontal disease is thought to be a cyclic process marked by extended periods of little activity with short bursts of destructive activity (Lindhe, 1989). Systemic conditions such as diabetes mellitus and local factors such as calculus also influence this inflammatory process.

Prepubertal periodontitis and juvenile periodontitis are two forms of periodontal disease that occur in children and young adults. Both types occur in localized and generalized forms. The pattern and severity of these varieties of periodontal disease are characterized by the absence of inflammation and local factors that might be expected (Lindhe, 1989). Regardless of the type of periodontal disease, the sequelae are loss of attachment, bone, and sometimes teeth.

Benefits and limitations of radiographs. Radiographs are a component part of periodontal disease assessment. When periodontal disease is evidenced clinically, radiographs should be taken to supplement the information obtained from a thorough clinical examination. When radiographs are obtained for this purpose, the clinician should use the paralleling periapical technique with vertical bitewings and long-scale contrast, high kilovoltage (80 to 90 kVp) exposure factors. Optimal radiographic, exposure, and processing techniques will yield the best possible results.

Radiographs offer the clinician the following types of information about periodontal disease:

1. The condition of the interproximal bony crests—approximate height and density
2. Root length and shape
3. The tooth crown-root ratio
4. Widening of the periodontal ligament space
5. The position of the maxillary sinus relative to a periodontal deformity
6. The condition of the bone surrounding the tooth root
7. Advanced furcation involvement
8. Local irritants—calculus and improperly contoured restorations

Although radiographs offer real benefits to the clinician, they do have limitations. Generally those aspects of periodontal disease that can best be demonstrated clinically are not readily seen radiographically. Radiographs are not effective in demonstrating these aspects of periodontal disease:

1. Incipient bone loss
2. The presence or absence of periodontal pockets
3. The precise morphology of bone deformities
4. Buccal and lingual bone status

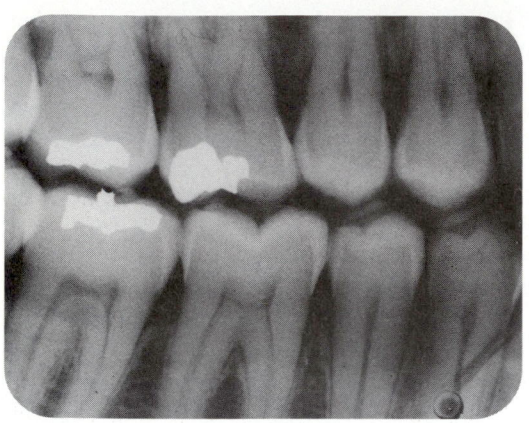

Fig. 10-36. Note loss of crestal shape and density as well as slight mesial and distal widening of periodontal ligament spaces.

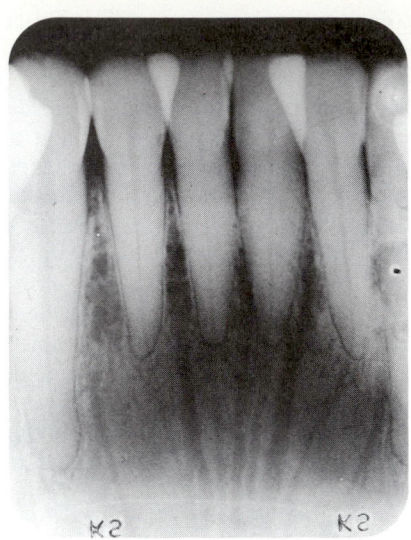

Fig. 10-37. Vertical radiolucent lines are widened vascular channels.

5. Tooth mobility
6. Level of the epithelial attachment
7. Early furcation involvement

Early disease observations. Some of the radiographic changes that may be observed in early periodontal disease include changes in the crestal bone, periodontal ligament space, and interseptal bone (Langland et al, 1988).

Early crestal lesions usually are localized areas of bony destruction. The alveolar crests may lose their normal configuration and cortical borders, which produces an irregular, diffuse radiolucent appearance (Fig. 10-36).

Widening of the periodontal ligament may be visualized on the mesial and distal aspects of the bone crests. Loss of bone on the lateral aspects of the crest results in a wedge-shaped radiolucent widening of the periodontal ligament (see Fig. 10-36). The clinician must use discretion in evaluating this type of change, for the healthy periodontal ligament space is slightly wider in the coronal region.

Another possible observation is the presence of vertical fingerlike radiolucent projections in the interseptal bone (Fig. 10-37). These radiolucencies represent widened vascular channels that allow passage of inflammatory fluid and cells into the bone. This process reduces the volume of cal-cified tissue present and is the result of deeper extension of inflammation from the gingival tissues. These vascular channels or nutrient canals also can be a normal finding.

It must be remembered that radiographs are limited in their ability to demonstrate early periodontal lesions. Thus a thorough clinical examination is necessary.

Moderate disease observations. As periodontal disease progresses, more destruction of the supporting structures occurs. Radiographs are useful for evaluating the residual bone, general bony contour and some bony defects. The actual extent, location, and rate of disease activity are not apparent on radiographs.

Evaluation of bone loss. The pattern of bone loss is determined by comparing the bony margin to the plane of adjacent CEJs. Horizontal bone loss is crestal height loss with the bony margin maintaining its parallel orientation to the CEJ and perpendicular to the adjacent teeth (Fig. 10-38). Vertical bone loss is angular loss of the bony septa with the bony margin oriented diagonally to the CEJ and adjacent teeth (Fig. 10-39). Bone loss can be classified further as a localized or generalized condition depending on the number of areas involved, and as mild, moderate. or severe, depending on the degree of bone reduction. Clin-

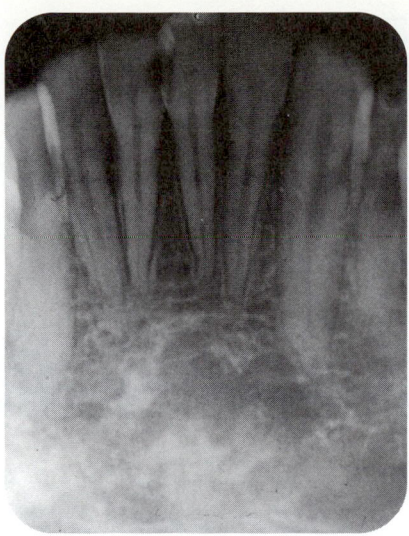

Fig. 10-38. Horizontal bone loss. Note widened periodontal ligament spaces on teeth Nos. 24 and 25.

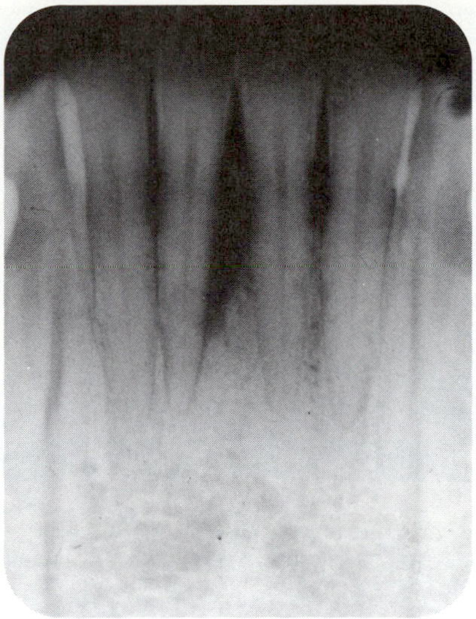

Fig. 10-39. Vertical bone loss. Note angular defect on mesial aspect of No. 25.

ical probing of the periodontium provides a more precise quantitative method of bone loss assessment.

Evaluation of bony defects. Radiographs may suggest the presence of bone deformities other than horizontal and vertical bone loss that result from progressed disease. Often bony defects are difficult to observe on radiographs because of their location or superimposition of structures over the deformity. Although radiographs cannot demonstrate the true morphology of bony defects, certain features of these lesions are displayed on radiographs.

In general, bony defects are areas of decreased density that vary in shape, size and location. Goaz and White (1987) describe five general types of bony defects: the interproximal crater, interproximal hemisepta, proximal intrabony defect, inconsistent bony margins, and bony pockets. Often these lesions are difficult to differentiate from one another radiographically. A brief summary of each type of lesion follows and serves as a guideline to further classify bone loss.

Interproximal crater. The interproximal crater is the most common defect in periodontal disease. It appears as a radiolucent troughlike depression in the crestal bone between two adjacent teeth. The crest of the defect may have a linear band of reduced density with a more opaque apical margin

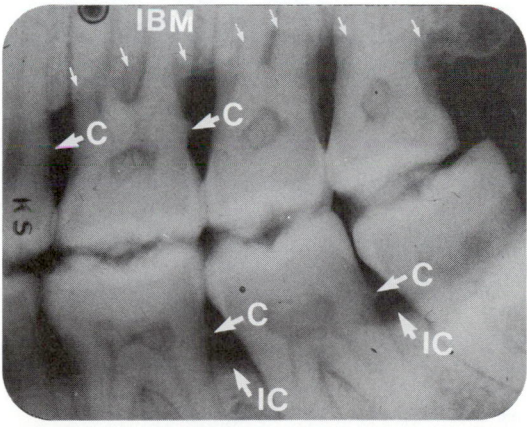

Fig. 10-40. Calculus *(C)* deposits are depicted as calcified points or ledges on the teeth. Interproximal deposits are present on teeth Nos. 13 to 16 and 17 to 19. A cervical deposit is found on tooth No. 17, distal. Interproximal crater *(IC)* is a troughlike depression in the crestal bone between two adjacent teeth. Irregular bony margins *(IBM)* or a scalloped appearance of the crestal bone results from uneven resorption of the buccal or lingual plates of bone.

(Fig. 10-40). The interproximal crater is classified as a two-walled bony defect formed between the buccal and lingual cortical plates.

Interproximal hemisepta. The interproximal hemisepta is a vertical V-shaped radiolucent defect that occurs on the mesial or distal aspect of

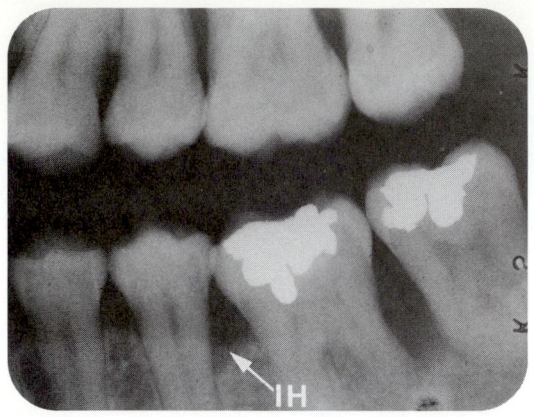

Fig. 10-41. Interproximal hemisepta *(IH)* is a v-shaped radiolucent defect on the mesial or distal aspect of the interproximal septum.

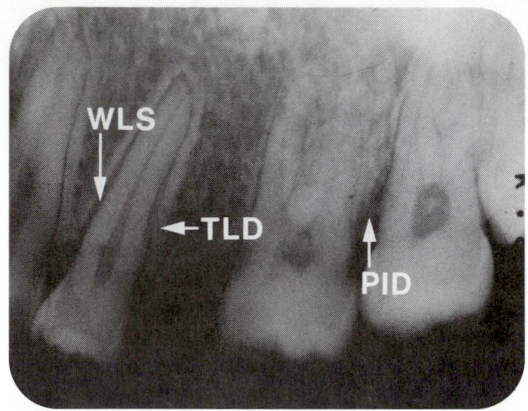

Fig. 10-42. Widened ligament space *(WLS)* and/or thickened lamina dura *(TLD)* may result from traumatism or periapical disease. In this radiograph, both of these structures are enlarged beyond their normal size. Also seen on this film, proximal intrabony defect *(PID)* is a three-walled vertical defect that extends apically from the alveolar crest. This defect occurs more commonly on distal aspect of teeth.

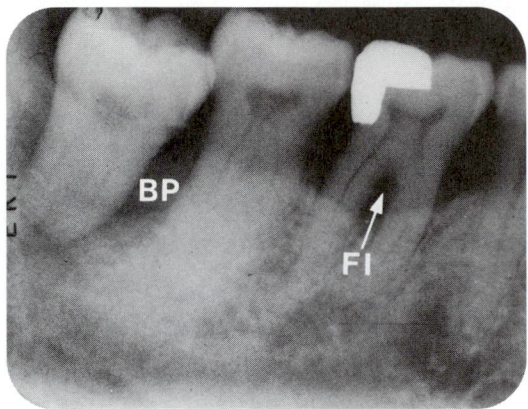

Fig. 10-43. Bony pocket *(BP)* occurs in the buccal or lingual bone overlying tooth roots. With advanced bone loss, furcations of multirooted teeth may become involved *(FI)* and reveal a radiolucent area between the roots.

the interproximal septum (Fig. 10-41). A hemiseptum is formed by resorption of one or both of the cortical plates or walls.

Proximal intrabony defect. The proximal intrabony defect generally is a sharply outlined, V-shaped defect in bone immediately adjacent to the root surface of the involved tooth (Fig. 10-42). This vertical defect extends apically from the alveolar crest and is surrounded by three walls: a hemisepta and the buccal and lingual cortical plates. This type of defect occurs more commonly on the distal aspect of teeth, usually in association with open contacts, attachment loss, and increased tooth mobility (Nielsen, Glavind, and Karring, 1980).

Inconsistent bony margins. Uneven resorption of either the buccal or lingual aspect of the cortical plates results in a scalloped or irregular appearance of the crestal bone (see Fig. 10-40). Careful inspection of the radiographs is necessary to see the subtle outlines of the buccal or lingual edges of the bone that superimpose over the root structure.

Bony pockets. Bony defects that occur in the buccal or lingual bone over tooth roots may be recorded on periapical radiographs (Fig. 10-43). Often these lesions are an extension of proximal bony defects. These lesions can only be seen if there is sufficient contrast between the area of resorption and the remaining bone.

Other observations. Radiographs may reveal other factors pertinent to the periodontal assessment such as calculus deposits, faulty restorations, occlusal traumatism, and the crown-root ratio. The essential features of each factor are discussed later.

Calculus deposits on the interproximal surfaces and sometimes on the buccal and lingual surfaces may be seen on dental radiographs. In general, interproximal deposits have a radiopaque spurlike

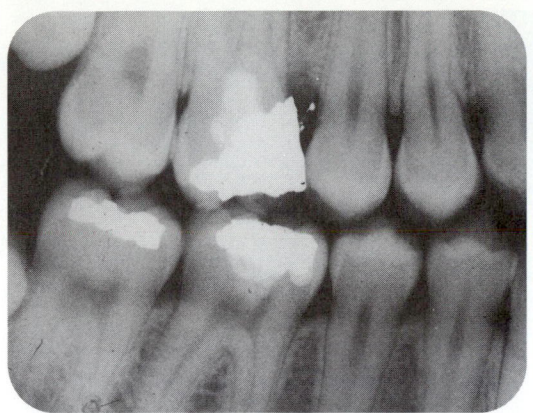

Fig. 10-44. Faulty restoration on tooth No. 3 with resultant crestal bone loss.

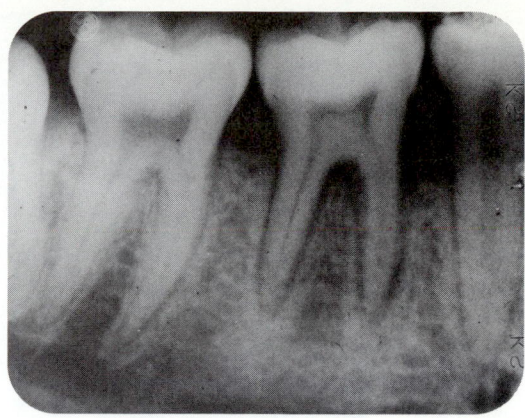

Fig. 10-45. Widened periodontal ligament space on tooth No. 30.

appearance (see Fig. 10-40), whereas buccal and lingual deposits have a more diffuse radiopaque ringlike appearance. As the deposits increase in size, the radiographic shape changes. Although heavy calculus deposits usually are demonstrated radiographically, smaller and less calcified deposits may not be imaged. Radiographs alone do not give the total picture of the presence or amount of calculus.

Faulty restorations such as those with overhanging margins or poor proximal contours may precipitate localized periodontal problems. Food and bacteria are attracted to these sites and cause localized areas of bony destruction, as seen in Fig. 10-44.

Occlusal traumatism may result in the radiographic appearance of a widened periodontal ligament space and a thickened lamina dura of the involved tooth. A widened periodontal ligament space is not always accompanied by a thickened lamina dura; each may result separately from occlusal traumatism. These changes may be observed on radiographs (Fig. 10-42 and 10-45), but occlusal traumatism must be established clinically. Bruxism, high restorations, or drifted teeth may contribute to this condition.

The crown-root ratio is the amount of tooth structure above the bone (the clinical crown) versus the amount of tooth structure in the bone (the root). The more root supported by bone, the more stable the tooth and vice versa. Also, the shape and length of the tooth play a role in this evaluation. For instance, patients with long roots may

be able to sustain more bone loss than those with short or resorbed roots. Therefore the crown-root ratio and tooth root morphology play a role in periodontal assessment and prognosis.

Advanced disease observations

As one might expect, radiographic findings of advanced disease include more extensive destruction of the supporting structures and may include severe bone loss and large bony defects. With advanced bone loss, the furcations of multirooted teeth may become involved. If the bone resorbs beyond the furcation on one aspect or the other, the radiograph may reveal an area of decreased density in the furcation itself (see Fig. 10-40). Radiographs, however, cannot demonstrate whether the resorption occurred on the buccal or lingual cortical plate or if the interradicular bone is involved. If the defect involves both the buccal and lingual bone, the furcation area will have a more pronounced radiolucent appearance (see Fig. 10-43). This type of defect is more difficult to observe on the maxilla than the mandible because of the superimposition of the palatal root over the furcation area.

Prepubertal and juvenile periodontitis

Prepubertal and juvenile periodontitis are two forms of periodontal disease peculiar to children and young adults. Prepubertal periodontitis usually involves the primary dentition but may extend into the permanent dentition. The localized form usually affects one or more of the primary

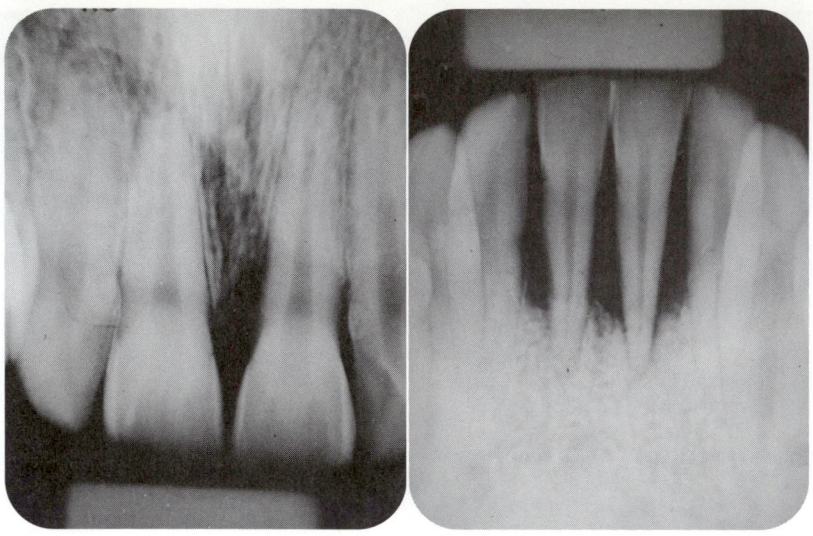

Fig. 10-46. Localized juvenile periodontitis.
(Courtesy Dr. Charles Redish, Indianapolis, In).

molars that have lost alveolar bone. The generalized form of this disease results in widespread destruction of alveolar bone and early loss of the primary teeth. Radiographs may assist the clinician in evaluating either form of prepubertal periodontitis.

Juvenile periodontitis is a form of periodontal disease that occurs in the adolescent. The generalized and localized forms of juvenile periodontitis follow patterns similar to prepubertal periodontitis. The localized form affects certain teeth, specifically first permanent molars and incisors (Fig. 10-46). Radiographs of the affected teeth reveal angular bone loss. The molar defects are often observed bilaterally. The generalized form is more extensive and involves more teeth than the first molars and incisors. As such, the radiographs will reflect the same angular defects but involve more teeth. It is not known whether the localized and generalized forms are separate diseases or if the localized disease progresses to the generalized disease.

Periapical disease

The radiographic assessment is not complete without thorough inspection of the apical regions of the teeth. The most common periapical lesions are those which result from irreversible damage to the pulp with subsequent apical infection.

Generally acute periapical infections show little or no radiographic changes. The patient will be symptomatic, but the radiograph may show only a slightly widened or thickened apical periodontal ligament space. On the other hand, chronic periapical infections such as the periapical granuloma, periapical cyst, periapical abscess, and condensing osteitis manifest changes that can be identified on radiographs. Although there are other types of periapical lesions, the following discussion is limited to the more common chronic periapical lesions.

Periapical granuloma. The periapical granuloma is one of the most common aftermaths of pulpitis. A localized mass of granulation tissue forms in response to the pulpal infection. The earliest radiographic indication of its presence is a thickened apical periodontal ligament space. As the lesion enlarges, more bone is resorbed and a radiolucent area at the root apex can be detected. Other radiographic features include a rounded and well-circumscribed border, often with a thin radiopaque periphery or zone of sclerotic bone (Fig. 10-47). These lesions vary in size and may show trabeculations in the central body. The involved teeth are non-vital and usually asymptomatic.

Periapical cyst. The periapical cyst or apical periodontal cyst is frequently the sequela of the periapical granuloma. In most instances the involved tooth is asymptomatic, and the lesion is the result of long-standing inflammation. Its ra-

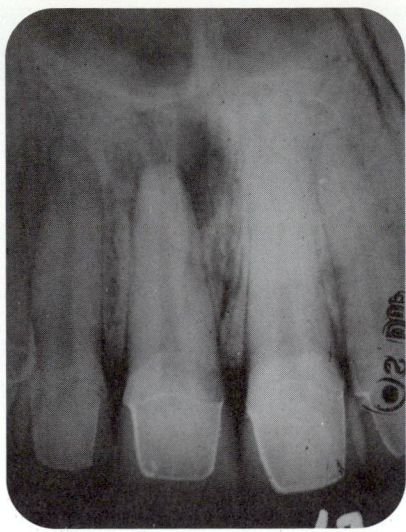

Fig. 10-47. Periapical granuloma.

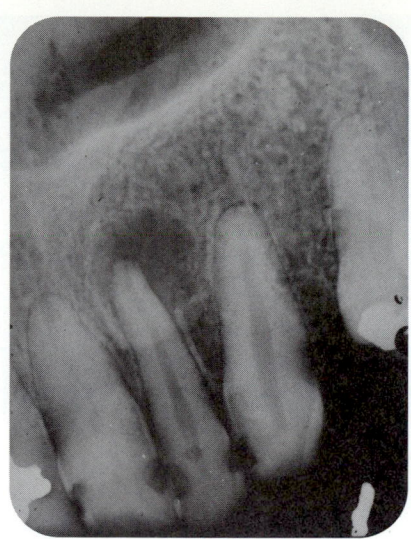

Fig. 10-48. Periapical cyst.

diographic presentation is identical to the periapical granuloma. Often the periapical cyst is a larger, more radiolucent lesion with fewer central trabeculations and may involve more than one tooth (Fig. 10-48). Histologic study of the periapical tissue is necessary for lesion differentiation.

Chronic periapical abscess. The chronic periapical abscess may develop after an acute periapical abscess or in an existing periapical granuloma. This radiolucent lesion has diffuse, irregular borders that tend to blend into the bony pattern (Langland et al, 1988), as seen in Fig. 10-49. Often the radiolucency extends beyond the tooth apex to involve the lateral aspects of the root or roots. In most instances the involved tooth is asymptomatic. A fistulous tract may be observed adjacent to the tooth on clinical examination of the area.

Condensing osteitis. Condensing osteitis, or chronic focal sclerosing osteomyelitis, is a reaction of the bone to infection. This lesion usually occurs in young individuals and frequently involves the mandibular first molar. Its radiographic presentation is a well-circumscribed radiopaque mass of sclerotic bone surrounding the root or roots of a carious tooth or a heavily restored tooth (Fig. 10-50). The root outline is apparent, and the sclerotic mass may have either a distinct or dif-

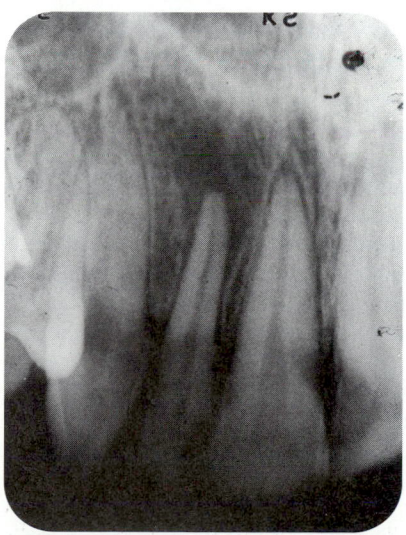

Fig. 10-49. Chronic periapical abscess.

fuse border that fades into the adjacent bone. The area of sclerosis may remain even if the tooth is removed, then known as *osteosclerosis* (Fig. 10-51).

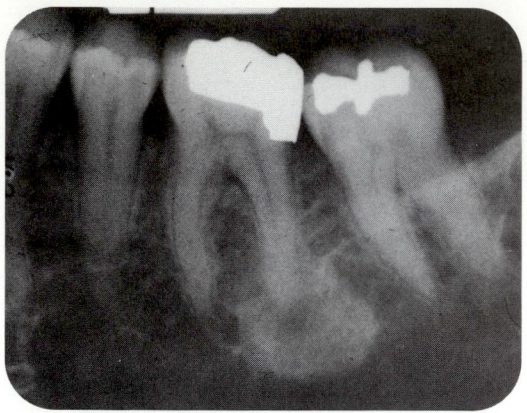

Fig. 10-50. Condensing osteitis.

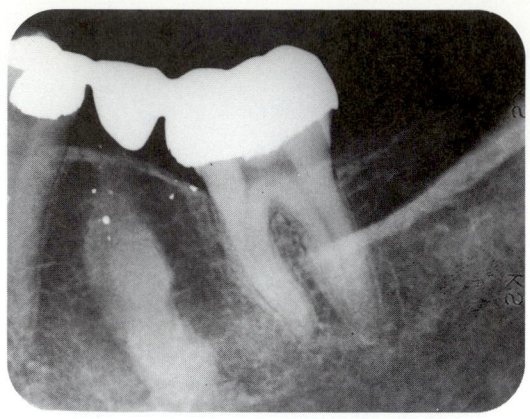

Fig. 10-51. Osteosclerosis.

RADIOGRAPHIC DESCRIPTION OF PATHOLOGIC LESIONS

Radiographs often reveal disease processes of which the patient may or may not be aware. As seen in some periapical lesions, the patient may be asymptomatic yet have radiographic evidence of disease.

The dental hygienist may observe conditions other than the more common periapical lesions. In such instances it would be useful to write a description of the lesion for further review and evaluation by the dentist. An organized radiographic description will help the dentist establish a differential diagnosis and select an appropriate course of action for the patient.

The following approach is a systematic means of describing the radiographic presentation of a lesion. The clinician answers a standard series of questions that together form the basis of the descriptive summary (Table 10-3). The end product is a formal description that incorporates the essential radiographic features of the lesion. After consultation with the dentist, the descriptive summary may serve as a framework for lesion documentation in the patient's record.

The presentation of certain combinations of radiographic features suggests an aggressive or possibly malignant lesion. The dentist and dental hy-

Table 10-3. How to write a radiographic description

Questions to answer

1. **Where is the lesion?**
   Maxilla or mandible?
   Anterior or posterior?
   Specific region?
2. **What size is the lesion?**
   Small, medium, large?
   Estimate in millimeters or centimeters.
3. **Is it single or multiple?**
   One or more locations?
4. **What is its overall shape?**
   Round, ovoid, pear/heart-shaped, irregular?
   Unilocular (One compartment)?
   Multilocular (Many compartments)?
5. **Is the body of the lesion radiopaque, radiolucent, mixed?**
6. **What do the borders look like?**
   Ill-defined or well-defined?
   Smooth or irregular? Continuous?
   Corticated or non-corticated?
7. **Are other structures involved?**
   Teeth: resorbed? displaced? impacted?
   Lamina dura: thin? absent? thickened?
   Periodontal ligament space: lost? enlarged?
   Bone: expanded? eroded? perforated? thinned?
   Specific anatomy involved?
   Maxillary sinus? nasal cavity? lower border of the mandible? mandibular canal?
8. What is your descriptive summary?

(Adapted from Miles et al, 1991.)

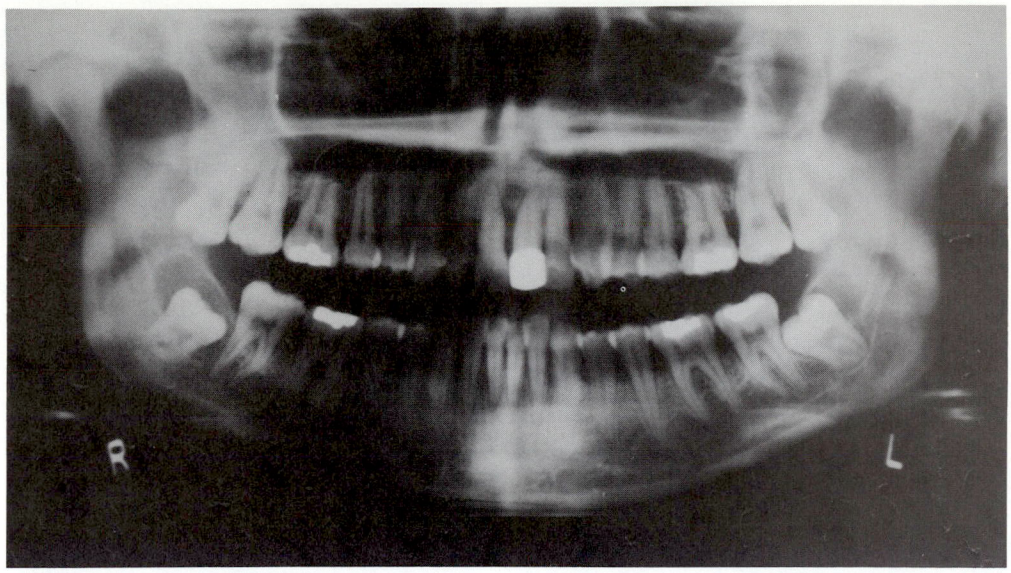

Fig. 10-52. Generalized moderate to severe periodontal disease with bilateral dentigerous cysts associated with impacted third molars, Nos. 17 and 32.

gienist should be especially concerned if a radiographic lesion appears as a single, radiolucent lesion with ill-defined borders that has resorbed tooth roots and eroded the cortical plate.

Following are several descriptive summaries along with their associated radiographs. The first radiographic summary includes a comprehensive description of all radiographic findings.

Assume that the dental hygienist has taken the panoramic radiograph in Fig. 10-52 during a new patient examination. At the end of the appointment, the dentist asks the hygienist to report the radiographic findings. The dental hygienist's assessment includes the following observations:

Restorations:	Occlusal amalgams are present in teeth Nos. 3, 14, 15, 18, 19, 30 and a porcelain-metal crown covers tooth No. 9.
Periodontal:	Moderate horizontal bone loss is present in the maxillary premolar regions and mandibular posterior regions with possible incipient furcation involvement of teeth Nos. 18, 19, 30, 31. Severe horizontal bone loss is present in the maxillary and mandibular anterior regions and maxillary molar areas. Localized areas of reduced bone density are present between Nos. 2 and 3; 14, 15 and 16; 19, 20, 21 and 22. A vertical defect involves the mesial of No. 8 and possibly the tooth apex.
Bone lesions	Two medium-sized pericoronal lesions involving the impacted mandibular third molars, Nos. 17 and 32, are present. The lesions are oval, unilocular radiolucencies with smooth, continuous, well-defined, corticated borders that have enlarged the follicular space. The inferior borders of the lesions approximate the superior border of the mandibular canal.

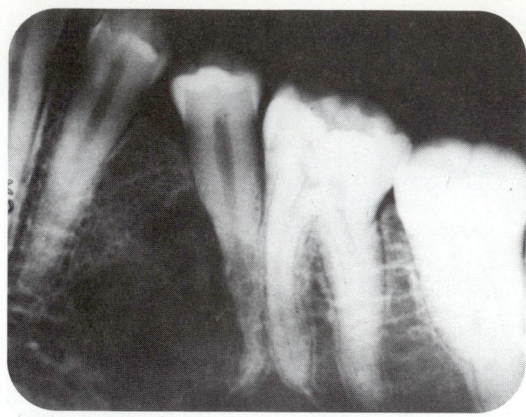

Fig. 10-53. This lesion was diagnosed as osteosarcoma, a malignancy of bone.

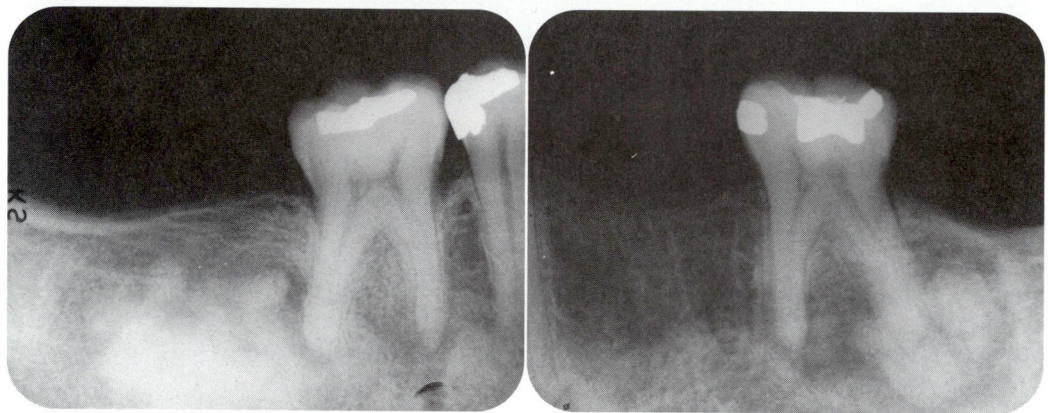

Fig. 10-54. Typical presentation of florid osseous dysplasia.

The final clinical diagnosis rendered by the dentist is bilateral dentigerous cysts.

The next lesion is recorded on a periapical radiograph as seen in Fig. 10-53. This lesion is located in the left posterior mandible between the first and second premolars, Nos. 20 and 21. It is a single, medium-sized, triangular, unilocular, mixed (primarily radiolucent with small calcifications in the central body) lesion with ill-defined, noncorticated, irregular borders that has displaced the premolars, destroyed the periodontal ligament space and lamina dura, and partially eroded the mesial aspect of the root of tooth No. 20. The mental foramen appears to be involved. Note the combination of descriptive terms. The radiographic presentation of this lesion corresponds to the radiographic characteristics of an ominous type of lesion. This lesion was diagnosed as an osteosarcoma, a malignancy of bone.

The third descriptive summary corresponds to the periapical views in Fig. 10-54. Multiple, medium-sized lesions of the posterior mandible apical to the first molars, Nos. 19 and 30, are present. The right lesion is oval, unilocular, and mixed with a noncontinuous, smooth, defined, corticated border on the mesial and distal aspects and an ill-defined, noncorticated border on the superior aspect. (The inferior aspect of the lesion is not shown on the radiograph.) The distal root of No. 30 has an intact periodontal ligament space but is surrounded by a mass of diffuse radiopacities with a radiolucent periphery. The left lesion is round, unilocular, and mixed with noncontinuous, smooth, defined, corticated borders on the

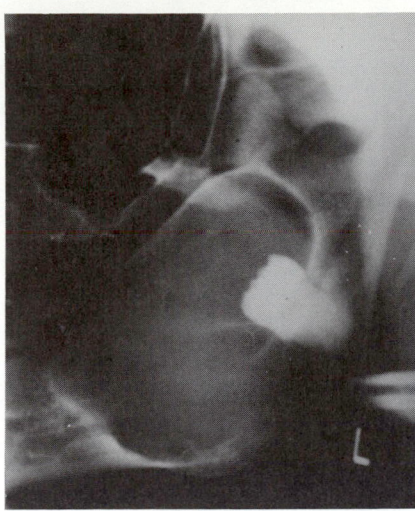

Fig. 10-55. This large lesion involving impacted tooth No. 17 was diagnosed as dentigerous cyst. Left untreated, these lesions can become quite large and destructive.

lateral and inferior aspects and an ill-defined, noncorticated border on the mesial aspect. The distal root of No. 19 has an intact periodontal ligament space but is surrounded by diffuse radiopacities with a radiolucent periphery. This appearance is consistent with the radiographic presentation of florid osseous dysplasia, a disease closely related to chronic diffuse sclerosing osteomyelitis and sclerotic cemental masses.

The final lesion, presented in Fig. 10-55, serves as an exercise for the reader. Work through the description questions (Table 3) and write a descriptive summary. A descriptive summary for this lesion is included in the answer section for review and comparison (Suggested Response, No. 12, Chapter 10).

ADVANCES IN DENTAL RADIOGRAPHY

The dental hygienist of the future will image dental structures with devices and techniques different from those used today. Conventional dental radiography and film processing procedures will become obsolete as these systems are replaced by computer-assisted image technology. The advances in computer technology and medical radiology have opened new horizons in dental radiology.

Digital radiography

Digital radiography (DR) has been the most common technology applied to dentistry thus far. In DR the x rays form an electronic image on a radiation detector rather than a film. The electronic image is received by a television camera, and the subsequent output signal is transmitted to a computer for translation into a digital form. The output of the computer converter is temporarily stored in the computer memory. The digital image is formed by a matrix of image cells, or pixels. The brightness of each pixel is determined by the computer-generated numerical value in each cell. These images can be displayed on a video screen or be recalled for further manipulation. The advantage of DR is that this numerical data provide the information necessary to perform image subtraction techniques. The most frequently employed subtraction technique is called temporal subtraction. In this technique, an image that was obtained previously is subtracted from an image obtained at a later time. The subtracted image demonstrates structural changes that may have occurred in the intervening time because of disease.

Conventional radiographs can be converted into digital images by use of a TV camera or a slide scanner system supported by the appropriate computer and display components (Hildebolt et al, 1990). Once the conventional images are digitized, the images can be manipulated and subtracted to reveal disease changes. The most important prerequisite of digital subtraction radiography is the projection of identical or nearly identical radiographic images. Dental researchers have conducted studies using digital subtraction techniques to evaluate carious, periodontal, and periapical lesions and to investigate devices and methods for image standardization. This type of research is ongoing.

The most recent development in digital imaging is a system for direct intraoral video recording and digitizing of the radiographic image, Radio-VisioGraphy (RVG) (Trophy U.S.A., Inc., Marietta, Georgia), as shown in Fig. 10-56. A solid state detector called a charge coupling device (CCD) allows lower x-ray dose image production and image display on a video monitor. The video monitor image can be manipulated in various ways to enhance the image and improve disease detection. An archival record of the displayed image can be printed onto thermal paper (Fig. 10-57) and viewed in reflected light, much like a

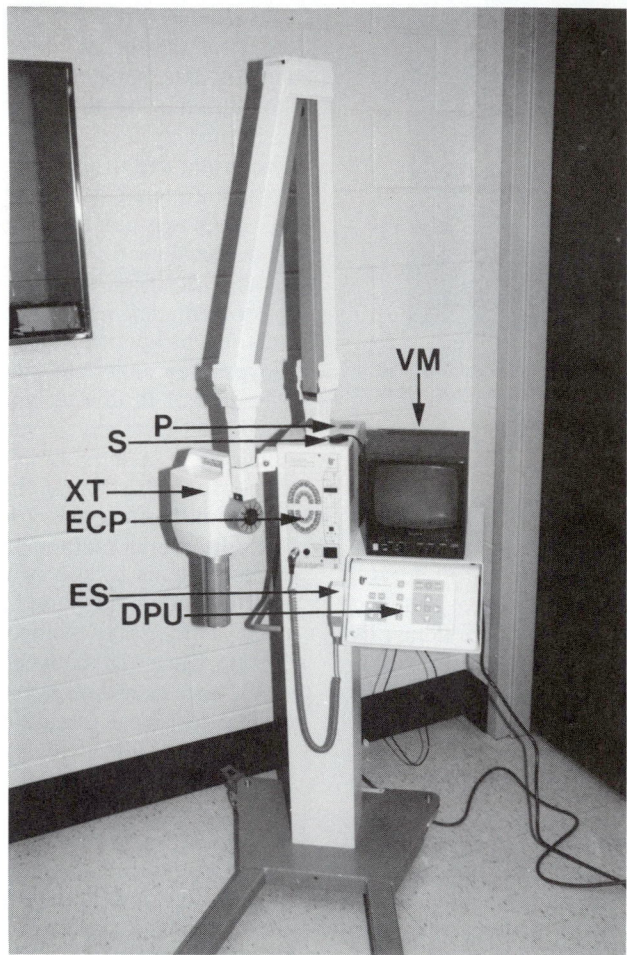

Fig. 10-56. X-ray tube *(XT)* is conventional and operates at an 8 mA and 70 kVp setting. Exposure control panel *(ECP)* allows for variation in exposure times and selection of conventional radiography or RadioVisioGraphy. Exposure switch *(ES)* is conventional; its insertion permits exposure of the sensor or a film. *(S)*, Sensor, or intraoral image receptor, is an 18 mm x 26 mm rare-earth intensifying screen, CCD device, which is connected via cable to the data processing unit. *(DPU)*. The DPU digitizes the electronic signals captured by the sensor and displays the image on the video monitor *(VM)*. Also DPU allows the operator to format and manipulate the image in various ways. Printer *(P)* can be attached to the RadioVisioGraphy unit to make hard copies of the dignitized, stored, and displayed images.

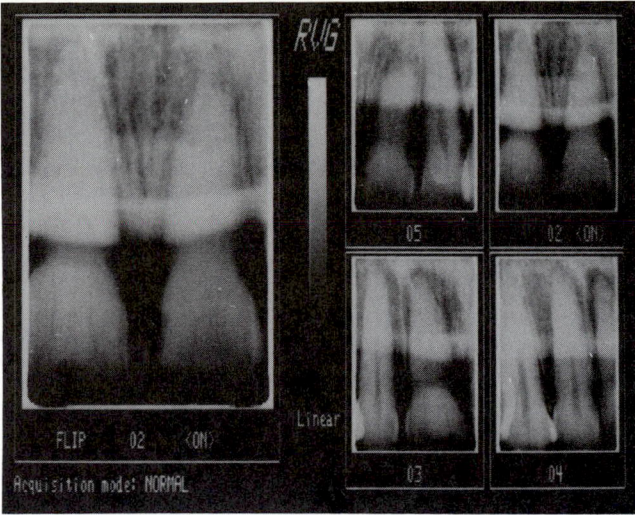

Fig. 10-57. RadioVisioGraphy printed images displayed in the five-window format, one large vertical window and four small vertical windows.

black and white photograph. This system can be used for conventional intraoral radiography as well. RadioVisioGraphy is the only commercially available system that provides direct digital intraoral radiography.

Dental hygienists will probably be operating this type of system or a similar digital imaging system in the future. A discussion of the basic components of the RVG system follows as an introduction to this new technology.

RadioVisioGraphy

The RVG system (see Fig. 10-56) is composed of four main components: an x-ray generator with a special electronic timer, an intraoral sensor, a display processing unit with a video monitor, and a printer (Trophy, 1991).

X-ray generator. The x-ray generator is a conventional type that operates at an 8 mA and 70 kVp setting. The selected exposure time is measured through a special electronic device to ensure short exposure accuracy. The x-ray head is equipped with an 8-inch cylinder cone or position-indicating device.

Intraoral sensor. The intraoral image receptor is composed of an 18-by-26 mm rare-earth intensifying screen sensor, fiberoptics, and a miniature charged coupling device housed in a larger, plastic casing. A long flexible cord connects the sensor to the display processing unit. Because this device cannot be sterilized, the clinician covers it with a disposable latex sheath before placing it in the patient's mouth. The sensor can be secured in the mouth by the patient or with specially designed holders that the patient stabilizes externally. As in conventional radiography, the operator must be proficient in paralleling and bisecting angle techniques for successful imaging.

The image is produced when x-rays cause intensifying screen fluorescence and the resultant light is conducted by the fiberoptics to the CCD. The CCD detects the light pattern and translates it into an electronic signal that is received by the data processing unit.

Data processing unit. The data processing unit captures the electronic signals from the sensor. The signals are stored, digitized, and displayed almost immediately on the video monitor. Four different display modes are available: one large vertical window along with a four-window format (see Fig. 10-57), two large vertical window formats, one large horizontal window format, and a four horizontal window format. The image can be manipulated further by contrast enhancement functions, negative-to-positive conversion (Fig. 10-58), and brightness and contrast video monitor adjustments. A zoom feature is available to enlarge a particular area of interest.

Printer. Different hard copy systems can operate with the RVG unit to make referral or chart

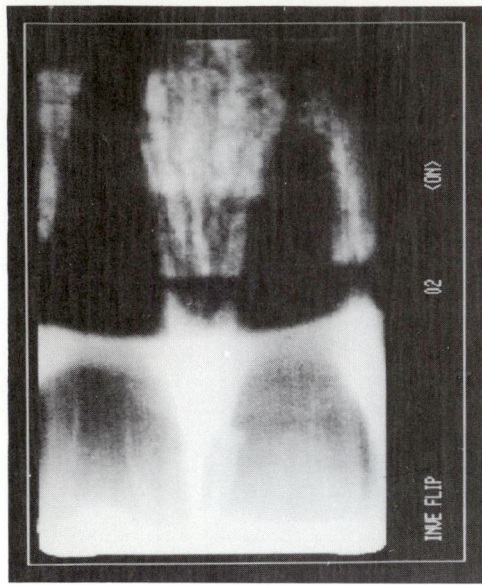

Fig. 10-58. One of the RadioVisioGraphy enhancement functions allows contrast reversal from negative-to-positive. This is an example of a reverse-contrast printed image.

copies of the images produced. The manufacturer recommends the use of a 3M Dry Silver System for high-quality copies.

Initial evaluation of this imaging system has generally been favorable; however, some drawbacks have been identified. The system is capable of producing clinically acceptable images at lower dose levels than film, but image resolution is somewhat less than that of conventional film (Benz and Mouyen, 1991; Horner et al, 1990; Mouyen et al, 1989). Some of the less desirable features identified were the size and thickness of the receptor, the extreme precision required for sensor placement, lack of rectangular collimation, density and contrast differences between the video image and the printed image, and unconventional displayed and printed image orientation (Horner et al, 1990). Further studies of this system and its capabilities are needed.

ACTIVITIES

1. In pairs, create four profiles of patients with different ages, dental histories, and clinical presentations. Then use selection criteria to determine an appropriate radiographic survey for each patient.
2. View a series of radiographs with ceiling or room light. Then view the same survey under ideal viewing conditions. Compare the two in terms of the ability to see detail. Next use a magnifying glass to view structural detail.
3. Make a chart of anatomic landmarks. Include the name, shape, location, and radiographic description of each landmark.
4. Practice mounting dental radiographs and check for correct film mounting using your landmark chart.
5. Observe an advanced student charting restorations, caries, periodontal findings, and periapical disease from dental radiographs.
6. Review chapter figures that show dental restorations and carious lesions. Chart your own findings on a separate piece of paper.
7. Assess the bone loss on the radiographs in the periodontal section. Use a small piece of paper to connect the CEJs of adjacent teeth. Then compare the plane of the paper to the crestal bone. Is the bone loss horizontal or vertical? Is it mild, moderate, or severe?
8. Refer to the periapical disease figures. Using the radiographic description questions, write a descriptive summary for each lesion.
9. Select one of the RadioVisioGraphy articles from the reference list and read it. Write a summary of the information presented in the article.

REVIEW QUESTIONS

1. Consider the following case scenario. An 18-year-old woman arrives for her yearly recall appointment. At her last recall appointment with the dental hygienist, she had no clinical or radiographic caries and was in good periodontal health. Your patient interview and oral examination reveal excellent general health, marginal gingivitis, fair oral hygiene, and several small occlusal carious lesions. Her only dental complaint was tissue tenderness distal to the second molars.
   What radiographic survey would you recommend for this patient?
   a. No radiographs at this time
   b. Posterior bitewings for caries evaluation
   c. Selected periapicals or a panoramic for third molar evaluation and posterior bitewings for caries evaluation
   d. A panoramic radiograph for third molar evaluation
   e. Complete full mouth periapical and bitewing

survey to evaluate the bone and apical regions of the teeth

2. Consider the typical landmarks that are recorded on maxillary molar periapical views. Of the landmarks listed, which ones would you expect to able to view on a molar film?
   a. Zygomatic process
   b. Coronoid process
   c. Lingual foramen
   d. Tuberosity
   e. Nasal septum
   f. Sinus cavity

3. Consider the primary anatomic landmarks of the mandible. Which of the following landmarks is a radiolucent landmark of the mandible?
   a. Inferior border of the mandible
   b. External oblique ridge
   c. Mental foramen
   d. Genial tubercles
   e. Mental ridge

4. Dental restorative materials have different radiographic presentations. Of the materials listed, which one would be most radiopaque on dental radiographs?
   a. Amalgam
   b. Cement base
   c. Porcelain
   d. Gutta percha points
   e. Composite resin

5. What is the typical radiographic presentation of root caries?
   a. Cervical crescent-shaped radiolucency
   b. V-shaped radiolucency at the contact points
   c. Triangular radiolucency in pits and fissures
   d. Wedge-shaped radiolucency at the CEJ
   e. Saucer-shaped radiolucency below the CEJ

6. During your oral and radiographic assessment, you observe an interproximal lesion on the maxillary left lateral incisor. On the radiographs the lesion has penetrated the enamel, and you see a vertical radiolucency along the DEJ. What is the correct classification of this lesion?
   a. Class II moderate lesion
   b. Class III advanced lesion
   c. Class V incipient lesion
   d. Class IV moderate lesion
   e. Class I severe lesion

7. In the radiographic assessment of periodontal disease, what information *cannot* be obtained from radiographs?
   a. Crown-root ratio
   b. Faulty restorations
   c. Tooth mobility
   d. Presence or absence of periodontal pockets
   e. Incipient bone loss
   f. Approximate bone height
   g. Morphology of bone deformities

8. What is the point of reference used for assessing bone loss on dental radiographs?
   a. Occlusal plane
   b. Curve of Spee
   c. Gingival margin
   d. CEJs of adjacent teeth
   e. Contact points of adjacent teeth

9. The effects of periodontal disease may be depicted on dental radiographs as changes in the alveolar bone level as well as in bone density. Is this true or false?

10. What is the first radiographic manifestation of periapical disease of pulpal origin?
    a. Widened periodontal ligament space
    b. Sclerotic bone at the tooth apex
    c. Periapical radiolucency
    d. Loss of bone density
    e. Fistulous tract

11. Examine the lesion in Fig. 10-55. Use the radiographic description questions (Table 10-3) to formulate a descriptive summary. Complete this process on a separate piece of paper.

12. What are the advantages of the direct digital radiography system?
    a. Reduced exposure levels
    b. Image enhancement features
    c. Optimal image receptor size
    d. Image orientation
    e. Immediate image display
    f. Conventional processing eliminated
    g. Superior image resolution compared with conventional film

REFERENCES

Benz C, Mouyen F: Evaluation of the new RadioVisioGraphy system image quality, *Oral Surg Oral Med Oral Pathol* 72:627, 1991.

Bodak-Gyovai LZ, Manzione JV: *Oral medicine patient evaluation and management,* Baltimore, 1980, Williams & Wilkins.

Bushong SC: *Radiologic science for technologists,* ed 4, St. Louis, 1988, CV Mosby.

Ettinger RL: Dental care and management of the aging dental patient, *J Tenn Dent Assoc* 69:10, 1989.

Fedi PE, editor: *The periodontic syllabus,* Philadelphia, 1985, Lea & Febiger.

Goaz PW, White SC: *Oral radiology principles and interpretation,* ed 2, St Louis, 1987, CV Mosby.

Hildebolt CF et al: Quantitative evaluation of digital dental radiograph imaging systems, *Oral Surg Oral Med Oral Pathol* 70:661, 1990.

Horner K et al: RadioVisioGraphy: an initial evaluation, *Br Dent J* 168:244, 1990.

Katz RV: Assessing root caries in populations: the evolution of the root caries index, *J Public Health Dent* 40:, 1980.

Langland OE, et al: *Radiology for dental hygienists and dental assistants,* Springfield, Ill, 1988, CC Thomas.

Lindhe J: *Textbook of clinical periodontology,* ed 2, Copenhagen, 1989, Munksgaarden.

Miles DA et al: *Oral and maxillofacial radiology,* Philadelphia, 1991, WB Saunders.

Mouyen F et al: Presentation and physical evaluation of RadioVisioGraphy, *Oral Surg Oral Med Oral Pathol* 68: 238, 1989.

Nielsen IM, Glavind L, Karring T: Interproximal periodontal intrabony defects: prevalence, localization and etiological factors, *J Clin Periodontol* 7:187, 1980.

Nyvad B, Ferjerskov O: Root surface caries: clinical, histopathologic and microbiological features and clinical implications, *Int Dent J* 32:312, 1982.

Shafer WG, Hine MK, Levy BM: *A textbook of oral pathology,* ed. 4, Philadelphia, 1983, WB Saunders.

Sturdevant CM, editor: The art and science of operative dentistry, ed 2, St Louis, 1985, CV Mosby.

The selection of patients for x-ray examinations: dental radiographic examinations, Rockville, Md, 1987, US Department of Health and Human Services (HHS Put. FDA 88-8273).

Tilliss TSI, Cross-Poline GN: Dental hygienists' performance of procedures emphasized in school: frequency and barriers, *J Dent Hyg* 63:134, 1989.

Trophy RVG user's manual USA, Fredericksburg, Va, 1991, Trophy, USA, Inc..

White S: An update on the effects of low-dose radiation, *AAOMR Newsl,* 17(4):1, 1990.

ACKNOWLEDGMENTS

The author wishes to thank Drs. Thomas Razmus and Don John Summerlin for their review of the manuscript and Mrs. Alana Barra, Mr. Mike Holloran, and Mr. Mark Dirlam for their assistance in preparation of the radiographic illustrations.

11 COMPREHENSIVE DENTAL CHARTING

Irene Woodall

LEARNING OUTCOMES

The dental hygienist will be able to

1. Include comprehensive dental charting procedures for assessing new patients and monitoring continuing care patients.
2. Select an appropriate charting form and method given the objectives of the charting and the records system used by the practice.
3. Given examples of tooth numbering systems, including universal, international, and Palmer's notation, identify to which tooth the example refers and specify from which system the notation is derived.
4. Given a variety of carious lesions or restorations, identify the proper classification number using G.V. Black's classification system.
5. Complete comprehensive chartings for a variety of patients, including identifying and recording the following from clinical findings:
   a. Sound teeth
   b. Missing or unerupted teeth
   c. Removable prostheses
   d. Restorations (including all classifications of single-tooth restorations, crowns, bridgework, sealants, and endodontic treatment)
   e. Caries
   f. Decalcification and hypocalcification
   g. Developmental anomalies
   h. Attrition, abrasion, erosion
   i. Malposed teeth
   j. Calculus
6. Read aloud recorded notations concisely and accurately, using proper dental terminology for verification by a second clinician.

A comprehensive dental charting provides an accurate description of the patient's dental status. It is a valuable tool in the assessment phase of care because it provides, in most instances, a graphic representation of the active or repaired disease process and the unique clinical problems of the patient's teeth. As a combined record of clinical and radiographic findings, it is a comprehensive diagnostic tool. Dental chartings are valuable legal records, as they show the patient's dental conditions at the beginning of care and a pictorial review of how those conditions changed over a period of months and years.

Depending on the format and manner in which a patient's treatment is documented, the dental charting can depict the maintenance of health or the progression of disease.

It also provides a useful check against financial records. Entries in financial records indicating the placement of specific restorations should be reflected in the updated charting of the patient's teeth.

Because the comprehensive charting is most often used to establish a basis of entering needs for purposes of treatment planning, the most comprehensive charting procedures are done at the initial patient visit. The initial data should be updated as treatment progresses and at subsequent recall visits when the patient returns for periodic diagnosis of new needs.

CHARTING FORMS

Fig. 11-1 is an example of an anatomic charting form. The anatomy of the crown and root(s) of each tooth is shown with facial, occlusal, and lingual views. Anatomic charting provides the most realistic graphic description, as the anatomic features of each tooth can be used to denote specifi-

cally the presence of lesions and restorations. This particular form allows for charting both permanent and primary teeth.

Fig. 11-2 provides an example of a geometric charting, with stylized "anatomy." The tooth surfaces are divided by lines to indicate marginal ridges and line angles so that the extent of disease

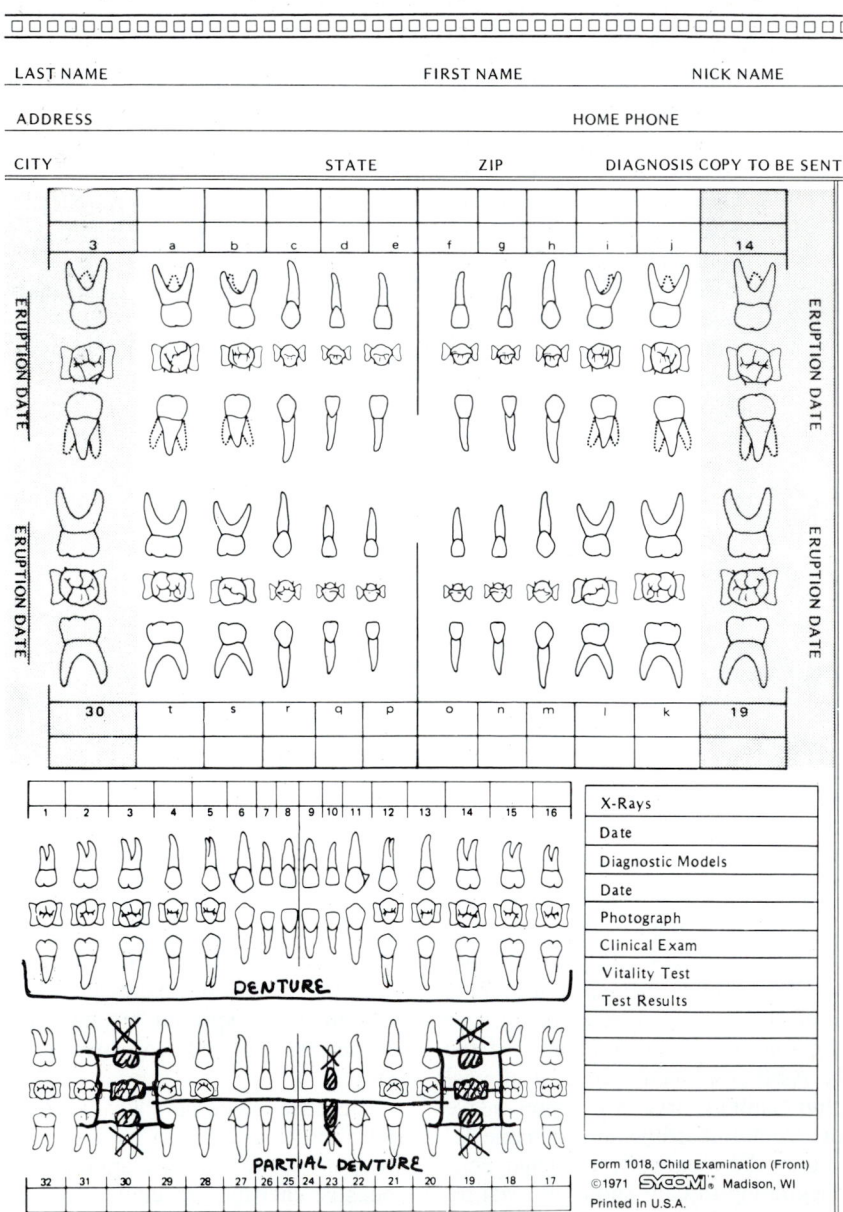

Fig. 11-1. Anatomic charting form that accommodates chartings of adult, primary, and mixed dentitions. A complete maxillary denture and mandibular partial denture are charted to illustrate one method of symbol use. (Courtesy Sycom, Madison, Wis.)

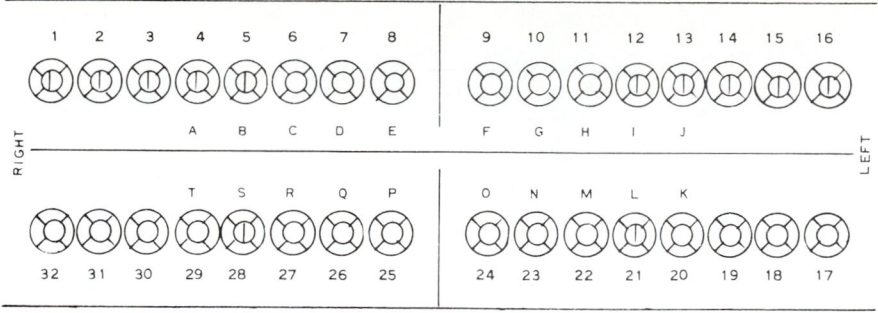

Fig. 11-2. Geometric charting form with stylized teeth. This form accommodates charting of adult, primary, and mixed dentition.

or a restoration can be shown without attempting to replicate the exact design. Because it does not require precise anatomic drawings of restorations and other characteristics, this is usually a neater, more easily read charting.

To follow the patient's progress, a comprehensive charting must be completely redone at each 6-month visit, or changes at each visit will become lost in the original charting. The original generally becomes increasingly cluttered and unreadable if there are many clinical changes. One way to preserve the original charting, to show progress at each assessment visit, and to avoid the time-consuming and tedious process of recharting the entire dentition is to photocopy the original charting. Findings at the second visit can be marked in colored pencil or pen on the photocopy to highlight recent changes. At the beginning of a third course of treatment in which a charting is indicated, the charting from the second course is photocopied and the new photocopy updated in color. This procedure results in a highly specific time line of conditions and care. It also results in many additional pages in the patient record. Eventually, microfilm or microfiche will be necessary to permit long-term storage.

The numeric coding system requires less paper for showing progress through time. Because this system uses number codes rather than drawings to indicate conditions of the teeth, the pictorial quality of anatomic and geometric chartings is lost. Fig. 11-3 shows a numeric code charting. As conditions change, markings are made in the next line above (for the maxillary teeth) or below (for the mandibular teeth). The lines are dated so that changes are identified along a time line.

TYPES OF CHARTINGS

The vast majority of chartings focus on the presence of caries, restorations, and missing teeth. Depending on treatment protocols in a given practice setting, the routine charting may be limited to these three conditions or expanded to include malposed teeth, attrition, erosion, abrasion, developmental anomalies, and other findings.

In addition to chartings of the clinical and radiographic conditions of the teeth, protocols may call for charting calculus deposits, periodontal conditions, plaque and hemorrhage points, and occlusal assessment. This section focuses on charting clinical findings of the teeth. Charting of other conditions is explained in subsequent chapters.

AUTOMATED CHARTINGS

Identifying oral conditions and writing them down or drawing them on a form is time consuming and prone to inaccuracy, especially if a single clinician is responsible for both identification and recording. A more serious problem for the unassisted clinician is controlling cross-contamination during the charting procedure. The pen, unless it is autoclaved, will carry bacteria to the gloved hand and then into the mouth. The bacteria from the mouth will be carried back to the pen and ultimately to the paper charting form.

One way to increase accuracy and efficiency and to minimize cross-contamination is to use a computerized charting program. One system, the Victor, developed by Avanti Computer Systems, uses voice activation. The clinician wears a headset and calls off the findings. The computer "hears" the calls and enters them in an electronic

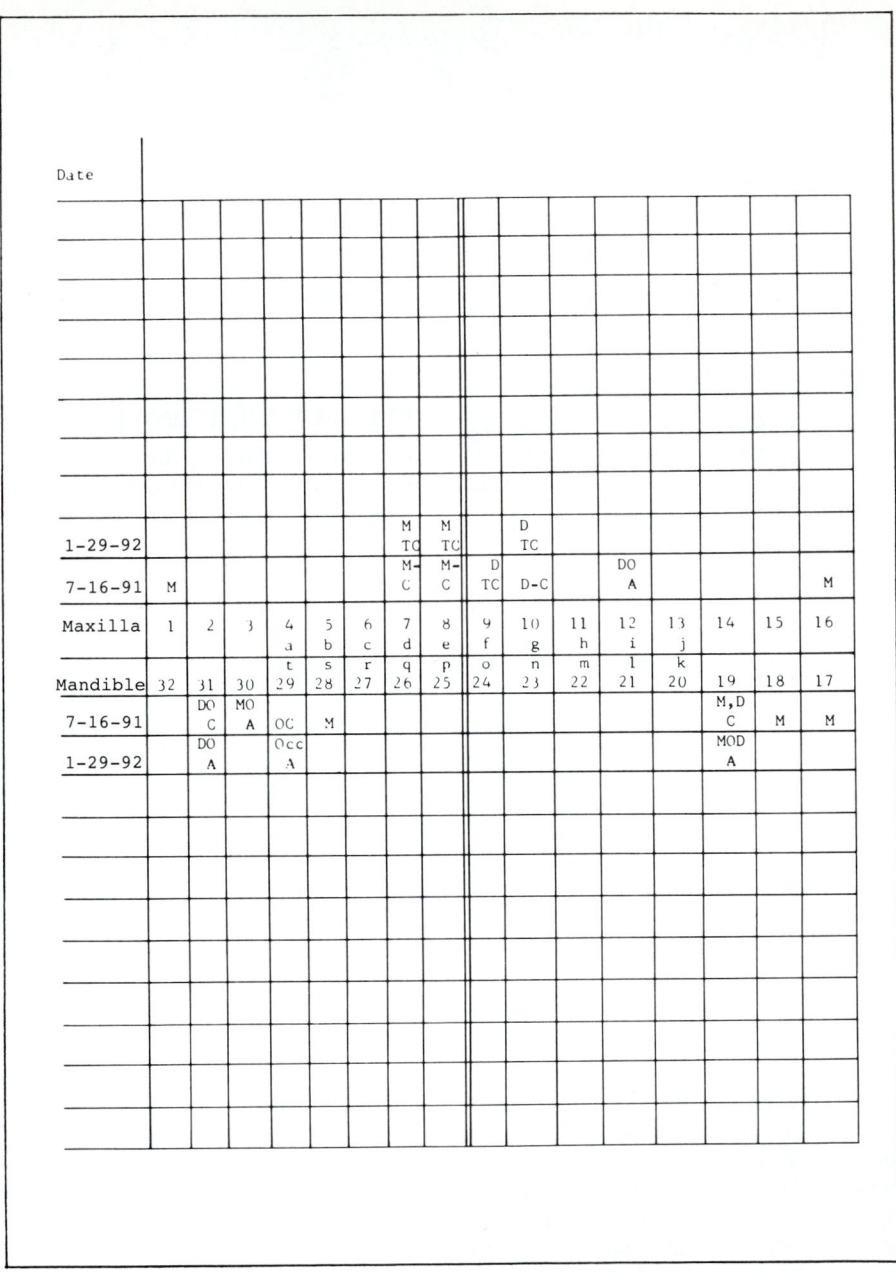

Date																
								M	M		D					
1-29-92								TC	TC		TC					
								M-	M-	D			DO			
7-16-91	M							C	C	TC	D-C		A			M
Maxilla	1	2	3	4 a	5 b	6 c	7 d	8 e	9 f	10 g	11 h	12 i	13 j	14	15	16
Mandible	32	31	30	t 29	s 28	r 27	q 26	p 25	o 24	n 23	m 22	l 21	k 20	19	18	17
		DO	MO											M,D		
7-16-91		C	A	OC	M									C	M	M
		DO		Occ										MOD		
1-29-92		A		A										A		

Fig. 11-3. Numeric code charting form. As each examination is performed, charting symbols are entered in the boxes above the maxilla entry and below the mandible entry. As defects are treated, corrections are entered in the next row of boxes above or below the corresponding teeth. As no anatomic drawings of caries and restorations are used, charting symbols must be explicit as to locations of specific condition.

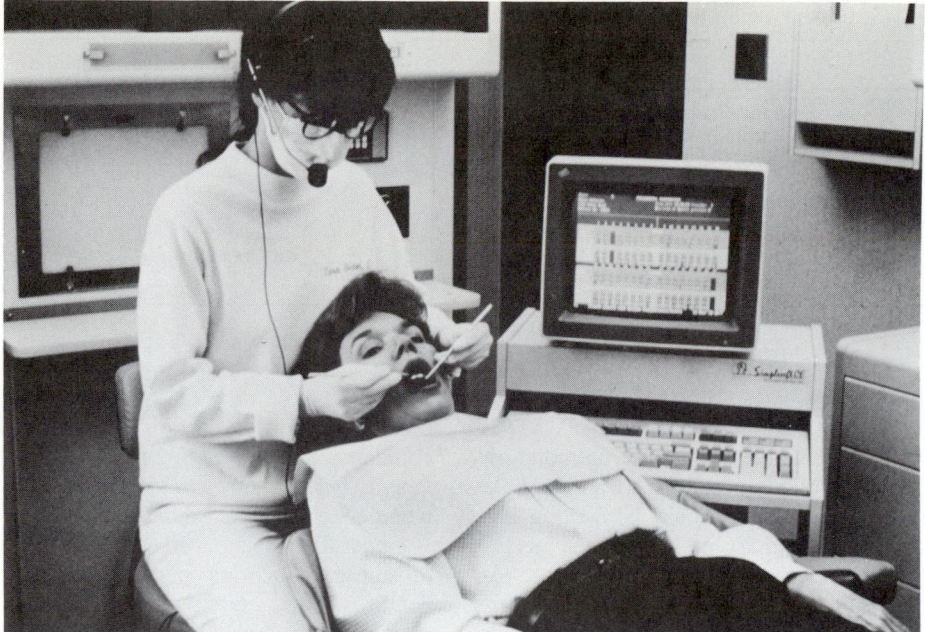

Fig. 11-4. Victor system in use.

file which can then be printed, producing a clear, concise picture of the patient's oral status. Fig. 11-4 shows the system in use. Fig. 12-10 shows an example of the printed form. Yet another system, the Autochart, uses a mouse to move among the graphic display of the teeth on the screen and to enter findings. The mouse can be barrier protected by a plastic bag or wrap and placed near the bracket tray for easy access by the clinician or the assistant.

TOOTH NUMBERING SYSTEMS

Regardless of the selection of anatomic, geometric, or numerically coded chartings and whether or not a computerized system is used, it is essential to adopt a consistent method of denoting the teeth. The *universal* system numbers each of the permanent teeth from *1* to *32* and the primary teeth from *a* to *t*, beginning with the last molar on the maxillary right quadrant and progressing sequentially around the arch to the last molar (Project ACORDE, 1974). The next tooth counted (or lettered) is the last molar on the mandibular left quadrant, progressing sequentially around the mandible to the last molar on the man-

dibular right. The "last molar" for permanent dentition (1 to 32) is the third molar; for children (a to t) it is the second primary molar. This system is widely accepted in the United States. (See Figs. 11-1 and 11-2 for the numbering of each tooth.)

An older system, *Palmer's notation,* numbers or letters each of the teeth in the quadrant from *1* to *8* for permanent dentition and from *a* to *e* for primary teeth. Therefore a permanent central is always No. 1. A permanent cuspid in any quadrant is labeled No. 3. The quadrant position of the tooth under consideration is identified by using the appropriate quadrant of a graph created by two intersecting perpendicular axes. Using the quadrant denotation, the second permanent premolar in the maxillary left quadrant would be written ⌊5. The second primary molar on the mandibular right would be written e̅⌉.

The *international system* is similar to Palmer's notation in that each tooth in the quadrant is numbered *1* to *8* from central to third molar. However, the quadrant location is designated by a prefix number *1, 2, 3,* or *4* for the maxillary right, maxillary left, mandibular left, and mandibular right, respectively. The quadrant prefix is fol-

Table 11-1. Summary of tooth numbering systems

System	Permanent dentition	Primary dentition
Universal	Each tooth is designated by a number (*1* to *32*)	Each tooth is designated by a letter (*a* to *t*)
International	Each tooth is designated by a quadrant number prefix (*1* to *4*) and a tooth number suffix (*1* to *8*) $$\frac{1|2}{3|4}$$	Each tooth is a designated by a quadrant number (*5* to *8*) and a tooth number (*1* to *5*) $$\frac{5|6}{8|7}$$
Palmer's notation	Each tooth is numbered (*1* to *8*) and positioned within intersecting axes to designate the quadrant	Each tooth is lettered (*a* to *e*) and positioned within intersecting axes to designate the quadrant

lowed by the tooth number (Project ACORDE, 1974). Thus the second permanent premolar in the maxillary left quadrant shown as an example in the previous paragraph would be written $\underline{25}$. For distinguishing primary and permanent teeth, primary quadrants are numbered *5, 6, 7,* or *8,* respectively, with numbers (not letters) used for primary teeth. Therefore the second primary molar on the mandibular right, given as an example in the previous paragraph, would be written $\overline{85}$.

Table 11-1 summarizes the differences among the three numbering systems. In practice it is important to determine what system has been adopted to enable all coworkers to identify the tooth under discussion. Because the universal system is still the most widely understood and used, the detailed procedures for preparing a charting are described with *1* to *32* and *a* to *t* tooth designations. To ensure an accurate, complete charting, a sequence moving from the maxillary right third molar to the mandibular right third molar (1 to 32) will be followed.

PROCEDURE FOR CHARTING

To prevent confusion and error, the first condition that should be charted is *missing teeth.* The teeth may have been extracted or may not yet have erupted. It is also possible that the tooth buds for the teeth were missing congenitally. In most instances it is not possible, with clinical data alone, to determine why the tooth is not present. A radiographic series can add data; a patient's dental history also provides information on the cause of missing teeth.

Missing teeth should be crossed out with a single vertical line or an *X.* Some practitioners prefer to box or color in missing teeth.

A partially erupted tooth can be marked so that

it is obvious which portion of the tooth is exposed clinically. (See tooth No. 16 in Fig. 11-5.) Marking *all missing teeth first* is especially important when charting mixed dentition.

Once all missing teeth are marked, removable prostheses, such as partial dentures, complete dentures, and removable bridges should be marked with brackets. Fig. 11-1 (on the adult dentition) shows a maxillary denture and a mandibular partial denture replacing Nos. 23, 30, and 19. The clasps are shown on Nos. 31, 29, 18, and 20.

After marking all missing teeth and removable prostheses, the clinician should return to the first chartable tooth in the maxillary right quadrant. The tooth number should be identified, and the tooth should be examined for existing restorations.

Marking restorations

The basic shape of the restoration should be drawn on the appropriate tooth on the charting form. There are a number of ways to further designate that the area defined is an existing restoration. These include filling in the area with a designated color or simply leaving the restoration outlined and using a letter code to indicate the material used in the restoration, such as amalgam, resin, gold foil, cast gold, or silicate.

For a precise charting, these letter designations for the type of restorative material may be used even if shading or otherwise filling in the outline is the preferred method. Thus an amalgam restoration may be designated by an anatomic outline of its shape, which is shaded in a color and marked *A* for amalgam. (See tooth No. 2 in Fig. 11-5 for an example.)

To draw and identify single-tooth restorations,

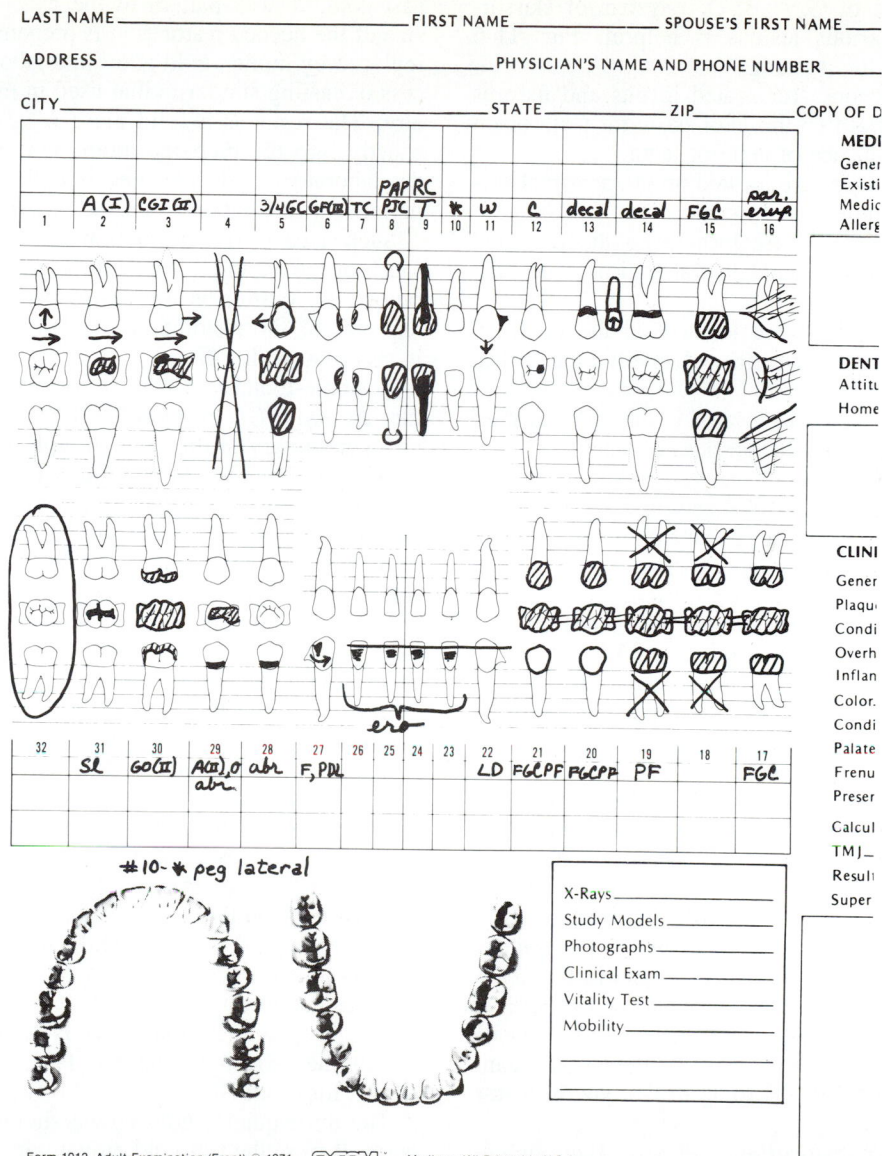

Form 1012, Adult Examination (Front) © 1971, SYCOM. Madison, WI Printed in U.S.A.

Fig. 11-5. Composite charting showing most commonly used charting symbols with provisions for clinical and radiographic findings.
(Courtesy Sycom, Madison, Wis.)
Key to symbols (numbers refer to teeth): 1—Facially inclined; drifted mesially 2—Occlusal amalgam; drifted mesially 3—Mesioocclusal, gold inlay; caries on distobuccal margin; mesially inclined and drifted mesially 4—Missing 5—Three-quarter gold crown; distally inclined 6—Class III, mesial gold foil 7—Class III, distal tooth-colored restoration 8—Porcelain jacket crown; periapical disease 9—Temporary crown; root canal 10—Peg lateral 11—Lingually inclined; watch for distal caries 12—Distal pit caries 13—Decalcification in gingival third on facial aspect; supernumerary tooth between 13 and 14 14—Decalcification in gingival third on facial aspect 15—Full gold crown 16—Partially erupted 17—Abutment tooth for fixed bridge; full gold crown 18—Pontic 19—Pontic with porcelain facing 20—Full gold crown with porcelain facing 21—Full gold crown with porcelain facing 22—Attrition; loss of continuity of lamina dura 23—Attrition; erosion 24—Attrition; erosion 25—Attrition; erosion 26—Attrition; erosion 27—Facet on distal third of facial surface; distal surface rotated toward facial; widened periodontal ligament (PDL) 28—Abrasion 29—Abrasion; mesioocclusal amalgam; overhang on mesial surface 30—Mesioocclusodistal gold onlay 31—Sealant 32—Unerupted.

a knowledge of G.V. Black's system of classification of carious lesions is helpful. Fig. 11-6 summarizes this system.

Class I lesions are located in pits and fissures of the occlusal two thirds of posterior teeth or on the lingual surface of anterior teeth.

Class II lesions are located on the proximal surfaces of premolars and molars.

Class III lesions are located on the proximal surfaces of central and lateral incisors and cuspids.

Class IV lesions are located on the proximal surfaces of anterior teeth and involve the incisal edge.

Class V lesions are located at the gingival third of the facial or lingual surfaces of anterior or posterior teeth.

Class VI lesions are located on cusp tips.

The same classification system applies to restorations that replace the tooth structure lost to dental caries.

In identifying restorations for chartings, the classification of restoration (I, II, III, IV, V, or VI) is noted, especially where idealized drawings are used. When verbally describing the restorations to an assistant who is recording the data on the charting, describing the classification of restorations helps the recorder picture the likely shape. Because restoration shape and size depend largely on the physics of retention and resistance to masticatory stress and strain, as well as to the maintenance of esthetics, restorations follow predictable patterns, most of which are shown in the comprehensive charting (see Fig. 11-5) and in Fig. 11-6. Therefore the procedure for marking a restoration is to outline its shape according to G.V. Black's classification system, shade in the outline carefully, and label it according to the type of restorative material.

Amalgam restorations. Plate 4, *F* through *G*, illustrates a variety of amalgam restorations. They are identifiable by their dark gray (unpolished) or bright silver (polished) appearance. Amalgam is commonly used for Class I, II, and V restorations.

Gold restorations. Gold is easily distinguished from amalgam by the obvious color difference. Gold has no gray cast; it resembles gold jewelry in color and shine. It is designated with a *G*. (Compare the restorations in Plate 4, *E* and *F*.)

The most frequently seen gold restoration is cast gold. A wax pattern of the exact shape and size of the needed restoration is prepared and then replaced by molten gold alloy in a laboratory process of casting similar to that used in making jewelry. The result is a solid piece of gold that fits exactly into the prepared tooth. It is polished in the laboratory and cemented into the tooth as a permanent restoration when the fit is exact.

Such a cast gold restoration feels hard to the touch of the explorer. As with the amalgam restoration, the outline is drawn to match the shape and size of the restoration, shaded, and labeled, in this case with a *G*.

A single-tooth cast gold restoration can be either an *inlay (GI)* or an *onlay (GO)*, so more detail is necessary to differentiate gold restorations. Tooth No. 3 in Fig. 11-5 has a gold inlay. It lies within the marginal ridges of the occlusal table, except where it crosses the mesial marginal ridge to include the mesial surface. It is a Class II gold inlay. Tooth No. 30 shows a Class II *mesioocclusodistal (MOD)* gold onlay, which includes all cusp tips and thus covers all the marginal ridges of the tooth. However, the onlay rarely extends below the occlusal third of the facial or lingual surfaces of the tooth. (See Plate 4, *J*, for two gold onlays, a DO inlay, and an MO amalgam.)

The three-quarter crown, in contrast, includes the full occlusal table and extends to the gingiva on the mesial, distal, and lingual aspects of the tooth. The facial marginal ridge is included, along with a small portion of the facial surface, to ensure strength and retention while allowing the natural tooth structure on the facial aspect to preserve esthetics.

The three-quarter gold crown is designated with an outline, shading, and the label *3/4 GC*, as shown for tooth No. 5 in Fig. 11-5.

The three-quarter gold crown should be differentiated from the full gold crown with a porcelain or acrylic facing. The full gold crown covers and replaces all visible enamel tooth structure and considerable underlying dentin. It is used to restore badly broken-down teeth. Although it is stronger than the three-quarter gold crown, it may result in less than desirable esthetics if the facial aspect is visible when the patient speaks or smiles. Thus when the crown is cast, an area is created on the facial aspect in which white porcelain or acrylic may be added to simulate white tooth structure. A full gold crown is outlined, shaded, and labeled *FGC*. (See tooth No. 15 in

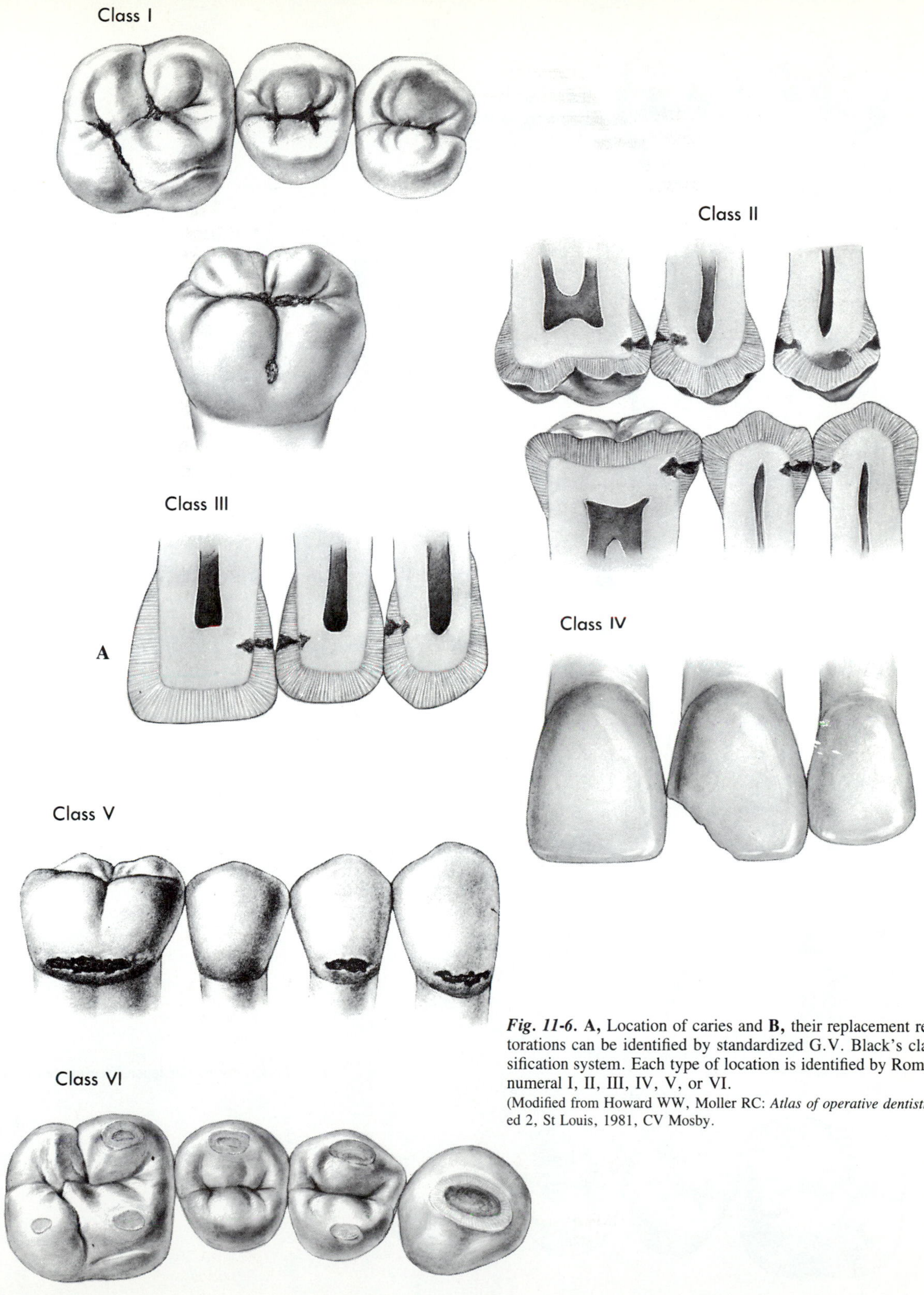

Class I

Class II

Class III

A

Class IV

Class V

Class VI

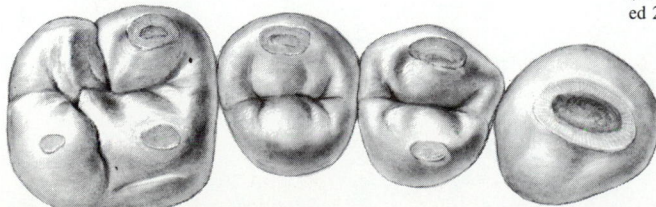

Fig. 11-6. A, Location of caries and **B,** their replacement restorations can be identified by standardized G.V. Black's classification system. Each type of location is identified by Roman numeral I, II, III, IV, V, or VI.
(Modified from Howard WW, Moller RC: *Atlas of operative dentistry*, ed 2, St Louis, 1981, CV Mosby.

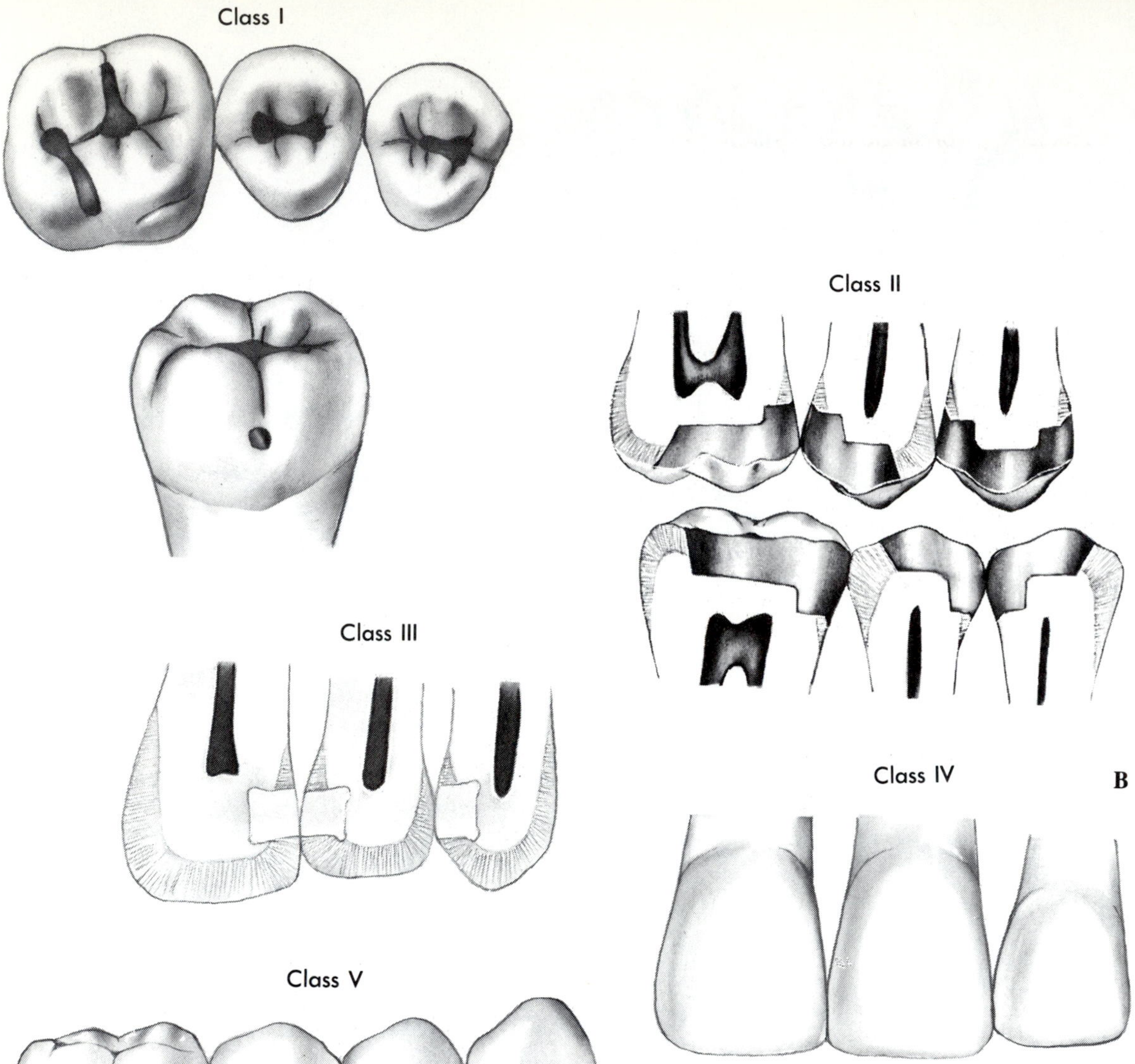

Class I

Class II

Class III

Class IV

B

Class V

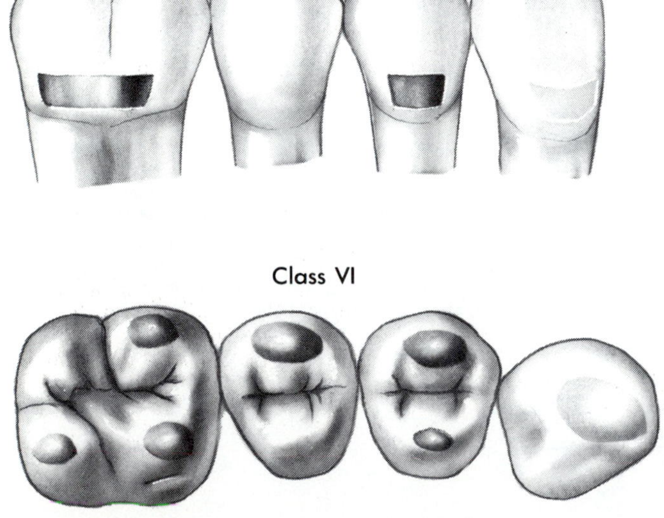

Fig. 11-6, cont'd. For legend see previous page.

Class VI

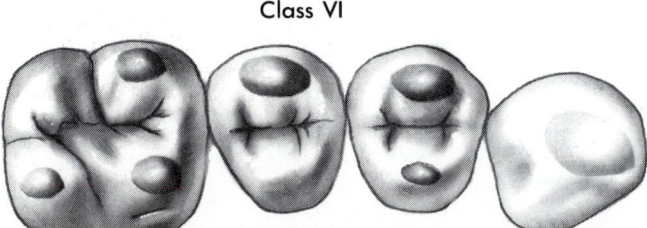

Fig. 11-5.) A gold crown with a facing is labeled *GCPF* for porcelain and *GCAF* for acrylic.

Another type of single-tooth gold restoration is *gold foil*. This restorative material is quite different from cast gold. It lacks the strengthening alloys that make cast gold hard and able to endure stress and strain. Gold foil is soft and is condensed or packed into the tooth preparation until the void area is completely filled and the anatomy can be carved. The material (1) feels softer to the touch of an explorer than does cast gold, (2) is a lighter or more yellow gold color because of the purity of the material, and (3) is used in Class I, II, III, IV, V, or VI restorations with minimal occlusal wear. When identified on a tooth, the outline should be drawn, shaded, and labeled *GF*. (See tooth No. 6 in Fig. 11-5.)

Gold is also used for multiple-tooth restorations such as *fixed bridges* (fixed partial dentures) that replace one or more missing teeth or *splints* that join several teeth together with a series of soldered or cast-together gold crowns intended to strengthen the ability of individual teeth to absorb occlusal forces. The teeth absorb the forces collectively by virtue of their joined crowns.

A bridge enables two or more healthy adjacent teeth to support a *pontic* (dummy tooth) so that an open space in the arch can be preserved with a functional tooth replacement. Usually the supporting teeth have full crowns or three-quarter crowns. The crowns to which the pontics are attached are *retainers*. They are seated or anchored on *abutment* teeth. The pontics are made of cast gold also; they can be distinguished from the abutment teeth because they have no roots. They are either cast in one piece with the abutments or soldered to the abutment teeth. In either case, the contacts are sealed together.

Another way to support multiple-tooth restorations is with *implants*. These fixtures are imbedded in bone in areas where there is insufficient support from natural teeth to support fixed prostheses. Once the implant is secure in the bone, a superstructure of replacement teeth is prepared and fitted onto the implants and remaining teeth, depending on the case. Implants require special attention by the patient and need careful professional monitoring. Therefore it is important to note their existence on the charting.

The easiest way to locate and chart a bridge is first to identify the location of the missing teeth. The roots of the missing teeth should be charted

as absent (by a vertical line, an *x*, or boxing the roots). The crowns replaced by pontics can be outlined and shaded. The abutment teeth or implants are then identified by examining the location of permanently joined contacts. The crown restorations on the abutment teeth are outlined, shaded, and labeled (¾ GC, FGC, GCPF, etc.). Then horizontal lines should be drawn between the attached abutments and pontics to show the size and location of the entire bridge. Fig. 11-5 shows a five-unit bridge (three abutments and two pontics) extending from Nos. 17 to 21. No. 17 has a full gold crown; Nos. 18 and 19 are pontics, with No. 19 having a porcelain facing; and Nos. 20 and 21 are full gold crowns with porcelain facings.

If the pontics are in close contact with the gingiva and cannot easily be differentiated clinically from rooted teeth, reference to a radiographic survey will quickly identify pontics and abutments. Also, when threading dental floss underneath one of the closed contacts, the clinician should be able to pass the floss under the pontics, thus identifying the absence of the root. Palpating the alveolar process should also help distinguish between edentulous areas where pontics replace the teeth and areas where supporting structure is present. The shape of the roots of the natural teeth and implants can be felt in the alveolar bone.

Tooth-colored restorations. Tooth-colored restoration (designated *TC*) is the generic term for silicate (a material used before the 1970s), composite, and resin single-tooth restorations that restore the tooth functionally and esthetically. They are used primarily in anterior teeth but may be also found in posterior teeth, depending on the location and size of the area to be restored. If it is possible and desirable to distinguish the material used, the labels *S* for silicate, *R* for resin, and *CR* for composite resin can be used in conjunction with the shaded-in outline of the restoration. Otherwise, the label *TC* is sufficient. (See tooth No. 7 in Fig. 11-5.)

In addition to tooth-colored restorations that restore a portion of a tooth, porcelain and acrylic jacket crowns (designated *PFC* and *AJC*) provide full coverage of teeth, usually where maintenance of esthetics is critical. (See tooth No. 8 in Fig. 11-5; for a clinical example, see tooth No. 9 in Plate 4, *A, B,* and *D*.)

Temporary restorations. Temporary restorations are usually easily identified as a chalky yellow, white, or pink substance placed in a prepared tooth or by an aluminum preformed or nonanatomic "can" fitted over a posterior tooth prepared for a full crown. Sometimes relatively crude-looking acrylic crowns are used as temporary restorations also, particularly for anterior teeth undergoing crown preparation. The label *T* is used to designate a temporary restoration. It is usually outlined and shaded as a permanent restoration would be (See tooth No. 9 in Fig. 11-5.)

Sealants. Sealants are thin, transparent plastic coatings that are chemically and physically bonded to posterior teeth with pits and fissures that would be highly susceptible to decay (caries). Therefore sealants are usually found on occlusal surfaces of posterior teeth. They are detected as a shiny narrow clear filling when felt with the tip of an explorer. Sealants can be clear or light pink, yellow or some other shade that enhances detection. When detected, they should be outlined, shaded, and labeled *Sl*.

Sealants are being used with increasing frequency, both for prevention of caries and for restoration of areas with beginning caries. The clinician can simply remove the carious portion of the tooth, without having to remove any additional tooth structure, to make a boxlike preparation as is commonly done for the previously introduced restorations. Research has shown that, if the teeth and type of sealant are carefully selected, these preventive resin restorations (PRR) give excellent results (Simonson, 1980, 1982).

Using the abbreviations described and being anatomically specific about the size and location of restorations and sealants leads to an accurate, detailed charting of the clinical conditions of the teeth.

Charting for other conditions

As each tooth is charted for the presence of restorations, the margins of each restoration should be explored for the presence of *recurrent caries* or an open area that may eventually become carious. *Overhanging margins* should be identified (with an *O*), as the overhangs should be removed or the restoration replaced. The prefix of *C* for caries or *D* for defective should be added to the letter label for the restoration. Therefore a carious amalgam would be labeled *C-A*. (See tooth No. 3 in Fig. 11-5 for a carious gold inlay.) A defective composite resin would be labeled *DCR*. When colored pencils are used to differentiate carious areas from

existing restorations, the carious margin can be marked simply with the color designated for caries, and the prefix letter is then unnecessary.

Likewise, all the exposed surfaces of the teeth should be felt for soft, *carious areas,* particularly in pits and grooves, at contact points, and on exposed root surfaces. If the sharp explorer tip sticks in a pit (it seems to be retained by the pit or groove) and the area feels soft, then it should be marked for caries with either the designated color or by outlining the area of caries, shading it in, and marking it *C*. Incipient or beginning caries or suspicious pits and grooves can be marked "watch," *W*. (See Nos. 11 and 12 in Fig. 11-5.)

Obvious areas of tooth breakdown, such as large craters, do not require exploration, and exploring them may cause the patient considerable pain.

Closely related to caries are areas of *decalcification*. These areas show evidence of demineralization of the tooth structure with an enamel surface that is whiter than the surrounding tooth and may be chalky and soft. If such an area is likely to become carious or needs to be noted for some other reason, such as esthetics, it can be noted on the chart by shading in the area and labeling it *decal*. *Hypocalcification,* which rarely is clinically significant and thus is rarely charted, can be labeled *hycal*. (See Plate 3, *D,* for a clinical example.)

A *supernumerary tooth* can be drawn in its general location (See Fig. 11-5 in the maxillary left quadrant.) Other developmental *anomalies* are usually marked with an asterisk near the tooth involved, with a full notation on the charting page to explain the observed characteristics. (See tooth No. 10 in Fig. 11-5.)

Attrition, the loss of tooth structure resulting from normal mastication, is often seen on the incisal edges of anterior teeth (see Fig. 11-5). This can be noted with a horizontal line drawn across the facial aspect of the drawings of the teeth to illustrate the amount of lost tooth structure. (See the mandibular anterior teeth in Plate 4 for a clinical example.) Closely related to attrition, but far more clinically significant, is the presence of *wear facets*. These highly polished wear areas often show the pattern of wear associated with malocclusion. Wear facets are boxed in to show the plane of wear on each tooth. They are marked with an *F*.

Abrasion is caused by mechanical wear other

than that associated with mastication. Vigorous horizontal strokes with a toothbrush cause abrasion, as does improper flossing, opening hairpins with the teeth, and other habits that wear the tooth structure. The area is outlined and shaded and marked *abr.* Colored pencils are useful to distinguish this characteristic from a Class V restoration or other defect. (See Plate 3, *H,* especially the maxillary right quadrant, for a clinical example.)

Erosion, in contrast to attrition and abrasion, is caused by chemical wear of the teeth. Sucking lemons, for instance, can cause generalized erosion of the anterior facial surfaces. It also is a characteristic of bulimia (vomiting to control weight). Because this feature is generalized over a broad surface and involves several teeth, the teeth involved can be bracketed and marked *ero.* (See Fig. 11-5 for a graphic description of these characteristics on Nos. 22 to 29 and Plate 1, *A.*)

Malposed teeth should be charted, including rotated, extruded, and inclined teeth. Rotated teeth are marked by drawing an arrow from the proximal surface that is rotated towards the facial, then arcing the arrow across the facial view of the tooth to suggest the direction of rotation. Fig. 11-5 shows No. 27 as having its distal suface rotated towards the facial. The arrow starts on the distal and arcs across the facial surface. It would be just as valid to show an arrow starting on the mesial surface and arcing across the lingual view; for consistency, however facial views are used for rotations. Because of the different perceptions persons have when viewing a two-dimensional drawing and attempting to visualize a three-dimensional characteristic, all persons who may record or interpret a dental charting should agree on one way to chart malpositions.

This is true not only for axial rotations, but also for lingual and labial versions (inclinations), which may cause equal confusion if a variety of methods are used to chart the condition. One easily understood rule is to place a vertical arrow pointing from the incisal edge away from the facial aspect of the tooth to show a *lingual version* (see tooth No. 11 in Fig. 11-5) and to place a vertical arrow starting at the incisal edge and traveling vertically up or down the facial aspect of the drawing of the tooth to depict *labial version.* Mesial inclination is shown with a straight, horizontal arrow pointing towards the midline of the arch from the mesial surface. The arrow points poste-

riorly from the distal surface to show distal inclination.

Drifting of the teeth, either mesially or distally and with or without rotation or inclination, is shown with a horizontal arrow pointed in the direction of the drift, above the occlusal table or incisal edge. Fig. 11-5 shows the distinction in recording version and drifting. Tooth No. 5 is distally inclined; tooth No. 3 is mesially inclined and drifted; and Nos. 1 and 2 are positioned mesial to their usual locations but are not inclined. This is probably because of the loss of tooth No. 4.

All these malpositions are located by sitting in a rear position (e.g., 11 o'clock) and observing the curve of the maxillary arch in the dental mirror. Careful observation should help contrast rotations and versions from the natural curvature of the maxillary arch. The curve of the arch on the mandible should reveal deviations from normal arch curve. (See the anterior rotations evident in Plate 4, *C,* and the more obvious malpositions in Plate 3, *F* and *G.*) Having the patient close his or her teeth and retracting the cheeks should reveal patterns of drift and version.

Radiographs are a necessary and helpful adjunct to the clinical examination. The radiographs provide information about the teeth and supporting structures that cannot be collected during a clinical examination. The next chapter will describe how to review the radiographic survey and how to record the findings.

All teeth to which none of the clinical or radiographic characteristics apply are described as *sound.*

Fig. 11-5 describes all the usual charting symbols, with the key to each symbol given in the legend. All will probably never be used for any one patient. However, in charting the dental conditions of a wide variety of patients, each symbol will prove useful.

Describing the charting orally

In some instances the person observing the oral conditions will also mark the symbols on the charting form or use a computer system for charting, which, of course, does not involve an oral description of the characteristic noted. Far more frequently, an assistant will record what is described aloud. In addition, the observer or the recorder will often need to describe each of the recorded findings to another person for verification.

To expedite the charting and/or verification system, an explicit and systematic approach should be used to describe each charted characteristic aloud.

Moving sequentially from 1 to 32 or a to t is the best organizational guideline, with all charted characteristics for each tooth described completely as each tooth is identified. The *tooth number* should be called first. If a restoration is present, the classification, the type of restorative material, and its anatomic location should follow. For example, "Tooth No. 2 has a Class I occlusal amalgam." In identifying anatomic locations, the basic structure (MOD, DO, MO) should be followed by a description of lingual or buccal extensions and the inclusion of complete cusps. For example, "Tooth No. 2 has a Class II MO amalgam with a buccal extension."

Any defective or carious margins should be described following the description of the restoration in question. For example, "Tooth No. 3 has a Class II MO gold inlay with recurrent caries on the distobuccal margin."

When describing a bridge, it is best to first call the number of units (abutments plus pontics) and then call each involved unit as an abutment or pontic and state the type of restoration present on the unit. For example, "There is a five-unit bridge from tooth No. 17 to tooth No. 21. No. 17 is an abutment with a full gold crown. Nos. 18 and 19 are pontics with gold crowns and a porcelain facing on No. 19. Nos. 20 and 21 are abutments with full gold crowns with porcelain facings."

Caries, decalcification, hypocalcification, attrition, facets, erosion, and abrasion are located anatomically. For example, "Tooth No. 12 has caries in the distal pit. Nos. 13 and 14 have decalcification on the gingival third of the facial surface. No. 27 has a vertical facet on the distal third of the labial surface."

Anomalies are called as the tooth is encountered. For example, "No. 10 is a peg lateral."

Malposed teeth are described by naming the tooth and indicating the direction in which it is inclined. For example, "No. 1 is buccally inclined (or verted)." Rotations are described by stating the proximal surface that is directed facially and describing the rotation. For example, "No. 27—the distal surface is rotated labially."

Proceeding around the mouth in this fashion allows for rapid, precise cross-evaluation of findings.

PEDODONTIC CHARTINGS

For most purposes, the preparation of pedodontic chartings is similar to that of adult chartings. Differences include the fact that primary dentition chartings usually use the lower case letters of the alphabet (*a* to *t*). Also, mixed dentition chartings may pose a challenge, as permanent teeth must be differentiated from primary teeth and described with the *1* to *32* system. For instance, a 6-year-old child may have four permanent first molars (Nos. 3, 14, 19, and 30) and four permanent centrals (Nos. 8, 9, 24, and 25), with all the rest being primary teeth (a, b, c, d, g, h, i, and j on the maxilla and k, l, m, n, q, r, s, and t on the mandible). It should be apparent that assessment of present and missing teeth *must* precede the attempt to mark restorations, caries, and other characteristics. A guideline never to be forgotten is that *the first permanent molar appears posterior to the second primary molar; it does not replace a primary molar, and it closely resembles the second primary molar.*

Tooth characteristics that may be encountered in pedodontic findings include space maintainers and preformed stainless steel crowns. A space maintainer should be identified by drawing the retaining band on the abutment tooth and drawing a bar to show the space being saved. Stainless steel crowns are marked like full gold crowns, except they are labeled *SSC*.

Practice in reading mixed dentition chartings aloud is particularly helpful, as it is easy to confuse the sequence of teeth described and to err in identifying teeth.

In all cases, precision in identifying and recording comprehensive chartings is extremely important, because the chartings serve as legal records and as one basis for treatment planning.

ACTIVITIES

1. Practice reading aloud from a completed anatomic or geometric form a variety of comprehensive chartings to a partner who will record the described findings on a blank form. Compare the chartings for accuracy.

2. Record comprehensive chartings for an advanced student who is assessing his or her patient's oral conditions. Read the findings back to a clinical instructor for verification.

3. In groups of three, take turns (1) observing and describing aloud each tooth's significant characteris-

tics, (2) recording the findings on a charting form, and (3) sitting as a patient observing in a mirror.

4. Translate anatomic or geometric charting symbols to a numerically coded charting form.

5. Read Johnson GK, Silvers JE: Attrition, abrasion, and erosion: diagnosis and therapy, *Clin Prev Dent* 9(5):12, 1987. Find clinical evidence of each of these phenomena among the group members or clinical patients.

6. Visit the commercial exhibits at a dental meeting and collect information about each of the computerized systems for charting and samples of charting forms for manual preparation. Compare the benefits of each of the systems and forms.

REVIEW QUESTIONS

1. Identify at least four basic uses of a comprehensive dental charting.

2. Give one advantage of each of the following charting formats:
   a. Anatomic
   b. Geometric
   c. Numerically coded
   d. Computerized (voice activated or mouse)

3. Following are three columns for the three types of systems used for numbering the teeth and a column to describe the designated tooth. How would the remaining blanks be filled in to identify the designations for a given tooth according to each system and to include a description of the tooth?

	Universal	Palmer's notation	International	Description
a.	–	6⌋	–	–
b.	29	–	–	–
c.	–	–	28	–
d.	–	⌈6	–	–
e.	–	–	–	Maxillary left second premolar

4. What is the likely Black's classification for a restoration on the following:
   a. DO #12
   b. M #6
   c. B #28
   d. O #18
   e. Cusp tip of #5
   f. MI of #24

5. Identify each of the following commonly used symbols in charting:
   a. A
   b. T
   c. TC
   d. FGC
   e. GF
   f. C
   g. SSC
   h. DGO

6. Describe how each of the following findings should be marked:
   a. Tooth anomaly
   b. Pontic
   c. Drifting
   d. Rotation
   e. Attrition
   f. Unerupted teeth
   g. Overhang

REFERENCES

Brand RW, Isselhard DE: *Anatomy of orofacial structures,* ed 3, St Louis, 1986, CV Mosby.

Ekstrand K, Qvist V, Thylstrup A: Light microscope study of the effect of probing in occlusal surfaces, *Caries Res* 21:368, 1987.

Johnson GK, Silvers JE: Attrition, abrasion and erosion: diagnosis and therapy, *Clin Prev Dent* 9(5):12, 1987.

Project ACORDE: *Restoration of cavity preparations with amalgam and tooth-colored materials: instructor's manual,* Washington DC, 1974, US Department of Health, Education, and Welfare.

Simonson RJ: Preventive resin restorations: three-year results, *JADA* 100:535, 1980.

Simonson RJ: Preventive resin restoration: innovative uses of sealants in restorative dentistry, *Clin Prev Dent* 4(4):27, 1982.

12 PERIODONTAL ASSESSMENT

Laura Mueller-Joseph
Irene Woodall
Nancy Stutsman Young

LEARNING OUTCOMES

The dental hygienist will be able to

1. Differentiate nonmineralized deposits of pellicle, materia alba, food debris, dental plaque, and mineralized calculus.
2. Describe the nature and formation of dental plaque and its importance in the etiology of periodontal disease.
3. Explain the relative importance of calculus in the initiation and progression of periodontal disease.
4. Locate and identify various types and formations of calculus intraorally and radiographically.
5. Summarize current theories of calculus formation.
6. Integrate the periodontal examination into the assessment, planning, and evaluation phases of dental hygiene therapy.
7. Evaluate the following factors associated with the periodontal assessment and determine their significance to periodontal disease:
   a. Pocket depths and periodontal attachement level
   b. Gingival height/recession
   c. Masticatory mucosa
   d. Attached gingiva
   e. Mobility
   f. Furcation involvement
   g. Suppuration
8. Describe the limitations of various types of data collected during the periodontal assessment to document and predict periodontal disease.
9. Monitor the periodontal health status of patients using diagnostic tests and clinical parameters.
10. Perform an effective periodontal probe evaluation in terms of adaptation, angulation of the tip, amount of pressure needed, and number and location of probe readings on each tooth.
11. Identify the significance of the following factors to the periodontal assessment: missing teeth; unerupted, impacted, or supernumerary teeth; malpositioned teeth; open contacts; poorly contoured restorations and crowns; prosthetic devices; and carious lesions.

Periodontal assessment is an important part of dental hygiene care. Its purpose is to correlate the clinical signs and patient symptoms with the presence of or potential for periodontal disease. The information you collect is the basis for diagnosis, treatment plan development, subsequent treatment, follow-up treatment or referral, and continuing care. Knowledge of the periodontium and the clinical indicators of periodontal disease helps you to properly evaluate the patient's periodontal health status.

ETIOLOGY

The complete etiology of inflammatory periodontal diseases is multifaceted. It involves *local factors* that relate to the extent and nature of irritants and *systemic factors* that determine the body's response to the irritants (Fig. 12-1).

Local irritants are those in the immediate environment of the periodontium. They initiate inflammation. *Acquired pellicle, plaque, materia alba,* and *food debris* are the terms used to de-

CHALLENGE:
(shift in bacterial load)

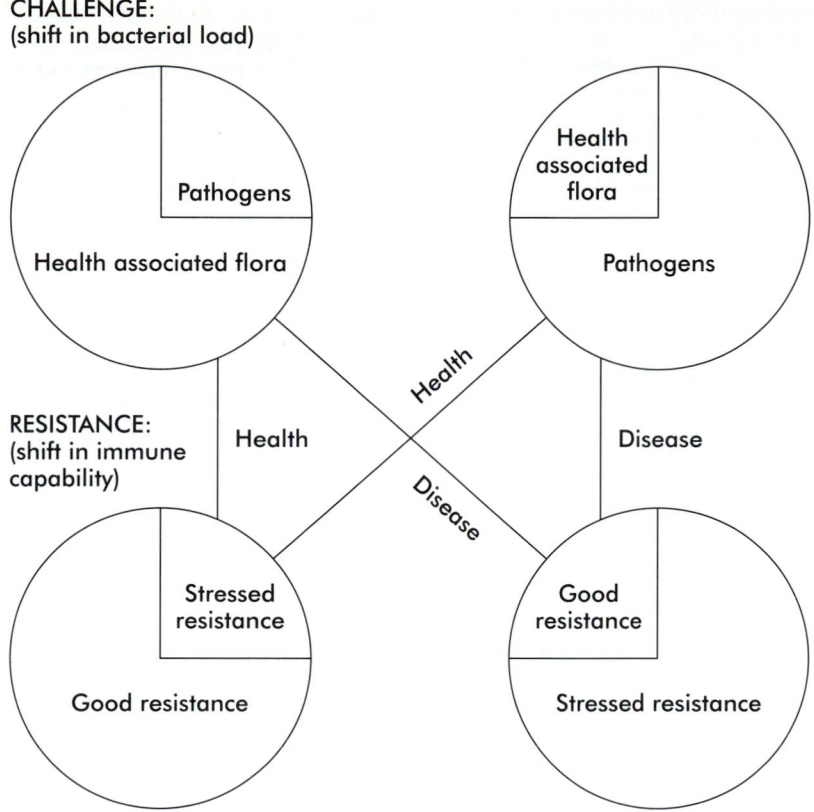

RESISTANCE:
(shift in immune
capability)

Fig. 12-1. *Health* exists when (1) there are few pathogens and/or (2) there is a sufficient host response to control the challenge. *Disease* occurs when (1) there are numerous pathogens and/or (2) there is a compromised or stressed host response to the challenge.

scribe the soft, nonmineralized deposits of the oral cavity. *Calculus* is calcified plaque and described as a hard, mineralized deposit. Although various materials accumulate on the tooth surface, dental or bacterial plaque is considered the primary etiologic factor in the initiation of periodontal disease. Table 12-1 lists the characteristics of each deposit.

Dental plaque

Plaque is a structured, yellow-gray, nearly transparent mass of colonizing bacteria that adheres firmly to the teeth. Microorganisms from the oral environment attach firmly to the salivary glycoproteins and extracellular polysaccharides to form a matrix. This intermicrobial matrix or plaque consists of inorganic and organic components. Initially, plaque is composed of gram-positive cocci. As the plaque matures, an increased number of gram-negative filamentous bacteria and rods appear (Löe et al, 1965). When oral hygiene practices are insufficient or discontinued, the existing microorganisms multiply and different types of bacteria begin to form within the existing microbial matrix.

Microorganisms forming supragingival plaque, coronal to the gingival margin, differ from those in subgingival areas, apical to the gingival margin. Gram-positive bacteria are more predominant in supragingival plaque, whereas more than 75% of the microorganisms in subgingival plaque are gram-negative. On a relatively clean tooth surface, more than 90% of the bacteria are gram-positive. As the plaque matures, the gram-positive microorganisms proliferate, and it is unusual for more than 25% of the plaque sample to con-

Table 12-1. Nonmineralized and mineralized dental deposits

Tooth deposit	Characteristic
Acquired pellicle	A translucent film composed of salivary glycoproteins. The pellicle cannot be removed by rinsing or brushing. It can be removed by professional prophylaxis; however, these acellular deposits will reform within minutes to hours. A disclosing agent will stain the pellicle; it appears much lighter than disclosed plaque or calculus. The acquired pellicle is the initial attachment site for bacteria that will eventually form the organized matrix defined as plaque.
Plaque	A dense coherent mass of bacteria in an organized intermicrobial matrix that adheres to surfaces of the teeth or restorations and remains attached despite muscle action or water rinsing. The primary sources of microbial plaque are oral microorganisms, their toxins, and salivary components.
Materia alba	A loosely adherent complex of bacteria and cellular debris that covers plaque deposits. It is white or gray in color with no uniform structure. Materia alba can be removed by vigorous water rinsing or irrigation.
Food debris	Loosely attached particulate matter that can be dislodged by muscular movements, water rinsing, and proper home care. Food debris can become impacted in plaque, between the teeth, or subgingivally and can be broken down by enzymes from plaque or saliva.
Calculus	A tenacious material formed by the calcification of dental plaque. The calcification process uses minerals found in saliva and sulcular fluid. Dental calculus is classified according to its location on the tooth as supragingival or subgingival.

tain gram-negative flora. In the subgingival plaque, the percentage of gram-negative organisms generally increases in rapidly progressing lesions (Löe et al, 1965; Loesche et al, 1985; Ritz, 1985).

Supragingival plaque, 1 to 2 days old, is composed of mainly *Streptococcus mutans, Streptococcus sanguis,* and *Actinomyces* (gram-positive cocci). *Streptococcus mutans* is considered an acidogenic microorganism and is responsible for enamel caries. It synthesizes carbohydrates into extracellular polysaccharides (dextrans, glucans, and fructans) and intracellular polysaccharides. The dextrans facilitate the plaque's adherence to the tooth's surface.

Plaque that is 3 to 4 days old consists primarily of cocci. There is a significant increase in filamentous bacteria that adhere to the surface of the colonized cocci at the gingival margin. These microorganisms eventually become the predominant species. As the supragingival plaque matures (6 to 10 days later), more complex forms of mixed bacterial flora that are gram-negative and anaerobic begin to appear. Fusobacteria, rods, and spirilla increase in numbers during this time; eventually vibrios and spirochetes will prevail as the plaque becomes older. Ten- to twenty-one-day-old plaque is composed of densely packed spirochetes and vibrios. Inflammation of the gingivae becomes apparent (Listgarten, 1988, Rateitschak et al, 1989).

The subgingival region provides a different environment for microorganisms. When the plaque extends beneath the gingival margin it exists in two forms, adherent and nonadherent plaque. Although both gram-positive and gram-negative microorganisms exist in this area and the microbial composition is similar to that of supragingival plaque, these organisms can be identified by their location on the tooth surface. Adherent plaque develops within the sulcus on the root surface. It is composed primarily of filamentous *Actinomyces,* with decreased numbers of gram-positive cocci. Nonadherent plaque consists of gram-negative anaerobic microorganisms, some of which are motile, including *Porphyromonas, Prevotella, Fusobacterium, Treponema, Campylobacter, Selenomonas,* and *Actinobacillus.* These organisms move around freely near the soft tissues and play an important role in inflammatory lesions (Fine et al, 1978; Slots and Taubman, 1992).

Microorganisms have been found to invade tissues and bone not as colonies but as separate organisms. Individual microorganisms are often seen in histologic sections of tissue and bone. Therefore the disease is referred to as an infection rather than simple inflammation. Toxins produced by subgingival microorganisms adhere to the surface of the cementum, impeding healing and reattachment. The host's response to the presence of microorganisms is a critical factor in the progression of the disease from gingivitis to periodontitis. In rate of healing, a person with impaired abilities to combat the virulent pathogens will be more susceptible to disease (Christersson et al, 1986, 1987; Genco et al, 1990).

Anatomic, physiologic, and iatrogenic factors are also considered local factors and include the following:

1. Supragingival and subgingival calculus provide an ideal foundation for plaque retention because of its surface irregularities and roughness.
2. Tooth malalignment, such as crowded, rotated, or partially erupted teeth, contributes to the accumulation of plaque.
3. Mouth breathing produces drying of the gingiva and teeth. This causes the plaque to be adhesive.
4. Tooth contours, such as the cementum overlapping the enamel, altered tooth structure, abrasion, and erosion, make removing plaque more difficult.
5. Restorative dentistry affects plaque retention if restorations and clasps are not contoured properly.
6. Gingival recession and enlarged, inflamed gingiva favor plaque accumulation.

CALCULUS

One of the technical functions you will perform in providing comprehensive care is the debridement of the teeth. This will include the removal of calculus, subgingival plaque, and endotoxin. *Calculus* is a term used to describe the hardened dental plaque that has accumulated supra-gingivally or subgingivally and is adhering to the teeth. Its primary clinical significance is that it harbors dental plaque on its rough surface, which can impair healing and make it more difficult for the patient to routinely disrupt dental plaque, particularly interdentally and subgingivally. Therefore detecting and removing calculus deposits is an important skill. Other chapters in this text will focus on using instruments to accomplish this goal.

Before periodontal research focused attention on bacterial pathogens, their toxic byproducts, and the host's immune response, the removal of calculus was the central focus of periodontal instrumentation. It was believed that calculus was the cause of periodontal disease. This belief persists among many clinicians, who continue to define the dental hygiene appointment as scaling and polishing augmented by oral hygiene instruction.

For them, the technical skill of thorough calculus removal is central to the performance of dental hygiene care. You will be learning the significance of calculus from a different perspective. You will learn the important skills of exploring for and removing calculus, but this procedure will be positioned differently in terms of importance from the way most of your predecessors have learned it.

This chapter will introduce you to the rationale for these changes and prepare you for further discussion in later chapters.

To locate and identify deposits, it is helpful to examine the different forms calculus can take.

Types of deposits

Calculus deposits vary in shape, size, and color. They may be chalky and relatively soft, or they may be extremely hard and firmly attached to the root structure (Schroeder, 1969). Calculus is frequently found in children. From 56% to 85% of children examined in one study had supragingival deposits; 30% to 67% had subgingival deposits. The occurrence was greater for children 12 to 14 years old than for those 9 to 11 years old. Calculus is more extensive in adults, particularly in those over 30 years old. In children as well as adults, calculus is most commonly found on the lingual aspect of mandibular anterior teeth and on the facial aspect of maxillary molars (Turesky, 1970).

The most common visible deposits are chalky yellow or white, rough *crustaceous* deposits located on the lingual aspect of the mandibular anterior teeth and on the facial aspect of maxillary molars (Alexander, 1971; Baumhammers et al, 1973). These two sites are adjacent to major salivary ducts. As many of the elements known to exist in calculus are found in saliva, the flow of saliva over the teeth is believed to influence the deposition of the hard material on the teeth (Alexander, 1971; Listgarten and Ellegaard, 1973; Mandel, 1972; Mislowsky and Mazzella, 1974). Drying the teeth with air and feeling them with the side of the explorer or probe will make it possible to find these deposits.

Patients who have not had professional scaling for extended periods of time may have a bridge of calculus covering the lingual surfaces of the mandibular teeth, filling the interdental spaces and literally splinting the teeth from cuspid to cuspid. Similar large deposits are sometimes seen on the facial aspect of the maxillary molars as well (Alexander, 1971). (See Plate 2, *A,* and Plate 5 for clinical examples.) One case in the literature reports a calculus deposit so large that a referring dentist mistook it for a bone tumor; it actually aided the patient's mastication (Subash, 1985).

Other unusual formations include a block of calculus in the lower anterior teeth observed in a patient who had not received dental care for 30 years (Walker, 1990). When this deposit was removed with the fingers, two teeth were removed with it. The deposit measured 6 cm in length. A similar mass revealed a horizontally positioned incisor completely encased in the deposit and with no attachment whatsoever to bone or soft tissue (Chuong and Starns, 1990). Another case revealed a stalactite formation of calculus that was so large it caused sores on the opposing tissues (Ackerman, Smith, and Pierce, 1989). During your years as a clinician you will probably provide care for a patient who has such large deposits, but the typical patient has considerably less accumulation.

Visible deposits are referred to as *supragingival,* or *supramarginal,* calculus because they are located coronal to the gingiva. In many instances, a deposit that is visible extends subgingivally into the sulcus or pocket and therefore is both supramarginal and submarginal in location.

Visible deposits are usually softer than subgingival deposits. They are usually amorphous or follow a pattern on the teeth that is molded by the pressure of the tongue or cheek. Efforts to remove the deposits often cause them to crumble. Complete removal of these types of deposits depends on persistence, good visibility, and frequent use of a stream of air to dry the teeth so that remaining particles are apparent. These fine residual deposits will often be visible only with a disclosant solution. If polishing does not remove the disclosant solution and the surface feels rough, the surface of the tooth should be scaled, as the remaining deposit is calculus and not plaque or stain.

Subgingival or submarginal deposits take on a variety of characteristics. They usually are dark brown, green, or black in appearance. They are usually harder than supragingival deposits, and they have a more identifiable form. Their microscopic structure is quite different from that of supragingival calculus (Mislowsky and Mazzella, 1974; Schroeder, 1969).

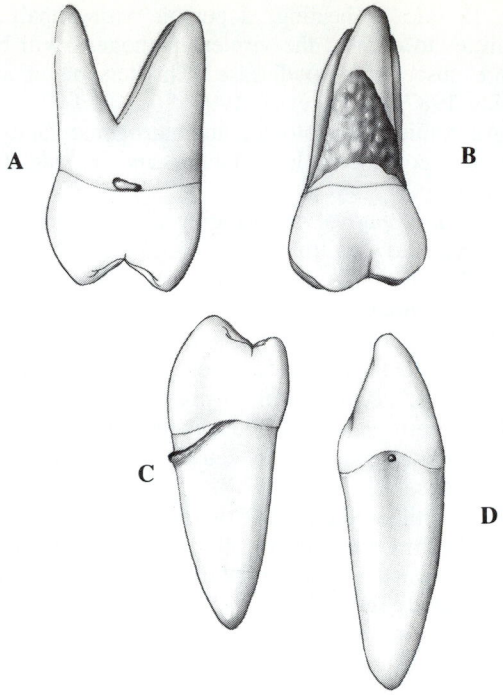

Fig. 12-2. Subgingival calculus can take many forms, including **A**, small spicule or portion of a ledge of calculus in depression on root, especially at cementoenamel junction; **B**, fingerlike or fernlike projection of calculus down the root; **C**, ledge or ring of calculus surrounding all or part of tooth; and, **D**, small nodules of calculus.

Calculus deposits can be long *fernlike* or *fingerlike projections* that are relatively flat against the root surface. They can also be hard spurlike *spicules* that extend outward from the tooth. A deposit can be a ledge or ring of calculus that encircles all or a part of a tooth. Deposits can also be found as hard *nodules* on the tooth surface (Turesky, 1970) (Figs. 12-2 and 12-3). In most instances the calculus is firmly embedded in the tooth surface (cementum) (Singh, Manhold, and Volpe, 1972) and is removed in chunks rather than in crumblings. Deposits can be found deep in periodontal pockets, and usually about halfway into the depth of intrabony defects (Richardson, Chadroff, and Bowers, 1990).

Because the deposits are subgingival, they are rarely visible. It is sometimes possible to direct a stream of air into the sulcus and see subgingival calculus deposits if the tissue is loose around the tooth. If the tissue is relatively tight to the tooth

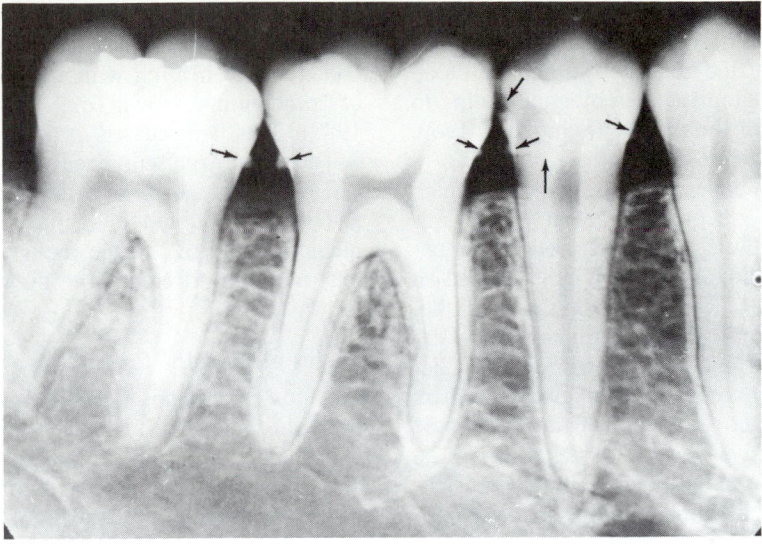

Fig. 12-3. Calculus is observable as spicules extending outward into proximal spaces and as ring around crown of second premolar.Compare radiopacity of calculus with radiolucency of caries on distal aspect of premolar.
(From Wuehrmann AH, Manson-Hing LR: *Dental radiology,* ed 5, St Louis, 1981, CV Mosby.)

and is not overly fibrous, the shadow of the dark calculus can sometimes be seen through the tissue. This is a particularly useful observation when a patient is being seen for a final evaluation of deposit removal and the tissue is healing well. The signs of localized continued inflammation and the dark "shadow" on the tissue stand out as signals that calculus remains in that particular area.

Veneer, or burnished calculus, is a subgingival deposit that has been shaved away rather than fractured away from the tooth in a chunk. With dull instruments or insufficient pressure against the tooth, it is possible simply to shave away the rough parts, leaving a very thin sheet of calculus that is still firmly attached to the tooth and now more difficult to engage and remove with a hand instrument. Two studies that reviewed the problem of residual calculus, (Kepic, O'Leary, and Kafrawy, 1990) showed that while instrumentation greatly reduced the volume of calculus, (Sherman et al, 1990) even the most consciencious instrumentation misses deposits. Robertson, in an editorial review of several studies, concludes that calculus is not the primary etiologic concern in instrumentation, especially since most remaining deposits are veneered and may be relatively inert in the disease process (1990).

In considering calculus deposits and the challenges of complete removal, you will find it helpful to examine the deposits on extracted teeth and to inspect those observable in dental radiographs. It is particularly enlightening to observe the root surfaces during an open flap surgical procedure for your patients after you have completed subgingival instrumentation.

Clinical significance

The presence of calculus is an important part of data gathering in assessing a patient's needs. This information helps you plan appropriate time for periodontal debridement including calculus removal. Calculus has long been associated with diseases of the periodontium, although there is continuing controversy regarding its role in the initiation and/or advancement of disease (Baer, 1970; Hazen, 1970; Mandel, 1986; Robertson, 1990; Schroeder, 1969; Turesky, 1970).

It is undisputed, however, that one phase of reducing and eliminating gingivitis and periodontitis is complete removal of calcareous deposits. These rough deposits harbor volumes of active microorganisms in a covering of dental plaque. The microorganisms irritate the adjacent soft tissues with their by-products (Baumhammers et al, 1973;

Turesky, 1970). Researchers believed that the bulk of the deposit limited the free flow of gingival/sulcular fluids and reduces the natural blood circulation to the gingiva, thereby contributing to the advancement of the disease (Schroeder, 1969; Turesky, 1970).

However, in an experiment using rats in which 2% chlorhexidine gluconate, together with brushing and interdental cleaning, was used over a period of time, junctional epithelial cells formed an attachment to the calculus deposits, perhaps because of decreased plaque formation and decreased toxicity of calculus (Listgarten and Ellegaard, 1973). More recently, Fujikawa and others (1988) demonstrated that clinical and histologic measures of gingival health in dogs could be maintained even in the presence of retained calculus. These are comforting findings that corroborate the clinical observation that patients treated with debridement heal despite the inability of clinicians to remove 100% of deposits. Indeed, though we teach and treat to perfection, calculus remains whether scaling is performed "blind" with a closed flap or with flap surgery to provide visibility and access to the root structure. Caffessee, Sweeney, and Smith (1986) showed that deep deposits remained on 68% of surfaces after closed-flap treatment compared with 50% of surfaces treated with open flaps. Buchanan and Robertson found that 40% of surfaces at deep sites treated with closed flaps, and 18% of those treated with open flaps, had residual calculus. Evaluating multirooted teeth instrumented by experienced clinicians only, Fleischer et al. (1989) found 75% of deep sites treated with closed flaps had residual deposits, compared with 45% of those sites treated with open flaps.

Patients with calculus typically undergo scaling (ultrasonic or hand instruments) before other periodontal or preventive procedures are begun. Instrumentation, in addition to removing a substantial amount of calculus, disturbs the bacterial plaque colonized subgingivally. Historically, scaling procedures (to remove chunks of subgingival calculus) were augmented by definitive root planing to remove "necrotic" cementum and curettage to reduce granulation tissue with the goal of enhancing healing and connective tissue reattachment. A complete review of the findings has caused many researchers to challenge and alter this clinical approach. The research suggests that removing calculus and using a chemical wash or light ultrasonic debridement of the tooth structure will remove endotoxin and create an environment conducive to healing without the "overtreatment" of cementum removal (e.g., see Blomlof et al, 1989). This is discussed in detail in Chapter 25.

Therefore you will need to be able to detect and remove deposits in order to debride the area and disrupt subgingival plaque; however, the methods you use and the focus of your treatment may be quite different from the strategies used in the past.

Stages of calculus formation

Calculus is composed of an organic matrix of bacterial plaque in which calcium (Ca^{2+}) and phosphate (PO_4^-) ions crystallize to form a hard mass (Armitage, 1974; Goldman and Cohen, 1980; Lustmann, Lewis-Epstein, and Shteyer, 1976; Schroeder, 1969). This formation is not simply a precipitation of ions, but rather an orderly deposition of layers of crystals into the matrix (Armitage, 1974; Goldman and Cohen, 1980; Lustmann, Lewis-Epstein, and Shteyer, 1976; Mislowsky and Mazzella, 1974; Schroeder, 1969). Mineralization occurs with the initiation of crystal growth at nucleation sites in the organic matrix (Lustman, Lewis-Epstein, and Shteyer, 1976; Mislowsky and Mazzella, 1974; Schroeder, 1969). The bacteria themselves may calcify intracellularly. Scanning electron photomicrographs show the patterns of microorganisms, which are both hollow and solid with hydroxyapatite and other calcium-phosphate minerals (Lustmann, Lewis-Epstein, and Shteyer, 1976; Schroeder, 1969; Ruzicka, 1984; Sakae, Yamamoto, and Hirai, 1985).

Filamentous organisms are layered over supragingival calculus, whereas subgingival calculus is covered by a mixture of cocci, rods, and filaments. These forms can be seen by examining calculus with a scanning electron microscope. When the filamentous organisms are destroyed with sodium hypochlorite, the calculus shows the patterns of attachment of those microorganisms, which further supports the conclusion that bacteria serve as a matrix for calcification (Friskopp and Hammarström, 1980).

The plaque layer contains small "islands of calcified material"; in some observations, a thin band of calcified plaque material is separated from the calculus by a layer of soft, noncalcified plaque. When viewed with polarized light, supragingival calculus shows "large crystals arranged in rosettes." The border of the calculus shows microorganisms surrounded by needle-shaped crystals (Friskopp, 1983).

Subgingival calculus is not stratified but homogeneous. It is covered with a thin layer of microorganisms, that is not as densely packed as supragingival plaque. It does not contain the crystals characteristic of supragingival plaque associated with calculus (Friskopp, 1983). The mineral content of supragingival calculus is approximately 37% by volume; subgingival calculus mineral content is approximately 58% (Friskopp and Isacsson, 1984).

Hydroxyapatite constitutes approximately 55% of the inorganic components, with octacalcium phosphate (31%), whitlockite (25%), and brushite (5%) being the remaining salts (Armitage, 1974). Supragingival calculus comprises mainly platelet-shaped crystals of octacalcium phosphate and needle-shaped crystals of hydroxyapatite. Subgingival calculus comprises mainly bulk crystals of whitlockite (Sundberg and Friskopp, 1985). A wide variety of trace elements have been identified in calculus (McDougall, 1985; Retief et al, 1972, 1973); including copper (Knuuttila, 1983). Supragingival and subgingival calculus have about the same amounts of calcium, but subgingival calculus has greater zinc and strontium concentrations and supragingival calculus has higher concentrations of manganese (Knuuttila et al, 1979).

The first stage of calculus formation requires, according to many researchers, the presence of acquired pellicle on the teeth (Canis et al, 1979; Schroeder, 1969). Schroeder (1969) has defined the pellicle as the *exogenous dental cuticle* and describes it as an unstructured, homogeneous layer that adheres directly to and penetrates into the crystalline tooth structure, as well as to all other firm surfaces in the oral cavity, and to old dental calculus. It is rapidly formed and renewed constantly. It is presumably formed by microbially altered salivary glycoproteins and is thin (Schroeder, 1969). Bacterial plaque attaches to this exogenous dental cuticle. Given the appropriate conditions, calcification begins. When the plaque pH rises above the pH in the saliva, calcification occurs. The rise may result from production of urea, ammonia, and amines through protein breakdown in the plaque (Driessens et al, 1985). Bacteria become encased in the forming

calculus. Gram-negative cocci have been seen to contain "spherules of amorphous calcium phosphate within the cytoplasm" as they are converted to the hard calculus substance (Sidaway, 1980).

Brushite is formed during the initial stages of calcification. It is slowly transformed into the less porous form of calculus, whitlockite. Thus calculus close to the tooth is harder and less porous, whereas that at the outer layers which is exposed to saliva is porous (Kani et al, 1983). Calculus close to the cementum often is hardly distinguishable from the tooth structure when viewed microscopically because of its solid structure and its mechanical interlocking with the microscopic topography of the cementum (Canis et al, 1979).

Hard deposits may be detected as early as 2 days after thorough cleansing, although it may require 12 days or more for undisturbed deposits of plaque to calcify and mature (Schroeder, 1969). There is great variability among individuals regarding how rapidly deposits form (Mandel, 1972). The saliva of calculus formers seems to have a higher phosphate precipitation rate (Mukherjee, 1986). Higher levels of calcium ions and urea in the saliva of the submaxillary salivary gland correlate with rapid deposit formation (Mandel, 1972; Schroeder, 1969). Studies indicate that smokers are more likely to have calculus deposits than nonsmokers (Feldman, Alman, and Chauncey, 1987; Kowalski, 1971).

As the calculus matures, the deeper layers of microorganisms calcify. Additional layers of plaque accumulate, and the process continues as the deposit grows. Subgingival calculus contains fewer microorganisms than supragingival deposits. The current theory, as originally suggested by Black about 1900, is that subgingival calculus draws its calcium phosphate crystals from the exudate of the inflamed tissue that covers it rather than from saliva (Schroeder, 1969). As mentioned earlier, subgingival calculcus is extremely hard and is often dark green or brown in color in contrast to the yellow color of most supragingival calculus.

Microorganisms are directly related to calculus formation. Greater numbers of microorganisms are associated with the presence of calculus (Singh, Manhold, and Volpe, 1972). The role of microorganisms appears to be largely one of providing a matrix of mineralization (Mislowsky and Mazzella, 1974). Devital microorganisms calcify more readily, because acid by-products of microorganisms are antagonistic to crystal nucleation (Schroeder, 1969).

One study suggests that calculus formation is enhanced by the enzymes contained in the layers of dental plaque that cover the forming deposit (Friskopp and Hammarström, 1982). Protease activity (perhaps derived from epithelial cells in salivary sediment rather than from plaque microorganisms) seems to be higher in subjects who tend to form supragingival calculus (Morita and Watanabe, 1986).

People who are heavy calculus formers show about 60% more lipid weight in their saliva compared with light calculus formers. Light calculus formers have much higher levels of free cholesterol and triglycerides in their saliva, whereas the saliva of heavy calculus formers contains more free fatty acids and cholesterol esters. Thus researchers suspect that salivary lipids play a role in calculus formation (Slomiany et al, 1981). The calculus matrix actually contains fatty acids, probably contributed by saliva and microorganisms (Slomiany et al, 1983).

Two distinct types of mineralization centers are seen in calculus: type A centers, which are initiated by and formed with microorganisms, and adjacent type B centers, which appear unrelated to microorganisms (Lustmann, Lewis-Epstein, and Shteyer, 1976; Schroeder, 1969).

Calculus can form without the presence of any microorganisms, but its nature is quite different. Such sterile calculus is much like mother-of-pearl and does not have the extremely rough surface characteristics of naturally occurring calculus (Theilade, Fitzgerald, and Scott, 1964).

Calculus deposits penetrate the irregularities of the tooth surface, creating a mechanical lock between the deposit and the tooth (Canis et al, 1979; Selvig, 1970). This is particularly true in areas where a preceding carious process, resorption lacunae, planing grooves, and other defects have created pathways for attachment. One investigator found "minute, atypical crystals within the surface layer of enamel and carious dentin immediately underneath calculus . . . [that] were similar in size to the crystals seen in the adjacent concrement, and characteristically different in size and orientation from the normal crystals of these hard tissues" (Selvig, 1970). When the calculus was chipped off, long needlelike crystals remained. This explains the difficulty frequently encountered in removing mature deposits.

Research into the causes and clinical significance of calculus continues. As the many questions about it are finally answered, the clinician's role continues to be, in part, to locate and remove the deposits in combination with helping the patient achieve a high degree of personal control over factors affecting calculus reaccumulation.

Several dentifrices and oral rinses are available for consumer use to minimize calculus formation. Pyrophosphate (Schiff, 1987) and zinc chloride (Lobene et al, 1987) are demonstrated to have an anticalculus effect if used daily as a part of normal oral hygiene. These ingredients do not reduce plaque formation; rather, they inhibit the calcification of the plaque. They can be recommended to patients who have a propensity for heavy calculus buildup.

Detecting calculus

Calculus can be seen in dental radiographs (see Chapter 10). Reviewing a radiographic survey can assist in locating deep deposits and those near margins of restorations, which might be easily missed.

Clinically, calculus can be detected most easily with a periodontal probe or an explorer. Ensure that the instrument tip traces the entire subgingival area from attachment to margin of gingivae. Move the instrument sufficiently across the proximal surface to ensure that the center of the proximal surface is explored from both aspects of the tooth (facial and lingual). Calculus tends to attach in the furrows and other indentations on the teeth, particularly on the mesial and distal aspects. Exploring short of the midpoint of the proximal surface will probably result in undetected deposits (Fig. 12-4).

Also, thoroughly explore the corners or line angles of the teeth. A clinician frequently will explore the proximal surfaces thoroughly and then, when turning the instrument to explore the direct facial and lingual surfaces, missing the corner of the root (Fig. 12-5). Spicules of calculus are then left uncharted.

When patients have a low prevalence of plaque and gingivitis, the role of irregular or malposed teeth in the formation of calculus becomes more obvious. There is a positive correlation between malposed teeth and calculus formation (Buckley, 1980, 1981); thus careful exploration for calculus in these areas is important and often challenging because of the limited access caused by the mal-

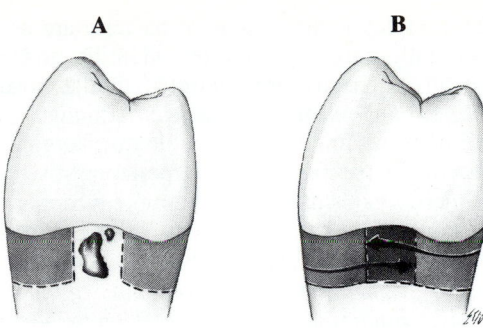

Fig. 12-4. When proximal area is being explored, explorer must cover tooth surface past midpoint of proximal surface. **A,** If exploratory strokes are stopped short of midpoint, calculus in furrows of root and directly below contact area will not be detected. **B,** Exploring past midpoint of tooth from both facial and lingual aspects will ensure that this critical portion of the tooth is thoroughly examined.

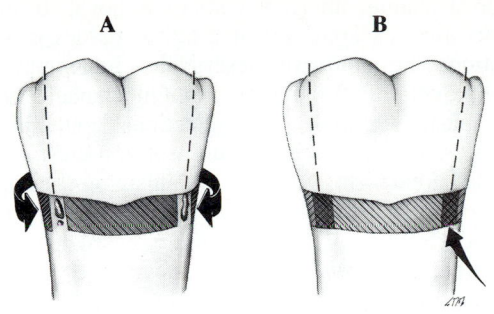

Fig. 12-5. A, Calculus remains undetected on line angles of teeth, **B,** unless exploratory strokes used to cover facial aspect overlap with strokes covering proximal aspects. Undetected calculus at "corners" of teeth is a common error of beginning clinicians.

positions. Even for patients who practice good oral hygiene, deposits are likely to form in these areas.

As each tooth is explored, it should be examined for the presence of supragingival calculus as well, using air and light and by tracing the tip of the explorer over the visible tooth structure. After determining the overall location and extent of deposits, you can determine which instruments are appropriate for deposit removal and debridement (see Chapters 25 and 26). After thoroughly treating the areas, explore to detect remaining deposits. As you locate each deposit, select the appropriate instrument to remove it before continuing.

Scoring calculus

If you function as a research clinician, you may find it necessary to quantitate the amount of calculus present on teeth. The most widely used indices in epidemiologic studies are the Periodontal Disease Index (PDI) (Ramfjord, 1959) and the Oral Hygiene Index (OHI) (Greene and Vermillion, 1960) or OHI-simplified index (OHIS) (Greene and Vermillion, 1964) in which only six teeth are scored. Calculus is an important component in these indices. In the PDI, presence of calculus is described as *slight, moderate,* or *abundant* for grades *1, 2,* and *3,* respectively. In the OHI indices, both supragingival and subgingival calculus are evaluated. Both the PDI and OHI require the use of an explorer to detect the amount and/or location of calculus deposits. These indices

are recommended for routine use because of their widespread acceptance and reproducibility (Volpe, 1974).

These and other methods have been developed to quantitate calculus on specific tooth surfaces. When they were compared in determining the effect of unsupervised toothbrushing on calculus formation after 1 to 2 weeks, all scoring methods showed significant effects; the greatest reduction was scored using the Volpe-Manhold probe method (Turesky, 1970).

This method measures the extent of a supragingival deposit in three planes (vertical and diagonally across the deposit from the mesioincisal and distoincisal edges) on the lingual surfaces of the six mandibular anterior teeth with a periodontal probe graduated in millimeters. The Volpe-Manhold probe method is most useful in doing clinical surveys; but it is of limited value in planning dental care for individual patients, because it assesses only selected teeth, does not address subgingival deposits, and requires that the examiner be highly trained (Volpe, 1974).

PATHOGENESIS

Periodontal disease's two main forms are gingivitis and periodontitis. *Gingivitis* is described as inflammation of the gingiva with no apparent attachment loss. Its primary cause is the presence and composition of bacterial plaque in and around the gingival sulcus. Secondary causes include factors that contribute to the accumulation of supragingival plaque, interfere with its removal, or enhance the susceptibility of gingival tissues to infection. *Periodontitis* is described as inflammation and infection of the periodontium characterized by apical migration of the junctional epitheilium with associated loss of attachment and crestal alveolar bone. The biologic and histologic events that occur in the tissues during the process of conversion from a healthy state to a diseased state are referred to as *pathogenesis*.

The process of gingival and periodontal inflammation has been described in terms of four progressive phases. The first phase is called the *initial lesion* and is the normal response of these tissues to the early plaque colonization. It occurs within 4 days of plaque accumulation. It includes increased vascular response and increased permeability of tissues to allow the passage of fluid and cells from the blood into the affected area. As almost everyone normally has some plaque accumulation in the mouth, there is some disagreement as to whether or not this category can be said to include healthy tissues as well as the initial stages of inflammation. Clinically, there is no clear-cut line of demarcation between the two situations. The *early lesion* is the second phase. It begins about 1 week after the formation of plaque. It includes the clinical signs of gingivitis in addition to the presence of lymphocytes and macrophages. The *established lesion* follows and is characterized by the further destruction of connective tissue fibers, the formation of a gingival pocket, and a predominance of plasma cells in the tissues. Some cases of established gingivitis remain stable and do not progress for months or even years, while other cases may rapidly convert to progressive destructive lesions. The last phase of inflammation, the *advanced lesion,* is characterized by the destruction of supporting tissues as well as gingival tissues and is also known as *periodontitis*. Although these levels of disease are described as stages, it is important to remember that activities within these stages can stabilize for long periods or even cease altogether, and that reversals can occur either spontaneously or as a result of treatment.

Chronic gingivitis and periodontitis are associated with the presence of microbial plaque. As periodontal disease progresses, the composition of the microbial plaque begins to change. Bacteria associated with a healthy sulcus are predominantly nonmotile, gram-positive cocci and rods.

More complex compositions of bacteria are associated with gingivitis and periodontitis and include an increasing proportion of motile, gram-negative, and anaerobic species. Although evidence does not implicate a specific microorganism as the major pathogen in adult periodontitis, certain microorganisms seem to be more strongly associated with this disease than others. Among these are *Prevotella intermedia* (formerly *Bacteroides intermedius*), *Porphyromonas gingivalis* (formerly *Bacteroides gingivalis*), *Campylobacter rectus* (formerly *Wolinella rectus*), *Actinobacillus actinomycetemcomitans*, *Treponema denticola*, and *Bacteriodes forsythus* (Loesche et al, 1985; Shah and Collins, 1988, 1990; Slots, 1986; Slots and Taubman, 1992). These pathogenic microganisms contain or release substances that cause inflammatory responses in the gingival and periodontal tissues (Lindhe, 1983). Even a healthy gingival sulcus has some pathogenic bacteria and a slight inflammatory response (connective tissue infiltrate) at all times (Page and Schroeder, 1976). However, the body's defense mechanisms and the ability of the microorganisms to cause infection are in balance; in other words, an equilibrium exists that allows both entities to coexist without a battle. When this equilibrium is maintained, there is no need for the body to initiate a full-scale inflammatory reaction to control the microorganisms; therefore, there are no overt inflammatory signs within the tissues (Listgarten, 1988).

However, if the host response is compromised, fewer bacteria may be tolerated, causing severe destruction and an opportunity for proliferation. Likewise, even in the absence of an infection, the body may persist in fighting the imagined invasion, causing progressive self-destruction from an unchecked inflammatory reaction. Understanding the biologic mechanisms of the pathogenesis underlying the periodontal disease, coupled with clinical observations, permits improved clinical investigations that ultimately will improve therapeutic approaches (Suzuki, 1988).

Host response

The body has three major biologic mechanisms for controlling and responding to infection: (1) the nonspecific defense mechanisms, (2) the specific defense mechanisms, and (3) the body's process of repair and regeneration.

The *nonspecific defense mechanisms* are activated when the host is challenged by a specific invader for the first time. When the defenses of salivary chemistry and flow and mucous membrane barriers are insufficient to stop the bacterial challenge, an army of inflammatory cells, polymorphonuclear leukocytes, and macrophages localize, engulf, and destroy the pathogens. The complement system (a group of serum proteins) assists in the removal of bacteria from the infected area, using two distinct mechanisms. The first is the *classical pathway*, which directly destroys the pathogens by attaching complement components to the invaders. When only some of the complement components are attached they act as a homing device for the phagocytes, making it easier for the phagocytes to engulf and kill the bacteria; this is the *alternate pathway*. Physical barriers, phagocytosis, and the complement system all cooperate in the generalized inflammatory response that usually characterizes the nonspecific defense mechanism.

In addition there is a generalized inflammatory response. An increase in blood flow and capillary permeability causes the cardinal signs of imflammation to appear: redness, swelling, heat, and pain (or a change in tactile sensitivity).

The *specific defense mechanisms* are activated when an invader appears subsequent to an initial infection by a bacterial pathogen or other foreign substance. This specific immune response is divided into two parts: the cellular immune response associated with the production of T-lymphocytes (T-cells) and the humoral immune response associated with the production of B-lymphocytes (B-cells).

The T-cells of the cellular immune response act as helper cells; suppressor cells, which regulate the immune response; and cytotoxic lymphocytes, which are capable of destroying cells. The B-lymphocytes from the humoral response mature into plasma cells that produce antibodies classified as immunoglobin G (IgG), IgM, IgA, IgD, and IgE, according to their form and function. These antibodies are involved in bacterial toxin neutralization.

The final biologic mechanism for controlling infection is the varying ability of tissues to undergo repair and/or regeneration to restore their natural barriers and functions, which may have been damaged as a result of infection and the inflammatory process. Both the specific and nonspecific defense mechanisms can damage cells that are infected or just innocent bystanders. This

can result in death of the host cells as well as pathogens. When these cells die, their contents are released into the host and can be measured in the gingival crevicular fluid. This knowledge has sparked a new area of research relating to the diagnosis of periodontal disease and will be discussed later in the chapter.

It is important to note that the equilibrium between existing microorganisms and body tissues can be maintained over an indefinite time as long as both the host tissue and the bacteria remain balanced in strength. However, a situation that overchallenges these mechanisms or a weak link in the system upsets the equilibrium established between pathogens and the body, resulting in infection, inflammation, and associated tissue destruction.

PERIODONTAL DISEASES
Gingivitis

Gingivitis can be either *acute* or *chronic*. An acute inflammation is one which occurs suddenly, is associated with pain, and is of short duration. Acute necrotizing ulcerative gingivitis and acute herpetic gingivostomatitis are examples of acute inflammatory reactions in the gingiva. Chronic gingivitis, in contrast, begins slowly, lasts a long time, and is usually painless unless the tissues become secondarily infected. Gingivitis may also be *recurrent,* meaning that it returns following treatment or disappears spontaneously and then reappears.

Gingivitis may vary in severity at different sites in the mouth and show varying patterns of distribution within the mouth, depending on the presence and composition of bacterial plaque. *Localized gingivitis* is confined to a specific area of the mouth, whereas *generalized gingivitis* involves the entire mouth. *Papillary gingivitis* involves the interdental papillae and may extend onto adjacent marginal gingiva. Most gingivitis develops first in the interdental papilla and then spreads to adjacent tissues. *Marginal gingivitis* involves the gingival margins of the teeth in addition to the papillae and may also include a portion of the attached gingiva. *Diffuse gingivitis* involves inflammation of all involved gingival tissues including papillae, marginal gingiva, and attached gingiva.

Epidemiology. Marginal gingivitis may appear in early childhood, increases in prevalence and severity through the teenage years, and then levels off and becomes less severe in young adults.

Table 12-2. Gingival assessment: clinical characteristics

Clinical characteristic	Ideal/Normal	Abnormal
Color	Uniformly coral pink Variations may occur depending on patient's complexion and race	Acute—bright red Chronic—red, bluish red, dark pink Color changes may be restricted to papilla or extend to marginal and attached gingiva.
Contour	Margins are knifelike Contour of free margin forms regular parabolic curve as it goes around teeth Papillae are pointed and fill embrasure space	Margins become rolled, bulbous, enlarged; irregular contour may be noted; clefting, festooning Papillae may be flattened, bulbous, blunted, or cratered
Size	Free margin is near cementoenamel junction (CEJ) Margin adheres closely to tooth	Enlarged because of excess fluid in tissues (edematous) or buildup of collagen fibers (fibrotic) Margin may be retracted away from tooth with air or instrument
Consistency	Firm	Edematous, soft, spongy; pressure on tissues with an instrument will leave a dent Fibrotic, firm, hard tissue
Surface texture	Smooth free gingiva Stippled attached gingiva	Acute—loss of stippling; smooth, shiny Chronic—stippling present; may increase in occurrence
Position of gingival margin	1 to 2 mm above CEJ in fully erupted teeth	May be enlarged so that margin is more coronal than CEJ May show apical recession so that root surface is exposed
Position of junctional epithelium	At CEJ in fully erupted teeth	Apical migration onto root surface
Mucogingival junction	Clear distinction between appearance of attached gingiva (pink, stippled, immobile, firm) and alveolar mucosa (red, shiny, smooth, mobile)	Lack of attached gingiva determined by 1. loss of junctional line 2. Mobility of all existing tissues 3. Probing extends beyond mucogingival junction
Bleeding	No bleeding detectable with palpation or probing	Spontaneous bleeding Bleeding resulting from probing
Exudate	No exudate with palpation or probing	Increase in amount of clear crevicular fluid Presence of white fluid (pus) with palpation

Data from Goldman and Cohen, 1980; Wilkins, 1989.

Although there are very few data regarding the prevalence of gingivitis in adults, estimates are that it affects from 50% to 100% of adults who still have natural teeth. The elderly do not appear to have higher prevalence rates than the rest of the adult population. Overall, the prevalence of gingivitis appears to be declining.

Males usually have higher levels of gingival inflammation than females, although a significant number of women experience more severe gingivitis during pregnancy (*pregnancy gingivitis*). African-Americans tend to have a higher prevalence of gingivitis than whites, although these higher rates are likely related to factors such as oral hygiene, socioeconomic status, and access to dental care (Stamm, 1986).

Clinical signs. Clinical detection of gingivitis depends on recognition of inflammatory signs within the gingival tissues. In the early stages of inflammation, these signs may be subtle and difficult to discern; they become more obvious as the inflammation becomes established. The gingival tissues should be examined for signs of bleeding, exudate, or abnormal color; size; contour; consistency; surface texture; position; or pain. Table 12-2 lists characteristic signs of normal and abnormal (inflamed) gingival tissues. The significance of each of these clinical characteristics to the periodontal examination will be discussed in detail later in this chapter.

Acute forms. Although chronic gingivitis is the more common type of gingival inflammation, you should also be able to recognize signs and symptoms of acute gingival inflammation. The presence of pain and rapid destruction of affected tissues makes it imperative that these conditions are promptly diagnosed and treated. It is your responsibility, as a dental hygienst, to recognize acute infections during the periodontal examination, gather assessment information, record significant findings in the patient's record, and report those findings in the diagnosis and treatment plan.

Acute necrotizing ulcerative gingivitis. Acute necrotized ulcerative gingivitis (ANUG) is an acute gingival inflammation also known as trench mouth, Vincent's gingivitis, Vincent's gingivostomatitis, and necrotizing gingivitis. It is most prevalent in young adults between the ages of 17 and 35 and is associated with factors other than those which cause chronic gingivitis. This is a complex disease and not a simple infectious process; although it is believed not to be communicable, the pathogenic mechanisms are still somewhat unclear. It can occur repeatedly in some patients, resulting in extensive periodontal destruction, referred to as necrotizing ulcerative periodontics (NUP). Currently implicated bacteria include spirochetes, fusiform bacteria, and *Prevotella intermedia*. However they seem to act as opportunistic pathogens that require the presence of underlying changes in the tissues to produce disease. Among the specific factors most frequently implicated in the occurrence of ANUG and NUP are (1) lowered host resistance as a result of diseases such as blood dyscrasias, malnutrition, Down's syndrome, or terminal cancer or associated with the use of steroids; (2) acute emotional stress and anxiety as occurs during war, examinations, or marital trouble; and (3) poor oral hygiene in the presence of an existing chronic gingivitis and smoking. Some evidence indicates that ANUG is an autoimmune disorder, because these conditions (poor oral hygiene, gingivitis, emotional stress, and lowered host resistance) can exist in individuals who never develop ANUG.

The most obvious clinical sign of ANUG is ulceration of the marginal gingiva and interdental papilla. This destruction begins with the appearance of a necrotic ulcer on the papilla that rapidly progresses until the entire papilla is destroyed, leaving a central depression or crater where the intact papilla once stood. The necrosis spreads to the adjacent marginal gingiva and other papillae. The affected gingiva is often covered with a grayish or yellowish "pseudomembrane," composed of necrotic tissue, bacteria, and destroyed blood cells, which forms over the red, raw, exposed connective tissues. This lesion is extremely painful and exacerbated by a continued lack of plaque control (see Plate 3, *I*). Spontaneous bleeding and a characteristic foul odor are common. In advanced cases swelling of the regional lymph nodes (regional lymphadenitis) may also be present.

The initial treatment of ANUG involves relief of the acute symptoms by removing local etiologic factors. Gross scaling, preferably accomplished with an ultrasonic scaler, will help relieve the acute symptoms. This initial debridement can be followed at a later appointment by more definitive instrumentation when the pain and discomfort have been reduced. Patients should be instructed to perform gentle but thorough plaque control in all areas. As it is painful to touch the inflamed tissues, brushing and frequent rinsing should be instituted first, followed by flossing or other interdental cleansing after some healing has occurred. The patient should rinse the mouth frequently with equal parts of hydrogen peroxide and warm water as a supplement to plaque control.

Following removal of all local etiologic factors, the other cause-related factors (such as poor oral hygiene habits, smoking, and stress) must be addressed to avoid recurrence. After initial therapy has been completed, periodontal surgery may be indicated to restore the anatomy of the area; this will support the patient's plaque removal efforts (Goldman and Cohen, 1980; Johnson and Engel, 1986; Lindhe, 1983).

Acute herpetic gingivostomatitis. Acute herpetic gingivostomatitis is an infection of the oral tissues caused by the herpes simplex virus. Clinically, this infection appears as diffuse redness of the mucosa with associated edema, gingival bleeding, and pain. Vesicles form initially and later rupture to form small painful ulcers, which make chewing, eating, or drinking extremely uncomfortable for the patient until they have healed. The disease runs a course of about 7 to 10 days, with the most acute stages lasting for 2 to 3 days.

This disease is seen most commonly in children under the age of 6, but it can also occur in older children and adults.

Desquamative gingivitis. Desquamative gingivitis is the term used to describe the gingival manifestations of a variety of systemic disturbances, most notably lichen planus or mucous membrane pemphigoid. Mild forms occur most often in girls and young women and appear as diffuse painless redness (erythema) of the gingival tissues. Moderate forms occur most often in persons between the ages of 30 and 40 and are accompanied by burning sensations and sensitivity to temperature changes. Individuals with desquamatine gingivitis may be unable to tolerate spicy or rough-textured foods or may experience pain during toothbrushing. Clinically, the tissues may appear smooth and shiny, with patches of bright red and gray. The surface epithelium may peel away from the underlying tissues, exposing a raw, bleeding, and extremely painful surface. These signs and symptoms become worse as more severe forms of the infection develop.

Treatment of this condition is mainly palliative and involves careful plaque control with a soft brush and oxidizing mouthwashes (such as one part hydrogen peroxide to two parts warm water) (Carranza and Perry, 1986). Careful examination of the patient's medical history and oral conditions is necessary to identify the exact nature of the infection or infections contributing to the symptoms. Once the contributing factors have been identified, the dentist can determine the need for systemic therapy or other treatment.

Pericoronitis. A localized gingivitis that occurs around a partially erupted tooth, such as an erupting third molar, is called pericoronitis. The gingival tissue overlying the partially erupted crown is a prime area for accumulation of plaque and food impaction. The nature of the inflammation may be acute, subacute, or chronic. Acute inflammation of these areas is characterized by swelling, redness, exudate, and pain which may radiate to areas in the ear, throat, or floor of the mouth. Tenderness of lymph nodes, facial swelling, inability to close the mouth, fever, and malaise may also be associated with acute pericoronitis.

Treatment involves local removal of the bacterial and other irritants and use of antibacterial or antiseptic rinses. Systemic symptoms may require antibiotic treatment.

Acute gingival abscess. A gingival abscess is a localized, painful, and rapidly progressing lesion that develops suddenly and appears as a red, swollen, smooth, shiny, and painful area. Within 24 to 48 hours, the inflammatory process results in a localized accumulation of pus, causing the lesion to "point" so that exudate can be expressed from its orifice. An abscess can develop in response to a puncture or irritation by a sharp object, such as a toothbrush bristle, or when foreign substances, such as popcorn hulls, become embedded in the tissue. These lesions usually rupture spontaneously, expel the foreign materials, and heal.

Inflammation caused by systemic factors. The following systemic factors may cause inflammation of the gingival tissue.

Pregnancy gingivitis. Changes in the hormonal balances and tissue metabolism during pregnancy can result in exaggerated responses of gingival tissue to local irritants and plaque. The clinical response to irritants under these conditions may result in generalized signs of gingivitis, including gingival enlargement, redness, and bleeding, either on probing or spontaneously. Gingivitis related to pregnancy may also be manifested as localized enlargements of gingiva, known as "pregnancy tumors." These tumors appear as raised spherical lesions that extend from the gingival margin or the interdental papillae and are attached by a sessile or pedunculated base to the underlying tissues. Treatment includes removal of local irritants through professional and personal plaque control methods.

Puberty gingivitis. Enlargement of gingival tissues may also occur as an exaggerated response to local irritation in both boys and girls during puberty. The interdental papillae are the areas most often affected. Treatment involves individual plaque control and professional removal of calculus and other local irritants. Once the hormonal changes associated with puberty have moderated, the exaggerated response of the gingival tissues to plaque and calculus subsides.

Other systemic factors that may affect the gingival response to inflammation include use of oral contraceptives, diabetes mellitus, diseases that affect the immune response, nutritional deficiencies, allergy, and metal poisoning.

Gingival hyperplasia. Use of the anticonvulsant drug phenytoin (Dilantin) can lead to chronic enlargement (hyperplasia) of the gingiva. The lesion begins as a firm, pale pink, resilient enlargement of the gingival margin and interdental tissues that shows no bleeding tendency unless aggravated by secondary inflammation. Enlargement occurs gradually and can continue until a large portion of the crowns of the teeth are covered by tissue overgrowth, which can interfere with occlusion. Local irritants need not be present for this enlargement to occur, but they can result in a secondary inflammation that further complicates the existing hyperplasia. When gingival hyperplasia becomes a functional or esthetic problem the tissue can be surgically removed; however, the condition will recur unless use of the drug is discontinued.

Periodontitis

When the destruction reaches the level of the connective tissues that form the attachment to the root of the tooth, gingivitis becomes periodontitis. It is important to note: that not all sites affected by gingivitis will progress to periodontitis. Periodontal disease is an inflammation and infection that causes destruction of the supporting tissues of the tooth, including loss of connective tissue attachment to the root surface; loss of periodontal ligament fibers, and loss of alveolar bone. Over time, continued periodontal destruction is associated with the development of deep pockets, gingival recession, exposure of furcations, mobility, secondary occlusal traumatism, and the ultimate consequence of tooth loss. Periodontal disease is a chronic condition that is progressive and destructive. The severity of the condition increases with age.

Although most cases of periodontitis fall into the category of *adult periodontitis,* a number of other categories of periodontitis affecting younger individuals have been categorized as *juvenile periodontitis, prepubertal periodontitis,* and *rapidly progressing periodontitis* (Page and Schroeder, 1976). Table 12-3 lists the categories of periodontal disease (American Academy of Periodontology, 1989).

Periodontal disease is currently considered to be a group of infections rather than a single infection with a single cause. Each periodontal infection is associated with different and specific groups of microorganisms (Newman, 1985). No single bacterial species has been identified as the primary cause of active periodontal disease. Instead different bacteria already present in the

Table 12-3. Classification of periodontal diseases

I. Adult periodontitis
II. Early onset periodontitis
   A. Prepubertal peridontitis
      1. Localized
      2. Generalized
   B. Juvenile periodontitis
      1. Localized
      2. Generalized
   C. Rapidly progressive
III. Periodontitis associated with systemic disease
IV. Necrotizing ulcerative periodontitis
  V. Refractory periodontitis

From American Academy of Periodontology, 1989.

mouth appear to combine to produce the pathogenic potential necessary to initiate the progression from gingivitis to destructive periodontitis (Theilade, 1986). The exact nature of these microbial combinations is likely to differ depending on the person and the specific site. Pathogenicity is also related to the host response, so bacteria that are pathogenic in one person may not be destructive in another. Because of the complex interrelationships of all these factors, it is difficult to determine the exact bacterial cause of periodontal disease and the conditions that must exist to predict disease activity (Socransky et al, 1987).

Active periodontal destruction occurs with differing levels of severity and at different rates in selected sites in the same person. Periodontal disease is site specific, meaning that the onset of the disease can occur in some areas of the mouth without affecting others (Haffajee et al, 1983; Socransky et al, 1984). The disease is cyclical in nature and does not progress in a linear fashion over time. Instead, it occurs in short bursts of intense activity and destruction followed by periods of remission, which can last months or years (Lindhe, 1983). Each burst of activity, however, results in additional destruction of the periodontal tissues, so that over a long period of time the apparent result is a steady progression of disease.

The progression from health to gingivitis to periodontitis is characterized by long periods of remission and spontaneous reversals of disease interspersed with short bursts of destructive activity

(Lindhe 1983; Page 1986). Some individuals are more susceptible to periodontal disease, as are specific sites within the mouth of the same individual. Even after treatment, some individuals remain more susceptible than others to recurrence of the disease, as only a small percentage of treated patients account for most of the recurrences.

The prognoses for gingivitis and periodontitis are quite different. The damaged epithelium and connective tissues that form the gingival unit can regenerate if the cause of the inflammation, called the *etiologic agent,* is removed from the soft tissue environment. Therefore simple gingivitis can often be treated quite successfully and the tissues brought back to normal form and function. Supporting bone does not have the same ability to repair and restore itself after being destroyed by the inflammatory process. Restoring bone and connective tissue fibers typically requires special surgical procedures that create an environment for bone fill and regeneration. The prognosis for periodontally involved teeth greatly depends on the extent of bone loss. Another result of periodontal disease is apical migration of the junctional epithelium and loss of connective tissue attachment, which result in the formation of deep periodontal pockets that are difficult, if not impossible, for the patient to maintain free of plaque. The preferred method of preventing periodontitis and restoring the tissues to complete health is to recognize early signs of gingival inflammation and to eliminate the etiologic factors that cause it. It is especially important to teach the patient to control etiologic factors, mainly dental plaque, before the condition develops into periodontitis. Guided tissue regeneration is a relatively new surgical procedure, that stops the apical migration of the epithelium during healing, allowing the connective tissues to fill and repair the area.

Occlusal traumatism. Another form of periodontal disease is not inflammatory but degenerative in nature. In this condition, known as *occlusal traumatism,* the supporting structures of affected teeth are damaged because they cannot withstand the occlusal forces acting on them. The result is a breakdown of the periodontal ligament fibers, loss of supporting bone, widening of the periodontal ligament space, and tooth mobility. When this destruction is caused by excessive occlusal forces acting on an otherwise normal periodontium, the condition is referred to as *primary occlusal trauma*. The sources of the pressure may include bruxism, night grinding, malocclusion, or poorly constructed dental restorations. These factors can produce more stress than the supporting structures can withstand, and the result is slow destruction. *Secondary occlusal trauma* is the result of normal occlusal forces on an attachment apparatus that has already been damaged and weakened by periodontitis. Some of the clinical signs of occlusal trauma include a widened periodontal ligament space, root fractures, loss of lamina dura, mobility, and signs of attrition or facets on the crowns of teeth (Grant et al, 1988), (see Chapter 14).

THE PERIODONTAL EXAMINATION

The information gathered and recorded during the periodontal examination will assist you in correlating all factors that might aid in assessing and describing each patient's level of periodontal health or disease. Without the information from a complete periodontal examination, diagnosis and treatment planning are a hit-and-miss proposition, based on conjecture and not on reliable observed data.

In addition to the periodontal charting, many other diagnostic aids contribute vital information, including medical and dental histories, head and neck examinations, dental chartings, radiographs, study models, bite registrations, photographs, and plaque and gingival indices. These assessment tools provide a total picture of the patient's periodontal condition and permit comprehensive treatment planning. Exact descriptions of these other components are contained elsewhere in this text. The information they provide is supplemental to the periodontal examination, and specific situations in which they may be used are mentioned as the periodontal examination is described.

Periodontal charting

The data collected and recorded in a periodontal chart serve multiple purposes for both the patient and clinician. As part of an initial examination, periodontal charting provides a record of *baseline data* describing the patient's periodontal condition before initial therapy. These data will later serve as a means for evaluating the success of treatment and preventive practices. Over time, changes in the patient's periodontal status can be noted to trace the control of disease and restoration of health. The periodontal charting provides *infor-*

mation that is necessary to establish a diagnosis of the patient's condition. It consolidates a comprehensive collection of clinical data that, along with other components of the periodontal examination, allow for a careful analysis of all observable conditions so that an accurate diagnosis can be made. Because the periodontal charting represents the clinical conditions in written form, this analysis can take place without the patient's presence. The accumulation of all available clinical signs and symptoms will help identify early signs of inflammatory disease while it still may be reversible.

After a diagnosis is made and confirmed, the periodontal charting continues to serve as a *resource for treatment planning*. Its information assists in establishing treatment priorities and in answering the following questions:

1. What areas show the most acute signs of disease and appear to have the highest potential for causing pain and/or destruction?
2. Which conditions demand additional examination or testing?
3. What types of treatment might be most effective?
4. What etiologic factors are present?
5. What combination of patient and professional efforts will be necessary to restore the tissues to health?

Data recorded as part of a complete periodontal charting can be used to formulate treatment plans for restorative, periodontal, and preventive therapy. During the presentation of the treatment plan, the periodontal charting and other diagnostic aids provide visual evidence of the clinical findings to the patient so that he or she can understand the diagnosis and its treatment.

The periodontal chart also serves as a valuable aid during *implementation of the treatment plan*. During probing, scaling, and subgingival debridement, the chart is a road map for instrumentation. Information such as the depth of pockets, root morphology, exposure of furcation areas, and mobility will affect your choice of instruments and the approach to scaling and debridement. When you know from the chart that deep and complex pocket morphologies are present, you will be alert to tactile cues during exploring and probing and can plan effective approaches to areas in which access may prove challenging. Information recorded during the periodontal charting helps identify the need for special treatment procedures,

such as temporary ligation of mobile teeth to facilitate subgingival debridement. It may also identify a need to recontour restorations to eliminate or at least reduce plaque-retentive characteristics. The description of the pocket morphology and degree of destruction incurred by the soft and hard tissues will assist you in determining indications for subsequent scaling procedures.

After treatment is completed, the periodontal chart serves as a valuable *reference for evaluating treatment success*. A posttreatment charting, when compared with pretreatment records, indicates where the soft tissues have been restored to some degree of normal form and function. It also serves as a point from which referrals for more advanced treatment, such as periodontal surgery, may be made. The periodontal chart should be updated during recall appointments to document the patient's periodontal status over time. If the gingiva remains healthy and shallow probing depths are maintained, it is an indication that personal oral hygiene, the patient's immune response, professional treatment, and recall intervals have been effective in health maintenance. If, on the other hand, subsequent chartings show that periodontal destruction is continuing, this signals that one or all of these elements require additional assessment and modification.

In addition, periodontal charting can be useful as *legal evidence* to support a diagnosis and to justify subsequent treatment. It also can provide information about the rationale for proposed or actual treatment in cases involving a third-party payer such as an insurance carrier. A less familiar use of dental records, including periodontal charts, is their application in *forensic dentistry*. A periodontal chart may be used to identify people who have died. Their dental and periodontal conditions are as specific to them as their fingerprints; thus, dental records can be invaluable for making positive identification.

Preappointment charting. Before the actual clinical examination, many factors relevant to the periodontal diagnosis may be assessed and charted from study models and radiographs. The advantage of studying these records is twofold. First, they provide information that can be reviewed when the patient is not present, thereby allowing time to examine both the study models and radiographs carefully and in detail for possible etiologic factors that might affect the periodontal diagnosis and final treatment plan. Second, information from the study models and radiographs will alert you to search for particular clinical signs and symptoms that might otherwise be overlooked. This preparation can save time during the appointment and allow a quicker diagnosis. The following paragraphs identify factors of the periodontal charting and examination that can be assessed in advance with the aid of radiographs and study models. The significance of each factor to the periodontal examination is described. Many of these factors have already been identified as components of comprehensive charting (see Chapter 11).

Missing teeth may indicate a history of periodontal disease. Areas left vacant by missing teeth create imbalanced forces that can result in periodontal breakdown and occlusal trauma (Goldman and Cohen, 1980).

Malpositioned teeth are not only susceptible to occlusal trauma but may also point to previous destructive disease, because shifting may result from breakdown of periodontal support (see Plate 3, *F* and *G*). Other signs of abnormal occlusal stresses or wear can be detected in radiographs and study models. The radiographs reveal signs of occlusal trauma such as periodontal ligament spaces that are abnormally wide because of increased pressures on the teeth. There may be signs of root fracture or loss of lamina dura. Attrition patterns on occlusal or incisal surfaces (wear facets) may be detectable on radiographs but can be seen more clearly on the study models as flattened areas on the cusp tips or occlusal surfaces resulting from constant wear of opposing teeth. Wear facets are charted by shading, on either the facial or occlusal views of the teeth, the worn portion of the tooth.

Impacted or *supernumerary* teeth can be detected in radiographs. An unerupted tooth is one that is incompletely formed or not yet visible in the mouth. An impacted tooth may be completely formed but is obstructed from normal eruption by an adjacent tooth or by its position in the dental arch. A supernumerary tooth is an "extra" tooth. These teeth usually form after the permanent dentition and remain apical to the erupted teeth in the alveolus. A common area for supernumerary teeth is apical to the maxillary central incisors. The significance of these conditions is that unerupted teeth can develop infections affecting the surrounding tissues. The constant pressure of an unerupted or impacted tooth against other hard tis-

sues, such as an adjacent tooth or bone, can cause resorption or permanent destruction of these tissues. *Partially erupted teeth* should also be noted on the charting form. If, for some reason, full eruption is not completed (as in impaction), it becomes difficult for the patient to keep these teeth clean and to keep the surrounding soft tissues healthy. These areas become prime sites for food impaction and gingival inflammation (e.g., pericoronitis).

An *open contact,* called a *diastema,* can be detected on radiographs and study models. A good radiograph shows the space between the adjacent teeth, and this can be confirmed by the study models. Clinically, the presence of a diastema can be determined visually if the diastema is wide (see Plate 3, *F* and *G*). Open or deficient contacts can also be detected by passing a piece of dental floss between the teeth. When the contact areas do not offer sufficient resistance to the floss, a deficient contact should be charted. Open or deficient contacts may be significant because of their potential for food impaction. They may also indicate tooth movement from periodontal destruction if the patient reports that development is recent. The presence of *plunger cusps* should also be noted during the periodontal examination. In this situation, cusps of teeth in one arch fit directly into the area between two teeth in the opposing arch. The significance of this phenomenon is that the plunger cusps can push food directly into the space between the opposing teeth, causing trauma to the soft tissues in the area (Pennel and Keagle, 1977). A plunger cusp should be detectable in the study models if the occlusal relationships have been properly reproduced in the wax bite (see Chapter 15).

Abnormal crown and root morphologies may be detected radiographically or on the study models and should be charted by drawing the existing anatomic shape over the symbol of the affected tooth. The drawing should represent reality as closely as possible. Examples of these deviations are teeth that are exceptionally large or small in relation to other teeth, teeth with dilacerated roots, teeth with abnormal distances from the cementoenamel junction to furcations, and teeth with roots that are spread abnormally or have more or fewer roots than normal. The discovery of any of these deviations is significant for the determination of a tooth's susceptibility to disease, its roots' "anchoring" ability, and how its roots should be treated during scaling or surgical procedures.

Two anomalies that may affect a tooth's susceptibility to disease are the *distopalatal groove* and *cervical-enamel projections*. The former is a groove that extends apically along the root on some maxillary incisors. Most distopalatal grooves are found on maxillary lateral incisors (Withers et al, 1981). Their presence as plaque-retentive areas increases the chances of periodontal destruction. Enamel projections occur in mandibular furcation areas, causing a lack of normal attachment and a predisposition for the buildup of plaque in those locations (Pennel and Keagle, 1977). Areas affected by *abrasion* or *erosion* are also significant in the periodontal examination because of their potential to harbor plaque. This loss of tooth structure affects the normal self-cleansing abilities of the dentition.

Other plaque-retentive conditions that serve as etiologic factors include *poorly contoured crowns and restorations, prosthetic devices,* and *carious lesions.* Until these problems are either removed, replaced, or restored, the patient will find it difficult to practice optimal plaque control and periodontal disease will persist.

The quality of the proximal tooth surface plays an important role in the periodontal condition of adjacent soft tissues. Proximal surfaces that have caries or poorly contoured restorations are more likely to experience plaque accumulation and increased probing depths than similar, intact proximal surfaces (Claman et al, 1986).

Periapical conditions should be carefully examined on the radiographs and charted where they appear. Any radiopacities or radiolucencies in the periapical regions or supporting bone should be noted, and a tentative diagnosis should be made. Additional tests and questioning of the patient during the clinical examination may be necessary to reach a final diagnosis.

Bone levels and the appearance of *bony defects* should be carefully examined on the radiographs. The topography of the bone should be scrutinized for the presence of vertical or horizontal defects. The extent of these defects should be estimated to guide periodontal probing during the clinical appointment. At that time, the clinical readings and the appearance of bone levels on the radiographs should be correlated to ensure that deep bony defects have not been overlooked. The crestal bone patterns should be examined for loss of definition or loss of lamina dura to determine the level of bone destruction. The presence of bony craters can also be observed on the radiographs (Newman and Moran, 1980).

However, it has been shown that radiographs, especially bite-wings, cannot be depended upon to identify early periodontal disease and bone loss (Mann et al, 1985).

Many of the aforementioned conditions may have already been charted as part of the comprehensive charting. If so, they need not be included on the periodontal chart. These elements are used in a periodontal examination to ascertain a restorative treatment plan, determine the causes of periodontal conditions, and select the best sequence of priorities to meet patient needs during comprehensive treatment planning.

After the radiographs and study models have been closely examined and all pertinent findings have been reviewed from the restorative chart and/or charted on the periodontal charting form, you will conduct the clinical periodontal examination. Make notes to indicate any special evaluations or tests that might be helpful in verifying diagnoses suggested by the initial assessment of data. When the patient is seated, the clinical examination assesses all characteristics of the soft and hard tissues that could not be evaluated from other sources.

Clinical examination

Before the periodontal examination begins, the patient's medical history should be reviewed and confirmed to detect any potential complications in treatment. Information gathered from the medical history can assist in identifying medical reasons for certain gingival and periodontal conditions. Systemic diseases such as diabetes, blood dyscrasias, and hormonal imbalances can affect the ability of the body to resist and repair damage resulting from inflammatory conditions. These patients may be more susceptible to periodontal destruction. Medications may also affect the periodontal tissues. Patients who take phenytoin sodium for control of seizures often exhibit hyperplasia or fibrotic overgrowth of gingival tissues. Patients who use oral contraceptives may exhibit gingival changes similar to those seen during pregnancy. Corticosteroids are antiinflammatory drugs, and their use can mask the usual signs of inflammation in the gingival soft tissues. Poor nutrition and emotional stress can also exacerbate the inflam-

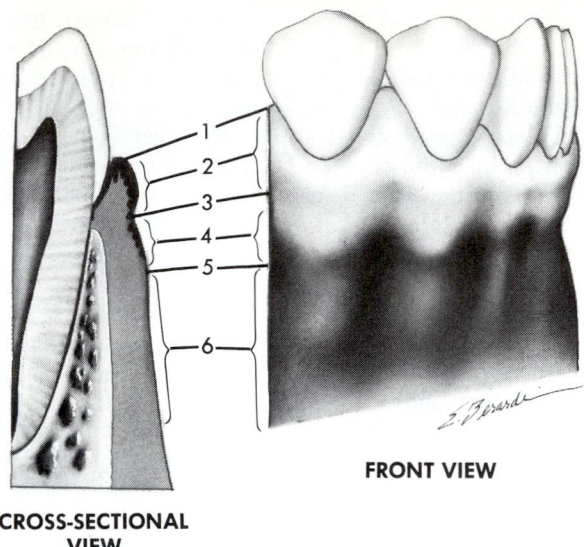

FRONT VIEW

CROSS-SECTIONAL
VIEW

Fig. 12-6. Normal landmarks and boundaries of gingiva and aveolar mucosa. *1*, Free gingival margin; *2*, free gingiva; *3*, free gingival groove; *4*, attached gingiva; *5*, mucogingival junction; *6*, aveolar mucosa. Clinician should be able to relate these landmarks to their appearance in patient's mouth.

matory response in the gingival and periodontal tissues.

Patients who require antibiotic premedication to prevent infection caused by bacteremias should be premedicated for all periodontal procedures. Periodontal probing can cause a bacteremia in a susceptible patient, as can any other periodontal or dental procedure that manipulates the soft tissue.

Information from the dental history indicates past dental or periodontal treatment that might affect the present periodontal examination, such as surgical treatment or explanations of tooth loss. The dental history also reveals information about the patient's attitudes regarding periodontal and preventive therapy; this information aids in treatment planning and can generate a list of risk factors that suggest relative susceptibility to disease. These include incidences of the disease in the family, previous periodontal treatment, and history of smoking.

The purpose of the periodontal examination and charting should be discussed with the patient and the procedure explained. He or she should understand that this is an exacting procedure. Explain that there may be discomfort and provide pain control (either topical, local, or nitrous oxide). After the examination has been explained and consent obtained, the procedure can begin.

Gingival assessment. The first area to be studied during the clinical examination is the gingiva, free and attached. Fig. 12-6 and Plate 3, *A,* show the normal structures of the gingiva and alveolar mucosa. The clinical appearance of the gingiva in all parts of the mouth should be closely examined for signs of inflammation. Table 12-2 contrasts the appearance of normal and inflamed gingiva. A careful examination is necessary to determine subtle changes in the gingiva, because the patient's prognosis for treatment is much improved if gingivitis is recognized and treated in its earliest stages. Deviations from normal should be noted and described as part of the periodontal examination. This description should also include the location and extent of the condition.

You should assess the condition of the gingiva by examining it for each of the following characteristics: color, contour, consistency, and texture. You should know the normal characteristics and changes that may be visible as a result of inflammation so that you can record exact descriptions of the character of the gingiva. The extent of gingival change caused by inflammation can vary. Signs of inflammation may extend into all attached and free gingiva, or they may be restricted to the marginal gingiva or interdental papillae. Specific changes may also be localized around one or several teeth, or generalized to an entire arch. Evaluate the degree of inflammation and extent of tissue involvement to determine if the inflammation is slight, moderate, or severe in quality.

The *color* of normal gingiva is usually a uniform, coral-pink shade. The light pink color should extend all the way from the mucogingival attachment to the gingival margin (see Plate 3, *A*). Shade variations occur among individuals, much the same as facial complexions differ. The amount of normal melanin pigmentation in the gingiva also varies. This pigmentation may be visible as brown patches of color distributed in varying degrees throughout the tissue. It is prevalent in African-Americans. An example of melanin pigmentation is shown in Plate 3, *B* and *F*.

The earliest color change associated with gingival inflammation often begins as a subtle change in the interdental papilla from light pink to a darker pink or red. This color change extends to the marginal gingiva and into the rest of the free and attached gingiva as the inflammation becomes more severe. Acutely inflamed gingiva will have a red color (see Plate 3, *G*), whereas chronically inflamed gingiva may take on a bluish (cyanotic) cast. This blue color change may be discernible around the margins of poorly contoured crowns (see Plate 4, *D*, No. 8). In many cases the color of fibrotic, chronically inflamed gingiva may be close to normal in appearance. Both chronic and acute signs of gingival inflammation may exist simultaneously in the same patient.

The *contour* of normal gingival tissues also can be seen in Plate 3, *A*. The interdental papillae fill the embrasure spaces and come to a sharp point at the contact area. The free gingival margins are knife-like and hug the coronal surface of the tooth. The margins also create a regular series of parabolic curves as the eye moves from tooth to tooth. The level of the free gingival margin should be at or slightly coronal to the cementoenamel junction of the tooth.

A number of changes in the contour of the gingiva result from inflammation. The interdental papillae become swollen and edematous. In later stages of the disease, they may become flattened, blunted, or cratered. This "punched-out" appearance caused by loss of papilla is characteristic in patients who have had ANUG. The marginal gingiva may also appear bulbous and swollen with rolled margins. As the edema increases, other gingival changes may occur such as clefting (see Plate 3, *E*) or festooning. The inflamed marginal gingiva also loses its elastic ability to adhere closely to the contour of the tooth. The inflamed tissues may stand away from the tooth, or they can be easily displaced with air or instrument retraction (see Plate 3, *G*). When gingival tissues undergo a change in the inflammatory response from acute to chronic inflammation, the constant destruction of tissues results in scar or fibrotic tissue that appears extremely firm and often enlarged and irregular in contour (see Plate 3, *D*).

Normal gingival tissues have a *consistency* that is firm and resilient. With the onset of inflammation, they become edematous, soft, and spongy. This situation can be detected by applying slight pressure on the dried tissues with the tip or side of a probe or other blunt instrument. A "dent" will remain. Chronically inflamed, fibrotic tissues are very firm, hard, and unyielding in consistency because of the buildup of excessive repair or scar tissue.

The *surface texture* of normal free gingiva is smooth. The attached gingiva may exhibit a smooth or stippled appearance. Stippling appears as tiny indentations in the surface of the attached gingiva, similar to the appearance of an orange peel (see Plate 3, *A* and *B*). Although many individuals display this normal characteristic, its absence does not necessarily indicate disease (Goldman and Cohen, 1980). Stippling may be easily detected if the tissues are dried with a stream of air. Acute inflammation usually results in the loss of stippling because of the increase in tissue edema. The surface texture becomes very smooth and glossy (see Plate 3, *C* and *F*). Stippling is often present during chronic inflammation, and may actually be more prevalent.

Evaluation of the external appearance of the gingiva is a useful assessment tool for describing the presence of gingival inflammation. However, it is not highly reliable. Waerhaug (1978a, 1978b) demonstrated that inflammatory changes affecting the marginal gingiva may occur independently of inflammatory changes in the sulcular areas. Patients who performed effective supramarginal plaque control had normal-appearing gingiva despite the presence of submarginal plaque and sulcular inflammation. Waerhaug warned clinicians not to be misled by the overt appearance of the gingival tissues, especially when the patient has effectively controlled plaque.

Although assessment of the clinical signs of gingival inflammation may help in determining the presence of gingivitis, these measures are of little help in identifying periodontitis, and their presence cannot predict the onset of periodontitis (Morrison et al, 1982; Ryan, 1985). The clinical signs of inflammation have been shown to be poor indicators of ongoing periodontal disease activity. Even during active periodontal destruction in the supporting tissues, the gingival tissues may exhibit no clinical signs of inflammation (Haffajee et al, 1983). An additional problem with the use of clinical signs is that it requires subjective interpretation of the appearance of the tissues rather than objective measures, leading to disagreements and variations in the interpretation of these signs. More objective methods of clinical assessment, such as noting the presence of bleeding or exudate from the pocket or sulcus, host response evaluations, and microbiologic monitoring should complement the gingival assessment.

The soft tissue that covers the supporting bone should be examined for signs of swelling, such as might be caused by periapical or periodontal abscesses, granulomas, or cysts. Initial signs of bone destruction caused by these lesions might have been detected during the radiographic examination, and the clinical examination can confirm the tentative diagnosis. Never rely solely on radiographs to diagnose these lesions, as they are not always detectable radiographically. Signs of openings or breaks in the gingiva or mucosa (such as draining fistulas) should be carefully examined and noted.

Gingival bleeding. The presence of sulcular bleeding can be detected during periodontal probing and is the result of an ulcerated sulcular epithelial lining. An acutely inflamed sulcus bleeds spontaneously from finger pressure against the tissue or from probing. Bleeding from incipient gingival inflammation may not be apparent at the surface of the free gingival margin for as long as 30 seconds after complete probing of the entire sulcular area (Carter and Barnes, 1974). Tissues that have become fibrotic because of a long-standing inflammation may bleed little or not at all. All areas of gingival bleeding should be charted according to where they occur in the mouth as a method of assessing the extent and location of the inflammation. In Fig. 12-7, a red dot indicates the presence of bleeding for each area probed. The amount of gingival bleeding may also be trans-

lated into a bleeding index by assigning a numeric value to its occurrence (see Chapter 13).

The presence of bleeding on probing is a good clinical indicator of gingival inflammation (Polson and Goodson, 1985). It also permits assessment of inflammation at the base of the lesion, which is a critical area to evaluate. Presence or absence of bleeding on probing is a somewhat more objective means of assessing inflammation compared with the interpretation of clinical inflammatory signs. Correlations of the presence of clinical bleeding with histologic evidence of the presence or absence of inflammation indicates that bleeding is an accurate indication of the presence of inflammation within the periodontal tissues (Abrams et al, 1984; Greenstein, 1984; Polson and Caton, 1986; Ryan, 1985). However, it does not differentiate gingivitis and periodontitis. Although the presence of bleeding on probing is associated with sites losing periodontal attachment, it is frequently noted at sites that do not progress. Continued absence of bleeding on probing is, however, a reliable predictor of health (Lang et al, 1990).

If a bleeding index is to be taken, it is wise to incorporate it with the periodontal probing and to record signs of gingival bleeding as they occur. It is also important to use this opportunity to explain the cause and significance of bleeding to the patient so that he or she does not associate it with the probing technique but rather with the inflammatory state of the soft tissues. This method of assessment is one that the patient should be encouraged to use at home to detect areas in which home care may not be optimal. Many patients experience bleeding from toothbrushing or flossing and regard it as a normal occurrence rather than a sign of inflammatory disease (see Chapter 20). This is an excellent opportunity to educate patients by showing them which areas need special attention during their home care practices.

Suppuration. The presence of inflammatory exudate or pus is an obvious sign of acute inflammation and infection. This exudate is composed of white blood cells and other inflammatory debris. Exudate may be noticed during probing, or it may be expelled from the pocket by applying gentle finger pressure to the adjacent gingiva. The presence of exudate should be noted for each tooth involved as part of the periodontal assessment. When pus is seen, this is good evidence that periodontal destruction is occurring. How-

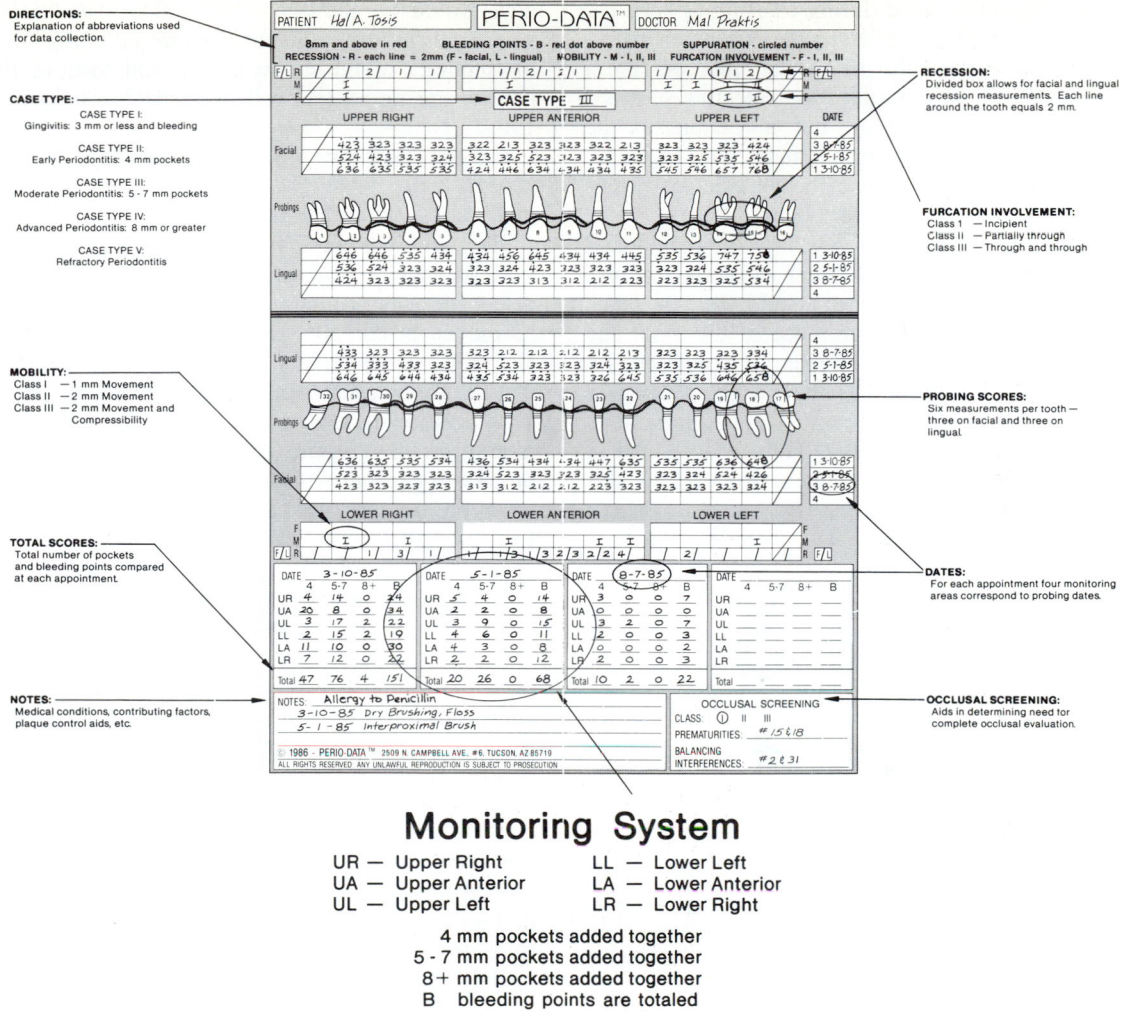

Monitoring System

UR — Upper Right	LL — Lower Left
UA — Upper Anterior	LA — Lower Anterior
UL — Upper Left	LR — Lower Right

4 mm pockets added together
5 - 7 mm pockets added together
8+ mm pockets added together
B   bleeding points are totaled

Fig. 12-7. Periodontal charting form.

ever, low level suppuration is not always clinically detectable.

Peridontal probing. The standard, hand-held probe is calibrated in millimeters to facilitate clinical measurements. There is a wide variety of probe designs, with the choice based mainly on individual preference. The diameter of the working end is important for detection during insertion into tight pockets. It should be long and narrow enough to be easily inserted without causing undue distension of the sulcular soft tissue. The tip, however, should be blunt or have a ball-tipped end so as not to puncture or damage the junc-

tional tissues at the base of the sulcus.

Calibrations of probes vary; some are calibrated at each millimeter up to 10, and others are calibrated in millimeter increments, with the markings at 4 and 6 deleted for ease of reading. An even less complex probe has calibrations only at 3, 6, and 8 mm. Some clinicians prefer color-coded probes to assist reading. Examples of several different probe designs are shown in Fig. 9-12. No matter what type of probe you choose, the accuracy of probing pocket depths depends on your skill and clinical judgment.

A saliva ejector and trisyringe (air-water syringe) should be used during charting to keep the field clear of saliva and blood. Two other instruments that are helpful in special situations are a shepherd's hook explorer, for detecting exposed furcation areas that are not accessible to the straight design of the periodontal probe, and a curette, for gross removal of heavy calculus pieces that might interfere with probing.

Six probe readings are taken for the periodontal charting (Fig. 12-8). Although only six readings are recorded, the probe should be "walked" around the entire circumference of the tooth and record the greatest depth reading for each area recorded. If, for instance, the pocket reading is deeper near the distobuccal line angle on the buccal surface of the tooth than on the exact center of the buccal surface, the correct reading for this

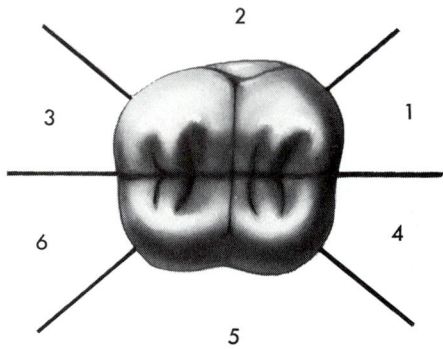

Fig. 12-8. Occlusal view of molar shows areas in which periodontal pocket depth readings are usually taken. Highest reading in each area is the one that should be recorded on charting form.

area would be the deeper one. This "walking" technique allows you to explore carefully the morphology of the entire pocket and to note all defects are noted (Hassell et al, 1973; Tibbetts, 1969).

For the most part, the probe's working end is kept as close to parallel to the long axis of the tooth as possible. The tip should be kept in close contact with the tooth surface at all times to prevent damage to soft tissues. As the mesial and distal surfaces are approached, the probe should be moved proximally until it touches the contact and then angled slightly into the proximal area so that the tip measures directly beneath the contact. This position is shown in Fig. 12-9, *A*. A common error is keeping the working end of the probe too parallel with the long axis of the tooth when the interproximal area is reached and therefore failing to measure the entire proximal surface adequately (Fig. 12-9, *B).* (To review correct adaptation of the probe to the tooth, see Chapter 9). Success with this adapation depends on tactile sense when keeping the tip against the tooth. The *col* area, which is apical to the contact, is a frequent site for periodontal breakdown and destruction (Goldman and Cohen, 1980), and it is important to probe it carefully from both facial and lingual aspects. When the procedure is done correctly, there will be a slight overlap between the area probed for the mesiofacial and the area probed for the mesiolingual. In Fig. 12-9, *A,* the probe has gone slightly beyond the midline of the tooth to obtain its reading. If a choice must be made, it is better that the probe be slightly

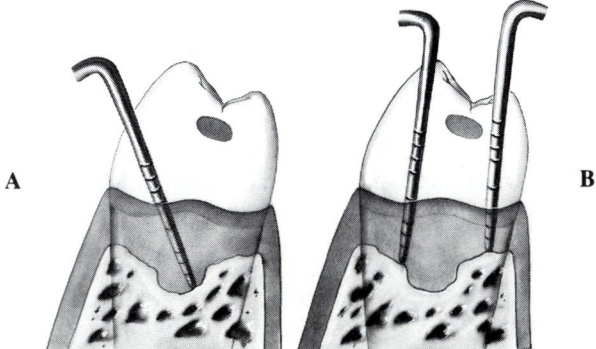

Fig. 12-9. A, Correct interproximal adaptation of probe. Both facial and lingual readings should detect crater if probe is angled in this manner. **B,** Deep interproximal bony defects are missed if probe is not angled below contact area interproximally. No matter how hard this clinician tries, neither facial nor lingual reading will accurately represent disease present in this area.

overangled than underangled. With the former there is a slight risk of getting a deeper-than-accurate pocket reading, but with the latter there is the possibility of missing a deep vertical defect altogether. With some clinical judgment and practice, you will be able to visualize the distance and angle that will ensure thorough exploration and accurate measurement of this vital area.

When the probe is being maneuvered around the tooth and a reading is taken, it is easiest to read the correct pocket or sulcus depth by evaluating the markings at the free gingival margin. Fig. 12-10 shows pocket depths recorded for the buccal and lingual surfaces of all teeth rounded up to the greater millimeter depth when the measurement falls between two whole number readings. Do not try to estimate within less than a millimeter.

Too much pressure on the probe causes pain. Another source of pain may simply be the normal response of acutely inflamed tissues to any type of contact by the probe which is entirely unrelated to poor technique. Inflamed tissues are ulcerated and bleeding, and they have an exaggerated response to any kind of instrumentation, whether it be probing or scaling. In situations such as this, be prepared to give an anesthetic for patient comfort. An alternative is to postpone probing and give home care instructions that may lead to healing of the acutely inflamed tissues.

Visibility is important during probing. Keep the area clear of saliva and use the trisyringe to help clear the area of blood and dry the teeth and tissues that are being examined.

Calculus can inhibit periodontal probing, too. If the deposits are small and scattered throughout the mouth, it is usually possible to move the probe away from the deposit and then to continue apically into the pocket. Do not mistake a calculus deposit for the pocket base (Fig. 12-11). Good tactile sense helps determine the difference between the hard resistance of the calculus and the more elastic resiliency of the pocket or sulcus base. If large calculus deposits that inhibit access are encountered, remove them, then probe.

Electronic probing systems. In 1979 the National Insitute of Dental Research issued a challenge to manufacturers to develop a periodontal probe that could accurately measure pocket depths and attachment levels. Since that time manufacturers have developed at least 2 electronic probing systems that accurately measure periodontal pocket depths and attachment levels with an additional function of computerized recording.

Interprobe. The Interprobe (Bausch and Lomb Oral Care Division, Tucker, Ga.) is an electronic probing system consisting of a control unit, memory card, down-loading recorder and dot matrix printer (Fig. 12-12). The control unit houses a handpiece similar to a traditional periodontal probe that electronically scans and reads pocket depths. The probe consists of a plastic handpiece and a filament that are discarded after each patient. The control unit also has a key pad and digital display area indicating tooth location and measurement scanned. The clinician places the probe and activates the measurement. To record the measurement on the memory card the operator taps a foot control. When the periodontal probing is complete, the memory card is inserted into the down loader and a graphic charting is printed (Fig. 12-13). A limitation of this system is the flexibility of the probing fiber. Tactile sensitivity is diminished and the probe cannot be "walked" around the tooth.

Florida Probe. Another computer-assisted probing device is the Florida Probe (Florida Probe Corp., Gainesville, Fla.). This system uses an IBM-compatible computer to record data measurements. Unlike the Interprobe, the Florida Probe includes a metal probe and handpiece that are autoclavable and thus reusable. Measurements taken with the Florida Probe are highly accurate.

Both of these systems save valuable time and provide a precise graphic representation of the periodontal conditions in the patient's mouth. The printouts are filed in the patient's chart and used for insurance and patient education purposes.

• • •

Several other computer-assisted, controlled-force probes have been used in research (Birek et al, 1987; Jeffcoat et al, 1986). One of these, developed at the University of Alabama, automatically read the location of the cemetoenamel junction enabling the clinician to measure changes in clinical attachment levels with an accuracy of 0.2 mm (Jeffcoat et al, 1986).

Significance of pocket depth measurements. The periodontal probe is a valuable clinical tool for exploring and measuring the extent of the healthy gingival sulcus and its pathologic counterpart, the periodontal pocket. For years it was assumed that this measurement of a clinical sulcus

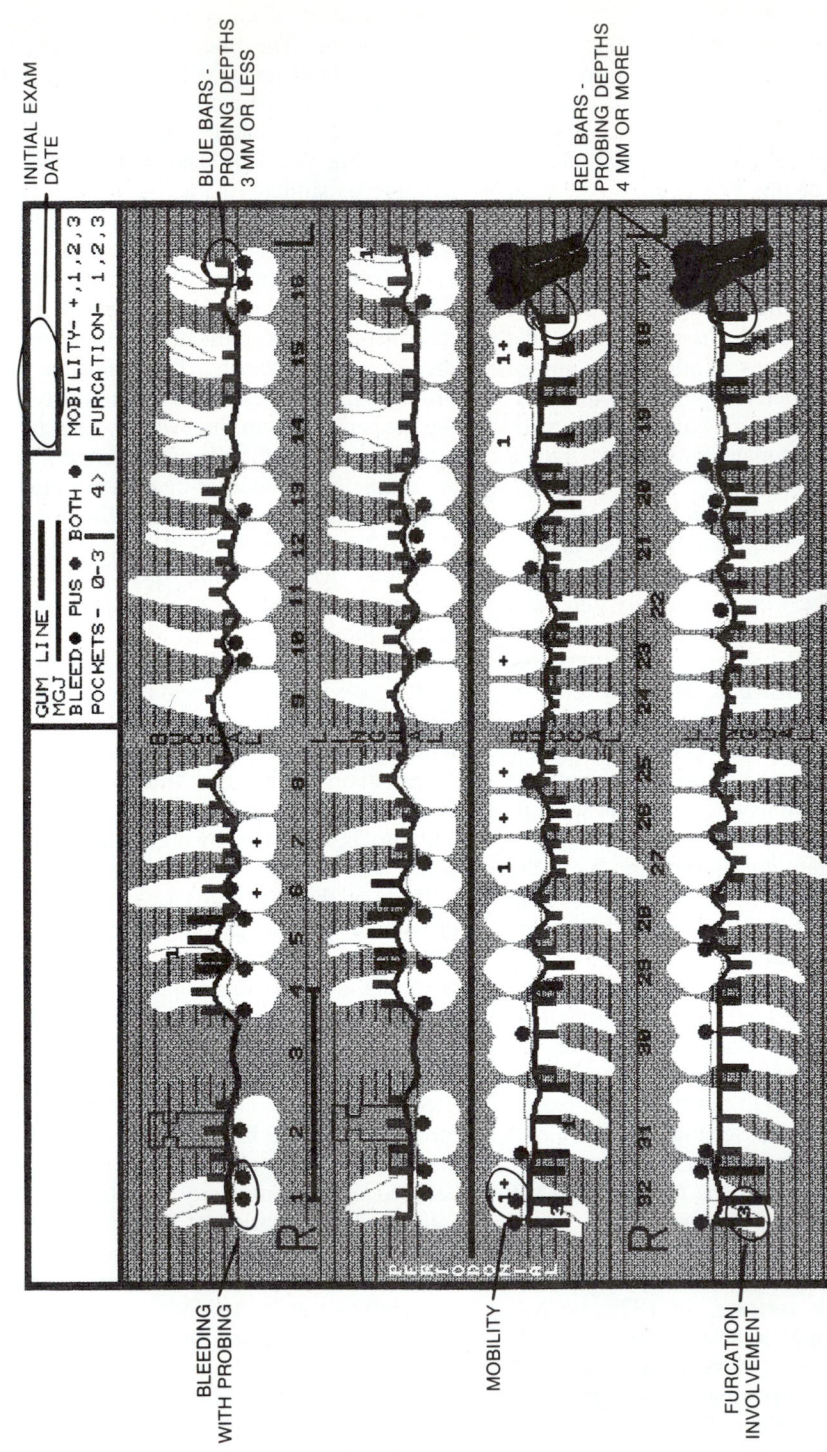

PERIODONTAL EXAM 1

Intial Exam Date:

Dr. J.M. Matthews
633 Lawrence Street
Batesville, Ar 72501   1-800-228-5595

(c) Copyright 1987,91 Avanti Corp.

Fig. 12-10. Victor voice-activated system: periodontal chart printout.

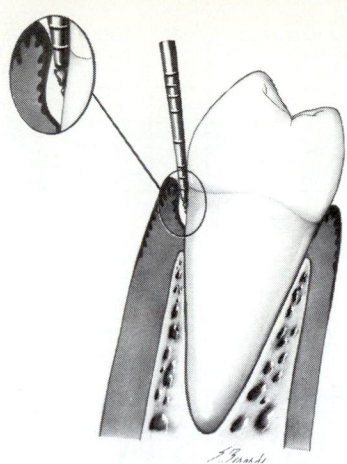

Fig. 12-11. Calculus ledges often prohibit tip of probe from reaching base of pocket. An inexperienced clinician may mistake hard, unyielding pressure offered by calculus as pocket base. If piece is small enough, it may be possible to navigate probe out and around it and continue on down to more resilient pocket base. If calculus piece is too large, it must be removed before accurate probing can be done.

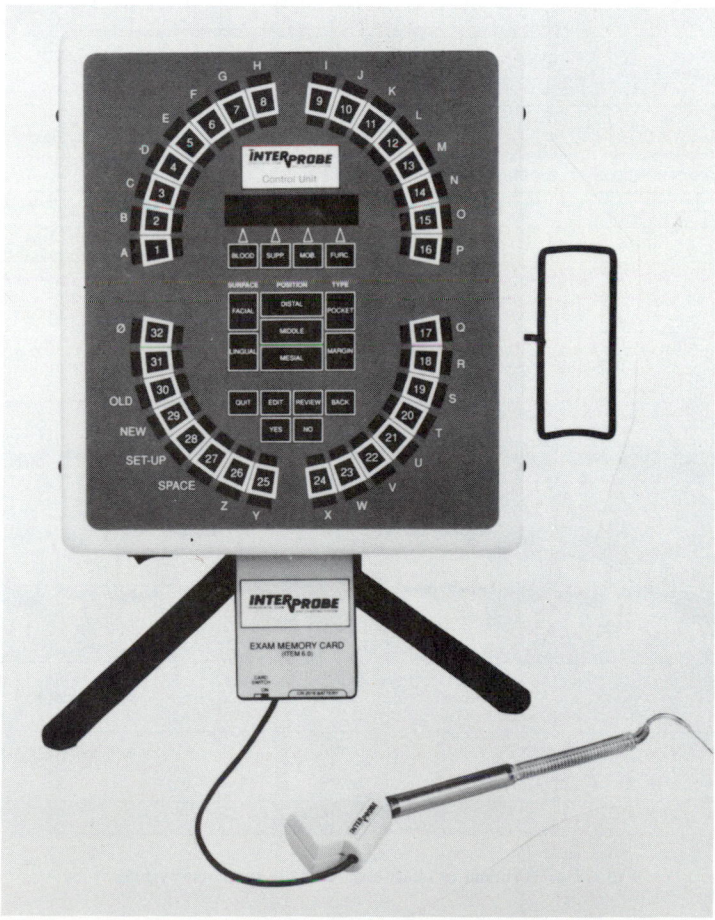

Fig. 12-12. Interprobe system.

INTERPROBE — PERIODONTAL EXAM AND CHARTING SYSTEM

BAUSCH AND LOMB
5243 ROYAL WOODS PARKWAY
TUCKER GA   30084

PATIENT   ANDERSON WM
SOCIAL SECURITY
EXAMINED BY
DATE   10/31/89

		1	2	3	4	5	6	7	8	9	10	11	12	13	14	15	16
MOBILITY		0	0	0	0	0	0+	0+	0	0	0	0	0	0	0	0	0
FURCATION	MESIAL					0							0				
	MIDDLE	0	0	0											0	0	0
	DISTAL					1							0				
POCKET	MESIAL	B 2.5	2.0	2.0	S 3.5	B 4.5	3.0	1.5	1.0	0.5	B 0.5	1.5	1.5	S 2.0	1.0	1.5	B 2.0
	MIDDLE	B 2.0	S 2.5	2.0	3.0	4.0	B 2.5	1.5	1.5	1.0	B 1.5	2.0	1.5	2.5	1.0	1.5	B 2.5
	DISTAL	2.0	2.0	2.5	B 3.0	4.0	2.0	1.5	1.5	1.0	1.0	2.0	2.0	2.0	2.0	1.0	S 2.0
RECESSION	MESIAL	B- 0.5	- 1.0	0.0	S- 2.0	B- 1.5	0.0	0.0	- 1.0	- 1.5	B- 0.5	0.0	- 0.5	S- 1.5	0.0	0.0	B- 1.5
	MIDDLE	B- 1.0	S- 1.0	0.0	- 1.5	- 1.5	B 0.0	0.0	- 1.0	- 1.0	B- 0.5	0.0	0.0	- 1.0	0.0	0.0	B- 1.0
	DISTAL	- 1.0	- 1.0	0.0	B- 1.5	- 1.5	0.0	0.0	- 1.0	- 1.0	- 1.0	0.0	0.0	- 1.0	0.0	0.0	S- 1.0

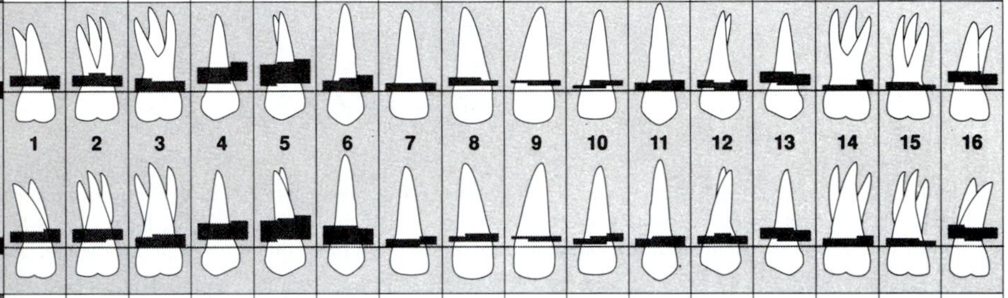

FACIAL — CEJ

1 2 3 4 5 6 7 8 9 10 11 12 13 14 15 16

LINGUAL — CEJ

		1	2	3	4	5	6	7	8	9	10	11	12	13	14	15	16
POCKET	MESIAL	B 2.5	2.0	2.5	* 3.5	B 4.5	* 3.0	1.5	1.0	0.5	B 1.0	1.5	1.5	S 2.0	1.5	1.5	B 2.5
	MIDDLE	B 2.0	* 2.5	2.5	3.0	4.0	3.5	1.5	1.5	1.0	1.5	2.0	B 2.0	2.5	1.5	1.5	2.5
	DISTAL	2.0	2.5	2.0	B 3.0	4.0	3.5	1.5	1.5	1.0	1.5	2.0	1.5	2.0	2.0	1.0	S 2.0
RECESSION	MESIAL	B- 1.0	- 1.5	0.0	*- 1.5	B- 1.5	*- 0.5	- 0.5	- 1.0	- 1.5	B- 0.5	0.0	- 0.5	S- 1.5	0.0	0.0	B- 1.5
	MIDDLE	B- 1.0	*- 1.0	0.0	- 1.5	- 1.5	- 0.5	0.0	- 1.0	- 1.0	- 0.5	0.0	B- 0.5	- 1.0	0.0	0.0	- 1.0
	DISTAL	- 1.0	- 1.0	0.0	B- 1.5	- 1.0	- 0.5	0.0	- 1.0	- 1.0	- 1.0	0.0	- 0.5	- 1.0	0.0	0.0	S- 1.5
FURCATION	MESIAL	0	0	0		0							0		0	0	0
	DISTAL	0	0	0		0							0		0	0	1

ANNOTATION CODE: B = BLOOD   S = SUPPURATION   * = BOTH

		32	31	30	29	28	27	26	25	24	23	22	21	20	19	18	17
MOBILITY		1+	0	0	0	0	1	0+	0+	0	0+	0	0	0	1	1+	1
FURCATION	MIDDLE	3	0	0											0	1	2
POCKET	MESIAL	5.0	3.5	2.5	2.5	1.5	2.0	2.5	1.5	1.0	2.0	2.5	S 2.0	3.0	4.0	4.5	5.5
	MIDDLE	6.0	3.5	B 3.0	3.5	2.0	2.0	2.5	1.5	1.0	2.0	2.5	2.0	3.5	4.5	B 4.0	4.5
	DISTAL	6.0	B 4.5	2.5	3.5	1.5	2.0	1.5	B 1.5	1.5	2.5	- 1.5	1.5	3.5	4.5	4.0	* 5.0
RECESSION	MESIAL	- 0.5	- 1.5	- 1.0	- 1.0	- 0.5	- 0.5	- 1.0	0.0	- 0.5	- 0.5	- 1.0	S- 0.5	- 1.5	- 1.0	- 1.5	- 1.5
	MIDDLE	- 1.0	- 1.0	B- 1.0	- 1.0	- 0.5	- 0.5	- 1.0	0.0	- 0.5	- 0.5	- 1.0	- 1.0	- 1.5	B- 1.5	- 1.5	- 1.5
	DISTAL	- 1.0	B- 0.5	- 1.0	- 1.0	- 0.5	- 0.5	- 1.0	B 0.0	0.0	- 0.5	- 1.0	- 1.0	- 1.0	- 1.5	- 1.5	*- 2.0

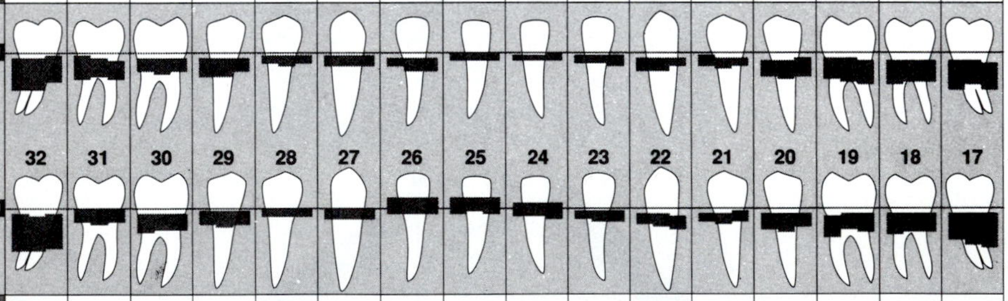

FACIAL — CEJ

32 31 30 29 28 27 26 25 24 23 22 21 20 19 18 17

LINGUAL — CEJ

		32	31	30	29	28	27	26	25	24	23	22	21	20	19	18	17
POCKET	MESIAL	* 6.5	2.5	3.0	B 2.5	1.5	2.0	3.0	3.0	2.5	1.5	2.0	1.5	* 3.0	B 4.0	4.0	* 5.0
	MIDDLE	6.5	3.0	S 3.0	3.0	1.5	2.0	3.0	S 2.5	2.5	2.0	* 2.5	2.0	* 3.5	3.0	3.5	B 6.0
	DISTAL	* 7.0	B 2.5	3.5	2.5	* 1.5	2.0	3.0	3.0	3.0	2.0	2.5	2.0	2.5	3.5	3.5	S 6.5
RECESSION	MESIAL	*- 1.0	- 1.0	- 1.0	B- 0.5	0.0	0.0	2.0	2.0	1.0	- 0.5	- 1.0	- 1.0	*- 1.0	B- 1.5	- 1.0	*- 1.0
	MIDDLE	- 1.5	- 1.0	S- 1.0	- 0.5	0.0	0.0	2.0	S 2.0	1.0	- 0.5	*- 1.0	- 1.0	*- 1.0	- 1.0	- 1.0	B- 1.0
	DISTAL	*- 1.0	B- 1.0	- 1.0	- 0.5	* 0.0	0.0	2.0	2.0	1.0	- 0.5	- 1.5	- 0.5	- 1.0	- 1.0	- 1.0	S- 1.0
FURCATION	MIDDLE	2	0	0											0	0	1

IP-414-119

Fig. 12-13. Printout of chart electronically prepared by InterProbe.

or pocket was an accurate representation of the actual histologic attachment of soft tissues to the tooth surface at the dentogingival junction. Based on this assumption, clinicians measured the depths of inflamed pockets before treatment and compared these measurements with those obtained afterwards. The resultant decrease in pocket depth was interpreted and described as a gain in attachment level. However, we now know that the probe does not measure the exact extent of the dentogingival junction in either health or disease (Listgarten, 1980). A number of factors contribute to this discrepancy: the degree of inflammation, the amount of probing pressure, and the probe's diameter (Polson and Goodson, 1985; Ryan, 1985).

As the inflammatory lesion of chronic periodontitis advances from early to established to advanced stages, there is a progressive disruption in the soft tissues of the dentogingival attachment. The junctional epithelium becomes more permeable to inflammatory cells and eventually loses its attachment to the tooth surface. The underlying and adjacent connective tissue fibers undergo destruction of their dense collagen network of supportive tissues. These inflamed tissues cannot resist the normal forces of probing, so that the probe tip usually penetrates the junctional epithelium and rests only when it reaches the increased resiliency of healthy connective tissue fibers. The probe tip penetrates through the partially destroyed fibers and stops approximately 0.25 to 0.40 mm apical to the termination of the junctional epithelium (Armitage, 1977; Hancock et al, 1978; Hancock and Wirthline, 1981; Listgarten et al, 1976; Powell and Garnick, 1978; Saglie et al, 1975; Sivertson and Burgett, 1976; Spray et al, 1978). Because you cannot feel the presence of the inflamed tissues that are being penetrated, the measurement of the pocket depth might be overestimated (Listgarten, 1980).

When pockets are treated with nonsurgical conservative methods and daily plaque removal, the inflammatory conditions subside and the soft tissues of the dentogingival junction undergo repair. The clinical result, when measured by the periodontal probe, may be a decrease in probing depth caused by an apparent gain in the level of the attachment and tissue shrinkage. Investigators have taken a closer look at the reported "gain" of attachment and have found that a decrease in pocket depth does not necessarily represent a gain

of new attachment. Instead, the healed periodontal tissues can regain their dense collagen network and provide resistance to the penetration of the probe (Fowler et al, 1982; Magnusson and Listgarten, 1980). In addition, a common healing response to initial therapy is the formation of a long junctional epithelium that forms a new biologic attachment to the tooth. The length of the new junctional epithelium has been estimated in one study to range from 1.0 to 4.5 mm (Listgarten and Rosenberg, 1979). The long junctional epithelium resists penetration by the probe in a healthy sulcus or pocket. Clinical pocket measurements following initial therapy are more likely to estimate the actual anatomic or histologic pocket depths than those made in the presence of inflammation.

Pocket depth alone does not predict future attachment loss. Okamoto et al. (1989) analyzed attachment loss, recession, and pocket depth and found that the majority of sites losing attachment (78%) were associated with pocket depth plus recession (43%) or recession only (35%). Pocket depth, however, can be a significant risk factor for attachment loss (Haffajee et al, 1991).

PerioTemp. The PerioTemp (Abiodent, Cambridge, Mass.) probe is a device that measures the temperature of the sulcus or pocket and compares it with the patient's core temperature while adjusting for the natural differences in temperature for the location of the various teeth. Increased temperature correlates well with inflammation and is a risk factor for periodontal breakdown. The probe also has millimeter markings so pocket depths can be measured simultaneously. When the electronic probe measures the temperature, a foot switch locks in that reading. The clinician reads the depth on the probe and signals that number to the computer with the foot switch. The printer then reports the temperature as low, medium, or high for each site and the corresponding pocket depth. A panel lights up with green, yellow, or red lights for each site corresponding with the three levels of temperature. This is helpful for involving the patient in assessing the level of health or disease.

Gingival enlargement or recession. Another measurement that must be made and recorded on the periodontal charting form is the height of the gingival margin on each tooth. The gingival height is the distance of the free gingival margin

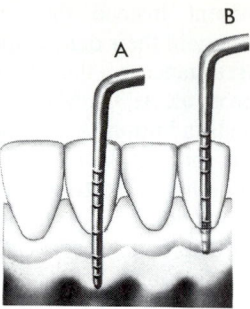

Fig. 12-14. The two measurements necessary to estimate amount of attached gingiva present. Probe *A* is measuring from mucogingival junction to free gingival margin on the facial aspect of the tooth (6 mm). Probe *B* is measuring pocket depth (3 mm). Comparison of these two readings, both taken on facial aspect of same tooth, will indicate amount of attached gingiva that is present (6mm − 3 mm = 3 mm).

from the cementoenamel junction (CEJ). If the height of the gingival margin is coronal to the CEJ, it is measured by placing the tip of the probe at the CEJ and measuring in millimeters to the free margin of the gingiva. If the free gingival margin has receded apically from the CEJ, the amount of recession is measured by placing the probe tip on the level of the free gingival margin and measuring to the level of the CEJ. Areas of gingival enlargement are recorded by noting a plus sign (+) in front of the number; areas of apical recession are recorded by placing a minus sign (−) before the number. Areas where the free gingival margin lies at the level of the CEJ are noted as zero (0) recession. Usually only one reading is taken on the buccal surface of each tooth, and another one is taken on the lingual surface. The highest readings obtained for each of these two areas are then recorded in the appropriate box on the charting form (see Fig. 12-7).

Pocket depth readings alone have little or no significance unless they can be compared with the level of the free gingival margin. For instance, a pocket reading of 3 mm on the buccal surface of a mandibular first molar may not sound significant by itself, unless the same area has 4 mm of apical recession, exposed root surfaces, possible furcation involvement, and bone destruction. Adding 3 mm to the 4 mm provides 7 mm of *loss of attachment*. The periodontal charting needs to show both the height of the gingival margin and the pockets measured from that landmark.

Masticatory mucosa measurements are also necessary. Place the tip of the probe at the mucogingival junction and measure to the free gingival margin. This measurement is shown by probe *A* in Fig. 12-14. Usually it can be made by simply identifying the difference in the appearance of the darker, shinier alveolar mucosa and the light pink, stippled attached gingiva (see Plate 3, *C* and *H*). If this line is not clear because of lack of attached gingiva or color changes resulting from inflammation, it may be helpful to retract the lip or cheek and move it coronally. Freely movable tissue is alveolar mucosa, and fixed tissue is attached gingiva (Kopczyk and Saxe, 1974; Vincent et al, 1976). This test is also valuable in determining whether or not frena or muscle attachments are pulling attached gingiva and causing recession. After the junction has been identified, one measurement can be taken for the buccal surface of each tooth and another for the lingual surface. The measurement representing the smallest amount of masticatory mucosa for any one tooth surface should be recorded on the charting form. This measurement is not necessary on the palatal surfaces of maxillary teeth because the attached gingiva is continuous with the masticatory mucosa of the hard palate. Subtract the pocket depth reading from the masticatory mucosa reading at each site to calculate the measure of attached gingiva. These two measurements are depicted in Fig. 12-14 as they are being taken on two different teeth. To be maintained in a healthy state, a tooth must have an adequate amount of attached gingiva. Experts disagree on exactly how much is "adequate," but studies have shown that as little as 1 mm may be sufficient to maintain gingival health. Less than that may be a significant factor in the etiology of periodontal destruction. The delicate, moveable, elastic alveolar mucosa cannot easily withstand the rigors of mastication and the trauma of brushing. If forced to do so, the result will be loss of gingival height and destruction of periodontal tissues (Hall, 1977, 1981; Lang and Löe, 1972).

Your clinical findings should be organized on a charting form such as the one shown in Fig. 12-7. The chart highlights comparison data for four separate evaluation periods. The monitoring system combines charted information and assesses the amount of inflammation according to sextants, assisting in tracking patient progress and differentiating case types.

Use an assistant to record the findings as they are detected clinically. This enables you to work more efficiently and makes it easier to prevent cross-contamination, because it avoids the necessity to keep moving from the mouth to the chart and back again. If an assistant is not available, you should minimize cross-contamination by disinfecting the writing implement before and after each patient. The Perio-pen (see Fig. 9-2) is an autoclavable pen with a calibrated probe at the other end.

Victor, a computerized charting system marketed by Pro-Dentec Inc. (Batesville, Ark.) removes the need for paper and pencil and eliminates cross-contamination altogether. Charting is accomplished by voice activation and produces graphic documentation on a comprehensive chart that can be filed in the patient's record. Fig. 12-10 is an example of the periodontal chart printout. This complete dental examination, diagnosis, and presentation system can be a valuable asset to any dental practice. Other computerized systems, with or without voice activation, are available to assist recording and archiving findings, both electronically and on paper.

The amount of attached gingiva on each tooth is also an important factor when considering treatment choices. Extensive instrumentation is frequently contraindicated in areas of inadequate attachment. Surgical techniques may be necessary for successful treatment of these areas.

Mobility

After completing the periodontal probing and soft tissue measurements, the clinician should continue to document the degree of bone destruction and loss of periodontal support by checking the mobility of all teeth. This can be accomplished with two single-ended instruments by placing the flat end of the handle of each instrument against opposite sides of the tooth and moving them alternately in a buccolingual and then a mesiodistal direction. Any more than normal mobility should be noted on the charting in the following manner (Periodontal Syllabus, 1975):

1 — Slight mobility
2 — Mobility of up to 1 mm in any direction
3 — Mobility of greater than 1 mm in any direction; tooth may be depressed in the socket

The amount of mobility should be noted in the box for each tooth on the charting form (see Fig. 12-7). This box should be left empty if no pathologic mobility is detected.

Furcation involvement

The presence of furcation exposure is a significant factor for both you and the patient. The patient should be aware of the presence and location of furcations that are exposed to the oral cavity and shown supplementary methods for plaque removal that can gain access to these concavities, such as wooden toothpicks, interproximal brushes, and irrigation. Instrumentation must be precise in these areas to disrupt and remove the plaque and endotoxins not accessible to the patient. Teeth with exposed furcations are highly susceptible to disease and frequently are lost as a result.

Use your knowledge of root morphology and your tactile sense to detect furcation involvements. It may be helpful to use a curved instrument such as a curette or a Shepherd's hook explorer, or Naber's probe (Fig. 12-15) to enter these areas. Fig. 10-43 depicts furcation involvement seen radiographically. The extent of destruction should be classified and recorded as follows:

Class 1. The explorer or probe can detect the concavity of the furcation but cannot enter it. This amount of involvement cannot be detected radiographically.

Class II. The explorer or probe can enter the furcation area but not extend through to the opposite side. A slight radiolucency in the furcation area may be detected with this amount of involvement.

Class III. The explorer or probe can pass all the way through the furcation to the opposite site. An obvious radiolucency should be visible, showing the total destruction of bone in the furcation area.

The classification Roman numeral I, II, or III should be placed in the appropriate box on the charting form (see Fig 12-7).

Limitations of current periodontal assessment methods

Most of the currently available assessment tools indicate with varying degrees of accuracy the presence of gingival inflammation or provide evidence of periodontal destruction. None of these measures can reliably predict the onset of periodontitis or the presence of actively destructive periodontal disease (Stark, 1992). There is no "gold standard" of measurement. Consider the limitations of each measure that is commonly used in the documentation of gingival and periodontal disease. (See Table 12-4 for limitations and Table 12-5 for emerging tests.)

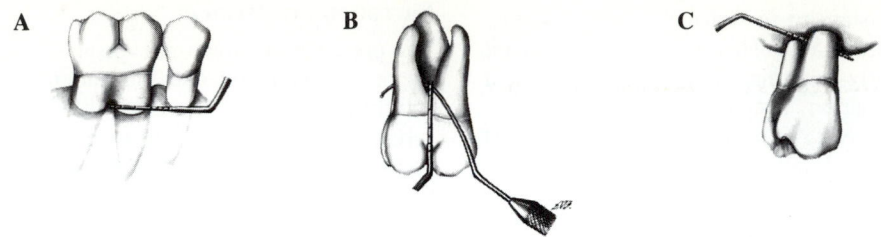

Fig. 12-15. Three teeth with furcation involvements. **A,** Tooth shows class I involvement in which probe can barely detect entrance to furcation. **B,** Tooth shows advantage of using a curved instrument, such as Naber's probe, to detect furcation. **C,** Tooth has class III involvement going all the way through to other side. (From Matarazzo R, Casullo D: *Continuing dental education*, University of Pennsylvania School of Dental Medicine, 1980.)

Table 12-4. Limitation of traditional measures of periodontal disease

Method	Measures history of disease	Detects current disease activity	Differentiates current gingivitis and periodontitis	Risk factor for periodontal breakdown
Probing depth attachment level	√			√
Gingival color, form, texture		√		
Bleeding on probing		√		√
Mobility	√			
Radiographic evidence	√			
Suppuration		√	√	√

Table 12-5. Emerging diagnostic techniques for periodontal disease

Method	Measures pathogens (cause)	Measures host response (effect)	Measures history of disease	Detects current disease activity	Differentiates current gingivitis and periodontitis	Rick factor for periodontal breakdown
Darkfield monitoring	√			√		
Culture	√			√		√
DNA testing	√			√		√
BANA hydrolysis	√			√	√	√
Aspartate aminotransferase		√		√	√	√
Collagenase		√		√		
β-glucuronidase		√		√		
Elastase		√		√		
Prostaglandin E₂		√		√	√	√
Interleukin-1		√		√	√	√
Perio temp		√		√		√

Measuring the putative cause

Darkfield monitoring measures the bacterial composition of specific periodontal sites to determine the presence and/or load of microorganisms believed to cause disease.

Listgarten and Hellden (1978) investigated the use of dark-field microscopy to examine the bacterial composition of submarginal plaque in both healthy and diseased periodontal pockets. They found that the distribution of bacteria in the healthy sites was primarily cocci (90%) and straight rods, with a small percentage of spirochetes (1.8%). In addition, most of the bacteria at these healthy sites were nonmotile rather than motile. When periodontally diseased sites were examined, the distribution of bacteria was very different. In these sites, spirochetes made up 37.7% of the total bacterial flora of the pocket, whereas cocci and rods made up only 40%. There were also equal numbers of motile and nonmotile bacteria. These investigators proposed that the simple technique of collecting bacterial samples from the pocket areas, examining them under the darkfield microscope, and counting the relative distribution of different types of bacterial cells would allow clinicians to determine exactly which sites had active periodontal disease at any given time. Listgarten and Hellden (1978) found that the numbers of spirochetes were reduced in pockets following treatment with tetracycline and/or scaling, as were other clinical parameters of disease. This demonstrated that identifying the proportion of spirochetes and motile rods by darkfield microscopy could be used as a means of evaluating treatment effectiveness. Singletary and others (1982) confirmed that microscopic evaluation of the subgingival flora was an accurate and convenient means of evaluating periodontal disease activity and monitoring the progress of treatment.

Darkfield monitoring is not considered an accurate predictor of periodontal disease activity. Although it does yield information about the presence of certain types of bacteria associated with diseased and healthy periodontal sites, the pathologic potential of these microorganisms and the thresholds or numbers of these bacteria needed to cause disease are still undetermined (Greenstein and Polson, 1985). Furthermore, some of the pathogens believed to be responsible are nonmotile and would not be counted on the negative side with darkfield monitoring. Until investigators can identify the bacterial levels or combinations most likely to result in disease in a given person or a given site, the results of microbial monitoring with phase contrast and darkfield microscopy are limited (Greenstein and Polson, 1985).

Culturing. Improvements in anaerobic techniques and in taxonomic classification of oral microorganisms in the past 20 years have made it possible to detect significant qualitative differences in the microbial compostion of healthy and diseased sites using culture techniques. By applying these techniques to clinical diagnosis, Slots (1986) identified a number of species associated with periodontal lesions. These species, referred to as the marker bacteria, are *Actinobacillus actinomycetemcomitans, Prevotella intermedia,* and *Porphyromonas gingivalis.* Though this method of detecting pathogens is still considered the "gold standard," it has been challenged for accuracy by DNA probes, ELISA, and immunofluo-

rescence assays (Loesche, 1992). It is highly variable and relies on bacterial samples that can survive 2 or more days' transport to the laboratory.

Deoxyribonucleic acid (DNA) probing. DNA assay detection of periodontal pathogens is at least equivalent and often superior to culture methods (Loesche, 1992; Savit, 1988). In contrast to cultural methods, these assays do not depend on the presence of living bacteria. Therefore they require no special media for bacterial samples and no special packaging.

DNA probe-based technology requires a plaque sample from a site under consideration or a pooled plaque sample from several sites. The sample is placed in a vial and mailed to a reference laboratory for testing. Three bacterial species present in the plaque are identified according to their specific DNA sequences and reported as high, medium, or low amounts of each pathogen. A study by Savitt and others (1990) showed that site selection should be based on clinical parameters such as probing depths of 5 mm or more and evidence of bleeding on probing. A specific test for *Actinobacillus actinomycetemcomitans* can help identify juvenile periodontitis in children and adolescents (Omnigene, Boston, Mass.). A device for in-office DNA testing is under development (Microprobe, Seattle, Wash.).

New techniques for assessing and monitoring periodontal disease

In medicine, a physician will use a variety of blood, urine, and other clinical patient samples to arrive at a diagnosis. Although this is not the case in dentistry, researchers are exploring other ways to assess and monitor periodontal disease. The objective is to find measures that can detect current disease activity, differentiate gingivitis and periodontitis, and/or identify sites likely to experience periodontal breakdown (sites at risk). As previously discussed, two factors are necessary for the initiation of periodontal disease: the causative agent or etiologic factor, bacterial plaque, and an insufficient or inappropriate host response. Both elements can be monitored to help identify sites of current and future disease activity.

Some clinicians will opt to use these tests at the beginning of treatment to establish a baseline result to which posttreatment measures can be compared. However, the more likely use is to help *identify a treatment endpoint following subgingival debridement where periodontal sites can be judged to be biologically compatible with health or to require further treatment*. These tests will also assist clinicians in general practice in *identifying patients whose lack of progress warrants referral to a periodontist*. In both general and periodontal practices, the results will help *determine sites at risk of further breakdown at recall or continuing care visits*.

Microflora: new diagnostics

(BANA). Benzoyl-DL-arginine-naphthylamide testing. Microbiologic testing can also be accomplished by evaluating the by-products of pathogenic organisms in the plaque sample. Three pathogens (*Porphyromonas gingivalis*, *Bacteroides forsythus*, and *Treponema denticola*), and only these, produce a trypsinlike enzyme that can be detected by an in-office biochemical chromogenic reaction test. A plaque sample is placed in contact with a reagent (BANA) that is hydrolyzed by trypsin; one of the resulting chemicals reacts with a colorant and appears as a blue blotch at sites on the test card that have plaque samples with one or more of these three pathogens (Perioscan, Oral B Laboratories, Redwood City, Calif.). BANA-positive test sites are associated with clinical signs of disease (Syed et al, 1984; Schmidt, 1988; Riviere et al, 1992), track the reduction and repopulation of periodontal pathogens following treatment (Simonson, 1992), and identify sites at risk for periodontal breakdown, including attachment loss (Loesche et al, 1990). The test requires approximately 15 minutes.

Filter separation enzyme immunoassays (FSEIA). Recently Eastman Kodak (Rochester, N.Y.) announced a FSEIA developed at the State University of New York at Buffalo. The test can identify antigens to *Actinobacillus actinomycetemcomitans*, *Prevotella intermedia*, and *Porphyromonas gingivalis*. The clinician mixes a plaque sample (taken with a paper point) with a reagent to produce a color reaction read as positive or negative. The test requires approximately 10 to 15 minutes of office time.

Enzyme-linked immunosorbent assays (ELISA) and immunofluroescence (IMF). Research laboratories have used ELISA to test for antibodies produced by specific pathogens and direct and indirect IMF techniques to tag specific species for microscopic identification. Neither of these is presently suited for routine office use.

Host response

As previously discussed, when the host is challenged by specific pathogens, the body responds.

Researchers have been studying various enzymes that are released from the host cells in response to periodontal infection. These include aspartate aminotransferase, collagenase, β-glucuronidase, lactate dehydrogenase, arylsulfatase, and elastase. Most of the effort in this area has been on the development of diagnostic tests that would measure the response of these enzymes in gingival crevicular fluid (GCF).

Aspartate aminotransferase (AST). AST is an intracellular enzyme responsible for cell metabolism. It is released into extracellular fluid on cell death. AST has been used as a marker of tissue destruction in liver and heart disease for many years. Animal studies (Chambers et al, 1984; Cohen et al, 1991) show a strong link between AST and tissue destruction in periodontal disease. Longitudinal human studies show a significant relationship between elevated AST levels and attachment loss in chronic periodontitis patients (Persson et al, 1990; Chambers et al, 1991). A rapid chairside test for AST is under development. It uses samples of GCF collected on filter paper strips that are placed in a test well and reacted with a liquid substrate to produce a color reaction that is eye readable as positive or negative.

Elastase. Elastase is one of several enzymes that is released by neutrophils as a result of tissue damage and bacterial infection. Studies have shown (Wells et al, 1990) that elastase levels in GCF are elevated in periodontitis as compared with healthy patients. A longitudinal clinical study (Palcanis et al, 1992) demonstrated significantly higher GCF elastase levels in sites with attachment and bone loss assessed 6 months later. A chairside elastase test is under development that uses GCF samples taken with impregnated substrate strips that are read using an ultraviolet view box.

β-glucuronidase (BG), arylsulfatase (AS), and alkaline phosphatase (AP). Alkaline phosphatase has been associated with bone metabolism and neutrophilic granulocytes. In a study by Binder and others (1987), levels of AP (73%) were associated with periodontal disease activity, although 36% of inactive sites were also identified. β-glucuronidase and arylsulfatase both demonstrate elevated levels in inflamed versus healthy sites (Lamster et al, 1985, 1986, 1989). BG levels have been correlated with increasing pocket depths and associated with subgingival bacteria including spirochetes, *Porphyromonas gingivalis*, and *Prevotella intermedia* (Harper et al, 1989). Further studies showing a relationship to attachment and bone loss are needed.

Collagenase. The collagenases are part of a group of enzymes know as metalloproteinases that are responsible for a majority of tissue destruction in periodontal disease (Page et al, 1991). Latent metalloproteinases are activated as part of the host response. Techniques for the measurement of latent metalloproteinases exist and could be adapted to chairside use. Long-term studies showing a relationship between levels of these molecules and active disease have not yet been published. A test kit based on nonspecific neutral proteases (of which collagenase is one) has been developed (Bowers et al, 1989) and approved for sale by the FDA. GCF is sampled with a filter paper strip that is placed on a collagen gel, incubated, and the resulting color reaction scored for quantity and intensity.

Inflammatory mediators. A significant number of inflammatory mediators are produced during gingivitis and periodontitis. To date two cytokines, tumor necrosis factor-α and interleukin-1 β have been studied. Prostaglandin E_2 is a product of the cyclooxygenase pathway of the metabolism or arachidonic acid and is a potent mediator of inflammation and bone resorption. A strong association between levels of PGE_2 in GCF and attachment loss has been demonstrated (Offerbacher et al, 1986). An in-office test has not yet been developed.

Other areas of study. A large body of data exists on the humoral immune response of patients (Ebersole et al, 1990). A number of researchers are engaged in the development of antibody assays to the putative periodontal pathogens. Although this information is unlikely to be of value on a site-specific basis, it may provide valuable information in assessing host susceptibility.

Much work still remains to be done in this area of host response tests. It is likely that there will be an integration of microbial and host response diagnostic information together with traditional clinical signs and symptoms to arrive at better initial diagnosis, monitoring of treatment, and patient prognosis.

LEGAL CONSIDERATIONS OF PERIODONTAL ASSESSMENTS

Bailey (1987) reported that the failure to diagnose and properly treat periodontal disease may be one of the leading causes of dental malpractice. The most common claim arising out of periodontal treatment procedures is negligence, indicating a failure on the part of the dentist or hygienist to meet a standard of care that is ordinarily used under similar circumstances by other members of the profession who are in good standing. Bailey also noted that dental hygienists are commonly named as codefendants with the dentist based on the failure of both to diagnose and treat periodontal disease.

A number of suggestions for protecting dentists and hygienists against lawsuits as a result of periodontal treatment have been given. Dentists and dental hygienists are legally responsible to detect, diagnose, and treat (or refer to specialists) periodontal disease in their patients. They must perform these duties in ways that are consistent with the current standards of care set forth by the dental profession. As research continues to modify the standards you need to evaluate and integrate these changes. You will probably work with dentists and hygienists who are not aware of these changes. In such cases, you need to consider your options and act responsibly (see Chapter 38).

SUMMARY

Periodontal assessment using traditional and emerging techniques is one of the most important functions you will perform as a clinician. The thoroughness and accuracy of your assessment have a major impact on the quality of the diagnosis and treatment planning that will precede treatment and on your ability to monitor patients who are in continuing care. Each aspect of the assessment helps complete the picture of health or disease and will reveal risk factors that will help you pinpoint areas of progressing breakdown and sites that are responding favorably to care. With the plethora of research regarding both the microbiologic and host response aspects of periodontal disease and healing, new diagnostics will be introduced in the coming decade that will help your decision making.

ACTIVITIES

1. View slides of actual clinical cases and describe and record as accurately and specifically as possible the gingival assessments. Discuss your descriptions in small groups and resolve discrepancies by reviewing the slides and discussing the most appropriate descriptions.
2. Examine extracted teeth for the presence of calculus, identifying each type of deposit for its shape, location, consistency, and color.
3. Explore the calculus on extracted teeth, tracing its shape and differentiating it from the cementoenamel junction and margins of restorations. Compare the feel of calculus with the feel of cementum and enamel.

4. Review the case descriptions of patients with unusual calculus formation noted in the text.
5. Review Moskow BS, Tannenbaum P, Bloom A: *J Periodontal* 56:223, 1985, which shows the periodontium with serial thin-section contact radiography. Note the calculus shown in Figs. 14 and 15 of that article.
6. Debate the issue: "Calculus must be removed for the periodontium to heal." Select references to support both sides of the argument. Include currently practicing clinicians on a panel to discuss the significance of this issue to clinical practice.
7. Watch slides depicting various factors that should be included on the periodontal charting form, such as the clinical appearance of tissues, radiographic findings, and study model records. (Study models could also be available for inspection.) Chart what you see individually while a faculty member does likewise on an overhead transparency. When the faculty member projects the transparency and slides together, check the accuracy and consistency of your chartings.
8. Assemble a variety of charting forms and compare samples for ease of use and completeness. Compare voice activated and direct-input (keyboard, electronic mouse, or probe-tip activated) charting systems for ease of use, cost, and completeness.
9. In small groups, discuss the many different ways in which periodontal findings can be recorded. For example, in how many different ways can the periodontal pocket depths be depicted? Use the same approach for gingival height, mobility, masticatory mucosa, and furcations. After the discussion, analyze these alternative methods in terms of *clarity* (could anyone understand what was being depicted?), *simplicity* (how complicated is it to reproduce?), and *efficiency* (can it be charted quickly?).
10. Identify all current and investigational diagnostic test and categorize each as a measure of cause (pathogens) or effect (host response). Review supporting research literature to specify whether the test can detect current active disease and/or predict breadown of specific sites.

REVIEW QUESTIONS

1. Identify seven uses of the periodontal examination and charting.
2. How is the amount of attached gingiva on a given tooth surface measured?
3. Describe the shape and location of the following types of calculus:
   a. Ledge
   b. Veneer
   c. Crustaceous
   d. Fingerlike projections
4. What is the role of calculus in the progression of periodontal disease?
5. True or false
   a. Calculus forms a mechanical lock with the cementum by molding itself to the irregularities of the tooth.
   b. Plaque is mineralized to form the hard deposit, calculus.
   c. Hard deposits can form within 2 days of a thorough debridement.
   d. The single most important skill for a dental hygienist is the ability to detect and remove calculus deposits.
   e. Plaque and gingival crecivular fluid contain enzymes that can help predict periodontal breakdown.
   f. BANA testing evaluates the presence of trypsin, produced by three periodontal pathogens.
   g. AST is a by-product of *Porphyromonas gingivalis*.
   h. The most important use for diagnostic tests for pathogens and host reponse is their ability to diagnose periodontal disease at the beginning of therapy.
6. Is it better to overangulate or underangulate the probe in interproximal areas?
7. On a charting, are pocket depths alone sufficient to describe the presence or absence of disease?
8. True or false:
   a. The calibrated end of the probe is adapted exactly parallel to the long axis of the tooth in all areas of the mouth.
   b. Periodontal charting will always be completed before any scaling is performed.
   c. Periodontal pocket readings are taken at the same points on every tooth.

REFERENCES

Abrams K et al: Histologic comparisons of interproximal gingival tissues related to the presence or absence of bleeding, *J Periodontol* 55:629, 1984.

Ackerman VH, Smith ES, Pierce LJ: "Stalactite" calculus formation, *Oral Surg Oral Med Oral Pathol* 67:613, 1989.

Alexander AG: A study of the distribution of supra and subgingival calculus, bacterial plaque and gingival inflammation in the mouths of 400 individuals, *J Periodontol* 42:21, 1971.

American Academy of Periodontology: *Proceedings of the World Workshop in Clinical Periodontics,* Chicago, 1989.

Armitage GC: *Selected lectures in periodontology,* San Francisco, 1974, University of California.

Armitage GC et al: Microscopic evaluation of clinical measurements of connective tissue attachment levels, *J Clin Periodontol* 4:173, 1977.

Baer PN: What is the role of subgingival calculus in the etiology of and progression of periodontal disease? *J Periodontol* 43:284, 1970.

Bailey BL: Malpractice and periodontal disease, *JADA* 115:845, 1987.

Barrington EP, Nevins M: Diagnosing periodontal diseases, *JADA* 121(4):460, 1990.

Baumhammers A et al: Scanning electron microscopy of supragingival calculus, *J Periodontol* 44:92, 1973.

Binder TA, Goodson JM, Socransky SS: Gingival fluid levels of acid and alkaline phosphatase, *J Perio Res* 22:14, 1987.

Birek P, Muculloch CA, Hardy V: Gingival attachment level measurements with an automated periodontal probe, *J Clin Periodontol* 14:472, 1987.

Blomlof L et al: Influence of granulation tissue, dental calculus and contaminated root cementum on periodontal wound healing, *J Clin Periodontol*, 16:27, 1989.

Bowers GM, Zahradnik RT: Evaluation of a chairside gingival protease test for use in periodontal diagnosis, *J Clin Dent* 1:106, 1989.

Buchanan SA, Robertson PB: Calculus removal by scaling and root planing with and without surgical access, *J Periodontol* 58:159-163, 1987.

Buckley LA: The relationships between irregular teeth, plaque, calculus and gingival disease, *Br Dent J* 148:67, 1980.

Buckley LA: The relationships between malocclusion, gingival inflammation, plaque, and calculus, *J Periodontol* 52:35, 1981.

Canis MF et al: Calculus attachment, *J Periodontol* 50;406, 1979.

Caffessee RG, Sweeney PL, Smith BA: Scaling and root planing with and without periodontal flap surgery, *J Clin Periodontol*, 13:205, 1986.

Carranza FA, Perry DA: *Clinical periodontology for the dental hygienist*, Philadelphia, 1986, WB Saunders.

Carter HC, Barnes GP: The gingival bleeding index, *J Periodontol* 45:801, 1974.

Chambers DA et al: A longitudinal study of aspartate aminotransferase in human gingival crevicular fluid, *J Perio Res* 26:65, 1991.

Chambers DA et al: Aspartate aminotransferase increases in crevicular fluid during experimental periodontitis in beagle dogs, *J Periodontol* 55:526, 1984.

Cohen RL et al: Association of gingival crevicular fluid aspartate aminotransferase levels with histopathology during ligature induced periodontitis in the beagle dog, *J Dent Res* 70:984, 1991.

Chaves ES et al: Diagnostic discrimination of bleeding on probing during maintenance periodontal therapy, *Am J Dent,* 3(4): 176, 1990.

Chuong R, Starns DL: Unusual calcareous bridge. *Oral Surg Oral Med Oral Pathol,* 70:681, 1990.

Claman LJ et al: Proximal tooth surface quality and periodontal probing depth, *JADA* 113:890, 1986.

Driessens FCM et al: On the physiochemistry of plaque calcification and the phase composition of dental calculus, *J Periodont Res* 20:329, 1985.

Ebersole JL: Systemic humoral immune responses in periodontal disease, *Crit Rev Oral Biol Med* 1:238, 1990.

Feldman RS, Alman JE, Chauncey HH: Periodontal disease indexes and tobacco smoking in healthy aging men, *Gerodontics* 1:43, 1987.

Fleischer HC et al: Scaling and root planing in multirooted teeth, *J Periodontol* 60:402, 1989.

Fowler C et al: Histologic probe position in treated and untreated human periodontal tissues, *J Clin Periodontol* 9:373, 1982.

Friskopp J: Ultrastructure of nondecalcified supragingival and subgingival calculus, *J Periodontol* 54:542, 1983.

Friskopp J, Hammarstom L: A comparative scanning electron microscopic study of supragingival and subgingival calculus, *J Periodontol* 51:553, 1980.

Friskopp J, Isacsson G: A quantitative microradiographic study of mineral content of supragingival and subgingival dental calculus, *Scand J Dent Res* 92:25, 1984.

Fujikawa K, O'Leary TJ, Kafrawy AH: The effect of reatined subgingival calculus on healing after flap surgery, *J Periodontol* 59:170, 1988.

Genco RJ, Goldman HM, Cohen DW: *Contemporary periodontics*, St. Louis, 1990, Mosby-Year Book.

Grant DA et al, editors: *Periodontics in the tradition of Gottlieb and Orban*. St. Louis, 1988, CV Mosby.

Greene JC, Vermillion JR: The oral hygiene index: a method for classifying oral hygiene status, *JADA* 61:171, 1960.

Greene JC, Vermillion JR: The simplified oral hygiene index, *JADA* 68:7, 1964.

Greenstein G: The role of bleeding upon probing in the diagnosis of periodontal disease—a literature review, *J Periodontol* 55:684, 1984.

Greenstein G, Polson A: Microscopic monitoring of pathogens associated with periodontal diseases: a review, *J Periodontol* 56:740, 1985.

Haffajee A et al: Clinical risk indicators for periodontal attachment loss, *J Clin Periodontol* 18:117, 1991.

Haffajee AD et al: Comparison of different data analyses for detecting changes in attachment level, *J Clin Periodontol* 10:298, 1983.

Hall WB: The current status of mucogingival problems and their therapy, *J Periodontol* 52:569, 1981.

Hancock EB: Determination of periodontal disease activity, *J Periodontol* 52:492, 1981.

Hancock EB and Wirthlin MR: The location of the periodontal probe tip in health and disease, *J Periodontol* 52:124, 1981.

Hancock EB et al: Histologic assessment of periodontal probes in normal gingiva, *J Dent Res* 57(special issue A):309, 1978.

Harper DS, Lamster IB, Celenti R: Relationship of subgingival plaque flora to lysosomal and cytoplasmic enzyme activity in gingival crevicular fluid, *J Clin Periodontol* 16:164, 1989.

Hassell TM et al: Periodontal probing: interinvestigator discrepancies and correlation between probing force and recorded depth, *Helv Odontol Acta* 17:38, 1973.

Hazen SP: What is the role of subgingival calculus in the etiology and progression of periodontal disease? *J Periodontol* 43:285, 1970.

Jeffcoat MK et al: A new periodontal probe with automated cemento-enamel junction detection, *J Clin Periodontol* 13:276, 1986.

Johnson BD, Engel D: Acute necrotizing ulcerative gingivitis: a review of diagnosis, etiology and treatment, *J Periodontol* 57:141, 1986.

Kani T et al: Microbeam x-ray diffraction analysis of dental calculus, *J Dent Res* 62:92, 1983.

Kepic TJ, O'Leary, Kafrawy AH: Total calculus removal: an attainable objective? *J Periodontol* 61:16, 1990.

Knuuttila M et al: Concentrations of Ca, Mg, Mn, Sr, and Zn in supra- and subgingival calculus, *Scand J Dent Res* 87:67, 1979.

Knuuttila M et al: Copper in human subgingival calculus, *Scand J Dent Res* 91:130, 1983.

Kopczyk RA, Saxe SR: Clinical signs of gingival inadequacy: the tension test, *J Dent Child* 41:22, 1974.

Kowaslski C: Relationship between smoking and calculus deposition, *J Dent Res* 50:101, 1971.

Kung R et al: Temperature as a periodontal diagnostic, *J Clin Periodontol,* 17:557-63, 1990.

Lamster IB et al: The effect of sequential sampling on crevicular fluid volume and enzyme activity, *J Clin Periodontol* 16:252, 1989.

Lamster IB, Hartley LJ, Vogel RI: Development of a biochemical profile for gingival crevicular fluid. Methodological considerations and evaluation of collagen-degrading and ground substance-degrading enzyme activity during experimental gingivitis, *J Periodontol* 56:13, 1985.

Lamster IB, Mandell RD, Gordon JM: Enzyme activity in human gingival crevicular fluid: considerations in data reporitng based on analysis or individual crecivular sites, *J Clin Periodontol* 13:799, 1986.

Lamster IB, Oshrain RL, Gordon JM: Lactate dehydrogenase activity in gingival crevicular fluid collected with filter paper strips: analysis in subjects with non-inflamed and mildly-inflamed gingiva, *J Clin Periodontol* 12:153, 1985.

Lang NP et al: Absence of bleeding on probing: an indicator or periodontal stability, *J Clin Periodontol* 17:714, 1990.

Lang NP, Löe H: The relationship between the width of keratinized gingiva and gingival health, *J Periodontol* 43:623, 1972.

Lindhe J: *Textbook of clinical periodontology,* Copenhagen, 1983, Munksgaard.

Listgarten MA: Periodontal probing: what does it mean, *J Clin Periodontol* 7:165, 1980.

Listgarten MA: A perspective on periodontal diagnosis, *J Clin Periodontol* 13:175, 1986.

Listgarten MA: The role of dental plaque in gingivitis and periodontitis, *J Clin Periodontol*, 15(8):485-7, 1988.

Listgarten MA, Ellegaard B: Electron microscopic evidence of a cellular attachment between junctional epithelium and dental calculus, *J Periodont Res* 8:143, 1973.

Listgarten MA, Hellden L: Relative distribution of bacteria at clinically healthy and periodontally diseased sites in humans, *J Clin Periodontol* 5:115, 1978.

Listgarten MA, Levin S: Positive correlation between the proportions of subgingival spirochetes and motile bacteria and susceptibility of human subjects to periodontal deterioration, *J Clin Periodontol* 8:122, 1981.

Listgarten MA, Rosenberg M: Histological study of repair following new attachment procedures in human periodontal lesions, *J Periodontol* 50:333, 1979.

Listgarten MA, Schifter C: Differential dark field microscopy of subgingival bacteria as an aid in selecting recall intervals: results after 18 months, *J Clin Periodontol* 9:305, 1982.

Listgarten MA et al: Periodontal probing and the relationship of the probe tip to periodontal tissues, *J Periodontol* 47:511, 1976.

Listgarten MA et al: Comparative differential dark-field microscopy of subgingival bacteria from tooth surfaces with recent evidence of recurring periodontitis and from non-affected surfaces, *J Periodontol* 55:398, 1984.

Lobene RR et al: Reduced formation of supragingival calculus with use of fluoride-zinc chloride dentifrice, *JADA* 114:350, 1987.

Löe H et al: Experimental gingivitis in man, *J Periodontol* 36:177, 1965.

Loesche WJ: Chemotherapy of dental plaque infections, *Oral Sci Rev* 9:65, 1976.

Loesche WJ et al: Bacterial profiles on subgingival plaques in periodontitis, *J Periodontol* 56:447, 1985.

Loesche WJ et al: Comparison of various detection methods for periodontopathic bacteria: can culture be considered the primary reference standard? *J Clin Microbiol* 30:418, 1992.

Loesche WJ, Giordano J, Hujoel PP: The utility of the BANA testing for monitoring anaerobic infections due to spirochetes (*Treponema denticola*) in periodontal disease, *J Dent Res* 69:1696, 1990.

Lustmann J, Lewis-Epstein J, Shteyer A: Scanning electron microscopy of dental calculus, *Calcif Tissue Res* 21:47, 1976.

Magnusson I, Listgarten MA: Histologic evaluation of probing depth following periodontal treatment, *J Clin Periodontol* 7:26, 1980.

Mandel ID: Biochemical aspects of calculus formation, *J Periodont Res* 10 (suppl):7, 1972; also 9:211, 1974.

Mandel ID: Calculus revisited: a review, *J Clin Periodontol* 13:249, 1986.

Mandel ID et al: Clinical immunologic and microbiologic features of active disease sites in juvenile periodontitis *J Clin Periodontol* 14:534, 1987.

McDougall WA: Analytical transmission electron microscopy of the distribution of elements in human supragingival dental calculus, *Arch Oral Biol* 30:603, 1985.

Meyerov RH et al: Temperature gradients in periodontal pockets, *J Periodontol,* 62(2):95-9, 1991.

Mislowsky WJ, Mazzella WJ: Supragingival and subgingival plaque and calculus formation in humans, *J Periodontol* 45:823, 1974.

Morita M, Watanabe T: Relation between the presence of supragingival calculus and protease activity in dental plaque, *J Dent Res* 65:703, 1986.

Morrison EC et al: The significance of gingivitis during the maintenance phase of periodontal treatment, *J Periodontol* 53:31, 1982.

Moskow BS, Tannenbaum P, Bloom A: Visualization of the human periodontium using serial thin section contact radiography, *J Periodontol* 56:223, 1985.

Mukherjee: The state of calicum phosphate in saliva of caries susceptible and calculus susceptible children and adults, *J Periodontol* 11:76, 1986.

Newman MG: Current concepts of the pathogenesis of periodontal disease—microbiology emphasis, *J Periodontol* 56:734, 1985.

Newman PS, Moran JM: Aspects of bone in periodontal disease, *Dent Update* 7:453, 1980.

Offenbacher S, Odle BM, Van Dyke TE: The use of crevicular fluid prostaglandin E2 levels as a predictor of periodontal attachment loss, *J Perio Res* 21:101, 1986.

Okamoto H, Haffajee A, Socransky SS: Longitudinal changes in peridontal subjects, *J Clin Periodontol* 14:662, 1989.

Page RC: Gingivitis, *J Clin Periodontol* 13:345, 1986.

Page RC: The role of inflammatory mediators in the pathogenesis of periodontal disease, *J Perio Res* 26:230, 1991.

Page RC, Schroeder HE: Pathogenesis of inflammatory periodontal disease: a summary of current work, *Lab Invest* 33:235, 1976.

Palcanis KG et al: Elastase as an indicator or periodontal disease progression, *J Periodontol* 63:237, 1992.

Pennel BM, Keagle JG: Predisposing factors in the etiology of chronic inflammatory periodontal disease, *J Periodontol* 48:517, 1977.

Periodontal syllabus, Bethesda, Md, 1975, Naval Graduate Dental School, US Navy Dental Corps.

Persson R et al: Relationship between levels of aspartate aminotransferase in gingival crevicular fluid and gingival inflammation, *J Periodont Res* 25:17-24, 1990.

Perrson GR, DeRouen TA, Page RC: Relationship between gingival crevicular fluid levels of aspartate aminotransferase and active tissue destruction in treated chronic periodontitis patients, *J Perio Res* 25:81, 1990.

Polson AM, Caton JG: Current status of bleeding in the diagnosis of periodontal diseases, *J Periodontol* 57:1, 1986.

Polson AM, Goodson JM: Periodontal diagnosis: current status and future needs, *J Periodontol* 56:25, 1985.

Powell B, Garnick JJ: The use of extracted teeth to evaluate clinical measurements of periodontal disease, *J Periodontol* 49:621, 1978.

Ramfjord SP: Indices for prevalence and incidence of periodontal disease, *J Periodontol* 30:51, 1959.

Randalls SA, Cohen ME: Problems in identifying "bursts" of periodontal attachment loss, *J Periodontol* 57:746, 1986.

Rateitschak KH et al: *Color atlas of periodontology*, vol 1, ed 2, New York, 1989, Thieme.

Retief DH et al: Quantitative analysis of Mg, Na, Cl, Al, and Ca in human dental calculus by neutron activation analysis and high resolution gamma spectrometry, *J Dent Res* 51:807, 1972.

Retief DH et al: The quantitative analysis of Sb, Ag, Zn, Co, and Fe in human dental calculus by neutron activation analysis and high resolution gamma spectrometry, *J Periodont Res* 8:263, 1973.

Richardson AC, Chadroff B, Bowers GM: The apical location of calculus within the intrabony defect, *J Periodontol,* 61:118, 1990.

Riviere GR et al: Relative proportions of pathogen-related oral spirochetes (PROS) and *Treponema denticola* in supragingival and subgingival plaque from patients with periodontitis, *J Periodontol* 63:131, 1992.

Ritz H: Population shifts in developing human dental plaque, *Arch Oral Biol* 12:15, 1985.

Robertson PB: The residual calculus paradox, *J Periodontol* 61:65, 1990.

Ruzicka F: Substructure of sub- and supragingival dental calculus in human periodontitis: an electronic microscopic study, *J Periodont Res* 19:317, 1984.

Ryan RJ: The accuracy of clinical parameters in detecting periodontal disease activity, *JADA* 111:753, 1985.

Saglie R et al: The zone of completely and partially destructed periodontal fibres in pathological pockets, *J Clin Periodontol* 2:198, 1975.

Sakae T, Yamamoto H, Hirai G: Scanning electron microscopy of dental calculi, *J Nipon Univ Sch Dent* 27:181, 1985.

Savitt ED et al: Comparison of cultural methods and DNA probe analysis for the detection of Aa, Bg, Bi in subgingival plaque samples, *J Periodontol* 59:431, 1988.

Savitt ED et al: DNA probes in the diagnosis of periodontal microorganisms, *Arch Oral Biol* 35:153-9, 1990.

Schiff TG: The effect of a dentifrice containing soluble pyrophosphate and sodium fluoride on calculus deposits, *Clin Prev Dent* 9:13, 1987.

Schmidt EF et al: Correlation of the hydrolysis of benzoyl-arginine naphthylamide (BANA) by plaque with clinical parameters and subgingival levels of spirochetes in periodontal patients, *J Dent Res* 67:1505, 1988.

Schroeder HE: *Formation and inhibition of dental calculus.* Bern, Switzerland, 1969, Hans Huber.

Selvig KA: Attachment of plaque and calculus to tooth surfaces, *J Periodont Res* 5:8, 1970.

Shah H, Collins M: Proposal for reclassification of bacteroides asaccharolyticus, bacteroides gingivalis, and bacteroides endodontalis in a new genus, *Prophyromonas, Int J Systemic Bacteriol* 1:128, 1988.

Shah H, Collins M: *Prevotella,* a new genus to include *Bacteroides melaninogenicus* and related species formerly classified in the genus *Bacteroides, Int J Systemic Bacteriol* 4:205-8, 1990.

Sherman PR et al: The effectiveness of subgingival scaling and root planing. II. Clinical responses related to resid calculus, *J Periodontol* 61:9, 1990.

Sidaway DA: A microbial study of dental calculus IV. An electron microscopic study of in vitro calcified microorganisms, *J Periodont Res* 15:240, 1980.

Simonson LG et al: *Treponema denticola* and *Porphyromonas gingivalis* as prognostic markers following periodontal treatment, *J Periodontol* 63:270, 1992.

Singh S, Manhold JH, Volpe AR: Definitive determination of clinical relationship between dental plaque and calculus, *J Periodontol* 43:39, 1972.

Singletary MM et al: Dark-field microscopic monitoring of subgingival bacteria during periodontal therapy, *J Periodontol* 53:671, 1982.

Sivertson JF, Burgett FG: Probing of pockets related to the attachment level, *J Periodontol* 47:281, 1976.

Slomiany A et al: Lipid composition of human parotid saliva from light and heavy dental calculus-formers, *Arch Oral Biol* 26:151, 1981.

Slomiany A et al: Lipids of supragingival calculus, *J Dent Res* 62:862, 1983.

Slots J: Bacterial specificity in adult periodontitis—a summary of recent work, *J Clin Periodontol* 13:912, 1986.

Slots J, Taubman MA: *Contemporary microbiology and immunology*, St Louis, 1992, Mosby-Year Book.

Socransky SS et al: Changing concepts of destructive periodontal disease, *J Clin Periodontol* 11:21, 1984.

Socransky SS et al: Difficulties encountered in the search for the etiologic agents of destructive periodontal diseases, *J Clin Periodontol* 14:588, 1987.

Spray JR et al: Microscopic demonstration of the position of periodontal probes, *J Periodontol* 49:148, 1978.

Stark DE, Hoover JN: Markers of periodontal disease susceptibility and activity—a review, *J Can Dent Ass* Feb 57(2):127, 1991.

Stamm JW: Epidemiology of gingivitis, *J Clin Periodontol* 13:360, 1986.

Subash G: An unusual deposition of calculus—a case report, *J Indian Dent Assoc* 57:180, 1985.

Sundberg M, Friskopp J: Crystallography of supragingival and subgingival human dental calculus, *Scand J Dent Res* 93:30, 1985.

Suzuki JB: Diagnosis and classification of the periodontal diseases, *Dent Clin North Am* 32:195, 1988.

Syed SA et al: Diagnostic potential of chromogenic substrates for rapid detection of bacterial enzymatic activity in health and disease associated periodontal plaques, *J Periodont Res* 19:618, 1984.

Theilade E: The non-specific theory in microbial etiology of inflammatory periodontal diseases, *J Clin Periodontol* 13:905, 1986.

Theilade J, Fitzgerald RJ, Scott DB: Electron microscopic observation of calculus in germfree and conventional rats, *Arch Oral Biol* 9:97, 1964.

Tibbetts LS: Use of diagnostic probes for detection of periodontal disease, *JADA* 78:549, 1969.

Turesky SS: What is the role of subginvial calculus in the etiology and progression of periodontal disease? *J Periodontol* 43:285, 1970.

Vincent JW et al: Assessment of attached gingiva using the tension test and clinical measurements, *J Periodontol* 47:412, 1976.

Volpe AR: Indices for the measurement of hard deposits in clinical studies of oral hygiene and periodontol disease, *J Periodont Res* 9(suppl 14):31, 1974.

Waerhaug J: Healing of the dento-epithelial junction following subgingival plaque control II. As observed on extracted teeth, *J Periodontol* 49:119(b), 1978.

Walker LG: Case report: unusual dental calculus. *J Can Dent Assoc* 56:847, 1990.

Wells B et al: Crevicular fluid elastase in healthy and periodontitis patients, *J Dent Res* 69(abstract):201, 1990.

SUGGESTED READINGS

Aeppli DM et al: Measuring and interpreting increases in probing depth and attachment loss, *J Periodontol* 56:262, 1984.

Allen D, Kerr D: Tissue response in the guinea pig to sterile and nonsterile calculus, *J Periodontol* 36:121, 1965.

Amato R et al: Interproximal gingival inflammation related to the conversion of a bleeding to a nonbleeding state, *J Periodontol* 57:63, 1986.

Armitage GC et al: Relationship between the percentage of subgingival spirochetes and the severity of periodontal disease, *J Periondontol* 53:550, 1982.

Caton JG, Polson AM: The interdental bleeding index: a simplified procedure for monitoring gingival health, *Compend Cont Educ Dent* 6:88, 1985.

Examination and diagnosis of periodontal disease, Bethesda, Md, 1975, US Department of Health, Education and Welfare.

Feldman RS et al: Periodontal disease indices and tobacco smoking in healthy aging men, *Periodontics* 1:43, 1987.

Fine DH, Mandel ID: Indicators of periodontal disease activity: an evaluation, *J Clin Periodontol* 13:533, 1986.

Fischman SL, Picozzi A: Review of the literature: the methodology of clinical calculus evaluation, *J Periodontol* 40:607, 1969.

Friskopp J, Hammarström L: An enzyme histochemical study of dental plaque and calculus, *Acta Odontol Scand* 40:459, 1982.

Gabathuler H, Hassell T: A pressure-sensitive periodontal probe, *Helv Odontol Acta* 15:114, 1971.

Gibbs CH et al: Description and clinical evaluation of a new computerized periodontal probe, The Florida Probe, *J Clin Periodontol* 15(2):137, 1988.

Giddon DB et al: Acute necrotizing ulcerative gingivitis in college students, *JADA* 68:381, 1964.

Goldhaber P, Giddon DB: Present concepts concerning the etiology and treatment of acute necrotizing ulcerative gingivitis, *Int Dent J* 14:468, 1964.

Goodson JM: Clinical measurements of periodontitis, *J Clin Periodontol* 13:446, 1986.

Green JC: Discussion: natural history of periodontal disease in man, *J Clin Periodontol* 13:441, 1986.

Haffajee AD et al: Clinical risk indicators for periodontal attachment loss, *J Clin Periodontol* 18: 117, 1991.

Hancock EB, Wirthlin MR: Histologic assessment of probing in the presence of gingivitis, *J Dent Res* 58(Special Issue A):239, 1979.

Hangorsky U: Early detection of periodontal disease by the general practitioner, *Compend Cont Dent Educ* 1:409, 1980.

Lang NP et al: Bleeding on probing: a predictor for the progression of periodontal disease? *J Clin Periodontol* 13:590, 1986.

Lang N, Hill RW: Radiographs in periodontics, *J Clin Periodontol* 4:16, 1977.

Listgarten MA: Pathogenesis of periodontitis, *J Clin Periodontol* 13:418, 1986.

Listgarten MA: A rationale for monitoring the periodontal microbiota after periodontal treatment, *J Periodontol* 7:439, 1988.

Mann J et al: Investigation of the relationship between clinically detected loss of attachment and radiographic changes in early periodontal disease, *J Clin Periodontol* 12:247, 1985.

Meitner SW et al: Identification of inflamed gingival surfaces, *J Clin Periodontol* 6:93, 1979.

Moskow BS: What is the role of subgingival calculus in the etiology and progression of periodontal disease? *J Periodontol* 43:283, 1970.

Moskow BS: A case report of unusual dental calculus formation, *J Periodontol* 49:326, 1978.

Muhlemann HR, Son S: Gingival sulcus bleeding—a leading symptom in initial gingivitis, *Helv Odontol Acta* 15:107, 1971.

Parr RW: *Examination and diagnosis of periodontal disease,* DHEW Pub No (HRA) 74-36, Washington, DC, 1975, US Government Printing Office.

Ralls SA, Cohen ME: Problems in identifying "bursts" of periodontal attachment loss, *J Periodontol* 57:746, 1986.

Ramfjord SP, Ash M: Significance of occlusion in the etiology and treatment of early, moderate and advanced periodontitis, *J Periodontol* 52:511, 1981.

Repine KD: Periodontal procedures for the general practitioner, I. Periodontal diagnosis, patient education, and referral procedures, *Compend Cont Dent Educ* 4:125, 1983.

Rodriguez-Ferrer HJ et al: Effect on gingival health of removing overhanging margins of interproximal subgingival amalgam restorations, *J Clin Periodontol* 7:457, 1980.

Schifter CC, Levin SI: Dark field microscopy: adjunct in assessment, *RDH* 4:52, 1984.

Setchell DJ, Shaw MJ: The graduated periodontal probe, *Dent Update* 7:431, 1980.

Singh S et al: Definitive determination of clinical relation between dental plaque and calculus, *J Periodontol* 43:39, 1972.

Spencer AJ et al: Periodontal disease in five and six year old children, *J Periodontol* 54:19, 1983.

Spindel LM et al: Plaque reduction unaccompanied by gingivitis reduction, *J Periodontol* 57:551, 1986.

Suomi JD et al: Oral calculus in children, *J Periodontol* 42:341, 1971.

Thielade J: An evaluation of the reliability of readiographs in the measurement of bone loss in peridontal disease, *J Periodontol* 31:143, 1960.

Van der Velden U, de Vries JH: Introduction of a new periodontal probe: the pressure probe, *J Clin Periodontol* 5:188, 1978.

Vanooteghem R et al: Bleeding on probing and probing depth as indicators of the response to plaque control and root debridement, *J Clin Periodontol* 14:226, 1987.

Villa P: Degree of calculus inhibition by habitual toothbrushing, *Helv Odontol Acta* 12:31, 1968.

Waerhaug J: Subgingival plaque and loss of attachment in periodontosis as evaluated on extracted teeth, *J Periodontol* 48:125, 1977.

Wilkins E: *Clinical practice of the dental hygienist,* ed 5, Philadelphia, 1989, Lea & Febiger.

Withers JA et al: The relationship of palato-gingival grooves to localized periodontal disease, *J Periodontol* 52:41, 1981.

13 PLAQUE AND GINGIVAL INDICES

Laura Mueller-Joseph
Irene Woodall

LEARNING OUTCOMES

The dental hygienist will be able to

1. Select the appropriate plaque or gingival index for evaluating plaque thickness, plaque area accumulation, gingival inflammation, and gingival bleeding.
2. Given a research article that reports plaque and/or gingival index data, describe the limitations of the measurements used and thus the limitations on the conclusions of the trial.
3. Integrate plaque and gingival inflammation measurement in daily clinical practice for the assessment, planning, and evaluation of dental hygiene therapy.
4. Use plaque and gingival indices during patient education and case presentation.
5. Perform the procedures associated with the evaluation of a particular index.

Plaque and gingival indices are used during the assessment, planning, and evaluation phases of dental hygiene care to gather information regarding the patient's oral hygiene practices and gingival health status. In addition, epidemiologic studies and clinical research investigations use plaque and gingival indices for data collection. It is important that you are familiar with these indices when reviewing scientific literature and selecting data collection measures for clinical practice or clinical research.

Indices range from simple to complex and each one has its limitations. The index you choose should be based on the question you are trying to answer. If you are selecting an index to motivate and monitor preventive home care programs then you need one that the patient can easily visualize and understand. If you find yourself in an alternative practice setting involving clinical research, you will be using a more discrete index that helps you quantify subtle differences.

USING INDICES IN CLINICAL TRIALS

In a research setting one or more of the indices described in this chapter may be used to quantitate plaque or gingival inflammation. You will use the indices during clinical trials (experiments) to identify appropriate subjects for the planned test and to measure each subject's status before the subjects begin their assigned regimens (baseline), at intervals during the study, and at the completion of the trial. The different regimens as-

signed to the different groups can be evaluated for their relative effectiveness by comparing the scores obtained from the various groups at each interval and at the conclusion.

For instance, if you wished to evaluate an antimicrobial rinse for its ability to reduce plaque and gingivitis, you would arrange for a colleague (so you remain "blind") to randomly assign one group to the active test rinse and the other group to a placebo rinse that has no active agent. You would score everyone's plaque and gingivitis at baseline and again at several time points during the trial and at the end. One or more statistical tests will determine whether the differences between the groups are statistically significant. The size of the differences between the groups, the amount of variability within each group, and the number of subjects tested contribute to this mathematical determination. You will use your professional judgment to determine whether the differences are clinically meaningful, in addition to their statistical significance.

Calibration

All examiners in clinical research trials must be calibrated with an experienced "gold standard" examiner before starting the trial and at intervals during studies of several months or more. If there is more than one examiner in a given trial, they must be calibrated with each other as well as with the gold standard examiners.

Calibration is performed in several phases.

First, the index is explained and discussed using the original documentation for the index as a reference. The examiners discuss, score, and resolve their judgments of intraoral color slides of the various conditions. The gold standard examiner is the arbiter of all calls that are not unanimous. Once the examiners reach agreement using the slides, the clinical evaluations commence. Subjects with a wide range of oral conditions are selected so that the full range of scores for a given index can be observed and scored. Each subject is scored by each of the examiners. Scores are compared among examiners to determine their percentage agreement.

All new examiners must have a high percentage agreement with the gold standard and all other examiners scoring in the same trial (inter-examiner agreement). Ninety percent and above provides confidence that each examiner will be viewing the conditions similarly, reducing error (noise) in the trial. Agreement below 80% introduces a greater likelihood of error in scoring among multiple examiners and less consistency with the definitions used for the index.

The last phase requires each examiner to be calibrated with him or herself (intra-rater agreement). Subjects are scored and rescored approximately 30 to 60 minutes later. The lag time allows the examiner time to forget how given areas were scored the first time. However, the lag should not be so long that oral conditions may have changed due to eating, drinking, brushing, etc. Again, 80% is a reasonable minimum target for intra-oral agreement; the higher the percentage obtained the better.

The most sensitive variable in a research trial is the outcome measure. If an examiner is poorly calibrated, the data that person gathers will be unlikely to show real differences that may exist between the groups.

Some of the following indices described present difficulty for calibration. Invasive indices that remove plaque or stimulate bleeding are problematic because once an examiner performs the index, the area is changed for the next examiner; thus the examiners' scores will vary. In such instances examiners are calibrated by making greater use of intraoral slides and then viewing the clinical sites together, scoring their results separately and silently. Others indices require extensive time for calibration because the judgment calls separating the various scores reflect subtle differences in plaque or tissue.

Review each of the following indices for the characteristic each is measuring and for the degree of subtlety each index measures.

PLAQUE INDICES

Dental plaque is positively correlated with periodontal disease. It is important for you to identify the presence or absence of plaque in the individual patient's mouth in clinical practice. Plaque indices provide more specific criteria to evaluate the presence or absence of plaque, plaque area accumulation, and plaque thickness and are used in research.

Plaque indices that identify plaque area accumulation use disclosing solutions to help see the deposits. The patient rinses with the dye or the clinician applies it directly to the teeth using a cotton swab or pellet. Several plaque-disclosing preparations have been accepted by the American Dental Association: erythrosine, or Food, Drug, and Cosmetic (FD & C) red No. 30; FD & C green No. 30; a combination of FD & C red No. 30 and FD & C blue No. 1, and fluorescein.

Erythrosine is the most widely used disclosing agent. However, care must be taken when applying the solution to the teeth because erythrosine can stain silicate fillings, clothing, and silk materials. It also temporarily stains oral soft tissues, including the lips, making it difficult to distinguish between stained deposits and stained gingiva. Patients do not find the staining a pleasant consequence.

Another visible colorant is FD & C green No. 30 (Mandel, 1974). Although this agent readily distinguishes plaque deposits from gingiva, it has the same staining potential as erythrosine. There are no commercially available products containing this colorant, and 2% to 5% solutions must be prepared by the clinican.

A commercially available combination of FD & C red No. 30 and FD & C blue No. 1 differentiates between old and newly formed plaque (Block, Lobene, and Derdivanis, 1972; Gallagher, Fussell, and Cutress, 1977). This is possible because of the differences in the plaque permeability of these two colorants. The red No. 30 distinguishes newly formed plaque, while old plaque is disclosed by blue No. 1. However, this agent also has the disadvantages of undesirable staining and discoloration of oral soft tissues.

A different type of plaque disclosing system is Plak-Lite (Brilliant International, Bala-Cynwyd,

Pa.). This system uses sodium fluorescein, which is visible only under a properly blue filtered light source (Lang, Ostergaard, and Löe, 1972). In laboratory studies, uptake of sodium fluorescein by plaque bacteria has been shown to be more specific than uptake of erythrosine (Landay et al, 1974).

Because the soft tissues are not stained, and the fluorescein is easily brushed from the teeth, patients view its use more favorably.

Once the disclosant of choice has been applied, the plaque is readily visible. You can show the stained plaque to the patient so he/she can see the extent of the deposits. This becomes a target for improving oral hygiene procedures. You can recommend that your patient use disclosants weekly to evaluate their efforts (see Plate 5 and Chapter 20).

Silness and Löe plaque index (PLI)

The Silness and Löe index evaluates the presence or absence of plaque and its thickness at the gingival margin. It is intended for use with the gingival index to help correlate the presence of dental plaque with gingival inflammation (Silness and Löe, 1964). No disclosant is used. To examine the plaque, the teeth are carefully dried with air. The examiner first looks to see if plaque is visible; if so, it is scored as either 2 or 3 (Table 13-1). If plaque is not visible, the examiner runs a periodontal probe along the tooth at the margin of the gingiva and examines the probe tip for plaque. If the probe is clear, the score is 0. If there is plaque on the probe, the score is 1. This index is useful for epidemiologic studies and clinical trials. However, calibration of the index examiner is difficult because the plaque is removed by the probe.

Turesky modification of the Quigley-Hein plaque index

The Turesky modification of the Quigley-Hein plaque index evaluates plaque area on the crown of the tooth without addressing plaque thickness. The plaque is disclosed and dried with air. The examiner looks at the area covered and scores the surface on a scale of 0 to 5, using the scoring criteria in Table 13-2. This index is designed to evaluate plaque area from the buccal and lingual aspects. It is widely used in clinical trials where more than one data collection period is needed without disruption of the plaque. Fig. 13-1 demonstrates the scoring criteria.

Table 13-1. Silness and Löe plaque index criteria

Score	Criteria
0	No plaque
1	A film of plaque adhering to the free gingival margin and adjacent areas of the tooth; the plaque may be seen in situ by using a probe on the tooth surface
2	Moderate accumulation of soft deposits within the gingival pocket or on the tooth and gingival margin that can be seen with the naked eye
3	Abundance of soft matter within the gingival pocket and/or on the tooth and gingival margin

From Silness J, Löe H: *Acta Odont Scand* 22:121, 1964.

Table 13-2. Criteria for the Turesky modification of the Quigley-Hein plaque index

Score	Criteria
0	No plaque
1	Separate flecks or a discontinuous band of plaque at the gingival margin
2	Thin (up to 1 mm) continuous band of plaque at the gingival margin
3	Band of plaque wider than 1 mm but covering less than 1/3 of the gingival third of the tooth surface
4	Plaque covering more than 1/3 but less than 2/3 of the tooth surface
5	Plaque covering 2/3 or more of the tooth surface

From Turesky S, Gilmore ND, Glickman I: *J Periodontol* 41:41, 1970.

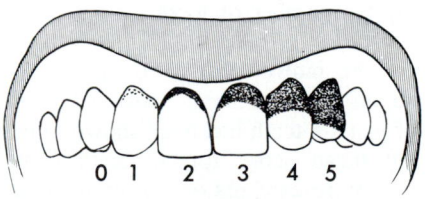

CROWN AREA COVERED BY PLAQUE

0 — None

1 — Separate flecks

2 — Continuous band to 1 mm

3 — >1 mm and <1/3

4 — >1/3 and <2/3

5 — >2/3

Fig. 13-1. Plaque area scoring method for the Turesky modification of the Quigley-Hein plaque index.

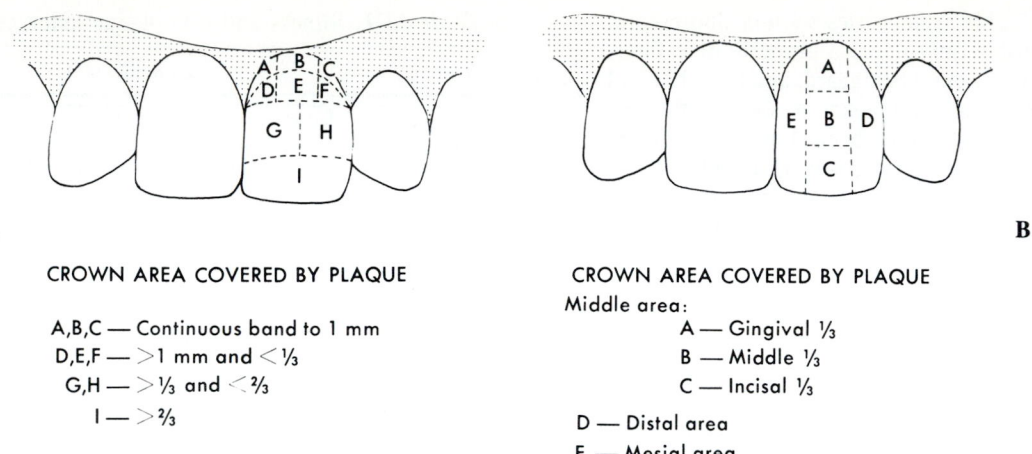

A

B

CROWN AREA COVERED BY PLAQUE

A,B,C — Continuous band to 1 mm
D,E,F — >1 mm and <⅓
G,H — >⅓ and <⅔
I — >⅔

CROWN AREA COVERED BY PLAQUE
Middle area:
A — Gingival ⅓
B — Middle ⅓
C — Incisal ⅓

D — Distal area
E — Mesial area

Fig. 13-2. **A,** Modified Navy plaque index. **B,** Martens and Meskin adaptation of Podshadley and Haley index.

• • •

Two other area scoring indices that emphasize the gingival margin and the interproximal areas are the *modified Navy plaque index* (Elliott et al, 1972) (Fig. 13-2, *A*) and the *Martens and Meskin* (1972) adaptation of the *Podshadley and Haley index* (Fig. 13-2, *B*). In these modified indices, each tooth is divided into nine or five segments, respectively, and each segment is assigned a letter and a score of 0 to 1. Numbers are totaled to provide a tooth score. Tooth scores are added and divided by the number of teeth for a whole mouth score.

All of the indices discussed up to this point evaluate all teeth present. However, the mean score of just six teeth has been shown to correlate with the mean score for all teeth (Ramfjord, 1959). Many researchers opt to score all teeth, although epidemiologic studies that are prohibitively large—500 to 2000 subjects—use these six teeth, the Ramfjord teeth, to provide an adequate sample of whole-mouth scores. The Ramfjord teeth are the maxillary right first molar, maxillary left central incisor, maxillary left first premolar, mandibular left first molar, mandibular right central incisor, and mandibular right first premolar.

O'Leary plaque index

The O'Leary plaque index is ideal for monitoring the patient's oral hygiene performance (O'Leary,

Drake, and Naylor, 1972). This index indicates the location of plaque and allows both the patient and the professional to visualize exactly where plaque exists. This visualization is valuable during plaque control instruction because specific problem areas can be pointed out and discussed with the patient, along with possible solutions. In addition, both the professional and the patient can see visual evidence of progress at recall appointments when improved plaque records are compared with the initial record.

The record is scored by applying a disclosant agent to the patient's teeth and then examining each tooth surface with an explorer or the tip of a probe. Only the cervical one third of the tooth at the dentogingival junction is evaluated; no attempt is made to quantify the amount of plaque on the tooth surfaces. Every tooth is divided into four sections (mesial, distal, buccal, and lingual) at the anatomic line angles (Fig. 13-3). If a soft deposit is visible, the corresponding surface is marked on the plaque control record by placing a dash on or shading the appropriate area. Missing teeth should be crossed out on the recording form; however, the pontics of fixed bridges should be evaluated because plaque can accumulate on these surfaces just as on natural teeth.

After all teeth have been examined, an index is calculated by dividing the number of plaque-containing surfaces by the total number of available

Name _____

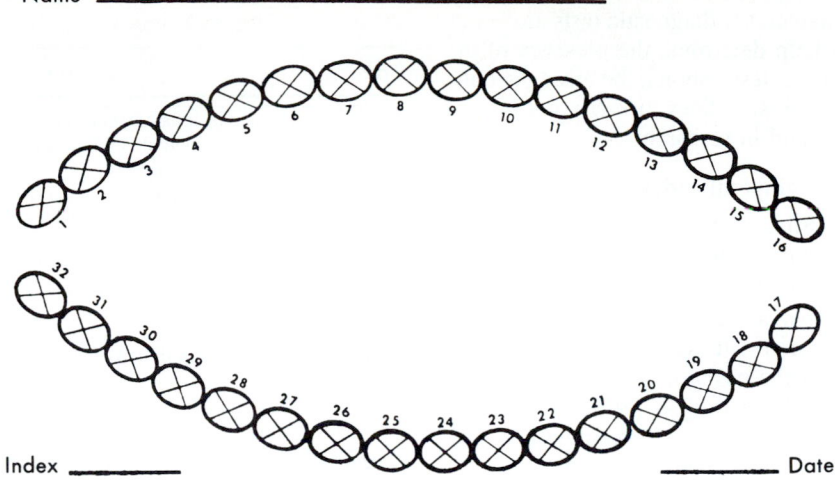

Index _____   _____ Date

Fig. 13-3. O'Leary plaque control record.
(From O'Leary TJ, Drake RB, Naylor JE: *J Periodontol* 43:38, 1972.)

surfaces (total number of teeth × 4 surfaces). This procedure is repeated at each appointment; the percentages of plaque-covered surfaces are compared to determine the patient's progress. O'Leary and coworkers have stated that a suitable goal in teaching plaque control is to reduce the plaque index to 10% or less of the available tooth surfaces.

Simplified oral hygiene index (OHI-S)

Greene and Vermillion developed the Oral Hygiene index in 1960 and modified it as the Simplified Oral Hygiene index in 1964. This index is very useful for large-scale epidemiologic studies; however, it is not sensitive enough to measure the oral hygiene status of an individual patient nor to look for subtle changes caused by variations in oral hygiene, which must be observed in many clinical trial designs. The index evaluates soft and hard deposits, plaque, materia alba, food remnants, and calculus on the facial and lingual surfaces of six teeth: the maxillary first molars, maxillary right central incisor, mandibular left central incisor, and mandibular first molars. The soft deposit score is added to the hard deposit score to determine the total OHI-S score, which is then divided by the number of surfaces examined to calculate the average oral hygiene score. The criteria used to evaluate this index are found in Table 13-3.

Table 13-3. Criteria for the Simplified Oral Hygiene index (OHI-S)

Score	Criteria
0	No debris or stain present
1	Soft or hard debris covering not more than one third of the tooth surfaces
2	Soft or hard debris covering more than one third but not more than two thirds of the tooth surface
3	Soft or hard debris covering more than two thirds of the tooth surface

From Greene JC, Vermillion JR: *JADA* 68:7, 1964.

GINGIVAL INDICES

Gingival indices are used in both private practice and clinical research. These indices evaluate the visual signs of inflammation, redness and swelling, and/or bleeding on probing. The examiner compares each papilla and gingival margin with color, form, and texture criteria and assigns the corresponding score. Some researchers have suggested that bleeding on probing is an easier and more sensitive indicator of inflammation (Hirsch et al, 1981; Meitner et al, 1979; Mühleman and Son, 1971). However, some inflamed gingival sites do not bleed when probed and other apparently healthy sites do (Ciancio, 1986). Therefore many researchers use both methods realizing that they are measuring two different variables. As discussed in Chapter 12, diagnostic tests are being developed that help determine the presence of inflammation. These tests should be used in conjunction with gingival indices to verify findings in clinical practice and in research.

Löe and Silness gingival index

The Löe and Silness gingival index measures bleeding tendencies, color, form, and texture of the gingiva. Just as the Silness and Löe plaque index separated that scale on the basis of visible plaque, the Löe and Silness gingival index separates the score of the basis of bleeding. If the site bleeds it is a 2; if bleeding is profuse, it is a 3. Although bleeding is the most important criterion of inflammation in this index, the distinction between normal and mild inflammation (on the low end of the scale) is based on tissue appearance.

The gingival condition of each tooth is examined by inserting a probe into the sulcus (approximately 1 mm) and sweeping the gingival margin. The intent is not to assess the depth of a pocket, to determine loss of attachment, nor to assess deep pocket ulceration but only to evaluate gingival health at the margin. If no bleeding occurs, then a score of 0 or 1 is given according to tissue appearance. If bleeding is present, a score of 2 or 3 is selected. The criteria for evaluating this index are found in Table 13-4. The patient's gingival index is determined by scoring the mesial, distal, buccal, and lingual gingival area of each tooth and dividing the sum by the total number of areas examined.

The Löe and Silness gingival index is invasive because the gingival tissue is manipulated by the periodontal probe at each examination point. Although this index is frequently used in clinical trials, its invasiveness represents a limitation. When the gingival tissue is manipulated, the microflora can be disrupted thereby stimulating a change in the gingival condition toward health during the course of the trial.

Lobene modification of the Löe and Silness gingival index

The Lobene modification of the Löe and Silness gingival index is noninvasive and focuses on color and form. The papillary unit along with the marginal gingiva is evaluated according to the criteria listed in Table 13-5. This index is highly sensitive with respect to subtle changes in gingi-

Table 13-4. Criteria for the Löe and Silness gingival index

Score	Criteria
0	Absence of inflammation, normal gingiva
1	Mild inflammation: slight change in color and little change in texture
2	Moderate inflammation: moderate glazing, redness, edema and hypertrophy; bleeding on probing
3	Severe inflammation: marked redness and hypertrophy; tendency to spontaneous bleeding; ulceration

From Löe H: *J Periodontol* 38:610, 1967.

Table 13-5. Criteria for the Lobene modification of the Löe and Silness gingival index

Score	Criteria
0	Absence of inflammation
1	Mild inflammation; slight change in color, little change in texture of any portion of, but not the entire, marginal or papillary gingival unit
2	Mild inflammation: criteria as above but involving the entire marginal or papillary gingival unit
3	Moderate inflammation: glazing, redness, edema and/or hypertrophy of the marginal or papillary gingival unit
4	Severe inflammation: marked redness, edema and/or hypertrophy of the marginal or papillary gingival unit; spontaneous bleeding, congestion, or ulceration

From Lobene RR et al: *Clin Prev Dent* 8:3, 1986.

val inflammation. Because it is a subjective measure, calibration is more difficult and time-consuming.

Papillary-marginal-attached (PMA) gingival index

The PMA gingival index is also considered noninvasive and is subject to the examiner's interpretation. The basis of this index is that gingival inflammation begins in the papilla, spreads around the gingival margin, and progresses to involve the attached gingival tissues (Schour and Massler, 1948; Massler, 1967). This index scores the severity of inflammation on a scale ranging from 0 to 4, as demonstrated in Table 13-6. It should be noted that there is controversy in the literature as

Table 13-6. PMA gingival index scores for the inflammation of the dental papilla, gingival margin, and gingival tissues

Score	Criteria
0	Normal, no inflammation
1	Mild papillary engorgement, slight increase in size, mild inflammation with slight change of color, and little loss of contour
2	Obvious increase in size, hemorrhage on pressure, moderate inflammation with swelling, glazing, and redness; tendency to bleed on slight pressure; papillae or margins become blunt and rounded; slight extention of inflammation to adjacent tissues.
3	Excessive increase in size with spontaneous hemorrhage; severe inflammation with more swelling and redness, pocket formation, spontaneous bleeding, and involvement of adjacent tissues
4	Necrotic changes, very severe inflammation, including ulceration and sloughing (as in acute necrotizing ulcerative gingivitis)

From Massler M: *J Periodontol* 38:592, 1969.

Table 13-7. Criteria for the sulcular bleeding index

Score	Criteria
0	Healthy appearance of P and M, not bleeding on sulcus probing
1	Apparently healthy P and M, showing no change in color and no swelling, but bleeding from sulcus on probing
2	Bleeding on probing and change of color due to inflammation; no swelling or macroscopic edema
3	Bleeding on probing and change in color and slight edematous swelling
4	(1) Bleeding on probing and change in color and obvious swelling; (2) bleeding on probing and obvious swelling
5	Bleeding on probing and spontaneous bleeding and change in color; marked swelling with or without ulceration

P, Papillary gingivae; *M,* Marginal gingivae.
From Mühlemann HR, Son S: *Helv Odontol Acta* 15:107, 1971

Table 13-8. Criteria for the papillary bleeding index

Score	Criteria
0	No bleeding after probing
1	One singular point of bleeding after bleeding
2	Several points of bleeding after probing
3	The interdental triangle fills with blood after probing
4	Blood flows immediately along the gingival groove after probing

From Mühlemann HR: *J Prev Dent* 4:6, 1977

to the validity of this index, and its usage has diminished (Ciancio, 1986).

Sulcular bleeding index (SBI)

Bleeding on probing is an essential part of the periodontal assessment and is a significant indicator of gingival inflammation (Greenstein, 1984). The SBI evaluates the presence or absence of bleeding by inserting the periodontal probe to the base of the sulcus and walking it mesiodistally and buccolingually. A score of 0 to 5 is recorded according to the criteria shown in Table 13-7. If only the identification of bleeding is desired, then the index may be evaluated using the scores 1 and 0, respectively. Bleeding on probing is easily assessed, and a more objective diagnostic sign.

Papillary bleeding index (PBI)

Another indicator of gingival inflammation is papillary bleeding. The PBI has been demonstrated to be useful in the dental office (Craig and Duhamel, 1981), public health programs, and school-based surveys (Saxter, Turconi, and Elsasser, 1977).

The PBI is performed by sweeping the papillary sulcus on the mesial and distal aspects with a periodontal probe. The mouth is divided into quadrants, with the maxillary right and mandibular left quadrants probed lingually and the maxillary left and mandibular right quadrants probed buccally (Fig. 13-4). Each papilla is scored according to the criteria listed in Table 13-8.

Bleeding measurement accuracy is affected by the width of the probe, angulation of insertion, and application of force. Each of these variables needs to be considered when analyzing index scores.

Gingival bleeding index

The gingival bleeding index evaluates the interproximal gingival unit for the presence or absence of bleeding, using unwaxed dental floss rather than a probe (Carter and Barnes, 1974). Unlike the periodontal probe, the floss provides a means of quickly evaluating a larger area of the sulcus. It is readily available, disposable, and can be

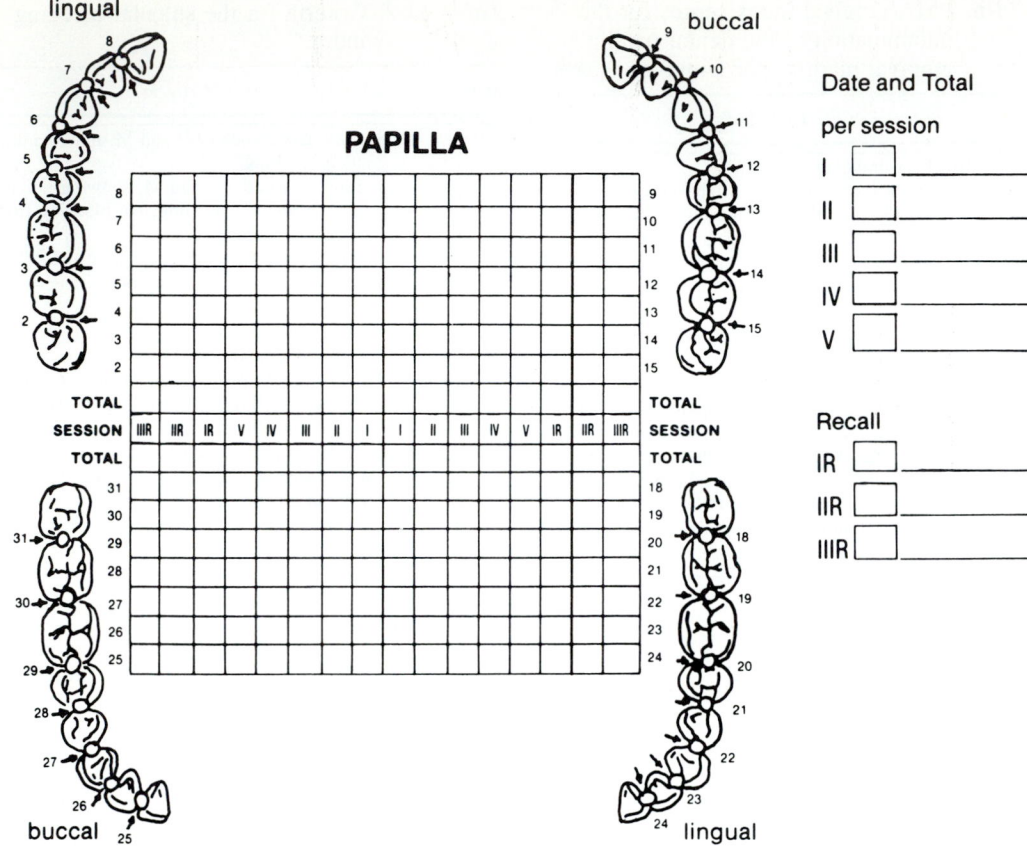

Fig. 13-4. Papillary bleeding index form.
(Courtesy of University of Pennsylvania, Philadelphia.)

used by the patient for self-evaluation.

No attempt is made to quantify the degree of bleeding with the gingival bleeding index. Floss is passed interproximally into the gingival sulcus, and the presence or absence of bleeding is recorded. Each interproximal area is considered one unit.

Caton and Polson (1985) modified the index to use wooden interdental cleaners (Stim-U-dents, Johnson & Johnson Products, Inc, New Brunswick, N.J.) instead of dental floss as the index instrument and renamed it the Eastman Interdental Bleeding Index. The Stim-U-dent is inserted between the teeth from the facial aspect, depressing the papilla 1 mm to 2 mm. This process is repeated 4 times, and the presence or absence of bleeding within 15 seconds is recorded. Both of these indices have demonstrated good validity and

reliability and serve as excellent self-evaluation instruments for the patient.

In reviewing clinical research that evaluates the efficacy of oral hygiene products such as floss, brushes, interdental devices, irrigators, dentifrices, and oral rinses, it is important to note which index was used for each parameter and to identify how those choices may have affected the outcome of the trial. For example, Glavind and Zeuner (1986) evaluated the effectiveness of a rotary electric toothbrush on oral cleanliness in adults. The investigators divided 40 adult subjects into two groups, matched according to dentogingival plaque. The control group was given a conventional toothbrush, an interdental brush, toothpicks, disclosing tablets, and home care instructions via an oral hygiene self-instructional manual. The experimental group received an electric toothbrush and instruction in its use from a dental hygienist. No additional home care devices were provided. Oral cleanliness and gingival health were assessed by evaluating (1) the presence or absence of plaque on each tooth from the facial and lingual aspects after disclosing with the Plak-Lite system, and (2) gingival bleeding following gentle probing. Measurements were taken at baseline and 3 months. Results showed similar improvements in oral hygiene in both groups, indicating that in the hands of patients, the electric toothbrush was just as effective as the comprehensive oral hygiene kit.

Although these results conclude that both home care systems were effective, data collected from the plaque index did not indicate the quantity of plaque present (thickness or area covered). Even if subjects from the control group had heavy plaque accumulation on certain teeth and subjects in the experimental group had minimal accumulation they would have been scored the same. Assessment of gingival inflammation was scored only with bleeding on probing, not accounting for changes in the appearance of the soft tissues. Also, some areas might have had profuse bleeding while others had only slight bleeding, yet both received the same score. The results of this trial might have shown superiority of one home care system over the other if the indices used evaluated the quantity of plaque and gingival bleeding instead of just their presence or absence.

SUMMARY

Familiarity with the available plaque and gingival indices is necessary when reviewing the literature, implementing independent research in private office settings, and monitoring patient home care progress. When choosing an index, remember to consider its limitations and your objective for evaluation. Base your choice on the ability of the index to provide clear and easily understood criteria, relative numeric values, and practical application.

Plaque and gingival indices are an important part of dental hygiene care to help determine the patient's present state of oral health. Previous chapters discussed diagnostic measures as they relate to the host response and the causative agent. All of these diagnostic tools are used in combination to provide the practicing dental hygienist with the information necessary to make accurate diagnoses and appropriate treatment choices.

ACTIVITIES

1. Use each of the described plaque and gingival indices on a student partner. Determine which methods are most easily incorporated in clinical practice for purposes of documentation and patient instruction.
2. Use a variety of disclosing solutions and evaluate each for its effectiveness, acceptability to the patient, and ease of use.
3. Conduct a patient education session using one of the plaque indices described.
4. Determine the success of your treatment by evaluating your patient using both plaque and gingival indices.
5. Select five articles that use plaque, gingival, and bleeding indices. Determine how results might have been different if a different index had been used.

REVIEW QUESTIONS

1. In gingival indices, the primary determinant in scoring is usually_____ and/or_____ in several aspects of each tooth or in each tooth as a unit.
2. Why should plaque and gingival indices be incorporated routinely into clinical practice?
3. What are the limitations of three gingival indices?
4. Identify the limitations of three plaque indices.
5. At what point in the dental hygiene process would indices be taken? Why?

REFERENCES

Block PL, Lobene RR, Derdivanis JP: A two-tone dye test for dental plaque, *J Periodontol* 43:423, 1972.

Carter HG, Barnes CP: The gingival bleeding index, *J Periodontol* 45:801, 1974.

Caton JG, Polson AM: The interdental bleeding index: a simplified procedure for monitoring gingival health, *Compend Cont Ed Dent* 88:89, 1985

Ciancio SG: Current status of indices of gingivitis, *J Clin Periodontal* 13:375, 1986.

Craig D, Duhamel L: The papillary bleeding index: a new aspect in motivation, *Eighth International Symposium on Dental Hygiene*, Brighton, England, 1981.

Elliott JR et al: Evaluation of an oral physiotherapy center in the reduction of bacterial plaque and periodontal disease, *J Periodontol* 43:332, 1972.

Gallagher IHC, Fussell SJ, Cutress TW: Mechanism of action of a two-tone plaque disclosing agent, *J Periodontol* 48:395, 1977.

Glavind L, Zeuner E: The effectiveness of a rotary electric toothbrush on oral cleanliness in adults, *J Clin Periodontal* 13:135, 1986.

Greene JC, Vermillion JR: Oral hygiene index, *JADA* 61:172-79, 1960.

Greene JC, Vermillion JR: The simplified oral hygiene index, *JADA* 68:7, 1964.

Greenstein G: The role of bleeding upon probing in the diagnosis of periodontal disease, *J Periodontol* 55:684-688, 1984.

Hirsch RS: The effect of locally released oxygen on the development of plaque and gingivitis in man, *J Clin Periodontol* 8:21, 1981.

Landay MA et al: A fluorescent microscopic study of human bacterial plaque smears stained with the plaklite fluorochrome, *Calif Dent Assoc J* 2:60, 1974.

Lang NP, Ostergaard E, Löe: A fluorescent plaque disclosing agent, *J Periodont Res* 7:59, 1972.

Lobene RR et al: A modified gingival index for use in clinical trials, *Clin Prev Dent* 8:3, 1986.

Lobene RR: Discussion: current status of indices for measuring gingivitis, *J Clin Periodontol* 13:381, 1986.

Löe H: The gingival index, the plaque index, and the retention index systems, *J Periodontol* 38:610, 1967.

Löe H, Theilade E, Jensen SB: Experimental gingivitis in man, *J Periodontol* 36:177, 1965.

Mandel ID: Indices for measurement of soft accumulations in clinical studies of oral hygiene and periodontal disease, *J Periodont Res* 9:7, 1974.

Martens LV, Meskin LH: An innovative technique for assessing oral hygiene, *J Dent Child* 39:12, 1972.

Massler M: The PMA index for the assessment of gingivitis, *J Periodontal* 38:592(part II), 1967.

Massler M: The PMA index for the assessment of gingivitis, *J Periodontal* 38:592, 1969.

Meitner SW et al: Identification of inflamed gingival surfaces, *J Clin Periodontol* 6:93, 1979.

Mühlemann HR: Psychological and chemical mediators of gingival health, *J Prev Dent* 4:6, 1977.

Mühlemann HR, Mazor ZS: Gingivitis in Zurich schoolchildren, *Helv Odontol Acta* 2:3, 1958.

Mühlemann HR, Son S: Gingival sulcus bleeding—a leading symptom in initial gingivitis, *Helv Odontol Acta* 15:107, 1971.

O'Leary, TJ, Drake RB, Naylor JE: The plaque control record, *J Periodontol* 43:38, 1972.

Ramfjord SP: Indices for prevalence and incidence of periodontal disease, *J Periodontol* 30:51, 1959.

Saxer UP, Turconi B, Elsasser CH: Patient motivation with the papillary bleeding index, *J Prevent Dent* 4:20, 1977.

Schour I, Massler M: Prevalence of gingivitis in young adults, *J Dent Res* 27:733, 1948.

Silness J, Löe H: Periodontal disease in pregnancy. II. Correlation between oral hygiene and periodontal condition, *Acta Odontol Scand* 22:121, 1964.

Turesky S, Gilmore ND, Glickman I: Reduced plaque formation by the chloromethyl analogue of vitamin C, *J Periodontol* 41:41, 1970.

SUGGESTED READINGS

Albino JE et al: Comparison of 6 plaque scoring methods for assessing oral hygiene, *J Periodontol* 49:419, 1978.

Barnes GP et al: Indices used to evaluate signs, symptoms, and etiologic factors associated with diseases of the periodontium, *J Periodontol* 56:643, 1986.

Bollmer BW et al: A comparison of 3 clinical indices for measuring gingivitis, *Clin Periodontol* 13:392-395, 1986.

Fischman SL: Current status of indices of plaque, *J Clin Periodontol* 13:371, 1986.

Marthaler TM: Discussion: Current status of indices of plaque, *J Clin Periodontol* 13:379, 1986.

Osterberg SK-A, Sudo, SZ, Folke LEA: Microbial succession in supragingival plaque of man, *J Periodont Res* 11:243, 1976.

Socransky SS et al: Bacteriological studies of developing supragingival dental plaque, *J Periodont Res* 12:90, 1977.

14 THE ROLE OF OCCLUSION IN DENTAL HEALTH AND DISEASE

Thomas G. Berry
Judith C. Berry

LEARNING OUTCOMES

The dental hygienist will be able to

1. Describe Angle's classification system.
2. Define overbite and overjet and demonstrate how to measure each.
3. Explain the importance of examining a child's occlusion with primary or mixed dentition.
4. Define the following terms:
   a. Occlusal trauma
   b. Occlusal traumatism
   c. Primary occlusal trauma
   d. Secondary occlusal trauma
   e. Centric stops
   f. Centric relation and centric occlusion
   g. Lateral and protrusive excursions
   h. Working and nonworking interferences
5. Recognize the differences between periodontitis and occlusal traumatism.
6. List, recognize, and record etiologic factors of occlusal trauma.
7. List, recognize, and record the subjective, clinical, and radiographic signs and symptoms of occlusal trauma.
8. Complete an occlusal screening for a partner.

Occlusion is important throughout life. Even a newborn has an occlusal relationship. When the infant closes his or her mouth, occlusion is obtained by placing the tongue between the maxillary and mandibular gum pads (Borell, 1980). From infancy onward, occlusion is important in such functions as suckling, swallowing, chewing, speaking, and even smiling. Many common complaints, such as headaches, sore muscles, toothaches, and tooth sensitivity to temperature changes, can be traced to occlusal or temporomandibular joint (TMJ) problems.

Occlusal relationships are important in each dental specialty—pedodontics, orthodontics, periodontics, prosthodontics, restorative dentistry, oral surgery, and endodontics. Pedodontists examine children's occlusion and growth patterns. If a primary tooth is lost prematurely, the pedodontist will recommend placement of a space maintainer to preserve the needed room for the succeeding permanent tooth (see Fig. 23-4), to maintain normal occlusal relationships. Pedodontists

and orthodontists evaluate the growing child's occlusion to detect early signs of malocclusion. If it is detected early, treatment is possible with a minimal amount of therapy. More severe malocclusions are treated by orthodontists. Periodontists are interested in occlusion because some patients' occlusion can damage the supporting structures of the teeth, which complicates periodontal treatment. Dentists performing prosthetic and restorative dentistry are concerned because each restoration placed will affect and be affected by the patient's occlusion either positively or negatively. Prosthodontists replace missing teeth to restore occlusal relationships. These occlusal relationships must be compatible with the patient's TMJ and neuromusculature to ensure comfort and function. Dental implants must have favorable occlusion to prevent bone loss, fracture of the prosthesis, or loss of the implant itself. Oral surgeons must be aware of these relationships when performing facial reconstruction procedures. Even endodontists must be careful to avoid traumatic occlusion on an endodontically involved tooth.

If you are to work with patients and clinicians in the various specialties to identify and help solve the problems related to occlusion, you need to examine the anatomy of the teeth, supporting structures, TMJ, muscles of mastication, and the blood and nerve supply to those areas. The hygienist's role is to detect potential or current occlusal problems and to alert the dentist to the findings. This chapter provides you with basic information about occlusion and methods for detecting problematic occlusal conditions.

APPROACHES TO OCCLUSION

The study of occlusion can be confusing because it is complex and can be approached through various means. Commonly accepted approaches to the study of occlusion and treatment of occlusal problems are the prosthetic concept, the orthodontic concept, and the concept of dynamic individual occlusion (Mosteller, 1980; Ramfjord and Ash, 1983). Each of these approaches to, or concepts of, occlusion has a particular set of guidelines for occlusal treatment.

The *prosthetic concept* of balanced occlusion was developed to guide the construction of full dentures. The word *balanced* is very crucial to this approach. The underlying principle is that there should be simultaneous, bilateral contact of the teeth during lateral and protrusive movements of the mandible to prevent the dentures from tilting or becoming dislodged. This approach is applicable for full dentures, rather than for natural dentitions (Mosteller, 1980; Ramfjord and Ash, 1983; Weisgold, 1975).

The *orthodontic concept* of occlusion is most concerned with tooth-to-tooth, particularly cusp-to-fossa, relationships between the teeth. Angle's classification and the positions of supporting cusps, discussed later in this chapter, are elements of the orthodontic concept. When orthodontia is performed, teeth are moved to approximate preestablished concepts of ideal occlusal relationships, such as a Class I molar relationship (Mosteller, 1980; Perry, 1976; Ramfjord and Ash, 1983). There is concern that excessive focus on cusp-to-fossa relationships, without enough regard for the neuromuscular and vascular components of occlusion and the TMJ, could lead to occlusal problems (Perry, 1976).

The concept of *dynamic individual occlusion* considers each person's particular occlusion and

recognizes that systems affecting occlusion are in a continual state of flux. Dynamic individual occlusion considers all factors, such as the neuromusculature and vascular systems associated with the TMJ and occlusion; stress and other psychologic conditions; tooth-to-tooth relationships; and other oral conditions, such as restorative, periodontal, and endodontic health (Mosteller, 1980; Ramfjord and Ash, 1983).

The dynamic individual concept of occlusion is presented in this chapter. Discussion of the relationship between occlusal and periodontal health, the occlusal screening examination, and the occlusal analysis are all drawn from this concept. Occlusal screening and analysis are beginning steps to evaluating the patient's occlusion. Other elements such as Angle's classification, overjet, overbite, and positions of supporting cusps are widely accepted measures of occlusion.

ANGLE'S CLASSIFICATION: IDEAL OCCLUSION

In 1899 Dr. E.H. Angle proposed a classification system designed to identify occlusions in need of treatment (Jago, 1974). This system evaluates the mesiodistal relationship between the maxillary and mandibular first molars (Thurow, 1977). Currently practitioners evaluate the cuspid relationship as well. There are three classifications in this system—I, II, and III. Class II is subdivided into division 1 and division 2. (See Figs. 14-1 to 14-3

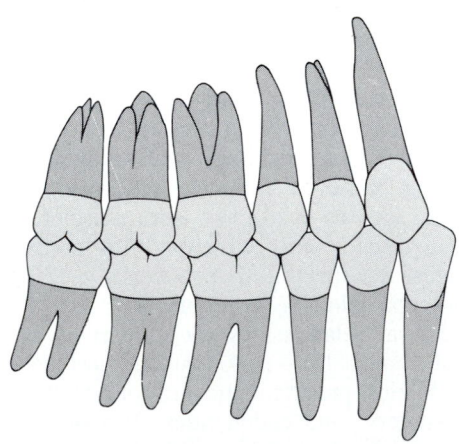

Fig. 14-1. Class I occlusal relationship. Mesiobuccal cusp of maxillary molar aligns with buccal groove of mandibular molar; maxillary cuspid rests between mandibular molar; maxillary cuspid rests between mandibular cuspid and first premolar.

(From Thurow RC: *Atlas of orthodontic principles,* ed 2, St Louis, 1977, CV Mosby.)

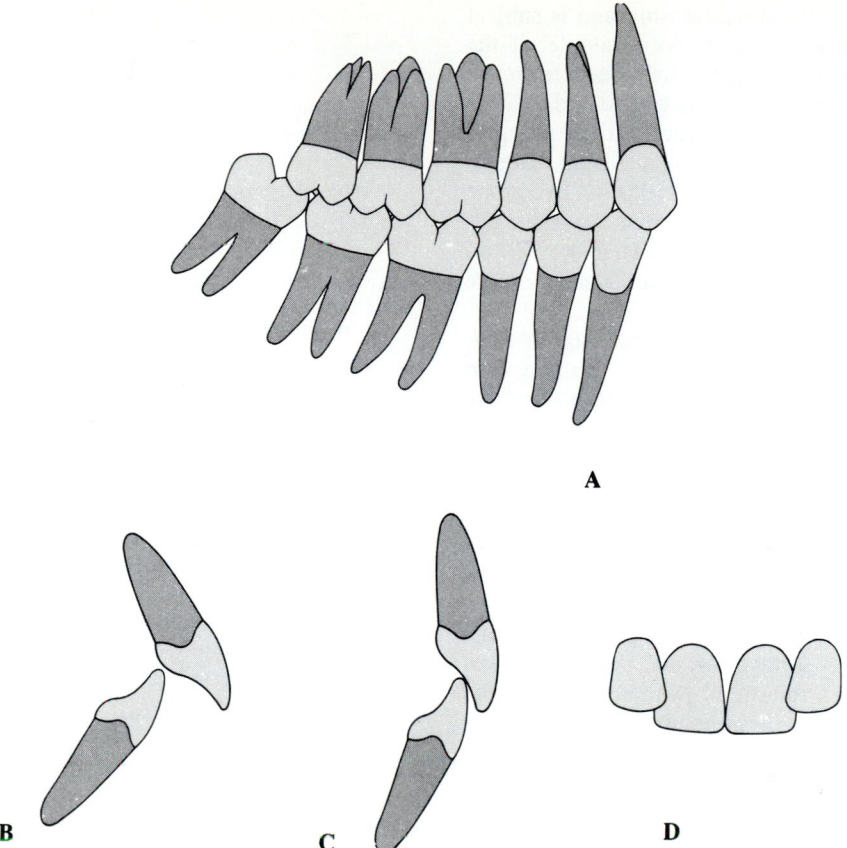

A

B   **C**   **D**

Fig. 14-2. **A,** Class II occlusal relationship. Mesiobuccal cusp and maxillary cuspid are mesial to mandibular landmarks. **B,** Class II, division 1. Anterior teeth are flared. **C** and **D,** Class II, division 2. Anterior central teeth are verted lingually.
(From Thurow RC: *Atlas of orthodontic principles,* ed 2, St Louis, 1977, CV Mosby.)

for a description of the classifications.) According to this classification system, Class I is the ideal occlusion. Any other type is considered a malocclusion that could require treatment. The terms *occlusion* and *malocclusion* are sometimes used synonymously for Class II, division 1; Class II, division 2; and Class III. The terms can also be used synonymously, although they usually are not, for Class I. It is possible for a patient to exhibit ideal first molar and cuspid relationship and to have crowded anterior teeth. This type of condition could be called a *Class I malocclusion,* although calling it *Class I occlusion with anterior crowding* would be more descriptive.

Angle's classification has limited meaning. It uses information about only a few teeth to clas-

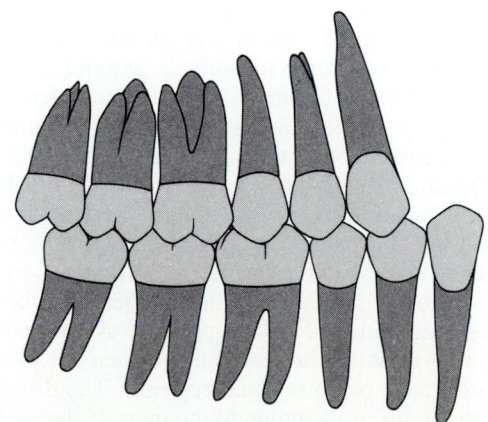

Fig. 14-3. Class III occlusal relationship. Mesiobuccal cusp and maxillary cuspid are distal to mandibular landmarks.
(From Thurow RC: *Atlas of orthodontic principles,* ed 2, St Louis, 1977, CV Mosby.)

sify the entire occlusal relationship and is subject to the clinician's judgment. For example, if the first molars are more than a half cusp from the ideal Class I, the occlusion is considered a Class II or Class III. Practitioners vary in their interpretation of half a cusp. Attempts have been made to develop new classification systems to overcome the shortcomings of Angle's system, but none has received universal acceptance (Thurow, 1977). Angle's system continues to be used until a more descriptive system is developed.

Angle's classification can also be used to evaluate the molar relationship in the primary and mixed dentitions. The primary second molars are used to determine the relationship in primary and mixed dentitions until the permanent first molars are sufficiently erupted.

During the clinical examination, Angle's classification should be noted and the patient's overjet and overbite should be measured with a periodontal probe. *Overjet* is the distance between the labial or lingual surface of the maxillary incisors and the facial surface of the lower incisors (Thurow, 1977) measured while the teeth are fully occluded. The probe is placed perpendicular to the long axis of the teeth with the point against the facial surface of the lower incisor and the side resting against the incisal edge of the maxillary incisor. Measurement may be made from the facial surface of the mandibular incisors to the labial or lingual surface of the maxillary incisor, depending on preference. If the measurement is to the labial surface of the maxillary incisor, the labiolingual width of the incisal edge is included (Fig. 14-4, *A*).

Overbite is the amount that the maxillary anterior teeth overlap the mandibular anterior teeth in a vertical plane (Thurow, 1977). If a patient has an edge-to-edge relationship between the maxillary and mandibular teeth, the amount of overbite is 0 mm. Usually the overbite is 2 to 3 mm. In a severe overbite the incisal edge of the mandibular teeth may occlude with the soft tissue of the hard palate. Overbite is measured in two steps. First, the probe is placed as if the overjet were being measured and held in that position as the patient slowly opens his or her mouth. When the mouth is open, the probe is placed upright. The distance from the tip of the probe to the incisal edge of the lower incisors is the amount of overbite (Fig. 14-4, *B*). Malaligned teeth may cause overjet and overbite to vary, so more than one measurement

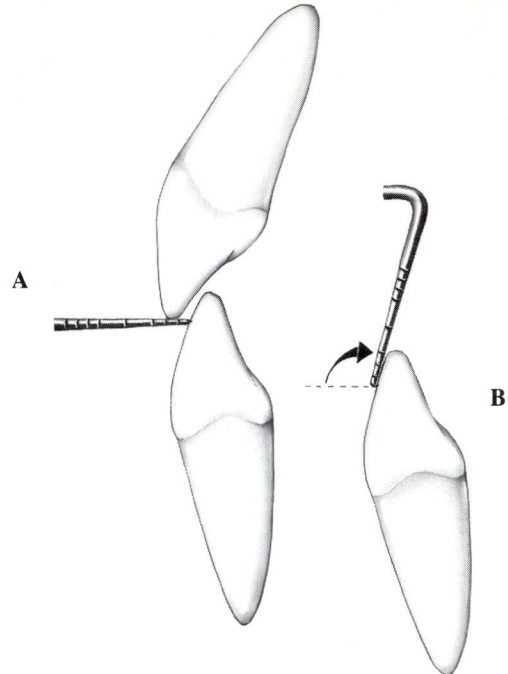

Fig. 14-4. **A,** Overjet is measured. **B,** Overbite is measured.

may be taken and recorded.

Overjets and overbites are measured the same way for the primary and mixed dentitions. Severe overbite is more common in the primary dentition than in the permanent dentition and is not necessarily significant unless accompanied by other problems.

DEVELOPMENT OF OCCLUSION

As previously stated, infants have an occlusal relationship. From infancy thorough old age, occlusion is important. This section briefly describes the development of occlusion from birth through the primary, mixed, and permanent dentitions. The characteristic occlusal relationships during each of these periods are discussed. Several influences on the development of occlusion must be kept in mind: biologic, anatomic, physiologic, pathologic, and environmental (Levine and Pulver, 1979).

Biologically, jaw size, tooth size, and the pattern of growth are inherited. Development of a person's occlusion will be affected by genetic endowment, but environmental and other factors play an important role (Levine and Pulver, 1979).

Anatomic influences include the craniofacial, vascular, muscular, neural, and endocrine structures and systems. All the systems composing the head, neck, face, and TMJ are of concern.

Physiologic influences include differential growth patterns. Chronologic and physiologic ages do not always coincide. Differential growth is a concern in evaluating development because the maxilla and mandible grow at different rates. At birth it is normal for a child to have a retrognathic mandible because mandibular growth is slower in utero. The coincidence of chronologic and physiologic age is to be considered in evaluating eruption of the teeth. Tooth eruption varies for each person. So, even though permanent first molars are "6-year" molars, very few children's molars erupt on schedule. It is necessary to consider the child's overall physiologic development when assessing occlusal development (Levine and Pulver, 1979).

Pathologic influences include physical and developmental disabilities or abnormalities that may interrupt, accelerate, or delay growth and development. These can range from minor problems (e.g., congenitally missing tooth) to more complex problems (e.g., a cleft lip and palate). Both would affect the occlusion, but to different extents (Levine and Pulver, 1979).

The final influence is *environmental,* including factors such as habits, carious lesions, traumatic injuries, improper dental treatment, and systemic disease. Habits such as finger or thumb sucking, improper swallowing, mouth breathing, bruxism, or tongue thrusting can affect the alignment of the teeth and growth of the jaws. Carious lesions cause tooth breakdown, which encourages tooth migration and loss of adequate space for succeeding teeth. Teeth can drift and tilt, contributing to abnormally directed force on the teeth. Traumatic injuries can cause tooth fracture or loss with sequelae similar to those of carious lesions. Iatrogenic problems, such as improperly placed restorations, interfere with occlusion. Systemic diseases can retard the growth and development of the jaws, teeth, or the entire skeletal system (Levine and Pulver, 1979).

In summary, these influences should be considered in assessing a child's or adult's occlusion. A thorough medical history is most important to fully understand a patient's condition.

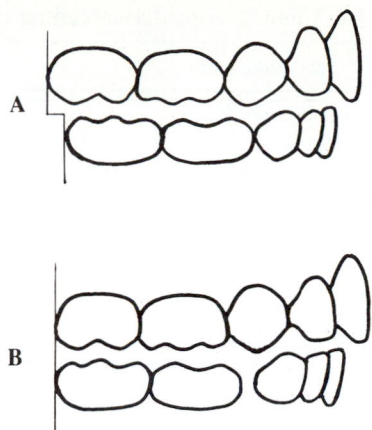

Fig. 14-5. Terminal plane is relationship between distal surfaces of maxillary and mandibular primary second molars. **A,** Mesial-step terminal plane: mandibular molar is mesial to maxillary molar. **B,** Straight terminal plane: molars are even. (From McDonald RE, Avery DA: *Dentistry for the child and adolescent,* St Louis, 1983, CV Mosby.)

Primary dentition and occlusion

By 2½ years a full set of primary teeth should have erupted. Eruption usually begins at 4 to 6 months. A deep overbite and overjet are common (Borell, 1980) because the growth rate of the mandible is slower. The growth of the mandible should be sufficient by the time the primary second molars erupt to reduce the overbite and overjet to approximately normal ranges. If not, the Class II molar relationship is likely to persist into the permanent dentition (Borell, 1980). The primary dentition usually includes spaces between the maxillary lateral incisor and the canine and between the mandibular canine and first molar. These spaces are called "primate spaces" (Moyers, 1988). In addition to the primate spaces, the primary dentition also includes upright teeth and either a straight or mesial-step terminal plane between the opposing second molars (Borell, 1980; McDonald and Avery, 1983). Fig. 14-5 illustrates the difference between a straight and a mesial-step terminal plane. The planes are important. The permanent first molars are guided into position by the distal surfaces of the second primary molars. The configuration of the plane, in conjunction with the presence or absence of the primate space, influences the likelihood of the development of a Class I molar relationship in the per-

Table 14-1. Centric stops during centric occlusion

Supporting cusps	contact with	Fossae or marginal ridges
Maxillary lingual cusps		*Mandibular ridges or fossae*
Lingual cusps of premolars		Marginal ridges of second premolar and first molar
Mesiolingual cusps of molars		Central fossae of mandibular molars
Distolingual cusps of molars		Marginal ridges of mandibular molars
Mandibular incisal edges and buccal cusps		*Maxillary ridges or fossae*
Incisal edges		Lingual fossae of incisors
Cusp of canine		Mesial marginal ridge of first premolar
Buccal cusps of premolars		Marginal ridges of premolars
Mesiobuccal cusps of molars		Distal marginal ridge of second premolar and marginal ridges of molars
Distobuccal cusps of molars		Central fossae of maxillary molars

Compiled from Ramfjord SP, Ash MM: *Occlusion,* Philadelphia, 1983, WB Saunders.

manent dentition (Borell, 1980; McDonald and Avery, 1983). A Class I relationship can develop with any combination of terminal plane and the absence or presence of the primate space, but it is most likely if there is a mesial-step plane and a primate space (McDonald and Avery, 1983).

Mixed dentition and occlusion

The mixed dentition is composed of both primary and secondary teeth. Permanent teeth are either *successional* (replacements for primary teeth) or *accessional* (new additions to the dental arches) (Borell, 1980). The mixed dentition covers the period from 6 to 12 years of age. This period is of great importance to the development of normal occlusion. Children should have their dentitions and occlusions evaluated, and steps should be taken to enhance normal development. Eruption patterns should be assessed and primary teeth should be extracted in a timely fashion. *Leeway space* (the sum of the mesiodistal widths of primary teeth from the cuspid to the second molar) should be evaluated. The leeway space is usually wider than the successional teeth. Maxillary leeway space is greater than the mandibular space. This enhances the development of a normal molar relationship in the permanent dentition (Borell, 1980).

The path of closure and the lateral and protrusive movements of the mandible should also be evaluated. These characteristic movements are likely to continue with the permanent dentition. If problems or interferences are present, they should be detected and treated (Borell, 1980). Evaluation of the path of closure and movements of the man-

dible will be described in the section on occlusal analysis.

Permanent dentition and occlusion

By age 12, the permanent dentition, excluding the third molars, is usually present. Normally there are no interproximal spaces. There are axial tilts to the teeth to foster a trituration chewing stroke (Borell, 1980). There is a Class I molar relationship. "Normal" is not synonymous with "ideal." The previous description of normal is close to ideal, but it covers a wide range. Occlusal screening and analysis determine if the patient's occlusion can be considered normal (i.e., not causing damage to the supporting structures). Many dentists refer to such an occlusion as a physiologic occlusion.

Centric occlusion, or maximum intercuspation, is the position of the mandible guided by the teeth (Ramfjord and Ash, 1983). Centric occlusion occurs when the patient closes his or her mouth "as usual." It is the position in which the teeth best fit together and usually is the position of the mandible during the last stages of chewing and swallowing. The buccal cusps of the mandible posterior teeth and the lingual cusps of the maxillary posterior teeth are called the *supporting cusps.* They occlude with either the marginal ridges or fossae of the opposing teeth. These occluding surfaces—cusp tips, marginal ridges, and fossae—are referred to as *centric stops* (Ramfjord and Ash, 1983). Table 14-1 lists the centric stops. To visualize the relationships among the centric stops, look at a set of study models of a normal occlusion.

Centric relation is the most retruded position of the mandible (Mosteller, 1980; Ramfjord and Ash, 1983). It is guided by ligaments and the structure of the condyles, articular disks, and glenoid fossae. Because centric relation is guided by anatomic structures other than the teeth, it is said to be a reproducible relationship between the jaws. Centric relation is routinely used to determine the occlusion when full or fixed partial dentures are constructed. In most persons centric relation and centric occlusion are not the same; rather, centric occlusion is usually slightly anterior to centric relation (Mosteller, 1980; Ramfjord and Ash, 1983). A discrepancy between centric relation and centric occlusion is noteworthy for the patient's chart, but it does not denote occlusal problems in and of itself (Mosteller, 1980; Ramfjord and Ash, 1983).

Protrusive excursion is the forward movement of the mandible from centric relation or centric occlusion until the anterior teeth are in an edge-to-edge relationship. Once the anterior teeth are edge to edge there should be no contact between the posterior teeth (Mosteller, 1980).

Lateral excursion is the movement of the mandible from centric occlusion or centric relation to the right or left until the cuspids on that side are in a cusp-to-cusp relationship. Some persons will be able to achieve contact between the cuspids only; others will have cusp-to-cusp contact with the premolars and molars as well. In lateral excursion the teeth on the opposite side, the *nonworking side,* should be out of occlusion. For example, a jaw movement to the right is a right lateral excursion. The right side is the *working side,* and the left side is the *nonworking side*. If any teeth other than the right cuspids are occluding, they may be *interferences: working interferences* if they are on the right side and *nonworking interferences* if they are on the left. Nonworking interferences are much more likely to cause destruction of the supporting structures than are working interferences. However, if several of the teeth in addition to the cuspid occlude evenly on the working side, the effect is not detrimental (Mosteller, 1980; Ramfjord and Ash, 1983).

Thus far the development of normal occlusion has been described and its characteristics discussed. Many patients have occlusal problems that cause great pain, discomfort, and tooth loss. The remainder of the chapter addresses occlusal trauma and assessment of occlusion.

TRAUMA FROM OCCLUSION

Ideally the teeth are well aligned within each arch; proximal contacts are present between adjacent teeth; marginal ridges of adjacent teeth are even; there are no rotated or malposed teeth (Krauss et al, 1969); and the teeth occlude in a Class I relationship (Thurow, 1977). This ideal arrangement permits occlusal forces to be directed along the long axis of the teeth and to be shared by adjacent teeth (Carranza, 1979; Goldman and Cohen, 1980; Krauss et al, 1969; Ramfjord and Ash, 1983; Thurow, 1977). The supporting structures of the teeth, the periodontal ligament, cementum, and the bone absorb the forces directed along the long axis of the tooth. The supporting structures can be damaged from forces that are in an oblique or horizontal direction to the long axis. In addition to directing the forces along the long axis, this ideal arrangement balances the forces applied to the teeth by the tongue with the forces applied by the lips and cheeks (Carranza, 1979; Goldman and Cohen, 1980; Krauss et al, 1969; Ramfjord and Ash, 1983; Thurow, 1977). Forces applied to a less desirable arrangement may damage supporting structures; this damage is called *occlusal traumatism* (Glossary of Terms, 1992). *Occlusal trauma* is a force capable of producing pathologic changes in the periodontium (Glossary of Terms, 1992).

There are two types of occlusal trauma: primary and secondary. *Primary occlusal trauma* is excessive occlusal force applied to a tooth with normal supporting structures (Glossary of Terms, 1992). *Secondary occlusal trauma* is defined as normal occlusal forces causing trauma to the attachment apparatus of a tooth or teeth because of inadequate support structure (Glossary of Terms, 1992).

Occlusal trauma is a noninflammatory, destructive disease that affects the supporting structures. It is independent from periodontitis. Occlusal trauma does not cause periodontal pockets (Carranza, 1979; Chasen, 1990; Goldman and Cohen, 1980; Zander and Polson, 1977). However, a tooth that is periodontally involved may be adversely affected by occlusal trauma. Occlusal traumatism is reversible if the etiologic factor or factors are removed or if the tooth moves away from the forces (Ramfjord and Ash, 1981). Therefore it is important to recognize and record the possible etiologic factors of occlusal trauma.

There are many possible etiologic factors of occlusal trauma. Any disturbance that interferes with normal direction of occlusal forces or is frequent and excessive, especially if exerted on one or a few teeth, can cause destruction of the supporting structures (Carranza, 1979; Goldman and Cohen, 1980). Etiologic factors that may affect occlusion include (Carranza, 1979; Goldman and Cohen, 1980; Krause et al, 1969):

1. Tooth position
   a. Rotated teeth
   b. Malposed teeth
   c. Extruded or submerged teeth
   d. Drifted teeth
   e. Missing teeth
   f. Other malocclusion
2. Tooth-to-tooth habits
   a. Clenching
   b. Grinding
3. Foreign object-to-teeth habits
   a. Biting pipe, pen, pencil, or other objects
   b. Biting or chewing fingernails
   c. Sucking thumb or fingers
4. Oral musculature habits
   a. Tongue thrust
   b. Tongue resting position
   c. Lip or cheek biting or sucking
   d. Mouth breathing
5. Iatrogenic factors
   a. Improperly contoured restorations
   b. Improperly fitted removal appliances

Factors causing occlusal traumatism or having the potential to cause it should be noted in the record during the examination. In addition to etiologic factors, specific subjective, clinical, and radiographic signs and symptoms of occlusal traumatism should be detected and recorded by the clinician using an occlusal screening form, such as illustrated in the sample.

OCCLUSAL SCREENING

Subjective signs and symptoms reported by the patient are important in detecting occlusal traumatism. The patient may notice aching muscles, tooth mobility, pain when biting or pain with temperature changes. It is important to question the patient about habits such as grinding or clenching the teeth, holding a pipe, chewing objects in one area, biting the lip, sucking a finger or thumb and about specific times of day that symptoms are noticeable. Sometimes a patient may be unaware of a habit or its significance until questioned.

SAMPLE
Occlusal Screening Form

Patient's subjective findings

1. Are you pleased with the way your teeth look?
2. Have you noticed if any of your teeth have moved?
3. Do you have any problems speaking or eating because of your teeth?
4. Are any of your teeth bothering you? Are any of your teeth sore?
5. Do you clench or grind your teeth?
6. Do you bite or chew your lips, cheeks, or fingers?
7. Do you bite or chew any objects such as pencils or pipes?
8. Do you feel a "click" or "bump" when you open or close your jaw?

Clinical findings: record the tooth number of any tooth that exhibits

1. Mobility
2. Wear patterns
3. Malposition
4. Faulty restoration

and note the presence of

5. Pain or clicking in TMJ
6. Excessive overjet or overbite
7. Malocclusion

Radiographic findings: record the tooth number of any tooth that exhibits

1. Widened periodontal ligament space
2. Loss of continuity of lamina dura
3. Bone or root resorption

Clinical and radiographic signs and symptoms should also be recorded (see box). Important findings are tooth mobility; wear patterns; changes in tooth position; poorly contoured or occluded restorations; plunger cusps; excessive overbite or overjet; overdevelopment of the muscles of mastication; clicking, pain, or improper movement of the TMJ; and tooth sensitivity (Carranza, 1979; Goldman and Cohen, 1980; Ramfjord and Ash, 1983). The presence of one or more of these signs does not mean that occlusal traumatism is present. All are indicators of potentially destructive forces, but the intensity, duration, and frequency of these forces and the resistance of the host are important factors in the development of occlusal traumatism. A force destructive of the supporting structures of one person may not affect those of another person. The key is whether the force is causing or is likely to cause damage to the supporting structures and if the destruction is progressive. The destruction can be detected radiographically and observed over time (Carranza, 1979; Goldman and Cohen, 1980; Zander and Polson, 1977).

Ramfjord and Ash (1981) have emphasized the role of plaque as an etiologic factor in periodontal disease associated with occlusal trauma. Destruction of the supporting structure from plaque must be differentiated from occlusal traumatism.

The destruction from occlusal trauma includes widening of the periodontal ligament space, necrosis of the periodontal ligament, cemental tears, loss of the lamina dura, bone resorption, and root resorption (Carranza, 1979; Goldman and Cohen, 1980; Greenstein and Polson, 1988; Zander and Polson, 1977). Widening of the periodontal ligament spaces, loss of the lamina dura, and bone or root resorption can be detected radiographically and should be recorded (see Chapter 10).

If these signs and symptoms are detected, they should be recorded and brought to the attention of the dentist. A sample format for occlusal screening suggests questions for gathering the subjective data from the patient. Once an occlusal screening has been completed, the dentist and/or dental hygienist may perform an occlusal analysis that examines the tooth-to-tooth relationships, the TMJ relationship, and the movements of the mandible.

OCCLUSAL ANALYSIS

Several formats for performing an occlusal analysis are available (Nasedkin, 1978; Ramfjord and Ash, 1979; Rieder, 1975; Shore, 1980). An analysis involves palpation and auditory examination of the TMJ using a stethoscope, palpation of the muscles of mastication, and examination of the tooth-to-tooth relationships. The occlusal analysis is presented here in a step-by-step format (see box on p. 306). An occlusal analysis form such as the one shown in the box should be used to record findings. The patient's subjective and radiographic findings, discussed in the section on occlusal screening, are also included in the occlusal analysis. It is necessary to use a recording procedure that avoids cross contamination, which is likely to occur when the clinician moves from the patient's mouth to the record, writing instrument, and so on, then back to the patient's mouth. An assistant to record the findings or a voice-activated tape recorder is most helpful (Baumgarten, 1988; Rothwell and Dinsdale, 1988).

Extraoral findings

You can examine the TMJ by placing your fingers over the joint and having the patient open and close his or her mouth. Record any clicking or excessive lateral movement of the TMJ. You can also palpate by placing your little fingers into the patient's ears and having the patient open and close; you can feel the posterior portion of the TMJ as the patient opens and closes (Nasedkin, 1978).

The lateral pterygoid muscle is palpated in two steps, although there is some question as to whether this muscle can truly be palpated (Johnsstone, 1980). First, have the patient open the mouth, and palpate the soft tissue posterior to the maxillary tuberosity. If a patient is experiencing TMJ dysfunction, the lateral pterygoid muscle may be extremely sensitive. Then palpate buccal to the maxillary tuberosity. The patient may have to close part way. If the muscle is in spasm, the patient will experience pain during the palpation. Record any pain or tenderness. Other muscles of mastication—the temporalis, masseter, and buccinator—can be palpated more easily. Again, record any tenderness, swelling, or spasm.

Also note if the swallowing pattern is normal. If the mentalis muscle is used during swallowing, the patient may have an abnormal swallowing pattern that can affect the occlusion.

Intraoral findings

The patient's Angle's classification, overbite, and overjet should be determined and recorded. The patient's *maximum opening* must be recorded with the mouth open as wide as possible. The opening from incisal edge to incisal edge is measured (Fig. 14-6). A range between 40 and 55 mm is considered good. Less than 35 mm is considered limited. The usual maximum opening is about 40 mm (Nasedkin, 1978). As the patient closes his or her mouth, the path of the mandible should be observed to note any deflection to the right or the left. An unusually small maximum opening or a large deflection may indicate a problem in the TMJ.

SAMPLE

Occusal Analysis Form

Extraoral findings

1. TMJ
   a. Pain
   b. Clicking
   c. Lateral movement
2. Lateral pterygoid muscle
3. Other muscles
   a. Masseter
   b. Buccinator
   c. Temporalis
   d. Mentalis
4. Swallowing pattern

Intraoral findings

1. Angle's classification
2. Overbite
3. Overjet
4. Maximum opening
5. Pathway of closure
6. Amount of movement from centric relation to centric occlusion
7. Direction of movement from centric relation to centric occlusion

Initial contact(s) in centric relation

1	2	3	4	5	6	7	8	9	10	11	12	13	14	15	16
32	31	30	29	28	27	26	25	24	23	22	21	20	19	18	17

Right lateral excursion

1	2	3	4	5	6	7	8	9	10	11	12	13	14	15	16
32	31	30	29	28	27	26	25	24	23	22	21	20	19	18	17

Left lateral excursion

1	2	3	4	5	6	7	8	9	10	11	12	13	14	15	16
32	31	30	29	28	27	26	25	24	23	22	21	20	19	18	17

Protrusive excursion

1	2	3	4	5	6	7	8	9	10	11	12	13	14	15	16
32	31	30	29	28	27	26	25	24	23	22	21	20	19	18	17

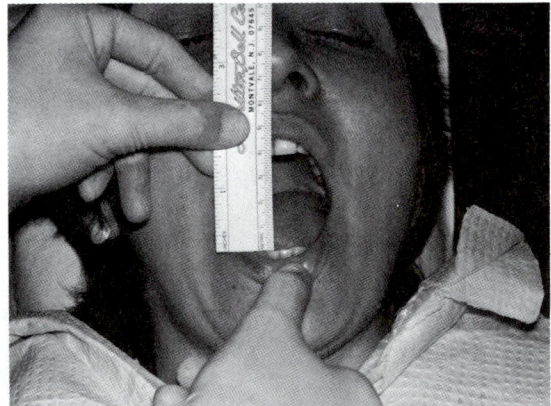

Fig. 14-6. Patient's maximum opening of mandible is measured.

Centric relation must be determined next. If a patient is having occlusal problems, the muscles and ligaments guiding the mandible into centric relation may be in spasm, so centric relation is difficult to determine. It can be reached if the patient relaxes the lower jaw to allow you to guide it into centric relation. First, stabilize the patient's head by holding the maxillary arch and grasping the chin to guide the mandible (Fig. 14-7, *A*). Then move the mandible gently up and down until it feels relaxed. Once the mandible is relaxed, guide it upward and backward into centric relation (Fig. 14-7, *B*). Then watch the mandible and direct the patient to bite together into centric occlusion. If the jaw shifts position as tooth contacts slide from centric relation into centric occlusion, note and record the approximate distance and direction from centric relation to centric occlusion. Other methods of guiding the patient into centric relation may be used if desired. (Dawson, 1990).

Guide the patient into centric relation and ask him or her to indicate which teeth contact first. Dry the indicated area(s) with a stream of air (Fig. 14-8, *A*) and place articulating paper between the teeth. Again, guide the patient into centric relation with the paper in place to mark the teeth that contact first. Note these initial contacts with areas colored from the paper (Fig. 14-8, *B, C*), then record them on the occlusal analysis form (see box on p. 306).

The lateral excursions are examined next. The patient starts from centric occlusion. Guide him or her into a left lateral excursion (Fig. 14-9), observing which teeth contact on the working as well as on the nonworking side. Mark any interferences with articulating paper and record them (Figs. 14-10 and 14-11). The same procedure is repeated for the right lateral and protrusive excursions (Fig. 14-12).

Once the teeth have been examined, the occlusal analysis is complete and ready to be studied. All of the findings must be considered as a whole. An interference may or may not be significant. If the interference is accompanied by other findings, such as bone loss, widened periodontal ligament space, tenderness of the lateral pterygoid muscle, soreness of the tooth, or tooth mobility, it is probably significant.

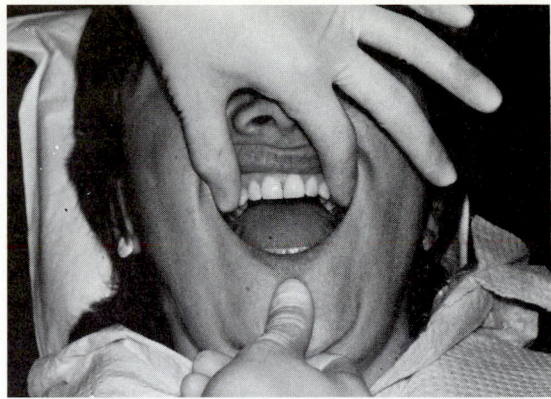

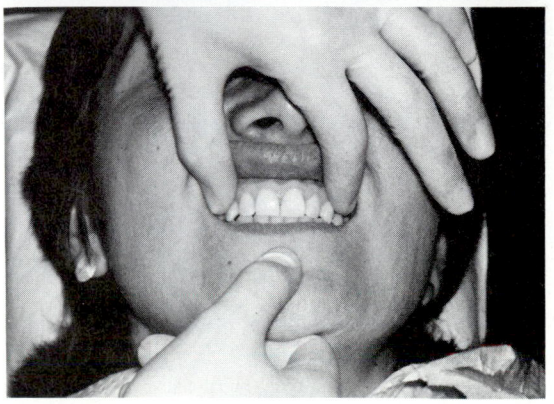

A

B

Fig. 14-7. Establishing centric relation. **A,** Patient's head is stabilized. **B,** Mandible is guided into centric relation.

SUMMARY

Occlusion is a complex human system that must be examined and considered as a whole. This chapter has presented information about the development of normal occlusion, the procedure of occlusal analysis, and the recognition of signs and symptoms of occlusal trauma. Knowledge of these aspects enables the hygienist to further contribute to the examination and evaluation of the patient's oral health. Patient complaints during hygiene procedures such as muscle fatigue, muscle discomfort, soreness of the teeth, and so forth are strong indicators of the need for further evaluation.

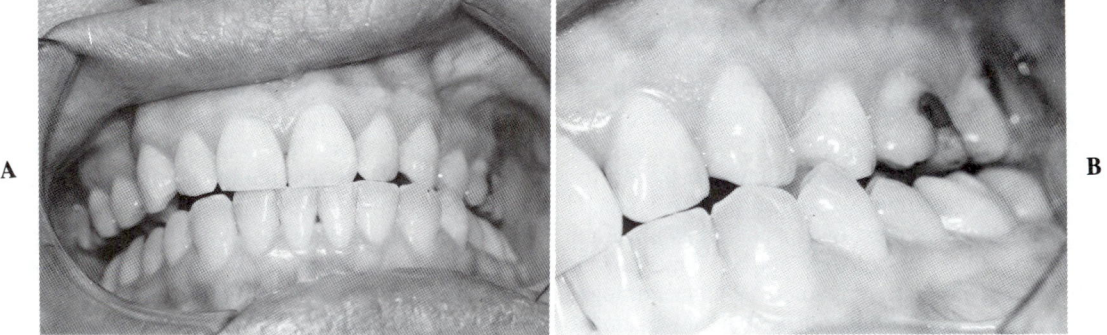

Fig. 14-8. Identifying initial contacts in centric relation. **A,** Drying teeth. **B,** Placement of articulating paper. **C,** Initial contact identified by markings.

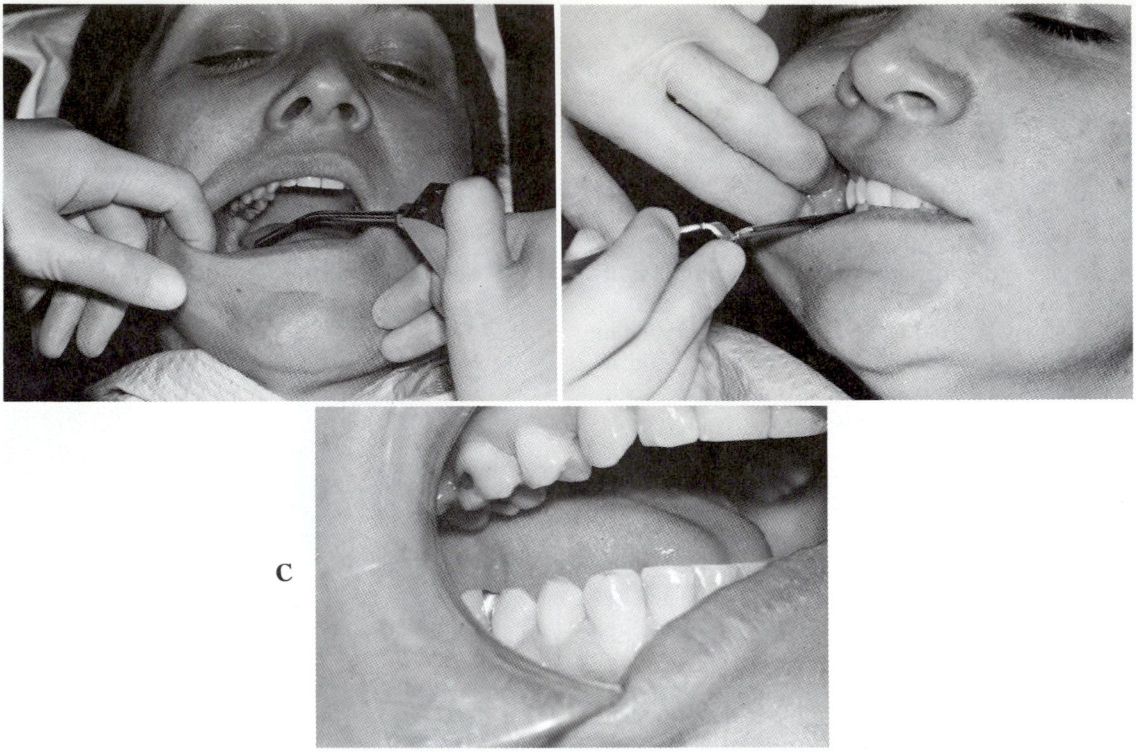

Fig. 14-9. Left lateral excursion. Mandible is shifted to left, **A,** until cuspids are edge to edge, **B.**

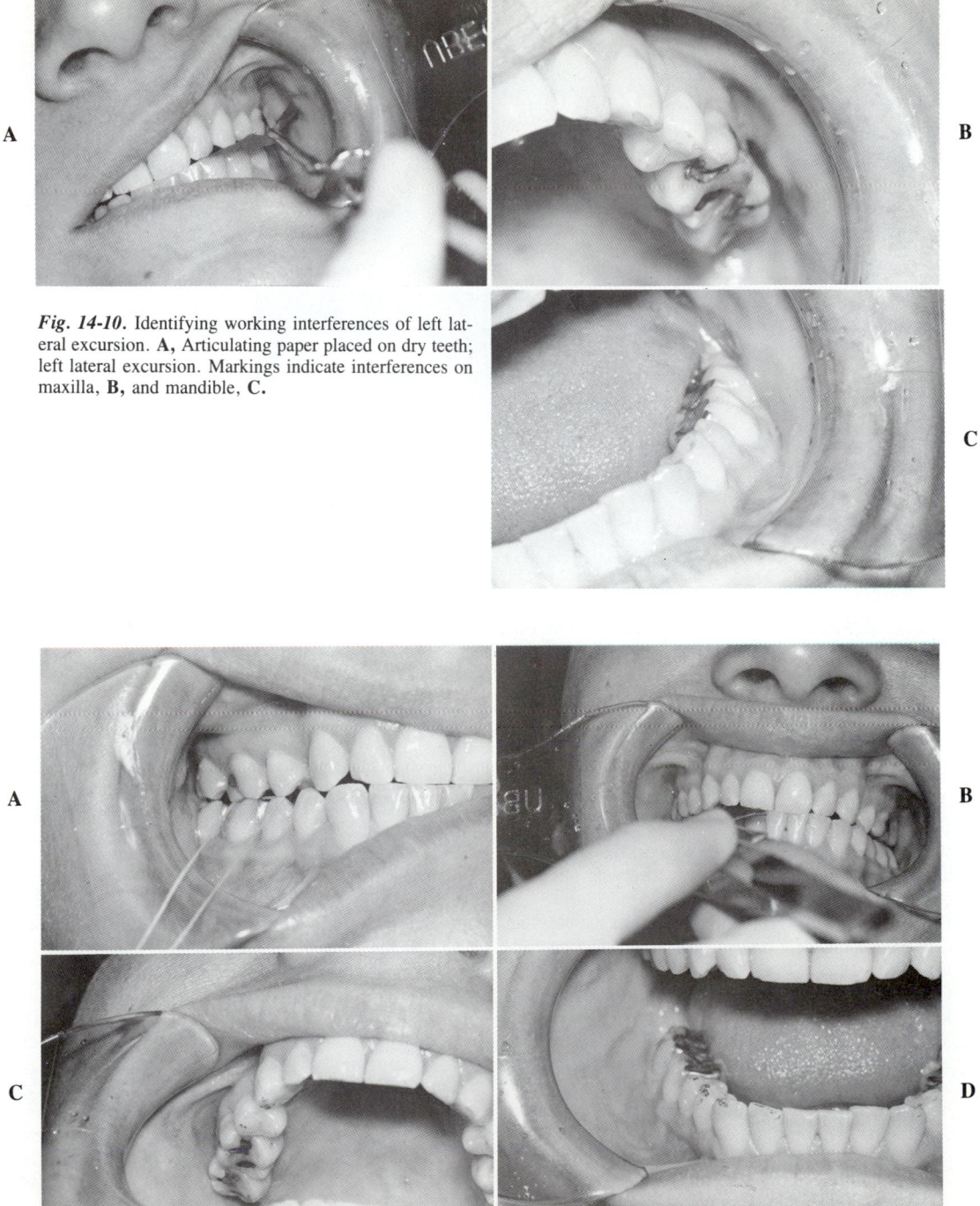

Fig. 14-10. Identifying working interferences of left lateral excursion. **A,** Articulating paper placed on dry teeth; left lateral excursion. Markings indicate interferences on maxilla, **B,** and mandible, **C.**

Fig. 14-11. Identifying nonworking interferences for left lateral excursion. **A,** Loop of floss is pulled from posterior to indicate interference. **B,** Articulating paper is placed. **C and D,** Interferences are shown by markings.

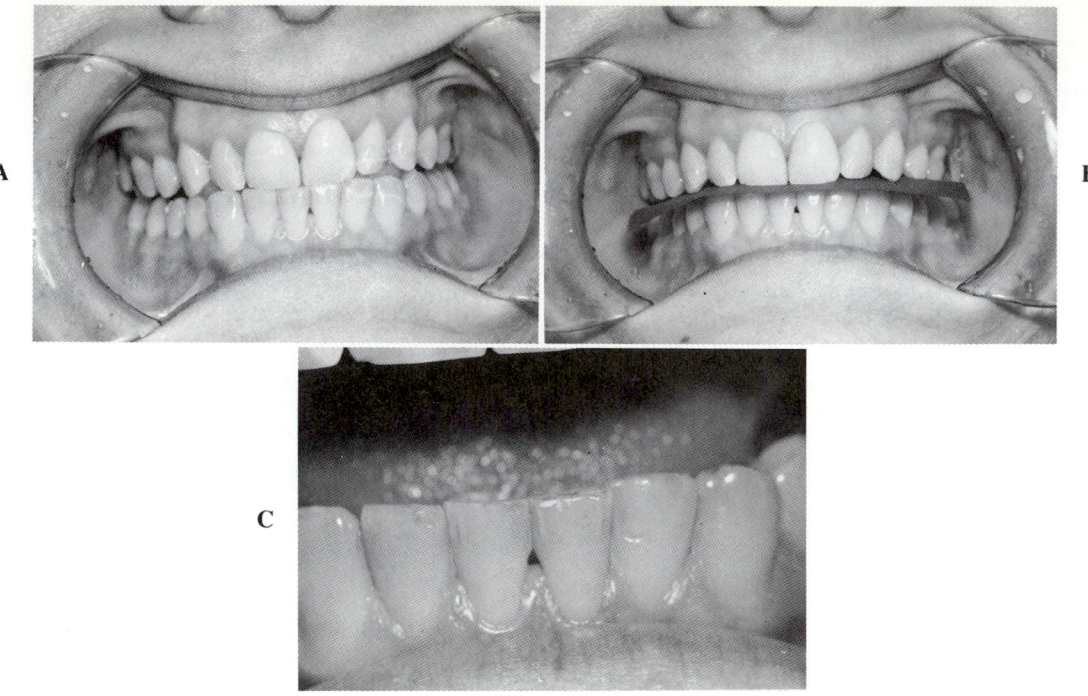

Fig. 14-12. **A,** Protrusive excursion. Articulating paper, **B,** shows markings of interferences, **C.**

ACTIVITIES

1. In groups of three, perform an occlusal screening with one person acting as the patient, one as the examiner, and one as the recorder, observing infection control guidelines.
2. Perform an occlusal screening as part of the baseline data collection for a patient observing infection control guidelines.
3. Complete an independent project on any of the following topics:
   a. Demonstrate, using study models and an articulator, the difference between centric relation and centric occlusion
   b. Using models or pictures, show the relationship of TMJ anatomy and occlusion
   c. Using pictures or models, show the interrelationships among the TMJ, muscles of mastication, nerve supply, and teeth
4. In groups of three, perform an occlusal analysis on a partner/patient using infection control guidelines.

REVIEW QUESTIONS

1. Define the following terms:
   a. Overbite
   b. Occlusal trauma
   c. Occlusal traumatism
2. List five etiologic factors of occlusal traumatism.
3. List the subjective, clinical, and radiographic signs and symptoms of occlusal traumatism.
4. True or false (correct each false statement):
   a. A patient may suffer from occlusal traumatism even though there is no damage to the supporting structure.
   b. Occlusal traumatism is serious because it causes the formation of periodontal pockets.
   c. If the force causing occlusal traumatism can be removed from the tooth, the supporting structures will in many instances repair themselves.

REFERENCES

Ash MM, Ramfjord SP: *An introduction to functional occlusion,* Philadelphia, 1982, WB Saunders.

Borell G: The development of normal occlusion, *Alpha Omegan* 73:15, 1980.

Bumgarten HS: A voice input computerized dental examination system using high resolution graphics, *Comp Cont Educ Dent* 9:446, 1988.

Carranza FA: *Glickman's Clinical periodontology*, Philadelphia, 1979, WB Saunders.

Chasen AI: Controversies in occlusion, *Dent Clin North Am* 34:1, 1990.

Dawson PE: *Evaluation, diagnosis, and treatment of occlusal problems*, St Louis, 1990, CV Mosby.

Glossary of terms, *American Academy of Periodontology*, ed 3, Chicago, 1992.

Goldman HC, Cohen DW: *Periodontal therapy*, St Louis, 1980, CV Mosby.

Greenstein G, Polson A: Understanding tooth mobility, *Comp Cont Educ Dent* 9:470, 1988.

Jago JD: The epidemiology of dental occlusion: a critical appraisal, *J Pub Health Dent* 34:80, 1974.

Johnsstone DR: Feasibility of palpation of the lateral pterygoid muscle, *J Prosthet Dent* 44:318, 1980.

Krauss BS et al: *Dental anatomy and occlusion*, Baltimore, 1969, Williams & Wilkins.

Levine N, Pulver F: Guiding the developing occlusion in children, *Alpha Omegan* 72:29, 1979.

McDonald RE, Avery DR: *Dentistry for the child and adolescent*, St Louis, 1983, CV Mosby.

Mosteller JH: Occlusion of the natural dentition, *J Ala Dent Assoc* 64:36, 1980.

Moyers R: *Handbook of orthodontics*, Chicago, 1988, Year Book Medical.

Nasedkin JN: Occlusal dysfunction: screening procedures and initial treatment planning, *Gen Dent* 26:52, 1978.

Perry HT: Temporomandibular joint and occlusion, *Angle Orthod* 46:284, 1976.

Ramfjord SP, Ash MM: *Periodontology and Periodontitis*, Philadelphia, 1979, WB Saunders.

Ramfjord SP, Ash MM: Significance of occlusion in the etiology and treatment of early, moderate, and advanced periodontitis, *J Periodontol* 52:511, 1981.

Ramfjord SP, Ash MM: *Occlusion*, Philadelphia, 1983, WB Saunders.

Rieder CE: Development of a simplified system for clinical evaluation of occual interrelationships: Part I, acquisition of information, *J Prosthet Dent* 33:264, 1975.

Rothwell TS, Dinsdale RC: Cross-infection control in dental practice: Part I, the practicability of a zone system to reduce cross-infection risks in conventionally designed dental surgeries, *Brit Dent J* 165:185, 1988.

Shore NA: Temporomandibular joint dysfunction: a review of successful diagnostic and therapeutic techniques, *Alpha Omegan* 73:67, 1980.

Thurow RC: *Atlas of orthodontic principles*, St Louis, 1977, CV Mosby.

Weisgold AS: Occlusion: review of various concepts, *Probe* 16:373, 1975.

Zander HA, Polson AM: Present status of occlusion and occlusal therapy in periodontics, *J Periodontol* :540, 1977.

SUGGESTED READINGS

Ash MM, Ramfjord SP: *An introduction to functional occlusion*, Philadelphia, 1982, WB Saunders.

Ericsson I, Lindhe J: Effect of long standing jiggling on experimental marginal periodontitis in the beagle dog, *J Clin Periodontol* 9:947, 1982.

Glaros AG, Rao SM: Effects of bruxism: a review of the literature, *J Prosthet Dent* 38:149, 1977.

Hoople S: *Occlusal evaluation module*, Seattle, 1976, University of Washington.

Ramfjord SP, Ash MM: *Periodontology and periodontitis*, Philadelphia, 1979, WB Saunders.

Robinson et al: Nocturnal teeth-grinding: a reassessment for dentistry, *JADA* 78:1308, 1969.

Schifter CC: *Occlusal analysis module*, Philadelphia, 1979, University of Pennsylvania.

Stallard RE: Periodontal disease and its relationship to pulpal pathology, *Periodontol Acad Rev* 2:80, 1968.

Waerhaug J: The angular bone defect and its relationship to trauma from occlusion and downgrowth of subgingival plaque, *J Clin Periodontol* 6:61, 1979.

Weinberg LA: The role of stress, occlusion and condyle position in TMJ dysfunction-pain, *J Prosthet Dent* 49:532, 1982.

Wirth CG: Occlusions. In Boundy SS, Reynolds NJ, editors: *Current concepts in dental hygiene*, vol 1, St Louis, 1977, CV Mosby.

Woerth JH: Detecting occlusal dysfunction, *Dent Hyg* 53:456, 1979.

15 PREPARATION OF STUDY MODELS

Thomas G. Berry
Judith C. Berry

LEARNING OUTCOMES

The dental hygienist will be able to

1. List and describe the four uses of study models.
2. Select the armamentarium used for making alginate impressions and gypsum models.
3. Discuss the health hazards associated with alginate, alginate impressions, and gypsum casts
4. Briefly describe the significance of each of the following factors for alginate and for gypsum:
   a. Water-to-powder ratio
   b. Water temperature
   c. Method of manipulation
5. Prepare a patient for an alginate impression.
6. Assist a patient with a gagging problem.
7. Determine if a tray is the proper size and prepare the tray.
8. Describe and use the steps for making maxillary and mandibular impressions.
9. Define the term *border molding*.
10. Properly remove an alginate impression from a patient's mouth.
11. State the rationale for making an interocclusal record and describe the technique.
12. Identify three methods for producing a properly formed base.
13. List the steps for pouring an alginate impression with plaster or stone.
14. Describe the effects of separating the impression too soon or too late from the cast.
15. Describe and follow the steps for trimming maxillary and mandibular casts.

STUDY MODELS

Study models, or diagnostic casts, are exact plaster or dental stone replicas of the patient's mouth. The models are constructed from impressions of the patient's mouth that are filled with plaster material. When the hardened plaster is separated from the impression, the resulting model is referred to as a study model or a diagnostic cast (Fig. 15-1). These models can be used as permanent records or diagnostic and educational aids, and for fabrication of temporary appliances (Craig, O'Brien, and Powers, 1987; Goldman and Cohen, 1980).

Study models may be included in the initial records to document the conditions existing in a patient's mouth at the beginning of treatment. These three-dimensional records of the patient's mouth are a helpful addition to the charts and radiographs normally included in an initial set of records. Study models document the progress of involved and/or long-term treatment. Models are made periodically during treatment and again at the conclusion of treatment. Several of the dental specialties (orthodontics, prosthodontics, periodontics, and oral surgery) as well as general dentistry routinely include models in patient records. Models may also be used in forensic cases.

Diagnostic aids

Study models permit the clinician to examine conditions in the patient's mouth from all views, including those impossible during a clinical examination (as from the lingual or the direct distal aspects) (see Fig. 15-1). The relationships between adjacent and opposing teeth can be examined, measured, and analyzed without discomfort to the patient. The clinician can draw or perform pro-

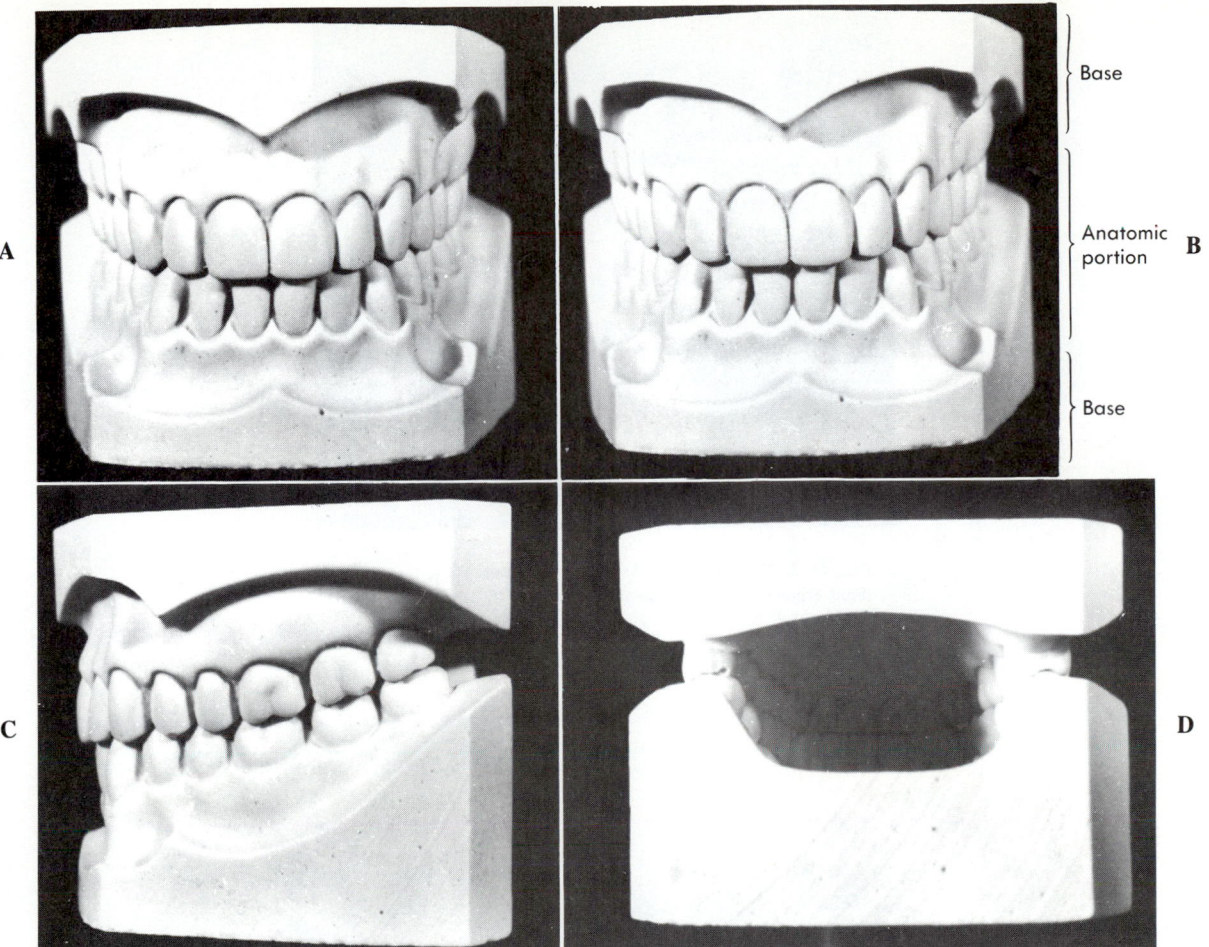

Fig. 15-1. Trimmed study models. **A,** Anterior view. **B,** Anterior view with anatomic portion and bases indicated. **C,** Side view. **D,** Posterior view.

posed treatments on the study models. Occlusal relationships can also be examined on the models by mounting the models on an articulator (Rudd, 1968) (Fig. 15-2). The dentist can consider mandibular movements when designing appliances and restorations.

Study models are also useful during charting procedures, particularly periodontal chartings (Goldman and Cohen, 1980). Wear facets, open contacts, rotated teeth, tissue recession, and other such findings viewed on the models can be recorded on the chart. The use of study models can save valuable chairside time.

Educational aids

During case presentations and patient education sessions, study models are a useful educational tool to illustrate the patient's existing conditions and possible treatments. The patient is able to view the mouth in the same way the clinician does. They are an excellent tool for describing and demonstrating individualized home care procedures. Patients can use the models to practice the techniques.

Fabrication of temporary appliances

Study models can be used in the making of tem-

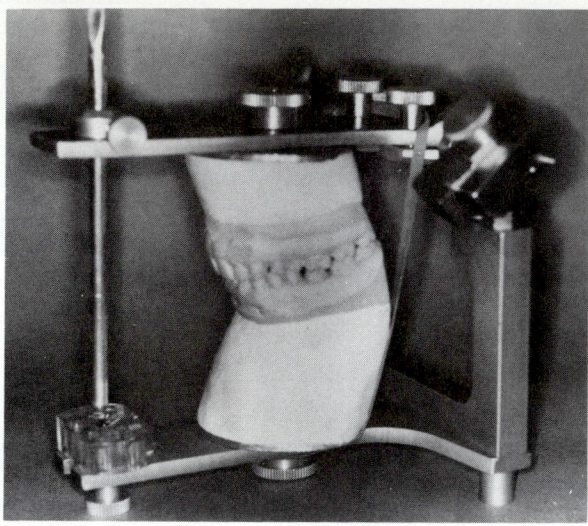

Fig. 15-2. Models mounted on an articulator.
(From Gilmore HW et al: *Operative dentistry,* ed 4, St Louis, 1982, CV Mosby.)

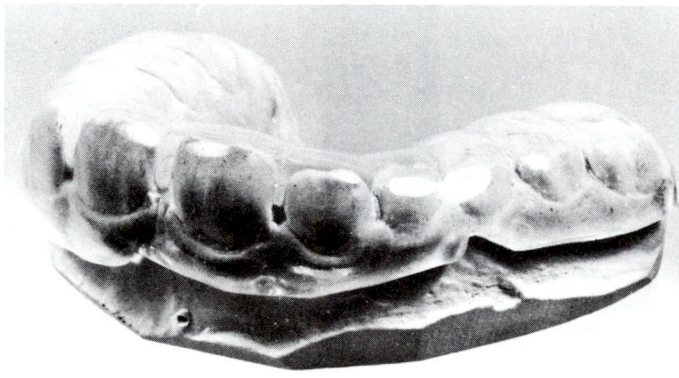

Fig. 15-3. Working model with clear plastic mouth protector in place.
(From Craig RG, O'Brien WJ, Powers JM: *Dental materials: properties and manipulation,* ed 3, St Louis, 1983, CV Mosby.)

porary appliances such as mouth guards and orthodontic appliances (Craig, O'Brien, and Powers, 1987). When used for this purpose, they may be called *working models*. They are usually constructed of a harder gypsum product than regular study models (Fig. 15-3).

Several states have dental practice acts permitting hygienists and assistants to make impressions and construct study models. This chapter describes these procedures. Brief descriptions of the materials used are presented. The reader should consult a dental materials textbook for in-depth discussions.

OVERVIEW OF THE PROCEDURES

The making of study models includes assembling the armamentarium, preparing the patient, making the alginate impressions and the interocclusal record, pouring, trimming, and finishing the models. It is a process that should be mastered in stages.

Assembling the armamentarium

The armamentarium needed is as follows:

Making the impression	*Pouring the model*
Rubber bowl and spatula	Rubber bowl and spatula
Alginate with powder and water measures	Plaster or stone
	Vibrator
Impression trays	Buffalo knife
Beading wax	Model base formers or boxing wax, glass slab, or other material(s) to form the base
Baseplate wax	
Buffalo knife	
Antiseptic mouthwash	
	Model trimmer
	Disinfectant spray or solution

Alginate is a flexible, irreversible hydrocolloid impression material. It is composed of sodium alginate salt (derived from marine kelp); calcium sulfate; potassium sulfate, zinc fluoride, silicates, or borates; sodium phosphate, diatomaceous earth or silicate powder; and flavoring and coloring agents (American Dental Association [ADA] Council, 1983; Craig, 1989). The material is supplied as a powder in either premeasured pouches or in a bulk-pack can to be measured as used. A scoop is used to measure the powder and a vial to measure the water in the proper proportions. When the powder is mixed with water, it forms a gel that will flow around the oral structures and then harden. When the alginate is removed from the mouth, it deforms slightly to pull over the structures and then springs back to the form it had in the mouth. Alginate is relatively pleasant tasting, easily mixed, inexpensive, and relatively accurate, making it the material of choice for study model impressions (Craig, O'Brien, and Powers, 1987).

Important factors to keep in mind when manipulating alginate are water-to-powder ratio, water temperature, and mixing method (Craig, O'Brien, and Powers, 1987; Roswick and Simon, 1974). It is important to follow the manufacturer's directions for best results.

Too much water results in a runny, slow-setting, weakened mix; too little produces a stiff, fast-setting, hard-to-manipulate mix. Water temperature also affects the setting time of the alginate mix. The mixing procedure should minimize the amount of air incorporated into the mix. This is accomplished by adding the powder to the water and by a mixing motion that wipes the spatula against the side of the bowl while the bowl is slowly rotated in the other hand (Fig. 15-4). A

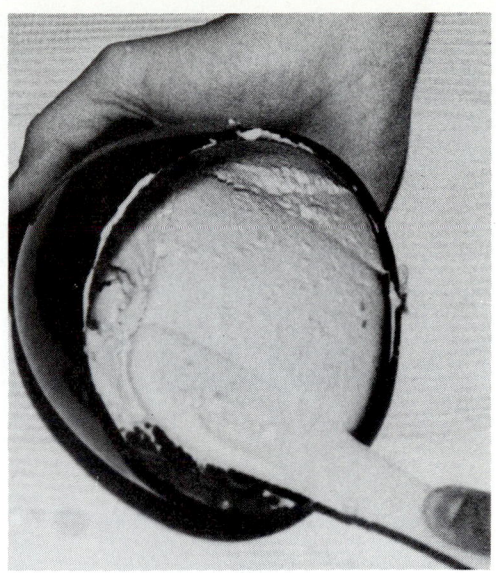

Fig. 15-4. Spatula is wiped against side of bowl to minimize air bubbles during mixing.

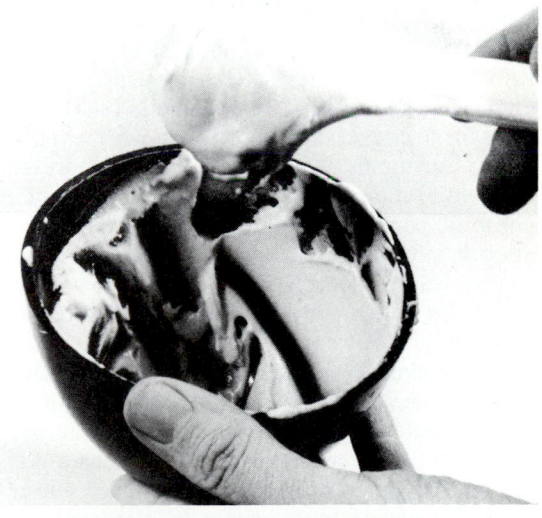

Fig. 15-5. Proper consistency of mixed alginate.
(From Craig RG, O'Brien WJ, Powers JM: *Dental materials: properties and manipulation,* ed 3, St Louis, 1983, CV Mosby.)

well-mixed alginate should be homogeneous, smooth, and creamy (Fig. 15-5).

Alginate is available in fast-set or normal-set formulas. Fast-set alginate gels in 1 to 2 minutes from the beginning of the mix; normal-set alginate gels in 2 to 4½ minutes (ADA Council,

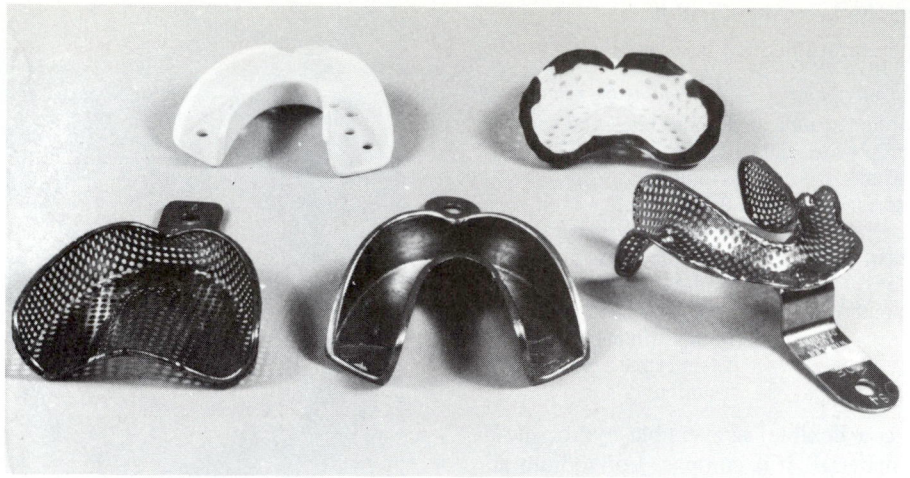

Fig. 15-6. Examples of impression trays: disposable and Styrofoam trays are also available. Note beading wax applied to upper right plastic tray.

(From Craig RG, O'Brien WJ, Powers JM: *Dental materials: properties and manipulation,* ed 3, St Louis, 1983, CV Mosby.)

1983). Fast-set alginate is indicated for patients with a gagging tendency and for children. Both types of alginate should remain in the mouth for at least 2 minutes, whenever possible, to allow sufficient flow of the material around the structures and time to gel (ADA Council, 1983).

Alginate impressions lose water when exposed to air, causing the impression to shrink and eventually to become very brittle. If plaster or stone is not to be poured into the impression immediately after disinfection, it should be sealed in a plastic bag or wrapped loosely in a wet paper towel until the plaster is poured (ADA Council, 1983; Craig, O'Brien, and Powers, 1987).

Impression trays. Various types of metal, plastic, and Styrofoam trays are available for use with alginate (Fig. 15-6). The type of tray used depends on convenience and the clinician's preference. The metal trays can be sterilized and reused; the plastic trays cannot be sterilized with heat. To avoid the potential of disease transmission, no tray should be used that has not been properly sterilized. (Greenlee, 1983). Styrofoam trays are designed to be used once and then discarded. The trays can be imperforate or perforated, as long as there is some means of mechanically locking the alginate into the tray to prevent dislodgement. Some Styrofoam trays may require use of an adhesive to ensure the impression is secure in the tray. Trays are available in several

sizes to accommodate any size mouth.

Beading wax. Beading wax, a soft wax available in strips, may be placed around the edges of a metal or plastic tray (see Fig. 15-6): this is done to extend the tray to include the vestibular and posterior areas in the impression. The wax also may make the tray more comfortable for the patient (Craig, O'Brien, and Powers, 1987).

Plaster and/or stone. Plaster and stone are two materials used to construct study models. They are derived from the mineral gypsum, the dihydrate form of calcium sulfate (Craig, O'Brien, and Powers, 1987). Plaster is less dense and easier to trim and finish. Stone is stronger and less likely to fracture or abrade. It is important to remember the following three factors when working with plaster and/or stone: water-to-powder ratio, water temperature, and mixing technique (Craig, O'Brien, and Powers, 1987; Roswick and Simon, 1974). Follow the manufacturer's recommendations for the water-to-powder ratio. The recommended ratio for plaster ranges from 40 to 50 ml of water for each 100 g of plaster; the range for stone is 30 to 40 ml of water for each 100 g of stone (ADA Council, 1983). Use scales and vials to correctly measure each component. Clinicians may learn to recognize the proper consistency through experience. Too much water increases the setting time and produces a weak final product. Too little water decreases the setting time and produces a stronger final product; however, the mix is extremely difficult to manipulate, and will not flow into the impression readily. Water temperature below 70° F (21° C) increases the setting time, and water between 70° F (21° C) and 98.6° F (37° C) decreases the setting time; however, a reaction will not occur in water above 98.6° F. Water temperature and water-to-powder ratio are very important when mixing plaster and/or stone (Craig, O'Brien and Powers, 1987; Roswick and Simon, 1974b).

The gypsum product is mixed by placing the water in the rubber bowl and adding the powder. Craig, O'Brien, and Powers (1987) recommend that the powder be allowed to sit in the water, undisturbed, for about 30 seconds before mixing to decrease the amount of air incorporated into the gypsum. The mixing technique uses rotary and wiping strokes similar to those recommended for alginate. Once the material is mixed, the bowl can be placed on the activated vibrator so that air bubbles will rise to the surface and burst. Eliminating air bubbles from the gypsum lessens the possibility of voids in the models. The mixed material should be homogeneous, smooth, and about the consistency of sour cream (see Fig. 15-17).

Vibrator. The vibrator helps to flow the mixture into the impression, spreading it evenly to eliminate air bubbles. The vibrator is discussed further in connection with pouring the model.

Model trimmer. The model trimmer is used to trim the base and border of hardened gypsum into the proper form. None of the anatomic structures recorded on the model are trimmed.

Considering health hazards

Seemingly harmless materials such as alginate and gypsum models present possible health risks that must be considered and guarded against. These hazards fall into three categories: cross-contamination from gypsum models, release of fluoride from alginate, and airborne particles from alginate.

Cross-contamination can occur between patients and dental personnel by means of gypsum models. Microorganisms have been recovered from stone casts, showing that the casts may be a medium for transmitting disease from patients to dental personnel, especially personnel working in a laboratory (Leung and Schonfeld, 1983). The specifics of infection control for impression materials are covered in Chapter 3.

Fluoride is a component of alginate that is released from the alginate and absorbed by patients (Hattab, 1981, 1987), which has caused concern because high blood levels of fluoride can be toxic. This, however, seems to be a highly unlikely consequence. If a large amount of alginate is swallowed, the fluoride level increases significantly. This is particularly important in children. Caution patients not to swallow the material.

The final health hazard to be considered is exposure to *airborne particles* from alginate. Most manufacturers recommend that alginate be shaken before it is measured, but shaking introduces particles into the air when the can or pouch is opened. Dental personnel are thus exposed to powder, lead, and silicone (Brune et al, 1978). Masks do not filter out all of the particles; no adequate protection is available. The concentration of the airborne particles is greatly reduced after 10 minutes. The precise effect of breathing these particles is unknown, but working in a well-ventilated area is recommended (de Freitas, 1980). Hattab (1981) measured the amount of fluoride absorbed by personnel exposed to alginate during mixing and found it to be negligible.

Preparing the patient

An important key to obtaining a good impression and, ultimately, an acceptable study model is proper patient management. A brief explanation of what will be done and how the patient can help is appropriate. This is important for both adult and pedodontic patients. Children want to know what is to be done and how they should help. It is helpful to liken the materials to objects with which the child is familiar—for example, the tray is like a big spoon (Hill and Gellin, 1970). Point out that, unlike with a spoon, the material in the tray *should not* be swallowed.

The patient may be positioned in either an upright or supine position for the impression procedure. When working without an assistant, an upright position may help to prevent the patient from gagging (Chasteen, 1988). With four-handed dentistry procedures, the patient can be placed in a supine position. Gagging may actually be less of a problem in this position because the tongue is in a relaxed position resting against the soft palate, which closes off the oropharynx (Hill and Gellin, 1970). If gagging is a problem for some patients, several approaches can be used to minimize it.

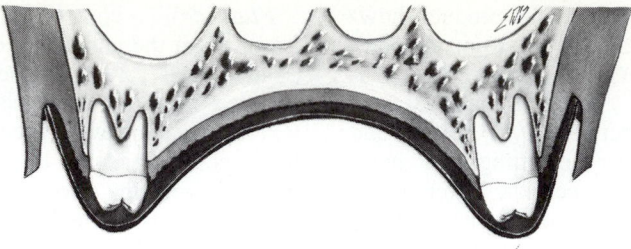

Fig. 15-7. Alginate flows between tray and oral structures. Note that there is about ¼ inch (6 mm) of material between tray and structures. Some of the alginate extends into mucobuccal fold area.

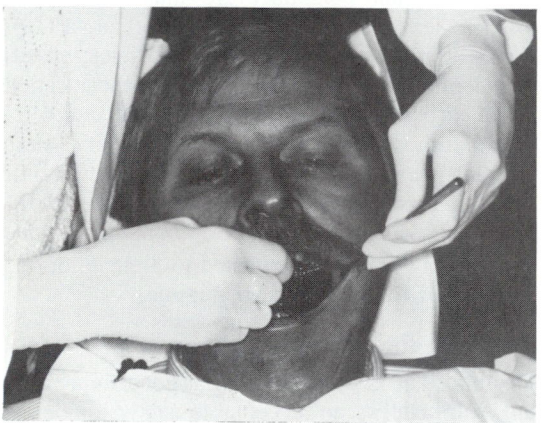

Fig. 15-8. After initial fitting of tray, beading wax has been applied to lower tray and tray is fitted once more.

Insertion of the impression tray can be delayed until shortly before the setting time if the clinician knows the working and setting times precisely (Craig, 1989). This will decrease the time in the mouth and the likelihood of material flowing onto the soft palate or throat.

Another approach to prevent gagging is for the patient to concentrate on breathing through the nose rather than through the mouth when the tray is seated. The patient can practice this before tray placement. This may help the patient feel less panicky if gagging occurs. The patient can also hold an ice cube in the mouth or rinse with an anesthetic mouthwash to produce a slight numbing effect. A topical anesthetic spray is not usually recommended (see Chapter 32) because a patient with a numb soft palate may experience a gagging

sensation. In addition, the gagging reflex helps prevent aspiration of a foreign object, so its elimination can be dangerous. For patients with a severe gagging problem, the dentist may prescribe an agent such as nitrous oxide sedation for the procedure (Chasteen, 1988). Another approach is to reduce the patient's concentration on the gagging sensation by focusing on something else, such as a spot on the wall or holding one leg up. It is very important for the clinician to remain calm and to reassure the patient. Alginate should not be removed until set; removing it too soon would worsen the situation, as the unset material will not produce an adequate impression and the procedure will have to be repeated.

Making the impression

Select a tray large enough to permit ¼ inch (6 mm) of alginate to flow between the tray and the oral structures (Fig. 15-7); however, if it is too large, it may impinge on the soft tissues or cause pain to the patient (Fig. 15-8). Beading wax may be added to the borders of the tray if greater tray dimension is necessary to capture detail in the muccogingival sulcus area or around muscle attachments. Wax extending more than 5 to 6 mm beyond the borders might prevent insertion and complete seating of the tray.

While the alginate is being mixed (or before), the patient should rinse with an antiseptic mouthwash to decrease the microorganisms present and reduce surface tension (Graber, 1972). The tray should be filled to the level of the beading wax and smoothed with damp fingers (Fig. 15-9) to produce a better surface on gypsum models (Morris et al, 1983). Overfilling the tray will cause material to flow out of the tray into the patient's

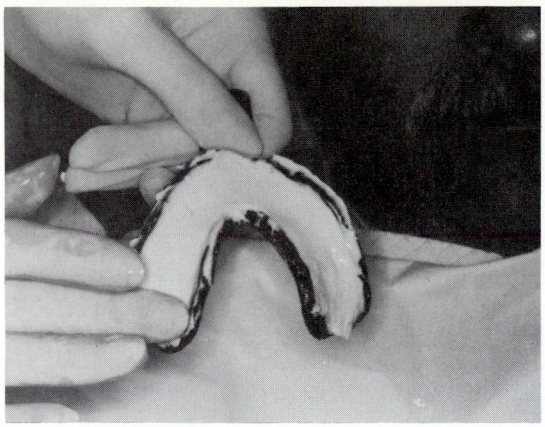

Fig. 15-9. Tray is filled to level of beading wax with alginate and smoothed with a damp finger.

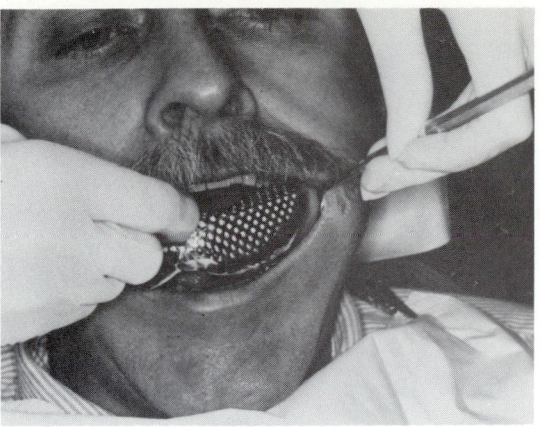

Fig. 15-10. Tray is inverted; one side is used to retract patient's right cheek while clinician retracts left cheek with a finger and rotates tray into mouth. Note that clinician is between 10 o'clock and 12 o'clock positions.

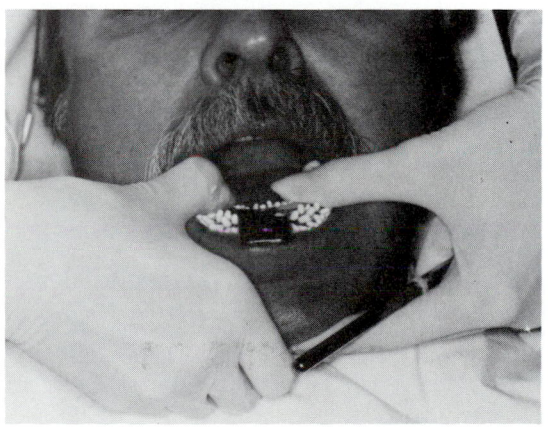

Fig. 15-11. Tray is centered, posterior border is seated, and tray is completely seated and stabilized until alginate sets.

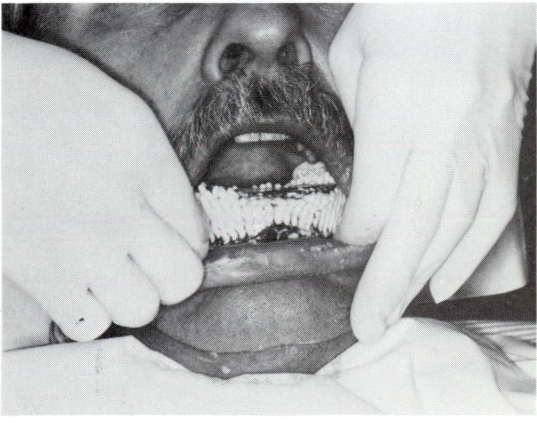

Fig. 15-12. Seal is broken with index fingers, and tray is removed with thumbs protecting upper teeth from contact with tray.

mouth; underfilling may result in voids in the impression. When the mandibular tray is properly filled, invert the tray, use the side of the tray to retract the cheek, and then rotate the tray into the mouth while retracting the opposite cheek with a mirror (Fig. 15-10). Once the tray is centered in the mouth and the posterior borders are positioned over the teeth, ask the patient to raise the tongue. The tray can then be seated first in the posterior area and then rotated down over the anterior area until completely seated (Fig. 15-11). Do not push the tray against the teeth, as this would displace

all the material, resulting in an inaccurate impression. The tray is held in position with light pressure while the lip is pulled up to ensure the inclusion of the frenum and the muscle attachments. This procedure of pulling the patient's lip is called *border molding* and is performed to record the patient's muscle attachment and mucobuccal fold. (Roswick and Simon, 1974).

The alginate is set when it is no longer "tacky." It is advisable to allow the impression to remain in place an additional 2 minutes to acquire greater resistance to tearing or deformation (Craig,

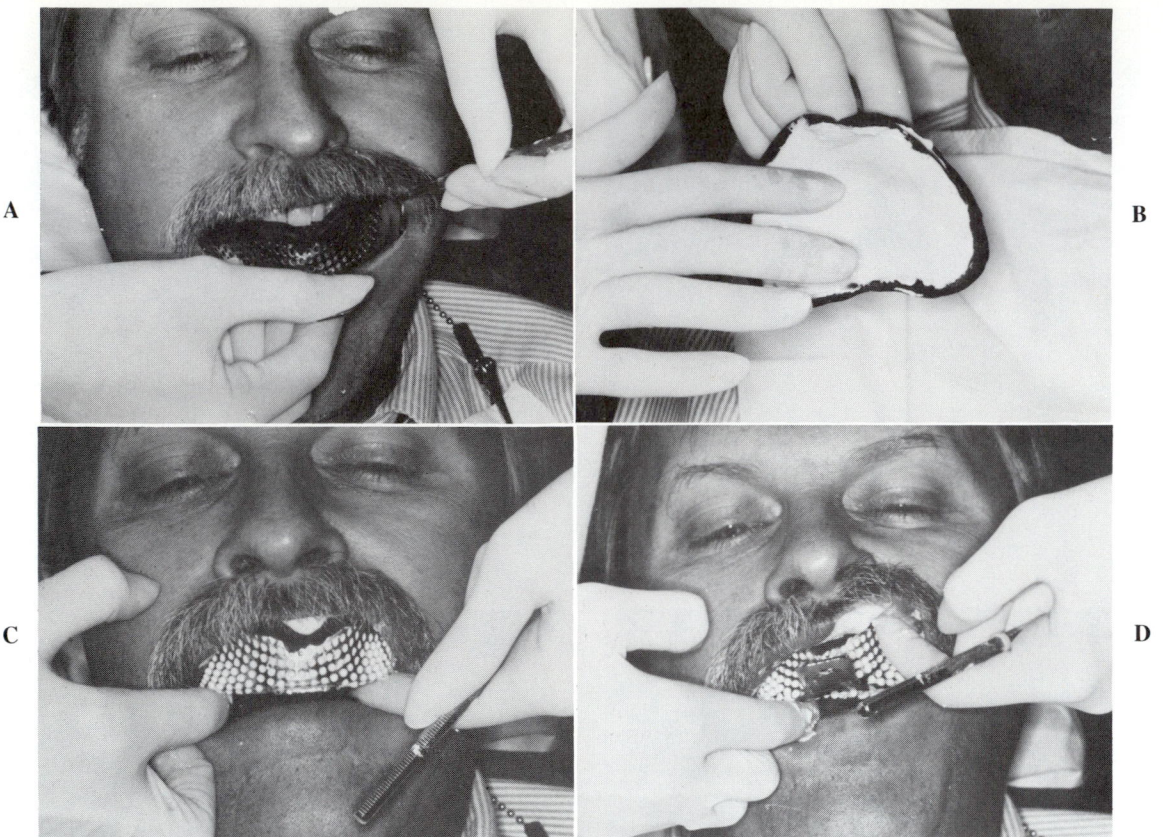

Fig. 15-13. Making maxillary impression. **A,** Tray is fitted. **B,** Alginate is wiped into tray and smoothed with damp fingers. **C,** Tray is rotated into mouth and posterior border is seated; then remainder of tray is seated. **D,** Clinician muscle molds by pulling lip downward.

O'Brien, and Powers 1987.) After the alginate is set, place the index fingers in the vestibule to break the seal and then lift the tray upward with a quick, steady motion (Fig. 15-12). Place the thumbs on the occlusal portion of the tray to protect the opposing teeth from the tray. An alternative method of removal uses the handle to pull the tray upward and the fingers from the other hand to protect the opposing teeth. It is important to use a quick motion to reduce distortion of the material. Rocking the alginate impression during removal causes permanent distortion of the material (Craig, O'Brien, and Powers, 1987; Roswick and Simon, 1974). Immediately on removal from the mouth, the impression should be sprayed with or soaked in disinfectant solution.

Similar techniques (Fig. 15-13) are employed to make and remove the maxillary impressions. The possibility of gagging is greater for the maxillary procedure. It is especially important to avoid excess alginate in the posterior region to lessen chances of gagging.

An acceptable impression is shown in Fig. 15-14. Always lay the tray down with the impression side up. If it is laid on the impression side, the weight of the tray could cause distortion (Craig, O'Brien, and Powers, 1987). The impression should be poured within 1 hour and properly stored to prevent dessication during that one hour.

Making the interocclusal record

An interocclusal bite record is needed to correctly relate the mandibular model to the maxillary model. Many techniques and materials are avail-

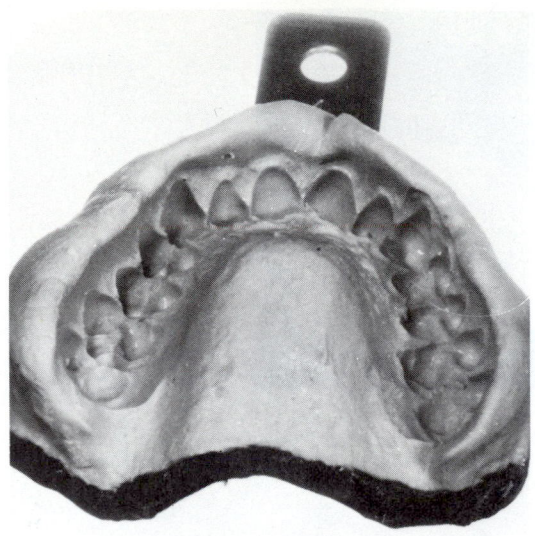

Fig. 15-14. Acceptable alginate impression.
(From Craig RG, O'Brien WJ, Powers JM: *Dental materials: properties and manipulation,* ed 3, St Louis, 1983, CV Mosby.)

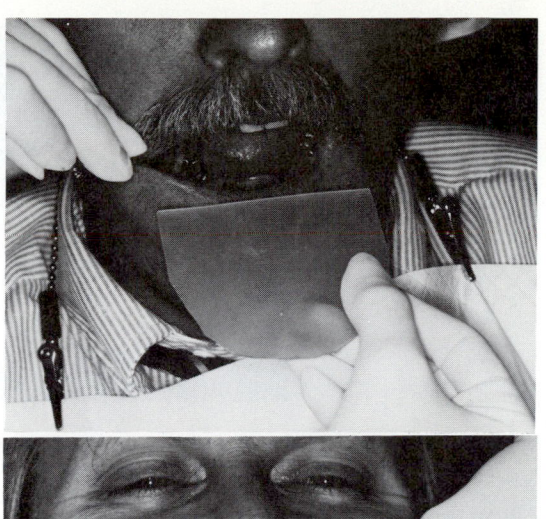

A

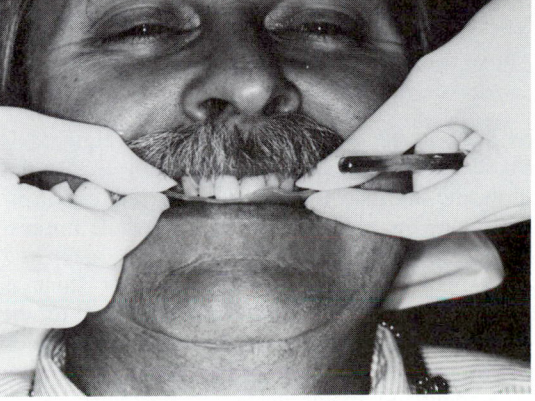

B

Fig. 15-15. Making interocclusal record. **A,** Trimmed baseplate wax. **B,** Softened wax is held against upper arch as patient bites.

able for making the bite record; one common technique uses a soft, moldable wax such as pink baseplate wax. The wax is folded double and trimmed to the shape of the patient's dental arch using a knife. The wax is softened in warm water and held against the maxillary arch while the patient is guided into the desired occlusal relationship (Fig. 15-15). The patient's occlusion is recorded by the indentations in the wax. The patient should be told to bite on the back teeth (check to be sure the patient is biting "as usual"). The patient may benefit from practicing this maneuver a few times before insertion of the wax to ensure he or she recognizes "biting as usual." While the patient is biting on the wax, use a cold water spray to harden the wax to avoid distortion when it is removed (Graber, 1972). As previously recommended for the impression, spray the bite record with a disinfecting solution.

Pouring the study models

Study models are composed of a base and an anatomic portion. The anatomic portion, formed by the impression, consists of the teeth and the soft tissues. The base can be formed by using a base former and/or boxing wax, with either a single-pour or a double-pour technique. Base formers, boxing wax, and the single-pour technique are de-

scribed in this section. The base formed should be large enough to give the trimmed models a ½-inch (12.5 mm) base and borders that extend about ¼ inch (6.0 mm) beyond the recorded vestibule.

Before pouring, the disinfected impression can be gently rinsed with soapy water to remove any possible debris and saliva. The surface of the impression can be dried gently with air to reduce the excess moisture. Water or saliva in the impression can cause air bubbles and/or voids in the final model.

The interarch portion of the mandibular tray must be filled in with alginate before the model is poured (Fig. 15-16). The tray is placed on a flat surface, with a folded damp paper towel placed between the flanges of the tray at a level about

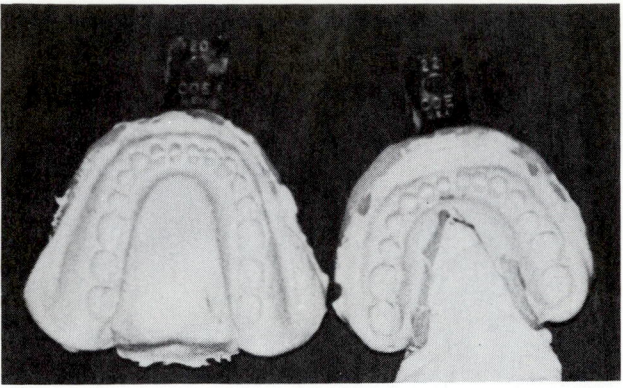

Fig. 15-16. Mandibular impression on left has had tongue area filled in with alginate; impression on right is ready for alginate to be smoothed into tongue area. This procedure eliminates void area in mandibular impression and prepares it to accept stone or plaster during the pouring process.

one-half its height. One measure of alginate is mixed and placed over the paper towel. Do not allow the alginate to flow into the impression itself. Once the alginate has set, the whole impression is ready to be poured.

A small increment of the plaster or stone is flowed from one end of the impression to the other by rolling the tray on the vibrator (Roswick and Simon, 1974) (Fig. 15-17). Small increments are added and manipulated, as described previously, until all of the indentations of the teeth are filled. Press the tray against the vibrator to eliminate air bubbles in the gypsum (Fig. 15-18). Throughout mixing and pouring, try to prevent and/or eliminate air from the mix. Once all of the teeth indentations are filled, larger increments can be added. The base can be formed as described below (Fig. 15-19).

A *base former* is a simple means of obtaining a base of acceptable shape and size. The base former is filled with the gypsum and placed on the vibrator for a few seconds to remove any air bubbles (Fig. 15-20). It is then moved to a flat surface away from the vibrator. The gypsum-filled impression is inverted, centered, and gently pressed into the gypsum in the base former (Fig. 15-21). The tray should be placed so that the occlusal plane of the impression is approximately parallel to the table. The tray and base former should be inspected to be sure that the gypsum in the tray has joined the gypsum in the base former but does not extend up and around the sides of the impression tray. If it does, the tray will be

"locked into" the gypsum and difficult to separate from the hardened model.

A *single-pour technique* is commonly used to form the base. After the tray is filled, the remaining gypsum is formed into a ¾-inch thick mass approximating the tray dimensions and placed on the glass slab. The tray is then inverted and pushed into the mass of gypsum. Adjust the tray so that the occlusal plane of the teeth is approximately parallel to the glass slab (Figs. 15-22 to 15-24).

A third way to form the base is with *boxing wax*. This method is popular to create working casts used to construct dentures or bridges. Before the impression is poured, a row of beading wax is attached to the outside of the tray. It may be necessary to trim the posterior portion of the alginate to allow close adaptation of the wax to this area. Use care not to remove any anatomic features. Once the beading wax is applied, boxing wax is molded around the tray, extending above the tray to hold the gypsum to form the base (Figs. 15-25 to 15-27). The gypsum is then flowed into the "boxed" tray.

Once the base is formed, the model should be left undisturbed for approximately 45 to 60 minutes while the gypsum sets. When the gypsum is no longer warm (the setting process is exothermic) to the touch, the model can be separated. If removed too soon, the model may break; if left in the impression too long, its surface will be rough (Craig, O'Brien, and Powers, 1987; Phillips, 1982). The dehydrated impression will harden,

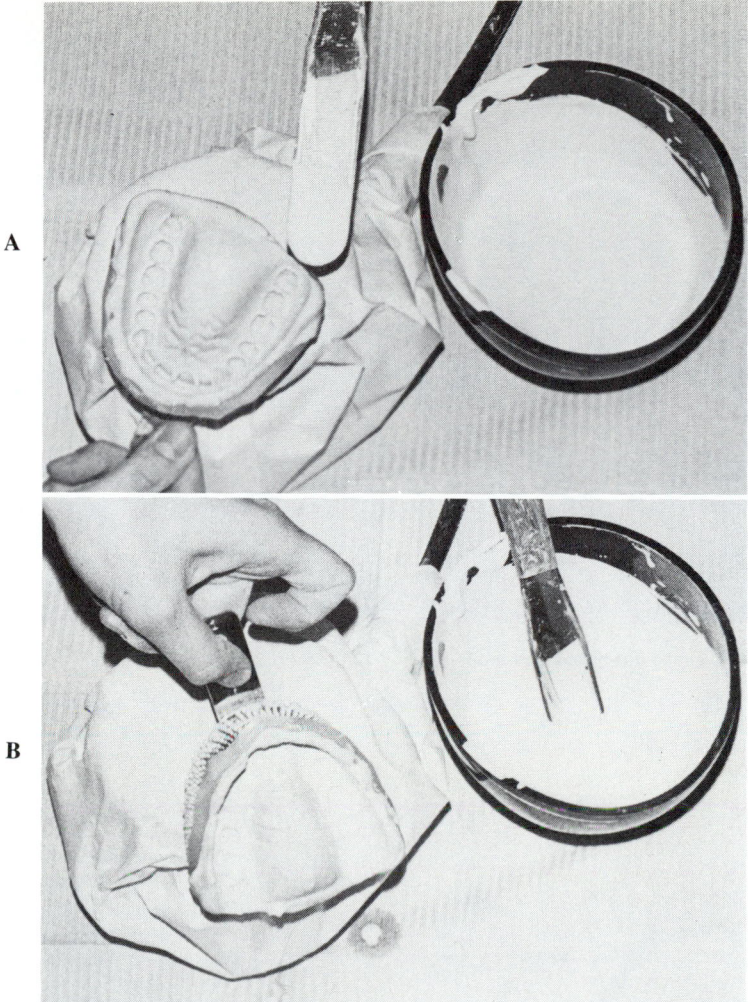

Fig. 15-17. A, Small increment is flowed into maxillary impression. **B,** Gypsum has been flowed around tray to fill all teeth. Note sour cream consistency of gypsum.

making it more difficult to separate the model without fracturing or abrading the surface. The models should be sprayed with a disinfectant spray such as iodophor or hypochlorite.

Trimming and finishing the study models

If no base former is used, the base and borders of the models are trimmed to form the shapes illustrated in Fig. 15-28. Some practitioners recommend very specific guidelines for trimming models, (Robson, 1973; Roswick and Simon, 1974). The generally accepted recommendations of Thurow (1977) are described in the accompanying illustrations. The degree of precision in the shape of the bases depends on the specific use for which the models are intended. Those used for treatment planning presentations, patient education, and orthodontic records need to be carefully formed. Those to be mounted on an articulator for occlusal analysis, appliance fabrication, and so forth do not require an elaborate base form.

The models should be soaked in water before trimming (Fig. 15-29). The maxillary cast is trimmed first, then the mandibular cast is trimmed

(Text continued on p. 329).

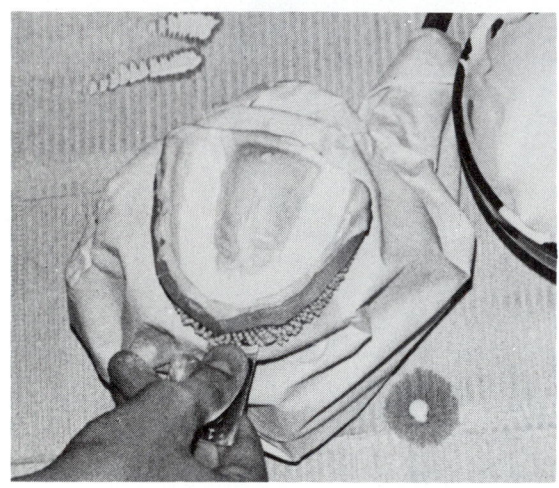

Fig. 15-18. Gypsum is added, and downward pressure is applied to tray on vibrator.

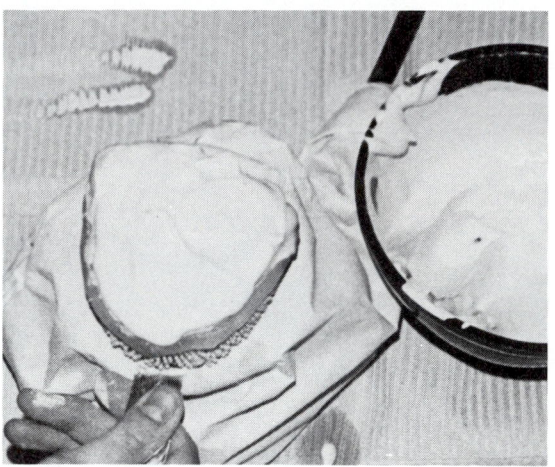

Fig. 15-19. Larger increments are added to fill tray.

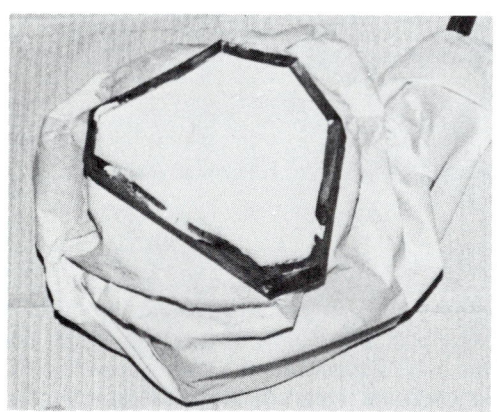

Fig. 15-20. Base former is filled with gypsum and vibrated to remove bubbles.

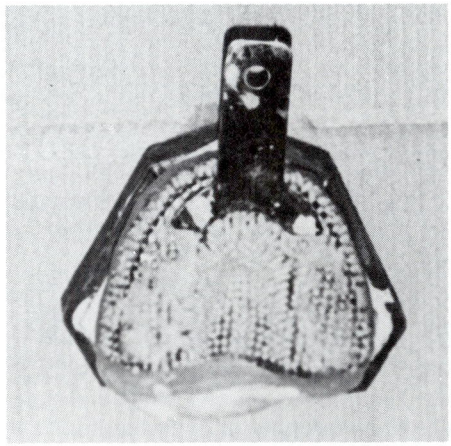

Fig. 15-21. Impression is inverted and joined with gypsum in base former.

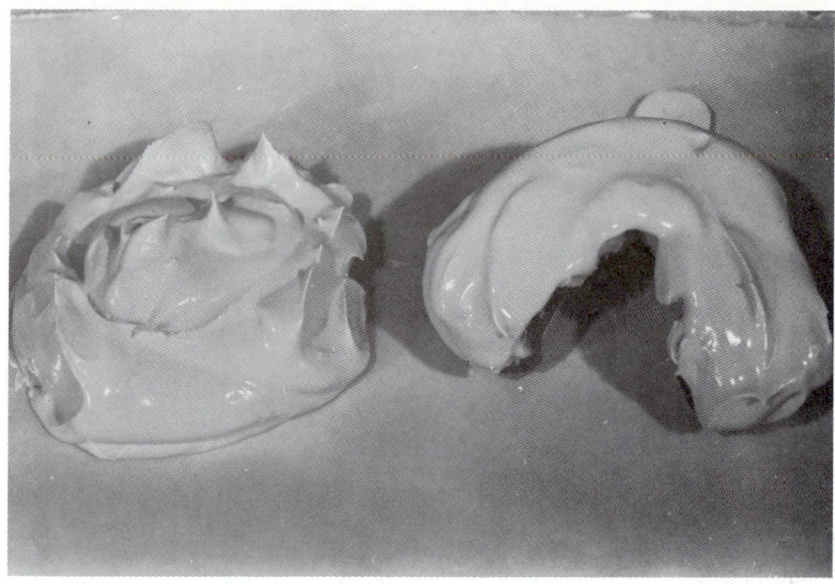

Fig. 15-22. Single-pour method. A mound of gypsum approximating shape of tray has been formed. Filled tray on right is ready to be inverted and joined to base.

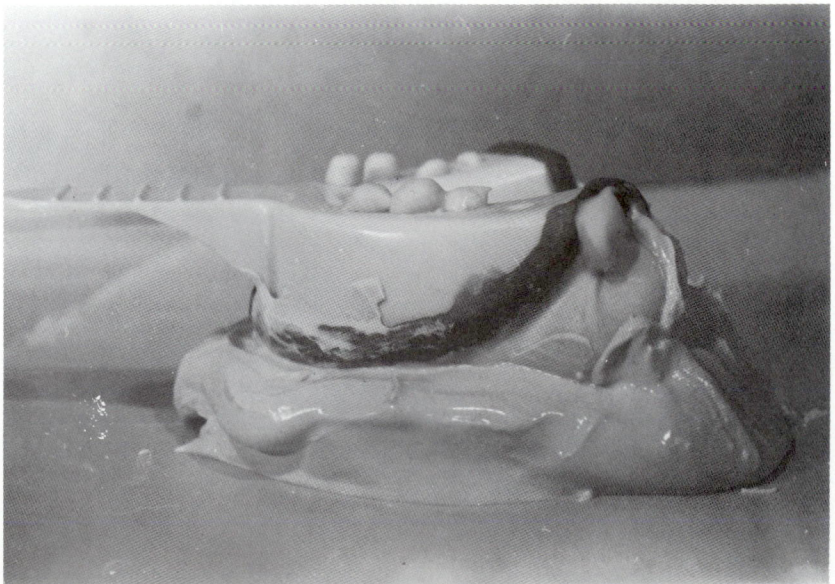

Fig. 15-23. Filled tray is joined to base so that tray and occlusal plane are parallel to table.

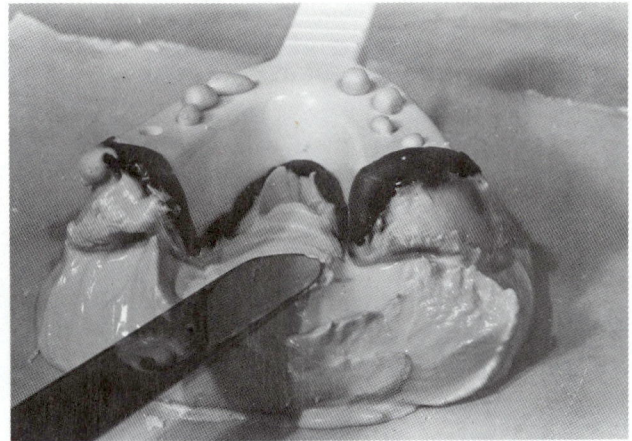

Fig. 15-24. As tongue area was not filled in with alginate, gypsum from that area is cleared with spatula.

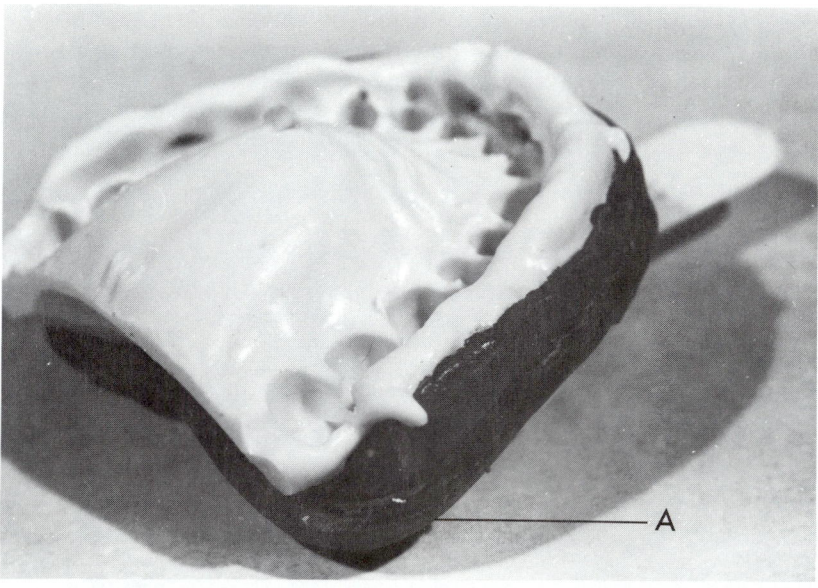

Fig. 15-25. Boxing wax method: an extra row of beading wax *(A)* has been applied to tray.

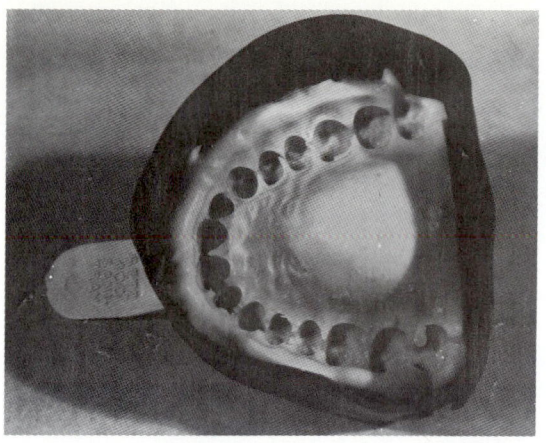

Fig. 15-26. Boxing wax is molded around tray and joined to beading wax.

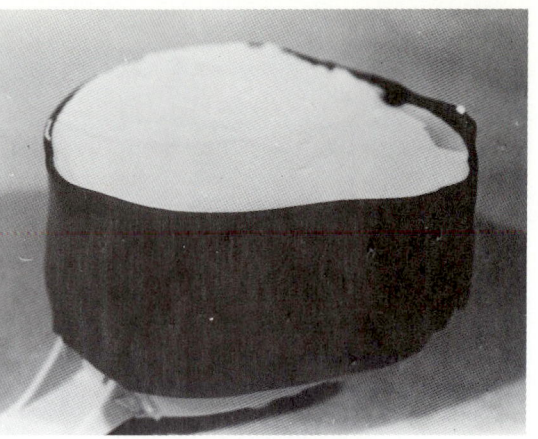

Fig. 15-27. Tray with boxing wax is filled with gypsum.

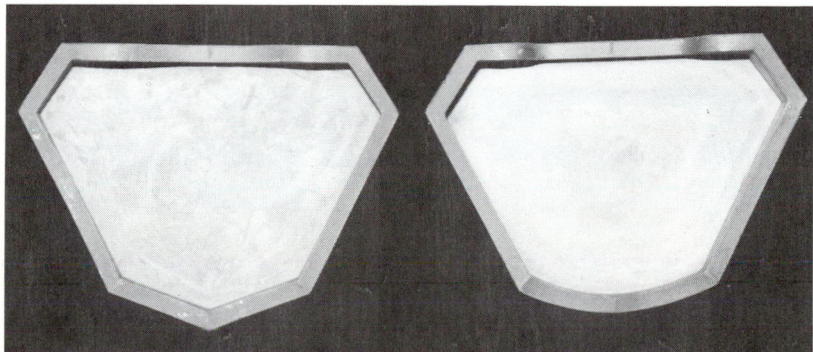

Fig. 15-28. These base formers show outline shapes of properly shaped models. Pointed former on left is shape of maxillary model. Rounded former on right is shape of mandibular model.

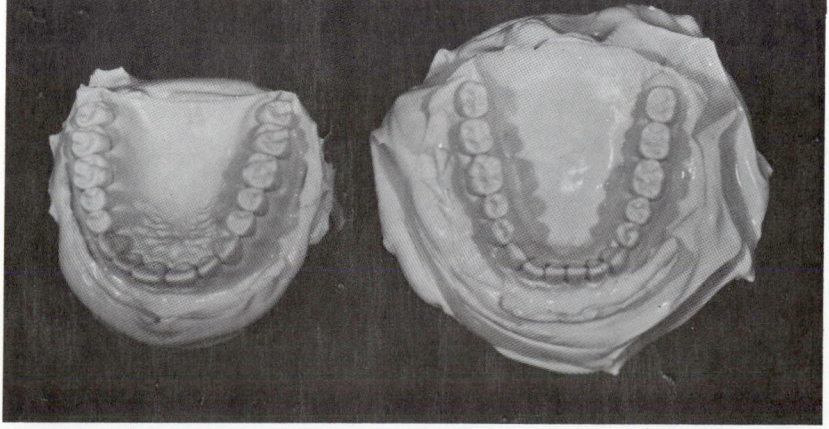

Fig. 15-29. Models removed from alginate impressions and ready to be soaked in water before being trimmed.

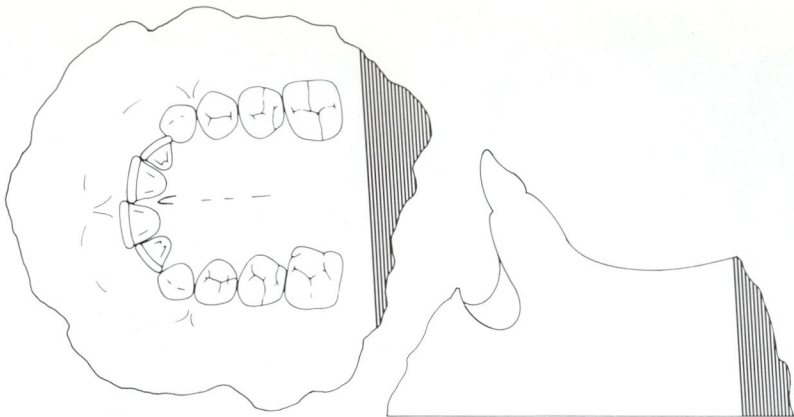

Fig. 15-30. Back surface of maxillary model is trimmed flat.
(From Thurow RC: *Atlas of orthodontic principles,* ed 2, St Louis, 1977, CV Mosby.)

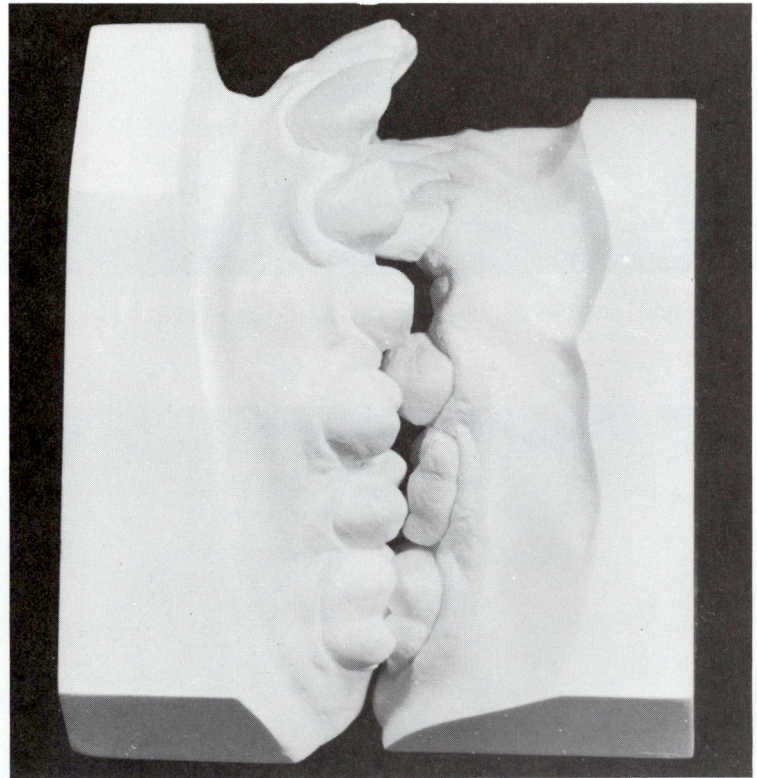

Fig. 15-31. Casts are trimmed so that they will occlude correctly when resting on posterior surfaces.
(From Thurow RC: *Atlas of orthodontic principles,* ed 2, St Louis, 1977, CV Mosby.)

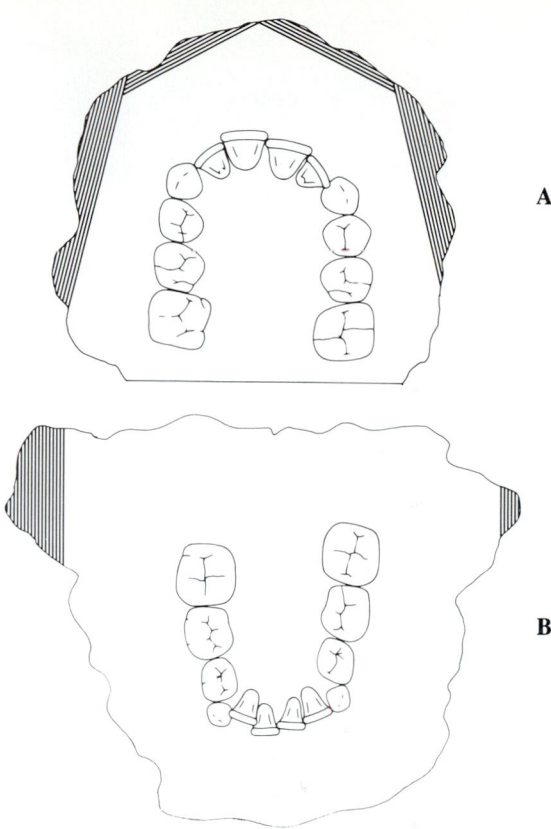

A

B

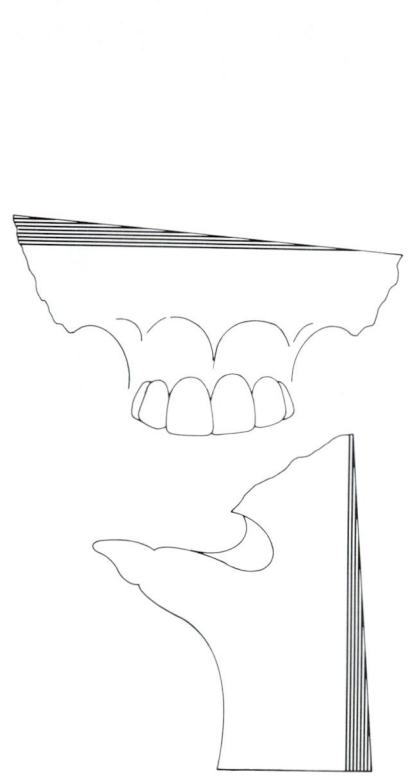

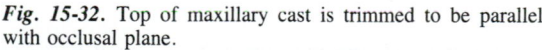

Fig. 15-32. Top of maxillary cast is trimmed to be parallel with occlusal plane.
(From Thurow RC: *Atlas of orthodontic principles,* ed 2, St Louis, 1977, CV Mosby.)

Fig. 15-33. Sides of maxillary (**A**) and mandibular (**B**) casts are trimmed.
(From Thurow RC: *Atlas of orthodontic principles,* ed 2, St Louis, 1977, CV Mosby.)

to match it. Only the base is trimmed; the anatomic portions are not trimmed. The posterior border of the maxillary cast is trimmed so it is flat and perpendicular to the midline of the palate (Fig. 15-30). The models will be able to stand on end without moving out of occlusion when correctly trimmed. (Fig. 15-31). Next, the top of the maxillary cast is trimmed parallel with the occlusal plane (Fig. 15-32). Then the sides of the cast are trimmed to remove the excess and to shape the base (Fig. 15-33). The shapes of the bases of the maxillary and mandibular casts are shown in Figs. 15-1 and 15-28. Note that the posterior borders and the sides of both casts are the same shape—the posterior borders are perpendicular to

the midlines; the posterior angles are trimmed to be parallel with the opposite cuspids; and the sides are parallel to a line through the tips of the cuspids and the central grooves of the posterior teeth. On the maxillary cast, the anterior border forms a point over the midline; each side is parallel to a line through the incisal edges of the anterior teeth. The anterior border of the mandibular cast is rounded from cusptip to cusptip of the cuspids. After the maxillary cast is shaped, the mandibular cast is trimmed to the rough outline. The first step is to trim the excess width of the mandibular cast (see Fig. 15-33). Place the interocclusal record between the teeth during this step to prevent damage to the teeth. Trim the wax so it

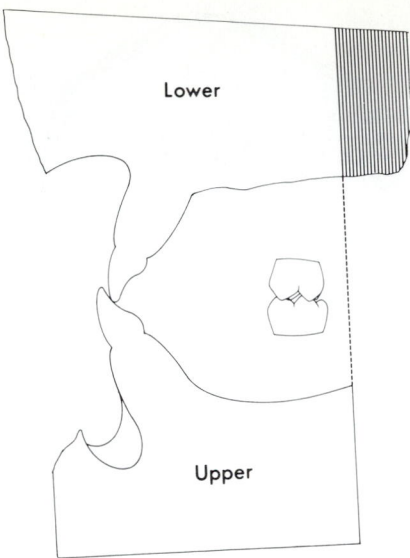

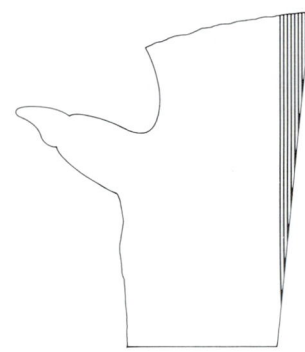

Fig. 15-34. Posterior border of mandibular model is trimmed to match maxillary model.
(From Thurow RC: *Atlas of orthodontic principles,* ed 2, St Louis, 1977, CV Mosby.)

Fig. 15-35. Bottom of mandibular model is trimmed.
(From Thurow RC: *Atlas of orthodontic principles,* ed 2, St Louis, 1977, CV Mosby.)

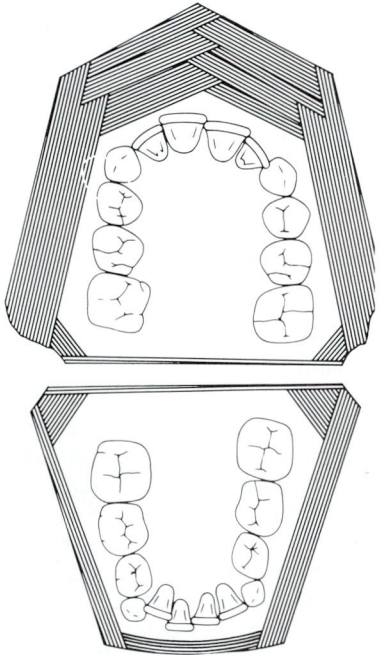

Fig. 15-36. Final shapes of both casts are achieved.
(From Thurow RC: *Atlas of orthodontic principles,* ed 2, St Louis, 1977, CV Mosby.)

does not touch the trimmer wheel. Then trim the posterior border of the mandibular cast even with the posterior border of the maxillary cast (Fig. 15-34). Next, trim the bottom of the mandibular cast parallel with the top of the maxillary cast (Fig. 15-35). The top of the maxillary cast and the bottom of the mandibular cast should be parallel to the occlusal plane. The casts should sit on a flat surface with the bottom of the mandibular cast, the occlusal plane, and the top of the maxillary cast all parallel to the flat surface (see Fig. 15-1). Gradually trim each cast to its final shape (Fig. 15-36). Fig. 15-37 shows casts being trimmed.

Study models can be smoothed and polished with fine sandpaper and then soaked in a soap solution and buffed or sprayed with model spray if they are to be used for presentation. Mark each model with an identifying number or the patient's name in case the models become separated. They can be stored in a box labeled with the patient's name and chart number.

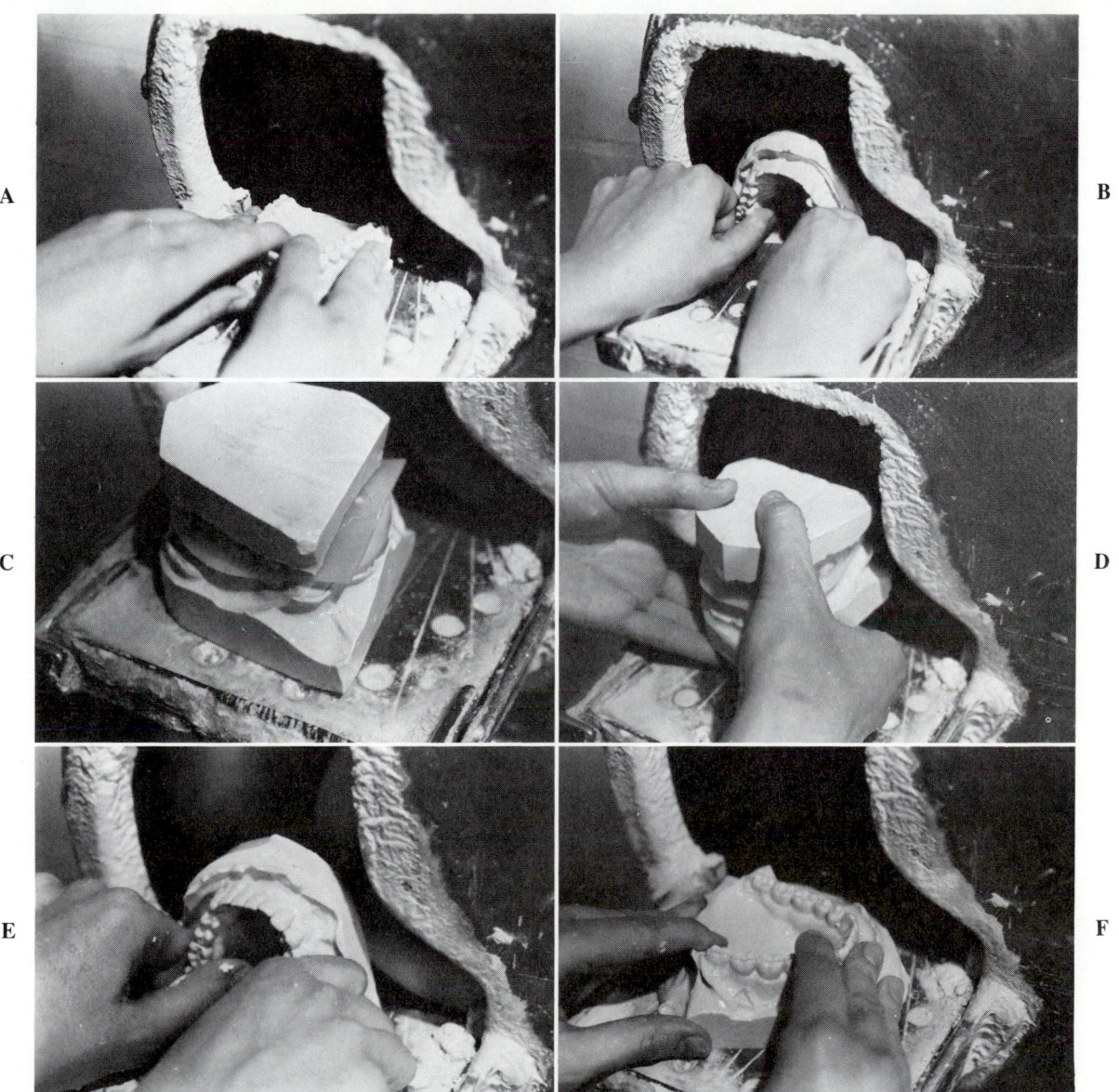

Fig. 15-37. Trimming casts with model trimmer; note firm grip used to hold cast against blade. **A,** Back surface of maxillary cast is trimmed flat. **B,** Top of maxillary cast is trimmed. **C,** Maxillary and mandibular casts are related with interocclusal record. **D,** After posterior border of wax is removed, casts are trimmed together. **E,** Bottom of mandibular cast is trimmed. **F,** Sides of mandibular cast are trimmed.

Continued.

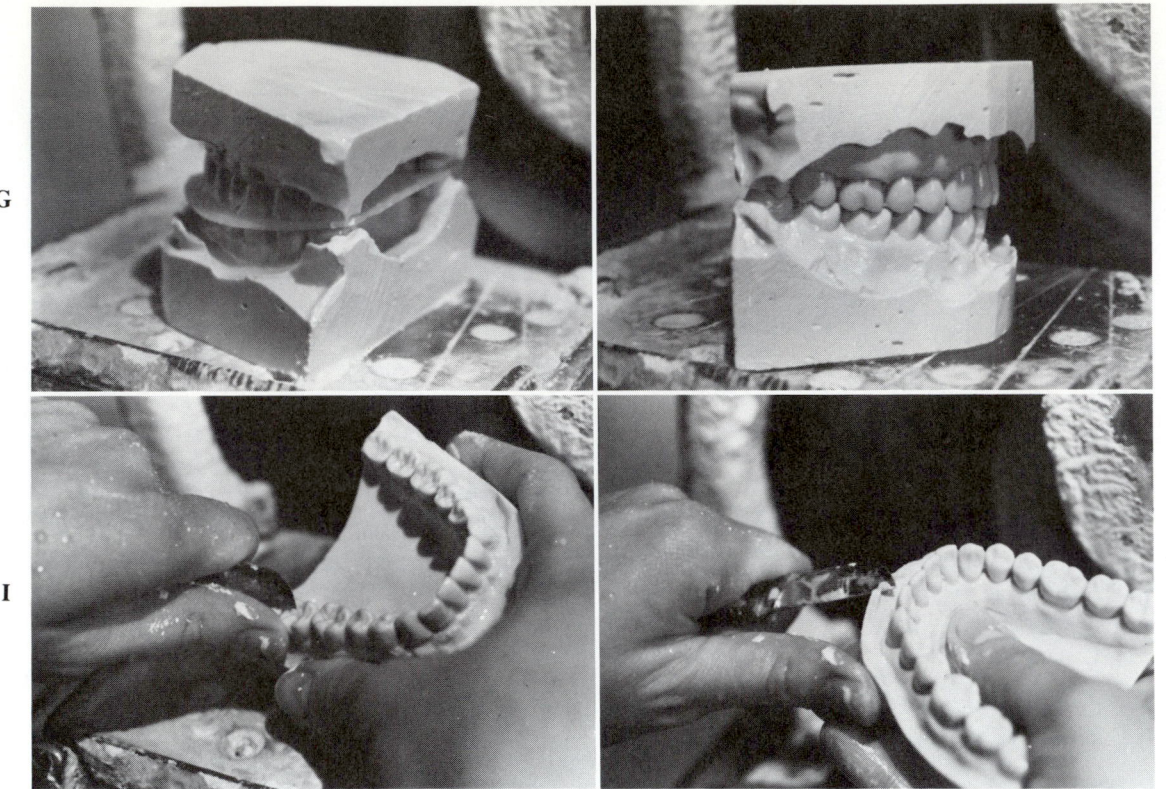

Fig. 15-37, cont'd. **G,** Mandibular casts are related to each other to see if further trimming is needed. **H,** Basic outline is achieved; top, occlusal plane, and bottom are parallel. **I,** Occlusal blebs are removed with Buffalo knife. **J,** Extensions of gypsum are removed.

ACTIVITIES

1. View videotapes demonstrating the making of an impression and trimming of casts.
2. Watch an experienced clinician make impressions and pour and trim models.
3. Prepare a set of alginate models for a partner; pour and trim the models (see check-off sheets). Use recommended infection-control procedures.
4. After being a patient for the procedure, discuss what it was like. In light of this experience, would you like to modify your technique?
5. Secure a set of study models and chart as many findings as possible on a caries or periodontal chart.

REVIEW QUESTIONS

1. What are the four uses of study models?
2. What three factors are important to remember when manipulating alginate and gypsum?
3. What are the criteria for determining if a tray is the proper size?
4. Describe how to place a maxillary tray filled with alginate into a patient's mouth.
5. What is border molding, and why is it performed?
6. What can the clinician do if a patient gags while the impression is being made?
7. What is the problem with removing an alginate impression from the mouth with a slow rocking motion?
8. What is the purpose of an interocclusal record?
9. How should gypsum be flowed into the impression during the pouring procedure?
10. Explain the infection-control procedures involved in making an impression and a model.

Making an Alginate Impression

Suggested check-off sheet

Mark **S** for satisfactory completion or **U** for unsatisfactory completion of each criterion in the appropriate space

PERFORMANCE CRITERIA:	FACULTY	STUDENT
1. Assemble the armamentarium		
2. Prepare the patient		
3. Select the proper tray		
4. Apply beading wax		
5. Have patient rinse with antiseptic mouth rinse		
6. Mix alginate properly		

Mandibular impression

	FACULTY	STUDENT
7. Fill the tray to the level of the beading wax		
8. Insert the tray properly by retracting one cheek with the mirror and the other with the side of the tray		
9. Have the patient raise his or her tongue		
10. Seat posterior portion of tray and then anterior portion		
11. Border mold		
12. Control gagging if necessary		
13. Remove the tray with a quick motion while protecting the opposing teeth		

Maxillary impression

	FACULTY	STUDENT
14. Fill the tray to the level of the beading wax		
15. Insert the tray properly by retracting one cheek with the mirror and the other with the side of the tray		
16. Border mold		
17. Control gagging if necessary		
18. Remove the tray with a quick motion while protecting the opposing teeth		
19. Make the interocclusal record		
20. Spray impression and interocclusal record with disinfectant		

EVALUATION:	FACULTY	STUDENT
21. Impressions free of voids and tears		
22. All necessary structures included		

ADDITIONAL COMMENTS

Pouring the Impressions

Suggested check-off sheet

Mark **S** for satisfactory completion or **U** for unsatisfactory completion of each criterion in the appropriate space.

PERFORMANCE CRITERIA:	FACULTY	STUDENT
1. Assemble the armamentarium		
2. Mix the gypsum properly		

Mandibular impression

	FACULTY	STUDENT
3. Fill in the tongue area		
4. Flow a small increment into the teeth		
5. Gradually flow larger increments into the teeth and impression		
6. Fill the base former		
7. Invert the impression into the base former, and set it away from the vibrator		

Continued.

Maxillary impression

		FACULTY	STUDENT
8.	Flow a small increment into the teeth	___	___
9.	Gradually flow larger increments into the teeth and impression	___	___
10.	Fill the base former	___	___
11.	Invert the impression into the base former, and set it away from the vibrator	___	___
12.	Allow the casts to completely harden before separating the impressions from the casts	___	___

EVALUATION:

13.	Impressions free of excessive voids, fractures, and/or air bubbles	___	___
14.	Impressions smooth and hard	___	___

ADDITIONAL COMMENTS:

Trimming the Casts

Suggested check-off sheet

Mark **S** for satisfactory completion or **U** for unsatisfactory completion of each criterion in the appropriate space.

PERFORMANCE CRITERIA:

		FACULTY	STUDENTS
1.	Spray casts with disinfectant spray	___	___
2.	Soak the casts in water	___	___

Maxillary cast

3.	Trim the posterior border to be perpendicular to the midline	___	___
4.	Trim the top of the cast to be parallel to the occlusal plan	___	___
5.	Trim the top of the cast to be parallel to a line from the cuspid to the last molar	___	___
6.	Trim the anterior portion from the cuspids to form a point over the central incisors	___	___

Mandibular cast

7.	Place interocclusal record between the cast as guide	___	___
8.	Trim the excess width	___	___
9.	Trim the posterior border to be even with the posterior border of the maxillary cast	___	___
10.	Trim the bottom of the cast to be parallel to the occlusal plane and the top of the maxillary cast	___	___
11.	Trim the sides to be parallel to a line from the cuspid to the last molar	___	___
12.	Trim the anterior portion to be rounded from cuspid to cuspid	___	___
13.	Trim the posterior angles of both casts to be even with the opposite cuspid	___	___

EVALUATION:

14.	Proper outline form	___	___
15.	Anatomic structures undamaged	___	___
16.	Adequate base—width and thickness	___	___
17.	Models remain occluded when positioned on posterior borders	___	___

ADDITIONAL COMMENTS:

REFERENCES

American Dental Association Council on Dental Therapeutics and Council on Prosthetic Services and Dental Laboratory Relations: Guidelines for infection control in the dental office and the commercial dental laboratory, *JADA* 110:969, 1985.

American Dental Association Council on Materials, Instruments, and Equipment: *Dentist's desk reference,* ed 2, Chicago, 1983, The Association.

Brune D et al: Levels of airborne particles resulting from handling alginate impression materials, *Scand J Dent Res* 86:206, 1978.

Chasteen JE: *Four-handed dentistry in clinical practice,* St Louis, 1988, CV Mosby.

Craig RG, editor: *Restorative dental materials,* ed 6, St Louis, 1989, CV Mosby.

Craig RG, O'Brien WJ, Powers JM: *Dental materials: properties and manipulation,* ed 4, St Louis, 1987, CV Mosby.

de Freitas JF: Potential toxicants in alginate powders, *Aust Dent J* 25:224, 1980.

Goldman HM, Cohen DW: *Periodontal therapy,* ed 6, St Louis, 1980, CV Mosby.

Graber TM: *Orthodontics: principles and practice,* ed 3, Philadelphia, 1972, WB Saunders.

Greenlee JS: Review of currently recommended aseptic procedures II. Dental instrument preparation, *Dent Hyg* 57:12, 1983.

Hattab F: Absorption of fluoride following inhalation and ingestion of alginate impression materials, *Pharmacol Ther Dent* 6:79, 1981.

Hattab F: The release of fluoride from alginate impression materials, 6:273, *Dental Materials* 3: 67, 1987.

Hill CJ, Gellin ME: Impression taking for the young child who gags, *JADA* 81:161, 1970.

Leung RL, Schonfeld SE: Gypsum casts as a potential source of microbial cross-contamination, *J Prosthet Dent* 49:210, 1983.

Morris JC et al: Effect on surface detail of casts when irreversible hydrocolloid was wetted before impression making, *J Prosthet Dent* 49:328, 1983.

Phillips RW: *Skinner's science of dental materials,* ed 8, Philadelphia, 1982, WB Saunders.

Robson E: Preparation of orthodontic study models, *Dent Tech* 26:50, 1973.

Roswick NA, Simon WJ: The pouring of models, *Dent Assist* 43:9, 1974.

Rudd KD: Making diagnostic casts is not a waste of time, *J Prosthet Dent* 20:98, 1968.

Sanad ME et al: The repair of gypsum casts, *J Prosthet Dent* 48:492, 1982.

Thurow RC: *Atlas of orthodontic principles,* St Louis, 1977, CV Mosby.

SUGGESTED READINGS

Appelbaum MB: Abused and misused—the alginate impression technique: a timely reminder, *Quintessence Int* 12:1051, 1981.

Buchanan S, Peggie RW: Role of ingredients in alginate impression compounds, *J Dent Res* 45:1120, 1966.

Carlyle LW: Compatibility of irreversible hydrocolloid impression materials with dental stones, *J Prosthet Dent* 49:434, 1983.

Durr DP, Novak EV: Dimensional stability of alginate impressions immersed in disinfecting solutions, *J Dent Child* 54:45, 1987.

Eisner S: *Morphodynamics of the human dentition,* Philadelphia, 1976, University of Pennsylvania.

Firtell DH et al: Sterilization of impression materials for use in the surgical operation room, *J Prosthet Dent* 27:419, 1972.

Hollenback GM: A study of the physical properties of elastic materials (the linear overall accuracy of reversible and irreversible hydrocolloids). IV, *J South Calif Dent Assoc* 31:403, 1963.

Knapp JG et al: Syringe application of alginate impression material, *J Mich Dent Assoc* 63:220, 1981.

Jarvis RG, Earnshaw R: The effects of alginate impressions on the surface of cast gypsum. I. The physical and chemical structure of the cast, *Aust Dent J* 25:349, 1980.

Lorton L: A method to facilitate impressions of orthodontically bonded teeth, *J Prosthet Dent* 48:356, 1982.

Miller JB, Burch JG: Criteria and procedures for cast trimming, *J Prosthet Dent* 30:843, 1973.

Pouring study casts, Lexington, 1977, Dental Auxiliary Education, Department of Dental Hygiene, University of Kentucky.

Selection and preparation of the impression tray for alginate impression, Lexington, 1977, Dental Auxiliary Education, Department of Dental Hygiene, University of Kentucky.

Skinner EW, Hoblit NE: A study of the accuracy of hydrocolloid impressions, *J Prosthet Dent* 6:80, 1956.

Stankewitz CG et al: Bacteremia associated with irreversible hydrocolloid dental impressions, *J Prosthet Dent* 44:251, 1980.

Storer R et al: An investigation of methods available for sterilizing impressions, *Br Dent J* 151:217, 1981.

Taking an alginate impression. Lexington, 1977, Dental Auxiliary Education, Department of Dental Hygiene, University of Kentucky.

Taking an impression, Haywood Calif, 1976, Quercus.

Thompson EO: Constructing and using diagnostic models, *Dent Clin North Am* 7:67, 1963.

Trimming study casts, Lexington, 1977, Dental Auxiliary Education, Department of Dental Hygiene, University of Kentucky.

16 INTRAORAL PHOTOGRAPHY

Bonnie Dafoe

LEARNING OUTCOMES

The dental hygienist will be able to

1. Discuss how intraoral photography can be used in dentistry.
2. Select the components of a clinical camera system which will be appropriate for a particular clinical setting or goal.
3. Use a clinical camera system to compose satisfactory images of all areas of the oral cavity.
4. Describe the composition of an intraoral series consisting of 12 views.
5. State the criteria for evaluating a photographic image.
6. Handle photographic equipment properly.
7. Display concern for the patient through:
   a. Gentle insertion of intraoral mirrors and retractors
   b. Considerate direction and communications
   c. Efficiency in time required to take intraoral images

Clinical photography has become an important part of standard dental practice. Clinicians in both general practice and specialty areas have found the pictorial representation of a patient's conditions to be an invaluable part of the patient's record.

As a communications tool, intraoral photography facilitates the delivery of comprehensive care. Photographic images capture the actual state of the patient as no other diagnostic aid can. For example, chartings of patient's restorations are useful for patient identification and reference, but these are time consuming to complete and may be inaccurate because of human error. The patient's actual tooth morphology and alignment configuration are difficult to illustrate on a diagrammatic chart. Study models are a diagnostic aid that captures the form of the teeth and adjacent soft tissues but are limited because not all areas of the oral cavity can be subjected to the impression technique. Radiographs have an important place in the patient record because they are excellent for assessing bony anatomy, caries, and restorations. However, though they provide a look at underlying conditions, an accurate representation of the soft tissue is lost.

The strength of intraoral photography is that the images capture the color, shape, texture, and characteristics of the oral cavity. The camera ob-

jectively records its subject, revealing conditions that may be lost in written notation or impossible to obtain by any other means.

Once you learn the technique, it becomes an integral part of clinical care that is extremely helpful in tracking clinical success.

A complete series of intraoral photographs is found in Plate 4.

Intraoral photography enhances dental practice in the following areas:

- Patient identification
- Record keeping
- Diagnosis
- Clinician and patient communications
- Treatment planning
- Case presentation
- Case documentation
- Patient education and/or motivation
- Professional peer review or instruction

Photographs for purposes of patient identification are part of the basic chart. A head-and-neck view in addition to selected intraoral images provides instant recognition of the patient as well as a record of past dental care or proposed treatment. When photographs are included in the record, the office staff can review the chart and consider treatment needs very easily with the exact patient in mind.

As an aid for diagnosis or confirmation of a diagnosis, photographs can be especially useful. If a patient presents with a questionable lesion on the buccal mucosa, the clinician may feel a biopsy is indicated. Before the biopsy, a photograph is made to document the exact color, size, and location of the lesion. The patient's record will be more accurate with visual documentation to accompany the pathology report.

Intraoral photographs are useful for treatment planning. The series can be referred to at the clinician's convenience. With this and other diagnostic aids, the patient's presence may not be necessary to assess, plan or review treatment needs. The ability to plan treatment in this way allows the dental team to organize the records and carefully prepare a detailed plan for a case presentation or consultation appointment.

Photographic images improve the communication process between the clinician and patient, changing the concept of case presentation. No longer is the clinician in the position of trying to describe complicated oral conditions to a patient who cannot visualize them. Suggesting the appropriate comprehensive or expensive treatment can occasionally create an awkward situation for both parties. The photographic series and other imaging techniques allow the clinician and patient to discuss treatment needs while studying the oral conditions together. With the help of intraoral imaging, the patient is able to see the the oral conditions from " the outside." This may encourage the patient to ask questions or discuss therapy from a more objective position. The patient can grasp and appreciate the scope of dental care and the need for a particular clinical solution. Case acceptance may be increased while actually decreasing the amount of consultation time required per patient.

If the clinician has photographic records of other completed treatments, the patient can study the before and after pictures. Although identical results cannot be guaranteed, the photographs help the lay person visualize the proposed treatment. As a bonus, the visual communication of the clinician's work may foster trust in the clinician's skills. In all cases, intraoral photography adds to the communication process between the dental staff and the patient.

Creating an accurate and thorough record is an absolute necessity. Intraoral photography becomes a major factor in documenting patient care. Images establish the patient's actual oral condi-

tions before treatment. Color images made during treatment record the progress of care (such as improvements in tissue or steps in restoration). At the completion of a phase of therapy, a final series establishes the treatment outcome. The entire series of images, which can be referred to at a future date, provides a detailed record of treatment and is an important step in practicing modern risk management. Too often, when recall is necessary, the memory is inadequate and written documentation is sketchy. Should a legal question concerning treatment arise, photographic records provide invaluable information. Case documentation procedures are described in Chapter 36.

As an educational resource, photography has endless possibilities. Clinical images can be used to motivate patients, personalize the office, or create instructional bulletin boards. Photographs can be used to create an office manual. Photos showing the contents of a storage cabinet or a tray setup quickly convey information to the staff.

When captured through photography, the results of treatment and home care regimens can reinforce satisfaction for both the clinician and the patient. Tissue changes occur slowly, making day-to-day appreciation of the healing process difficult, but patients can be motivated by seeing themselves in photographs before and after treatment (Fig. 16-1). The opportunity to be photographed makes most patients feel special and important. The patient can appreciate the results of successful restorative care through photographs and spread the word to family and friends. In this way a satisfied and enthusiastic patient becomes a practice builder for the dental office (Hook, 1987; Levin, 1990).

The clinician's slide collection rapidly becomes a resource for presenting information to groups of patients or peers for various instructional or educational purposes. Kodachrome slides can be made to create instructional series for professional seminars as well as interoffice purposes. Quality color or black-and-white prints can be made from slides. In this way the clinic or office can develop educational materials to suit its clinical philosophy. Series depicting the use of an auxiliary aid or the options of cosmetic treatment for certain conditions are examples of topics that can make interesting display presentations.

As the concept of peer review grows, photography will no doubt become an important dimension for assessing quality care. It is no longer possible

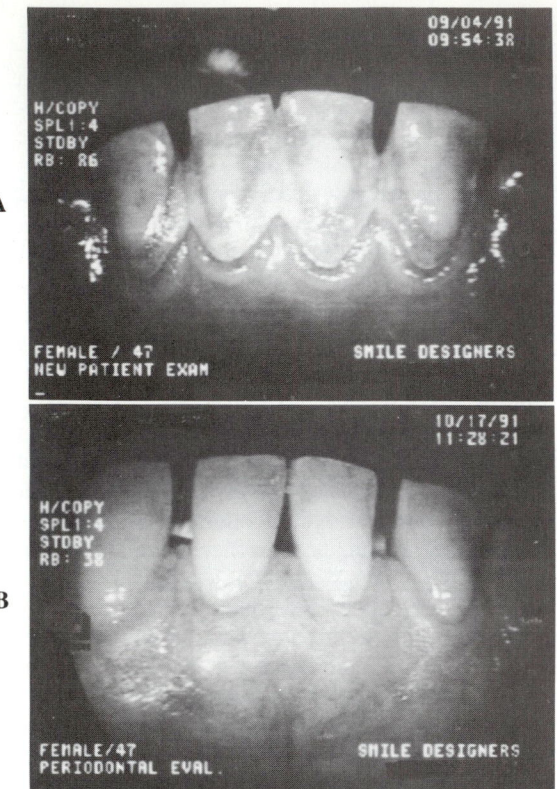

Fig. 16-1. **A,** Initial appointment: intraoral photograph showing calculus and inflammation prior to dental care. **B,** Follow-up appointment: intraoral photograph showing teeth and tissue after treatment and proper home care. Hardcopy photos made from video source.

to fully judge operating success by the use of explorers and radiographs alone. Restorations that may be acceptable by these standards could be deemed as failures by visual or photographic standards (Freedman, 1989). Visual documentation of initial oral conditions and treatment outcomes may be required as third-party payment mechanisms increase. In many cases, insurance companies will cover the cost of clinical photographs related to specific treatments.

In recent years, clinical photography has been enhanced by the development of intraoral video systems. Current photographic and computer systems allow patients to view not only existing oral conditions but also the possibility of a variety of treatment options simulated on images of their own teeth. As imaging technology improves, clinical applications for dentistry will continue to develop.

Intraoral photography has become a standard part of comprehensive oral health care. The degree of sophistication with which photographic imaging is integrated into every dental practice will vary, but a basic level of competency in photographic documentation is rapidly becoming an essential skill for all members of the dental team.

SELECTING A CAMERA SYSTEM

Many camera systems are available for use in dental practices. These range from simple instant-print cameras to the most recent innovations in intraoral video systems, which allow for extraoral cosmetic simulation and editing.

Daniels and Sherill (1975) have summarized the objectives of a clinical camera system that provides excellent quality and maximum flexibility for photographing all aspects of the oral cavity. The camera system is able to do the following:

1. Provide for a simple and repeatable clinical procedure requiring approximately 1 minute to take a photograph at any image size.
2. Provide for minimum manipulation (i.e., without the need for changing accessories or components) regardless of the subject area being photographed.
3. Provide for accurate focusing and composing of the subject.
4. Provide a continuous focusing range from very close (1:1) magnification to a "head-to-clavicle" size for maximum convenience and flexibility.
5. Provide for adequate working and lighting distance.
6. Provide for optimum photographic quality in the final result.

In general, four types of clinical camera systems are useful in dentistry. These are (1) an instant close-up camera, (2) a macrolens camera, (3) a bellows camera system, and (4) an intraoral video camera or combination intraoral video camera and extraoral cosmetic simulation system.

The instant close-up camera is designed to provide instant pictures for basic patient identification. The advantage is that these photos can be placed in the chart for the permanent record or given to the patient immediately. The patient may receive a photo for considering a proposed treatment or as part of his or her home care instruction program. The camera can make head-and-neck views and general intraoral views such as occlusal, buccal, or direct facial photos. Friedman

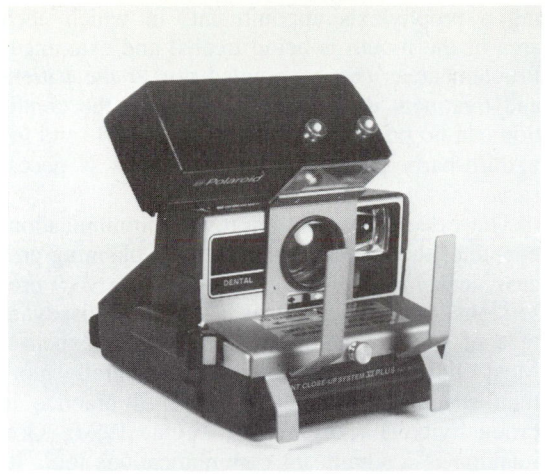

Fig. 16-2. Dental-Pro instant close-up camera.
(Courtesy Trojan Camera, Los Angeles, Ca.)

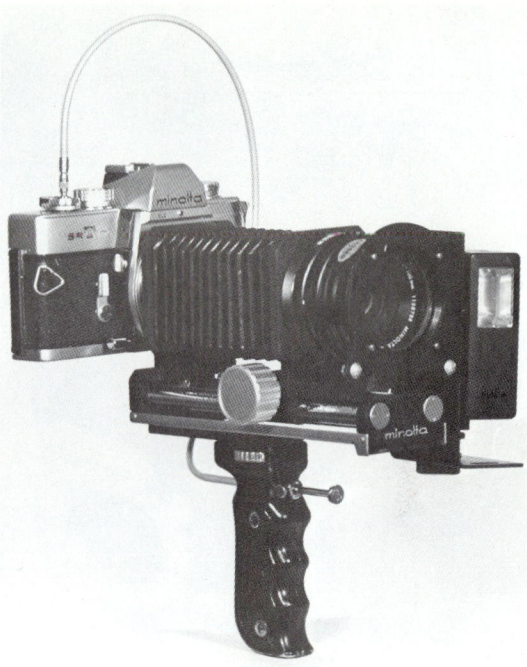

Fig. 16-3. Complete Minolta bellows clinical camera unit.
(Courtesy CL Freehe, Sumner, Wash.)

(1991) discusses the benefits of using instant photography to improve communications with patients about esthetic procedures. The instant photo can "freeze" the patient's smile, allowing the patient and the clinician the chance to discuss treatment options. Additionally, instant photographs are easily included in communications with the dental laboratory technician, greatly reducing the need for narrative descriptions while conveying important aspects of general scale, tooth size, color distribution, and lip relationship.

The instant camera generally does not produce finely detailed photographs, very close-up views, or images with lasting color quality. The photos are adequate for basic record keeping, for creating bulletin board displays, and as copies for the patient, laboratory, or insurance company. The cameras are very simple to operate (Fig. 16-2).

For documenting treatment with slides that show excellent detail and have professional color, select one of the other clinical camera systems. The macrolens system and the bellows camera are made up of component parts that require some manipulation and care but are quite easy to use (Figs. 16-3 to 16-5).

Though "still" cameras will remain popular because of their practical and relatively inexpensive nature, intraoral video imaging is the latest step in enhancing patient care through photography. Intraoral video technology consists of an advanced

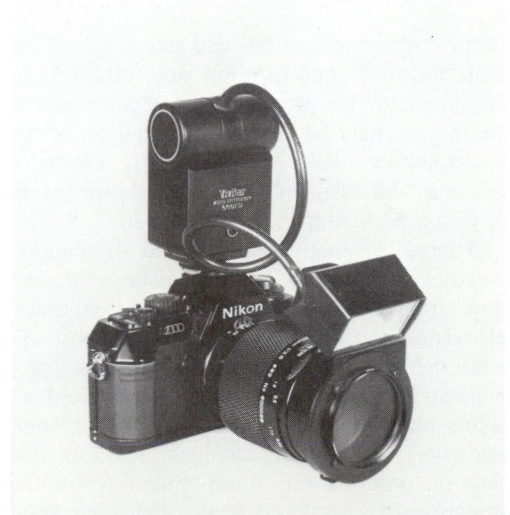

Fig. 16-4. Trojan clinical camera system. Auto system N2000, 90 mm-F/2.5 macro-lens with rotating point source flash unit.
(Courtesy Trojan Camera, Los Angeles, Ca.)

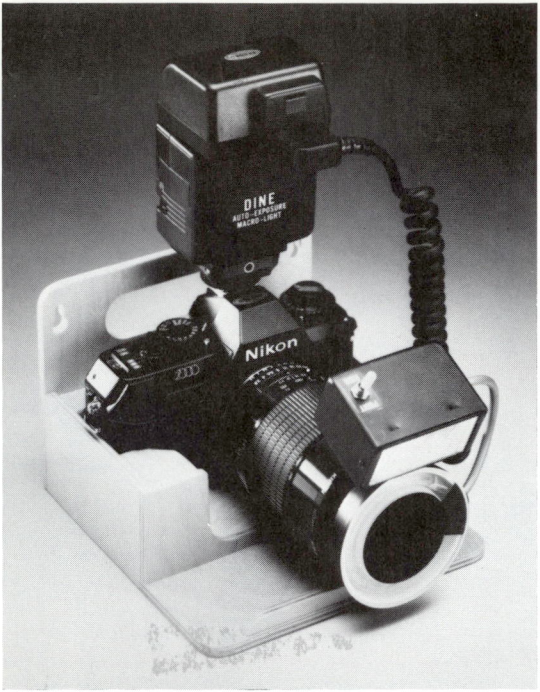

Fig. 16-5. Dine auto exposure system. Nikon N2000, 105 mm-F/32 macro-lens with ring light and point source flash combination lighting unit.
(Courtesy Lester A. Dine, Inc., Farmingdale, NY).

microcamera that can be held like a hand instrument and positioned to allow any intraoral or facial image to be projected on a color monitor. The images may be saved on videotape or stored on a computer disk. When desired, selected images may be "frozen" to create a printed hard copy of a particular view (Fig. 16-6).

Extraoral cosmetic imaging and simulation allow the clinician to edit or make changes on stored images of the patient's actual dentition to help visualize and select the treatment best suited to the patient's needs. Dental treatments that can be illustrated by cosmetic simulation include diastema closure, recontouring of teeth or gingiva, veneering, orthodontic changes, replacement of metal restorations with tooth-colored restorations, correction of discolored teeth, and other anomalies (Clinical Research Associates, 1991).

Intraoral video imaging equipment is relatively easy to learn to operate. The dental hygienist has the perfect opportunity to use the equipment during a prophylaxis appointment, in which each area of the mouth is being treated and examined. Problem areas can be pointed out to the patient and treatment discussed. A record of the condition can be printed for the patient's chart, and for a third-party payer if preauthorization is necessary.

The video equipment improves communication, expedites the examination-treatment planning process, and improves record keeping in a very professional and personal way. The main disadvantage of video imaging systems is their expense. Most clinicians report the cost is generally more than adequately offset by increased practice in productivity (Lackey, 1991; Levin, 1990). Oral imaging is a significant communications tool. Its impact on dentistry will evolve as microcamera and computer technology mature.

The companies listed at the end of the chapter are excellent sources for camera components, complete clinical systems, and a variety of photographic accessories.

INTRAORAL CLINICAL CAMERAS
Camera body and viewing system

A clinical camera system includes a 35 mm camera body. This number refers to the size of film that the camera holds.

The "viewing system" of the camera body is very important. A standard 35 mm camera often has a *range finder* viewing system. With this system, the photographer is not able to look directly through the lens to compose the view, because the view window is placed beside the lens. The photographer sees the general composition of the view, which is satisfactory for taking a picture of a large scene. It is not accurate when taking close-up views, when a few millimeters of difference could eliminate important details. The discrepancy between what the lens sees and what the photographer sees when using a range finder is called *parallax*. The viewing system for intraoral photography must be single-lens-reflex (SLR). This means the photographer is able to look directly through the lens, with the help of mirrors, to compose the image based on the actual view the lens sees. The accuracy of this viewing system makes it best suited for intraoral photography.

Lens

Clinical photography requires a camera lens between 90 and 135 mm in length. The standard 35

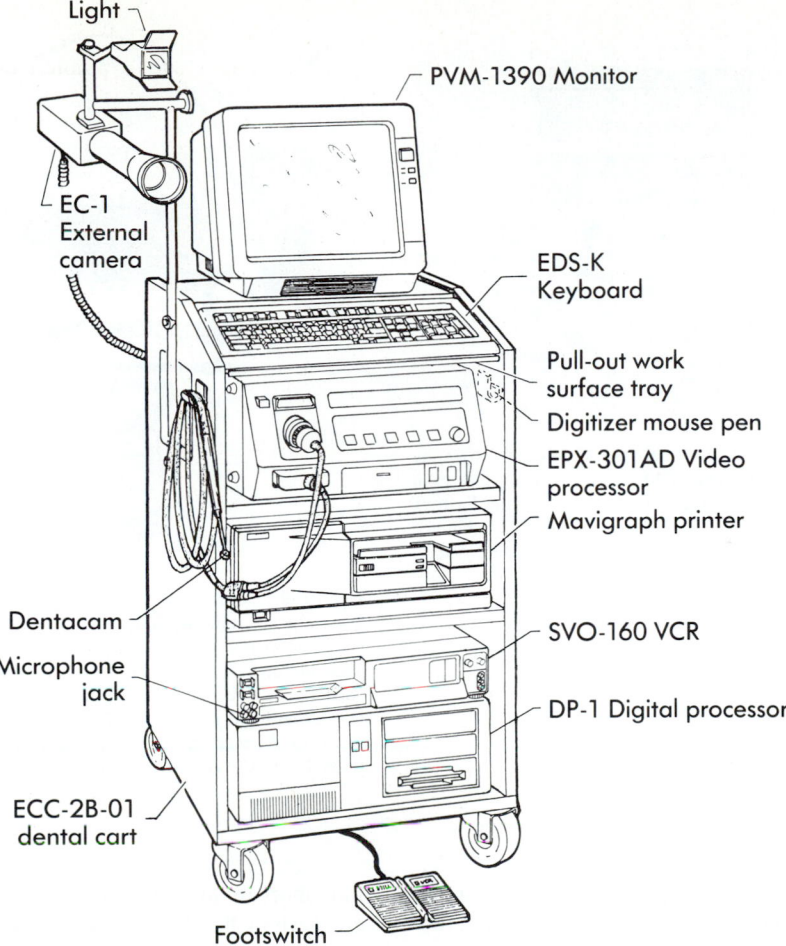

Light

PVM-1390 Monitor

EC-1
External
camera

EDS-K
Keyboard

Pull-out work
surface tray

Digitizer mouse pen

EPX-301AD Video
processor

Mavigraph printer

Dentacam

SVO-160 VCR

Microphone
jack

DP-1 Digital processor

ECC-2B-01
dental cart

Footswitch

Fig. 16-6. Combined DentaCam and VisionPlus System.
(Courtesy Fugi Optical Systems, Inc.)

mm camera usually comes equipped with a 50 mm lens. This lens is good for general, nonclinical photography because it "sees" approximately what normal vision sees. If used clinically for close-up photos, however, a 50 mm lens has to be placed about 4 inches from the subject. This does not allow enough working space or room for proper lighting. At best, in a close frontal view, the anterior teeth would appear distorted and wider than normal. Lenses between 90 and 135 mm do not distort the close-up subject and allow a working distance of approximately 8 inches between the camera lens and the subject. If images are made during a clinical procedure, this distance provides an adequate working field for dental in-

struments and photographic accessories such as mirrors and retractors. All 35 mm camera lenses between 90 and 135 mm are free of perspective distortion.

The lenses can be attached to the camera body or to an automatic bellows. A macrolens attaches to the camera body and allows focusing from infinity to close-up. Depending on the lens, an adapter extension may be necessary to achieve full life size (1:1) magnification. Some practice is necessary to become comfortable with the size and weight of the macrolens camera system. This and the need for occasional use of an adapter may be important in deciding whether this type of camera system is best suited to the clinician's needs.

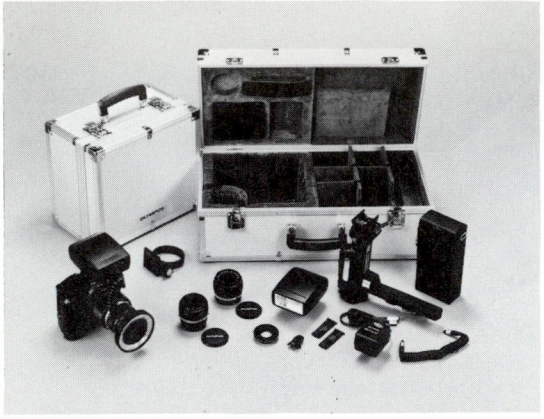

Fig. 16-7. Olympus medical/dental and scientific photography system. Components include: OM-2 Body Black, 135 mm/F4.5, 50 mm/F3.5, 80 mm/4.0 macrolenses, T10 ring flash, T power control, ring flash filter, electronic flash T32, bounce grip, power pace, TTL auto connector and cord, Macrophoto/Medical Case B.
(Courtesy Olympus Corporation, Woodbury, NY.).

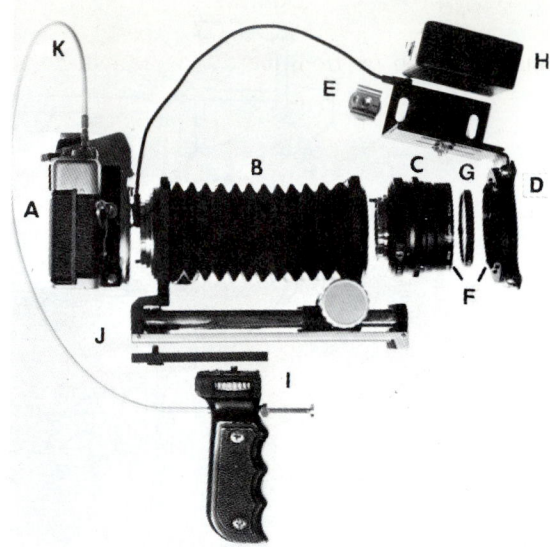

Fig. 16-8. Camera and parts needed for a fully automatic bellows clinical unit. *A*, Single-lens = reflex camera body; *B*, fully automatic bellows; *C*, 100 mm short-mount lens; *D*, Washington Scientific 180-degree rotating flash bracket; *E*, shoe and bolt for flash; *F*, S-7 lens adapter rings; *G*, S-7 color correction filler; *H*, vertical electronic flash unit; *I* to *K*, pistol grip with 20-inch cable release and balance bar.
(From Freehe CL: *Dent Clin North Am* 27:3, 1983.)

Fig. 16-7 shows a complete macrolens camera system. Components have been separated for display, along with a custom storage case.

Another intraoral camera system uses a 100 mm short-mount lens, attached to an automatic bellows system. The bellows is an adjustable accordion-type apparatus. The main characteristic of the bellows system is that it is continuously adjustable. The short-mount lens and bellows can focus from 4 ½ feet to 7 inches, achieving orthodontic views ranging from a head-to-clavicle view to one consisting of four to five anterior teeth. No other parts need to be added or adjusted.

The bellows apparatus attaches to a pistol grip, which is helpful in providing stability when handling the camera. A cable releases the shutter when the trigger in the pistol grip is pulled. This enables the free hand to adjust the bellows, aid in focusing the view, assist the patient, or place an instrument in the view. Some consider the size of the bellows system to be a disadvantage. The 100 mm short-mount lens and automatic bellows camera system has been specifically designed for intraoral photography. This camera can be recommended for use in other health, natural science, and research fields in which quality close-up photography is desired (Fig. 16-8).

Lighting units

Lighting is the most critical feature in photography. The direction and power of the lighting create the image of the subject. Lighting for clinical photography can be achieved by using a single point source flash mounted on a rotating bracket, a ring light flash unit, or a combination ring light and point source flash that can be used selectively.

A point-source flash is mounted on a rotating bracket at the front of the lens. When attached in this manner, the flash unit moves with the lens to provide correct lighting for the view and proper exposure. The light source can be rotated 180 degrees to adequately illuminate the field and cast a shadow for definition. The position of the flash close to the lens is important, as a horizontal placement too far from the lens will produce too much shadow, creating a poor image.

A ring light attachment encircles the lens. In this way the light source moves as lens focuses to adequately light the photographic field. Some ring lights have a rheostatic power control and require power adjustment to assure proper exposure of each view. These adjustments take time and may cause slight changes in slide color. The ring light produces an image that may lack definition, contrast texture, and good color. The center of the image has no shadow, whereas a hazy 360-degree shadow is cast around the subject. These images may appear flat when compared with point-source lighting, which provides a more natural, three-dimensional image because of the contrast created by lighting the subject from one side. All quality art or scientific images require some directed shadow to capture true form.

The bellows system uses a point-source light unit, and a macrolens system uses a ring light. In some systems, a ring light and point-source flash can be used together. The clinician's preference for lighting control and color and the adaptability of the camera/lens system will determine the best lighting solution.

Electronic flash units may be manual or automatic (through-the-lens [TTL]). An automatic flash is programmed for specific exposures at each camera setting, depending on the light sensitivity of the film. The light meter reads the light reflected off the film through the lens and adjusts the flash automatically. Manual systems set the flash for a specific exposure at each camera setting. As long as the film speed (ISO) is consistent, the exposure will be reliable.

The color output of the flash unit should be as close to 5500 kelvin (K) as possible. Most flash units have a color output of 5600 to 6400 K, which produces images with blue or purple tissue color. If the color output is below 5500 K, tissue color will be red to yellow. Depending on the flash unit and the type of lighting in the clinical setting, color correction filters over the lens and flash may be necessary to achieve ideal color. A light yellow filter is indicated if the films appear blue. A bluish filter will improve a yellow color on the films after processing. The dental light can affect the color tone of the slides and should be directed on the cheek, not on the area to be photographed.

Flash units can operate on alternating current (AC) or battery power. Using AC power offers convenience, but access to electrical outlets and maneuverability may be a consideration. Rechargeable batteries are recommended if battery operation is preferred. The flash should recycle within 5.7 seconds to aid in quickly taking a series of pictures. A flash duration of 1/800 to 1/1000 second is also recommended.

Once the camera system is selected, a roll of practice film should be exposed in the clinical setting to determine the necessary corrections in lighting and color filtration.

Camera adjustments

The shutter speed, aperture setting and film speed work together with the lighting to create high-quality images. Each of these factors requires specific settings on the camera.

The shutter speed is the period of time the shutter remains open, thus determining the amount of light that strikes the film. The shutter speed is usually recorded on the camera in fractions of a second: $\frac{1}{60}$, $\frac{1}{125}$, $\frac{1}{250}$. To set the shutter speed, simply rotate the shutter speed dial until the desired speed is aligned with the indicator on the camera body. The higher the shutter speed, the more efficiently it will "stop" the action of the subject. This concept is important to understand, but in clinical photography the need to stop action is rarely necessary. What is important, however, is that the shutter speed be synchronized with the flash unit. For intraoral photography, the shutter speed is 60, or $\frac{1}{60}$ of a second. This is the speed at which the electronic flash is automatically synchronized with the opening of the shutter. On some cameras the synchronized flash speed may be as high as $\frac{1}{125}$ of a second. Consult the camera and flash attachment information to determine the correct setting.

The aperture setting refers to the size of the lens opening. It is also called the f-stop. This setting is important because it determines the depth of field, or the area of the image in which all objects are in focus. A great depth of field is desired in intraoral photography to achieve sharpness of all objects in the picture. The smaller the aperture opening, the greater the depth of field. The smallest aperture opening is indicated by the largest f-stop number. The f-stops usually range from f-4 (lens wide open) to f-32 (very small opening). As the aperture is closed from each f-stop to the next smaller one, the light reaching the film is decreased by 50%.

Cameras with fully automatic lenses allow the photographer to compose the view by looking through the lens at the largest f-stop, (f-4). This allows enough light to see the view clearly, but the depth of field is very small. Only one tooth may be in focus. The photographer should compose the view by focusing one-third of the way into the scene. For a full direct facial view of the teeth in occlusion on a normally curved arch, this means focusing on the midline of the cuspid. When the shutter is tripped, the automatic lens closes the aperture to the preset f-stop. Using the example of the full direct view, the f-stop would be preset at f-19. Everything in the final image from the central incisors to the first molars would be in sharp focus.

For a normal head-to-clavicle view taken at a distance of 5 feet, the aperture setting would be f-8, with the focus on the eyes. For most intraoral views consisting of four to six teeth, the f-stop is set at f-22. Intraoral views of dark-skinned people should be set one-stop more open, at f-19. When photographing a pure white subject, such as a set of plaster casts, the aperture setting should be closed to f-27 (Freehe, 1983).

Film selection

The principal purpose of the photograph will determine the type of film to be used.

Color film available for slides is called *transparency film*; an example is Kodachrome film. Color print film, such as Kodak Vericolor (VPS-135 type III) professional film, is called *negative film*.

Color negative film can be used to produce color prints, black and white prints, or fair color slides, but with each generation of processing a small amount of photographic quality is lost. Kodachrome 64 film produces a grainless color transparency. The film exposed in the camera is processed and mounted to make the slide, thereby preserving the greatest resolution of the original quality. When necessary, color or black and white prints can be produced from the original color slide by making an internegative. These copies are of the same quality as those from any negative film, as Kodachrome is grainless. Kodachrome is the only permanent color film today. Its color can last 100 or more years. Ektachrome slides or negative film will last 4 to 20 years.

Photographic film is given an ISO number, which refers to its light sensitivity. This is the amount of time the film needs to be exposed to light to create a high-quality image and is referred to as film speed. A *fast* film with a high ISO number, such as 400 or 1000, indicates that the film is extremely sensitive to light. Less light is necessary to produce an acceptable image. Although useful in some types of photography, these films are not practical for intraoral photography, in which excellent color and detail are the main concerns. As film speed increases, grain size increases and contrast decreases. An intermediate film speed such as Kodachrome 64 is ideal for slide production or color print copy because of its high sharpness and lack of grain. Kodachrome 25 could be used, but it has too much magenta for dental photography unless the proper light filters are used to correct for excessive redness. When an electronic flash is used and color is corrected with a filter for 5500 K, color daylight film should be used. Kodachrome (ISO) 64 with the proper electronic flash is the correct choice for medical and dental photography.

PHOTOGRAPHIC ACCESSORIES
Cheek retractors

Cheek retractors are used to clear the lips and labial and buccal mucosa out of the area to be photographed. This improves visibility and allows the maximum amount of light to enter the oral cavity. Cheek retractors are available in clear plastic or metal (Figs. 16-9 and 16-10). Metal retractors are less attractive but can be autoclaved. Strict aseptic measures are as important during intraoral photography as in any other dental procedure in which infectious pathogens can be transmitted to dental personnel or between patients. The main use of the wire retractor is to hold the mirror for a buccal view. Only one wire retractor is necessary, as a plastic retractor is used for retracting the lips on the other side (Fig. 16-11). The transparent plastic retractors are esthetically most acceptable. Natural tissue color shows through them, limiting the potential for distraction.

Retractors are either single or double ended. Double-ended retractors provide both a small and large curvature. This feature allows adaptability to a variety of mouth sizes. The end of the retractor acts as a handle to aid retraction. Single-ended plastic retractors (Fig. 16-12) have longer, tapered handles. The curved end is larger for excel-

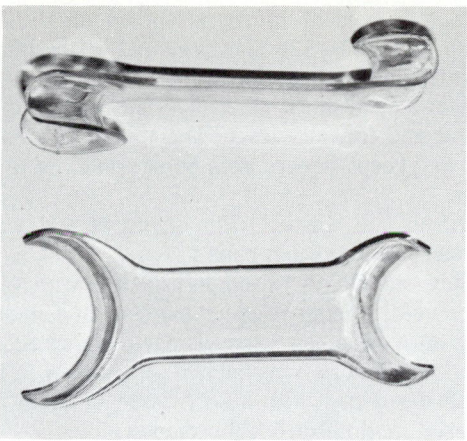

Fig. 16-9. Clear plastic cheek retractors, double ended.

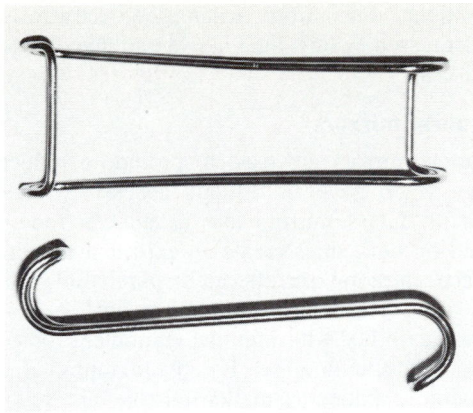

Fig. 16-10. Metal cheek retractors, double ended.

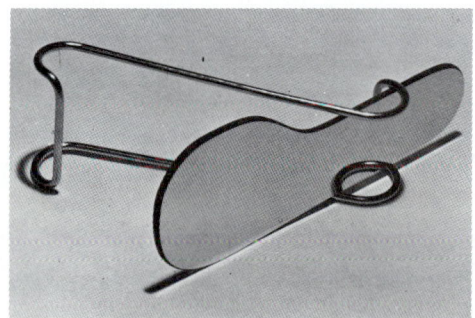

Fig. 16-11. Use of Columbia wire lip retractor with buccal mirror for posterior buccal view. Use one curved plastic lip retractor on opposite side.
(From Freehe CL: *Dent Clin North Am* 27:3, 1983.)

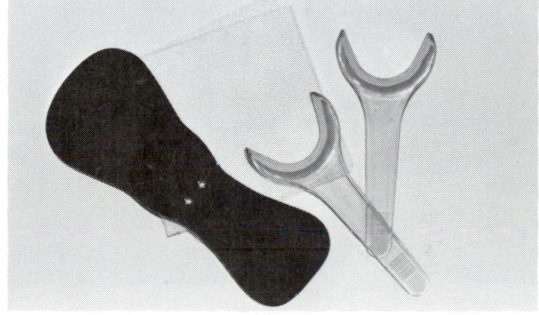

Fig. 16-12. Lester Dine mouth mirror and single-ended plastic cheek retractors.

lent lip retraction and can be cut down or modified to make smaller sizes.

Because plastic retractors cannot be autoclaved, chemical sterilization is necessary. After sterilization, the retractors should be rinsed well to remove all traces of the chemical, which could be irritating to the patient. Directions should be followed for the timing of chemical sterilization, because extended time in the solution may damage the plastic.

Technique for inserting retractors (Valentine, 1975)

1. Moisten the retractors in water.
2. Ask the patient to relax the lips and open the mouth slightly.
3. Place the rim of the retractor onto the edge of the lower lip (Fig. 16-13).
4. Rotate the handle of the retractor until it is parallel to the corner of the mouth (Fig. 16-14).
5. Repeat this for the other side of the mouth if necessary.
6. Instruct the patient to bite down on the posterior teeth. Pull out the retractors laterally and slightly forward (Figs. 16-14 and 16-15). Avoid pulling the retractor handles toward the ears. This will cause the buccal mucosa to be pressed onto the buccal surfaces of the teeth, as well as cause the pa-

tient discomfort when the retractor is pressed against the gingiva and alveolar process.

Intraoral mirrors

Intraoral mirrors are used to provide a reflected image when areas of difficult access are photographed. Glass mirrors that have been rhodium plated on both sides create an excellent reflective surface. Intraoral mirrors can be purchased in several sizes. The two mirrors shown in Fig. 16-16 allow flexibility with minimal equipment for general adult photography. For photography of the pedodontic patient, smaller mirrors are recommended, especially a child-size occlusal mirror.

Another type of mirror is shown on the tray set-up in Fig. 16-12. The large end of the mirror provides an excellent surface for capturing occlusal views, and the smaller end can be placed for palatal and lingual views. The mirror is easy to hold and keeps fingers from being too close to the scene.

Mirrors are washed with detergent and water and sterilized between patients.

They should be rinsed thoroughly with plain water before being used in the patient's mouth. Care must be taken when using mirrors because they can be easily scratched or broken. They should be wiped with a soft tissue or cloth and wrapped in cloth or felt for safekeeping.

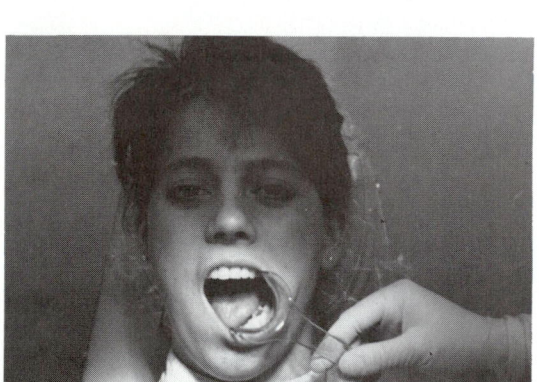

Fig. 16-13. Cheek retractor insertion. With patient's mouth open slightly and lips relaxed, place the rim of the retractor onto the edge of the lower lip. Gently rotate the retractor to the side.

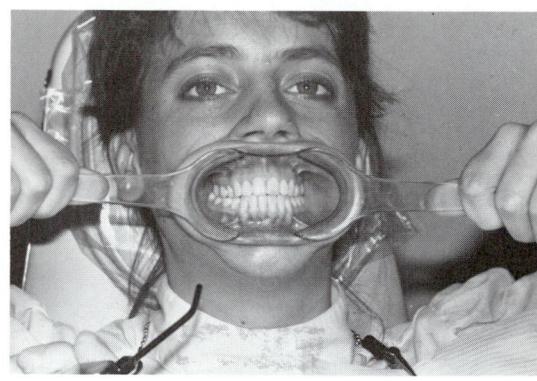

Fig. 16-14. Place the second retractor onto the lower lip and to the opposite side. Pull out laterally and slightly forward.

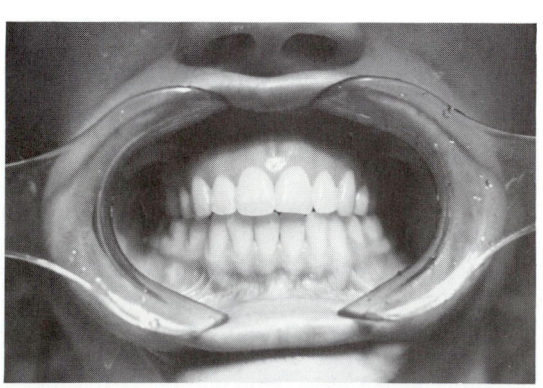

Fig. 16-15. Position for full direct facial views (see Plate 4, *A* and *B*).

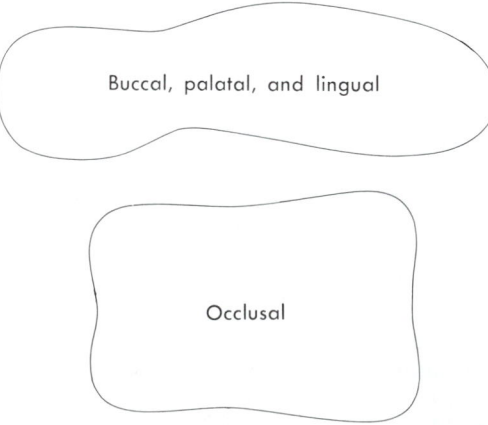

Buccal, palatal, and lingual

Occlusal

Fig. 16-16. Intraoral mirrors.

Technique for inserting mirrors

1. Place the mirror in warm water before use to prevent fogging. A small heating pad could also be used to keep mirrors warm.
2. Insert the appropriate cheek retractors.
3. Select the mirror and the appropriate end for the desired view.
4. Place the mirror flat into the mouth. As you retract with your fingers, rotate the mirror into position. Take care not to hit the teeth or press into the alveolar process, as this is annoying and uncomfortable for the patient.
5. Hold the mirror securely at the opposite end while maintaining retraction.
6. If fogging occurs, blow a gentle stream of compressed air onto the mirror.

Figs. 16-17 to 16-27 diagram that portion of the mirror used for the reflected image. Additional directions for mirror placement are given in the section on technique for individual views.

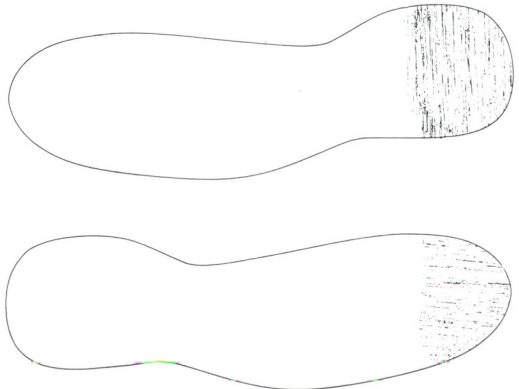

Fig. 16-17. Shaded area indicates portion of mirror that is used for the reflected image in anterior lingual views.

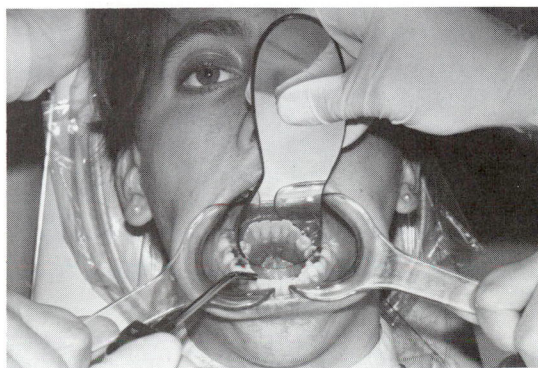

Fig. 16-18. Mirror and retractor placement for mandibular anterior lingual view (see Plate 4, *C*).

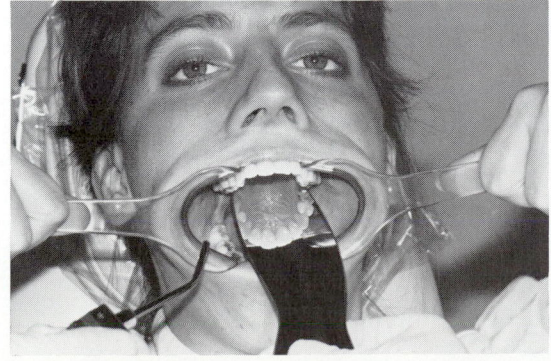

Fig. 16-19. Mirror and retractor placement for anterior palatal view (see Plate 4, *D*).

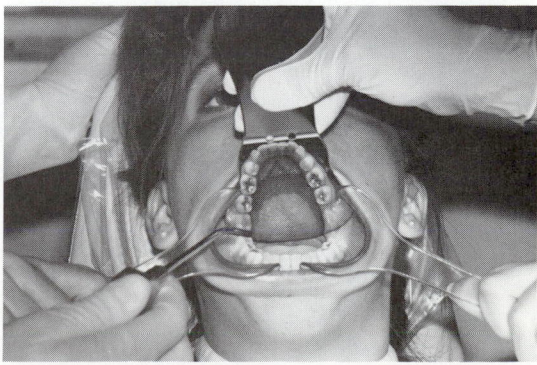

Fig. 16-20. Mirror and retractor placement for mandibular occlusal view (see Plate 4, *E*).

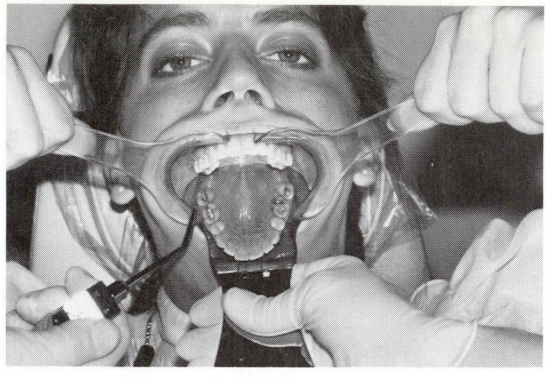

Fig. 16-21. Mirror and retractor placement for maxillary occlusal view (see Plate 4, *F*).

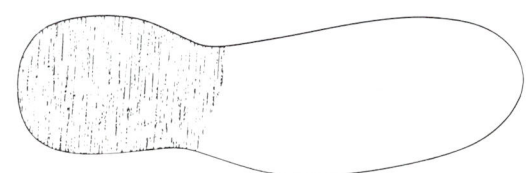

Fig. 16-22. Shaded area indicated portion of mirror used to reflect posterior palatal view.

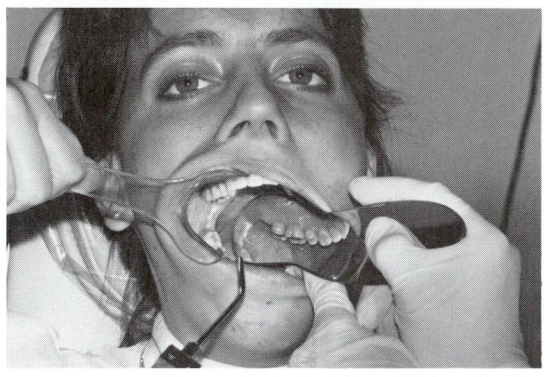

Fig. 16-23. Mirror and retractor placement for right posterior palatal view (see Plate 4, *G*).

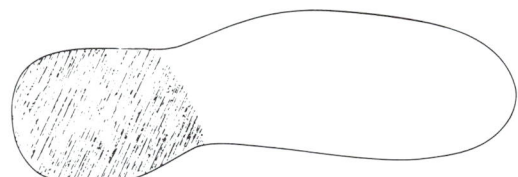

Fig. 16-24. Shaded area indicates portion of mirror used to reflect posterior lingual view.

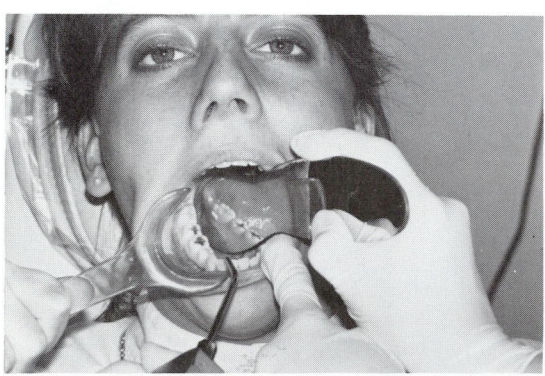

Fig. 16-25. Mirror and retractor placement for right posterior lingual view (see Plate 4, *I*).

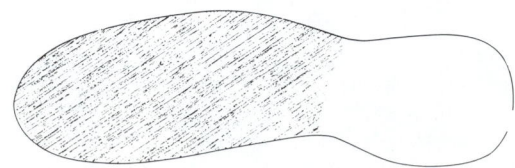

Fig. 16-26. Shaded area indicates portion of mirror used to reflect buccal view.

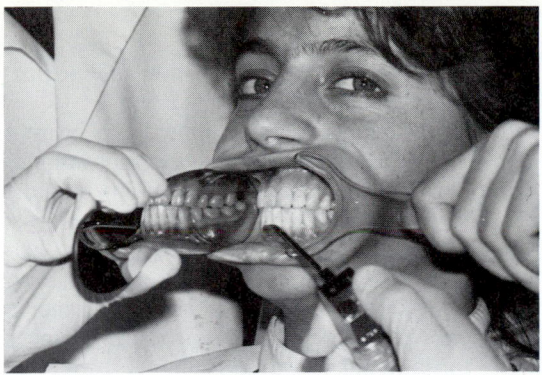

Fig. 16-27. Mirror and retractor placement for left buccal view (see Plate 4, *L*).

RECORD KEEPING AND STORAGE

Keeping track of camera use to ensure the proper distribution of slides or photos to a patient's chart requires careful and accurate records. A notebook can be placed in the case with the camera. This book consists of pages numbered to correspond with the exposures available on each roll of film. On the line that corresponds to the camera exposure number, record the patient's name and the view that was exposed. Other information may include the date, the photographer's name, or the camera setting if adjustments were made.

Recording the date and name of the person who loaded and unloaded the camera is helpful in determining the status of the film in the camera. When a film cartridge is unloaded, the camera is reloaded out of courtesy to the next user. This ensures that the camera is ready to be used at a moment's notice.

When the film is processed, the slides are sorted according to the notation in the record book. For identification, each slide is labeled with the patient's name and view. The clinician's name and the appointment at which the exposure was made are also helpful. The month the slide was processed is generally already printed on the side mount.

To store slides, clear plastic sheets that hold 20 or 36 slides are available to fit three-ring binders. The labeled slides are arranged according to the patient and either stored in a central location or incorporated in the patient's record (Barch, 1972). Slides should be projected or viewed on a color-corrected viewer. The radiographic viewbox will cause the slides to have poor color. Manual slide viewers that magnify the image are also available. As color slides may fade with time, they should be protected from unnecessary exposure or handling. Kodachrome film has permanent color, so slides need only to be protected from dirt, dust and finger oils.

GENERAL PHOTOGRAPHIC TECHNIQUE
Camera parts

Proper handling of a camera requires knowledge of its parts and their function. The maunfacturer's instruction booklet is most helpful in this regard. In general, it is important to be able to identify the following parts:

Shutter and ISO speed dial
Film advance lever
Shutter release button
Frame counter
Finder eyepiece
Aperture setting (f-stop)
Lens and lens cover
Electronic flash unit attachment
Flash plugs connecting at "X" on camera and on flash attachment
Flash "ready" light
Film rewind crank and back-cover release
Film cartridge chamber
Film take-up spool
Film pressure plate
Film rewind button on camera base
Battery cover and switch on camera

Loading the camera

Following are general principles of loading and unloading film. Consult the manufacturer's directions for specific steps suited to the particular camera.

1. Raise the back-cover release knob and "pop" the back open.
2. Place the film cartridge in the cartridge chamber at the left. Replace the back-cover release knob to hold the cartridge, and feed the film leader onto the take-up spool.
3. Operate the film advance lever. The film will begin to wind around the spool. Watch that the film perforations are engaged on the upper and lower teeth of the sprocket gears.
4. Press the shutter release button when the advance lever locks. After two shutter releases, the film should be well secured.

5. To make sure the film is flat against the pressure plate and attached to the take-up spool, carefully rotate the film crank in the top of the back-cover release knob to slightly increase the tension on the film. Always move the crank in the direction of the arrow. At this point the back of the camera can be closed.

6. Record your name and the date the camera was loaded.

Removing the film

1. Press the rewind button on the bottom of the camera base.

2. Rotate the rewind crank in the top of the back-cover release knob in the direction of the arrow. This winds the film back into the cartridge.

3. As you wind towards the end of the film, you will feel resistance on the crank. Usually after a click that signals the release of the film from the spool, the tension is then released and the crank will move effortlessly. You can then assume that all the film is back in the cartridge.

4. Raise the back-cover release knob, and the back will open.

5. Place the film in its protective canister and send for developing.

6. Record your name and the date of unloading. It is a courtesy to load the camera for the next person.

Making the photograph

Steps in making a photograph include checking the camera settings, placing the accessories, and composing the view.

1. Check the shutter speed—"60" for intraoral photography.

2. Check that the f-stop is set at 22, 19, or 8, depending on the view.

3. Check that the electronic flash "ready" light is on.

4. Check that the film has been advanced.

5. Hold the camera with the pistol grip in the right or left hand. If a macrolens is used with no pistol grip, place the safety strap from the camera body around your neck.

6. Insert the cheek retractors and mirrors if necessary.

7. When using mirrors and a rotating flash unit, make sure that the flash unit is on the same side as the mirror.

8. Dry the field with compressed air as needed.

9. Check the picture composition and the mirror reflection for any adjustments.

10. Look through the viewfinder. The bellows is used to obtain the correct composition of the picture. Adjusting the bellows to the most extended position provides the most magnified, close-up view. Change the bellows position for each view as necessary. The bellows does not focus the image; it only provides image ratio or size changes for intraoral views.

11. Correct the mirror placement if necessary. For the best image, position the mirror so that only the reflected image is seen through the viewfinder. Often the natural teeth are observed, which creates a confusing slide (Fig. 16-28). To correct this problem, move the entire mirror farther away from the subject. Although it is not always possible to clear the natural teeth from the view, particularly on occlusal or buccal views, it is generally beneficial to try. Often a movement of 1 or 2 mm is all that is necessary.

12. Focus the view. For maximum brightness during focusing, the automatic bellows lens is always at its largest opening (f-4). With the lens aperature set to f-19, for example, it is wide open during focusing but closes down to f-19 as the shutter is triggered. The view is focused by rocking the camera and the photographer's body back and forth until the center image in the viewfinder is sharp. Focus on a point one-third of the way into the scene of the subject. For example, use the mesial aspect of the first molar for focus on palatal or mandibular posterior lingual views.

13. Make a final check through the viewfinder for distracting fingers, mirror, or retractor edges, and natural teeth (Fig. 16-29). At this point, the photographer gives the assistant verbal directions for adjusting the accessories without taking his or her eyes away from the viewer. This eliminates additional time spent composing the view and focusing again (Fig. 16-30).

14. While steadying the camera, gently squeeze the shutter release.

15. If the correct exposure is uncertain, make the necessary adjustments and take an ad-

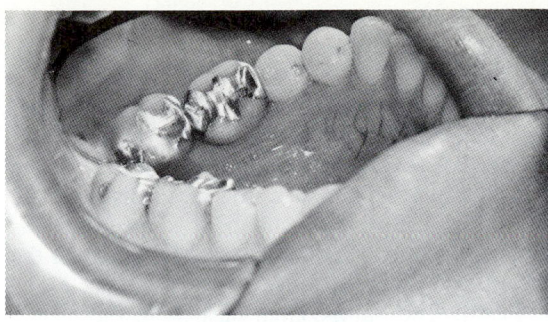

Fig. 16-28. Natural teeth and reflected image create a confusing picture. Capture only the reflected image. Use a stream of air to defog the mirror.

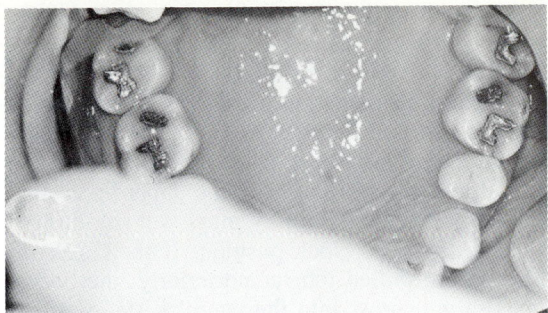

Fig. 16-29. Fingers can be distracting in final picture. As the edge of the view may not be in focus in the viewfinder, check the composition carefully before taking the shot.

ditional exposure. Film is inexpensive compared with the cost of setting up again or losing the record forever.

16. Record the exposure in the camera notebook.

THE PHOTOGRAPHIC SERIES

A complete series of intraoral photographs is shown in Plate 4. It consists of 12 views of the teeth and adjacent soft tissues. The series does not include a full face or profile view, which may be incorporated depending on the clinician's preference. If the slides identify a person and are going to be used for display or educational purposes, a permission or release form can be developed for the patient to sign (Steele, 1991). Usually views of "teeth only" provide necessary identification for dental personnel but do not provide easy recognition of the patient by others.

Implementing intraoral photography into a busy practice requires that the procedure be a simple, standardized routine. Documentation can be misleading if features on the photos are distorted by discrepancies in technique such as irregular lighting or positioning. A protocol that establishes the same camera and light positions, subject distance, and composition for each view will produce consistent quality in photography from patient to patient (Claman, 1990; Kumagai, 1988; Steele, 1991).

TECHNIQUE FOR INDIVIDUAL VIEWS
Anterior facial views

Composition. Full direct view: The photograph includes all teeth in occlusion as far posterior as possible. The incisal and occlusal plane

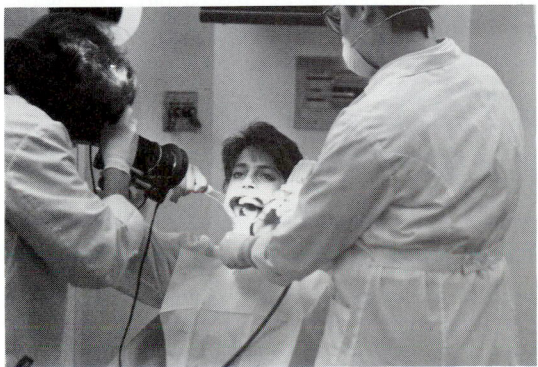

Fig. 16-30. Intraoral photography is a cooperative effort. While looking through camera, the photographer gives directions to the patient holding the retractors and to the person holding the mirror and compressed air.

should run in a straight line horizontally across the middle of the slide. The midline is centered (see Plate 4, A).

Anterior direct view: The photograph includes the area from the distal aspect of the right cuspid to the distal aspect of the left cuspid, as well as an adequate zone of gingiva. The incisal plane should run in a straight line across the middle of the slide. The midline is centered (see Plate 4, B).

Patient position. The patient sits upright in the chair, with the head resting securely in the headrest. The mandible is parallel to the floor when the teeth are in occlusion. The photographer approaches the subject from directly in front of the face. To prevent leaning over the dental chair, the photographer can ask the patient to turn his or her head toward the camera.

Retractors. Both retractors are pulled laterally when composing these pictures (see Fig. 16-15).

Mirror. None is required.

Flash. The point-source flash is in the 3 or 9 o'clock position for both the full direct view and the anterior direct view.

Helpful hints. Beware of the upper lip casting a shadow on the maxillary gingiva if the flash is used in the 12 o'clock position. If the cheek retractors are pulled too far posteriorly, the buccal mucosa will press into the buccal surfaces of the teeth.

Anterior lingual views: mandibular

Composition:. The photograph contains a lingual view of the mandibular anterior teeth and the gingiva from the distal aspect of the right cuspid to the distal aspect of the left cuspid. The incisal plane runs in a line horizontally across the slide, and the midline is centered (see Plate 4, C).

Patient position. The patient is tilted back slightly in the chair with the head resting securely in the headrest. The mouth is opened wide with the tongue relaxed in the floor of the mouth.

Retractors. Both retractors are used in retracting the lower lip.

Mirror. Either end of the tapered mirror can be used in composing this picture, depending on the width of the patient's mandibular arch (see Fig. 16-17). It is placed one tooth distal to the teeth that are to be photographed and held as close to parallel as possible to the long axis of the anterior teeth (see Fig. 16-18).

Flash. The point-source flash is in its top position for this view, or if more light contrast is desired, the flash can be placed in the 3 or 9 o'clock position.

Helpful hints. To avoid an excess of saliva in the composition, ask the patient to swallow first.

Anterior lingual views: maxillary anterior palatal

Composition. The photograph contains a palatal view of the maxillary anterior teeth and gingiva from the distal aspect of the right cuspid to the distal aspect of the left cuspid. The incisal plane runs in a horizontal line across the lower edge of the slide, and the midline is centered (see Plate 4, D).

Patient position. The patient should be tilted back slightly in the chair, with the head resting securely in the headrest. The mouth is opened wide, with the tongue resting against the mandibular anterior teeth.

Retractors. Both retractors are pulled straight out with a slight upward rotation to retract the upper lip.

Mirror. Either end of the mirror can be used in composing this picture, depending on the width of the patient's maxillary arch and the size of the palatal vault. It is placed one tooth distal to the teeth that are to be photographed and held as close to parallel as possible to the long axis of the teeth (see Fig. 16-19).

Flash. The point-source flash is in the 3 or 9 o'clock position for this view.

Helpful hints. To prevent inclusion of the patient's nostrils in the photograph, make sure the lower edge of the miror is depressed as far as possible against the mandibular teeth with the mouth opened wide.

Occlusal/soft tissue views: mandibular

Composition. The photograph includes the mandibular arch around the perimeter of the mirror (occlusal surfaces) and the floor of the mouth or the tongue (see Plate 4, E).

Patient position. The patient is tilted back in the chair, with the mandible pointed slightly upward. The occlusal plane is parallel to the floor when the mouth is opened wide. The tongue may be placed lightly on the soft palate or left to relax in the floor of the mouth.

Retractors. Both retractors are used for this view. Retract the lip downward as necessary.

Mirror. The occlusal mirror is used specifically for this view. Depending on the size of the patient's mouth, either the small or the large end of the mirror is inserted posteriorly until the borders of the mirror rest on the retromolar pad. The mirror is then adjusted until it rests at a 45-degree angle to the plane of the occlusion. Blow a stream of compressed air to defog the mirror before taking the photograph (see Fig. 16-20).

Flash. The flash is in the 3 or 9 o'clock position for this view.

Helpful hints. To avoid including the fingers or retractors in your composition, hold the mirror at its very edge. Tilt the chair back slightly if necessary. In some cases the cheek retractors do not have to be used if the lips are not obscuring the view. Have the patient swallow to prevent pooling of saliva.

Occlusal/soft tissue views: maxillary

Composition. The photograph includes the maxillary arch around the perimeter of the mirror (occlusal surfaces) and the palate (see Plate 4, *F*).

Patient position. The patient is sitting in the chair with the head resting securely in the headrest. The mouth should be opened wide and the tongue relaxed against the mandibular teeth.

Retractors. Both retractors are used in this view.

Mirror. The occlusal mirror is used specifically for this view. Depending on the size of the patient's mouth, either the small or large end of the mirror is inserted posteriorly until the borders of the mirror rest on the retromolar pad. The mirror is then adjusted until it rests at a 45-degree angle to the plane of the occlusion (see Fig. 16-21).

Flash. The flash is in the 3 or 9 o'clock position for this view.

Helpful hints. To avoid seeing the fingers or retractors in your composition, hold the mirror at its very edge. If the nostrils are still in view, depress the mirror more towards the mandibular teeth or have the patient open wider. Tilt the chair back slightly if necessary. In some cases the retractors do not have to be used if the lips are not obscuring the view.

Posterior palatal view (right and left)

Composition. The photograph includes a palatal view of the maxillary posterior teeth and gingiva from the distal aspect of the cuspid to the maxillary tuberosity. The occlusal plane runs in a straight line horizontally across the slide (see Plate 4, *G* and *H*).

Patient position. The patient is tilted back slightly in the chair, with the head resting securely in the headrest and usually slightly to the side being photographed. The patient's head is turned slightly to the side to permit the best view of the mirror.

Retractors. Both retractors are used to retract the lips and to provide access for the mirror on the specific side.

Mirror. The rounded end of the buccal mirror is preferred for this view (see Fig. 16-22). It is placed along the midline of the palate until its distal portion is adjacent to the maxillary tuberosity. The anterior end may rest on the incisal surfaces of the lateral incisor of the opposite quadrant. For a direct palatal view, the mirror is maintained as parallel to the long axis of the teeth as possible (see Fig. 16-23).

Flash. The flash is rotated to the same side as the mirror for this view.

Helpful hints. To avoid stimulating a gag re-

flex, do not rest the mirror on the soft palate. If the patient's natural teeth are in the composition, move the entire mirror toward the midline.

Posterior lingual view

Composition. The photograph includes the area from the distal aspect of the cuspid up to and including the retromolar pad. The view is a direct lingual view and shows as little of the occlusal surfaces as possible (see Plate 4, *I* and *J*).

Patient position. The patient is tilted back slightly in the chair with the head resting securely in the headrest. The mouth is opened wide with the tongue relaxed on the floor of the mouth.

Retractors. Both retractors are used to retract the lips and to provide access for the mirror on the specific side.

Mirror. The more rounded end of the mirror is preferred for this view, with the arc towards the floor of the mouth (see Fig. 16-24). The tongue is gently retracted away from the lingual surfaces of the teeth with the mirror as it is positioned just distal to the retromolar pad. The mirror will cross the arch diagonally, and the anterior portion of the mirror will rest as far posteriorly as possible on the bicuspids of the opposite quadrant. The mirror is held as vertically as possible to provide the best view. If the top edge of the mirror is tilted towards the teeth, too much of an occlusal view will be observed. The entire mirror is moved away from the teeth if the natural teeth are in view (see Fig. 16-25).

Flash. The flash is rotated to the same side as the mirror for this view.

Helpful hints. Work quickly with this view, as it may be uncomfortable and is taken in an extremely wet field. Be careful not to retract the tongue too harshly, stimulating the gag reflex.

Posterior buccal views (right and left)

Composition. The photograph includes the area from the distal aspect of the cuspids to the distal aspect of the most posterior tooth in each arch, as well as a glimpse of the retromolar pad or the maxillary tuberosity. The occlusal plane runs in a straight line horizontally across the midline of the slide. The view is as direct a buccal view as possible, rather than a mesial view (see Plate 4, *K* and *L*).

Patient position. The patient is sitting upright in the chair, with the head resting securely in the headrest. With the teeth in occlusion, the mandible is parallel to the floor.

Retractors. One wire retractor is used to hold the mirror for the best view. A plastic retractor is used on the opposite side to retract the lip.

Flash. The flash is rotated to the same side as the mirror for this view.

Mirror. The long tapered end of the buccal mirror is preferred for composing this picture (see Fig 16-26). The mirror is inserted into the frame of the wire retractor and placed between the buccal surfaces of the teeth and the buccal mucosa as far distal as the last tooth in the arch. It should be pulled laterally away from the alveolar process as much as possible (see Fig. 16-11). An alternative technique does not use a wire retractor. The mirror is placed and positioned as described. A secure grip should be kept on the mirror to prevent the buccal musculature from pushing the mirror anteriorly or medially (see Fig. 16-27).

Helpful hints. Retract the tissue firmly and as close to a 45-degree angle as possible from the natural teeth to provide the photographer with the best view.

SUMMARY

These directions are intended as a guide for the beginner. Depending on the camera system and the clinical environment, experience will help each clinician determine the best technique. Often, slight adjustments in chair position or cheek retractor and mirror placement need to be made according to the patient's oral conditions.

EVALUATION OF SLIDES

The student is encouraged to evaluate photographic slides according to the following criteria:
Above average
   1. Inclusion of all desired oral structures.
   2. Excellent photographic detail; excellent focus
   3. Excellent lighting and color
   4. No extraneous material
   5. Structures well centered
   6. Slide labeled properly
Average
   1. Inclusion of desired oral structures
   2. Adequate photographic detail
   3. Lighting and color improvement needed
   4. Extraneous material included, but not to distraction of slide's value
   5. Centering improvement needed
   6. Slide labeled properly

Unacceptable
   1. Omission of desired oral structures
   2. Inadequate photographic detail
   3. Inadequate lighting and color
   4. Obvious extraneous material included
   5. Subject completely off-center
   6. Slide incorrectly labeled

After the student has evaluated the photographic slides, the student and an instructor can discuss them. Focus on suggestions to improve technique for future photography sessions. Positive comments and encouragement are helpful, as hours of practice are necessary to reach competency in this psychomotor skill.

The criteria sheet on p. 355 is included for process evaluation of student progress during laboratory or clinic instruction.

CONCLUSION

Intraoral photography is a part of contemporary dental practice. With this skill, the clinician enhances communication with the patient regarding treatment planning and accurate documentation of care. This chapter has presented basic skills for handling a clinical camera system and composing a series of intraoral views.

ACTIVITIES

1. Identify the parts of a camera. Practice loading and unloading a "test" film cartridge.
2. View slides of the complete intraoral series, identifying the composition of each view. Unacceptable slides may be shown to illustrate common photographic errors.
3. Divide into laboratory groups of four students: photographer, patient, mirror holder, and an extra to assist with retractors, light position, dry field, and other tasks. Rotate being the photographer and practice taking the intraoral views (1 hour per session is suggested). One faculty member per group is ideal. Eight to ten sessions are suggested for mastering basic skills.
4. When slides are returned from processing, meet as a group to critique the views and plan new technique strategies.
5. Practice photographic skills by taking a complete series of intraoral photographs for clinical patients as a part of treatment and case documentation.

REVIEW QUESTIONS

1. Discuss at least four ways intraoral photography contributes to providing comprehensive dental care.
2. Match the terms in column 1 with those in column 2

that are most closely related.

a. single-lens reflex
b. aperture setting
c. focus
d. shutter speed
e. parallax
f. depth of field
g. film
h. 100 mm
i. point-source flash
j. bellows position

1. error in viewing
2. 60
3. controls photo composition
4. produces shadow for definition
5. "rocking" adjustment with body and camera
6. lens
7. ISO 64
8. plane of focus
9. mirror viewing system
10. f-22

3. Give the steps for placement of intraoral cheek retractors.
4. Give the composition of the following views:
   a. Mandibular anterior lingual
   b. Buccal of right side
   c. Anterior direct
   d. Maxillary occlusal
5. State the criteria for evaluating an *above average* photographic image.

Intraoral Photography

STUDENT: _____

DATE:

PERFORMANCE CRITERIA: COMMENTS

1. Prepare all equipment for intraoral photography (camera, sterile mirrors, retractors, film, record book)
2. Make all adjustments on the camera to ensure a successful exposure (1/60 shutter speed, electronic flash "ready", appropriate f-stop).
3. Position the electronic flash according to the area of the mouth to be photographed.
4. Insert cheek retractors with a minimum of trauma to the patient.
5. Correctly place the intraoral mirrors to obtain the desired composition.
6. Use compressed air to dry the area to be photographed.
7. Hold the camera securely.
8. Focus the camera by adjusting the bellows and body position, or by adjusting the macrolens.
9. Record all photos in the record book
10. Store the camera without cocking the trigger
11. Rack the bellows to the full "in" position for storage, or correctly position and store the macrolens
12. Sterilize and store the cheek retractors and mirrors appropriately
13. Care for the photographic equipment in a responsible manner
14. Load and/or unload the camera properly
15. Evaluate the quality of slides and recommend variations in photographic technique to correct inadequate exposure

COMPANIES TO CONTACT FOR CLINICAL CAMERA SYSTEMS AND PHOTOGRAPHIC ACCESSORIES

American Dental Camera
2600 West Big Beaver
Troy, MI 48084
(800) 359-1959

Competitive Camera Corporation
157 West 30th Street
New York, NY 10001
(212) 868-9175

Cosmetic Imaging Systems
309 Santa Monica Boulevard, Suite 315
Santa Monica, CA. 90401
(800) 258-2218

Densply/Equipment Division
570 West College Avenue
P.O. Box 870
York, PA 17405
(800) 877-0020

Dental Tools-THC Video and Electronics
2525 Bay Area Boulevard
Houston, TX 77058
(713) 488-3434

Envision Imaging Technologies
One College Park
8910 Purdue Road, Suite 690
Indianapolis, IN 46268
(800) 432-2442

Evaporated Metals Films (mirrors only)
701 Spencer Road
Ithaca, NY 14850
(607) 272-3320

Fugi Optical Systems
170 Knowles Drive
Los Gatos, CA 95030
(800) 634-6244

Lester A. Dine
351 Hiatt Drive
Palm Beach Gardens, FL 33418
(800) 237-7226

New Image International
212B Vanowen Street
Canoga Park, CA 91303
(800) 634-7349

Olympus Corporation
Crossways Park
Woodbury, NY 11797
(516) 364-3000

Pro/Vision-DIS
460 Division Street
Campbell, CA 95008
(800) 966-5123

Trojan Research and Development
15500 Erwin Street, Suite 1101
Van Nuys, CA 91411
(800) 338-9433

Washington Scientific Camera Co.
P.O. Box 88681
Tulwila, WA 98188
(206) 863-2854

ACKNOWLEDGMENT

Special thanks to Sharon Spotts at Fugi Optical Systems, Los Gatos, California; Terry Biggs at Patterson Dental Company, Sunnyvale, California; and Gayle Schmidt, R.D.H. and Professional Relations Director, SMILE Designers, San Jose, California; for their help and expertise with intraoral video systems.

The author is grateful to the Department of Dental Hygiene at Thomas Jefferson University, College of Allied Health Sciences in Philadelphia, Pennsylvania, and especially to Jaclyn Gleber, R.D.H., Ed.D., and dental hygiene students Kathleen O'Brien and Elizabeth Clark for providing the views of photographic technique presented in this chapter.

REFERENCES

Barch L: Storage and filing of dental color slides, *J Acad Gen Dent* 20:24, 1972.

Bengel W: Standardization in dental photography, *Int Dent J* 35:210, 1985.

Bernstein M: The application of photography in forensic dentistry, *Dent Clin North Am* 27:151, 1983.

Claman L et al: Standardized portrait photography for dental patients, *Am J Orthod Dentofacial Orthop,* 98:197, 1990.

Clinical Research Associates: Imagers, extraoral cosmetic simulation, *Newsletter* 15(3):1, 1991.

Daniels T, Sherill C: *Handbook of dental photography,* San Francisco, 1975, University of California School of Dentistry.

Freedman G: Standardization in dental photography, *Comp Cont Educ Dent* 10:682, 1989.

Freehe C: Photography in dentistry: equipment and technique, *Dent Clin North Am* 27:3, 1983.

Friedman M: Polaroid photography: an important tool for esthetic dentistry, *Calif Dent Assoc J* 19:23, 1991.

Hook S: The camera is a practice builder, *Dent Econ* 77:71,1987.

Kumagai T et al: Standardized intraoral photography for the dental team, *JADA* 116:677,1988.

Lackey A: Uses and features of intraoral video camera systems, *Dent Today* 10(4):44, 1991.

Levin R: Building your practice with an intraoral camera, *Comp Cont Educ Dent* 11:52, 1990.

Steele D: Dental photography with a professional approach, *J Indiana Dent Assoc* 70(3):12, 1991.

Valentine R: *Expanded duties: a self-determined pace laboratory program,* Philadelphia, 1975, Department of Dental Hygiene, School of Dental Medicine, University of Pennsylvania.

SUGGESTED READINGS

Baker I: Record taking in the orthodontic office, *Dent Asst* 60 (2):25, 1991

Bickley S et al: Use and effect of clinical photographic records on the motivation and oral hygiene practices of a group of mentally handicapped adults, *Dent Health* 29 (1)3, 1990.

Brackett W: Dental photography: getting started, *Compend Contin Educ Dent* 7:297, 1986.

Clinical Research Associates: Camera for clinical photography, *Newsletter* 7 (5):1, 1983.

Cooley R, Barkmeier, W: Adapting a flash unit for dental photography, *Dent Radiogr Photogr* 52(3):62, 1979.

Costello M: A simple and standardized approach to clinical photography, *Aust Orthod J* 7(5):1, 1981.

Faucher R: Dental photography in the graduate teaching program, *Dent Clin North Am* 27:109, 1983.

Fleming C et al: Photographic technique for the recording of children's teeth for signs of enamel mottling, *J Audio V Media Med* 12:16, 1989.

Freedman G: Dedicated camera makes clinical photography easy, *Dent Today* 9:48, 1990.

Freedman G: Photomarketing in dentistry: the instant photo option, *J Dent Pract Admin* 7:35, 1990.

Freehe C: Dental photography, *Funct Orthod* 1 (4): 41, 1984.

Gholston L: Reliability of an intraoral camera: utility for clinical dentistry and research, *Am J Orthod* 85:89, 1984.

Green K: High-tech dentistry spurs practice growth, *Dent Econ* 80):81, 1984.

Gregg T: A modified lighting system for dental photography, *J Ir Dental Assoc* 30:3, 1984.

Hamilton A: Preparing text, tables and illustrations for a journal editor, *Dent Clin North Am* 27:197, 1983.

Jordan R et al: A clinical lecturer's application of dental photography, *Dent Clin North Am* 27:121, 1983.

Lackey A: Intra-oral video photography: questions and answers, *Can Dent Assoc J* 19(3):29, 1991.

Nelson L: Photography: its uses in dental practice, lectures and the home, *Dent Clin North Am* 27:171, 1983,

Neuman K: Cosmetic imaging: a new level of communication, *J Dent Pract Admin* 7(3):94, 1990.

Nuckles D et al: Close-up photography in the dental office, *JADA* 90:152, 1975.

Osborne P: An evaluation of a 90 mm macro lens for use in intraoral photography, *Gen Dent* 35:193, 1987.

Palmer M: Using photography to gain case acceptance, *Dent Manage* 28(11):52, 1988.

Rayman M, Eilers A: Basic intraoral photography technique, *Can Dent Assoc J* 13(4):53, 1985.

Tilly D, Hagen A: Preparing graphics for visual presentation, *Dent Clin North Am* 27:75, 1983.

Tribe H: Selecting and preparing illustrations for publication and presentation, *Dent Clin North Am* 27:95, 1983.

Walker R: Guide to dental photography systems, *LDAJ* 43(3):17, 1984.

Zuckerman A: Utilization of instant closeup photography for the esthetic improvement of multiple full coverage restorations, *Quintessence* 15:545, 1984.

DIAGNOSIS

Even though dental hygenists have rarely used the term "diagnosis" to describe the decision-making procedures they follow, this process is an integral part of dental hygiene care. Whenever you use the information you and the dentist have gathered to determine a patient's health status and to decide which health goals and courses of treatment are best for a patient, you are diagnosing. Dental hygenists prepare a *dental hygeiene diagnosis* and sometimes a preliminary dental diagnosis. Because two opinions about a case are better than one, it is appropriate to discuss your dental hygiene diagnosis with a dentist colleague or employer or with dental hygiene colleagues whenever possible.

Because dental hygienists have practiced diagnosis for decades but not formalized the theory and process, this chapter emphasizes the theoretical basis for developing a diagnosis. It involves the general health and dental health data for the person so that the diagnosis can reflect all the apparent factors that influence the current state of health or disease. It is from this basis that goals and treatment are set.

17 DIAGNOSTIC DECISION MAKING

JoAnn R. Gurenlian

LEARNING OUTCOMES

The dental hygienist will be able to

1. Define the term *dental hygiene diagnosis*.
2. Describe the purpose of formulating a dental hygiene diagnosis.
3. Explain why dental hygiene diagnosis is a controversial issue in dentistry.
4. Appreciate the importance of the dental hygiene diagnosis in relation to the dental hygiene process of care.
5. Compare the dental hygiene diagnostic model with the diagnostic models of medicine, dentistry, and nursing.
6. Identify the components of the dental hygiene diagnostic decision making process.
7. Develop a list of resources that can be used during the initial review phase of the diagnostic decision making process.
8. Differentiate between the initial review and the problem synthesis phases of the diagnostic decision making process.
9. Describe the purposes of the hypothesis formulation phase of the diagnostic decision making process.
10. Identify the types of data collection procedures used during the inquiry strategy phase of the diagnostic decision making process.
11. Recognize the importance of self-directed learning in developing and refining dental hygiene diagnostic decision making skills.
12. Use the dental hygiene diagnostic decision-making process to analyze patient problems.

After assessment, the next phase of the dental hygiene process is determining the dental hygiene diagnosis. Arriving at this diagnosis is a multifaceted process that requires the development of clinical reasoning, decision making, and problem-solving skills; this determination is one of the most challenging and rewarding aspects of providing patient care. It serves as the basis for treatment planning, providing preventive and therapeutic services, and evaluating the achievement of goals to obtain patient health.

This chapter will highlight the development of the concept of dental hygiene diagnosis and compare it with other health care models of diagnosis. The diagnostic decision-making process will be described so that you can use a systematic framework to develop and refine your clinical evaluation skills.

HISTORICAL PERSPECTIVE

The concept of a dental hygiene diagnosis is relatively new. Discussion concerning its development began in 1982. At that time, it was proposed that dental hygienists needed to develop independent decision making with a focus on identifying patient problems requiring treatment within the dental hygiene process of care (Miller, 1982).

In 1985, the American Dental Hygienists' Association (ADHA) published the Standards of Applied Dental Hygiene Practice (ADHA, 1985). Four major categories were established: assessment, planning, implementation, and evaluation. The concept of a dental hygiene diagnosis is included in the assessment component of the standards. Specifically, standard 2 states that a dental hygiene diagnosis is formulated based on the patient's general health status and oral health status. The concept of dental hygiene diagnosis includes the identification of limitations to achieving optimum oral health. Further, the standards recognize that a dental hygiene diagnosis is related to the diagnoses of dentists and other health care professionals.

As the dental hygiene process of care continues to be refined, the concept of a dental hygiene diagnosis has grown in importance. Dental hygiene process models now include five major categories: assessment, dental hygiene diagnosis, planning, implementation, and evaluation (Darby, 1990.).

Literature relating to dental hygiene diagnosis in the professional journals is limited. Since the development of Applied Standards of Dental Hygiene Practice, the *Journal of Dental Hygiene* has included relatively few articles pertaining to diagnositic decision making or dental hygiene diagnosis. Before the standards of dental hygiene practice were developed, case studies of oral pathoses and decision making appeared sporadically in *Dental Hygiene* (Cohen, 1981; Davis et al, 1982a 1982b, 1983, 1984 Hlava et al, 1982, 1983a, 1983b; Nielson, 1983; Sprague et al, 1982a, 1982b, 1984). Recently, *RDH* has featured case studies of oral pathoses in each issue.

This paucity of literature on dental hygiene diagnosis and diagnostic decision making is related to political issues regarding the role of the dentist versus that of the dental hygienist. Traditionally dental hygiene students were taught to record abnormalities of the head and neck regions and report them to the dentist, who made the diagnosis. Dental hygienists were not expected to formulate a diagnosis; in fact, much of dental hygiene education focused on gathering all the necessary information and moving directly to a standardized treatment plan without pausing to consider the specific problems or goals for each patient. Yet a diagnosis must be developed to provide effective dental hygiene care, and this is a legitimate function of dental hygiene practice today. Dental hygienists have a professional obligation to their patients that includes providing a dental hygiene diagnosis and helping them understand the nature of the problems present, the causes of these problems, and the treatment protocols required to restore health. Diagnosis helps practitioners individualize patient care; it is not appropriate to provide the same procedures for every patient regardless of need.

DEFINITION

Diagnosis is a statement about an actual or potential problem. Diagnostic decision making is a process involving the ability to collect, analyze, and synthesize data. This process is used in health care as well as in a variety of occupations. Dental hygiene diagnosis requires a baseline of knowledge and a systematic approach to clinical evaluation, which are part of the learning process of dental hygienists. Acknowledging that dental hygienists diagnose health problems eliminates their frustrations about the artificial limitations imposed by dentistry and enhances patient care. It shifts the focus from control of one profession over another to the real focus, the patient's health and well-being. Further, it enables dental hygienists to use their skills to teach patients how to benefit from self-examination and the diagnostic decision-making process.

MODELS OF DIAGNOSIS

The diagnostic models most closely related to dental hygiene diagnosis are the medical model, the dental model, and the nursing model.

Medicine's perspective of diagnosis is the most familiar model and one that is widely used in health care settings. Medicine is primarily concerned with the diagnosis and treatment of disease. Practice is based on knowledge from the biomedical sciences, and with an emphasis on the need to describe, understand, manage, and predict pathophysiologic events. The scientific method is used to research disease entities and develop treatment modalities, as well as to formulate diagnoses.

The medical model of diagnosis evaluates data and classifies diseases according to major systems: cardiovascular, respiratory, gastrointestinal, genitourinary, and so forth. Diagnostic skills are highly valued in medicine. The process is standardized to maintain consistency in the clinical data base and among physicians.

Physicians use a deductive process to determine a diagnosis. This process involves observation and examination of the patient, generation of diagnostic hypotheses concerning clinical data, the use of laboratory tests to further evaluate the clinical problems, and use of cues to verify hypotheses (Balla, 1985; Barrows et al, 1991; Cutler, 1985; Eddy et al, 1982).

Dentistry uses a similar approach in dental diagnosis. The dental model emphasizes the identification of symptoms of dental disease and incorporates deductive reasoning to determine dental pathoses. The process consists of history taking related to the chief complaint, physical and radiographic examination of the patient, development of a working diagnosis, and use of laboratory tests to determine the definitive diagnosis (Hall, 1988; Ibsen, et al, 1992; Puskas, et al, 1991; Redding, et al, 1990; Somis, et al, 1984; Wood, et al, 1975). Both medical and dental diagnoses have been well established and used by health care professionals.

The nursing model of diagnosis is a newer concept that broadens the focus of diagnosis from disease entities to the health functioning of individuals and groups. Nursing diagnosis describes the actual or potential health problems that nurses are able and licensed to treat (Gordon, 1987). A nursing diagnosis contains the problem, cause, signs, and symptoms and is viewed as a product of assessment.

The nursing diagnostic model consists of direct observation of patient behaviors. The nursing history and examination serve as the basis of diagnostic labeling. The process involves information collection, information interpretation, information clustering, and naming the cluster (Carpenito, 1987; Curry, 1991; Dediarian, 1991; Gordon, 1979; Gordon et al, 1979; Gross, 1991; Kirsch, 1991; Lash, 1978; Mehmert, 1989; Ratliff, 1989).

Nursing diagnosis for a community involves a six-step reasoning process consisting of pre-encounter data, data gathering, clusters of information, diagnostic explanations, supporting the diagnosis, and testing the fit. Pre-encounter data relate to the specific demographic data of the community and the population's general health status. Data gathering is based on four types of cues: risks of health problems, strengths and resources, actual problems, and irrelevant problems. As data are gathered, they are grouped into clusters of information that are meaningful to the group. Diagnostic hypotheses or explanations are derived from the anaylsis of the clusters of information.

Table 17-1. Diagnostic focus and terminology

Medical		*Dental*		*Nursing*	
Focus	*Examples*	*Focus*	*Examples*	*Focus*	*Examples*
Diagnosis and treatment of disease	Myocardial infarction Multiple sclerosis Tuberculosis Pancreatitis Cholecystitis Meningitis Otitis media Osteosarcoma Hepatitis Asthma Leukemia Psoriasis Diabetes mellitus Rheumatoid arthritis	Identification of symptoms and determination of dental pathoses	Caries Juvenile periodontitis Recurrent herpes labialis Periapical abscess Gingivitis Dentigerous cyst Papilloma Candidiasis Pyogenic granuloma Geographic tongue Dilantin hyperplasia Recurrent aphthous stomatitis Ranula	Health functioning of individuals or groups	Injury, potential for Mobility, impaired physical Swallowing, impaired Noncomplicance (specify) Home maintenance, alterations in Nutrition, alterations in: less than body requirements Fear Communication, impaired verbal Infection, potential for Knowledge deficit (specify) Oral mucous membrane, alterations in Comfort, alterations in: pain Skin integrity, impairment of, actual Cardiac output, alterations in decreased

Data are then analyzed further to support or rule out the hypotheses. Finally, the fit between the diagnosis and the cues is tested based on a series of questions (Kneeshaw et al, 1989).

Nursing diagnosis is often documented through a charting system referred to as "SODA," consisting of *s*ubjective patient statements, *o*bjective data collected by the nurse, *d*iagnostic labels that describe the patient's health problem, and the nursing *a*ctions taken related to the diagnosis. (Durham, 1988).

Examples of medical, dental, and nursing diagnoses appear in Table 17-1. Note the difference between the disease orientation of the medical and dental diagnostic terms and the total-person focus of the nursing taxonomy.

DENTAL HYGIENE DIAGNOSTIC MODEL

The dental hygiene diagnostic model incorporates components and terminology from a variety of health care models including the medical, dental and nursing models. *Dental hygiene diagnosis is defined as a formal statement of the dental hygienist's decision regarding the actual or potential problems of a patient that are amenable to treatment through the dental hygiene process of care.* Dental hygiene diagnostic decisions include both the dental hygienist's and the patient's perceptions of the problem, and of the psychologic, social, ethical, and economic factors as well as the patient's value systems.

Dental hygiene diagnosis focuses on restoring total patient health and well-being. Dental hygienists cannot diagnose patient problems in a vacuum; they must use a broad knowledge base that incorporates health promotion and disease prevention concepts to prevent the occurrence and/or recurrence of oral diseases. The diagnostic process uses the patient as a partner in care to identify the actual or potential problems and to develop supportive therapy.

Dental hygiene diagnosis includes both process and product components. The process involves a standardized systematic approach based on scientific inquiry methods. The process is based on a series of assessment procedures, as described in previous chapters. Data provided in the assessment phase enable the dental hygienist to clarify perceptions of the problem and to label it. This outcome or label represents the end product, the dental hygiene diagnosis.

Dental hygiene diagnostic decisions are based on probability. A series of facts related to a perceived or potential problem are reviewed, and multiple hypotheses concerning the cause of the problem are generated. Assessment procedures guide the inquiry. As new facts are determined, they are analyzed in light of the proposed hypotheses. Data related to the problem are synthesized, and decisions are made based on the most probable cause of the problem.

Becoming a dental hygiene diagnostician requires knowledge, clinical reasoning and problem-solving skills, and self-directed learning. The bases of these skills are continual practice, monitoring, review, evaluation, and maintaining an open mind. Without these components, one can only achieve superficial decisions that are of limited benefit to the practitioner and, more importantly, to the patient.

As you gain knowledge from the biomedical, dental, and dental hygiene sciences, that information is stored within your memory. As you process information during the assessment phase of care, you begin to recognize patterns related to data collected. Through practice, you begin to associate patterns of information with specific patient problems. When reviewing patient information, your memory is triggered, thoughts are organized, patterns are determined, and ideas concerning patient problems are developed. This practice represents the training ground that enables the systematic process of diagnostic decision making to become automatic.

Throughout the process of diagnostic decision making, you must monitor your approach and review data carefully. You must ask yourself whether or not you have followed the systematic model, if you have remained open to information, whether biases have entered the picture, and whether you have used all the information presented.

When the process is complete and the diagnosis is determined, you need to evaluate your clinical reasoning and problem-solving skills. You must honestly consider how well you used the information presented and what other knowledge would have helped you derive the diagnosis. As practitioners and educators, dental hygienists cannot be expected to know in depth every systemic disease and its effects on the oral cavity or all the behavioral factors related to noncompliance. However, when new situations are encountered it is important to take the time to learn the circumstances of those situations. This new information will be helpful in determining future diagnoses.

Many available texts can be used to learn how to evaluate and treat various oral health problems (Eversole 1984; Ibsen et al, 1992; Shafer et al, 1983; Sonis et al, 1984; Wood et al, 1975). This chapter is not meant to be a review of oral pathology. Rather, it focuses on the process of diagnostic decision making so that the dental hygienist can evaluate patient problems and learn how to learn from patient experiences.

PROCESS OF DIAGNOSTIC DECISION MAKING

The process of diagnostic decision making involves six steps: (1) initial review, (2) hypothesis formulation, (3) inquiry strategy, (4) problem synthesis, (5) diagnostic decision making, and (6) learning from the process (Barrows et al, 1991). The dynamic nature of this process is illustrated in Fig. 17-1.

The *initial review* phase of the diagnostic process refers to the information gathered at the beginning of the patient encounter. When first greeting a patient, you are processing information about the patient's appearance, facial expression, posture, and mobility. While proceeding to question the patient about the chief complaint, you may notice other elements such as tone of voice, speech patterns, knowledge level, and communication style.

Data contributing to the initial review includes the following (Barrows et al, 1991; Eversole, 1984; Gordon, 1987) :

1. The patient's statement of the oral health problem and comments related to questions about the chief complaint (i.e., type of problem, location, duration, etc.)
2. The patient's physical appearance and mobility
3. The patient's speech characteristics
4. The appearance and conduct of the people with the patient (spouse, parent, legal guardian, significant other)
5. Prior medical records
6. Prior dental and dental hygiene records
7. Comments from related personnel such as parents, spouse, other relatives, school officials, social worker, nurse, director of a community agency, or any person with knowledge of the patient
8. Referral letters

The backbone of a diagnosis is the history; thus gathering information for the initial review is critical to determining an accurate dental hygiene di-

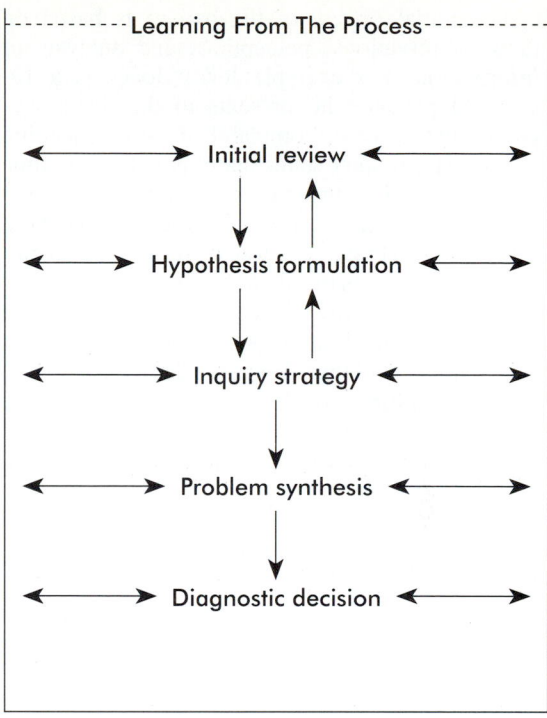

Fig. 17-1. Diagnostic decision-making process.

agnosis. Using the resources just listed gives the dental hygienist a broad picture of the patient versus an immediate focus on problems in or around the oral cavity.

Diagnostic decision making is often described as solving a puzzle or mystery. One must use clues to create a mental image that enables the puzzle to be solved. A wealth of clues exist within the resources as long as you are looking for them. We tend to see what is in focus in the center of our vision. If several people look at a photograph of a child playing in a park, each will see something different in the picture. One person may focus on the child's hair. Another may see the child's clothes. Someone else might focus on the expressions on the child's face, and another person might focus on the beautiful sky or the flowers in the park. Each of these is just one small element of the entire picture. You must make a conscious effort to step back and look at the entire picture, using all of the senses to evaluate the patient. If you do not look and listen for the clues, you will not see or hear them. (Barrows et al, 1991; Ibsen et al, 1992.)

The initial review of the patient is based on facts, observations, perceptions and analysis of information. For example Jenny Jones is a 10-year-old patient who presents to the dental hygienist with a chief complaint of "sore, bleeding gums." Her mother states that this is the first time she has heard Jenny complain about a problem with her mouth and felt that it should be checked. Jenny is of average height and weight. Her medical history is noncontributory. She appears to be healthy and mildly concerned about her oral health problem. Take a moment to picture Jenny Jones and her mother. Visualize Jenny sitting in a chair and telling you her chief complaint. Now write a description of your initial review.

If your initial review included a statement such as "gingivitis" or "periodontitis," you are attempting to diagnose without having sufficient information. Although it is tempting to leap to conclusions, allow yourself the opportunity to deal only with the facts, without generating ideas or hypotheses about the problem. The initial review should be a statement about the problem based on known facts and observations. Without having the benefit of an oral examination, you cannot include gingivitis as part of the initial review. Your initial review statement is limited to "a healthy, 10-year-old female presents with sore, bleeding gingiva."

Further questioning of the patient reveals that she began receiving orthodontic treatment 2 weeks ago. Because of the pain associated with adjusting to the braces, Jenny states that she no longer flosses; she brushes once each day. Mrs. Jones confirms that Jenny has complained about her mouth hurting from the braces, and that she seems less interested in her home care regimen. Take a moment and refine your initial review statement based on the additional information provided.

In formulating your initial review statement, be careful not to impose personal bias into the description or to misinterpret the problem. For example, Mrs. Jones stated that Jenny seems less interested in her home care regimen. Avoid interpreting that information as "Jenny is becoming lazy since she got her braces."

The initial review statement should include the following information:

A healthy, 10-year-old female presents with sore, bleeding gingiva associated with the initiation of orthodontia and a change in home care regimen.

Once the initial review has been completed, you are ready to *formulate hypotheses* about the information established. These hypotheses are derived automatically through associations triggered by the initial review process. They represent a working or differential diagnosis that provides a focus for the inquiry strategy phase of the decision-making process.

Hypotheses are based on the information gathered from the initial review. The hypotheses generated may differ according to the dental hygienist's experience and education. What are your initial hypotheses about Jenny Jones' problem? Write them down on a piece of paper.

Some plausible hypotheses include gingivitis, type I periodontitis, knowledge deficit related to lack of understanding about braces and appropriate home care regimens required to maintain health, noncompliance associated with gingival pain, and fear associated with inducing more gingival soreness by brushing and flossing.

The following exercise will illustrate how the hypotheses formulated depend on the nature of the initial review. When reviewing each of the following examples, write down the hypotheses that come to mind. Don't be afraid to guess!

Hypothesis formulation exercise

1. A middle-aged woman complains of multiple painful ulcers in her mouth. What hypotheses can be developed based on this initial review statement?
2. An 18-year old male college freshman complains of aching jaw pain. What hypotheses come to mind with this initial review statement?
3. A 45-year-old man presents with halitosis. What hypotheses can be formulated from this initial review statement?

Refer to Table 17-2 for plausible hypotheses related to each example illustrated above.

Some of the hypotheses in Table 17-2 are specific while others are broad. These hypotheses are labels that help to guide inquiry. Some may be easy to determine based on knowledge of the epidemiology of oral diseases. Others will require further investigation and inquiry to refine.

Some hypotheses are conventional diagnoses and can be specific, such as the following:

Caries

Gingivitis

Herpes labialis

Table 17-2. Hypothesis formulation exercise

Case 1.

Primary herpes
Recurrent aphthous ulcers
Contact stomatitis
Potential for infection

Case 2.

Wisdom tooth formation
Temporomandibular joint dysfunction
Bruxism
Stress

Case 3.

Oral infection
Abdominal disorder
Plaque accumulation
Poor oral hygiene related to knowledge deficit
Poor oral hygiene related to noncompliance

Some hypotheses may describe causes:

Fungal infection
Nutritional disorder
Drug/product reaction

Some hypotheses represent anatomic disorders:

Supernumerary tooth
Anodontia
Micrognathia

Some hypotheses represent psychologic or social considerations:

Fear
Poverty
Noncompliance

The purposes of formulating hypotheses are to broaden the concept of the patient's problem and to guide the collection of additional information necessary to determine the diagnosis. As additional information is discerned from the patient and examination procedures, some hypotheses may be rejected and others developed. The process of hypothesis formulation is meant to be dynamic and creative and should include the patient's ideas. Often the patient can generate many plausible hypotheses based on knowledge of his or her personal, social, and psychologic experiences (Balla, 1985; Barrows et al, 1991; Cutler, 1985; Eddy, 1982).

Once the hypotheses have been generated, the next step in diagnostic decision making is to determine the kinds of information from the physical examination and other tests that are needed to reject competing hypotheses and validate the correct hypothesis. This phase is referred to as *inquiry strategy*. Choosing the correct hypothesis or diagnosis will enable you and the patient to determine the appropriate treatment for the problem.

Examples of tests that can be used in inquiry strategy include follow-up questions related to the history of the problem as well as the medical and dental histories, extraoral and intraoral examinations, occlusal examination, periodontal charting, restorative charting, radiographs, blood assays, urinalysis, laboratory cultures, and excisional and incisional biopsies. Consultations with dentists, physicians, nurses, physical therapists, occupational therapists, and other health care professionals may be indicated for thorough patient evaluation (Eversole, 1984; Ibsen et al, 1992; Sonis et al, 1984; Wood et al, 1975).

Return to the example of Jenny Jones and those in the hypothesis formulation exercise. What elements of inquiry strategy would you employ for each example to determine the dental hygiene diagnosis? Write your ideas on a piece of paper.

The process used in inquiry strategy is deductive reasoning. Deduction involves making inferences or conclusions based on general principles. In formulating a diagnosis, you determine which data will help to support or refute the hypotheses generated. An important component of deductive reasoning is to use information to separate competing hypotheses so as to decide which is the most probable (Barrows et al, 1991; Redding et al, 1990; Sonis et al, 1984; Wood et al, 1975).

The inquiry strategy process may involve several steps. Sometimes the results of this data collection phase do not reveal specific information that rules out or separates competing hypotheses. Therefore you may have to reevaluate the tests used and consider alternative tests or examinations to help identify the correct hypothesis.

For example, for the 18-year-old college freshman with aching jaw pain, the dental hygienist may determine the most likely hypothesis is wisdom tooth formation. An intraoral examination and radiographic series will either confirm or eliminate this hypothesis. If these tests are noncontributory, then consider other tests to rule out a TMJ problem, bruxism, or stress.

The next step in the diagnostic decision-making process is referred to as *problem synthesis* (Barrows et al, 1991; Eversole, 1984). In this phase, data collected during inquiry strategy are compared with the information collected during the initial review phase. The problem synthesis summarizes all the facts relating to the hypotheses and eliminates extraneous information.

When consulting with another health professional about a patient problem, the dental hygienist must be able to present a summary statement that contains all of the significant data. This statement should not include irrelevant information. Data contained in the summary statement should be organized in a manner that suggests the underlying diagnosis. On reviewing the problem synthesis, another practitioner can formulate diagnostic ideas or make recommendations concerning further tests that might be relevant to the hypotheses.

Clarity is the key feature of problem synthesis. An endless narrative that includes every detail about the patient and the problem delays the effective processing of information by clinicians (Barrows et al, 1991; Cutler, 1985).

Refer to the first example cited in the hypothesis formulation exercise, the middle-aged woman with multiple painful ulcers in her mouth. Possible hypotheses include herpetic lesions, aphthous ulcers, contact stomatitis, and potential for infection. Your approach is to review the chief complaint and to conduct thorough medical and dental histories (initial review).

On completion of these steps, you learn that the patient has experienced no previous episodes of oral ulcers. She denies a history of primary herpes or herpes labialis. She denies any change in stress level at home or work. The patient denies using any medication and states that she is in good health and has a physical examination once each year and dental evaluations twice each year. She reports that she typically brushes with a fluoride toothpaste twice each day and flosses every evening. Examination of the oral cavity reveals multiple small ulcerations randomly dispersed throughout the gingiva, tongue and oral mucosa. The patient states that the ulcers developed over the past 2 days.

At this point in the examination, there is not enough data to separate the hypotheses so that one can be determined as the most likely cause of the problem. You must continue the inquiry strategy process to gather more information. You may decide to question the patient further about her oral habits and events that may have occurred before the onset of the ulcers. Further questioning reveals that the patient has changed toothpaste and mouthwash products. She states that she had coupons for new home care products and wanted to try them. She purchased and began using the new products 2 days ago. Additional questioning reveals no further changes in her home care regimen.

The information the patient provides on further inquiry helps to separate the hypotheses. You recall information about each hypothesis and match these data with each possible cause. The problem synthesis step enables you to determine the best fit between the available data and the hypotheses.

Using the example provided above, the problem synthesis might read:

Mrs. X, a middle-aged female, presents with a chief complaint of multiple painful ulcers of the oral cavity of 2 days' duration. Examination reveals small ulcers randomly dispersed throughout the gingiva, tongue, and oral mucosa. Patient presents in good health. Medical and dental histories are noncontributory. Patient reports using new toothpaste and mouthwash products concomitant with date of eruption of oral ulcers.

Notice how the problem synthesis condenses previously presented information to focus on the most critical elements of the initial review and inquiry strategy phases. The information in this problem synthesis enables the experienced dental hygiene diagnostician to determine which hypothesis is most likely to be correct.

Once the problem synthesis has been defined, the next step is to decide on the correct diagnosis. A *diagnostic decision* must be determined before treatment can be rendered. The dental hygienist must accept an element of risk in the decision-making process. Sometimes, the diagnosis will be readily determined (as in the case of contact stomatitis illustrated in the problem section on synthesis). Other times, you may be forced to choose among several plausible hypotheses. When faced with insufficient information or conflicting hypotheses, you be prepared to take a calculated risk to benefit the patient. Diagnosis is based on probability.

To gain experience in formulating diagnoses, take the time to write down your reasons for the diagnostic decision made. With each diagnostic encounter, you will attain increased confidence in decision making and clinical reasoning skills.

The last step of the diagnostic decision-making process is *learning from the process* (Barrows et al, 1991; Eddy et al, 1982; Gordon, 1987). Dental hygiene diagnosis is a dynamic process; there is much to be learned from each patient encounter. A good diagnostician recognizes the importance of self-education in an effort to increase diagnostic skills.

Learning from the process includes analyzing how the diagnostic decision making process was used, the accuracy of the diagnosis, and information about the patient problem itself. The novice dental hygiene diagnostician should relegate time in the daily schedule to review and evaluate each diagnosis made. Practice and experience enable the dental hygienist to appreciate that "potential for infection" is as important a diagnosis as is "periodontal abscess" to the patient with a history of diabetes mellitus.

CONCLUSION

Dental hygiene diagnosis is the second phase of the dental hygiene process of care. The dental hygiene diagnosis is derived through initial review, hypothesis formulation, inquiry strategy, problem synthesis, diagnostic decision making, and learning from the process. Diagnosis is a legitimate function of the dental hygienist. It provides the basis for decisions about dental hygiene treatment, evaluation, and referral. The challenge of dental hygiene diagnosis is in the development of clinical reasoning, problem-solving, and decision-making skills. Dental hygiene's professional credibility rests on development and refinement of this diagnostic skill.

LEARNING ACTIVITIES

1. Divide into small groups and develop a list of dental hygiene diagnostic terms that represent total patient care. Remember to consider terminology that goes beyond oral medicine and dental disease terms.
2. Conduct a class discussion on evaluating the need for a dental hygiene diagnosis. Focus on the relevance of the diagnosis to dental hygiene care, the relationship of the dental hygiene diagnosis to the Standards of Applied Dental Hygiene Practice, and the controversies surrounding the act of diagnosing patient problems. Discuss ways in which dental hygienists can educate the public and other health care professionals about the importance of the dental hygiene diagnosis.
3. Identify and describe the components of the dental hygiene diagnosis. Include a description of the differences between each phase of the diagnostic process.
4. Develop a list of resources that can be used during the initial review phase of the diagnostic decision making process. Challenge yourself to identify resources other than the ones listed in this chapter.
5. Maintain a professional journal for one month in which you describe each patient encounter and the dental hygiene diagnoses for each patient. Evaluate the diagnostic decision-making process used. Focus on practicing skills related to each phase of the process.
6. Develop a self-directed learning plan to refine your diagnostic decision-making and clinical reasoning skills. Evaluate your progress with the plan on a weekly basis.
7. A teenage boy presents with a fractured maxillary central incisor as the result of a baseball game. List three dental hygiene diagnoses that must be considered in addition to the obvious fractured tooth.
8. A 68-year-old woman presents with bilateral lymphadenopathy and a radiolucency around the apex of tooth No. 12. The patient states that tooth No. 12 has been "sore" for 6 weeks, but she was afraid to have it evaluated because she did not want the tooth to be extracted. List three hypotheses that relate to this scenario. Identify the inquiry strategies you would use to determine the dental hygiene diagnosis.
9. A 4-year-old girl and her mother present to you for a "regular checkup and teeth cleaning." The child states that she would like to use floss, but her mother will not let her. The mother reports that she believes that the child is too young to be flossing her teeth. Formulate three hypotheses that relate to this scenario. Restate this case in the form of a problem synthesis statement.
10. Develop a list of health care professionals (in addition to other dental hygiene colleagues) who can be used as resources and consultants for evaluating patient problems.

REVIEW QUESTIONS

1. Define the term *dental hygiene diagnosis*.
2. Explain why dental hygiene diagnosis is a controversial issue in dentistry.
3. Identify the components of the dental hygiene diagnostic decision making process.
4. List five resources that can be used as part of initial review.
5. List five resources that can be used as part of inquiry strategy.
6. What is the significance of the dental hygiene diagnosis?

REFERENCES

American Dental Hygienists' Association: *Standards of applied dental hygiene practice*, Chicago, 1985, The Association.

Balla JI: *The diagnostic process: a model for clinical teachers*, Cambridge, England, 1985, Cambridge University Press.

Barrows HS et al: *Developing clinical problem-solving skills: a guide to more effective diagnosis and treatment*, New York, 1991, WW Norton.

Carpenito LJ: *Nursing diagnosis: application to clinical practice*, ed 2, Philadelphia, 1987, JB Lippincott.

Cohen WL: Herpes simplex virus and oral cancer, *Dent Hyg* 55(11):31, 1981.

Curry J: Nursing diagnosis: communication, impaired, *J Emerg Nurs* 17:124, 1991.

Cutler P: *Problem solving in clinical medicine: from data to diagnosis*, ed 2, Baltimore, 1985, Williams & Wilkins.

Darby ML: *Theory development and basic research in dental hygiene: review of the literature and recommendations*, Chicago, 1990, American Dental Hygienists' Association.

Davis CC et al: Preliminary evaluation of extraoral and intraoral leasions, *Dent Hyg* 56(1):44, 1982a.

Davis CC et al: Preliminary evaluation of oral lesions: what is this unilocular radiolucency in the mandible? *Dent Hyg* 56(6):36, 1982b.

Davis CC et al: Preliminary evaluation of oral leasions: what is this superficial swelling? *Dent Hyg* 57(3):34, 1983.

Davis CC et al: Preliminary evaluation of oral lesions: what is this exophytic mass on the gingiva? *Dent Hyg* 58(5):217, 1984.

Derdiarian AK: Effects of using a nursing model–based assessment instrument on quality of nursing care, *Nurs Admin Q* 15(3):1, 1991.

Durham JD: SODA: a method of charting nursing diagnosis, *Nurs Manage* 19(11):74, 1988.

Eddy DM et al: The art of diagnosis: solving the clinicopathological exercise, *N Engl J Med* 306:1263, 1982.

Eversole LR: *Clinical outline of oral pathology: diagnosis and treatment*, Philadelphia, 1984, Lea & Febiger.

Gordon M: The concept of nursing diagnosis, *Nurs Clin North Am* 14:487, 1979.

Gordon M: *Nursing diagnosis: process and application*, ed 2, New York, 1987, McGraw-Hill.

Gordon M et al: Methodological problems and issues in identifying and standardizing nursing diagnosis, *Adv Nurs Sci* 2:1, 1979.

Gross DL et al: Nurse educator: development of a nursing process-based documentation system, *J Emerg Nurs* 17(3):173, 1991.

Hall WB: *Decision making in periodontology*, Toronto, 1988, BC Decker.

Hlava GL et al: Preliminary evaluation of extraoral and intraoral lesions, *Dent Hyg* 56(2):44, 1982.

Hlava GL et al: Preliminary evaluation of oral lesions: what is this white patch on the buccal mucosa? *Dent Hyg* 57(1):33, 1983A.

Hlava GL et al: Preliminary evaluation of extraoral lesions: what is this radiopacity? *Dent Hyg* 57(2):31, 1983B.

Ibsen AC et al: *Oral pathology for the dental hygienist,* Philadelphia, 1992, WB Saunders.

Kirsch E: Treating nursing's response to nursing diagnosis, *J Emerg Nurs* 17(3):125, 1991.

Kneeshaw MF et al: Nursing diagnosis: not for individuals only, *Geriatr Nurs* 10:246, 1989.

Lash AA: A re-examination of nursing diagnosis, *Nurs Forum* 27:332, 1978.

Mehmert PA et al: Computerizing nursing diagnosis, *Nurs Manage* 20(7):24, 1989.

Miller SS: Dental hygiene diagnosis, *RDH* 2(4):46, 1982.

Nielson NJ: Decision making associated with dental hygiene practice, *Dent Hyg* 57(12):24, 1983.

Puskas JC et al: Comparison of self-instruction methods for teaching diagnostic testing, *J Dent Educ* 55:316, 1991.

Ratliff CV et al: Computerized nursing diagnosis: applications for the surgical patient, *J Adv Med Surg Nurs* 1(3):63, 1989.

Redding SW et al: *Dentistry in systemic disease: diagnostic and therapeutic approach to patient management,* Portland, Ore, 1990, JBK.

Shafer WG et al: *A textbook of oral pathology*, ed 4, Philadelphia, 1983, WB Saunders.

Sonis ST et al: *Principles and practice of oral medicine*, Philadelphia, 1984, WB Saunders.

Sprague WG et al: Preliminary evaluation of oral lesions: what is this ulceration? *Dent Hyg* 58(11):307, 1984.

Sprague WG et al: Preliminary evaluation of extra and intraoral lesions, *Dent Hyg* 56(4):36, 1982a.

Sprague WG et al: Preliminary evaluation of oral lesions: what is this white patch on the tongue? *Dent Hyg* 56(12):37, 1982b.

Wood NK et al: *Differential diagnosis of oral lesions,* St Louis, 1975, CV Mosby.

PLANNING

Once the site is prepared and assessment data are gathered, it is time for logical *planning* for the patient. This includes (1) developing an action plan to solve the problems that have emerged from the assessment phase and the dental hygiene diagnosis and (2) setting goals for the patient's health progress.

Involving the patient in planning is an important key to ensuring active participation and shared ownership of the plan. Therefore, in Chapters 18 to 20, the patient is discussed as an integral part of the planning of care.

Some signs of implementation will begin to emerge in these planning chapters, as the line between planning and implementation is often difficult to define. The planning process in many ways triggers the patient's need to know and to receive care. The dental professional's responsibility is to ensure that planning is adequately defined and that the program moves into implementation at a point when the patient is most receptive.

18 FORMULATING A TREATMENT PLAN, CASE PRESENTATION, AND APPOINTMENT PLAN

Irene Woodall
Cheryl Wiles

LEARNING OUTCOMES

The dental hygienist will be able to

1. Assemble assessment data from a variety of patient cases (including medical history, vital signs, intraoral and extraoral examinations and chartings, radiographic surveys, diagnostic casts, and the patient's expectations).
2. Design a treatment plan best suited to the specific needs of each patient based on the established dental hygiene diagnosis.
3. Design at least one alternative plan for each case.
4. Design a case presentation format for each patient that meets (1) the legal requirements of *informed consent* and (2) the basic principles of *interpersonal communication*.
5. Design a logical sequence of planned appointments to fulfill the treatment plan for each case.
6. Identify priorities for treatment, including:
   a. Emergency needs.
   b. Prevention of disease.
   c. Therapy.
   d. Maintenance needs.

NATURE AND ROLE OF TREATMENT PLANNING

Treatment planning creates an individualized approach to dental hygiene care. It guides the health care provider in identifying specific *problems* and *health goals*. It helps identify treatment to solve the problems and to meet the health goals. Careful planning allows these two foci to be accomplished in tandem.

In addition, treatment planning provides an opportunity to specify the problems and goals so that they can be shared with the patient and explained in rational, understandable terms. It provides an opportunity to organize and plan the sequence of care so that the patient can identify with and participate in progress as it is made. Such organization maximizes efficiency and reduces frustration.

The written, agreed-on treatment plan is a legal contract that forms the basis of the legal relationship between the health care provider and the patient. It is an invaluable resource in a court of law as well as at the chairside. It provides a medium for discussing wants, needs, and expectations and for promoting a free exchange of perceptions (Clark and Morton, 1977).

PREPARING A TREATMENT PLAN

Once all of the assessment phases of care have been completed, the data from each assessment procedure should be analyzed carefully and synthesized into a comprehensive picture of the needs of the individual patient (Clark and Morton, 1977; Fechtner, 1978; Fishman and Ortiz, 1977; Wood, 1978).

The medical history, review of systems, and vital signs should point out precautionary measures to ensure the general well-being of the patient. The need for a physician's clearance or referral to a physician should have been identified clearly before intraoral examination. Be especially aware of general signs of fatigue, unrest, anxiety, or

373

other conditions based on this carefully collected data.

The significant findings from each examination and charting should be identified and compared. Clinical evidence of health and disease should be compared with radiographic evidence. Tests that quantify periodontal microflora and the host response to such a challenge should be compared with clinical and radiographic evidence. Evaluations of the conditions of the teeth should be compared with soft tissue findings in their respective areas of the dentition. Results of plaque indices should be laid alongside patterns of disease occurrence for the teeth and periodontium. A comprehensive picture of the patient's objective clinical needs should emerge, or further questions about health status should be raised (Barsh, 1981; Morris, 1983).

A logical way to design a treatment plan is (1) to review each assessment finding systematically in terms of its significance; (2) to identify each significant finding as a problem or goal; and (3) to identify an appropriate course of action. Once these three steps are complete, then (4) a priority should be established for each procedure; from this, (5) a specific sequence in care should be assigned; and (6) the time needed for each step should be estimated (Wood, 1978). The cases included in this chapter follow this approach to treatment planning.

As objective needs emerge to form a series of preventive or treatment procedures that are appropriate for the patient, more subjective needs are considered. Especially important are those expressd by the patient during the self-assessment of needs. The health care provider's attitudes toward these needs and expectations are apparent in the treatment plan. If the patient's desires are clearly noted, accounted for, and reflected in the plan, his or her role is validated. However, if they are ignored, the patient will feel ignored. This can have a significant effect on the patient's perception of how well-planned care meets his or her needs (Goldberg, Plume, and Nacman, 1973). Patients may not express their dissatisfaction verbally to the clinician; more likely they will show it nonverbally through canceled appointments and failure to comply with requests.

The assignment of priorities reflects the dental hygienist's philosophic approach to providing care. Most clinicians would agree that clinical problems that are causing pain or are likely to cause pain in the near future are *emergency treatment* procedures and should receive top priority. Therefore deep caries, the presence of an apical radiolucency, or a suspicious oral lesion will delay preventive care.

Differences in philosophy are more apparent among health care providers when deciding whether *preventive* procedures or *therapy* is the next highest priority and how they should be sequenced. Many clinicians believe that ensuring the patient's *control* of his or her dental health supersedes any treatment other than emergency procedures. Others believe that prevention should follow basic treatment procedures. Many combine these priorities by integrating preventive procedures into each treatment appointment. Clinicians also may elect to start with therapy or prevention based on the individual patient case—perhaps the most logical way to decide this issue. *Maintenance* care, which ensures long-term periodic examinations and preventive procedures, logically follows the completion of therapeutic procedures.

The sequence of treatment does not necessarily follow the priority assignment, as some high-priority elements are more effective if they follow other preliminary procedures. For instance, a patient may not be able to properly deplaque his or her teeth if heavy calculus deposits impede access. The higher priority is to help the patient establish a self-care approach to daily oral hygiene; however, the sequence may dictate that the teeth must be free of gross deposits of calculus first. Another example is a patient for whom the highest priority goal is to stop smoking; however, the sequence may require that the patient feels successful first about changes in oral hygiene health behavior.

Estimating the time needed to complete each procedure is an important step in treatment planning and should be noted while the assessment data are fresh in the clinician's mind. Large, subgingival calculus deposits noted on the charting and visible on the radiographic survey can prompt more realistic estimates of time needed for debridement than can later recollections. The actual time required will vary from clinician to clinician and with type of equipment used. For instance, a complete debridement of supragingival and subgingival calculus may require 1 hour with an ultrasonic instrument using fine tips. With hand instruments, four or more appointments of 30 to 45 minutes each may be required.

Once the treatment plan is complete, the dental hygienist should review the patient's wants, needs, and expectations to ensure that they are met, or at least addressed. A useful preliminary step is to imagine oneself as the patient who will soon learn about the treatment plan. The following series of questions may prove helpful in ensuring that the wants, needs, and expectations expressed at earlier appointments are met and in translating the treatment plan into a case presentation:

- Where in the plan are the patient's expressed needs addressed?
- Are the *course of action* for meeting those needs and their *priority* likely to be satisfactory to the patient? Why or why not?
- What additional phases of care included in the plan are related to needs of which the patient may be unaware?
- How can those needs be described simply and accurately for the patient? How can self-assessment data substantiate the findings?
- Is the patient likely to be alarmed or upset by these additional findings? Is the patient likely to view these plans as a luxury or as unnecessary?
- How can the proposed treatment and its likely outcomes be described so that the patient's confidence and trust are maintained? What questions is the patient likely to ask?
- What specific goals for health should be emphasized? How can the patient become involved in helping to realize those goals?
- What alternative plans for care could be followed and with what consequences?
- Is the patient likely to be concerned about appearance, pain, cost, and/or time? How does each of those concerns appear justified in terms of the proposed treatment plan?
- What would be the likely outcome if the patient refused care or selected a modified plan?

The treatment plan therefore requires considerable knowledge of the implications of the assessment data as clinical and radiographic signs are interpreted. It is a critical point in individualizing and personalizing care and in applying knowledgeable professional judgment (Wood, 1978).

DESIGNING A CASE PRESENTATION

After having completed the planning worksheet and answered the aforementioned questions regarding the patient's likely perceptions, the dental hygienist should be prepared to translate the plan into an understandable case presentation. The primary purposes of the case presentation are to solidify the understanding of needs and plans and to formalize the contractual relationship between the patient and the dental hygienist for the treatment phase of care. *Informed consent* is the legal reason for the case presentation (Miller, 1979; Rosoff, 1981). *Mutual understanding* and *cooperation* are the more personal reasons.

The guidelines for establishing informed consent form a natural framework for explaining the case to the patient. First, the nature of the patient's condition should be described in understandable terms. There should be ample opportunity to respond to the patient's concerns and requests for further explanation. It may be helpful to show the patient his or her study models and radiographs and to refer to other data gathered. The suggested plan or treatment should follow, including a discussion of the likely outcomes of the treatment. Risks should be described, as should the likely outcome of not proceeding with care. Finally, alternative treatment approaches should be offered, with a discussion of their advantages and disadvantages (Fishman and Ortiz, 1977; Miller, 1979; Rosoff, 1981).

If the patient is involved fully in the case presentation and agrees to proceed with care, informed consent is secured (Miller, 1979; Rosoff, 1981). The costs of care (usually expressed as a close estimate) and the time needed should also be discussed to minimize surprises and to further involve the patient in decision making (Miller, 1979; Rosoff, 1981). The time estimates and sequence identified in the treatment plan should enable the hygienist to identify an order and number of appointments most compatible with the patient's time constraints.

Although the practice of including the requirements of informed consent in the case presentation is an important preventive approach in avoiding litigation and misunderstanding, two additional points have important legal ramifications for the contractual relationship. First, if any additional procedures are to be included in treatment, the patient's informed consent must be obtained for them. If this is not done, the dental hygienist is liable for *technical assault* or *battery* (performing a procedure to which the patient did not consent) under tort law. Second, all procedures agreed to in the case presentation must be performed within a reasonable time and with a reasonable standard of care. If a procedure is to be omitted or delayed, the patient first must be informed and must agree. If this is not done, the dental hygienist is subject to a breach of contract suit (Fechtner, 1978; Miller, 1979; Rosoff, 1981).

More altruistic reasons for the case presentation are to decrease the patient's fear of the unknown, to build trust, and to form a helping relationship that maximizes positive outcomes. The case presentation should be thorough but simple and should be made with enthusiasm and sincerity. The thorough, thoughtful case presentation should improve the patient's desire to cooperate by appearing for appointments, following preoperative and postoperative instructions, and paying for services. A sense of participation in care promotes this cooperation; the patient develops a sense of ownership of his or her needs and the methods to meet them (Cohen, 1975; Keltner, 1973). Likewise, the dental hygienist may derive great satisfaction from having learned about and cared for a person who needed assistance.

The case presentation also helps the patient recognize the significance of the numerous assessment procedures in the beginning phases of care. He or she learns about good dentistry and good health care and experiences shared responsibility in care by having the opportunity to participate in the discussion.

No matter what the quality of the assessments of the patient's needs, the logic of the treatment plan, and the interest of the case presentation, the patient may decline treatment. A health care provider cannot force a patient to accept care (Fishman and Ortiz, 1977; Miller, 1979). Though it may be shocking to hear the patient say, "I really don't think I want all this dental work," that kind of honesty is preferable to a nonverbal expression of the refusal to accept care—the broken appointment. It can be risky to ask, "Would you like to proceed with treatment?" It can be difficult to hear the response, "No." However, the direct positive response is usually a strong indicator of the patient's commitment to cooperate in care. It indicates that he or she accepts the described health needs as real and the proposed course of action as appropriate. A negotiated or compromised treatment plan, although it may not be ideal in the health care provider's view, is usually an even more positive sign of a solid partnership, with mutual respect between the patient and the health

care provider (Clark and Morton, 1977; Keltner, 1973). With this kind of a relationship the "ideal" plan is more likely to be realized in the long run.

Hesitancy to accept the plan or a simple rejection deserves follow-up discussion (Fishman and Ortiz, 1977). Questioning the patient about his or her concerns may elicit perceived roadblocks (financial problems, fear of discomfort or altered appearance, lack of time) or apparent misunderstandings of the problem or the plan. The health care provider can help reduce or eliminate these obstacles by further clarifying the specifics of the treatment plan. In any case, if the patient declines treatment, the reasons should be fairly clear, and the health care provider should be able to accept that decision as the patient's right. "Good persuasion endures and allows people to make intelligent choices; it does not take advantage of people's weaknesses" (Keltner, 1973).

With acceptance of the final plan, the development of an appointment plan solidifies the agreement and defines a set of expectations: when and for how long the patient and health care provider agree to receive and provide treatment, respectively. A commitment is made.

APPOINTMENT PLANNING

Translating the treatment plan into specific appointments requires several considerations. Obviously, the estimated time needed for each procedure and the logic of grouping interrelated procedures are the primary determinants in designing appointments. Using 10- or 15-minute increments (for example) as appointment units simplifies blocking appointment time.

The patient's tolerance for long sessions in a dental chair (or for frequent trips to the dental office) is an important consideration. Children, for instance, usually should be scheduled for short appointments at a time of day when they are least fatigued. Some patients prefer a series of short appointments; others prefer fewer, longer appointments. For most treatment needs, procedures can be sequenced to accommodate patient preferences.

Beginning clinicians will define their time needs for treatment differently. Time needed to complete various procedures will decrease with greater skill and practice. Another important variable, regardless of the clinician's skill and experience, is the amount of time spent waiting or discussing the case with coworkers. In health care delivery systems that require patient evaluation in several different clinics or departments, the time requirements may be high in the beginning phases of care. In less complex systems, the time needed for activities such as consultations, preparing release forms, and referral procedures may be less. Therefore these examples are given primarily to illustrate how individual differences and needs can affect the planning of treatment and appointments and are not intended to reflect ideal time use.

Dental hygiene treatment planning should always question the appropriateness of "routine" care. It seeks out and responds to the individual needs of patients, whether they are startlingly apparent or elusive. Such planning is an essential professional responsibility of dental hygienists.

The ideal way to develop the ability to translate assessment data into a plan and then into an appointment sequence is to practice with a variety of hypothetical and real cases. Case presentations can then be role-played, with students serving as patients and observers. These students can then report whether informed consent requirements were met and whether the "dental hygienist" listened and responded to the expressed wants, needs, and expectations of the "patient." Such practice facilitates clinical application of these basic skills in synthesis, planning, and communicating.

TREATMENT PLANNING AND DIAGNOSIS: LEGAL AND PROFESSIONAL RESPONSIBILITIES

In an era when the dental hygienist's role and responsibilities are not uniformly defined by law, the use of the term *treatment planning* may raise concern in clinical practice settings or in educational programs that such a role is "beyond the scope" of the dental hygienist. Most licensing jurisdictions specifically reserve treatment planning and diagnosis for the dentist.

However, many dental hygienists sequence and schedule appointments specifically for the dental hygiene care to be provided. To do this, they must gather assessment data and translate them into a meaningful summary and conclusions to form a *dental hygiene diagnosis*. The rationale and procedures for this diagnosis were presented in the previous chapter.

Generally, the dental hygienist prepares this initial synthesis and then discusses and confirms findings requiring a *dental diagnosis* with the dentist responsible for the patient's overall dental needs. The dentist makes the dental diagnosis, and the dentist or hygienist informs the patient of the results of the assessment. The keys to remaining within the law and to building and maintaining a cooperative team relationship with the dentist are (1) to perform a thorough, reliable assessment; (2) to draw preliminary conclusions from the data; (3) to use the dentist as a resource and arbiter of decisions regarding the patient's status and proper treatment; and (4) to follow through with high-quality dental hygiene care, providing status reports for the dentist as the case progresses and ensuring that the patient receives follow-up care related to the dental diagnosis. In many dental offices, the dental hygienist serves as the patient advocate, coordinating the progression of care.

In this way the dental hygienist can use and expand his or her understanding of basic, behavioral, and dental sciences with each case while remaining within the bounds of professional responsibility and maintaining an interdependent relationship with the dentist. Maintaining this balance is critical, as the patient's well-being and the profession's credibility depend on it.

CASE #1: *MS. L. EVANS*

Long-term patient with chronic disease
New dental hygienist in established dental practice

Ms. Evans is a long-term patient in the dental practice. She has several oral problems that suggest a continuing downhill course despite regular dental care. The hygienist is new in the practice. The patient has been scheduled for a "standard 45-minute prophy-and-exam appointment." The patient expects to have her teeth cleaned and to have the care paid for in total by insurance.

The standard approach to care in this general dental practice is to see patients every 6 months on a recall program in which the teeth are scaled, polished, and examined for dental caries, and the dentist reviews those findings to determine whether a restorative appointment is necessary. The hygienist also asks the patients about their brushing and flossing habits and distributes a new toothbrush. All of this, along with bitewing radiographs and a fluoride treatment, must occur within the 45-minute appointment.

Thus, patients typically do not receive a complete head and neck examination or an intra-oral and periodontal examination at each visit. The hygienist has always complained, "There isn't enough time."

A new policy in the office is being introduced as a result of a continuing education seminar attended by the dentist and the hygienist. The seminar stressed comprehensive assessment as an important way to avoid malpractice litigation and to ensure that patients' needs are identified on a regular basis.

At this visit, you explain to Ms. Evans that it is time for a complete review of her general and oral health status, especially given her record of repeated needs for restorative care. The dentist has agreed that the appointment time should be spent completing a reassessment. Following are the results.

Personal data	Married, female. Travel agent. Mother of one child (female, born 11/24/73).
Date of birth	10/20/51
Medical history and review of systems	Periodic sinus infections (respiratory). Hypothyroid disease (endocrine). Vocal cord polyps in 1970 (respiratory). Two years since last physical examination.
Vital signs	BP: 130/86 (AM RAS). Pulse: 75.
Dental history	Seeking care in this dental office since 7/88. Regular visits, q 6 mos. Dental caries requiring tx, q 6 mos. Soft tissues bleed when she brushes. Teeth sensitive to touch and cold. Brushes once daily; no other oral hygiene aids. Uses "toothpaste on sale." Uses no mouthrinse.
Patient's wants, needs, expectations	Concerned about sensitivity near CEJ of Nos. 4, 5, 12, 13. Unhappy with the color of her teeth.
Dietary assessment	High intake of refined sugars (nibbles on cookies kept in desk; likes desserts).
Extraoral and intraoral examination	Crepitus in TMJ. All other structures appear normal. Halitosis.
Periodontal examination	Generalized bleeding on probing. Pocket depths 4 mm or less. Healthiest gingival areas: Nos. 9, 10, 11. Worst gingival areas: Nos. 18, 19, 30, 31. Moderate staining (coffee). Heavy anterior lingual calculus (supragingival). Heavy plaque at margin of gingivae (generalized).
Dental charting	Three areas of decalcification (DB Nos. 31, 14, 15). All posterior teeth have MO, DO, or MOD amalgams, often with lingual or buccal extensions. Anterior teeth have no restorations.
Radiographic evidence	No apparent bone loss. Overhanging restorations on Nos. 2, 3, 12, 28. Enamel radiolucency, D No. 10.
Guided self-assessment	Surprised at the number of "big fillings." "Can't believe" what is behind her front teeth (anterior calculus). "Did that blood come from my mouth?" "My front teeth sure are dingy looking."

Dental hygiene diagnosis	*Treatment goals*
Receptive patient	Home care should be achievable
Borderline dental health and a worsening situation	Establish health; do not let it worsen
Knowledge deficit: under the care of a dentist, but minimally aware of needs; did not realize she had a problem	Gentle, practical instruction
Gingivitis	Professional and daily at-home debridement of microbial plaque
Recurrent caries and decalcification	Fluoride rinse, nutrition counseling
Halitosis	Evaluate for relation to sinus infection or other systemic disease
Hypothyroid disease and vocal cord polyps	Recommend periodic re-evaluation with physician
Potential for infection: periodic sinus infection	Periodic re-evaluation; check for relation to oral health status
Hypersensitivity	Desensitization
Crepitus	Occlusal evaluation and possible referral for TMJ disorder
Nutritional deficiency: high intake of sugars	Nutrition counseling

TREATMENT PLANNING

Because the majority of the goals for this patient focus on reversing a long-term trend and you are the new hygienist, it is important to protect the integrity of previous clinicians while gently moving the patient to a more proactive role in her own oral hygiene. The patient's commitment to oral hygiene and her ability to implement it on a daily basis are more important than much of the hands-on instrumentation that will support her efforts.

SELF-QUESTIONS

If I simply perform extensive instrumentation, will this help Ms. Evans to reach her goals? Will she have postoperative pain that will compromise her cooperation? Also, will she begin to adopt the self-care behavior that is essential to achieve stated goals? If I remove the debris, calculus, and so forth, she may continue to believe that doing so is my periodic responsibility rather than her continuing responsibility. How do I help the patient to accept responsibility (at least in part)?

What is really important? Is it to remove the calculus and polish away plaque and stain? Or is it to help the patient make a commitment?

What is the best way to approach the patient? Is it a straight forward announcement of the problem and the ways to fix it? How do I present this situation and related goals without injuring the reputation of the dentist and previous hygienists? Is it better to inform the dentist about the situation and ask him or her to explain it to Ms. Evans for me? Or is it better for the dentist and me to work out a solution and jointly explain the situation, using the patient's current needs as the focus?

What treatment options does this patient have?
Continue as before, with periodic visits to "quick fix" the soft tissue problems and restore the new caries.

Customize an approach to meet her needs: more frequent care; more frequent follow-up for motivation and evaluation; self-evaluation techniques for plaque, gingivitis, and diet; varied home care techniques for plaque control, gingival health, and dietary improvement.

Refer to a specialist.

What are the priorities for this patient? How do her wants and needs fit with those priorities? How have the expectations for "dental hygiene care" under the scale-and-polish assumptions of recall visits affected the hygienist's, the dentist's, and the patient's willingness to attend to the real needs?

Do I have all the information I need to establish a plan? What else would I need? Do I clearly understand what the patient wants? Does she have enough information to understand the situation and help make related decisions? The patient needs to have enough information to make an intelligent decision about what is best to do; I need to make sure I account for her goals, concerns, and beliefs in presenting that information.

How do I schedule the time for this patient? I've used most of the time establishing what she needs at the first appointment. What can I accomplish with the remaining time? How much time should I schedule for the second appointment? How do I explain to the patient that she will need to return for a subsequent visit? And what about the need to see her after a few weeks to review her progress? Will that require a short appointment—or should I plan to spend at least 30 minutes reinforcing the earlier messages?

How will the patient pay for these appointments? Insurance coverage will usually pay for a portion of what she needs. Will I limit the care I provide to what insurance will cover? Or do I provide the care the patient really needs, with the patient being fully aware that she will need to pay directly for a portion of the care?

SAMPLE DIALOGUE

"Good morning, Ms. Evans. I'm Glenda North, the dental hygienist who works with Dr. Brown. I see from the appointment book that you are scheduled for a routine recall visit, but Dr. Brown and I have reviewed your chart and agree that it is time for you to have a complete dental assessment. When patients stay with one practitioner for a long time, the clinicians tend to build on the early data that they obtained years ago, and sometimes it is important to take a comprehensive look at where you are today and see if we are aware of all your oral health needs. Basically, we start over as if you are a new patient and gather fresh information. It gives us a new perspective, and it can help you see more clearly how your oral health is progressing. (Use charts, radiographs, etc. to reinforce the amount of information that has accumulated over the years.) Dr. Brown and I are suggesting that we take today to redo that complete assessment and then use the remainder of today's appointment and at least one subsequent appointment to complete your treatment needs. We'll use the information to ensure that we are on the right track with your oral care. How do you feel about that?"

There are several options at this point: (1) She agrees; you proceed; (2) She looks anxious; you ask what her hesitations are; (3) She asks to see Dr. Brown; you either ask Dr. Brown to join you or ask if there are questions you can answer and then bring in Dr. Brown; (4) She asks about finances; you provide the options; (5) She refuses; you engage in a discussion of the relative merits of continued recall versus a complete reassessment followed by appropriate care. It is essential to listen carefully to the patient's reasons for refusing before providing more information about why this course of action is necessary.

Once the decision to proceed is made, you can ask the patient how she feels about her teeth and about having dental care.

"Well, Ms. North, I want you to know that I'm the worst dental patient. I simply don't like coming here, even though Dr. Brown is always so good to me. Just be careful because my teeth are so sensitive."

"When are they sensitive? To hot or cold or both?"

"They are just sensitive. Sometimes I notice it when I drink iced tea. But when I put my fingernail right here (demonstrates with finger around the gingival margin of Nos. 4 and 12) and sometimes when I brush, it hurts."

"I'm glad you told me that. Is there anything else that is bothering you, Ms. Evans? (Continue to discuss other items the patient mentions, noting them for later reference. In this case the patient mentions that she does not like the color of her teeth. Then proceed to the rest of the assessment:) "Let me tell you what we would like to do for you today to start. I'll thoroughly review your medical and dental history, since it has not been completely updated since you first came to this practice in 1988. Then I'll do a head and neck examination for any growths or abnormalities that could be signs of cancer, take your blood pressure and pulse, check your gingivae (or gums) for periodontal disease, update your dental charts, and take necessary x-rays. Then Dr. Brown and I will review the findings and decide what else we should do with the remainder of your appointment time. I'd also like to update you on the latest dental research about how you can care for your mouth."

"Wow, all of that. Since when did you start checking for cancer? I think that's great."

"Most dental professionals do it all the time, but just never tell you that they are doing it. It's just my philosophy to tell my patients what I'm doing and educate them so they will be better dental consumers and know what to expect from their dental team. Shall we proceed?"

"With all that to do, I think we should."

"Let's start with your medical history. Are you presently on any medications?"

"No."

"Have you ever been hospitalized for any major illnesses or diseases?"

"No, not really."

"What do you mean by not really?"

"At one time I had a hypothryoid condition."

"Are you taking any medication for it?"

"No, not any longer."

And, thus you begin the assessment procedures, giving information and answering questions as appropriate to ensure that the patient is a partner in the data gathering and understands its significance. Once the data are gathered and you have conferred with Dr. Brown, explain the recommended procedures, including the need for additional appointments and the likelihood that insurance will help with a portion of the cost but probably not all. Consult with the insurance company for the extent of coverage to ensure that the information you give to the patient is accurate.

"It is a good thing we took the time to do a complete reassessment. It appears that you are walking a fine line between health and disease, and we want to make sure you move more securely over to the side of health. That will help you avoid falling into a costly pattern of gradually worsening problems."

A sample treatment plan for this patient follows.

JOINTLY DETERMINED TREATMENT PLAN

Today

Ultrasonically scale the teeth to remove calculus and irrigate the gingival area with an antimicrobial agent (to reduce the bacterial load). Review brushing (frequency, method, brushing to cleanse gingival area, type of brush). Recommend antimicrobial toothpaste and mouthrinse. Add fluoride rinse or gel for daily or weekly (higher concentration) use (for caries and hypersensitivity).

Second visit (10 days later)

Take blood pressure to assess borderline hypertension; refer to physician if necessary. Measure host response of tissues (sites at risk for periodontal loss of attachment). Assess caries susceptibility. Determine level of success in personal oral hygiene. Assess compliance with recommended procedures (frequency, methods, products). Help patient remove roadblocks to success. Suggest alternative oral hygiene procedures that will boost effectiveness (floss, oral irrigation, dental sticks). Confer with dentist regarding need for restorative care and temporomandibular joint or occlusal evaluation (schedule as needed).

Third visit (3 weeks later)

Take blood pressure and compare with previous measures; inquire regarding referral to physician if applicable. Determine level of success with oral hygiene care. Continue modifying recommendations and removing roadblocks. Complete removal of deposits and irrigate (if necessary). Give fluoride treatment. Jointly establish recall interval (1 month?) for thorough evaluation of patient progress toward goals.

CASE #2: *MR. J. BORG*

New patient in a general dental practice
Hygienist has 15 years experience in this practice

Mr. Borg has a history of dental problems, including orthodontics, endodontics, and crown and bridge work, as well as tender, bleeding gingivae. He has been referred to your office by a nondental colleague who is also a long-term patient in the practice.

Your responsibilities with new patients in this practice are to collect all pertinent assessment data for medical and dental histories; complete a head, neck, and oral examination; document vital signs; and assess the patient's wants, needs, and expectations. You are also responsible for diagnostic tools such as radiographic surveys and enzyme assays, initial periodontal therapy, oral prophylaxis, and home care techniques and tools, as well as for evaluation of patient progress toward health goals.

Personal data	Single, male. Account executive.
Date of birth	1/14/48.
Medical history and review of systems	No significant findings; all systems within normal limits. Health conscious; distance runner.
Vital signs	BP: 118/68 (PM, RAS). Pulse: 50.
Dental history	Unhappy with previous dentist. Last examination and oral prophylaxis—6 mos ago. Isolated areas bleed during flossing. Flosses regularly. Uses an antimicrobial mouthrinse: Viadent. Many restorations placed during teen years; some recently replaced.
Patient's wants, needs, and expectations	Dental checkup and "tooth cleaning." Not satisfied with "appearance of crowns on front teeth."
Dietary assessment	Health conscious; limited fat intake; high complex carbohydrate intake
Extraoral and intraoral examination	No significant findings other than maxillary torus.
Periodontal examination	Marginal bleeding and interproximal edema near posterior crowns. No pockets > 3 mm. Recession: facial and lingual of No. 29. 4 mm cement remaining on the lingual of No. 9 (near core buildup)
Dental charting	Crowns: Nos. 3, 7-10, 14, 19, 30.

Radiographic evidence	All remaining teeth have restorations except Nos. 6, 11, 22-28.
	No apparent horizontal bone loss.
	No enamel radiolucencies.
	All other features suggest health.
Guided self-assessment	"I've spent a lot of time in the dental office, and I want to keep this smile."

Dental hygiene diagnosis	*Goals*
Motivated patient	Respond to his interest; help him achieve optimal health
Works hard at oral hygiene but has numerous restorations that hamper effectiveness	Reinforce what he is doing well; help him understand the handicap of maintaining the tissues surrounding the defective restorations
Identify ways of maintaining areas near defective restorations that will not be replaced	Show personal and professional interest
Esthetic concerns of patient: crowns on front teeth	Possible referral to prosthodontist
Torus palatinus	No treatment required
Potential for infection: cement on lingual No. 9	Remove excess cement
Defective restorations	Recontour and/or refer to dentist to repair
Gingivitis	Debridement and home care instruction

TREATMENT PLANNING

Because the majority of the goals for this patient focus on maintaining optimal oral hygiene, the issue of the defective restorations (particularly on the posterior teeth) is central. However, the teeth are functional and there is no evidence of periodontitis or caries.

SELF-QUESTIONS

How can I help Mr. Borg maintain optimal oral health? What new equipment, methods, or strategies (documented by research) are available that could help his special needs? What is the best way to approach the topic of improving or replacing the current restorations? This is an issue that relates to preserving the integrity of the previous dental professionals and to the availability of new materials and methods that may meet his restorative needs.

Am I meeting the patient's expectations for this visit as well as introducing new ideas for him to consider? Maintaining this balance is important in establishing trust with a new patient. How will I evaluate whether what I (we) do in this practice meets his needs, given that he is dissatisfied with his former dentist?

Is the plan for Mr. Borg complicated or simple? What is the best way to approach a dental health education plan for him? How will I integrate this plan with the dentist's (likely) plans for further restorative care?

SAMPLE DIALOGUE

"Ms. Hart, I have spent a lot of time in the dental office, getting my teeth fixed. I want to keep my smile. I just didn't feel that the dental work I was getting at my previous dentist was up to par."

"So, you've spent quite a few hours in the dental chair, but are dissatisfied with the result. What's not up to par?"

"My front teeth don't look right and I keep getting food caught around the crowns in the back of my mouth. I have to carry dental floss with me all the time in order to clean the spaces. And the gums bleed everytime I floss there. It just can't be right."

"So, you are unhappy with the crowns in the front because they look bad to you and the ones in the back because they trap food. I can't blame you for being unhappy. How long have you had those crowns?"

"My last dentist started replacing my old fillings about 4 years ago. I get a crown every 6 months or so just to keep up with it."

"Why don't we have Dr. Dietz take a look at your crowns when we're finished here? He's very conservative and well versed in the new restorative materials available and the latest procedures. I think he'll be able to help you. In the meantime, I'd like to see if there are ways we can help the soft tissues around some of your crowns so they don't bleed. Today I'll completely assess your oral health so we can see if these bothersome crowns are the extent of your problem. Then, you and I can discuss the findings and decide what other care is appropriate for today."

(Complete all assessment procedures; results are shown above.)

"Just looking at the shape of the tissue around those crowns suggests we may want to attend to finding ways you can maintain those sites and remove the deposits around them that make it difficult for you to be successful. You noticed during the assessment that the tissues bled when I touched them with the probe and that there was an accumulation of plaque and calculus near the margins of the crowns. I'll use equipment that will thoroughly cleanse those areas and create a flushing action that helps reduce the bacteria. Then I have a great way for you to keep the gums healthy and flush away bacteria on a daily basis."

"I think I like it here already."

JOINTLY DETERMINED TREATMENT PLAN

Today

Ultrasonically scale the teeth. Remove calculus, stain, and residual cement from lingual No. 9. Se-

lectively polish to remove stain. Perform in-office irrigation with antimicrobial solution.

Review flossing as necessary. Introduce at-home, daily oral irrigation with an antimicrobial (Viadent or Listerine, depending on the patient's preference) to help resolve gingival bleeding.

Second visit (3 weeks later)

Evaluate effectiveness of oral hygiene routine; review procedures (flossing, irrigation). Finalize restorative treatment plan (dentist). Jointly establish recall interval (3 months).

CASE #3: *MR. M. WILLOFF*

Patient requiring premedication
Hygienist has 3 years experience in this general practice

Mr. Willoff has been a patient in this practice for 4 years. He has received regular, preventive-maintenance services and no additional dental treatment. Two years

ago he had a total left hip replacement as a result of arthritis. His orthopedic surgeon recommended that he be premedicated for any dental services that might result in a bacteremia.

Personal data	Married, male. Scientist. One child (male, born 12/22/89).
Date of birth	1/22/55.
Medical history and review of systems	Total left hip replacement (skeletal, cardiovascular).
	Arthritis, generalized (skeletal).
	Medication: Naprosyn.
	Previous hypertension (cardiovascular).
	Daily multivitamin supplement.
	Allergy to bee stings.
Vital signs	BP: 128/74 (AM, RAS).
	Pulse: 75.
Dental history	Satisfied with teeth.
	Orthodontic treatment as a teenager.
	Maxillary wisdom teeth congenitally missing.
	Flosses weekly.
	Uses mouthrinse sporadically.
	Familiar with proper brushing and flossing techniques.
Patient's wants, needs, expectations	"It's been 10 months since I've had my last cleaning and exam."
Dietary assessment	Dislikes vegetables; takes multivitamins to compensate.
Extraoral and intraoral examination	All structures appear normal.
Periodontal examination	Recession (2 mm) on Nos. 30, 31, 2, 3.
	No bleeding on probing.
	Moderate stain.
	Slight supragingival calculus (lower anteriors).
Dental charting	Six occlusal restorations.
	Two "watch" areas on Nos. 32 and 17 for occlusal caries.
Radiographic evidence	All structures appear normal.
Guided self-assessment	Considers himself to be in good health. "I've never had any major dental problems. I guess I've been lucky."

Dental hygiene diagnosis	_Goals_
Well educated, concerned patient	Reinforce prevention commitment
Healthy periodontally	Understands the rationale for premedication
Explain possible relationship between anti-inflammation medication for arthritis and lack of periodontal disease	Has had no serious dental problems
Arthritis and associated hip replacement	Premedicate as per physician's instructions
Potential health compromise: hypertension	Evaluate at each appointment and refer to physician if necessary
Potential for infection: caries Nos. 17, 32	Sealants
Potential for oral health compromise: attachment loss	Re-evaluate localized areas of attachment loss; possible referral to periodontist

TREATMENT PLANNING

This patient requires minimal treatment intervention. However, it is important to remember that he should receive a thorough assessment and careful monitoring at each visit to detect subtle changes. It is easy to become complacent with patients who regularly appear with good dental health and optimum oral hygiene techniques.

SELF-QUESTIONS

Does it matter that Mr. Willoff flosses only weekly, given that his soft tissues are healthy and there is no sign of periodontitis? Is it important to insist he floss more frequently? What oral rinse is he using? How often does he use it, and how likely is it to be contributing to his oral health?

What is the role of his medication in controlling inflammation—arthritic inflammation as well as periodontal? He has his mandibular third molars, which are difficult to maintain (with either brushing or flossing). Yet he shows no signs of inflammation in those areas. How can this be explained? What research is emerging to show the possible role of antiinflammatory medications in the treatment of periodontitis?

Should you use another measure of periodontal risk factors in addition to tissue observation, periodontal probing, and radiographs? Is it possible that the patient has the risk factors of periodontal pathogens, but that they are not causing observable destruction? Would a test of tissue inflammation (such as asparatate aminotransferase or the neutral proteases) show signs of tissue breakdown that are not observable clinically?

SAMPLE DIAGLOGUE

"Well, Mr. Willoff, you look great as usual. Everything looks healthy. It is such a pleasure to work with a person who has good dental and periodontal health. Whatever you are doing seems to be working; keep doing it.

"There are a couple of things we'd like to do today. First, I would like to seal your two lower third molars—the ones farthest back in your mouth. They are difficult for you to reach, and there is the possibility that the deep grooves may decay. So, we can seal the biting surfaces of those teeth and prevent decay. We seal them with a plastic material; it is easy to do and takes about 10 minutes. It may be that these teeth will never decay, but taking this precaution can save you considerable expense if they should start to break down. Your insurance company should be able to help you pay for it. I'll check with our office manager about that. But even if they do not cover sealants, I strongly suggest we place them. It is a good preventive procedure."

"I do have difficulty cleaning around those back teeth. I tend to gag when the brush reaches that far back. My son has sealants on his teeth; I didn't realize you could use sealants for adults."

"In your case, yes. Those areas are at risk. I'll need to apply the etching solution for a longer time for you since those teeth have been 'toughening' from the fluoride you consume. But the procedure is essentially the same.

"The other agenda item for today is to collect a sample of the bacteria around your third molars. The tissue looks very healthy, but that may be because you are taking antiinflammatory drugs for arthritis. Such drugs reduce inflammation throughout the body, including your mouth. As a result, you may not have any clinical signs of periodontitis—a nice side benefit of the medication you take for a different problem. But just to be on the safe side, I would like to see if you have any of the known periodontal pathogens populating the plaque around those teeth. It would be helpful to document whether you have bacterial flora that could cause you problems in the future. This is a simple chairside test that I perform by taking a sample from around the area and adding reagents to see if the pathogens are present. Shall we go ahead?"

JOINTLY DETERMINED TREATMENT PLAN

Before treatment

Premedicate to prevent adverse effects of bacteremia.

Today

Collect bacteriologic samples from maxillary molars and mandibular third molars. Seal Nos. 32 and 17. Remove calculus and selectively polish stains. Jointly establish continuing care interval (6 months).

CASE #4: *DR. C. BALSIGER*

Periodontal continuing care patient
New dental hygienist in established general practice

Dr. Balsiger has been receiving periodontal maintenance care for 2 years. The treatment and progress notes indicate "gross scaling mandibular anteriors" and "two quads of root planing with no anesthesia," followed by quarterly continuing care appointments. However, the patient has not been in for 1 year. All treatment was provided by the general dentist.

This patient requires a thorough evaluation of her periodontal status, as well as a thorough review of her medical and dental histories and home care techniques. It is important to assess her needs and expectations of you as a dental hygienist. Ask questions to get a feel for her values and impressions of her dental health.

It is possible that the patient is well maintained with no signs of active periodontitis. However, do not assume that there has been no activity since the last visit.

Personal data	Married, female. Computer scientist.
Date of birth	10/30/44
Medical history and review of symptoms	Uses aspirin daily (two tablets).
	Mother died of liver disease (digestive).
	Chronic sinus problems (respiratory).
	Hospitalized for hernia operation (muscular).
	Smokes 1½ packs of cigarettes daily (respiratory, cardiovascular).
Vital signs	BP: 124/74 (PM, RAS)
	Pulse: 84
Dental history	Last dental visit: 1 year ago.
	Problems with bleeding gums. Several large, posterior restorations placed during the 1950s and 1960s. Decalcification on buccal of Nos. 15 and 2.
Patient's wants, needs, expectations	Believes "periodontitis is behind me."
	Expects to have her teeth cleaned and examined with no additional radiographs.
Dietary assessment	Eats "on the run" with a reliance on fast food.
	Minimal intake of fruits and vegetables.
Extraoral and intraoral examination	Nicotine stomatitis.
	Leukoplakia on retromolar pads.
Periodontal examination	Spontaneous bleeding throughout entire mouth.
	Poor tissue contour, texture, color, consistency.
	Class I bifurcation, Nos. 2, 15, and 31.
	Inadequate attached gingiva on facial No. 11.
	Malposed teeth: Nos. 25 and 26.
	Generalized soft and hard deposits, including severe staining. Pocket depths range from 3 to 6 mm.
	Case type: Class II—maxillary and mandibular anteriors; Class III—maxillary and mandibular posteriors.
Dental charting	Multi-surface restorations on all posterior teeth.
Radiographic evidence	Generalized horizontal and vertical bone loss; severe in molar regions.
Guided self-assessment	"Thank goodness Dr. Levy cleaned my teeth so well last time, so I don't have any more gum problems."

Dental hygiene diagnosis	*Treatmemt goals*
Patient is unaware of periodontal condition	Raise awareness of current periodontal health and ramifications

Smoker	Ultimately: stop smoking; Intermediate goal: show relationship of smoking to periodontal disease Show personal and professional interest in patient's well being.
Knowledge deficit: patient is unaware of periodontal condition	False awareness
Periodontitis	Periodontal debridement
Potential for injury: aspirin intake	False awareness concerning long-term benefits and effects of aspirin intake
Potential for infection: chronic sinus infection and decalcification	
Nutritional deficiency	Nutritional counseling
Nicotine stomatitis	Oral cancer self-examination
Leukoplakia	Smoking cessation program Re-evaluate oral lesion for possible biopsy

TREATMENT PLANNING

This patient has recurrent, acute, active periodontal disease despite previous treatment, exacerbated by a smoking habit. The patient believes she is healthy and needs no further treatment. Her commitment to oral hygiene and her ability to control supragingival plaque are lacking.

SELF-QUESTIONS

Why does the patient believe that once her periodontitis was treated that there would be no further problems? Is she unaware of the signs of periodontitis that are obvious to the clinician? Has anyone taken time to educate her to observe her oral condition and participate in continuing care? What does she do for daily plaque removal, and how much does she know about what she should do? How do I/we inform her about her recurrent disease?

Does she know that smoking greatly increases her risk of periodontitis? Is she trying to stop smoking? Would she work to stop smoking if she knew it was related to her oral condition? What is the best method to investigate her attitudes about smoking cessation? What is the best motivational strategy to capture her attention?

What is the relevance of the family history of liver disease?

How do I investigate it further?

SAMPLE DIALOGUE

"Dr. Balsiger, it's been a while since we've seen you. How have you been doing?"

"I've been just fine since Dr. Levy cured my periodontal disease. That was just awful to go through all that treatment, but it's been just fine since then."

"What did he do for you?"

"He used this sharp instrument to dig deep into my gums to get rid of all that hard, old tartar. It must have been there for years."

"Did he tell you anything about what caused the tartar or why your gums bled?"

"Yes, but I can't remember. I think it runs in the family. Anyway, it is nice to have all that behind me."

"Well, let's see how they look today. Sometimes the problem can recur. We need to make sure there is no disease that we need to take care of. So let's start with a look around the mouth. You hold the mirror and I'll use mine to help us both."

"Why? Does something look wrong?"

"My preliminary examination indicates that there are some areas that are in trouble again. Let me show you."

(Show the patient the color and form of the tissue and compare it to the healthiest areas in the mouth or to a color photo of healthy tissue. Take a diagnostic test for bacteria and/or for host tissue response (inflammation) to identify activity in key areas. Then use the periodontal probe to measure several areas. Explain what the pocket depth of healthy areas should be and then show the patient how far the probe drops into several areas. As you do this, she will become aware that all is not well. You will at some point either confirm for the patient or introduce the idea that periodontal disease has recurred.)

"If you are interested in controlling this problem, there are several treatment options available. We can repeat what Dr. Levy did for you, ensuring that what you do at home helps in the success of therapy. Then we can assess how well the condition responds and see you more frequently to monitor the disease. We might have to refer you to a specialist, but let's try the conservative approach first. We'll see how successful we are on the basis of how your tissues respond."

"How did this happen? I thought I was cured."

"Some health problems tend to recur. It has to do with our ability to fend off disease, and in your case, with the presence of bacteria that actually infect the tissues. In some ways, this problem is like gaining weight. If you are not vigilant, the problem comes back. It takes daily commitment to keep it under control. We'll do everything we can to help you find a daily program that can work for you to keep things under control, and we'll do our part to bring the tissues back to health."

"So I have to start all over again."

"If we want to reverse the problem, yes. It sounds like this is upsetting for you. You thought the problem was solved, and now you hear it needs more attention."

"I'm really disappointed, and you're right—I'm upset. How do I know it won't come back again after this round of treatment is finished?"

"It could come back. But we will be able to monitor your tissues at more frequent intervals, and the approaches to treatment and home care have improved a great deal in the last few years. You may have a much better chance of keeping the disease under control given what we have recently learned about it. We'll do everything we can to help you. And we'll make sure you have a way to track your progress at home as well as here in the office."

JOINTLY DETERMINED TREATMENT PLAN

Today

Complete the oral assessment. Perform bacterial and host response enzyme assays. Discuss findings with dentist and patient. Discuss treatment plan. Commence home care plaque control procedures and smoking cessation program.

Second visit (1 week)

Institute initial therapy (ultrasonic scaling and subgingival debridement, including irrigation with antimicrobial agents).Reinforce home care plaque control. Assess compliance with recommended procedures. Suggest alternative oral hygiene procedures to boost effectiveness.

Third visit (1 week)

Complete initial therapy. Evaluate success of oral hygiene strategies.

Fourth visit (2 weeks)

Evaluate success of initial therapy (including microbiologic and host response monitoring tests). Consider referral to a specialist or jointly determine continuing care interval. Reinforce home care plaque control and smoking cessation program; consider referral for smoking cessation program.

CASE #5: *MS. C. TURNBULL*

Patient with dental implants
Hygienist with 35 years experience in a periodontal practice

Ms. Turnbull had such difficulty chewing with her dentures that she nearly starved to death. She was hospitalized, approximately 6 months after her husband's death, because she had wasted to a mere 70 pounds. She could not eat and was severely depressed, causing her to place little importance on preparing foods that she could properly digest and that would provide nutritional value.

She was treated by her physician for depression and weight gain, and he recommended that she see a periodontist for the placement of implants to provide stability for a denture or for full-mouth reconstruction.

This is the most unusual case the dental hygienist has ever dealt with. It is essential that the patient maintain the implants and that they be successful.

Personal data	Widowed, female. Housewife.
Date of birth	9/24/43.
Medical history and review of symptoms	Clinically depressed. Recent weight loss. Taking lithium carbonate for depression.
Vital signs	BP: 98/64 (AM, RAS). Pulse 78.
Dental history	Seeking care because of dissatisfaction with previous dentist; dentures fit poorly. Full-mouth extractions at age 25 because she thought her teeth were ugly.
Patient's wants, needs, and expectations	She can't use her dentures to eat. She wants something to replace them and wishes she had real teeth again.

Dietary assessment	Consumes as little as 500 calories per day.
	Often eats only gelatin or broth.
Extraoral and intraoral examination	All structures appear normal.
Periodontal examination	Not applicable.
Dental charting	Full dentures.
Radiographic evidence	Adequate alveolar ridge.
	No signs of pathology.
Guided self-assessment	"I simply cannot eat with these dentures. They do not work."
	"I am so depressed. I have many problems besides these false teeth. Can't we do something to fix at least this problem?"

Dental hygiene diagnosis	*Treatment goals*
An anxious, depressed person	Create safe, trusting, environment
Serious, life-threatening condition	Correct the problem; ensure the solution is maintained
Dental diagnosis confirms that implants would be successful and are indicated	
Nutritional deficiency and potential for injury: ill-fitting dentures, poor dietary habits	Nutritional counseling to correct the problem; ensure the solution is maintained
Edentulous dentition	Implant therapy

TREATMENT PLANNING

This difficult situation must be handled with patience and respect. The patient needs individualized attention and support to have successful treatment and to maintain the good results of therapy. She will need to be motivated through the process of surgery for implant placement, adjustment to the new prosthetic appliances, and prevention of periimplantitis.

SELF-QUESTIONS

Ms. Turnbull had her teeth extracted at a young age because she thought they were ugly. Will she place any more importance on implants than she did on her teeth? Is she motivated to maintain her implants, given this history? Given her clinical depression, will she be able to sustain the daily routine of cleansing the implants and the attached protheses?

What special attention will be required to provide support during surgery and recuperation?

What issues are important in developing the dental health education plan? Time? Careful deplaquing? Implements to be used to cleanse the areas? Use of antimicrobial agents? Use of daily irrigation?

How frequently should this patient be monitored to ensure that periimplantitis is prevented and identified early if it occurs?

How can the hygienist cooperate with the physician to help support nutritional improvement?

SAMPLE DIALOGUE

"How have you been doing, Mrs. Turnbull? You're looking terrific!"

"Thanks for asking. I feel so much better. These implants have really made a difference."

"What we want to do today at this appointment is to evaluate the tissue response around the implants. It's imperative that the gums stay very healthy for the stability of the prosthesis. I'll be using very special plastic instruments to cleanse the area while protecting the implant. How does that sound?"

"Fine, but I have one question. I want you to watch me clean these areas and see how I am doing. I want to make sure these implants stay in my mouth. For the first time in years I can eat."

JOINTLY DETERMINED TREATMENT PLAN

Today

Complete needs assessment. Joint discussion with periodontist regarding the likelihood of success of implants and the procedures necessary for implants to be placed and maintained. Suggest alternative soft foods to augment gelatin and broth (easily prepared, tasty, and nutritious); coordinate suggestions with physician's recommendations. Attend to the patient's attitude and behavior; provide trusting support; report observations to the physician as appropriate.

Postoperative/postprosthesis delivery

Introduce techniques necessary for daily maintenance of implants: irrigation, special brushing, special floss materials and fabrics (with antimicrobial agent), antimicrobial mouthrinses. Review diet; reinforce nutritious food choices; suggest additional alternatives (recipes; dietary support groups). Jointly establish continuing care interval (2 months).

Continuing care appointment

Evaluate success of oral hygiene regimen. Reinforce success. Evaluate soft tissue health. Deplaque implants and remove hard deposits (if necessary) with plastic scalers.

CONCLUSION

Treatment planning, case presentation, and appointment planning represent the integration of the patient's assessment information and mutually agreed on health care goals. Each patient evaluation and discussion of treatment options will be determined by individual needs. The information and documents generated create a legal relationship as well as establish the patient's condition and the plan of action to which the patient and dental team will be committed during care.

ACTIVITIES

1. Assemble assessment data from clinic patients who are receiving care from advanced dental hygiene students. Complete a treatment planning worksheet for three or more patients. Share your worksheets and appointment plans in groups of four or five and develop composite plans, and then share the plans with the entire class.
2. Role-play case presentations derived from the plans generated in the preceding activity. A "dental hygienist" should present the case to a "patient" while a third student serves as an observer. The observer should watch for the elements of informed consent and the presence of sensitivity to the patient's wants, needs, and expectations. Rotate roles to give each student the opportunity to act as an observer, patient, and dental hygienist.
3. Read Miller SS: Dental Hygiene Diagnosis, *RDH* 2(4):46, 1982. As individuals and then as a class, define dental hygiene diagnosis and develop a preliminary diagnostic nomenclature.

REVIEW QUESTIONS

1. What six elements must be included in a case presentation to meet the requirements for informed consent?
2. If a procedure is performed for a patient to which he or she did not give consent, the clinician may be charged with _____.
3. What is a critical reason for integrating the patient's wants, needs, and expectations in the treatment plan?
4. The first priority in the sequence of care is treatment to meet any _____ needs of the patient.
5. How can a dental hygienist function responsibly and legally as part of the dental team when performing treatment planning for dental hygiene care?

REFERENCES

Barsh LI: *Dental treatment planning for the adult patient,* Philadelphia, 1981, WB Saunders.

Clark JD, Morton JC: Behavioral assessment: an appraisal of beliefs and behaviors relating to treatment, *Dent Clin North Am* 21:515, 1977.

Cohen DW: Preventive periodontics, *J Indian Dent Assoc* (special issue), p 273, 1975.

Fechtner JL: Treatment planning, *Dent Clin North Am* 22:219, 1978.

Fishman SR, Ortiz E Jr: Effective case presentation, *Dent Clin North Am* 21:539, 1977.

Goldberg HJ, Plume M, Nacman M: The importance of attitude in the delivery of health services, *J Public Health Dent* 33:35, 1973.

Keltner JW: *Elements of interpersonal communication,* Belmont, Calif, 1973, Wadsworth Publishing.

Lynch MA: *Burket's oral medicine,* Philadelphia, 1977, JB Lippincott.

Miller SL: *Legal aspects of dentistry,* New York, 1979, GP Putnam's Sons.

Miller SS: Dental hygiene diagnosis, *RDH* 2(4):46, 1982.

Morris RB: *Principles of dental treatment planning,* Philadelphia, 1983, Lea & Febiger.

Rose L, Kaye D: *Internal medicine for dentistry,* St Louis, 1983, CV Mosby.

Rosoff A: *Informed consent,* Rockville, Md, 1981, Aspen Systems.

Wang CC: *Radiation therapy for head and neck neoplasms,* Boston, 1983, John Wright/PSG.

Wood K: *Treatment planning: a pragmatic approach,* St Louis, 1978, CV Mosby.

19 MODIFICATIONS OF DENTAL HYGIENE CARE FOR PATIENTS WITH SPECIAL NEEDS

Dianna Weikel
Hermine McLeran
Susan Barnard

LEARNING OUTCOMES

The dental hygienist will be able to

1. Identify patients with special needs for whom dental hygiene care should be modified.
2. Modify dental hygiene care for patients with special needs in the following areas:
   a. Communication.
   b. Appointment planning.
   c. Environmental considerations such as equipment positioning and patient positioning.
   d. Instruction for individualized home care.
   e. Safety precautions in treatment.
3. Identify the reasons for seeking specific resources to gain additional information regarding patients with sensory and physical limitations.
4. Define the following:
   a. Dental phobia.
   b. Shaping.
5. Describe common oral side effects associated with:
   a. Chemotherapy.
   b. Radiation therapy.
   c. Bone marrow transplantation.
6. Provide a treatment plan for prevention and/or palliation of oral side effects.
7. Discuss factors affecting the use of dental care by the elderly and suggest ways in which barriers to access can be eliminated.
8. Discuss the role of the dental hygienist in alternative practice settings such as a nursing home, hospital, home care program, or other institutional setting.

Every patient needs to be treated as an individual with a unique personality, set of senses, and physical self. In fact, modifications in dental care are made regularly for patients with special needs. This includes patients who are very tall, very short, pregnant, or very young, as well as overweight and extremely fearful patients, patients with busy schedules, older patients, and patients who live far from the office.

In general, the professional team deals with these patients by modifying communication, appointment planning, chair and equipment considerations, and individualized instruction for home care. This same attention applies to patients who are handicapped in a mental, physical, or sensory way.

COMMUNICATION

Communication differs with each person. For patients who can see, looking at pictures, reading information, looking at and handling equipment, and observing other patients during dental procedures does much to acquaint them with care. Patients without sight can use hearing, touch, smell, and taste to explore dentistry. Depending on the sensory limitation present, communication by way of the remaining senses helps the patient experience dentistry without fear. The clinician who takes time to reach out to these patients and to create a good dental experience will no doubt make friends as well as ensure the patient's cooperation.

Careful introductory procedures are useful for deaf or blind patients. These patients lack essential sensory cues for determining what procedures are about to occur. A deaf person may be able to lip-read. If so, the dental professional should speak only when the patient can see the professional's lips. It is usually annoying and embarrassing for the lip-reading patient if the dental professional accentuates mouth movements in speaking or shouts. Speaking slowly but normally is usually most acceptable. A helpful tool for communication is to know sign language for the deaf or to write out a series of descriptions and questions for the patient.

For the blind patient, it is possible to describe procedures and allow the patient to feel the components of the dental operatory. For obvious reasons, sharp instruments should be felt only with caution and careful direction or not at all. Disinfection should follow the guided tour of equipment, and sterile instruments should replace those handled by the patient. This process should be explained to the patient to avoid arousing concern over why the instruments are being changed.

Patients who may not understand the visual or verbal introduction to dentistry will need to take one step at a time. Every patient does better when surprises are minimized in a new and potentially frightening situation. Human qualities of friendliness, a calm manner, light touch, and gentle tone indicate in a universal language that the professional cares.

HOSPITALIZED, BEDRIDDEN, AND NURSING HOME PATIENTS

The oral health care of patients who are being cared for by others in the home, a hospital, nursing home, or other institution is all too often neglected. This is because of the magnitude of their other health problems, their inability to perform self-care, or the lack of time, knowledge, or motivation on the part of the individuals responsible for providing daily care. The dental hygienist can assist in the delivery of improved oral health care to patients who are bedridden and/or institutionalized by providing services directly to them and by

teaching family members or institutional staff members how to provide effective, daily oral hygiene. Although the hygienist's role will be discussed in the context of a nursing home, much of the information in this section is applicable to other settings as well, including care of the homebound, hospitalized, or any individuals who must depend on others for their care.

The United States government has specified certain requirements related to dental care that nursing homes must meet to receive Medicare funding. All skilled nursing facilities must retain the services of an advisory dentist who is responsible for performing annual oral examinations, arranging for dental in-service training, establishing written policies regarding dental care, and providing emergency dental care. In some cases the advisory dentist may be the provider of routine dental care, or the facility may make arrangements for obtaining routine care with other dental services in the community. Intermediate care (custodial care) facilities are not required to retain an advisory dentist, although facilities that provide both skilled and intermediate care must follow the regulations that apply to skilled nursing facilities. Regulations governing dental care delivery in nursing homes vary from state to state, as does the degree of compliance of individual nursing homes with federal regulations. Dental hygienists who wish to work in nursing homes should familiarize themselves with the regulations that govern the provision of dental care in institutional settings.

Depending on the requirements of state dental practice acts, the hygienist may be permitted to perform some or all clinical procedures associated with dental hygiene treatment, including oral screenings, complete dental examinations, periodontal assessments, prophylaxis, radiography, and oral hygiene instructions. Requirements for dental supervision of the hygienist in institutional settings vary from one state to another.

The delivery of care may occur in several different ways. Individuals who are mentally and physically capable of leaving the facility may be transported to private dental practices or public dental clinics. Some larger health care facilities may be equipped with a dental operatory for on-site dental care. When patients who are homebound or in long-term care facilities cannot be transported to a dental office, dental treatment can be provided on-site with the help of portable dental equipment or in mobile vans equipped for dental procedures.

The dental hygienist also may assume an administrative function. Dental hygienists, as skilled clinicians, may serve as liaisons between the facility, the advisory dentist, and the professional dental community to coordinate the provision of dental care to residents. Tasks include assessing the needs of residents and staff members; planning for the treatment needs of residents and the educational needs of both staff and residents; establishing dental protocols, records, and schedules; securing necessary resources; coordinating treatment and examination procedures; and evaluating the success of the dental program in improving the oral health of the patient population. Prerequisites for this role include knowledge of dentistry, communication skills, and skills related to assessment, planning, implementation, and evaluation of dental health programs.

The dental hygienist can provide oral health education to residents and in-service training to staff members. Residents who are capable of performing their own oral hygiene procedures should be taught proper plaque control and preventive skills and their relationship to overall health and well-being. The nursing home responsible for their care must also ensure that these individuals have access to regular oral screenings or dental examinations to ensure prompt diagnosis of dental problems.

Planning for the needs of residents who cannot perform oral hygiene care independently requires a different focus for the dental hygienist. Unless the dental hygienist is a full-time employee of the institution, his or her educational efforts are more effective if aimed at the care providers rather than the residents themselves. Time and resources should be directed towards teaching those staff members who are responsible for assisting residents with their oral hygiene care the importance of that task and how to perform it effectively.

In-service programs provided by the dentist and/or hygienist should attempt to teach care providers, usually nurses' aides, the importance of maintaining their own personal oral hygiene and effective plaque control and preventive methods. Once they are informed and motivated to meet these needs for themselves, they will be more likely to understand the importance of providing daily oral hygiene care for others. Topics that may be covered during in-service programs include oral cancer screening, periodontal disease, dental caries (especially root caries), care of dental appliances, identification methods for dental appliances, and daily oral hygiene care.

The majority of oral hygiene care for nursing home residents is provided or monitored by nurses' aides. For these individuals, providing oral hygiene care is just one of a long list of duties that they are assigned to perform or to assist the patient with daily. Time is a limiting factor in their ability to perform and/or monitor daily oral hygiene care. In addition, their understanding of the importance of oral health care and their motivation to maintain optimal oral hygiene may be limited. Many people, including other health care providers, may find it distasteful and unpleasant to clean someone else's mouth.

Therefore the challenge facing the dental hygienist is to share with these individuals the importance of performing or monitoring these tasks for the overall well-being of their patients or residents. Staff members also will be more interested and attentive when they understand how the information presented is relevant to their job performance and that they will find it helpful in solving day-to-day problems. They should be told why daily mouth care is important in terms of eating, speaking, socializing, and esthetics, as well as for health reasons. Planning educational experiences that will help them understand how they would feel if they traded places with the patient or resident may help motivate them to perform these tasks.

Information presented should be useful, simple, and interesting. Adult learners tend to prefer activities, such as problem-solving sessions, demonstrations, and hands-on practice, rather than lecture presentations. Effective use of visual aids will also enhance audience attention and understanding of the information presented. The American Dental Association and the American Dental Hygienists' Association are excellent resources for both written and audiovisual materials that can be used to plan and deliver effective in-service presentations.

Oral hygiene care

Before determining the appropriate oral hygiene care for a resident or patient, the hygienist must have a clear idea of the dental and medical status of the individual. Close consultation among the dental hygienist, supervising dentist, nursing staff, and physician is necessary to ensure that there are no medical contraindications to the prescribed dental hygiene treatment or oral hygiene procedures. Based on this information, the hygienist can tailor dental hygiene procedures to meet individual patient needs. The following suggestions for daily oral hygiene care may be helpful for these patients.

Care for dependent patients. Dependent patients include individuals who are bedridden or who must rely on nursing staff for daily oral care. They may be dependent because of mental incapacity, physical disability, or loss of consciousness. Oral hygiene care for these patients must be provided at least once and preferably twice daily.

If the patient is confined to an adjustable bed, position the bed at a 30- to 45-degree angle before performing oral hygiene procedures. The patient can also be elevated by propping several firm pillows behind the back. A towel should be placed over the patient's chest. Patients who can expectorate should have an emesis basin placed under their chin in which to empty the mouth. If the patient is unconscious or unable to expectorate, it is important that oral hygiene procedures do not introduce quantities of fluids that could be aspirated. Bedridden patients will also benefit from the use of portable oral evacuators to remove excess fluids during oral hygiene procedures. The patient's face should be turned toward the operator.

Patients who are not bedridden can be positioned for oral hygiene procedures in a chair or wheelchair located near a sink. The hygienist should stand behind the patient and lean the head back so that the oral cavity can be seen. Head support may be provided by the hygienist's arm or body or by a portable headrest attached to the chair. One hand is used to open the mouth and retract the soft tissues while the other hand is used to clean the teeth and soft tissues. Disposable gloves must be worn when any type of intraoral care is given.

The lips should be lubricated before oral hygiene procedures begin to prevent discomfort and cracking. If the patient cannot cooperate in opening the mouth, it may be propped open by a commercial mouth prop, a rolled washcloth, or a mouth prop made by wrapping several tongue blades together.

If the patient has natural teeth, they should be brushed and flossed thoroughly. If the patient is unconscious or bedridden, do not use a regular foaming-type dentifrice because of the risk of aspiration of fluids. Instead, clean the teeth with a brush that has been moistened in water, antimicrobial rinse, or sodium bicarbonate solution. If use of a regular toothbrush is contraindicated because of bleeding problems or danger of bacteremia, a disposable foam toothbrush (e.g., Toothette) or a gauze square wrapped around a finger may be substituted for more gentle cleaning. Patients who are conscious but bedridden may benefit from the use of a suction toothbrush, which is attached to oral evacuation equipment so that all excess fluids used during the brushing procedure are removed from the mouth through the head of the toothbrush (Fig. 19-1). A nonfoaming, ingestible dentifrice (e.g, NASAdent) may also be helpful for those patients. Teeth should be flossed by hand or with the help of a floss holder, unless interproximal cleaning procedures are contraindicated by the patient's medical status.

The tongue should be lightly brushed or wiped clean. Other soft tissues in the mouth should be cleaned with moistened gauze squares, disposable sponge applicators, or swabs saturated with an antimicrobial rinse. Use of a brush-on fluoride gel is recommended for prevention of dental caries in long-term care patients who can tolerate this procedure. After cleaning, patients who can rinse may do so with lukewarm water or an oral rinse. For patients who cannot rinse, the mouth can be wiped with gauze squares or a clean damp washcloth. Soft tissues may be lubricated with mineral oil or artificial saliva preparations. Massaging the gums with the fingers may help stimulate circulation in those tissues.

Patients who wear dentures should have them cleaned daily and removed from the mouth at night. Denture care should follow the guidelines discussed in Chapter 23. Patients who do not require their dentures for eating or talking (e.g., unconscious patients) should have all removable appliances taken out of the mouth.

Dentures should also be marked with the name of the individual or an identifying number so that they can be returned to the proper individual if they are misplaced. As this is a common problem in nursing homes, nursing home staff and dental consultants should be responsible for checking all dentures to make sure they are clearly labeled. Ways of doing this are discussed in Chapter 23.

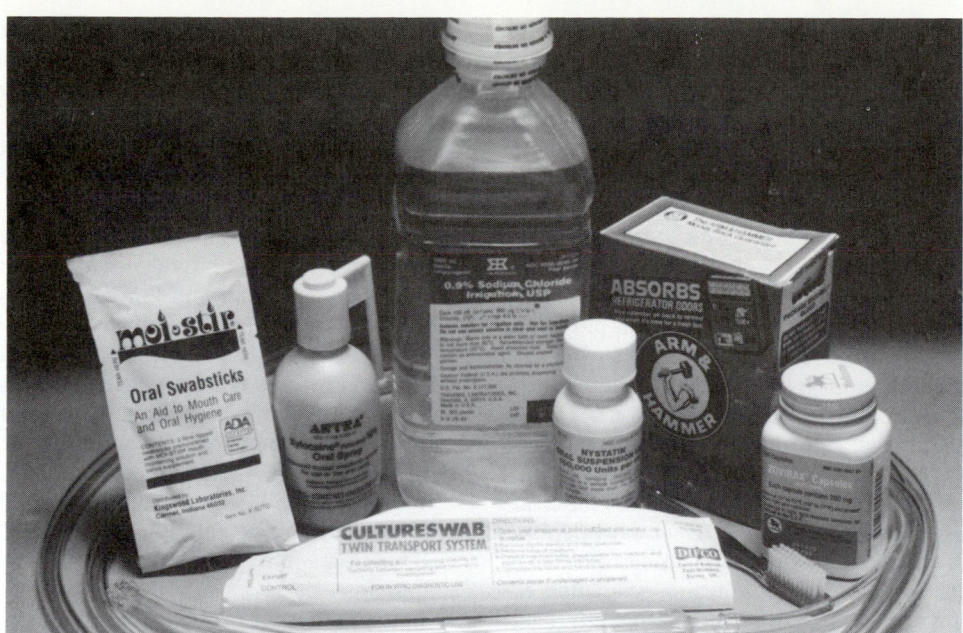

Fig. 19-1. Aids for plaque control for the chronically ill patient. *From left:* premoistened swabs, topical anesthetic, saline solution, antifungal suspension, sodium bicarbonate, soft toothbrush, and 50 ml syringe/suction tip.

These techniques should be discussed with nursing home staff so that they are able to perform this service themselves.

Care for those needing partial assistance. Patients who are capable of performing their own oral hygiene should have access to the supplies necessary for daily home care. Oral hygiene kits can be organized and distributed according to the patient's dental needs. Items that might be supplied include the following:

1. *For patients with natural teeth:* Toothbrush, floss, disclosing tablets.
2. *For patients with dentures:* Denture brush, denture cleaning tablets, denture cup, mouth swabs.
3. *For patients with both teeth and dentures:* A combination of the items listed above.
4. *For edentulous patients:* Toothbrush, mouth swabs, gauze.

These residents may need individualized oral hygiene instructions provided either by the dental hygienist or trained nursing staff members. Special adaptations of oral hygiene aids should be recommended to those with physical handicaps.

The interest of the nursing staff is a critical factor in ensuring that these residents are maintaining adequate oral hygiene and receiving positive reinforcement for their efforts. Oral hygiene care is one function that many patients can provide independently, and they should be encouraged to do so not only because it relieves the workload of the staff but especially because it reinforces the patient's self-esteem through the exercise of some independence and control. Because of the day-to-day contact that nursing staff have with institutionalized patients, they often are aware of factors likely to motivate individuals to maintain their oral hygiene. They may be more successful in encouraging behavior change than dental professionals who are not known by the patients.

Residents of long-term care facilities should receive regular screening examinations by nursing staff and complete oral examinations by dental professionals to detect problems that need treatment, including periodontal disease, caries, mobile teeth, soft tissue abnormalities, broken restorations or appliances, and poorly fitting dentures. Nursing staff who supervise and provide oral hygiene care should also be trained to recognize common oral problems and report them to a dental professional for prompt diagnosis.

Access to dental care must be provided for all individuals, including those who reside in institutions and those who are homebound. The dental hygienist can play an important role in providing access through the delivery of dental hygiene treatment and the provision of oral health education to care providers. Health promotion efforts to organize preventive programs where none exist and to involve other dental professionals in finding alternative ways to provide care for these individuals also are necessary. Dental hygienists' skills are needed in a variety of settings other than traditional private practice. Health promotion efforts should focus on educating community leaders, other health care providers, and legislators regarding the skills that dental hygienists possess. In this way, more of the access barriers separating dental consumers with special needs from professional dental hygiene care can be eliminated.

PREGNANT PATIENTS

A few modifications in care are necessary for pregnant patients. Women of childbearing age should be questioned about pregnancy through the medical history or recall history update before treatment. During the first trimester of pregnancy, the fetus is undergoing critical development of all organs and tissues. At this stage, called organogenesis, the unborn child is most susceptible to substances or events that could disturb normal growth. Exposure to certain medications and radiation could adversely affect the well-being of the mother and developing fetus. If there is a possibility that the patient may be pregnant, diagnostic radiographs should be delayed. Routine prophylaxis and examination can be performed if the patient is feeling well. Otherwise, all elective dental work can be postponed until the second trimester of pregnancy or until after the child is delivered.

It is best to provide treatment for the pregnant patient in the last half of the second trimester (fifth or sixth month). At this point, organogenesis is completed. The patient may be feeling quite well, and the weight and size of the fetus will generally not cause the patient discomfort when she is in the supine position. In later stages of pregnancy, the enlarged fetus puts pressure on major abdominal veins, blocking venous return from the legs when the patient is supine. Hypotension and syncope can result if the patient is in a reclining position for too long.

In general, all medications should be avoided throughout pregnancy. However, routine restorative dentistry can be provided with local anesthesia during the second and third trimesters. Additional vasoconstrictors are not necessary in anesthetic solutions. Nitrous oxide analgesia and general anesthesia are contraindicated. In emergency situations, many medications can be administered safely during pregnancy. The clinician should have full support of the patient's obstetrician before prescribing or administering any type of analgesic, sedative, or antibiotic.

If radiographic diagnosis is essential, radiographs may be taken late in the second trimester or in the early part of the third trimester. To limit radiation to the patient, only a single film of the area in question should be exposed. The x-ray unit should have proper collimation and shielding. High-speed film and a long-cone/high-voltage technique are recommended. The patient is also protected by the lead shield drape as usual (Gier and Janes, 1983).

Patient education is important for the pregnant patient. This is an ideal time for the clinician to lay to rest the myths about decalcification of the mother's teeth and loss of teeth resulting from pregnancy. It is an especially good time to review the need for good home care habits and plaque control. In 1963 Löe and Silness studied 121 prenatal and postnatal women for signs of clinical inflammation. Gingival changes occurred in all of the subjects. Changes were noted as early as 8 weeks' gestation and were most severe by 8 months' gestation. The accumulation of plaque paralleled the gingival changes. When complete removal of plaque was accomplished, gingivitis usually resolved. Other factors contribute to gingivitis and oral problems during pregnancy. For example, pre-existing periodontal conditions may be aggravated by hormonal changes. Home care habits may change as a result of general fatigue. Nausea and vomiting associated with "morning sickness" may make oral hygiene difficult. If the gag reflex is easily stimulated, the patient may avoid brushing and flossing. Vomiting will produce a temporary acidic state in the oral cavity, leaving the teeth more susceptible to attack. Providing understanding and support for the pregnant patient is as important as encouraging good oral hygiene habits and a noncariogenic diet.

The clinician should ask whether the patient is receiving nutritional information in conjunction with prenatal classes at the medical clinic or hospital. If not, this is something the dental staff should provide. The pregnant patient has increased demands for protein, calories, calcium, iron, and vitamins A, B-complex, C, and D (Williams, 1982). The function of these nutrients during gestation and the types of food or supplements in which they may be found in is important information to cover. (See Chapter 24 for more nutritional information.) The teeth begin to develop in the fetus at 6 weeks. Substances consumed during pregnancy can affect the development of the teeth. Overconsumption of fluoride during gestation can cause fluorosis of the deciduous teeth. Some antibiotics taken during pregnancy may stain developing teeth (Cheney and DePaola, 1979). A discussion of the importance of supplemental fluoride to prevent decay after the birth of the child can be mentioned at this time also. Ideally, the mother and child can be seen at a future appointment to review fluorides, eruption dates, and the beginnings of home care for the infant.

Review the role of plaque and the frequency of sugar consumption as they relate to tooth decay. This will be beneficial to the patient and will be useful information in feeding the child later. Baby bottle syndrome is a condition that fits in nicely with a discussion of sugar and decay. The patient may not be aware of the danger to the teeth when a child is put to bed with a bottle of milk or juice to nurse through the night. This practice can result in characteristic rampant decay on the facial surfaces of the teeth.

Usually the pregnant patient is very receptive to any information concerning the well-being of the expected child and having a safe and healthy pregnancy. The clinician should be ready to act as a resource for any questions the patient may have throughout this time. If gingival problems occur, an appointment to remove irritating calculus and review plaque control may be appreciated. A parent who is informed and motivated about dental health will be an excellent model for the child. Seemingly routine information provided to the pregnant patient may be more meaningful than ever before.

PATIENTS ENCOUNTERING DENTISTRY FOR THE FIRST TIME

Occasionally a dental professional sees an *adult who is encountering dentistry for the first time* or *who is frightened because of previous negative dental experiences*. If fear of pain was the primary reason the patient avoided dental care, the "day of reckoning," when the patient does appear, may be the zenith of anxiety for him or her. The very reason for the visit may be to alleviate the pain of a toothache or badly inflamed oral tissues; thus the patient is in pain and is fearing further pain. A situation such as this requires careful handling. Even if the patient's long delay in seeking dental care is not directly related to fear, the messages about dentistry that people see on television, in cartoons, in comic routines, and in other media frequently connote pain and discomfort for the patient.

The patient may expect that dental care will be close to the stereotypes depicted in the movies *Little Shop of Horrors, Marathon Man,* or *The In-laws* or in the comic routines of Bill Cosby and others. The object of the first and subsequent encounters is to disprove those negative images.

The process begins with the phone call to the office, which may be a difficult, tenuous step for the patient. When accepting calls from new patients, the hygienist must listen for signs of distress and follow up with reflective listening that clarifies the source of the patient's anxiety. The patient should hear comfort, concern, and encouragement. The patient could be reacting to anticipated pain and to cinematic or comedic stereotypes. The patient may also be recalling a horrendous experience with dentistry, usually one in which the clinician would not stop treatment despite repeated complaints of pain.

The patient may have had a negative encounter with dentistry that has resulted in a high level of anxiety and avoidance; this is called *dental phobia,* which is a fear of dentistry that "has ballooned all out of proportion." In this case, the office staff should move into a *shaping* mode, in which the patient is incrementally reintroduced to dentistry through a series of nonthreatening encounters with staff, environment, equipment, and finally dental procedures. This often includes a preliminary appointment at which the patient is guided through sequential muscle relaxation and breathing exercises and may listen to audiotapes designed to soothe and distract him or her from anxiety. Relatively noninvasive procedures such as oral hygiene instructions and a head and neck examination may be introduced early, followed by a dental and periodontal charting at a subsequent visit. For some patients, shaping must be broken down into even smaller steps, including time to examine and hold a dental mirror, followed by the patient placing it in his or her own mouth and then the clinician holding it in the patient's mouth with no other instruments in sight. Each instrument and procedure is gradually introduced, with the clinician emphasizing by words and actions that the procedures will not be uncomfortable and that the patient can stop the clinician at any time. The patient should be given a hand signal to use to stop the clinician if discomfort is experienced (Kroeger, 1987).

Early steps in working with dental phobics may occur away from the dental office or in the consultation room away from the dental chair and other equipment. For some people, getting into the dental chair will be the seventh or eighth shaping step. Remember to explain to the patient that the chair will be placed in a supine position; moving into the flat-on-the-back position can trigger a sense of vulnerability. Gradually, patients can be reintroduced to dental procedures, including local anesthesia ("the needle") and "the drill," two of the most dreaded procedures. The patient should be reassured that these procedures can and will be performed with little or no discomfort. Pain management techniques such as those suggested in Chapter 32 should be followed so that the implied promises of comfort are kept. When discomfort can be expected, the patient should be forewarned and the type of sensation described. Discomfort should never come as a surprise (Kroeger, 1987).

Similarly, if the patient has never had dental treatment, the emphasis is on introducing the patient to each item, describing its use, and then moving ahead with the least-threatening procedures. The patient may be terrified of the anticipated evils that can be inflicted with an innocent trisyringe; such terror can be avoided if the patient feels free to ask, "What is that?" The sequence for the first-time adult patient will typically move more quickly than that for the dental phobic.

Often the first-time adult patient or dental phobic will call for an appointment because he or she is in pain. The pain should be relieved promptly. This may require the use of a sedative, analgesia, or some other method that makes dental care possible and as pleasant as possible under the circumstances. Today's dentistry is unlikely to live up to the expectations of those who have avoided it because of fear, so even an uncomfortable procedure may be a pleasant experience in contrast to what the patient's mind has created or remembered.

A baffling experience for a clinician is the patient who complains of pain when the procedure typically does not create discomfort. A natural and typical reaction is one of disbelief. How could the patient complain about discomfort during a simple charting or polishing? An anxious patient has tense muscles. A person who has significant muscle tension is more likely to experience pain. Also, a person who believes a procedure will be painful will probably feel pain regardless of how benign the procedure may be. The memory bank of sights, sounds, smells, and feelings can be so vivid and so closely associated with pain that the patient reacts with pain as a conditioned response to those stimuli. If the patient can be relaxed and distracted from worry and negative stimuli, the psychologic or physiologic transmission of pain can be minimized. Any procedure that creates perceived pain should be halted and steps taken to distract, relax, or otherwise reduce the sensations. This may require anesthesia, analgesia, or other steps (Kroeger, 1987).

Introducing a *child patient* to dentistry follows many of the guidelines used for fearful or first-time adult patients. The dental hygienist has an integral role in providing a stress-free atmosphere that allows for continuous education and optimal dental hygiene care. The child should be introduced sequentially to pleasant, simple procedures using a guided, experiential approach.

Infants who have a developmental disorder or whose parents have poor dental health should see the dentist no later than 6 months of age. Other children should be seen for their first appointment between the ages of 18 and 24 months (Wei and Nowak, 1982). The American Academy of Pediatric Dentistry recommends in particular that children be seen by 1 year of age to ensure that baby bottle syndrome has not developed and to assess proper growth and development (American Academy of Pediatric Dentistry, 1991–92). Many clinicians follow the guideline of seeing children as soon as primary teeth appear. They use this appointment to introduce the parent to the day-to-day attention that should be given to the child's oral health so that the child grows up with good habits and an awareness of dental health.

The infant or toddler should be escorted into the operatory with the parent. Depending on the age of the child, a parent may sit on the dental chair first and place the child on his or her lap. The child's head should be placed in the crook of the parent's arm, with the other arm holding the child's body. This will help control the child's movements and prevent accidents (Wright, Starkey, and Gardner, 1983).

If the child elects to sit alone in the chair, invite the parent to sit close by and observe. The office philosophy may be to involve the parent in health education or to have the parent wait in the reception area. The clinician should obtain a complete medical history from the parent, in particular noting all immunizations (American Academy of Pediatric Dentistry, 1991–1992) (Fig. 19-2) as

well as allergies or medical conditions requiring antibiotic premedication. Emotional status, including any lifestyle changes, (e.g., the birth of a new sibling, parental separation or divorce, new school, new home, or new babysitter) should be noted. This information may prove relevant at a later time. The focus of this appointment is examining the oral structures for normal eruption patterns and overall proper growth and development. Counseling regarding diet, the use of pacifiers, the effects of finger- or thumb-sucking, and what to expect in the coming months with regard to eruption of teeth can also be done during these early-age appointments. The parent can be shown how to wipe plaque from the gum pads and how to brush the newly erupted teeth.

Before beginning the clinical examination, explain why you will be wearing gloves and a mask. Open the instrument packet while the patient is in the chair. Explain to the parent and child how you maintain proper infection control in your practice. All questions should be answered in simple terms. If a child of 2 or 3 years of age (or older) has never visited a dental office, time will need to be spent introducing the child to the dental equipment and procedures (Fig. 19-3).

A child should be introduced to the chair and instruments in a calm, matter of fact manner that may also prove to be fun. It should be an experience that touches all of the senses: sight, smell, touch, sound, and taste. Creating a magical atmosphere for the child helps to reduce anxiety. The use of visuals such as videotapes, handheld games, models, and pictures aids in capturing the child's attention.

Once the child has been shown the instruments, a generalized clinical examination may be completed. The child may watch with a hand mirror and help count the teeth (Fig. 19-4). Use creativity for the descriptions and explanations of any aspect of the dental hygiene appointment as long as they reflect the truth and do not produce anxiety. The clinician should always place a fingertip next to the sharp point of the explorer when moving in or out of the mouth or when moving from one tooth to another to prevent sticking the child.

Ask the child to open wide. If the child has a tendency to inadvertently close the mouth slowly, a mouth prop may be used. Often a child may have a prominent gag reflex. This is an uncontrollable reflex, and often the child becomes frightened. Gently calm the child and have the child

Immunization schedule recommended by The American Academy of Pediatrics

	DTP	Polio	TB Test	Measles	Mumps	Rubella	Hib-Conjugate	Tetanus-Diphtheria
2 months	✓	✓						
4 months	✓	✓						
6 months	✓							
1 year			✓					
15 months				✓	✓	✓		
18 months	✓	✓					✓	
4-6 years	✓	✓						
5-21 years				✓	✓	✓		
14-16 years								✓

Fig. 19-2. Chart represents immunization schedule recommended by the American Academy of Pediatrics 1991-1992.

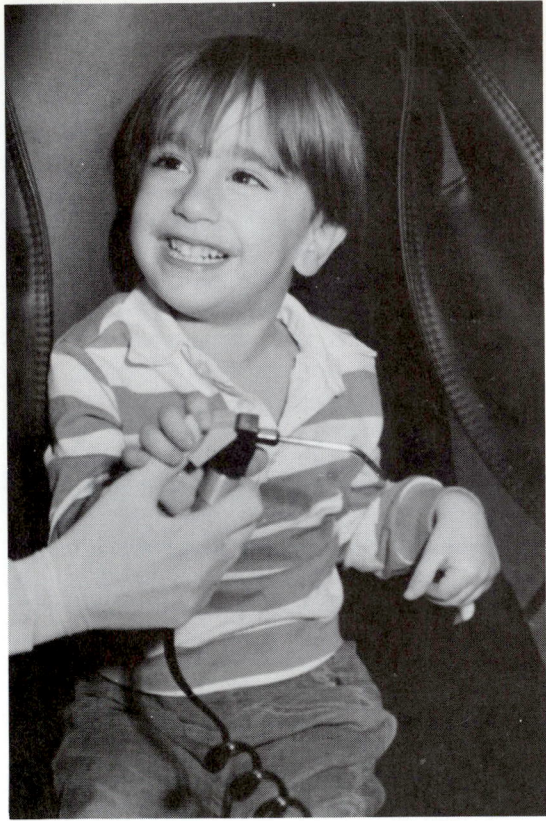

Fig. 19-3. A child's introduction to the dental environment should be experiential. Child may be given an opportunity to push buttons that cause the "spaceship chair" to rise and descend and to use the "squirt gun."

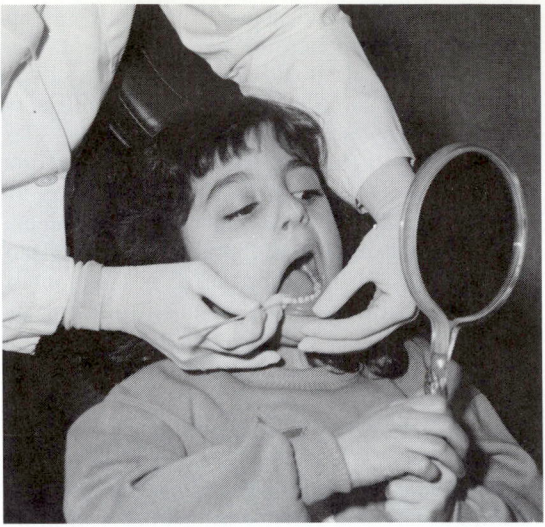

Fig. 19-4. Counting teeth with child observing in mirror involves child in beginning stages of care and familiarizes child with having a metal instrument and mouth mirror in mouth.

take deep breaths. Once relaxed, have the child open only halfway and complete the clinical examination on the mandibular. Next have the child gently tip the head back and open halfway again. Complete the examination on the maxillary. Praise the child for his or her cooperation. During any intraoral procedures, ask the child to maintain a limited opening. At times it may be difficult for you, but the rewards are immeasurable. Trust is established between you and the patient that is not easily forgotten. Assessment of occlusion and soft tissue should also be made at this time. The remainder of the dental hygiene appointment should be an individualized plan.

During the examination, small pieces of calculus may occasionally be found on the lingual surfaces of the mandibular anterior teeth and on the facial surfaces of the maxillary molars; these can be removed with a scaler or curette. If the child is comfortable with the explorer feeling the teeth, the scaler should be easily accepted also. It may be necessary to gently caution the child to sit very still during the critical moments of adaptation.

Often young children present with stains attributable to chronic use of antibiotics for ear infections or of iron supplements for iron deficiency anemia. Parents may be concerned that the child is not brushing properly. The hygienist can take this opportunity to educate parents about the long-term use of pediatric antibiotics that contain sweetener bases to ensure compliance (Hill, Flaitz, and Frost, 1988). These tend to stain the teeth extrinsically. The stain is not removed by daily brushing; it can, however, be removed by polishing with an abrasive.

If selected teeth are to be polished with an abrasive using a motor-driven handpiece, the instrument can be described as an electric toothbrush. An unattached rubber cup can be handed to the child to squeeze so he or she can see how soft it is. The unattached cup can then be rubbed first on the child's fingernail to prove its harmlessness and then on the front of a central incisor. Explaining that toothpaste goes in the rubber cup helps the child figure out why the "electric tooth-brush" has no brush.

It helps to show how the cup attaches to the prophylaxis angle and then to the handpiece. With all the parts assembled, the cup should again be rubbed on the tooth to show that it feels the same. A critical point is when the handpiece is activated and begins to hum or whistle. To prepare for that, it can be explained that the cup could be rubbed by hand on the teeth but that it would take a long time to do it. Most children have plans for some pleasant activity following a dental appointment, which they do not wish to delay—the electric toothbrush helps make sure they will not be late. The rotating cup should be applied with *light in-termittent pressure* on the fingernail and then on an incisor. Then polishing paste ("toothpaste") is added, and stains are polished off.

The saliva ejector attachment (a "straw") for high-volume suction should be used to evacuate saliva and the abrasive, as small children cannot easily control swallowing and expectoration.

In many cases neither calculus nor stain will be evident on the teeth. In these cases, both scaling and polishing are unnecessary. More appropriate is the use of a disclosant, with the child locating the plaque and brushing (and flossing with assis-tance) to remove it.

After plaque is removed, a topical fluoride treatment may be appropriate (see Chapter 21). Care must be taken that the child does not swal-low the fluoride. Ingesting the fluoride gel can cause nausea, vomiting, and illness. Large quan-tities can cause death.

Once the child is old enough to aim a tooth-brush into the mouth, dental appointments shift towards a shared parent/child responsibility for deplaquing the teeth. The child and parent are shown the evidence of plaque with disclosing so-lution, and a toothbrush and a pea-size portion of fluoride toothpaste are used to remove the plaque. The parent and the child are instructed in the proper use of the brush. The parent should be shown how to support the child's head while brushing his or her teeth, but the child should be given the opportunity to use the brush to imitate the proper motions. The goal is to remove all the plaque during the appointment and for the parent to ensure that it is removed daily, with both brush and floss, to minimize caries and gingival inflam-mation (Wei and Nowak, 1982).

It is vital that the parents minimize the child's exposure to fluoride toothpaste. Children tend to like the sweet-tasting paste and can be found eat-ing it or loading it onto the toothbrush. The fluo-ride levels in toothpaste, particularly in the higher-concentration formulas, can contribute to fluorosis (permanent spotting of the developing enamel) and even to a toxic reaction when they are used in combination with fluoridated water and other dietary sources of fluoride. Children should either brush under supervision, with only a minuscule portion of fluoride paste, or be given nonfluoride toothpaste to use. Most clinicians will recommend the former of those two alternatives, opting for the benefits of frequent low doses of fluoride to remineralize enamel.

Dietary evaluation is an important part of early dental care. Patterns of snacking and foods typi-cally eaten during mealtime should be examined for cariogenicity and for a good balance of essen-tial nutrients. Fluoride supplements should be pre-scribed if the water supply is not fluoridated (see Chapter 21).

Dental hygiene care procedures do not cause great discomfort; in many instances, they cause none at all. Therefore the dental hygiene ap-pointment can be an important opportunity to build a trusting relationship, free from fear, and develop good attitudes toward dental health and care.

Behavior management is an important aspect of pediatric dental hygiene care. Document the child's acceptance of care. This will aid appoint-ment scheduling, modification of treatment plans, and assessment of the child's accomplishment's.

The following general guidelines are helpful in preparing for a child patient (Andlaw and Rock, 1987; Bailey, 1979; Goose and Kurer, 1973; Huggins, 1973; McDonald and Avery, 1983; Pinkham, 1988; Roche, 1975; Wei and Nowak, 1982; Wright, Starkey, and Gardner, 1983):

1. Do not keep the child waiting.
2. Call the child by name, touch him or her gently, and give the child a big smile. Project that you are happy to see the child. The child's assessment of you is based on this first interaction.
3. Gently guide the child to the operatory or to the sink and plaque-counting area while holding his or her hand; this helps the child feel confidence in the clinician. For first visits it may be wise to start with plaque counting and finish with exploring and any necessary scaling, polishing, and fluoride treatment.

4. Your body language is very important. Use smooth, fluid movements. Short abrupt movements indicate an uncomfortable feeling. Accent the positive. If a child is apprehensive, focus on the accomplishments of the appointment and highlight what will be done at the next visit.

5. Be *truthful*.

6. Use a voice intonation that reflects calm, firm, gentle control and understanding— this is often more important than the content of what you say.

7. Obtain attention and establish communication before attempting behavior-shaping methods.

8. *Do not use baby talk.* Use a gentle adult-to-adult tone with simple words.

9. Use the "tell, show, do" method before every procedure.

10. Praise the child; take a genuine interest in the child's life, ideas, activities; help the child feel important.

11. If the child will not open his or her mouth, it can be useful to teasingly say, "I bet you don't have any teeth in there. Do you have teeth in there? Give me just a peek." As soon as the teeth peek out, praise them and exclaim, "I guess you *do* have teeth. How many?" The child will probably suggest a number such as 6, 7, or 58. Counting them answers the question and permits some preliminary inspection and caries detection.

12. Allow the child to wear sunglasses during the appointment. Sunglasses will decrease the glare of light, which is uncomfortable for children who have sensitive eyes. Sunglasses also protect the eyes from debris. Disinfect the glasses between appointments.

13. When working with a chairside assistant, be certain conversation is directed toward the child. The child should be the center of attention.

Meticulous recordkeeping is essential. The child's dental status will change from visit to visit, especially during the mixed dentition years. Note changes in eruption patterns, soft tissue occlusion, and dental charting. Behavior should also be noted.

The child's first encounter with dentistry, and all subsequent visits, should be positive and rewarding for both patient and clinician and should contribute to lifelong oral hygiene and prevention. They should form a bond of professional friendship that makes dental care a pleasure.

CANCER PATIENTS

Approximately 1 out of 3 adults now living in the United States will eventually have cancer (American Cancer Society, 1992). Of the 1,130,000 new cancer cases diagnosed in 1992, oral cancers were estimated to account for about 30,000. It is well documented that survival rates are higher when cancer is diagnosed early. Therefore it is important for the hygienist to educate all dental consumers to perform routine oral cancer self-examinations to improve the chances of diagnosing and thus treating an abnormal oral condition early (see Chapter 8).

Because of the length of some cancer therapies and the need for routine follow-up, the dental hygienist in a private practice will probably encounter patients who are undergoing or have recently completed cancer therapy. The dental hygienist plays a key role in preserving function of the oral cavity and preventing or palliating oral complications that may arise from cancer therapy. The purpose of this section is to review systemic treatment options for cancer patients, to detail the side-effects associated with each option, and to provide measures for controlling such side-effects. It is important to stress the need for regular dental examinations for all patients, especially those at high risk for oral cancer or at risk for infection.

Types of cancer therapy

Cancer treatment may involve one or a combination of the following methods: surgery, radiation, chemotherapy, or bone marrow transplant. Primary therapy for tumors of the head and neck involves excision of the affected area and surrounding tissue. Because a margin of healthy tissue is also excised to ensure complete removal of the malignant cells, this treatment may involve loss of a significant amount of healthy tissue. If a head and neck tumor extends beyond surgical application, ionizing radiation is implemented. Radiation can be delivered to the cancer site in one of four ways: (1) external irradiation, in which the source of radiation is outside the body; (2) perioral irradiation, in which the radiation beam is directed through a cone into the oral cavity, directly to the surface of the tumor; (3) interstitial irradiation, in which radioactive material is implanted directly into the tissues to be treated; or (4) surface irradiation, in which an applicator containing radioactive material is applied to the surface being treated (e.g., lip) and the patient wears the applicator until the desired dose is delivered (Chen, 1986). The size of the tumor determines the dose. To improve the effectiveness of radiation therapy and to minimize the damage to normal tissues, the total dosage is delivered in equal daily doses over several weeks. For instance, a common dose of 6000 to 7000 centrigray (cGy) is delivered in doses of 200 cGy per day, 5 days a week for 6 to 7 weeks (Chen, 1986).

Investigation now focuses on the timing of the radiation—that is, hyperfractionization of the total dose. For example, a dose of 6000-7000 cGy may consist of 160 cGy per fraction, 2 times daily with 4 hrs between fractions for 12 days, 5 days a week. After 3800 cGy, the patient is given a 2-week break for the side effects of acute oral mucositis to subside. He or she then resumes twice-a-day radiation therapy with similar fraction size for another 8 days, to bring the total dose to approximately 6400 cGy.

The use of chemotherapy in head and neck cancer is limited (Bloom and Hanham, 1987). It is used experimentally as adjuvant therapy following progression of disease after surgery and/or radiation. Chemotherapeutic protocols are used widely for hematologic malignancies and cancers other than those of the head and neck. It may be part of combination therapy for tumors involving breast, lung or central nervous system tissue. Chemotherapeutic drugs work by destroying rapidly growing and reproducing cancer cells. Unfortunately, these drugs are not selective in their effects and also destroy rapidly producing normal cells, including hair follicles, bone marrow cells, and epithelial cells.

In hematologic disorders such as leukemia, cytotoxic drugs such as daunorubicin and cytosine arabinoside are necessary to produce bone marrow aplasia (myelosuppression). Bone marrow suppression places the patient at risk for infection. Infection is a well-documented complication of cytotoxic antineoplastic therapy (Bodey et al, 1966). For patients with hematologic malignancies, controlling morbidity and mortality of such therapy is challenging. Comparatively, chemotherapeutic management of some solid tumors without bone marrow involvement may not be associated with marrow aplasia. The anticipated severity and duration of bone marrow suppression is of concern to the clinician.

Bone marrow transplantation is a process used to treat bone marrow failure. This may be considered the treatment of choice for severe aplastic anemia, acute leukemia, and immunodeficiency disorders. Age, disease status at the time of transplant, and histocompatibility of the donor are variables affecting the success of this therapy. Because of the aggressive nature of this treatment, morbidity and mortality are high.

Oral complications of cancer therapy

The oral complications of surgery may include facial disfigurement, speech impairment, need for a special prosthesis to restore function, or loss of function of the muscles of facial expression or mastication. Consider the extent of these complications for each individual and be prepared to adapt regular treatment procedures and home care instructions to accommodate any loss of function resulting from surgery. If the patient has been fitted with a special intraoral prosthetic device, consult with the maxillofacial specialist who designed the device regarding recommendations for its care. Thus you can reinforce instructions regarding the care of the appliance or prosthesis during regular dental visits.

Radiation treatment may cause mucositis, taste alteration, trismus, xerostomia, rampant caries, and osteoradionecrosis. The occurrence, severity, and duration of these side effects vary among individuals according to the area being treated; preexisting oral condition; and type, dosage, and duration of radiation treatment.

Oral side effects of chemotherapy include mucositis, dental neuropathy, xerostomia, dental caries, oral bleeding, and oral infections. Sonis, Sonis, and Lieberman 1978 found that 40% of all chemotherapy patients develop oral complications. The severity varies among individuals depending on the type, dosage, and duration of therapy (McClure et al, 1987a).

A number of other physical symptoms and problems may affect cancer patients. These conditions may result from the effects of the cancer itself, responses to cancer therapy, or psychologic reactions to the diagnosis of cancer or to its treatment. They include anemia, bleeding from skin or mucous membranes, constipation, diarrhea, fa-

Table 19-1. Dental appointment series for the cancer therapy patient

Treatment	Dental exam and treatment plan	Immediate dental treatment	Preventive care during cancer therapy	Oral evaluation during therapy	Frequency of postcancer therapy comprehensive dental care
Radiation (RT)	2 weeks before initiation of RT	Oral surgery: 2 wks before RT Restorative: before RT Endodontics: before RT Periodontics: before RT Oral hygiene instructions: before RT Fluoride: before RT Diet counseling: before RT	Oral hygiene care Fluoride therapy Diet management	Weekly	Months 1-2: at least once per month Months 4-6: at least every 6 weeks Months 6+: at least every 4 months
Chemotherapy (CT)	2 weeks before initiation of CT	Oral surgery: 2 wks before CT Restorative: before myelosuppression Periodontal (cleaning): before myelosuppression Oral hygiene instruction: before CT	Oral hygiene care	2-3 times weekly	Care begins immediately following recovery of bone marrow
Surgery	1 week before surgery	Oral surgery: before or at time of surgery Restorative: before surgery Endodontics: before surgery Prosthetics: before surgery Periodontics (cleaning): before surgery Oral hygiene instruction: before surgery	Oral hygiene care Diet management	Daily while inpatient	Frequency of care to be determined by patient's needs: e.g., prosthetics
Bone marrow transplant (BMT)	2 weeks before bone marrow transplant	Oral surgery: 2 weeks before BMT Restorative: 2 weeks before BMT Periodontal: 2 weeks before BMT Oral hygiene instruction: before BMT	Oral hygiene care Oral microbial suppression	2-3 times weekly	Care begins following recovery of bone marrow

Modified from Peterson DE et al: *Head and neck management of the cancer patient,* Norwell, Mass, 1986, Martinus Nijhoff.

tigue, hair loss, itchy skin, anorexia, nausea and vomiting, pain, respiratory problems, sexual and reproductive problems, and urinary tract problems. Awareness of these potential problems increases the dental hygienist's effectiveness in treating cancer patients.

Pretherapy management for the head and neck cancer patient

A dental consultation should be scheduled for all cancer patients before therapy begins. The chances of maintaining a healthy dentition and minimizing the side effects of cancer treatment are closely related to the health of the oral tissues before treatment and the patient's ability to maintain a thorough oral hygiene regimen during and

after cancer therapy. Dental professionals must be advised regarding the immediacy and type of cancer therapy planned. If cancer therapy must be immediate, the dentist, in consultation with the medical team, must address the most critical dental needs without compromising the cancer therapy schedule.

Dental treatment for patients who are about to begin radiation therapy should be discussed among the health professionals who will be providing treatment. Before radiation therapy, the dental professional, in conjunction with the radiation oncologist, should determine the site and dosage of radiation. When possible the necessary dental treatment should be completed before therapy begins (Table 19-1). This may include impressions for custom-fitted trays for fluoride application or as mucosal guards. Review the technique of home fluoride application and stress the importance of daily fluoride therapy. Nutritional counseling regarding intake of foods containing sucrose and increased fluid consumption is essential.

Pretherapy management for the non-head and neck cancer patient

Ideal preparation of the patient with cancers other than those of the head and neck includes procedures that will eliminate or reduce oral infections. A complete oral examination, including a radiographic series, is required to determine dental treatment needs and their priority. Sources of infection in the mouth may compound the potential for complications related to the chemotherapy (Peterson and Sonis, 1983). Therefore, whenever possible, all dental caries, abscesses, and periodontal infections should be treated before chemotherapy is initiated (see Table 19-1). In addition, any surfaces within the mouth that could irritate mucosal tissues, such as fractured teeth, broken or poorly contoured restorations or fixed prostheses, calculus, or poorly fitting dentures should be eliminated. Teeth with nonrestorable caries, periapical diseases, or serious periodontal involvement should be extracted before therapy because of their potential to cause life-threatening infections.

Stress the importance of frequent and effective plaque control both during and after treatment to reduce the potential for acute periodontal infection and other oral complications. Home care instructions should be adapted to each individual's needs, depending on dental conditions, medical treatment, treatment of potential side effects, patient's dexterity, and compliance levels. Specific recommendations for the management of oral side effects of each type of cancer therapy will be discussed to assist you in designing an appropriate preventive treatment plan.

Oral problems related to cancer therapy and their management

Oral complications of cancer therapy occur in varying degrees in patients treated for head and neck malignancies and in almost half of patients receiving chemotherapy for non–head and neck cancers (Peterson, 1984; Schubert, Sullivan, and Truelove, 1986; Silverman, 1990). Infections are responsible for nearly half of deaths in the general cancer population (McElroy, 1984). Infection remains the leading cause of morbidity and mortality among myelosuppressed patients with cancer (Schimpff 1979). Some drug therapies suppress bone marrow function, resulting in a reduction of white blood cells, specifically granulocytes, which are necessary for the body's defense against microbial infection. The oral mucosa, which normally acts as a physical barrier against the passage of pathogenic microorganisms into the bloodstream, may also be affected by the therapy. Thus mucositis occurs with associated thinning and ulceration of the mucosa (Plate 5, O). Breakdown of the mucosa allows pathogens to enter the bloodstream, placing the patient at risk for sepsis. Viral, bacterial, and/or fungal infections are frequently encountered in the immunocompromised host (Wade, 1986). The oropharyngeal flora of chronically ill patients shifts toward gram-negative organisms (Johanson, Pierce, and Sanford, 1969). The most common fungal infection is candidiasis. It appears clinically as a white elevated plaque on mucosa, tongue, or palate that can be rubbed off, exposing raw, bleeding areas (Plate 5, Q). The dentist or physician may prescribe an antifungal agent to treat this condition.

Herpes simplex is a commonly occurring viral infection in immunocompromised patients. It usually begins as small vesicles on the lips, which can spread to include gingival erosion and ulceration. Lesions may coalese to involve large areas of the oral cavity or surrounding tissues (Plate 5, P). Montgomery, Redding, and Lemaistre (1986) found that 48% of immunocompromised patients contracted herpetic infections during chemotherapy. Both gram-positive and gram-negative bacterial infections can occur in immunosuppressed patients as a result of increased virulence of normal oral flora, shifts in bacterial flora towards more pathogenic microorganisms, and lack of host defense mechanisms. Any of these oral infections may be life-threatening. Control of oral infections is a major concern. Perform a thorough scaling and polishing of teeth before therapy to enhance periodontal health. During therapy, patients may benefit from more frequent supragingival polishing with a rubber cup or soft toothbrush as a means of plaque control, unless this procedure is contraindicated because of the patient's medical status. Patients must know the importance of keeping the oral and dental tissues clean and demonstrate appropriate cleansing methods as a means of preventing infections.

Myelosuppressed patients may need antibiotic coverage before any type of dental treatment. The physician should always be consulted before dental treatment.

Thrombocytopenia is a decrease in the total number of circulating platelets (thrombocytes). Preventive practices are essential in caring for the thrombocytopenic patient. Specifically, invasive procedures in the mouth should be limited when platelet levels are below 50,000 cells/mm^3. Normal platelet counts range from 150,000 to 350,000 cells/mm^3. Spontaneous and prolonged bleeding are associated with platelet counts below 20,000 cells/mm^3 (Overholser et al, 1982). Procedures that must be performed during profound thrombocytopenia may require prophylactic platelet transfusion. This reinforces the importance of early dental consultation and treatment so that invasive oral procedures (e.g., extractions, scaling) are completed before the patient becomes thrombocytopenic. Oral factors that can predispose these patients to bleeding include trauma from poorly fitting dentures, improper toothbrushing or use of a hard-bristled toothbrush, plaque and calculus, mobile teeth, restorations, orthodontic appliances, and decayed or fractured teeth (Peterson and Sonis, 1983).

Prevention of oral bleeding requires removal of all rough surfaces in the mouth that might irritate or injure soft tissues before chemotherapy. Custom-fitted vinyl mouthguards should be constructed from impressions of the patient's teeth. These can later be used for both home fluoride therapy and, if necessary, for delivery of hemostatic agents to control bleeding. Patients who wear dentures may be advised not to wear them during chemotherapy or to wear them only while eating, always removing them at night to prevent denture-related irritation of soft tissues (DePaola et al, 1983; King and Martin, 1983). For patients currently undergoing chemotherapy, medical consultation to assess blood cell counts is recommended before any dental treatment, even prophylaxis or home care instructions.

Oral bleeding may be treated with pressure against localized bleeding sites with premoistened, sterile gauze sponges containing topical hemostatic agents such as Gelfoam, Surgicel, or Thrombostat until bleeding subsides. Hemostatic agents can also be placed in custom-fitted vinyl trays, like those used for fluoride application, which are held in the mouth until localized bleeding has stopped. In the nonmyelosuppressed patient, bleeding may also be controlled by placement of a periodontal surgical dressing (McClure et al, 1987a). Have the patient avoid vigorous rinsing, spitting, or use of drinking straws after oral surgery or in the presence of oral bleeding, as they may dislodge the clot.

Hemorrhage resulting from thrombocytopenia or coagulopathy is another complication of chemotherapy. Advances in platelet support therapy have minimized this consequence of chemotherapy and marrow aplasia (Aisner, Schiffer, and Wiernik, 1980). Sufficient levels of circulating, functioning platelets and prevention of mucosal injury remain the best techniques for control of hemorrhage.

Mucositis is an inflammation of the oral mucosa that is common during both radiation therapy and chemotherapy. It results directly from the cytotoxic effects of cancer therapies. Mild forms are characterized by erythema, leukoplakia or yellow patches, and mild discomfort. Symptoms of more severe mucositis include tissue thinning, ulcerations, sloughing tissue, or necrosis on any soft tissue surface. The pain and discomfort associated with these lesions often impair nutrition, oral hygiene, speech, and ability to take oral medications. Disruption of the mucosal barrier predisposes the patient to opportunistic infection (Shelton and Weikel, 1990). In cases of radiation-induced mucositis, the severity of this condition depends on the port, duration, and dosage of radiation given. Mucositis usually begins during the second week of treatment (Silverman and Greenspan, 1985). It is a reversible and temporary condition that is usually resolved by 1 to 2 weeks after the end of therapy (McClure et al, 1987b).

Plaque control procedures may have to be modified to reduce oral discomfort. The patient should be instructed to avoid extremely hot, spicy, acidic, coarse, or dry foods; tobacco; and alcohol. Commercial mouthwashes with alcohol, phenol, or astringents should also be avoided (Wescott, 1985).

Rinsing with a mixture of salt, sodium bicarbonate, and warm water (½ to 1 teaspoon of each in 1 quart of warm water) may provide some relief (McClure et al, 1987a; Sullivan and Fleming, 1986). This mixture should be used shortly after it is prepared, because the effervescence of the

Table 19-2. Agents used in the treatment of oral mucositis

Anesthetics	Coating agents
Dyclone hydrochloride 0.5%	Kaopectate
Benadryl-lidocaine solution	Maalox
Unflavored xylocaine HCl 2%	Mylanta
Tessalon Perles 100 mg/tab	Gelusil
Sucralfate suspension	

sodium bicarbonate lasts only about 20 minutes (McClure et al, 1987a). A solution of 0.5% hydrogen peroxide has also been suggested for cleaning oral tissues. Use of this agent should be limited to the removal of hardened debris attached to the dentition and debridement of acute periodontal infections. Long-term use may disrupt the normal oral flora. A 50% mixture by volume of Kaopectate and Benylin cough syrup may also soothe and reduce inflammation (Table 19-2) (Toth and Fleming, 1983; Toth and Frame, 1983).

Topical anesthetic preparations should be used in moderation. The irritating chemical qualities of many of these agents may intensify and prolong mucositis if they are used frequently or over a long period (Toth and Fleming, 1983; Toth and Frame, 1983). In a chronically ill patient who is unable to mobilize secretions, risk of aspiration is also of concern.

Radiation therapy for head and neck cancer frequently involves the major and minor salivary glands, resulting in partial or total loss of salivary flow (xerostomia), including changes in the quality and the quantity of saliva. Saliva may become thick and ropey, or its flow may be altered.

These changes usually begin 7 to 10 days after treatment begins and may become worse as treatment continues. They are usually irreversible (Sullivan and Fleming, 1986; Yasko and Greene, 1987). Some individuals may experience limited return of function within 6 to 12 months after treatment (Baum et al, 1985; Reynolds et al, 1980). Treatment of symptoms may need to continue indefinitely.

Patients treated with chemotherapy may also have xerostomia. However, this is a temporary condition, with normal function returning after the cessation of therapy (Vuolo, 1987). Treatment for drug-induced xerostomia and fluoride therapy to prevent xerostomia-related dental decay should be continued throughout chemotherapy and discontinued after normal salivary flow has returned and normal home care can be resumed.

Salivary changes can create problems for patients, the most serious of which is rampant dental caries. Other problems include inadequate digestion of starches; irritation of mucous membranes; difficulties with speech, taste, and nutrition; and problems with denture retention.

Suggested remedies for relief of xerostomia include use of artificial saliva preparations (e.g., Moi-Stir, Orex, Salivart, Xerolube) and frequent hydration with water. Use of sugarless mints, candy, or gum may also aid in stimulating salivary flow.

Patients can use a water-based lubricant (e.g., Surgilube, K-Y jelly, or hydrous lanolin), cocoa butter, or a lip balm to prevent drying and chapping (McClure et al, 1987a; Yasko and Greene,1987). Vaseline or petroleum jelly is anhydrous and will aggravate dryness (Barker, 1982; Debiase and Komives, 1983; Toth and Fleming, 1983; Toth and Frame, 1983). A cool mist vaporizer to increase room humidity and air filters to eliminate smoke may also help (Barker, 1982; Toth and Fleming, 1983; McClure et al, 1987a).

A special diet of foods from each of the food groups that are already moistened should be suggested to make chewing and swallowing easier. Patients should drink up to 8 to 10 glasses of water daily (Yasko and Greene, 1987). Resources are available to assist the patient in planning and preparing foods that are easy to eat and nutritious. Pamphlets containing additional suggestions are available from the American Cancer Society and the National Institutes of Health.

Many factors related to radiation therapy combine to favor development of rampant caries in patients. "Radiation caries" may appear as any combination of the following: (1) dark brown to black discolorations with no apparent demineralization, (2) cervical decay, which may encircle the entire tooth, or (3) decay that begins on the incisal or cuspal surfaces of the tooth (Reynolds et al, 1980). Radiation caries progresses rapidly and can occur at any time after the completion of therapy throughout the patient's lifetime. It can occur even in persons who have no history of decay if preventive methods are not employed both during and following radiation treatment. Xerostomia is a primary factor in the initiation of rampant decay. Changes in the quantity and viscosity of saliva decrease its lubrication and cleansing abilities. There is also a loss in the buffering effects of the saliva (its ability to neutralize acids), a reduction in output of the protective substances contained in saliva, and a decrease in remineralizing effect. Radiation treatment also initiates a shift in the bacterial flora of the mouth favoring the growth of cariogenic bacteria such as *Streptococcus mutans*. Increased bacterial acids reduce the pH of the saliva considerably. The patient's diet often contains less fiber and roughage because of the difficulty and pain of chewing these foods. Instead, the patient eats high-carbohydrate foods that are softer, easier to chew, and more adherent to the teeth. Prevention of rampant caries requires a rigorous program of strict oral hygiene and daily applications of fluoride. Patients should be taught proper and thorough means of mechanical plaque removal through use of a soft toothbrush, floss, and other appropriate aids. It should be impressed on patients that no amount of professional help can compensate for a lack of strict compliance in their own daily home care. Patients who cannot or will not exercise strict home care practices must be informed of the consequences. Development of rampant decay can destroy the existing teeth, and the resulting infections or treatment (e.g., extractions) can precipitate even more destruction as a result of osteoradionecrosis. The dentist may consider extraction of the teeth before therapy for patients with poor oral hygiene; this is done to eliminate the risks of further deleterious effects of the radiation therapy.

A second critical step in the prevention of radiation caries is daily use of a topical fluoride gel. Tested products of either 1% neutral sodium fluoride or 0.4% stannous fluoride gel unflavored have been recommended for this purpose (Ritchie et al, 1985; Rothwell, 1987; Schweiger and Salcetti, 1986; Sullivan and Fleming, 1986; Wescott, 1985; Wright, 1985). Selection of the product may be based on the pH that the patient can tolerate comfortably. Sodium fluoride gels have a higher pH than acidulated phosphate and stannous fluoride and are less likely to irritate inflamed tissues.

Place the fluoride in a custom-made vinyl tray. This ensures maximum adaptation of the gel to the tooth surfaces and minimizes leakage of the fluoride gel during the treatment. Trays should be applied once daily, preferably after the teeth have been cleaned, and left in place for a minimum of 5 to 10 minutes. After removal, the trays should be rinsed in cool water. The patient should expectorate excess fluoride and refrain from eating, rinsing, or drinking for at least 30 minutes to receive maximum benefit from the treatment. This method is recommended for patients with poor oral hygiene or those who suffer from moderate to severe xerostomia (Sullivan and Fleming, 1986). Depending on oral conditions, some patients may need to use topical fluorides more frequently than once a day, especially if decay is detected or if profound xerostomia exists. Use of a toothbrush or disposable sponge brush may also be indicated for fluoride application if the patient cannot tolerate fluoride trays. Sullivan and Fleming (1986) suggest an alternate method of fluoride therapy for patients who have excellent oral hygiene and minimal mouth dryness. Using a toothbrush, the patient should apply 0.4% stannous fluoride gel to all teeth for 1 minute. The solution should then be swished vigorously around the teeth, held in the mouth for 1 minute, and then expectorated. The patient should not eat, drink, or rinse for 30 minutes afterwards. Because this method of application may not allow the gel to contact the tooth surfaces directly for the recommended treatment time, it is not the method of choice for patients who show signs of beginning decay or for those with less than optimal oral hygiene.

Individuals suffering from radiation-induced xerostomia must continue daily fluoride treatments indefinitely. The conditions that render these patients susceptible to rampant caries are likely to be present for the rest of their lives.

Osteoradionecrosis (ORN). Osteoradionecrosis is the most serious complication of radiation therapy. When large doses of radiation are directed at bone, a number of changes occur. The blood supply to the bone is impaired, and the cells responsible for remodeling and repairing bone tissue are destroyed. Therefore irradiated bone tissue is much more susceptible to infection and has a reduced ability to repair and remodel itself after trauma. According to Marx (1983), ORN is a consequence of defective wound healing in which the tissue demands for oxygen, energy, and nutrients exceed the available supply.

After radiation therapy, this bone defect can occur spontaneously, although commonly it occurs as a result of trauma to the bone. It is characterized by acute inflammation and destruction.

Bone may be exposed to the oral cavity which causes severe pain.

This condition occurs more frequently in the mandible than the maxilla (Wescott, 1985) and represents permanent damage. Some cases of ORN have been reported to occur as long as 25 years after the actual radiation treatment (Westcott, 1985).

Osteoradionecrosis can have seemingly minor causes. Overzealous use of a toothbrush (Ritchie et al, 1985) or poorly fitting dentures can irritate the soft tissues to the extent that the underlying bone becomes infected. Destruction can also be precipitated by periodontal infections (Fattore, Strauss, and Bruno, 1987). Because of the possibility of introducing infection and the reduced healing capacity of irradiated bone, invasive dental procedures—including extractions, periodontal surgery, apicoectomies, or vigorous subgingival debridement—are strictly contraindicated for patients at risk of ORN.

Prevention begins before radiation therapy. Existing infections must be eliminated, and all conditions that could precipitate future infection of either soft or hard tissues must be controlled. The patient at risk must be educated about the potential for development of ORN, the seriousness of this side effect, and the importance of strict compliance with the recommended home care regimen to prevent dental infections. Patients who wear dental prostheses may be advised to wear them as little as possible during treatment and should be closely monitored to ensure that the prostheses do not cause any oral irritation.

If ORN does occur it should be managed as conservatively as possible, because surgical manipulation may make the situation worse. In addition to antibiotic therapy, good oral hygiene must be maintained; affected tissues can be irrigated with sterile saline solution and gently debrided to aid healing. Hyperbaric oxygen therapy has also been found to be useful for treatment of this condition (Myers and Marx, 1990). If conservative treatment fails to control the bone infection, radical resection of the affected jaw may be necessary to stop the destructive process (Wescott, 1985).

Loss of taste perception. A common side effect of radiation therapy, loss of taste perception usually begins during the second week of treatment. Damage to the taste buds and the microvilli of the tongue results in a loss of acuteness of the tastes of sweet, salty, bitter, and acidic sub-

stances. In many cases, this alteration is temporary, and varying degrees of taste perception return within a few months after the completion of therapy (Rothwell, 1987). Individuals who receive doses in excess of 6000 cGy may have a permanent problem (Friedman, 1990). This side effect contributes to a diminished appetite and thus poor nutrition. Individuals may also compensate for the loss of taste through overuse of salt, sugar, and other spices, which could compound other medical or dental problems (e.g., hypertension, dental caries, mucositis). Because proper nutrition is critical to the overall health and recovery of these patients, nutritional counselling is indicated. Zinc sulfate (220 mg tablets) twice daily with meals has been reported to improve taste sensation for some patients (Mossman and Henken, 1978; Silverman and Thompson, 1984).

Trismus. Irradiation of the temporomandibular joint or the muscles of mastication can cause muscle fibrosis and muscle spasms, which result in limitation of the patient's ability to open the mouth. This problem can prevent the patient from performing necessary oral hygiene and preventive procedures, and it interferes with eating. It can be treated by instructing the patient to perform a variety of exercises prescribed by the dental professional or a physical therapist.

Before treatment, the patient's maximal mouth opening should be measured and recorded. This measurement can then be used as a standard to identify a limitation of motion. Simple exercises to improve movement can be recommended such as opening the mouth to its maximum and then closing it 20 times in succession. This exercise should be repeated three times a day during and after radiation therapy (McClure et al, 1987b; Peterson, 1983). Another exercise is to insert a mouth prop (formed by putting several tongue blades together) between the teeth and then rotate the blades to gradually force the teeth further apart. This exercise should be repeated two to three times a day with more tongue blades added as needed (Rubin and Doku, 1976).

Sullivan and Fleming (1986) suggested two other exercises: placing the heel of both hands under the jaw and pushing up against the lower jaw while stretching the mouth open as wide as possible, and placing the middle and index fingers on the mandibular teeth and the thumb on the maxillary teeth and twisting the fingers to force the teeth apart for 2 seconds. This exercise should be performed ten times in succession with the right hand, then ten times with the left hand, and should be repeated four times daily.

Neuropathy. An oral side effect of chemotherapy is neuropathy. Certain drugs used in cancer therapy may affect nerve function in various parts of the body, including the oral cavity, causing symptoms of pain or numbness. Toxic effects of these drugs on the nerve tissues may result in the patient complaining of pain in the teeth, periodontium, or jaw for which no apparent cause is detected. Awareness of this complication and consultation with the oncologist will assist the dentist in diagnosing the source of the problem. Drug-induced neuropathy should cease after discontinuation of the drug.

Educating the cancer patient

The dental hygienist's most important role in helping patients who are about to undergo cancer therapy is that of educator and motivator. The hygienist should inform patients (or those responsible for their care) of the possible oral side effects of their treatment while emphasizing that not all individuals will experience the same side effects or to the same degree. The patient or care provider must also be taught how to prevent or alleviate these side effects effectively, and they must be motivated to comply with instructions. Cancer patients must understand the importance of their role in preventing or reducing oral complications and in preserving their general and oral health (Engelmeier, 1987).

Because of the emotional nature of their medical problem, these patients are likely to be distracted, confused, and fearful during consultation for dental treatment. Therefore it is wise to provide complete verbal instructions as well as written instructions for later reference.

Before therapy, patients should be instructed in a rigorous plaque control program to reduce inflammation. Patients should be shown sulcular brushing (the Bass method) using a soft-bristled nylon brush. Bristles can be softened further by rinsing or soaking them in hot water before use. After use, toothbrushes should be thoroughly rinsed and stored in a cool, dry area to reduce microbial contamination.

An approved fluoride dentifrice should be recommended. If tissue irritation is a problem during treatment, a less irritating preparation such as a baking soda paste or solution may be substituted. Proper use of dental floss and other interdental cleaning aids, as recommended by the hygienist, will help reduce bacterial plaque and control infection. Finger massage or rubber tip massage of gingival tissues may improve circulation following plaque removal. Oral irrigators may also be useful for cleansing and rinsing the mouth; these should be used on a low power setting (Rothwell, 1987; Yasko and Greene, 1987).

Home care procedures must be adapted for patients with compromised ability to fight infection, abnormal bleeding tendencies, or extreme oral discomfort. It has been recommended that a normally aggressive home care regimen is appropriate as long as the absolute neutrophil count is greater than $2,000/mm^3$ and platelet counts are greater than $20,000/mm^3$ (De Paola et al, 1986; Wright et al, 1985). Modifications in home care, however, are necessary if severe mucositis, low white blood cell counts, or spontaneous bleeding occur.

If use of a toothbrush is contraindicated, teeth can be cleaned using a 4- × 4-inch gauze sponge moistened with a sodium bicarbonate and water solution and wrapped around the finger. Disposable sponges (Toothettes) may also be used but are limited in effectiveness. These measures are also appropriate for individuals who are unable to tolerate the abrasiveness of a toothbrush. It has been suggested that lemon-glycerine swabs should not be used because they are anhydrous and can irritate friable tissues (Debiase and Komives, 1983). Flossing and use of any other sharp implement for plaque removal (e.g., toothpicks) should be discontinued until platelet counts return to normal. Dentures should be cleaned thoroughly every night with a stiff brush and soaked in a denture cleaning solution overnight.

Dentures should be thoroughly rinsed with water before being returned to the mouth to remove colonizing microorganisms. The container used for soaking should be cleaned daily and the solution replaced so that it does not serve as a bacterial reservoir.

Patients must also be educated regarding the need for frequent and regular recall appointments during and after their treatment to answer questions, provide additional remedies, and reinforce and monitor home care. Reinforcement is essential. Because many side effects of treatment are likely to be problems even after treatment for the cancer has been completed, continuous monitoring of the patient's oral health and prompt treatment of dental problems are important.

OLDER ADULTS

The percentage of elderly persons (65 years and older) in the United States population has been increasing steadily since 1900 and will increase even more dramatically in the years to come. In 1900 the elderly made up about 4% of the total population (US Senate, 1991). Since that time, birth rates and life expectancies have increased as a result of advances in science and medicine, improvements in health, and economic and environmental factors. In 1990 elderly persons comprised about 12.6% of the population (Aging America, 1991).

The percentage of elderly is predicted to rise to 13.0% by the year 2000 and then to 21.8% by the year 2030. Individuals born in the late forties and early fifties, known as the "baby boom" generation, will be reaching retirement age at that time. The youngest baby boomers will have passed their sixty-fifth birthday, and the number of people 85 and older will have grown from fewer than 600,000 in 1950 to over 8 million. The growth of this segment of the population indicates the need for society to redirect its focus towards the concerns and needs of the elderly. Health care providers must be aware of the needs of this population group and be prepared to meet the challenges of serving it.

It is a mistake to attempt to categorize or to stereotype all older adults as a homogeneous group in terms of their physical or mental capabilities. Older adults are unique as individuals and perhaps more heterogeneous as a group than any other age group. Aging is a great diversifier (Warren and Blandford, 1985). There is no such thing as a "typical" older adult, any more than there is a "typical" 18-year-old.

An important objective of this chapter is to impress the dental care professional with the understanding that all people, regardless of their special needs relative to age, physical condition or mental status, must be treated as unique persons rather than stereotyped because of one condition or situation affecting their lives. Although special needs can fall neatly into categories, people do not. The challenge to dental care professionals and to all health care providers is to meet the individual needs of each patient.

Physiologic changes related to aging

Warren and Blandford (1985) described aging as "a slow progressive decline in physiologic reserve during which the body loses some of its ability to adapt." Aging involves a complex interaction between the physiologic changes that occur as part of the aging process and age-related diseases. Multiple chronic diseases in older adults make them more vulnerable to stresses that would be considered minor in younger, healthier individuals.

Early studies of changes associated with "normal" aging indicated that changes often began in early adulthood but did not become functionally significant until the loss was fairly extensive. Andres and Tobin (1977) suggested that most organ systems seem to lose function at roughly 1% a year beginning around age 30. More recent studies (Svanborg, Bergstrom, and Mellstrom, 1982), in which the same people were followed longitudinally, suggest that the changes may be less dramatic and begin well after age 70.

Overall changes associated with aging are decreased height, weight, and total body water and increased fat-to-lean body mass ration (Kane, Ouslander, and Abrass, 1989). Sensory changes involve vision, hearing, taste, smell, and touch. The skin will exhibit increased wrinkling and atrophy of sweat glands. Functional changes in the cardiovascular system result in decreased cardiac output, decreased heart rate response to stress, and decreased compliance of peripheral blood vessels. The kidney has decreased creatinine clearance, renal blood flow, and maximum urine osmolality. In the respiratory system there is a decrease in vital capacity, maximal oxygen uptake, and the cough reflex. Changes in the gastrointestinal tract include decreased hydrochloric acid, saliva flow, and fewer taste buds. The immune system has decreased T-cell activity.

Though there may be some modest decrease in mental agility, most older adults remain alert with intact intellectual capabilities, sound judgment, and creativity in the absence of disease (Richardson, 1982). However, some declines in learning and memory are observed in most people after the age of 70 (Katzman and Terry, 1983).

The skeletal system may have some loss of bone substance and osteoarthritis. The endocrine system will show a decrease in free testosterone and an increase in insulin, norepinephrine, parathyroid hormone, and vasopressin.

Deterioration or debilitation often is attributed to physiologic changes when it is really caused by disease. For example, xerostomia (lack of salivary gland function) is a condition that is often present in older adults, but it is usually caused by pathologic changes or drug therapy rather than physiologic aging.

A genuine biologic outcome of aging can be distinguished from disease through the following criteria: (1) it is detectable in all human beings; (2) it occurs independent of outside influences; (3) it is progressive and irreversible in nature; and (4) it is harmful to survival (Viidik, 1986). When measured against these criteria, many conditions that were assumed to be part of normal aging are seen to be disease entities with a higher prevalence and incidence in the elderly.

Common diseases among older adults

The dental hygienist should expect that most of the elderly patients who seek dental care will be functioning at physical and mental levels comparable to those of other adult age groups. Dental care providers should assume that most older dental care consumers will be healthy and active, but that occasionally a patient will manifest significant changes in function or medical status that require modifications in the delivery of dental care.

Over the past 80 years the pattern of illness and disease has changed for older adults (US Senate, 1991). In the early 1900s acute conditions predominated, while today chronic conditions are the burden of older age. More than four out of five people age 65 or older have at least one chronic condition, and multiple conditions are common among older people, especially older women. In 1989 the leading chronic conditions were arthritis, hypertension, hearing impairments, and heart disease. The hygienist should be alert to those conditions which require medical consultation and prophylactic antibiotic premedication before dental treatment.

Heart disease accounts for more mortality and health care use by older adults than any other chronic condition. It is the leading cause of death and the leading diagnosis for short-term hospital visits for people over 65 (National Center for Health Statistics, 1985).

If the patient reports use of anticoagulant medications for treatment of cardiovascular problems, the patient's physician must be consulted before any treatment that could induce bleeding is performed, including periodontal probing and dental prophylaxis. Laboratory tests to determine bleeding time may also be indicated.

The second most common chronic condition is hypertension, which is the major risk factor for stroke, heart failure, and coronary artery disease. Individuals with a systolic blood pressure greater than 160 mm Hg and diastolic blood pressure greater than 95 mm Hg should be referred to their physician for further examination. In patients with severe hypertension, dental treatment should be postponed until the condition is under control. Drugs used to treat hypertension may also produce side effects, including xerostomia and postural hypotension.

Common nervous system disorders include cerebral vascular disease or stroke, development of tremors (Parkinson's disease) and dementias (Alzheimer's disease). Patients who have had a stroke may experience paralysis that affects their ability to move and walk. This disease may also affect their ability to understand others and to communicate their own thoughts. Home care instructions should be modified as appropriate so that these patients or those who care for them can perform effective oral hygiene procedures. Stroke patients may also be receiving anticoagulant therapy that requires special attention before dental treatment, as discussed previously. Persons with tremor disorders may have difficulty eating, which affects their overall nutritional status. They may also experience difficulty with performing daily oral hygiene procedures for themselves. While in the dental chair, these patients may have difficulty remaining still, swallowing, and keeping their mouths open.

A number of rheumatologic disorders are also prevalent in older adults including arthritis and osteoporosis. Arthritis affects the individual's ability to perform normal oral hygiene procedures and may require modifications of oral hygiene aids to facilitate their use. Some patients with severe osteoarthritis may have had joint replacement, and they should receive antibiotic premedication before dental treatment to prevent infection of those joints. Consultation with the patient's physician is recommended.

Osteoporosis is most common in postmenopausal women and leads to fractures of the long bones, the hip joint, and the vertebral bodies of the spine. Individuals suffering from osteoporosis need extra time for positioning. They may have difficulty remaining seated for long periods of time or may require extra cushioning while in the dental chair.

Hearing impairment, another common age-related problem, can occur as a result of both physiologic and pathologic changes. High-frequency hearing loss is first manifested near the age of 50 and is called presbycusis, or hearing loss of old age. Over age 65 approximately one fourth of the population has a clinically significant hearing loss (Horvath and Davis, 1990). Hearing disorders are probably the most common sensory disorder in older adults and require extra attention to communication skills by the dental professional.

For many of these patients, the hearing loss involves the frequency of different sounds rather than a loss of volume. High-pitched consonant sounds such as "k," "sh," "ch," "t," "p," "th," and "f" are difficult for these persons to distinguish. Raising one's voice may be helpful in some situations, but shouting is not. It is important to speak clearly and at a normal rate. Everyone finds it easier to converse when they can see the speaker's face. Instructing these individuals while seated in operating position at the side or rear of the dental chair or talking with a face mask in place makes it more difficult for them to understand. Reducing background noises—such as office music, ultrasonic scalers, dental drills, or suction devices—while speaking with the patient may improve communication. Patients who wear hearing aids may appreciate being advised when noisy equipment will be used so that they can adjust or remove their hearing aid rather than experience amplification of the noise.

Instructions should be written in large print for the patient whose vision is impaired. Vision problems including cataracts and glaucoma are common in older adults. Individuals with slight vision impairments may need more light to read or see demonstrations. Many cannot distinguish certain colors, especially blues, violets, and greens. Some may have difficulty perceiving distances and depths, especially in low-light environments. The eyes may require more time to adjust from high to low light intensities (Brock, 1985).

Drug use in older adults

Older adults are the biggest consumers of both prescription and nonprescription drugs within the population. Drug use increases with advancing age, with the average older person taking four or more drugs on a daily basis (Shapiro, 1986).

There are many problems associated with this high rate of drug use. Older adults are more susceptible to adverse drug interactions. Factors such as multiple drug use, age-related changes in bodily functions, and multiple illnesses all have the potential to interfere with the predicted action of a given drug in an older adult. Depending on the specific medical and drug history of the individual, the absorption, distribution, effects, metabolism, and excretion of drugs can be altered in older adults. Therefore, a complete medical and drug history is required (see Chapter 6).

If the dentist determines that drugs should be prescribed in the course of dental treatment, the patient should be completely informed as to its purpose, how it should be used, and its possible side effects. For older adults, instructions for use should also be communicated in writing and sent home with the patient. Since many older adults have difficulty managing containers with child-proof caps, that type of container should not be used.

Psychologic aspects of aging

Erik Erikson (1982) believed that every human being works through certain psychosocial stages during a lifetime of development from child to adult. He categorized these eight stages using terms that represent opposite ends of a continuum of development of the following life attitudes: (1) trust versus mistrust, (2) autonomy versus shame, (3) initiative versus guilt, (4) industry versus inferiority, (5) identity versus identity confusion, (6) intimacy versus isolation, (7) generativity versus stagnation (self-absorption), and (8) integrity versus despair.

By the time adults reach old age, they have spent a lifetime developing their social and personal identities. Old age often brings a series of losses or limitations in their lives, including loss of health, spouse, family, friends, work and career, income, and sometimes even loss of the independence to direct their own lives. These losses can contribute to an individual's perception that many of the accomplishments and developments of a lifetime are now being slowly taken away. This results in loss of identity and feelings ranging from anxiety, frustration, and confusion to depression, withdrawal, and anger. If the individual cannot adapt to these changes and resolve them to maintain a sense of identity and worth, the resulting conflict may cause a slipping away from the psychologic goals achieved in adulthood and a return to a more childlike outlook on life.

Of course, not all older adults will have difficulty in all areas, but the unique situations of each person's life combined with the individual's personality will affect how he or she handles these changes psychologically. Erikson's descriptions of developmental stages in terms of these bipolar attitudes of psychologic and social identity provide a useful framework for understanding how the individual may be affected by the losses and limitations that often accompany aging.

Trust versus mistrust. Older adults may have learned through a lifetime of experiences that there are some people who should not be trusted. As a result, they may "test" people before being able to trust them. Health care workers must demonstrate their trustworthiness to gain the cooperation and respect of these individuals.

Autonomy versus shame and doubt. Most adults have developed a valued sense of control over themselves and their lives. With aging, they may experience a loss of control in their lives. Losses extend to their life-style, income, health, family, friends, and a sense of being able to control their own fate. Instead of making their own choices, choices are made for them. This loss of independence can result in any number of negative feelings. Older adults need to feel that they have control over the decisions and the events that surround their dental treatment.

Initiative versus guilt. As children mature, they develop a sense of initiative toward behaviors and establish a conscience about their actions. If they perceive that their behaviors are "bad," feelings of guilt emerge. When initiative is blocked in older adults, feelings of apathy or frustration are likely to occur. They now must learn to conform to the expectations of others who are assisting them with their care and may feel "bad" or guilty if they attempt to exercise their own initiative and, as a result, displease those whose expectations were not met. Older adults should be encouraged to try new things and to exercise initiative in their lives without fear of reprisal or remediation.

Industry versus inferiority. As children become workers they become involved in producing rather than just consuming. They gain recognition for work and learn to work cooperatively and productively with other people. When older adults are no longer employed or find that they can no longer perform many of the tasks that made them feel productive, they may develop feelings of uselessness or of being a "burden" to others around them. Every adult needs to feel worthwhile and to

experience recognition for his or her efforts, yet these needs are often overlooked in the elderly. As a result, older adults may develop feelings of inferiority.

Identity versus identity confusion. A central task for all adults is to move through the process of acquiring a sense of identity that defines who they are and their place in society. Older adults may experience a loss of identity as a result of isolation from social contacts, loss of control over their lives, and loss of privacy. In the dental office, the staff should not converse with a family member about the older adult's care or refer to him or her using third-person pronouns (he, she) as if the person were not present. Use of first names or pet names may represent a lack of respect for the person's seniority.

Intimacy versus isolation. Once people have established their own identity they can begin to invest time and energy in developing intimate relationships and commitments to others. The older adult may become isolated from those with whom he or she has established intimate relationships, including family, friends, and coworkers. If new relationships and friendships are not formed, the result is isolation, self-absorption, and loss of ego. Many older adults enjoy the dental visit because it provides a source of social contact. Dental professionals should understand this need for contact and be interested and willing listeners.

Generativity versus stagnation (self-absorption). Generativity involves a person's concern for participation in the process of establishing and guiding the next generation. This process includes teaching one's own children or other young persons about the lessons of life and therefore contributing to their understanding and ability to deal with life situations. When older adults perceive that no one is interested in them, their knowledge, or their expertise, they can become bored, introverted, or withdrawn. They need opportunities to share their memories and experiences and to feel that something valuable can be learned from them.

Integrity versus despair. Integrity refers to a person's ability to accept that one has only one lifetime and that the events of the past were significant and meaningful. People who have developed integrity feel satisfied with their lives and can look back on life and feel no regrets; those who are despairing feel like saying, "If only I could start all over." As adults age, they have more and more time for introspection: for examining life, putting it into perspective, and coming to conclusions about how they have spent their time. These individuals need support as they work through this task, and they may need to talk and have someone listen as they attempt to sort out these issues.

• • •

An understanding of the relationship between a person's psychologic needs and development and the aging process is important for understanding the implications of our behaviors and attitudes as health care providers for the elderly. The dental hygienist should analyze each of the concepts discussed in terms of how they may affect the approach to providing dental hygiene treatment and patient education to older adults in a manner that will maximize their positive psychologic perceptions of themselves.

Dental needs of older adults

Older adults have a higher level of unmet dental needs than any other age group (Tyron, 1981). One encouraging trend is that edentulism rates are decreasing, meaning that people are retaining more of their teeth later in life. Recent data confirm that the prevalence of edentulism in the United States has continued to decline since the 1950s and that this trend can be expected to continue (Douglas and Gammon, 1985; Ismail et al, 1987). This trend results primarily from increased exposure to preventive measures and dental treatment. It also indicates, however, that significantly more teeth will be at risk for dental diseases in elderly populations.

Although the rate of edentulism is declining, the treatment needs and education needs of the edentulous population are still significant problems. The 1986 National Survey of Adult Health found that the prevalence of edentulism in the older adult U.S. population was 41% (National Institute for Dental Research, 1987). Warren and Blandford (1985) reported that 90% of those over 65 are partially edentulous. These individuals require regular dental examinations to evaluate their partial and complete dentures for proper fit, to examine soft tissues for the presence of disease, and to reinforce instructions for appliance care and oral hygiene.

The need for periodontal services for older adults will continue to escalate because of the decrease in edentulism and the increased retention of natural teeth (Suzuki, Niessen, and Fedele, 1991). Periodontal disease is estimated to affect 90% of the elderly who have natural teeth (Ettinger and Beck, 1982). Holm-Pedersen, Agerbaek, and Therlade (1975) demonstrated that the periodontal tissues of the older adult are more susceptible to microbial-related inflammation than those of younger individuals. They also found that older adults tend to accumulate more plaque and to develop gingivitis more rapidly and more severely. Greater plaque retention may be caused by gingival recession, resulting in exposure of more tooth structure and the increased difficulty of maintaining oral hygiene in these areas. Other factors affecting gingivitis in older adults may include medications and nutrition-deprivation states (Suzuki, Niessen, and Fedele, 1991). Page (1984), however, cautioned that even though older adults manifest more clinical evidence of periodontal destruction, these conditions may result from the cumulative effect of periodontal disease progression, rather than from enhanced susceptibility to the disease caused by aging. Furthermore, it is still not certain that this increased susceptibility actually results in higher prevalence and severity of active periodontitis in older adults (Page, 1984).

Recent studies indicate a low prevalence of advanced periodontal disease in older adults, while their prevalence and severity of moderate periodontal breakdown is relatively high (Hunt, Levy, and Beck, 1990; National Institute for Dental Research, 1987). A primary variable in the periodontal disease equation is oral hygiene, not necessarily age (Suzuki, Niessen, and Fedele, 1991). However, it is generally more difficult for older adults to practice effective self-care because of functional limitations such as those resulting from arthritis, stroke, or other debilitating disease. The preventive actions of the elderly may also be hindered by lack of understanding of the importance of preventive care or lack of knowledge regarding available preventive measures.

Dental caries continues into old age (Banting, 1991). However, coronal caries in the elderly is manifested primarily as secondary decay rather than primary decay (Goldberg et al, 1980; Banting, 1991).

Adults who have exposed root surfaces as a result of loss of periodontal attachment are also at increased risk of root caries. This is most commonly found on molar teeth, especially mandibular molars (Banting, 1991). It is generally agreed that prevalence rates increase with age, making root caries more common in the elderly (Banting, 1991; Beck, 1984).

Though the exact cause of root caries has not yet been established, it is generally agreed that unique interactions of diet and bacterial plaque are important factors. In addition, certain potential risk factors have been identified (Beck, 1990). The number of periodontal pockets greater than 3 mm and the number of teeth previously experiencing root caries were predictors. Onset of illness during the past year, current and former smoking status, and the use of smokeless tobacco were all positively associated with root caries. Measures of anxiety and the level of a person's social integration and social support were also associated with the incidence of root caries.

Currently recommended measures for prevention of root caries in older adults include elimination of the parasite, increasing the resistance of the host, and reducing the availability of substrate for the parasite (Banting, 1991). Elimination of the parasite can be achieved by most older adults with normal oral hygiene procedures. For those who cannot adequately perform these procedures, a chlorhexidine rinse may be recommended. Banting, Bosma, and Bollmer (1989) found a 35% reduction in supragingival plaque in adults using a 0.12% rinse twice daily over 2 years compared to controls. Fluoride has been effective in preventing root caries as well as coronal caries (Seichter, 1987). Root caries has been less prevalent in populations that benefit from fluoridated water supplies compared to those living in nonfluoridated areas (Stamm et al, 1980). Topical fluoride application in conjunction with recontouring and smoothing of shallow areas of root caries has been proposed as an acceptable alternative to restorative treatment in some cases. For patients with recurrent coronal caries, a regimen of semiannual topical application of 1.23% acidulated phosphate fluoride or 2.0% sodium fluoride gel is recommended. The recommendation for new or recurrent root caries is a semiannual topical application of 5.0% sodium fluoride varnish. For rampant coronal or root caries, the recommendation is a quarterly topical application of 5.0% sodium fluoride varnish and a daily 0.2% sodium fluoride rinse (Banting, 1991).

The role of diet and reduced salivary flow is also important in the caries process and should be included in a preventive program for older adults. Prevention of periodontal disease is the best means of preventing root caries.

Oral cancer is also prevalent in older adults. Cancer is the second leading cause of death in individuals aged 55 and over, with heart disease being the number one cause of death. Silverman and Greenspan (1985) reported that about 95% of all oral cancers occur in persons over 40 years old and that the average age at the time of diagnosis is about 60. The elderly account for nearly 50% of all oral cancer cases reported annually in the United States (Baranovsky and Myers, 1986).

Oral cancer occurs more frequently in men than in women at a ratio of about 2:1. The tongue is the most frequent site of oral cancer, followed by the lip, oropharynx, and the floor of the mouth. About 95% of all oral cancers are squamous cell carcinomas (Silverman, 1985).

Hygienists can perform a valuable function by educating elderly patients about the need for regular oral examinations. This must occur not only in the private dental office but also through community-wide efforts. Hygienists and dentists must promote preventive dental care for the elderly through educational in-services at retirement homes, nursing homes, and other institutions that serve the needs of the elderly. Educational programs should be presented in community centers that provide social activities and/or nutritional services to older adults. Oral cancer screenings can also be scheduled at these sites or at community health fairs through the combined efforts of dentists and hygienists. Effective use of mass media (newspaper, radio, and television) is another excellent way to promote the message that preventive oral care can help preserve the health and well-being of dental consumers of all ages.

Use of dental care by older adults

In spite of the tremendous need for dental care, use patterns for older adults reflect fewer regular dental visits than other segments of the population. Data from the National Survey of Oral Health in U.S. Employed Adults and Seniors indicated that in 1985 only 37.46% of adults aged 65 years and over who visited senior centers had gone to a dentist within 1 year, compared with 58.54% of employed adults.

However, the demand for dental care among socially active older adults may be increasing.

Edentulous persons are less likely to have regular dental visits than those who have teeth. Dentate individuals are four times more likely to have visited a dentist yearly than those who are edentulous (Ismail et al, 1983).

The National Institute for Dental Research (1987) also indicated that only 21% of the seniors mentioned "regular checkup" as the main reason for the last visit for dental care, compared with 41% of employed adults. There are a number of reasons why older adults do not use regular dental care, including the cost of dental care, the priority of dental care compared to other needs, lack of accessibility or availability of dental services, lack of perceived need on the part of consumers, negative attitudes on the part of both consumers and providers, and medical and psychologic problems of the elderly.

Only 36% of the seniors felt they needed dental treatment in one survey (National Institute for Dental Research, 1987). The issues of the perceived need for dental care, the perceived accessibility of dental care, and the priority assigned to dental care compared with other basic needs are all closely related to the cost of dental care. Dental care is expensive for older adults on a fixed income, and it must usually be paid for from out-of-pocket funds. Most older adults who may have previously enjoyed dental coverage from private insurance plans when they were employed are no longer covered by these plans. Of the two primary public assistance programs, Medicare offers no coverage for routine dental care, and coverage of dental services under Medicaid programs is extremely limited. The end result is that many older adults perceive that the cost of routine dental care makes it less accessible than other types of medical care and assign a lower priority to dental needs compared with other basic needs of living (Antczak and Branch, 1985; Blau, 1982; Bomberg and Ernst, 1986; Gooch and Berkey, 1987; Marinelli et al, 1982).

Some may not seek dental care because they perceive a lack of respect and consideration for their needs on the part of dental professionals. Studies have shown that medical, dental, and nursing students believe the erroneous and stereotypical myths about aging (Bomberg and Ernst, 1986). Solomon and Vickers (1979) noted that people hold these stereotypes regardless of socioeconomic or occupational status or age and despite the increasing amount of factual information

available regarding older adults. These myths include: most older adults are senile, frail, and dependent; aging is a "second childhood"; most old people live below the poverty level; people become less intelligent as they age; most older adults are institutionalized; "you can't teach an old dog new tricks"; and the elderly can no longer be creative, productive, and self-sufficient members of society.

Many older adults do not seek dental care because they do not feel that they have dental problems, or they believe that dental problems are an unavoidable consequence of aging or that their dental problems cannot be corrected.

Ettinger and Beck (1982) noted that the social, cultural, and historical experiences of the "old elderly" (75 years and over) led to the ideas that dentistry is a luxury and that loss of teeth is an expected and inevitable part of growing old. The concept of prevention of oral diseases was unknown to these individuals.

In contrast, the "new elderly" (aged 60 to 64) grew up in an environment that allowed them to be better informed, resulting in greater demand for prevention. The economic prosperity of the 1950s and improvements in dental technology also helped.

Ettinger and Beck went on to predict that the more positive attitudes of the "new elderly" towards dental care, coupled with the fact that more of them have retained more of their natural teeth, will result in an increase in the demand for dental services among this group.

Dental hygiene treatment planning for older adults

Appointment scheduling. When scheduling appointments for older adult patients, consider their health status and stamina. Whenever possible, schedule appointments for midmorning, when the patient's energy reserves are highest. Patients who are physically debilitated, those with serious medical problems, or those with short attention spans or who exhibit restlessness should be scheduled for several short appointments rather than longer ones. Appointments should not interfere with eating schedules of diabetic patients or those whose meals are provided only at certain times. Patients with arthritis may need late-morning appointments to limber up before the dental appointment. Some patients may not want to drive or take public transportation during busy traffic periods or after dusk. Schedules may also need to be coordinated with individuals who drive the patient to the office.

Medical and dental history. Obtaining and discussing the medical history is often the dental professional's first opportunity to establish effective rapport with the elderly patient. Bomberg and others (1985) noted that clinical success with an elderly patient depends more on the ability to communicate empathy for the patient through a positive attitude of caring and concern than on either clinical competence or technical skills.

A careful medical and drug history is imperative when treating older adult patients. Because some patients may not remember the exact names and dosages of their medications, suggest they bring the containers with them to the initial appointment or write down the information. Questions regarding the health history that the patient does not recall or cannot answer may be referred to family or friends or the patient's physician. Conditions that may contraindicate dental treatment should be discussed with the physician. It is also important to obtain a dental history from the patient or care provider to determine previous dental experiences and attitudes toward dental treatment.

Oral examination. An examination should be performed in the same way as for any individual but with particular care for the fragility of oral tissues and alertness to oral conditions that are more prevalent in older adults.

The patient should be taught how to examine his or her own oral structures properly. (See Chapter 8). The importance of regular professional examinations of hard and soft tissues of the mouth should also be stressed, especially for edentulous patients who may think they need not seek dental care.

It is important to determine how adequately the patient will be able to perform oral hygiene techniques as part of the oral examination. Older adult patients may be classified into the following categories for the purpose of developing oral hygiene care plans (McLeran, 1982):

Category I

Patient is completely self-sufficient and able to perform all oral hygiene techniques with the possible exception of flossing and other skills requiring fine motor skills. Mentally alert and able to comprehend and demonstrate motivation to perform hygiene procedures.

Category II

Patient is self-sufficient but unable to adequately perform techniques due to arthritis, limited range of motion, or limited use of hands. Needs some assistance. Mentally alert but may exhibit depression, forgetfulness, or little interest in self-care.

Category III

Patient is unable to care for daily needs and is dependent on others to perform oral hygiene procedures. Can cooperate with the caretaker but is mentally unable to comprehend or communicate; unable to care for self.

Category IV

Comatose patient; completely dependent.

Oral hygiene care plans. After completing the oral examination, the dental hygienist can develop an oral hygiene care plan (OHCP). The OHCP is essential for maintaining oral hygiene in the older adult patient.

In a private practice, the care plan should be given to the patient in writing (large print) and should contain clear and concise messages.

In a nursing home the OHCP will be incorporated into the patient's chart and can be referred to by the nursing home staff. Care plans are a part of each patient's record and provide specific instructions about the patient's daily care such as medications, physical therapy, and daily needs. Most care plans do not include oral hygiene needs; therefore a specific OHCP must be developed.

Oral hygiene care plans will differ significantly for each category of patient. The OHCP for a patient in Category I may not differ from that for a patient in other age groups if the patient has reasonable dexterity.

Communication with the older adult is one of the most important aspects in developing a care plan. The first essential point is that the dental hygienist must take time to LISTEN to complaints and accounts of past experiences. Sit at eye level and speak slowly and directly to the patient in a distinct voice. Look at the patient while speaking, since many are lip-readers. Provide the patient with eyeglasses while giving instructions and suggest they wear glasses when performing plaque control procedures. A magnifying mirror may also be helpful. Make suggestions gradually over a series of appointments. It is important not to institute a completely new method; rather, try to adapt a practice the patient is already using.

Older adult patients need to be encouraged and helped to gain a sense of accomplishment. They should be commended for any success, however minor, and rewarded with praise. Above all, the practitioner needs to have an optimistic attitude about the degree of oral health that the older adult patient can be expected to achieve.

Patients in Category II will vary greatly in their ability to be self-sufficient, depending on the nature of their disability. For some, adaptations to oral hygiene aids can make them totally self-sufficient, such as modified toothbrush handles or the use of electric toothbrushes. It may be necessary to include some help from a caregiver in the OHCP.

For patients in Category III, the OHCP will need to be developed for the caregiver; however, it is important to include the patient. The patient needs to feel a part of the planning process and to understand the rationale for the care plan to ensure cooperation.

Special procedures need to be implemented for patients in Category IV—the unconscious or acutely ill patient. The caregiver needs to understand how important oral hygiene procedures can be to the patient.

Patient education. Preventive education is especially important for people in this age group, because they may not have grown up with preventive attitudes. Because more and more older adults will be retaining their natural teeth, preventive strategies should be designed to reduce the risk of dental caries and periodontal disease. Awareness includes recognizing the signs of dental disease in one's own mouth as well as understanding what has caused it. Explanations should avoid complicated terminology. Emphasizing the positive aspects of preventive behaviors is more likely to create patients' interest in themselves than emphasizing negative possibilities. Motivating techniques should therefore stress the positive outcomes of healthy behavior rather than focus on the consequences of disease and the patient's own fears.

Older adults should be approached with the expectation that they are intelligent, responsible, and capable. It is also important for older adults to believe in their own abilities to be self-sufficient and to provide care for themselves. Encouraging them to depend on others for care decreases their self-esteem and sense of independence. Ignoring these abilities in older adults and treating

them or communicating with them as if they were dependent children is known as "infantilization." This process can lead to a loss of perceived ability on the part of the individual and result in a vicious cycle in which individuals become less competent and self-sufficient because that is the perceived expectation of those around them (Dolinsky and Dolinsky, 1984).

Techniques should be demonstrated in the patient's mouth and then by the patient under the hygienist's supervision. Techniques should be observed and reinforced to ensure that they are being performed properly. If the older adult is being assisted with oral health care, follow the same procedures with the person assisting.

Replacing old habits with new ones is difficult for an individual of any age. It requires patience and reinforcement. The hygienist must constantly evaluate the patient's progress and assess the reasons for lack of improvement in oral health. It is important to try to provide some positive comments before telling the patient how to improve. Failure to improve oral health through the use of self-care methods may be attributed to lack of motivation, lack of understanding or improper technique, or instructions that were not clear and concise.

Physically debilitating conditions may not permit use of normal oral hygiene aids. The hygienist should suggest appropriate modifications of the devices or a novel method of use that will compensate for the patient's problem. Manual toothbrushes may need to be modified to improve the access of the brush to all areas of the mouth. Dental floss is a valuable aid for removing plaque between the teeth; however, many older adult patients with dexterity problems will find floss difficult to use even with a floss holder, and tissue damage can result if floss is not used properly. For these reasons, flossing is generally not recommended unless the patient has the dexterity and can demonstrate the proper use. Flossing should be encouraged for patients who are sufficiently dextrous. Some patients may find the wider dental tape, the interproximal brush, yarn, or a pipe cleaner easier to use. Electric toothbrushes may also be helpful for these persons. Use of a pulsating oral irrigator may help in the control of supragingival and loosely attached subgingival plaque. Plaque control can be further enhanced through the supplemental use of tested antiplaque agents such as chlorhexidine, sanguinarine, sodium benzoate, and fluoride rinses and gels. These products can be used as mouthrinses or diluted in oral irrigators as additional measures of plaque control (see Chapter 28).

Treatment planning. Gordon and Sullivan (1986) proposed that each of the following factors should be evaluated when formulating treatment plans for older adult and/or compromised patients:

1. How the current dental situation affects the patient's quality of life.
2. Whether the current situation is likely to get better, worse, or remain the same without treatment.
3. The patient's desire for dental treatment.
4. The potential for additional medical or dental problems as a result of treatment.
5. The amount of time required to complete treatment and the length of time the treatment is expected to last.
6. The limitations of the dentist in terms of technique, equipment, and access to the patient.

After evaluating each of these factors, the dental hygienist presents as many viable treatment alternatives as possible to the patient or the patient's guardian. The clinician explains the benefits as well as the limitations or risks of each alternative so that the responsible party can give informed consent for the selected treatment plan.

Dental prophylaxis. Thorough debridement is an important part of preventive dental treatment and maintenance for older adults. Removal of supragingival and subgingival deposits is important in controlling and maintaining health. History of periodontal disease may result in oral conditions that challenge the hygienist, including gingival recession, pocket formation, root sensitivity, furcation involvement, tooth mobility, and other associated conditions. The esthetics of a dental prophylaxis are as important to an elderly patient as to a younger one.

There is no conclusive evidence that older persons have either a greater or lesser sensitivity to pain than their younger counterparts (Chapman, 1984). Therefore do not assume that older adult patients are likely to be more or less sensitive to the pain of treatment than anyone else simply because of their age. The need for careful manipulation of soft tissues during debridement is as important in these patients as in any other.

Nonsurgical periodontal treatment may be the treatment of choice in older adult patients who either cannot withstand surgical treatment or who are poor medical risks for such treatment. Because many reports indicate that periodontal disease can often be treated as successfully by nonsurgical means as by surgical interventions, thorough debridement can be an important part of periodontal therapy for elderly patients.

Individual assessments should be made as to the amount and length of treatment that should be rendered at any one sitting. The patient's comfort and ability to tolerate treatment procedures should be carefully considered when the treatment plan for each appointment is determined.

Use of fluorides. The use of professional and home fluoride therapy should be based on the same criteria for older adult patients as for other patients. Presence of primary, secondary, or root caries and reports of root sensitivity are all indications for active fluoride therapy. Selection of the type of fluoride to use should be based on the individual's unique dental needs.

Fluoride is an important part of the preventive regimen for dental caries in adults as well as in children. Both topical and systemic delivery of fluoride to susceptible tooth surfaces are effective means of preventing dental decay. Topical fluoride in the form of gels, varnishes, rinses, or dentifrices can play a significant role for the caries-prone older patient (Rounds and Papas, 1991). Studies have shown that daily application of a 1% fluoride gel can produce significant levels of remineralization and may be recommended for the older adult who is experiencing increased caries activity.

Determination of continuing care intervals. Regular dental visits for health monitoring and prevention are as important to older adults as to any other age group. Decisions about the amount of time between preventive visits should be based on the patient's current periodontal status, ability to control plaque through chemical and mechanical measures, and ability to gain access to dental treatment (e.g., transportation, mobility, financial considerations). Research has shown that the most beneficial recall interval for patients with periodontal disease activity is no longer than 3 months. Patients who have difficulty maintaining satisfactory plaque control may need to return for more frequent professional maintenance than those whose plaque control is optimal (see Chapter 38).

ACTIVITIES

1. Invite a panel of pedodontists and dental hygienists who work with children to discuss management of behavior problems associated with fear or resistance to care.
2. Prepare a report of the causes and characteristics of pregnancy gingivitis.
3. Invite a clinician who works with handicapped patients in private practice or in an institutional setting to discuss practical modifications in care.
4. Experience sensory deprivation during a clinic or classroom session by dimming the lights, wearing waxed paper over the lenses of prescription or safety glasses, wearing gloves, and putting cotton in your ears. After being a patient or a student under these conditions, discuss what frustrations you experienced as a result of the sensory deprivations. Relate these frustrations to those which an elderly or disabled patient might experience during treatment or patient education.
5. Review the "gate control theory," which describes the psychologic and physiologic transmission of pain, in Melzack R, Wall PD: *The challenge of pain,* New York, 1982, Basic Books.
6. Design a detailed shaping procedure for a dental phobic who needs a complete examination and dental prophylaxis. Specify each step and the criteria that will be followed in deciding to introduce the patient to each subsequent step. Use your knowledge of behavior modification in designing the procedure.
7. Prepare a report describing the types of sedatives or analgesics that can be used to help control fear, pain, or lack of cooperation among special patients. Identify risk factors and advantages of each. Detail precautions that must be taken when working with patients who have received each medication.
8. Make arrangements to visit a nursing home or retirement center. During your visit participate as a volunteer in assisting the older adults or interacting with them during social activities. Observe the atmosphere. Talk to staff members about different daily or weekly activities. If possible, discuss dental care with the dental consultant or members of the staff.
9. Ask to accompany a home health nurse or public health nurse on home visits in your community. Consult with the clients about their dental health needs and with the nurses regarding their assessment of the clients' oral health needs.
10. Invite a radiation therapist, maxillofacial surgeon, or oncologist to discuss procedures for management of complications arising from cancer therapy.
11. Increase your awareness of the achievements of older adults in society by looking for examples of individuals over the age of 65 who are still active contributors in the fields of politics, education, business, the arts, religion, or science. Get examples from newspapers, magazines, books, television, and movies.
12. Before class discussion, write down your answers to Palmor's Facts of Aging Quiz (1988). Use the answers to discuss the myths and stereotypes that society associates with aging. Discuss possible reasons for some of these attitudes and how they may affect the delivery of dental care to the elderly.
13. The American Dental Hygienists' Association curriculum guide *Dental Hygiene Care for the Geriatric Patient* provides ideas for class activities to help develop skills related to caring for elderly persons.
14. Review the American Association of Dental Schools' Geriatric Curriculum Resource Book for Dental and Dental Hygiene Educators. It contains 24 curriculum modules with lecture outlines, bibliography, activities, and assignments (AADS, 1990).

REVIEW QUESTIONS

1. True or false: If a child is reluctant to cooperate in receiving care, it is best to send the child home and suggest that he or she return when older.
2. In working with a patient who is new to dentistry (whether an adult or a child), it is wise to introduce the patient slowly with a thorough explanation of procedures. Give an example.
3. Describe several modifications in communication that are appropriate for treating a patient who is visually handicapped.
4. List four (or more) implements that can be used to ensure safe delivery of care for a mobile patient.
5. Identify several different modifications of treatment that should be assessed before treating the elderly patient.
6. At what age should a child first see a dentist or hygienist?
7. Should a child's teeth be polished as part of a dental hygiene appointment?
8. What type of brushing tool modification would be appropriate for a patient with limited arm movement?
9. List three areas of patient education to cover with a pregnant patient.
10. Which side effects of radiation therapy for cancer are permanent problems that require life-long preventive measures?
11. What remedies can be suggested for patients who suffer from xerostomia?
12. Describe the recommendations for topical fluoride therapy for patients undergoing radiation therapy.
13. State reasons why a complete drug history is an

important part of the assessment of older adult dental patients.

14. What dental problems are more prevalent in older adult populations than in their younger counterparts?

15. What three roles can a dental hygienist perform in a nursing home or other institutional setting?

16. Describe modifications in oral hygiene procedures for unconscious or bedridden patients.

REFERENCES

Aisner J, Schiffer CA, Wiernik PH: *Cell support*. In Spivak S, editor: *Fundamentals of clinical hematology,* Hagerstown, Md, 1980, Harper & Row.

American Academy of Pediatric Dentistry reference manual, 1991-92, Chicago, The Academy.

American Cancer Society: *Cancer facts and figures,* Atlanta, 1992, The Society.

Andlaw RJ, Rock WP: *A manual of paedodontics,* New York, 1987, Churchill Livingstone.

Andres R, Tobin JD: Endocrine systems. In Fince CE, Hayflick L, editors: *Handbook of the biology of aging,* New York, 1977, Van Nostrand Reinhold.

Antczak AA, Branch AA: Perceived barriers to the use of dental services by the elderly, *Gerodontics* 1:194, 1985.

Bailey BE: *Psychological management of the pedodontic patient*. In Boundy SS, Reynolds NJ, editors: *Current concepts in dental hygiene,* vol 2, St Louis, 1979, CV Mosby.

Banting DW: *Management of dental caries in the older patient*. In Papas AS, Niessen LC, Chauncey HH: *Geriatric dentistry: aging and oral health,* St Louis, 1991, CV Mosby.

Banting DW, Bosma M, Bollmer B: Clinical effectiveness of a 0.12% chlorhexidine mouthrinse over two years, *J Dent Res* 86 (special issue):1716, 1989.

Baranovsky A, Myers MH: Cancer incidence and survival in patients 65 years of age and older, *CA* 36:26, 1986.

Barker G: Radiation therapy to the head and neck, *Dent Hyg News,* 4:4, 1991.

Baum BJ et al: Therapy-induced dysfunction of salivary glands: implications for oral health, *Spec Care Dent* 5:274, 1985.

Beck J: The epidemiology of root surface caries, *J Dent Res,* 69:1216, 1990.

Beck JD: The epidemiology of dental diseases in the elderly, *Gerodontology* 3:5, 1984.

Blau ZS: Socioeconomic variations in dental status and behavior of today's elderly, *Spec Care Dent* 2:244, 1982.

Bloom HG, Hanham IF, editors: *Head and neck oncology,* New York, 1987, Raven Press.

Bodey GP et al: Quantitative relationships between circulating leukocytes and infection in patients with acute leukemia, *Ann Intern Med* 64:328, 1966.

Bomberg TJ, Ernst NS: Improving utilization of dental care services by the elderly, *Gerodontics* 2:57, 1986.

Bomberg TJ et al: Developing the health history of the elderly patient, *Gerodontics* 1:165, 1985.

Brock AM: Communicating with the elderly patient, *Spec Care Dent* 5:157, 1985.

Chapman CR: Pain perception in the elderly patient: an overview of the issues, *Gerodontology* 3:71, 1984.

Chen TY: Radiation. In Carl W, Sako K, editors: *Cancer and the oral cavity,* Chicago, 1986, Quintessence.

Cheney HG, DePaola DP: *Preventive dentistry,* Littleton, Mass, 1979, PSG/Wright.

Debiase CB, Komives BK: An oral care protocol for leukemic patients with chemotherapy-induced oral complications, *Spec Care Dent* 3:207, 1983.

DePaola LG et al: Dental care for patients receiving chemotherapy, *JADA* 112:198, 1986.

DePaola LG et al: Prosthodontic considerations for patients undergoing cancer chemotherapy, *JADA* 107:48, 1983.

Dolinsky EH, Dolinsky HB: Infantilization of elderly patients by health care providers, *Spec Care Dent* 4:150, 1984.

Douglass CW, Gammon MD: Implications of oral disease trends for the treatment needs of older adults, *Gerodontics* 1:51, 1985.

Engelmeier RL: A dental protocol for patients receiving radiation therapy for cancer of the head and neck, *Spec Care Dent* 7:54,1987.

Erikson EH: *The life cycle completed: review,* New York, 1982, Norton.

Ettinger RL, Beck JD: The new elderly: what can the dental profession expect? *Spec Care Dent* 2:62, 1982. Fattore LD, Strauss R, Bruno J: The management of periodontal disease in patients who have received radiation therapy for head and neck cancer, *Spec Care Dent* 7:120, 1987.

Friedman, Richard: Osteoradionecrosis: causes and prevention. *NCIM* 9:145, 1990.

Gier RE, Janes DR: Dental management of the pregnant patient: symposium on the patient with increased medical risks, *Dent Clin North Am* 27:419, 1983.

Goldberg PZ: *So what if you can't chew, eat hearty!* Springfield, Ill, 1980, Charles C Thomas.

Gooch BF, Berkey DB: Subjective factors affecting the utilization of dental services by the elderly, *Gerodontics* 3:65, 1987.

Goose DH, Kurer J: *A guide to children's dentistry,* London, 1973, Henry Kimpton.

Gordon SR, Sullivan TM: Dental treatment planning for compromised or elderly patients, *Gerodontics* 2:217, 1986.

's-Gravenmade EJ et al: Artificial saliva in the management of patients suffering from xerostomia, *Gerodontology* 3:243, 1984.

Hill EM, Flaitz CM, Frost GR: Sweetener content of common pediatric oral liquid medications, *Am J Hosp Phar,* 41:135, 1988.

Holm-Pederson P, Agerbaek N, Therlade E: Experimental gingivitis in young and elderly individuals, *J Clin Periodontol* 2:14, 1975.

Horvath TB, Davis KL: *Central nervous system disorders in aging*. In Schneider EL, Rowe JW, editors: *Handbook of the biology of aging,* San Diego, 1990, Academic Press.

Huggins B: *Practical paedodontics,* Edinburgh, 1973, Churchill Livingstone.

Hunt RJ, Levy SM, Beck JD: The prevalence of periodontal attachment loss in an Iowa population aged 70 and older, *J Public Health Dent* 50:251, 1990.

Ismail AI et al: Findings from the dental care supplement of the national health interview survey, 1983, *JADA* 114:617, 1983.

Johanson WG, Pierce AK, Sanford JP: Changing pharyngeal bacterial flora of hospitalized patients: emergence of gram negative bacilli, *N Engl J Med* 281:1137, 1969.

Kane RL, Ouslander JG, Abrass IB: Essentials of clinical geriatrics, New York, 1989, McGraw Hill.

Katzman R, Terry R: *Normal aging of the nervous system.* In Katzman R, Terry R, editors: *The neurology of aging,* Philadelphia, 1983, FA Davis.

King GE, Martin JW: Prosthodontic care of patients receiving chemotherapy and irradiation to the head and neck, *Curr Probl Cancer* 7:43, 1983.

Kroeger RE: *Managing the apprehensive dental patient,* Cincinnati, 1987, Heritage Communications.

Löe H, Silness J: Periodontal disease in pregnancy. Prevalence and severity, *Acta Odont Scand* 21:532, 1963.

Marinelli RD et al: Perception of dental needs of the well elderly, *Spec Care Dent* 2:161, 1982.

Marx RE: Osteoradionecrosis: a new concept of its pathophysiology, *J Oral Maxillofac Surg* 41:283, 1983.

McClure D, et al: Oral management of the cancer patient. I. Oral complications of chemotherapy, *Compend Contin Educ Dent* 8:41, 1987a.

McClure D et al: Oral management of the cancer patient. II. Oral complications of radiation therapy, *Compend Contin Educ Dent* 8:88, 1987b.

McDonald RE, Avery BS: *Dentistry for the child and adolescent,* ed 4, St Louis, 1983, CV Mosby.

McElroy TH: Infection in the patient receiving chemotherapy for cancer: oral considerations, *JADA* 109:454, 1984.

McLeran H: *Oral hygiene care of the elderly: module 13, geriatric curriculum series,* Iowa City, 1982, University of Iowa.

Montgomery MT, Redding SW, LeMaistre CF: The incidence of oral herpes simplex virus infection in patients undergoing cancer chemotherapy, *Oral Surg Oral Med Oral Pathol* 61:238, 1986.

Mossman KL, Henkin RI: Radiation-induced changes in taste acuity in cancer patients, *Int J Radiat Oncol Biol Phys* 4:663, 1978.

Myers RA, Marx RE: Use of hyperbaric oxygen in postradiation head and neck surgery, *NCI Monog* 9:151, 1990.

National Center for Health Statistics: *Data from the national health interview survey, health, United States, 1985,* DHHS pub no 86-1232, Washington, DC, 1985, US Government Printing Office.

National Center for Health Statistics: *Health United States, 1989,* DHHS pub no (PHS) 90-1232, Hyattsville, Md, 1990, Public Health Service.

National Institute for Dental Research, US Department of Health and Human Services: *Oral health of United States adults: national findings,* NIH Pub No 87-2868, 1987.

Overholser CD et al: Dental extractions in patients with acute nonlymphocytic leukemia, *J Oral Surg* 40:296, 1982.

Page RC: Periodontal disease in the elderly: a critical evaluation of current information, *Gerodontology* 3:63, 1984.

Palmor E: *The facts on aging quiz,* New York, 1988, Springer.

Peterson DE: Dental care of the cancer patient, *Compend Contin Educ Dent* 4:115, 1983.

Peterson DE: Toxicity of chemotherapy oral lesions. In Perry MC, Yarbro JW, editors: *Toxicity of chemotherapy,* New York, 1986, Grune & Stratton.

Peterson D, Sonis S: *Oral complications of cancer chemotherapy,* The Hague, Netherlands, 1983, Martinus Nijhoff.

Pinkham JR: *Pediatric dentistry: infancy through adolescence,* Philadelphia, 1988, WB Saunders.

Reynolds WR et al: Dental management of the cancer patient receiving radiation therapy, *Clin Prev Dent* 2(5):5, 1980.

Richardson EP Jr: Neuronal degenerations of aging, *Adv Neurol* 36:115, 1982.

Ritchie JR et al: Dental care for the irradiated cancer patient, *Quintessence Int* 12:837, 1985.

Roche JR: Preventive pedodontics. In Vernier JL, Muhler JC: *Improving dental practice through preventive measures,* ed 3, St Louis, 1975, CV Mosby.

Rothwell BR: Prevention and treatment of orofacial complications of radiotherapy, *JADA* 114:316, 1987.

Rounds MC, Papas AS: Preventive dentistry for the older adults. In Papas AS, Niessen LC, Chauncey HH, editors: *Geriatric dentistry: aging and oral health,* St Louis, 1991, CV Mosby.

Rubin RL, Doku HC: Therapeutic radiology: the modalities and their effects on oral tissues, *JADA* 92:731, 1976.

Schimpff SC: Infections in the compromised host. In Mandell GC, Douglas RG Jr, Bennett JE, editors: *Principles and practice of infectious diseases,* New York, 1979, John Wiley & Sons.

Schubert MM, Sullivan KM, Truelove EL: Head and neck complications of bone marrow transplantation. In Peterson DE, Elias EG, Sonis ST, editors: *Head and neck management of the cancer patient,* The Hague, 1986, Martinus Nijhoff.

Schweiger JW, Salcetti MA: Dental management of the geriatric head and neck cancer patient, *Gerodontology* 5:119, 1986.

Seichter U: Root surface caries: a critical literature review, *JADA* 115:305, 1987.

Shapiro S et al: Drug utilization by a non-institutionalized ambulatory elderly population, *Gerodontics* 2:99, 1986.

Shelton BK, Weikel DS: Alterations in the oral mucosa: assessment to intervention, *Proc NTI* 233, 1990.

Silverberg E, Lubera J: Cancer statistics, 1987, *CA* 37:2, 1987.

Silverman S, Greenspan D: Early detection and diagnosis of oral cancer, *Can Dent Assoc J* 13:29, 1985.

Silverman S Jr: *Oral cancer,* ed 3, Altalnta, 1990, American Cancer Society.

Silverman S et al: Occurrence of oral candida in irradiated head and neck cancer patients, *J Oral Med* 39:194, 1984.

Silverman S Jr, Thompson JS: Serum zinc and copper in oral/oropharyngeal carcinoma: a study of seventy-five patients, *Oral Surg* 57:34, 1984.

Solomon K, Vickers R: Attitudes of health workers toward old people, *J Am Geriatr Soc* 27:187, 1979.

Sonis ST, Sonis AL, Lieberman A: Oral complications in patients receiving treatment for non-head and neck malignancies, *JADA* 97:468, 1978.

Sonis ST et al: Oral complications in patients receiving treatment for malignancies other than of the head and neck, *JADA* 97:468, 1983.

Sreebny L, Swartz SS: A reference guide to drugs and dry mouth, *Gerodontology* 5:75, 1986.

Stamm JW, Banting DW: Comparison of root caries prevalence in adults with life-long residence in fluoridated and non-luoridated communities, *J Dent Res* 59A(abstract):552, 1980.

Sullivan MD, Fleming TJ: Oral care for the radiotherapy-treated head and neck cancer patient, *Dent Hyg* 60:112, 1986.

Suzuki JB, Niessen LC, Fedele DJ: Periodontal diseases in the older adult. In Papas AS, Niessen LC, Chauncey HH: *Geriatric dentistry: aging and oral health,* St Louis, 1991, CV Mosby.

Svanborg A, Bergstrom G, Millstrom D: *Epidemiological studies on social and medical conditions of the elderly,* Copenhagen, 1982, World Health Organization.

Toth BS, Fleming TJ: Oral/dental considerations for pediatric patients receiving anticancer treatment, *Mass Dent Assoc J* 63(3):33, 1983.

Toth BB, Frame RT: Dental oncology: the management of disease and treatment-related oral/dental complications associated with chemotherapy, *Curr Probl Cancer* 7:7, 1983.

Tyron AF: A model for integrating geriatrics into the dental school curriculum, *Spec Care Dent* 1:114, 1981.

US Department of Health, Education, and Welfare: *National health survey: prevalence of chronic conditions and impairments,* PHS pub no 10000, Ser 12,8, Washington DC, 1979, US Government Printing Office.

US Senate Special Committee on Aging: *Aging America: trends and projections,* Washington, 1991, US Senate.

Viidik A: The biological basis of aging. In Holm-Pedersen P, Löe H, editors: *Geriatric dentistry: a textbook of oral gerontology,* Copenhagen, 1986, Munksgaard.

Vuolo SJ: Oral complications of cancer chemotherapy and dental care for the cancer patient receiving antineoplastic drug therapy: a literature review, *NY J Dent* 57:50, 1987.

Wade JC: Principles of infection management. In Peterson DE, Elias EG, Sonis ST, editors: *Head and neck management of the cancer patient,* Boston, 1986, Martinus Nijhoff.

Warren GB, Blandford DH: Geriatrics and geriatric dental education in the United States, *Spec Care Dent* 5:150, 1985.

Wei SHY, Nowak AJ: Implementing a preventive pedodontics practice. In Stewart RE et al, editors: *Pediatric dentistry: scientific foundations and clinical practice,* St Louis, 1982, CV Mosby.

Wescott WB: Dental management of patients being treated for oral cancer, *Can Dent Assoc J* 13:42, 1985.

Williams SR: *Essentials of nutrition and diet therapy,* ed 3, St Louis, 1982, CV Mosby.

Williams TF: Patterns of health and disease in the elderly, *Gerodontics* 1:284, 1985.

Wright GZ, Starkey PE, Gardner DE: *Managing children's behavior in the dental office,* St Louis, 1983, CV Mosby.

Wright WE: Periodontium destruction associated with oncology therapy: five case reports, *J Periodontol* 58:559, 1987.

Wright WE et al: An oral disease prevention program for patients receiving radiation and chemotherapy, *JADA* 110:43, 1985.

Yarden J, Gedalia I, Kohn M: Fluoride concentration of dental calculus, surface enamel and cementum, *Arch Oral Biol* 8:697, 1963.

Yasko JM, Greene P: Coping with problems related to cancer and cancer treatment, *CA* 37:106, 1987.

Zack L: *The oral cavity.* In Rossman I, editor: *Clinical geriatrics,* ed 2, Philadelphia, 1979, JB Lippincott.

SUGGESTED READINGS

Bamberg TJ et al: Developing the health history of the elderly patient, *Gerodontics* 1:165, 1985.

Banting DW: Dental caries in the elderly, *Gerodontology* 3:55, 1984.

Bernhoft C, Skaug N: Oral findings in irradiated edentulous patients, *Int J Oral Surg* 14:416, 1985.

Brudevold F et al: Inorganic and organic components of tooth structure, *Ann NY Acad Sci* 85:110, 1960.

Burch GE: Fundamentals of clinical cardiology: interesting aspects of geriatric cardiology, *Am Heart J* 89:99, 1975.

Clark J et al: *Care document of the geriatric area health education center,* Baltimore, 1982, University of Maryland.

Daly KM, Boyne PJ: *Nutrition and eating problems of oral and head-neck surgeries: a guide to soft and liquid meals,* Springfield, Ill, 1985, Charles C Thomas.

Ernst et al: Pharmacological considerations for the elderly patient, *J Oral Med* 39:131, 1984.

Fay JT, O'Neal R: Dental responsibility for the medically compromised patient, *J Oral Med* 39:218, 1984.

Fischbach FT: *A manual of laboratory diagnostic tests,* Philadelphia, 1980, JB Lippincott.

Furseth R: A study of experimentally exposed and fluoride treated dental cementum in pigs, *Acta Odontol Scand* 28:833, 1970.

Gambert SR: Aging—an overview, *Spec Care Dent* 3:147, 1983.

Gambert SR: Drugs and the elderly, *Spec Care Dent* 4:102, 1984.

Gambucci JR et al: Dental care utilization: patterns of older adults, *Gerodontics* 2:11, 1986.

Gedalia I et al: Fluoride content of surface enamel, cementum, lamina dura and subperiosteal bone from mandibular angle of Hebrews, *J Dent Res* 44:452, 1965.

Rosenthal G: *Smooth food for all with dental problems. . .and everyone else,* Washington DC, 1980, Library of Congress.

Rubin RJ, Kruger B: Hearing loss in the elderly. In Katzman R, Terry R, editors: *The neurology of aging,* Philadelphia, 1983, FA Davis.

Schachtele CF et al: Diet and aging: current concerns related to oral health, *Gerodontics* 1:117, 1985.

Singer L, Varmstrong WD: Comparison of fluoride content of human dental and skeletal tissues, *J Dent Res* 41:154, 1962.

Spiro RH: Squamous cancer of the tongue, *CA* 35:252, 1985.

Stepnick RJ et al: The effects of age and fluoride exposure on fluoride citrate and carbonate content of human cementum, *J Periodontol* 46:45, 1975.

Waldman HB: Knowing more about the elderly can help if we want to provide needed services, *Gerodontology* 4:83, 1985.

Warren KL: Increasing access to dental care for the older patient: a special challenge, *Spec Care Dent* 2:248, 1982.

Wilson JR: *Non-chew cookbook,* Glenwood Springs, Colo, 1985, Wilson.

PART SIX

DISEASE PREVENTION AND HEALTH MAINTENANCE

Though a major part of dental hygiene care involves assessing oral health needs, developing a dental hygiene diagnosis, and providing treatment, an equally important part is providing oral health education for individual patients and for groups of people. The basis for oral health education is the concept of prevention. A strong prevention orientation is one of the key cultural characteristics of dental hygiene. It is a theme that runs through all of clinical practice.

Supporting oral health education are specific clinical procedures that will help your patients maintain good health, including using and prescribing fluoride, recommending and applying pit and fissure sealants, and helping patients maintain their restorative appliances.

The following five chapters will introduce you to the philosophy and methods of disease prevention and health maintenance. In many ways, these concepts and the attitudes that support them constitute the cornerstone of what makes dental hygiene valuable to the public.

ORAL HEALTH STRATEGIES: PREVENTING AND CONTROLLING DENTAL DISEASE

Irene Woodall
Cheryl Wiles

LEARNING OUTCOMES

The dental hygienist will be able to

1. Adopt a philosophy of prevention that
   a. Encompasses the total oral health of the patient
   b. Specifically targets the (1) health behaviors in the control of the patient, (2) the patient's life-style, and (3) those professional procedures which can enhance health maintenance.
2. Provide patient care that balances professional treatment and patient self-care.
3. Develop strategies to implement dental health educational programs for individuals and small groups for each of the main topics of prevention (fluorides and sealants, changes in normal oral structures, nutrition education, need for specialized dental care, blood pressure screening, oral habits, cessation of tobacco use, and plaque control).
4. Individualize prevention programs to enhance patient motivation and to identify and remove roadblocks to adopting good health behaviors.
5. Select oral hygiene procedures, products, and devices that specifically meet individuals' needs for plaque control.

Your most important asset is your ability to motivate patients into adopting a daily routine of good oral hygiene—to help them value their oral health and want their smile for a lifetime. Patients will adopt preventive behaviors based on their values, wants, needs, and expectations. The dental hygienist's role is to determine the best combination of information, timing, products, and practical applications for each patient to help him or her make personal oral health decisions.

A person who adopts good health behaviors and prevents disease from occurring is much better off than one who never learns or cares about health behaviors and thus needs extensive therapy. It is costly and unpleasant to undergo extensive dental care, and sometimes even the best treatment cannot repair the damage that has occurred. A person who learns to practice good oral hygiene is likely to be spared the multiple costs of extensive treatment or tooth loss. Likewise, a person with reversible advanced disease will benefit from learning to prevent its recurrence.

In many ways, providing solid information and skill development for your patients will be one of your most rewarding roles in dental hygiene. Though your prowess with subgingival instrumentation may be essential to help your patients reverse disease, you will contribute far more to their long-term health if you can find the magic motivating words to help them change their habits and enter into a partnership with you in keeping themselves healthy. Many patients who have their "teeth cleaned" every 6 months end up in the periodontist's office with a diagnosis of periodontitis. If the hygienist who performed the "cleanings" has not carefully monitored the patient for periodontal health and emphasized repeatedly the importance of daily oral hygiene, the referred patient has suffered "supervised neglect" (Dunbar, 1976). Such neglect by the hygienist can trigger legal action by the patient. Further, it is an ethical breach to lull the patient into believing appropriate care is being delivered when little more is being done than a routine removal of stain and calculus.

People change slowly and sometimes not

enough. Preventive oral health education requires good planning, persistence, frequent follow-up, flexibility, a wide array of reinforcement, and interpersonal skills. For many patients, the instrumentation procedures are relatively easy compared with the effort required to launch a workable, effective program of disease prevention.

No matter which oral health topic is most relevant to a given patient, you will have the greatest impact if the patient can learn that staying healthy requires periodic professional care and daily, personal health practices. Prevention requires a partnership between you and the patient.

ORAL HEALTH TOPICS: FOCI OF A PREVENTION PARTNERSHIP
Fluoride and sealants

The importance of fluoride in controlling caries should be included in the dental health education agenda for persons who (1) have a caries problem, (2) belong to a caries-prone family, (3) are entering caries-prone years, (4) are pregnant or will soon have a new child in the family, or (5) are voters who may someday consider a fluoride referendum in the community.

Chapter 21 discusses the importance of fluoride in prevention, so details will not be given in this chapter. However, it is important to plan to incorporate fluoride education into any prevention plan and to emphasize it for patients to whom its relevance is paramount. This is especially important during an era in which dental caries receives less attention than other oral problems, such as periodontal disease. Dental caries may have declined significantly in developed countries in recent decades, but it is still a major health problem for many people. Also, if fluoride is not emphasized for the patient groups listed, the prevalence of dental caries may begin to increase. Children need to learn to avoid sugared foods and to brush regularly to disrupt plaque. The most readily available source of fluoride—fluoridated communal water—needs continued community support.

The oral health partnership includes professionally applied fluorides, at-home fluoride therapy, dietary assessment, and regular examination and treatment of dental caries. The patient's half of the partnership is to use a fluoride toothpaste, avoid sugared foods, consume an otherwise healthful diet, obtain regular examinations and appropriate treatment, and continue support for communal fluoridated water.

While fluoride helps protect the smooth surfaces of the teeth (facial, lingual, proximal), sealants protect the occlusal surfaces by penetrating the pits and fissures, making them impenetrable by bacteria. Chapter 22 explains the research supporting the use of sealants and how to place them. Your health education role in this regard is to explain the availability and function of sealants to patients who could benefit from them.

Self-screening

Identifying changes in the normal structures of the mouth (commonly referred to as an oral cancer screening) is an essential component of oral health education. It is important for people to know what normal oral structures look like and to learn how to monitor those structures each month for changes in color, shape, size, tenderness, and tendency toward bleeding. The gingival tissues are also monitored for a tendency towards periodontal problems. The inspection goes beyond the gingivae to include the buccal mucosa, tongue, lips, soft palate, alveolar bone, floor of the mouth, and other structures. The oral cancer self-examination is described in Chapter 8. These procedures are especially critical for adults who smoke or chew tobacco, consume alcohol, or have personal or family histories of cancer. Just as women should perform monthly breast self-examinations and men should self-examine their testicles, all adults should evaluate their oral structures on the same schedule. It is an easy way to keep track of one's health, and it can mean the difference between normalcy and disfigurement or between life and death. The oral health partnership includes regular professional examinations coupled with monthly patient self-examinations and reporting of any observed change to the dental professional for evaluation.

Nutrition education

Nutrition education is receiving more attention in dentistry as the public emphasis on fitness and personal responsibility for general health rises. The link between diet and cardiovascular disease and cancer is becoming clearer, and medicine is taking nutrition education more seriously. Dentistry is shifting its emphasis from a narrow discussion of sugar consumption to an understanding that a visit to the dentist may be the ideal time to discuss nutrition and diet from the standpoint of general as well as oral health. Chapter 24 provides more detail on and strategies for this topic. Your role in the partnership is to help the patient identify good dietary choices and to remove roadblocks to them. The patient's role is to acknowledge the "right" choices, make them regularly, and, if necessary, record the influences affecting meal-to-meal decisions about food and drink. Patients with eating disorders will require special assistance; your role will be to help identify the disorder (often evident because of dental erosion) and to locate appropriate counseling for the patient.

Need for specialized dental care

Need for specialized dental care often falls within the dental hygienist's purview. Patients may have missing teeth, malocclusion, faulty or aged dental work, cosmetic problems, or other dental conditions that will require a dentist's attention. You can identify conditions that require dental diagnosis and discuss how they affect the patient's dental and general health and appearance. You also can discuss the fundamentals of procedures used to correct the problems and provide information about new options for treatment. Typically, this information occurs after a dental consultation, but often an informal discussion about the potential problems stemming from the oral conditions can help prepare the patient for the dental diagnosis and for some of the probable treatment options.

Careful coordination with the dentist(s) providing the care makes this preparatory phase of education particularly helpful to the dentist when he or she presents a complex treatment plan for the patient. Some dentists rely on their hygienists to present proposed treatment plans; others recognize the role of the hygienist in ferreting out patients' reservations and questions about procedures after the dentist has presented the plan. In any case, providing this kind of information is an important part of oral hygiene education. Your role in the partnership is to provide accurate information and to listen carefully to the patient; the patient's role is to provide honest reactions and questions.

Blood pressure screening

Another valuable prevention topic is routine blood pressure screening performed at each continuing care appointment and self-monitoring between visits if pressure is borderline. Having a hygienist (or a dentist) measure blood pressure may be a new experience for some patients. You may find yourself explaining its importance to every patient you see for the first time. As explained in Chapter 8, it is a simple and vital procedure for quick identification of patients whose blood pressure is borderline or high, who can then be referred for medical attention. Also, the recording tells you whether your patient is at risk of having a cerebrovascular accident while receiving dental care. Prevention education for such patients should include a recommendation that they frequently have their blood pressure measured at a pharmacy or other convenient location with reliable equipment.

Oral habits

Nail biting, thumb or finger sucking, pencil chewing, lip or cheek biting, or abnormal swallowing patterns are another focus of individualized oral health education. As you assess the patient, you will see signs that a patient likely has one or more of these habits. Working with patients to identify when and why they practice these habits and providing alternatives for them can help reduce the need for extensive orthodontic care or restorative repair to the teeth. You can form a partnership for identifying ways to reduce the frequency of the undesirable habit and eventually to eliminate it.

Addictive behavior

One of the most harmful oral habits is the use of tobacco. Numerous clinical and laboratory studies have shown the effect of nicotine on both epithelial and connective tissue cells (Hanes, Schuster, and Lubas, 1991). Nicotine's effect on the blood vessels including the fine capillaries that feed the periodontal tissues makes it more difficult for the patient to mount an appropriate immune reaction to microbial invasion (Danielsen et al, 1990). One of the cardinal signs of gingival inflammation, bleeding on probing, is masked in tobacco users because of nicotine's effect. People who use tobacco are at much greater risk of having periodontal disease (Bergstrom and Eliasson, 1987), and they do not heal as well after treatment (Preber and Bregstrom, 1990; Sweet and Butler, 1979). Other human and animal studies show that nicotine is a potent and powerful psychoactive drug that affects the human brain (Henningfield, 1990). Therefore it is essential to discuss tobacco use cessation techniques with patients. It is important to address the addiction as well as the habit in helping patients quit. Some of the strategies that can be useful in conducting such a program are included in this chapter.

Plaque control

Finally, and perhaps central to most oral health education, is plaque control. Plaque is the primary cause of dental caries and periodontal disease, and disrupting it regularly is an important part of oral hygiene. Patients cannot remove all of the plaque every day, but they can keep it under control by brushing, flossing, irrigating, using interdental cleaning devices, and augmenting this mechanical cleaning with antimicrobial solutions. The professional partnership in this case involves periodic debridement of subgingival areas and assessment of periodontal and tooth health. The patient implements daily plaque disruption and keeps regular dental appointments. A major portion of this chapter will address the various approaches to plaque disruption.

INTEGRATING PREVENTION IN CLINICAL PRACTICE

Prevention is not a "procedure" that happens during a given time of the appointment. It is integrated throughout every appointment and exists as a philosophic foundation for every clinical procedure you perform. It starts with assessment and weaves its way through all the subsequent phases of the cycle of care, including diagnosis, planning, implementation, and evaluation. Your philosophy should be to identify every aspect of the patient's oral health needs that deserves discussion, along with ways to preserve and restore health and to prevent disease recurrence.

For instance, during the assessment, as you examine each aspect of the head and neck, review the medical history, chart the teeth and the periodontium, and so forth, you should be looking for health and for deviations from health. You should show the patient each condition and explain its significance. Your purpose is to educate the patient to know the terminology and his or her own health status and to see the logical way in which your observations build toward a summary of the patient's needs as you see them. This discussion enables the patient to express concerns and ask questions. Ideally, when the assessment phase is complete, there will be no surprises for the patient in the diagnosis and treatment plan. The patient should look to you for suggestions regarding care that is needed to improve problem areas and for

ideas about how to maintain health. Your verbal and nonverbal concern for the patient's condition as you progress through each aspect of the examination will naturally convey the importance of the findings.

Sometimes, as indicated in Chapter 18, it is important to commence treatment to reduce pain or infection, or to sufficiently clean the mouth so that the patient can adequately care for the dentition. Other times, treatment should be delayed until the patient's primary educational needs are met. It may be far more important to talk about the effects of smoking and to determine the patient's interest in stopping smoking before progressing to periodontal debridement. An anorexic patient may be much better served by a discussion of that problem than by instructions on how to brush and floss. In all situations, the primary goal is to move the patient to a healthier set of habits and for him or her to hear your sincerity regarding the importance of changing specific behaviors in an incremental fashion.

In order to make oral health a partnership, the patient needs to feel that he or she is involved in the decision making and that it is acceptable to express concerns, ideas, disagreement, and feelings to you. Oral health education is not a lecture. It is more listening than talking. It is more problem solving than instruction.

If the patient is actively involved in the oral assessment, the discussion of what exists will naturally flow into a discussion of what to do about it. When the patient asks, "What can we do about this?" you should respond with a brief set of suggestions: "I can show you ways to keep those areas healthier and spend a few appointments disrupting the bacteria that are living there. This dual strategy would probably help a great deal." When you have given the brief synopsis of what you plan to do, wait for the patient's reaction. You will want to know immediately whether the patient is interested in hearing more and in proceeding or is turning you off mentally. Listen to both the nonverbal behavior and what the patient says. Reflect back what you have heard both from the words and physical movements: "Looks like you want to hear more" or "You are looking really uncomfortable." This kind of reflective listening allows patients to confirm whether you are correct in your observation and to say what they are thinking and feeling.

Use your listening skills to work through the issues surrounding the proposed program of care. Work with the patient to identify a program that he or she believes will work and that you believe makes sense, given the oral condition.

As each phase of care is commenced, remind the patient how much the two of you have accomplished already and where you are in the treatment plan. Emphasize the successes attributable to the patient's role in the partnership. Show the patient the improvements in the tissues. Take a moment to celebrate your joint successes at each visit. Revise the plan with the patient as necessary.

Helping the patient to adopt new health behaviors or to overcome addictive behavior is the common theme in health education. Maslow's hierarchy of needs (1970) provides a helpful and interesting framework for understanding motivation in general. His thesis is that patients must feel secure and free from physical discomfort before they can respond to higher-order motivators such as self-esteem and self-actualization. You will probably find that most patients are motivated by the desire to keep their teeth, to look nice, and to be socially acceptable. Many do not want to spend excessive sums of money on their teeth, and still others have no inclination to spend long hours in the dental chair. Much of your success as a health educator will hinge on your ability to determine which motivators apply to each of your patients.

Many clues about the specifics of an individual's motivators can be seen in your opening interview with the patient, in which you talk about why the person is seeking care and what the problems or goals are regarding oral health. During the assessment phase, you should listen carefully for comments such as, "How much will this cost?" "How long will it take?" "Will this make my gums look better?" "I think I have bad breath; will this help?"

How do you use this information about what motivates patients? It helps if you can emphasize how the proposed treatment will minimize their fears and enhance what will please them. If the patient is not terribly socially self-conscious and is having financial difficulty, it may be better to point out how having treatment now will minimize larger expenses later than to emphasize how much better the smile will look.

Once the patient has made a fundamental commitment to work with you on improving his or her oral health, you can begin with a few recommendations for behavior change, typically worded as a question. The recommendations should be concrete and specific: "Could you bring fruit with you to work instead of pastry for snacks?" For the patient who has no time for interdental cleansing but who likes to read at night: "How would you feel about using this interdental brush while you are reading?" For the person who brushes with a vigorous scrub: "Do you think you could shorten your stroke so you cover three teeth at a time instead of six?" Begin with a few simple, important changes.

Evaluate the patient's progress at the next visit by asking: "Which of the suggestions were you able to try since the last visit?" Listen for the patient's self-perceived successes and acknowledge the importance of this progress: "Cutting down from 20 to 10 cigarettes a day sounds like great progress." "Using that interdental brush every night for 10 minutes is bound to help your tissues."

Also listen for the unsuccessful efforts: "I tried that floss, but I just hate the feel of plaque all over my fingers." "I told myself I would skip that nightly hot fudge sundae, but when my wife and kids sat down to their bowls, I gave in and joined them." "Every time I get in the car, I find myself lighting a cigarette. I also notice I do that when the phone rings."

Your task when efforts are unsuccessful is to identify the smallest roadblocks or parts of roadblocks that can be reduced or removed: "Do you think this floss holder might make flossing more-acceptable? Or would you rather use an interdental brush like this? Which would be better for you?" "Can we come up with a snack that will let you join your family during treat time? Maybe the new frozen yogurt would be a reasonable substitute. And they even have fat-free hot fudge now. If you take a small portion of each you might still be able to join in, but you would be consuming a more healthful treat. Would that work for you?" "What could you substitute for a cigarette when you are driving or on the phone? How about having a dry toothbrush by the phone to play with and use between sentences? Can you think of anything else?" Work with the patient to jointly identify alternative approaches. If you provide all the suggestions, you may find yourself in a game of "Yes, but. . . ." with the patient, where everything you suggest has a complication. When this happens, the patient is telling you that he or she does not really want to change and that it is your task to come up with the nonexistent magical solution.

When a patient lacks motivation, you may be able to institute a program in which he or she practices the desirable behavior under supervision, which eventually translates into an attitude change. Attitude change does not have to precede behavior change. It helps if it does, but it is not essential. You may be able to make an agreement with the patient that he or she will visit the dental office every other day to brush and irrigate, for instance, with supervision and assistance. Practicing a habit over an extended period can eventually shift attitudes so that the person actually values the habit and feels at a loss if it is not carried out. Rarely will this approach be necessary, but it may prove helpful.

Successful health education relies upon a continuing respect for the patient and his or her beliefs, attitudes, and relative successes. It helps to be able to look the patient in the eye and say, "This is, after all, your body and your mouth. I know you will take care of it as well as you care to and as well as you can. If I can give you advice and guidance, I'll be glad to."

This approach to health education eliminates lecturing and judgment from the interaction. You do not have to adopt a parental authority role and the patient does not have to feel like a small child reporting in for your approval or disapproval. An adult-to-adult interaction in which you respect the patient's ideas and attitudes enhances the notion of a partnership rather than a dependency relationship.

Open interaction with patients requires considerable practice and experience. It also demands that you constantly examine your own motives. Are you feeling upset because you have no direct control over what the patient does? Are you frustrated because your good work is not being enhanced by the patient's efforts? Are you feeling good because *you* have succeeded or because *the patient* has?

If you are feeling upset, it often is good to share that feeling with the patient—not by being upset but by telling him or her: "I can feel myself getting upset because your efforts did not work out for you this week. I guess I was hoping the results would be better. It bothers me when the tissues don't seem to respond as they should and

our plans don't work out. I'm sorry if I seem grumpy." Not saying how you feel and not explaining the source of your feelings can backfire, because the patients usually can tell you are upset. They just do not know why, and they may be offended or misconstrue the message of your subtle nonverbal signals. Simply saying how you are feeling, and doing it in such a way that avoids laying blame on the patient, can stimulate the patient to respond with renewed enthusiasm or with a simple acknowledgement that you seem upset.

It is a fact of life that some patients are not yet ready to be helped or to help themselves. There is no need to be upset, although you will sometimes feel that way, especially if your hopes were high. If you avoid laying blame and look forward to another day when the patient may be ready, you will have a solid relationship from which to start.

STARTING A TOBACCO-USE CESSATION PROGRAM

In the past decade, several breakthroughs have occurred in the area of smoking cessation. The area most relevant to you is the focus on behavioral interventions with patients participating in an office-based smoking cessation program. Studies show that 67% to 72% of patients are interested in receiving help in tobacco cessation from their dental team (Severson, 1990). A study conducted at Kaiser Permanente Dental Health Care Program showed that 87% to 90% of the patients receiving advice to quit smoking from their dental team found it helpful and encouraging (Little, 1990).

How can you help your patients stop smoking? Dr. Jack Hollis of Kaiser Permanente Center for Health Research in Portland, Oregon describes the key components of a smoking cessation program this way:

S Show professional and personal concern to your patients. Ask questions to open the door to discussion and awareness.

T Talk about the reasons to quit, citing current professional research. Use published literature to show the patient tobacco-related oral health effects.

O Offer assistance and support to your patients. Express your confidence in their ability to quite smoking. Create strategies to help your patients between visits.

P Plan for future action with your patients. Simply setting a date to quit smoking has proven to be an effective strategy (Little and Stevens, 1991).

These strategies are obviously consistent with those suggested for implementing oral health education on any topic. In the area of smoking, patients may at first believe the topic is not relevant to oral health and thus may resent or question your interest in the topic. Therefore it is important to have good supporting literature to help your patients understand the direct relevance to oral health as well as general health. Smoking cessation efforts are an extension of all the other preventive oral health techniques dental hygeinists provide to their patients. Because the dental team sees patients at regular continuing care intervals, they have an ideal opportunity to individualize patient support, monitor progress, and reward success. Research shows that a team of health care professionals can be successful in helping people quit smoking (Christen and McDonald, 1986; Mecklenburg et al, 1989).

A plan developed at the Indiana University School of Dentistry uses the National Cancer Institute's basic guidelines which suggest that in-office strategies include five basic elements (The first national dental symposium on smoking cessation, 1990; Smoking cessation for the dental office, 1990):

1. Select a smoking cessation coordinator.
2. Create a nonsmoking office environment.
3. Note smoking status of all patients on their records.
4. Develop a patient-oriented smoking cessation program.
5. Generate a strategy for patient support and encouragement.

There are specific aids to help your patients quit. For instance, nicotine gum can be prescribed as a substitute for chewing tobacco or for smoking. Also, slow-release nicotine patches are commercially available by prescription. Both of these aids will help the patient cope with the nicotine addiction. Other approaches include a system of filters that reduce the available nicotine from the patient's usual cigarette. This approach permits the patient to continue the physical act of smoking and thus requires another step to substitute for the habit of lighting and and smoking a cigarette. The patient can also try switching brands from a strong cigarette to one with less nicotine and tar. The most successful methods, however, may be those which provide nicotine in a form other than cigarettes or chewing tobacco and which help the patient adopt behaviors that replace the physical act of smoking or chewing.

When commencing a cessation program, seek out the assistance of a trained substance abuse counselor with experience in smoking/chewing cessation. You will want to work with that person to design the specifics of the program, including selecting materials, working with individual patients' problems, and evaluating the success of the program. As smoking cessation becomes a routine part of dental practice, a variety of programs and materials will be available for adoption.

IMPLEMENTING A PLAQUE CONTROL PROGRAM

The patient's half of the partnership in controlling oral microbial flora is to disrupt plaque on a daily basis so that it is less likely to cause dental caries or to stimulate gingival inflammation leading to periodontitis.

To help the patient adopt a positive attitude and behaviors towards plaque control, it helps to clarify what plaque is and where it is present on the teeth. Start by showing the patient areas of plaque in his or her mouth that are sufficiently thick to be seen when the tip of a probe is run along the margin of the gingivae (Plate 5, A). Explain how it develops and accumulates and how it puts the teeth and soft tissues at risk if it remains undisturbed for more than a few days.

Then use one of the available disclosing solutions (preferably fluorescein dye and a PlakLite, since this dye does not stain the soft tissues) to identify all the plaque in the mouth (Plate 5, L to N) (Squillaro, Cohen, and Laster, 1975). Chapter 13 provides additional information about disclosants and their use. Show the patient where the accumulations are in the mouth, pointing out particularly heavy deposits and areas that are difficult for the patient to cleanse because of their location in the mouth or the complications of malposed teeth and restorations. Note the presence of stained plaque on the tongue.

Then ask the patient to use a toothbrush to remove as much of the plaque as possible. Wet the brush but do not use toothpaste. Watch the patient while he or she brushes, giving encouragement to remove as much of the stained plaque as possible. Point out that most of the plaque is near the margin of the gingivae; ask the patient how he or she might be able to best reach and disrupt that plaque. Help the patient think through the best way to get the brush to the critical area. If the handbrush works well, it may not be necessary to

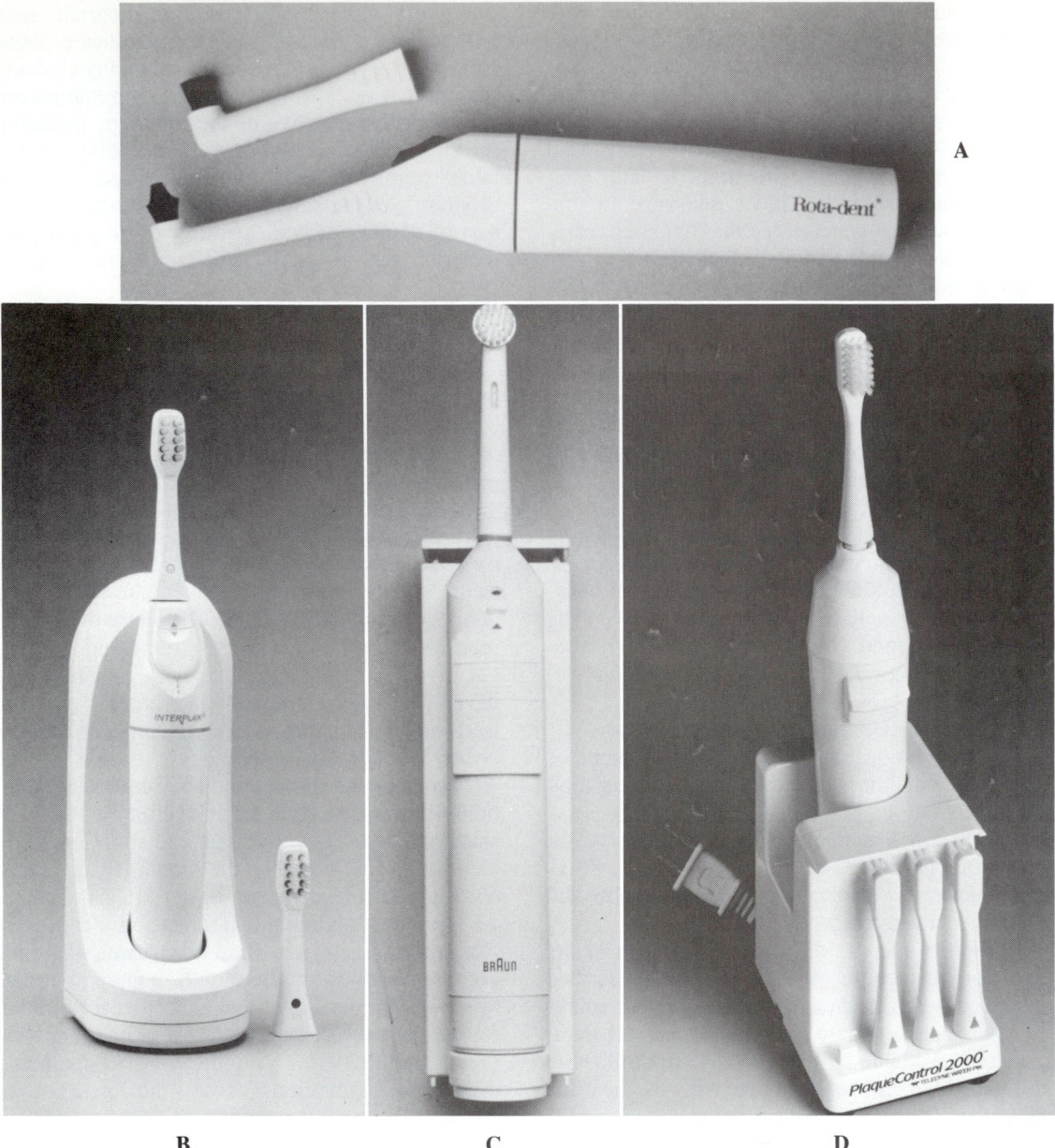

Fig. 20-1. Four electric toothbrushes that can enhance the patient's efforts at reaching marginal and interdental plaque. **A,** Rotadent; **B,** InterPlak; **C,** Braun Oral B Plaque Remover; **D,** Water Pik Plaque Control 2000.

recommend any other brushing devices. If the patient seems unable to direct it properly or to reach the essential areas of the mouth, suggest a powered toothbrush, such as the Rotadent, InterPlak, or the Oral B Plaque Remover (Fig. 20-1). Each of these brushes provides a rotating action that can be directed at the margin of the gingivae.

Have samples of those brushes in your operatory for the patient to try. See which one seems to disrupt the most plaque and which one the patient prefers. Ask the patient to scrape the brush over the tongue to loosen and reduce plaque. Redisclose when the patient believes the task is complete.

In most instances, plaque will be dramatically reduced on facial and lingual surfaces when a handbrush has been used. Proximal surfaces and the area directly adjacent to the margin of the gingivae are more likely to be cleaner if one of the motorized, rotating brushes is used. The Water Pik Plaque Control 2000 also provides good interdental access. Ask the patient to look for the sites that still have plaque. They likely will identify the proximal surfaces as needing more help.

Show the patient the options for cleaning the interdental area. This includes floss (all the various kinds), interdental brushes, and interdental sticks. Explain how each one is used, and let the patient try each one. Ask the patient to select the one that looks most acceptable and use it throughout the mouth to remove the remaining plaque. When the patient has finished, disclose the teeth again and see what remains. Remind the patient that it will not be possible to remove all plaque in a normal oral hygiene routine, but that the task is to disrupt and remove as much as possible and to do so thoroughly at least twice daily. Also, point out the difference between plaque and stained calculus, which may be making it difficult to cleanse interdental areas. Note that part of your role is to remove these hardened deposits so that it will be easier for the patient to maintain good oral hygiene.

In addition to focusing on visible, supragingival plaque, your oral hygiene assessment should include measures of subgingival plaque and enzyme evaluations of the health of the periodontal tissues. This is especially helpful for patients who have minimal visible plaque but whose periodontal disease progresses. The simplest approach is to show the patient the plethora of bacteria and their activity in a sample taken from the sulcus or periodontal pocket. You also can use one of the chairside tests for periodontal pathogens that are entering the market. A color change on a treated sample of plaque indicates the presence of certain putative periodontal pathogens. Taking a sample of gingival crevicular fluid and adding reagents to evaluate the host response to disease and the levels of tissue destruction can also provide valuable information, especially for periodontitis patients. Show the results to the patient and explain them in simple terms. Just as they can see the bleeding from probing they can see the sites in which disease activity is likely occurring. See Chapter 12 for further discussion of these tests.

With two simple implements (a brush and an interdental cleaner) most patients will be able to reduce and prevent gingivitis. This is, of course, dependent on their willingness and ability to perform a thorough cleaning on a regular basis. If the patient is successful, little more is needed for good plaque control and tissue health. However, if this simple mechanical disruption is not enough, other procedures must be substituted or added. The more important measure of successful oral hygiene is the condition of the tissues. If 10 days of oral hygiene measures do not reduce marginal inflammation, the approach to care should be altered.

Substitute a motorized brush for a handbrush if the total load of plaque is not adequately reduced with handbrushing. Suggest that the patient use a timer to ensure that adequate time is spent brushing. Add oral irrigation if the gingivae still appear inflamed. Irrigation will bathe the plaque with a pulsating stream of liquid that removes the loosely adherent toxins from the plaque. It also reaches farther into the sulcus than does the brush or floss. See Chapter 28 for a complete review of oral irrigation. Suggest a dilute solution of antimicrobial solution for use in the irrigator to help reduce plaque load. Patients should irrigate twice daily after brushing and interdental cleaning.

ORAL PHYSIOTHERAPEUTIC AIDS

As suggested in the description of the overall strategy of plaque control, there is a parade of physiotherapeutic aids that can help your patient control disease.

Toothbrushes

The primary tool in the disruption of dental plaque is the toothbrush (Bass, 1948). It is one of the best implements to use to control plaque.

Handbrushes. Though dental professionals have traditionally believed that a flat-headed, multitufted toothbrush with soft bristles is the most desirable style, there is minimal research to support this contention. There are many styles of head size, tuft configuration and shape, and handle shape and angle (Fig. 20-2). Selecting a brush is a highly personal choice, and more than one kind of brush should be available for patients to try. The bottom line in selecting a brush is that it can readily remove plaque without causing tissue damage.

Generally, professionals still recommend soft-bristled brushes. It is believed that soft bristles are gentler to the soft tissues and any exposed cemen-

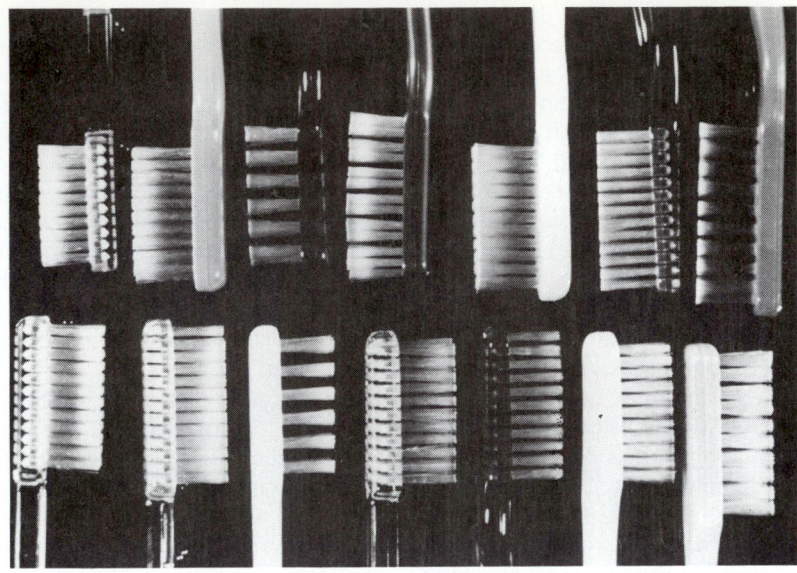

Fig. 20-2. Various acceptable brushing tools.

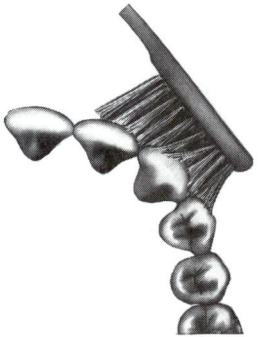

Fig. 20-3. Soft-textured brush adapts well to contours of dentition.
(From Yankell S, Emling R: *Contin Dent Educ* 1:18, 1978.

tum or dentin and that they are more likely to trap and remove plaque. They also adapt better to the contours of the tooth, cleansing more of it (Fig. 20-3). The diameter of each bristle dictates its softness. Length of the bristles is also a factor, since longer bristles have more flex and thus less resiliency to pressure. Recently there has been considerable emphasis on end-rounding of bristles. Magnify the tips of different toothbrushes and look at the very ends (Figs. 20-4 and 20-5).

Some are cut into saber shapes that could abrade tissue; others appear uniformly round.

Toothbrushes should be replaced as soon as the bristles show wear or splay outward. Typically this is every 8 to 12 weeks. Oral B markets brushes with several blue-colored bristles that fade when it is time to change brushes. Other ways of knowing when to change brushes will soon be introduced, including a dial that is set when the brush is first used to show the month in which it should be replaced. Since toothbrushes harbor bacteria from the mouth, it is wise to change toothbrushes after the patient recovers from an upper respiratory infection.

The "best way" to use a handbrush is another subject that is replete with tradition. During the 1950s and 1960s, the "roll" method was popular and the official choice of the American Dental Association. In this method, the patient grasps the brush so that the bristles are pointed apically and places the bristles on the gingiva. With a sweeping motion, the bristles are gently rolled over the gingiva and teeth towards the incisal edge or occlusal surface (Fig. 20-6). Ideally, the brusher should repeat the roll 4 or 5 times before moving to the next area. When all facial and lingual areas have been brushed, the occlusal surfaces are

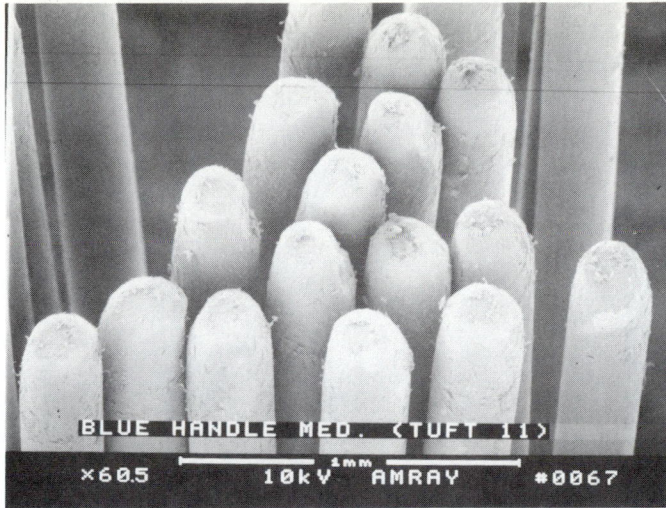

Fig. 20-4. Magnified bristles showing end-rounded and other unfinished bristle tips. (×60 magnified).

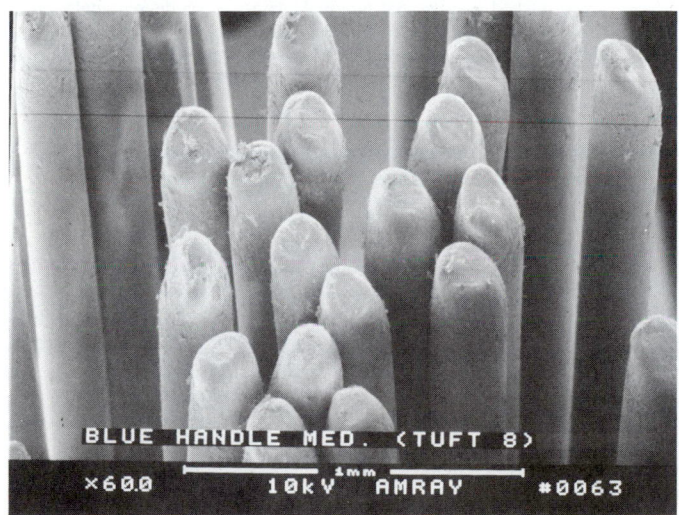

Fig. 20-5. Magnified bristles showing unfinished bristle tips. (×60 magnified).

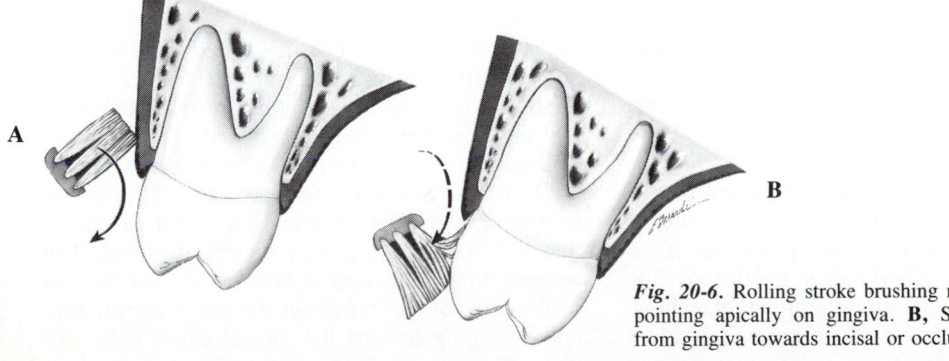

Fig. 20-6. Rolling stroke brushing method. **A,** Place bristles pointing apically on gingiva. **B,** Sweep bristles over teeth from gingiva towards incisal or occlusal surface.

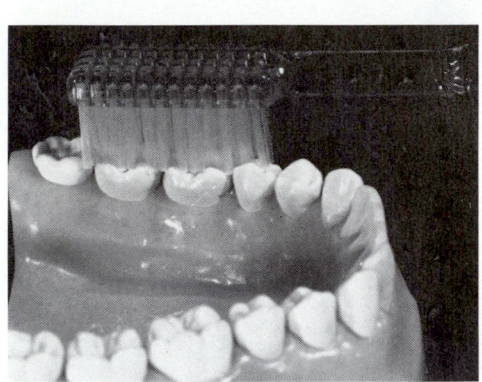

Fig. 20-7. Occlusal cleaning. Brushing bristles back and forth along occlusal surfaces.

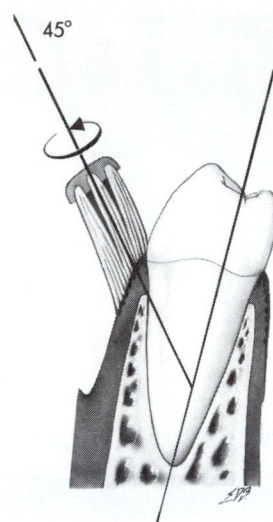

Fig. 20-8. Stillman brushing method. Place bristles on attached gingiva and gingival margin at 45-degree angle. Activate bristles with a small circular motion to stimulate tissues and clean cervical area. Following this step, roll bristles over the crown (modified Stillman method).

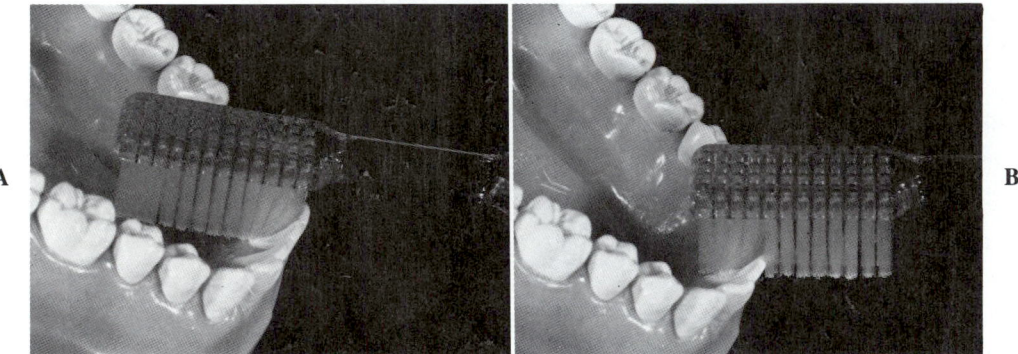

Fig. 20-9. Anterior lingual brushing. **A,** Place brush vertically into narrow anterior portion of arch. **B,** Sweep brush from gingiva toward incisal edge.

scrubbed with a back and forth motion (Fig. 20-7). The limitation of the roll method is that the bristles tend to miss the cervical area, where plaque is most likely to accumulate.

Another historically recommended method is the modified Stillman method. The patient points the bristles apically at approximately 45 degrees to the long axis of the tooth and places them on the attached gingiva. The bristles are flexed with enough pressure to cause slight gingival blanching and are activated with a small rotary (circular) motion (Fig. 20-8). The rotation is repeated eight

to ten times, then the brush is rolled from the gingiva towards the occlusal surfaces. With a soft-bristled brush, the bristles adapt to the interproximal areas as the roll is completed. The rotation/roll sequence is performed several times before the brush is moved to the next area. Care should be taken to overlap at least one tooth to ensure that the brushing sequence cleans all areas. The anterior lingual section is brushed by placing the heel or toe of the brush on the gingiva, rotating, and sweeping toward the incisal edges (Fig. 20-9).

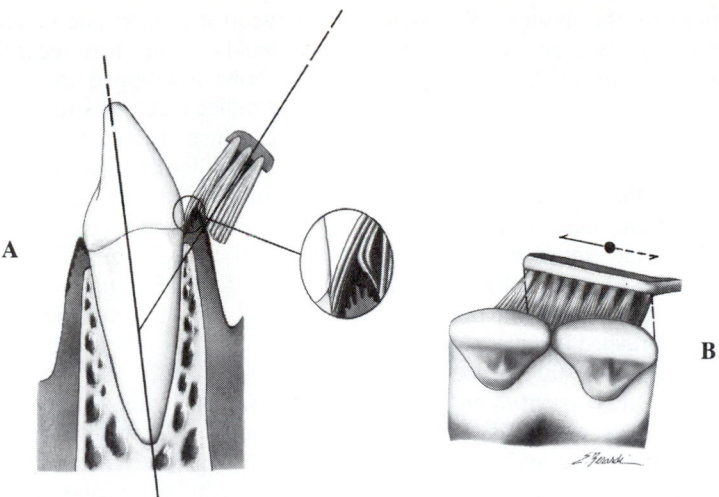

Fig. 20-10. Bass brushing method. **A,** Place bristles pointing apically at 45-degree angle to long axis of tooth. First row of bristles will approximate sulcus, and adjacent row will touch gingival margin. **B,** Activate brush with a short back-and-forth vibration to disorganize plaque at entry to sulcus. Following this step, complete rolling stroke to clean clinical crowns (modified Bass method).

The Bass method is the most generally recommended and accepted method for removing plaque from the sulcular area (Fig. 20-10). The method is similar to the modified Stillman approach, except that the bristles are placed at the margin of the gingiva rather than on the attached gingiva. The bristles are vibrated in place to disrupt the plaque and to move the bristles in the sulcus as far as practical. Some people recommend rolling the bristles towards the occlusal area once the vibratory motion is completed. The full length of the brush head is used on the facial and lingual surfaces, except on the anterior lingual surfaces. In this area, the brush is used vertically, starting with the heel of the brush at the margin of the gingiva. With ideal performance, the bristles slide into the sulcus and reach the interproximal area.

Regardless of the method you teach your patients, the majority will resort to the popular "scrub method." With this method, the bristles are placed at a 90 degree angle to the long axis of the tooth and the brush is moved back and forth or in a large circular motion, covering several teeth with each stroke. Unless a hard brush is used, this method removes plaque successfully from the direct facial and lingual surfaces of the teeth. Its drawbacks are 1) the potential damage to tooth structure and to the soft tissues if the mo-

tion is too vigorous, 2) the inability to reach proximal surfaces reliably. Often it is possible to modify this method for the patient so that fewer teeth are brushed with each stroke and a softer brush with gentle pressure is used. Generally, whatever method the patient is comfortable with and that safely disrupts plaque is acceptable. You can fine-tune procedures over a series of appointments.

Because the tongue is a reservoir for bacteria, it is also important for the patient to brush it. The simplest method is to place the brush at the back of the tongue and sweep forward several times across the dorsum.

When brushing is completed, the brush should be thoroughly rinsed and the handle tapped on the sink edge to remove excess moisture. It should be stored to permit air circulation and drying.

For patients who are particularly ineffective with a handbrush or who like to use motorized devices, electric toothbrushes are ideal. All electric toothbrushes can be expected to be as effective as a handbrush if they are applied in all areas of the mouth and given sufficient time to cleanse the teeth. The newer designs that feature rotating bristles or that simulate the modified Bass method have solid research showing their efficacy, even for reaching proximal and sulcular areas. For patients who can afford to purchase them, they may be the ideal solution to the issues of which method to teach, which method the patient actually uses, and how effectively the teeth are cleaned.

Interdental cleaners

Dental floss and tape are the primary aids for interdental plaque disruption. One study of 119 young adults showed that the groups who brushed and flossed each day for 10 days lowered their gingival bleeding scores by 67% compared with 35% for those who only brushed (Graves, Disney, and Stamm, 1987). This is probably because the floss can reach from the contact point to an area 1 to 2 mm subgingivally on the proximal surfaces. Used properly and regularly, floss and/or tape are effective.

Floss and tape need to fit easily through the tight contact areas to accomplish this goal. Because interdental spaces and patients' preferences about floss and tape vary, there are many kinds available. French and Friedman (1975) found that both waxed and unwaxed products clean effectively. Stevens (1980) and Lobene and Soparker (1982) have reported similar studies, in which variable-diameter and mint-flavored floss removed plaque as well as other floss products. Patient preference varies also. When 100 subjects were asked which floss they preferred, 80% preferred waxed and 20% preferred unwaxed. Sixty percent purchased waxed floss and 30% purchased unwaxed; 50% chose mint-flavored brands. Regardless of whether the product is waxed or unwaxed, thin or thick, teflon or nylon or Goretex, the important issue is whether the patient will faithfully floss every day to disrupt plaque. Therefore start by identifying the type of floss that fits the need and that the patient prefers.

Flossing is not easy. Unless you provide a floss holder (Fig. 20-11), the patient will need to secure the floss in the hands, manipulate it between each pair of teeth and scrape it down the proximal surface on each side of the papilla without harming the soft tissue, and then remove it and use a fresh section of the floss for the next pair of teeth. It takes time to learn this procedure, and it is awkward, particularly if the patient has large hands, tight contacts, rough restoration margins, or a sensitive gag reflex.

For patients in whom flossing is the first choice for interdental cleaning, follow this approach:

1. Cut an 18-inch (45 cm) section of floss and wrap it around one or more fingers on both hands so that it is securely held. Fig. 20-12 shows it wrapped around the little fingers. A simpler method is to tie the floss into a loop and use different sections of the loop at each interdental area (Fig. 20-13).
2. Stretch the floss over the thumbs or forefingers so that there is approximately 1 inch (1.9 to 2.5 cm) of floss between the two hands. This length of floss will be moved past the contact point to reach the full length of the proximal surfaces (Fig. 20-14).
3. Use the thumbs to press the floss past the maxillary contacts (Fig. 20-15); use the forefingers to press it downward past the mandibular contacts (Fig. 20-16).
4. Work the floss back and forth at the contact area until it passes (Figs. 20-17 and 20-18).
5. Once it has eased gently past the contact point, wrap the floss around the tooth and move it up and down against the tooth between the sulcus and the contact area of one tooth (Fig. 20-19). Clean the adjacent tooth surface the same way (Fig. 20-20), taking care not to cut the papilla as the floss is moved from one proximal surface to the other. Also, ensure that the floss is not snapped through the contact, which can damage the tissues (Fig. 20-21).
6. Hold the floss against the tooth and use the back-and-forth motion to remove it past the contact. If the contact is particularly tight, release one end of the floss and pull it through the interdental space. Also, a floss threader can be used to insert the floss through the embrasure to avoid tight contacts and to insert floss under bridge pontics (Fig. 20-22).
7. Wind the used section of floss onto one hand and use the next clean section for the next interdental area.

In addition to floss and tape, the patient may be helped by yarn, gauze strips, a shoestring, or a pipe cleaner (Figs. 20-23 to 20-26). These are usually chosen when there are large embrasure spaces or missing teeth adjacent to the site to be cleaned.

Flossing is nearly sacred to the dental profession and has been since the mid-1960s. It is especially helpful for cleansing the contact point and reducing the risk of interdental caries. Performed

Text continued on p. 445.

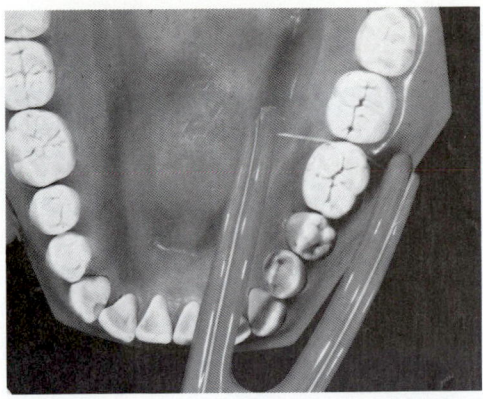

Fig. 20-11. Floss holder. Floss is stretched over frame and can be maneuvered for standard flossing with one hand.

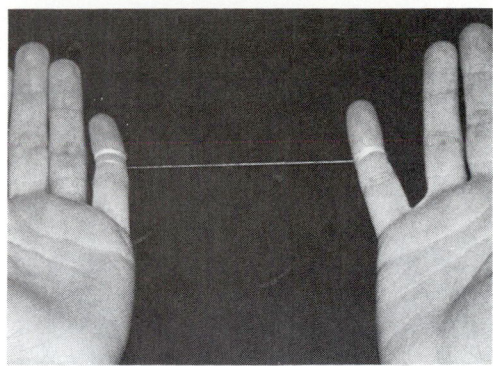

Fig. 20-12. Cut approximately 18 inches of floss. Wrap securely around one or more fingers.

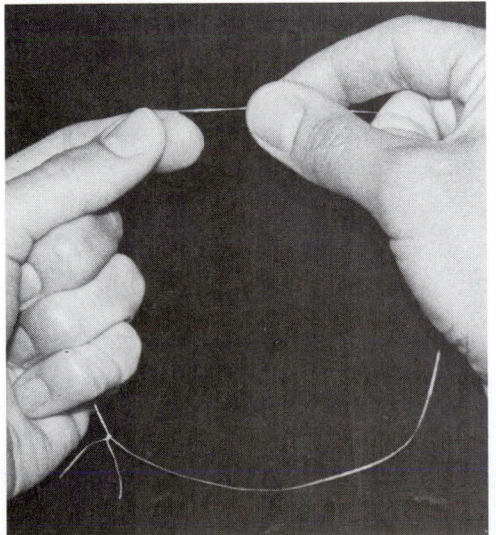

Fig. 20-13. Floss tied in a loop may be easier to maneuver for some patients.

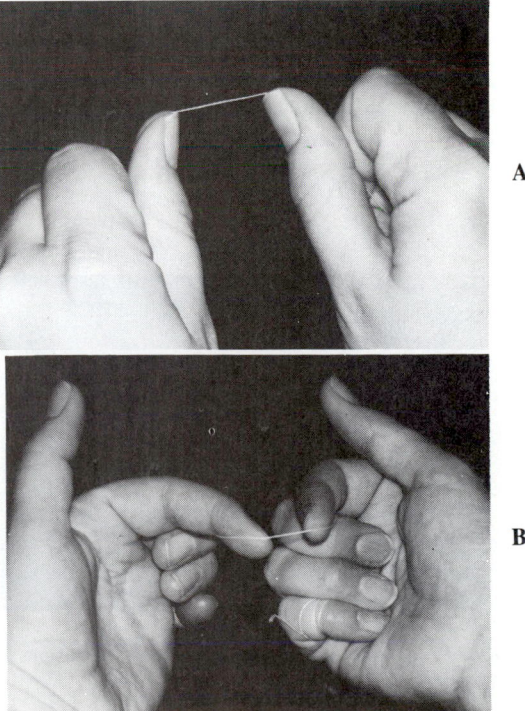

Fig. 20-14. Stretch floss over thumbs, **A**, or forefingers, **B**, to manipulate the floss.

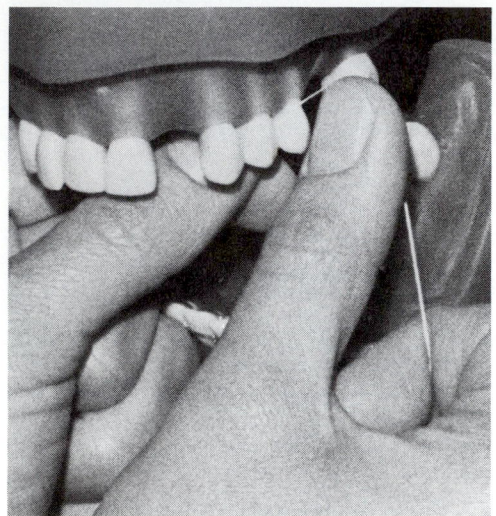

Fig. 20-15. Placement of thumbs and floss for maxillary technique. To clean proximal surfaces, one thumb is placed on lingual aspect of arch; other thumb is placed on facial aspect with approximately 1 inch (2.5 cm) or floss between thumbs.

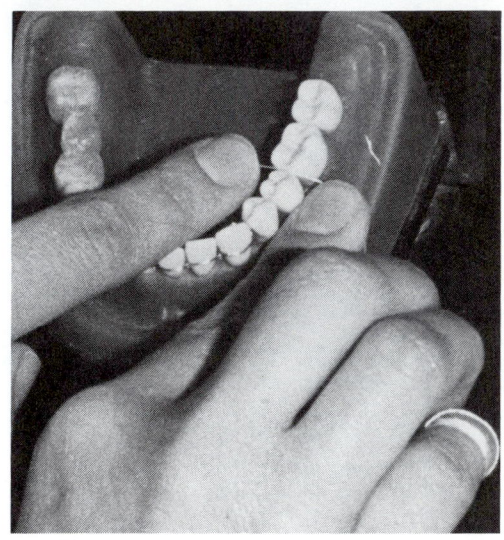

Fig. 20-16. Placement of index fingers for mandibular technique. To clean proximal surfaces, one finger is placed on lingual aspect of arch; other finger is placed on facial aspect.

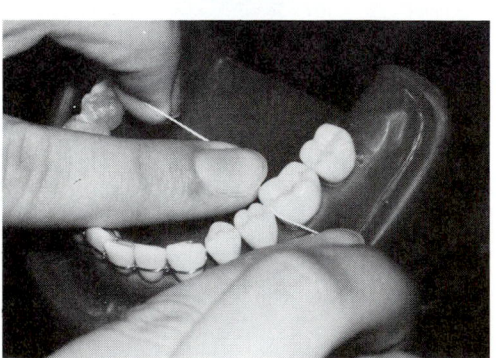

Fig. 20-17. Insert span of floss into contact area. Hold floss around one of the teeth to help ease past contact.

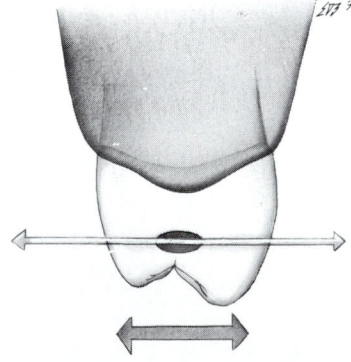

Fig. 20-18. Back-and-forth, seesaw motion helps move floss through contact area.
(From Corn H, Marks M: *Cont Dent Educ* 1:14, 1978.)

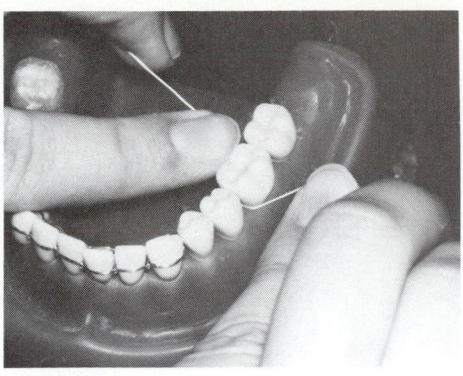

Fig. 20-19. Once past contact area, wrap floss around tooth and move floss up and down on proximal surface.

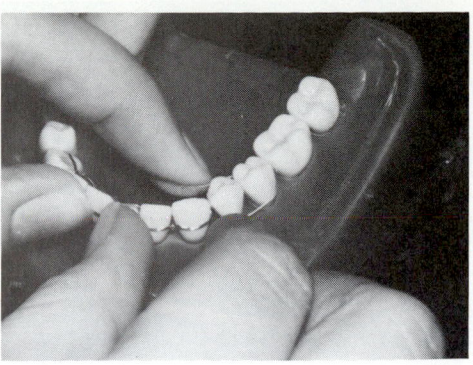

Fig. 20-20. When first proximal surface is completed, wrap floss around adjacent tooth, and use same vertical cleaning stroke.

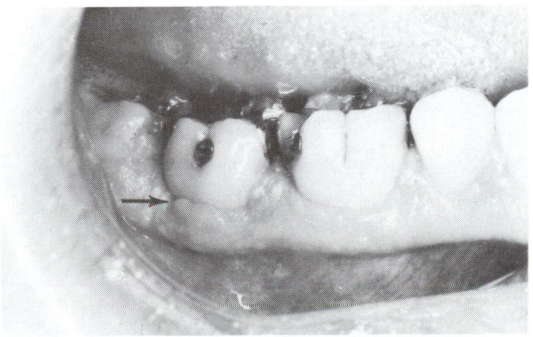

Fig. 20-21. With improper placement a gingival cleft may result from floss being continually forced into sulcus. (From Corn H, Marks M: *Cont Dent Educ* 1;16, 1978.)

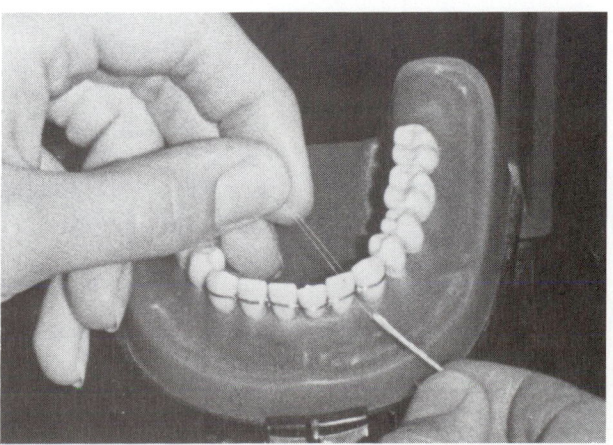

Fig. 20-22. Floss threader. Place floss through eye of clear plastic threader (Zons), and feed floss under appliance, tight contact, or bridge area.

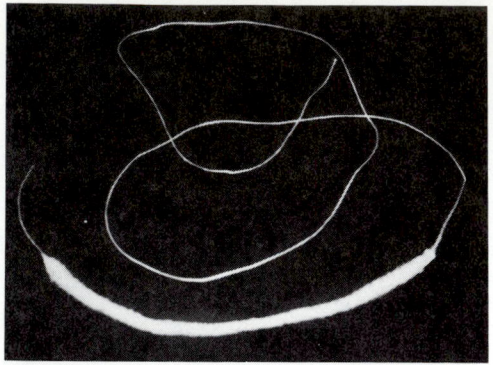

Fig. 20-23. Variable diameter ("Super") floss. This product contains a stiff end for threading, an area of yarn-type floss, and a large section of regular floss.

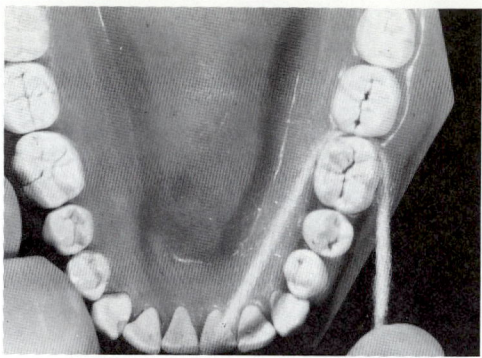

Fig. 20-24. White synthetic yarn makes excellent cleaner for wide interproximal areas.

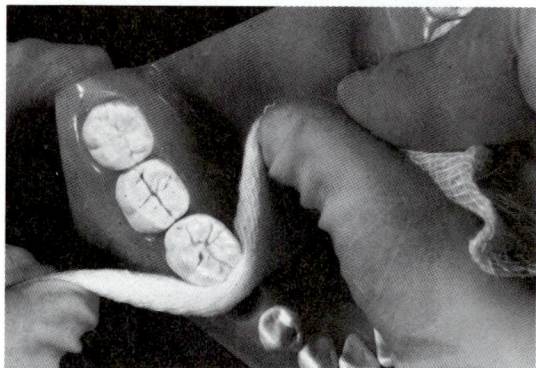

Fig. 20-25. Gauze strip can be folded and adapted to polish a wide interdental area.

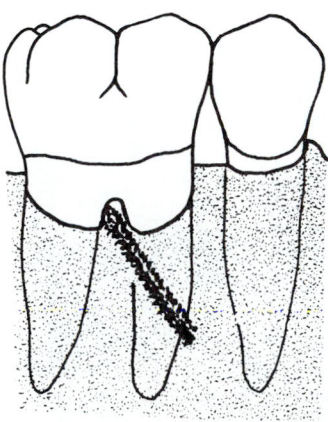
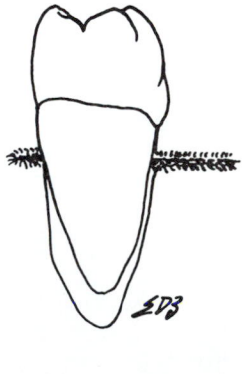

Fig. 20-26. Pipe cleaner can be bent and adapted to furcation area and other areas with limited access.

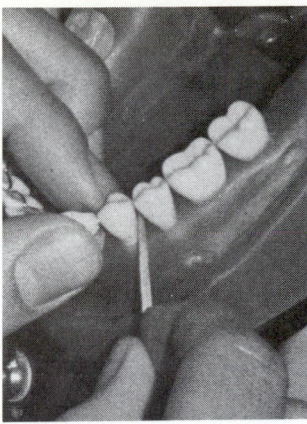

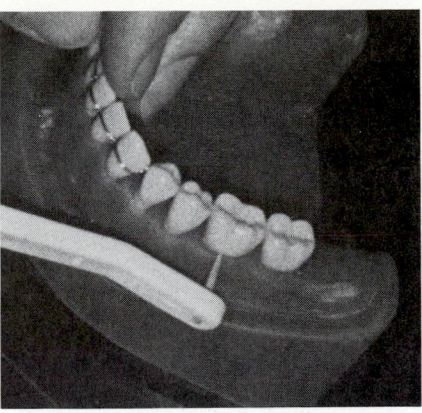

Fig. 20-27. Wood wedge interdental cleaner is softened and placed with base of wedge on tissue. Point wedge occlusally and clean proximal surface by sliding wedge against tooth.

Fig. 20-28. Periodontal aid is toothpick in plastic holder. Toothpick is softened by wetting and applying to gingival margin. Tip can be moved gently in sulcus at less than a 45-degree angle to remove plaque or adapted on cervical surface to burnish fluoride into the exposed roots to control sensitivity.

properly, it can help reduce gingival inflammation. However, for patients who cannot or will not floss, there are alternatives that can disrupt interdental plaque. It is important to have many approaches to help individual patients maximize their efforts and feel successful. Therefore it is not essential that all patients floss.

Interdental sticks, tips, and brushes remove plaque in the proximal areas. The most popular ones are sticks that are triangular in cross-section. The flat part of the triangle is rested on the interdental papilla and the stick is moved gently in and out of the embrasure space from the facial aspect (Fig. 20-27). Look at the sides of the stick after each use, and you will see that an accumulation of plaque has been removed from the proximal surfaces of the teeth. Interdental sticks are highly portable, and many patients will be willing to use them while driving or reading or watching television. As a result, they may be used more frequently or for a greater duration than flossing, depending on the patient's preference. People who regularly use sticks will have flattened papillae, a normal response to the procedure.

Some professionals recommend using round toothpicks to clean the proximal areas. They can be broken off and inserted in a Perio-aid plastic holder to allow access to posterior areas. With the tip directed at less than 45 degrees to the long axis of the tooth, it can be used to remove plaque

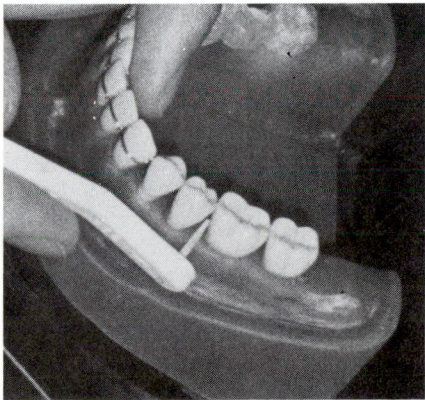

Fig. 20-29. Periodontal aid can be used to clean proximal surface of tooth. Tip is directed occlusally and moved along cervical area.

from the sulcular area as well as interdentally (Figs. 20-28 and 20-29). This implement is also ideal for burnishing fluoride into sensitive root surfaces.

The rubber tip also cleans tooth structure and massages the soft tissues. The tip is placed on the interdental area, with the end directed toward the occlusal surface. Use a rotating or back-and-forth motion with the side of the tip on the tissue (Fig.

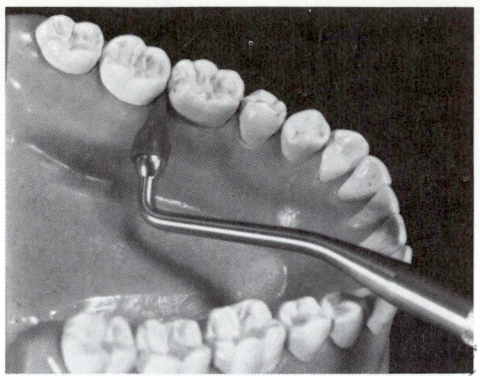

Fig. 20-30. Place rubber tip in interdental area, pointed occlusally. Massage tissue and remove plaque by rotating tip against tissue.

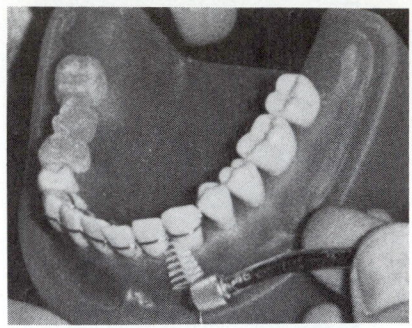

Fig. 20-31. Interproximal brush is spiral-shaped brush that can be placed in wide interdental areas to clean proximal surfaces and stimulate interdental tissue.

20-30). The rubber tip can also be used in open furcation areas.

A small, spiral-shaped interproximal brush or a single tuft of bristles on a handle is very effective in removing interdental plaque and in cleaning the sulcular area (Fig. 20-31).

Oral irrigation

Nearly all the devices just discussed are restricted to supragingival plaque control. Manual brushing can approach 1.5 to 3.0 mm subgingivally (Waerhaug, 1976), and flossing reaches to a maximum depth of 2 to 3 mm around a well-defined papilla (Reitman, 1980). Toothpicks, pipe cleaners, and interdental brushes have minimal access to subgingival plaque.

The oral irrigator, in contrast, can reach subgingival plaque even when the stream is applied supragingivally (Eakle, Ford, and Boyd, 1986). The flushing effect of a pulsating stream of water or an antimicrobial solution can reach subgingival plaque deposits, detoxifying the plaque and disrupting the microbial colonies (Cobb, Rogers, and Killoy, 1988). Supragingival oral irrigation used on a daily basis by the patient at home has been shown to reduce gingivitis, gingival bleeding, and the percentage of periodontal pathogens in subgingival plaque (Ciancio et al, 1989; Flemmig, Newan, and Doherty, 1990; Meis et al, 1992). Oral irrigation is an important part of oral hygiene for patients who cannot control their gingivitis with brushing and interdental cleansing or who are at risk of developing periodontal problems.

See Chapter 28 for further discussion of the research relating to oral irrigation.

When introducing the irrigator, provide supervised instruction in the office. Many professionals provide irrigators at the dental office, because a mere recommendation will not necessarily lead to a purchase and it allows them to instruct the patient in the use of the unit. Others keep one unit available and provide a new tip for the patient and a written recommendation about which irrigator to purchase.

Begin by identifying which supragingival tip you prefer. Many professionals are recommending the plastic SulcusTip or PikPocket tips, which are designed to carry the irrigant directly into the pocket but without using a cannula (blunt needle) (Figs. 20-32 and 20-33). Help the patient select the proper power setting (medium for SulcusTip or PikPocket; high for standard tip) and prepare the irrigant in the reservoir of the irrigator. Recommend warm water either for diluting an antimicrobial solution or using only water; warm water is more comfortable. Show the patient how to trace the tip around the teeth and the sequence to follow. With the tip in the mouth and the patient leaning over the sink with the mouth slightly open (in an "O" shape), turn on the irrigator. The patient should use the irrigator throughout the mouth until the solution is gone. Typically the patient can reach all areas of a full dentition in 1 minute. Irrigation should be done twice daily after brushing.

Many professionals recommend that their pa-

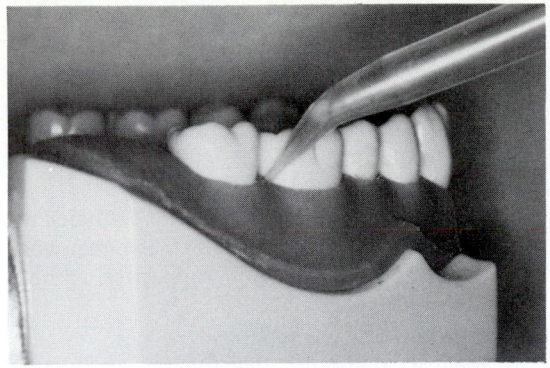

Fig. 20-32. SulcusTip is designed to carry water or antimicrobial agents to the gingival sulcus or the periodontal pocket.

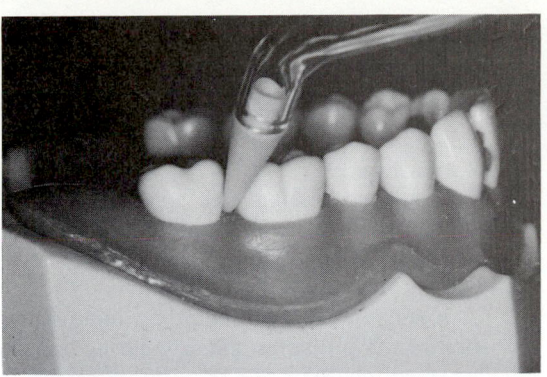

Fig. 20-33. PikPocket is designed like a rubber tip stimulator and used to reach subgingivally with water or antimicrobial agents.

tients who are attempting to maintain deep pockets use a subgingival cannula at home to irrigate (Fig. 20-34). Patients can use these safely if they are properly instructed. Show the patient the sites to irrigate and how to guide the cannula to the site and insert it 2 to 3 mm. Watch the patient's ability to direct the cannula properly, and ensure that the cannula is not being forced into the pocket. The irrigator should be set on the lowest power for this procedure so that the irrigant is carried but not forced into the pocket.

To judge which oral physiotherapeutic aids will work for your patients, you should evaluate them by disclosing the teeth and seeing how much plaque is removed and with which methods. Another important test is to probe the mouth to identify bleeding sites, institute the oral hygiene program you believe is best suited for the patient, and then re-evaluate for bleeding approximately 4 to 6 weeks later.

INDIVIDUALIZING ORAL HEALTH STRATEGIES: CASE ANALYSES

Individualizing strategies to fit the specific needs of the patient is the basis for success in oral health education. Refer to the case descriptions included in Chapter 18. Review each case description, and then review (and modify as necessary) the oral health strategies identified here.

Case #1: Ms. L. Evans

Goals for the patient.
  1. Adopt a more successful long-term approach to oral care.

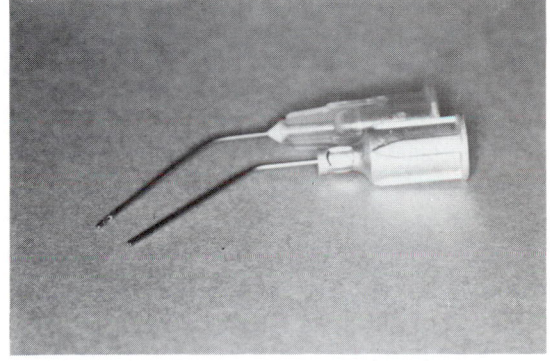

Fig. 20-34. Cannulas for subgingival irrigation.

  2. Understand her own oral condition.
  3. Adopt an "I want to be healthy" attitude.
Oral health education objectives.
  1. Establish professional rapport and trust with the patient.
  2. Maintain patient receptiveness.
  3. Jointly develop and implement an oral hygiene regimen for home and work.
  4. Help the patient see improvements and recognize their importance.
Oral hygiene recommendations.
  1. Sulcular brushing with soft brush,
  2. Densensitizing fluoride toothpaste or gel.
  3. Antimicrobial rinse (Peridex initially; then switch to Viadent or Listerine), daily, in an irrigator.
  4. Fluoride rinse (0.05% daily or 0.2% weekly).

5. Interproximal cleaning: choice of sticks or floss.
6. Substitution for sugared snacks: crackers, fruit, or vegetables; review total diet once trust is established and incremental success has occurred.
7. Schedule continuing care appointments for every 3 months, at least until oral hygiene is under control.

Motivational strategies.

1. Ask her how you can help her improve the oral health problems she saw during the assessment phase.
2. Integrate your recommendations into the discussion that ensues following #1.
3. Stress what she is presently doing well and reinforce positive change at subsequent appointments.
4. Ensure that she understands the ramifications of not adopting new behaviors versus making positive change (caries, gingivitis sequelae).
5. Listen to verbal and nonverbal messages regarding her understanding of information, acceptance of new ideas, and involvement in deciding which procedures will work best.

Clinician self-assessment.

1. Were the patient's wants, needs, and expectations addressed? Were they met?
2. Was the motivational plan realistic given her life-style?
3. Is the patient returning for her scheduled visits?
4. Is she making progress to reverse the pattern of continuing dental caries and gingivitis?

Case #2: Mr. J. Borg

Goals for the patient.

1. Maintain high expectations regarding oral health care and oral hygiene.
2. Understand that the faulty restorations are preventing effective oral hygiene.
3. Continue good oral hygiene habits.
4. Replace restorations as soon as financially and practically possible.
5. Evaluate the impact of previous dentistry logically and adopt a positive approach to resolving issues of responsibility.

Oral health education objectives.

1. Establish professional rapport and trust with the patient.
2. Maintain patient receptiveness.

3. Jointly review the patient's current oral hygiene regimen.
4. Reinforce relationship between the effort required for good physical health and the efforts required for good oral health.
5. Substitute or add other interdental cleaning devices for areas near faulty crowns
6. Allow the patient to discuss his attitudes regarding his previous dentist and the work that was performed; be supportive without placing blame.

Oral hygiene recommendations.

1. Electric toothbrush that focuses on sulcular and interdental cleansing; fluoride toothpaste.
2. Alternative interproximal cleaning for areas near faulty crowns: dental sticks; floss other areas or use sticks for all areas.
3. Daily irrigation with oral rinse, especially near faulty crowns.
4. Schedule continuing care appointments every 4 months to provide supportive therapy for crown areas until they are replaced.

Motivational strategies.

1. Ask him how you can help him improve the oral health problems he saw during the assessment phase.
2. Integrate your recommendations into the discussion that ensues following #1.
3. Stress that his approach to oral hygiene and his diligence are important; reinforce his positive efforts.
4. Ensure that he understands the ramifications of the current restorative dental procedures; provide sufficient support so that necessary delays will have minimal negative impact on oral health.
5. Listen to verbal and nonverbal messages regarding his understanding of information, acceptance of new ideas, and involvement in deciding which procedures will work best.

Clinician self-assessment.

1. Were his wants, needs, and expectations addressed? Were they met?
2. Was the motivational plan realistic given his life-style?
3. Is the patient considering or scheduling restorative care?
4. Is he making progress to control inflammation near the faulty restorations?
5. Are his attitudes towards his previous dentist in line with the scope of the problem?

Case #3: Mr. M. Willoff

Goals for the patient.
1. Maintain high expectations regarding oral health care and oral hygiene.
2. Continue or improve regular dental care.

Oral health education objectives.
1. Establish professional rapport and trust with the patient.
2. Maintain patient receptiveness.
3. Jointly review his current oral hygiene regimen.

Oral hygiene recommendation.
1. Continue current efforts.
2. Come regularly for examinations and needed care.

Motivational strategies.
1. Ask him if there is anything he needs you to do to help him maintain his good oral health.
2. Integrate your opinions and encouragement about his oral status in the discussion that ensues following #1.
3. Stress that his approach to oral hygiene and his diligence are important; reinforce positive efforts.
4. Ensure that he understands the possible relationship between his arthritis medication and his periodontal health.
5. Listen to verbal and nonverbal messages regarding his understanding of information, acceptance of ideas.

Clinician self-assessment.
1. Were his wants, needs, and expectations addressed? Were they met?
2. Are you becoming complacent about this person's health levels? Have you planned sufficient time to practice diligent assessment at continuing care intervals?

Case #4: Dr. C. Balsiger

Goals for the patient.
1. Recognize the partnership role between professional care and self-care in preventing the recurrence of periodontitis.
2. Adopt oral hygiene habits that are specific to the problems of periodontitis.
3. Recognize the strong relationship between nicotine and periodontitis.
4. Identify how work habits and life-style affect oral hygiene and smoking habits.
5. Make a commitment to reduce risk factors for periodontal disease and increase factors that prevent it.

6. Accept more frequent and thorough debridement of periodontally involved areas.
7. Continue to feel positively about the contribution of previous periodontal treatment.
8. Improve diet to maximize fruits and vegetables.

Oral health education objectives.
1. Establish professional rapport with the patient.
2. Maintain patient receptiveness.
3. Jointly review current oral health status and possible improvements in oral hygiene regimen; introduce more effective measures for plaque control.
4. Offer smoking cessation program; discuss current research findings regarding smoking and periodontal disease.
5. Discuss episodic nature of periodontal disease and the risk factors associated with it.
6. Review the purposes of subgingival debridement.
7. Review alternative "quick meals" that provide better nutritional value.

Oral hygiene recommendations.
1. Electric toothbrush that provides maximal access to marginal and interdental areas.
2. Interdental cleaning device: floss and/or interdental sticks.
3. Irrigation with antimicrobial solutions (Peridex, Listerine, or Viadent) daily.
4. When ready, enter into smoking cessation program.
5. Shorter continuing care interval: 3 to 4 months.

Motivational strategies.
1. Ask her how you can be of help in improving the signs of disease that were obvious in the guided self-assessment.
2. Integrate your suggestions and encouragement during the ensuing discussion following #1.
3. Reinforce positive efforts and focus on the areas in the mouth that look healthy.
4. Find ways to provide alternative habits to smoking during work and at home.
5. Listen to verbal and nonverbal messages regarding her understanding of the role of smoking in the progression of disease.

Clinician self-assessment.
1. Were the patient's wants, needs, and expectations addressed? Were they met?
2. Did she accept the necessary treatment and/or recommendations for improved oral hygiene?

3. Is she considering stopping smoking or has she actually started a smoking cessation program?
4. Does the patient still feel positive about the previous treatment she received?
5. Have her dietary choices improved?

• • •

Every patient case you review will suggest a wide variety of educational and treatment choices if you take the time to assess the patient's current status and look past a rote approach to oral hygiene care. Not everyone needs to learn to floss, not everyone needs nutritional guidance, and not everyone should appear for continuing care on the same schedule. Part of what makes dental hygiene a valuable and interesting field is the opportunity to think through the variables each patient brings and to identify appropriate choices with the cooperation of the patient. Using a structure like the one shown for the 5 patient cases can help you organize your thoughts and plan a solid approach to helping the patient regain and maintain health.

ADAPTING ORAL HEALTH EDUCATION TO SMALL GROUPS

Oral health education is addressed in this chapter primarily in terms of working with individual patients. However, the principles discussed also apply when working with groups of people in a variety of settings. Even hygienists who expect to work on a one-to-one basis rather than as community hygienists will have opportunities to meet with school groups, senior citizens, birthing classes, patients with special needs, and even other health care providers. The content of the teaching is often the same for groups as for individuals; so is the need to focus on the specific needs and characteristics of the persons involved and to evaluate the success of the program. However, several important different dimensions are involved in working with groups.

Though it may be relatively easy to engage an individual in conversation while sitting together at the dental chair or in a separate teaching area, it is not as easy in a group. As you lecture a small group, each person may be paying varying amounts of attention. When this occurs, you will have no clue regarding whether they need to hear what you are saying, whether they understand and agree, and whether there will be any effect on their subsequent oral health habits. Mentally, you need to believe you are speaking with everyone in the group and that you respect differing attitudes and beliefs. Your task, more than giving information, is to engage them in discussion.

To encourage discussion, it is better to sit at the level of the group, perhaps in a circle, or if it is a large group, to walk among them with your microphone. It helps to feel a part of the group rather than an outsider.

In beginning your discussion, speak briefly about the purpose of the session and what you hope to accomplish. Tell them a bit about yourself and why you have decided to meet with them. To move into the content of the session, ask a question for which there should be an array of answers. And then wait for an answer. For instance, if it is a smoking cessation group, you can begin with: "How many of you have tried to quit smoking before?" Hands should go up. Then ask, "How did you do it?" followed by, "How successful was it for you?" As each response is given, use active listening (repeating and rephrasing the information to show understanding) as your response to each comment. Convey respect and empathy for their efforts. Be supportive. If you can engage virtually everyone in the small group in the discussion, and their responses appear to be frank and sincere, you will have established the seeds of trust that will enable you to help them look at new ways of stopping smoking.

Sometimes, the group will be hesitant to respond to your opening question. Often, all you have to do is wait. It may seem like an eternity, but it usually is no more than 10 seconds. People need time to gather their thoughts and decide whether it is safe to risk answering. Give them that time. If they still do not respond, it may be helpful to add: "I really do want to know what has worked and what has failed for you. Then we can build on that." That tells them how you will use the information and may make them more responsive.

Working with small groups also involves the specialized skills of keeping the group on track and on time, ensuring that the shy ones are included and that the ones who believe they have all the answers are politely limited. Keeping the group on track can be managed by having a series of five or six questions that will move them from one phase of the discussion onward. For instance, for a group discussing the topic of selecting oral hygiene aids, you may begin with: "What are your favorite commercials about toothbrushes?" If you want to limit the amount of time on that topic, you may move the group along after a few comments by shifting the discussion to: "How many of you actually buy the brands of toothbrushes you see advertised? How do you know which brush is best for you?" You can introduce information about selecting brushes as the discussion progresses. Then you can move it ahead again by asking: "How often should you buy a new brush?" Each question carries the group through the agenda you have planned. Identify how much time and energy you want to spend on each topic so that the most important objectives receive the most attention.

Using a group discussion format that is based on a series of questions keeps the group and you alert. You never know what they will say to which you will need to respond. This carries an element of risk. However, you are more likely to be successful in meeting your goals for the group than if you opt for the "safe but boring" route of telling them what you think they need to know in a lecture format. Active listening is helpful because while you are repeating the essence of the other person's comment you can gather your wits about how to respond.

If you sense that a person is trying to carry too much of the discussion to the exclusion of the others, you may wish to reflect back what he or she says and then redirect your attention to the rest of the group to solicit a response to the person: "What do the rest of you think about that? How would you solve that problem?" "Has anyone else had a similar situation?" This helps you avoid getting into a back-and-forth discussion with one person who monopolizes your time and attention.

Drawing out shy people is a bit more difficult. It usually does not help to put that person on the spot. If you think he or she may want to participate but cannot seem to jump in, you can say: "You look like you have something to say, Judy. What do you think?" Some people will show nonverbal cues that say: "I don't want to be here; I'm bored." You can opt to ignore the person, which may confirm that you do not really care about what he or she thinks. Or you can risk saying: "I'd like to hear what you think about Harry's idea, Jim." In fact, you may not like to hear the response, if it is a harsh comment. If so, you can politely thank the person and resume with the

group. It is important to maintain a respectful, adult-to-adult response, even when you are greeted with one that begs for you to become authoritarian.

If you follow the interactive mode with small groups, the time will go quickly, and you will feel as if you have learned as much as you have taught. This will make you an even better health educator for the next group.

• • •

Working with groups effectively takes practice, and so does working with individuals. Developing these skills should be a focal point of your clinical education. Work with classmates and colleagues to develop a style that aligns with the basic tenets of effective communication and human relations. Role-playing, watching and critiquing videotapes of your interactions with patients and small groups of your peers, observing other clinicians' approaches, and asking your patients for their evaluation of your abilities as an agent for education and change will help you excel.

CONCLUSION

An integral part of dental hygiene is its preventive orientation. Central to this is oral hygiene education. It is important to adopt an adult-to-adult partnership style, research-based content, and individualized techniques and approaches to help each patient obtain and keep the best possible oral health. This can be the most rewarding and important aspect of dental hygiene care. See Chapter 5 for more discussion about building helping relationships with patients.

ACTIVITIES

1. Write your professional definition of prevention and the rationale for focusing on prevention throughout oral hygiene care. Describe your philosophy of oral health education. In a small group, discuss your definition and philosophy. Make a commitment to practice what you think!
2. Describe your encounters with dentists and dental hygienists and recount how they did or did not practice prevention as you now believe it should be practiced. Discuss what you would do differently to bring those encounters in line with a focus on prevention.
3. Despite dental hygienists' best efforts, patients will implement plaque control based on their values and desires. How can you determine and understand a patient's values, wants, needs, and expec-

tations? Write down questions that probe positively into the patient's life-style. List open-ended questions that generate conversation.

4. Videotape other dental hygiene students or graduate hygienists during their discussions of oral health with patients. Review those tapes with the clinicians involved and discuss what worked and what could be improved. Invite the patients to participate as well to learn their impressions of when they were learning and when they were distracted (boredom, anger, amusement).

5. List the preventive dental aids and equipment necessary in any dental setting for you to implement an individualized health education plan for a patient. Include toothbrushes, floss, an irrigator, and so forth. In small groups, demonstrate the use of the devices and explain the role of each. Develop communication techniques for introducing the devices to patients.

6. After sufficient practice with brushing techniques and the use of other aids, form small groups. Give each group an envelope filled with slips of paper asking for a demonstration of a particular oral hygiene technique. Select a slip of paper and demonstrate the designated technique for the group.

7. The following exercise may take several weeks to complete. It is designed to help each dental hygiene student bring his or her personal oral health to an optimal level. Complete a dental health assessment for a classmate. Jointly determine your classmate's values, wants, needs, and expectations. Work with your classmate to optimize his or her oral hygiene. Work closely with a faculty member during the assessment and planning stages. Reverse roles with your "patient." In small groups, discuss the variety of needs and the various choices and strategies considered for optimization.

8. Provide individualized preventive education for a clinical patient. Keep a journal of events documenting the initial assessment, educational plan, instruction sequence, and follow-up evaluation. Share this in a small group for feedback and evaluation.

9. Invite community hygienists, preventive therapists, or dentists to present a seminar on the preventive education format they use in their practice settings.

10. The focus of motivating patients has passed from selecting specific dental aids to determining the factors that will motivate the patient to adopt new behaviors. Life-style is central to this. How can differing life-styles determine the likelihood of success? How can they provide insights for suggesting compatible oral hygiene practices? In groups of 3 students, answer these questions individually and then discuss them as a group in terms of what health behaviors might be most appropriate to suggest:

a. Describe a typical day in your life. What events and activities do you value most?

b. What percentage of time do you spend in leisure activities? Do you work first and play later or the other way around?

c. Rank the following in order of their importance to you: social acceptance, financial success, health, intelligence, family, professional success, relaxation, contributing to society's needs, and fame. Discuss how your made your choices, giving examples of what each item means to you personally.

d. Identify one health behavior you have trouble adopting (using seatbelt, selecting low-fat foods, regular exercise, routine plaque control, avoiding tobacco, etc.). Discuss what it would take for you to adopt the proper behavior. Specify the roadblocks that prevent you from adopting the proper behavior.

REVIEW QUESTIONS

1. A patient you are treating has had her teeth "cleaned" every 6 months for years in another practice. She expects you will do the same for her at first appointment. When and how will you decide whether that service is important for her at that visit.

2. Another patient appears for care with healthy teeth and gingivae. A review of oral hygiene techniques reveals that the patient does not floss and uses a simple scrub method for brushing. What do you do for this patient?

3. Which brushing technique tends to miss the cervical portion of the tooth?

4. Which brushing technique is the generally recommended by clinicians and why?

5. What is the best way to deplaque the proximal surfaces?

6. Why is it better to use a discussion format in teaching good oral health behaviors?

7. Why is smoking cessation a legitimate concern of dental hygienists and dentists?

REFERENCES

Bass CC: The optimum characteristics of toothbrushes for personal oral hygiene, *Dent Items* 70:696, 1948.

Bergstrom J, Eliasson S: Noxious effects of cigarette smoking on periodontal health, *J Periodont Res* 22:513, 1987.

Christen AG, McDonald JL: Helping patients quit smoking: useful strategies for the dental health team, *Dentistry 86*, 6:16, 1986.

Ciancio SG et al: The effect of a chemotherapeutic agent delivered by an oral irrigation device on plaque, gingivitis, and subgingival microflora, *J Periodontol* 60:310, 1989.

Cobb CM, Rogers RL, Killoy WG: Ultrastructure examination of human periodontal pockets following the use of an oral irrigation device in vivo, *J Periodontol* 59:155, 1988.

Danielsen B et al: Effect of cigarette smoking on the transition dynamics in experimental gingivitis, *J Clin Periodontol* 17:159, 1990.

Dunbar S: Term coined for continuing education course for dental hygienists, 1976.

Eakle WS, Ford C, Boyd RL: Depth of penetration in periodontal pockets with oral irrigation, *J Clin Periodontol* 13:39, 1986.

The First National Dental Symposium on Smoking Cessation: helping dental patients to quit smoking, *J Dent Assoc* (supp):41, Jan 1990.

Flemmig T, Newman MG, Doherty FM: Supragingival irrigation with 0.06% chlorhexidine in naturally occurring gingivitis: 6 month clinical observations, *J Periodontol* 61:112, 1990.

French CI, Friedman LA: The plaque removal ability of waxed and unwaxed dental floss, *Dent Hyg* 49:449, 1975.

Graves R, Disney J, Stamm J: Comparative effectiveness of flossing and brushing in reducing interproximal bleeding, *J Periodontol* 58:243, 1987.

Hanes P, Schuster G, Lubas S: Binding, uptake and release of nicotine by human gingival fibroblasts, *J Periodontol* 62:147, 1991.

Henningfield J: Understanding nicotine addiction and physical withdrawal process, *JADA*, special supplement, January 1990.

Little SJ, Stevens VJ: Dental hygiene's role in reducing tobacco use, *J Dent Hyg* 65:346, 1991.

Lobene R, Soparker P: Use of dental floss, effect on plaque and gingivitis, *Clin Prevent Dent* 4(1):5, 1982.

Maslow AH: *Motivation and personality*, New York, 1970, Harper & Row.

Mecklenburg R et al: *How to help your patient stop using tobacco: a National Cancer Institute manual for dental professionals*, Bethesda, Md, 1989, US Public Health Service.

Meis P et al: Supragingival irrigation in gingivitis: 8 week clinical and microbiological findings, *J Dent Res* 70(abstract 1554):1554, 1992.

Preber H, Bergstrom J: Effect of cigarette smoking on periodontal healing following surgical therapy, *J Clin Periodontol* 17:324, 1990.

Reitman WB et al: Proximal surface cleaning by dental floss, *Clin Prevent Dent* 2:7, 1980.

Severson HH et al: Dental offices practices for tobacco users: independent practice and HMO clinics, *Am J Public Health* 80:1503, 1990.

Smoking cessation for the dental office, *Indiana University School of Dentistry*, Marion Merrell Dow, Inc, Kansas City, MO, 1990, p 17.

Squillaro RC, Cohen DW, Laster L: A comparison of microbial plaque disclosants after personal oral hygiene instruction and prophylaxis, *J Prevent Dent* 2:3, 1975.

Stevens AW Jr: Comparison of effectiveness of variable diameter versus unwaxed floss, *J Periodontol* 51:666, 1980.

Sweet J, Butler D: The relationship of smoking to localized osteitis, *J Oral Surgery* 37:732, 1979.

Waerhaug J: The interdental brush and its place in operative and crown and bridge dentistry, *J Oral Rehabil* 33:107, 1976.

ACKNOWLEDGMENT

Thanks to Ann Brecht, Teledyne WaterPik, RT for her consultation and expertise on oral irrigation.

21 FLUORIDE THERAPY

Irene Woodall
James Wefel
Nancy Stutsman Young

LEARNING OUTCOMES

The dental hygienist will be able to

1. Describe what causes dental caries.
2. Describe how fluoride inhibits dental caries, including the following factors:
   a. The formation of fluorapatite.
   b. Its effect on microorganisms and plaque.
   c. Its function in the outermost layer of enamel.
   d. Its role in calcium and phosphorus remineralization.
3. Distinguish between the benefits of systemic and topical fluoride in preventing caries.
4. Specify the optimal level of fluoride in communal water supplies.
5. Describe dental fluorosis and how it is caused.
6. Define posteruption maturation.
7. Describe the logic and results of the Grand Rapids/Muskegon and Kingston/Newburgh studies.
8. Administer a professional topical fluoride treatment using the following:
   a. Sodium fluoride.
   b. Stannous fluoride.
   c. Acidulated phosphate fluoride.
9. Describe the recommended regimen for fluoride rinses containing 0.025%, 0.05%, and 0.20% sodium fluoride.
10. Outline and follow procedures designed to minimize toxic reactions to fluoride during the following:
    a. Daily use of fluoride supplements.
    b. In-office topical fluoride treatments.
11. Outline the current controversies and trends relating to the following:
    a. Using high concentration topical fluorides.
    b. Excessive exposure to fluorides from dietary and professional sources.
    c. Polishing teeth before topical fluoride application.
    d. Using frequent, low-dose fluorides.
    e. Using higher-concentration fluorides in dentifrices.
    f. Water fluoridation.
12. Outline a fluoride therapy program for caries-prone patients.

FLUORIDE AND DENTAL CARIES

Until the last decade, more teeth were lost to dental decay than to any other dental problem. In the past several years, however, caries incidence has dropped dramatically (Burt, 1983; Downer, 1983; U.S. Public Health Service, 1981). Fluoride is cited as one of the primary reasons for this decline (Granath and McHugh, 1986). Fluoride is found in many public water supplies, in toothpastes, in oral rinses, in lozenge form, in concentrated topical gels, and even in foods. Frequent exposure to multiple forms of fluoride undoubtedly has had a positive effect on tooth enamel's resistance to dental decay. Most dentists and hygienists consider fluoride to be the most reliable preventive agent for caries (Isman, 1984).

Dental plaque, as pointed out in earlier chapters, is rich in microorganisms. *Streptococcus mutans* is believed to be the principal bacterium in caries formation, even in root caries (Keltjens et al, 1987). When *S. mutans* is exposed to simple carbohydrates, such as those in sucrose, glucose, or fructose, it metabolizes those sugars and produces acid. The acid is held against the enamel, resulting in a loss of mineral content from the tooth.

This mineral loss is balanced by the remineralizing ability of saliva when the pH is raised. Thus an equilibrium is established between the episodic demineralization and remineralization cycles occurring in the mouth. A carious lesion develops when the numerous pH drops produced by plaque overcome the protective effects of saliva.

Fluoride itself cannot remineralize the tooth, but it acts as a catalyst to promote calcium and phosphate precipitation, thus aiding in the repair of demineralized tooth structure. This cyclic flow of mineral to and from the tooth is detected clinically when a white spot lesion forms. This lesion has a relatively intact surface layer and significant subsurface demineralization (Wefel, Silverstone, and Clarkson, 1982). Fluoride has been shown to be most effective in maintaining this hard outer layer and thus preventing the need for a restoration. Scanning election microscopy of the surface reveals focal holes that allow entrance to deeper layers (Driessens et al, 1985). The subsurface demineralization may therefore continue towards the dentin unless remineralization is able to repair or at least arrest lesion progression. Otherwise, the relatively intact surface layer breaks down, allowing greater access to the remaining mineral. When the demineralization reaches dentin, it advances more rapidly towards the pulp and laterally along the dentinoenamel junction (DEJ).

FLUORIDE'S MECHANISMS OF ACTION

Fluoride is unique in its ability to affect both the microflora and the hard tissue in a positive way for caries reduction. It acts both systemically during tooth formation and topically once the tooth has erupted. During tooth formation the presence of fluoride has been claimed to produce shallower pits and fissures and to be incorporated into the forming enamel. It may assist in the transformation of precursor calcium phosphate phases into the more stable hydroxyapatite and fluorapatite mineral phases. Once the tooth has erupted into the oral environment, fluoride may also be incorporated into enamel during posteruptive maturation and/or remineralization (Wefel, 1981).

In addition to enamel incorporation, fluoride may disrupt plaque formation and metabolism. At low concentrations, fluoride can inhibit enolase, an enzyme involved in glycolysis and sugar transport. This can result in less acid production and a less acidogenic plaque (Harper and Loesche, 1986). At high concentrations, fluoride can be bactericidal and may affect many more metallodependent enzyme systems. Thus intracellular and extracellular polysaccharide synthesis may be disrupted. High fluoride concentrations may also prevent salivary pellicle formation and/or adherence of bacteria to the tooth surface (Newbrun, 1986). This unique ability of fluoride to affect the hard tissue and microflora and to function both systemically and topically has helped its universal acceptance as a caries preventive agent.

Water fluoridation has generally been shown to reduce caries by 50% to 60%, but a great deal of this effect has now been attributed to the topical effects of fluoride. Although fluoride is incorporated into developing enamel, no clear correlation between enamel fluoride content and caries reduction has been established on an individual basis (Clarkson et al, 1988; Mellberg et al, 1985; Retief, Harris, and Bradley, 1987). Thus increased enamel fluoride content from systemic fluoride is insufficient to explain the extent of caries reduction afforded by fluoride. The topical effect of fluoride on the demineralization/remineralization equilibrium process may help to explain these results. Fluoride's ability at low concentrations (less than 1 part per million [ppm]) to inhibit demineralization or enhance remineralization is thought to be one of its most important mechanisms of action. In this regard, fluoride decreases enamel demineralization by its presence in the acid milieu produced by bacterial metabolism in the plaque. As little as 0.1 ppm fluoride in a partially saturated buffer can decrease mineral dissolution (Manly and Harrington, 1959; ten Cate and Duijesters, 1983). Small amounts of fluoride also act to enhance remineralization once the plaque acids have been neutralized. In this regard, fluoride acts as a catalyst for the precipitation of hydroxyapatite or fluorapatite and enhances the gain in mineral. This mineral is less soluble because it is more crystalline and purer than the original enamel mineral that has dissolved. Although enamel is described as hydroxyapatite (Ca_{10} $[OH]_2$ $[PO_4]_6$) in its composition, we now realize that a great many impurities exist in this hard tissue (Featherstone and ten Cate, 1988). Enamel should not be considered a pure crystalline form but a carbonate and magnesium-containing calcium-deficient apatite. Thus remineralization produces a more perfect crystal by merely eliminating the natural impurities within enamel.

The mechanisms of action of fluoride are manifold; no single mechanism is responsible for all of its reported effects. Several mechanisms probably act at the same time or in concert with one another. For example, professionally applied topical fluorides may affect bacterial metabolism, adherence, polysaccharide production, enamel fluoride uptake, inhibition of demineralization and enhancement of remineralization, and calcium fluoride formation. The effects associated with high fluoride concentrations are quickly lost as the fluoride is cleared from the oral cavity. That which remains must operate via mechanisms requiring much less fluoride. Salivary fluoride levels are normally 0.01 to 0.03 ppm and too small for most known mechanisms. Plaque, however, may accumulate fluoride and release it during times of acidity (Charleton et al, 1974; Schamschula et al, 1982).

ENAMEL/FLUORIDE INTERACTION

The interaction of fluoride and enamel first occurs developmentally. Fluoride may be incorporated into the enamel crystals and/or may assist in the transformation of precursor phases to apatite. Even in areas where the water is highly fluoridated, there is only a partial substitution of fluoride for hydroxyls. Pure fluorapatite would contain 38,000 ppm of fluoride, but the levels found in enamel from a fluoridated area range from 1000 to 3000 ppm at the surface. The high surface fluoride levels must result from pre-eruptive and posteruptive maturation, since inner enamel fluoride values are in the hundreds, not thousands of parts per million (Iijima and Katayama, 1985; Nakagaki et al, 1987). The high surface fluoride content coupled with the topical effects of fluoride have resulted in significant caries reduction (50% to 60%) for lifelong residents. Children who lived in a fluoridated community for at least 3 years during tooth development had 26.8% fewer carious lesions in their permanent teeth than their counterparts living in nonfluoridated communities

(Burt, Eklund, and Loesche, 1986). These results indicate that a significant systemic, as well as topical, effect may occur. Similarly, Stephan, McCall, and Tullis (1987) showed that when fluoride was removed from a water supply, decayed, missing, and filled surfaces (DMFS) increased by 39.6% over a 5-year period. This suggests that the loss of fluoride's topical effect is quite significant.

If the concentration of fluoride in the water is too high (twice optimal levels) the teeth may develop with white patchy areas of increased porosity. This very mild dental fluorosis increases in severity with increased fluoride ingestion during tooth development. Severe dental fluorosis produces pitting, brown staining, and widespread disfiguring of the enamel. Since dietary sources of fluoride, water fluoride, and inadvertent ingestion of topical fluorides (e.g., toothpaste and rinses) may contribute to the problem, children must be monitored to ensure that they are not overexposed (Heifetz and Horowitz, 1984). The improper use of fluoride supplements in optimally fluoridated areas is a major risk factor in dental fluorosis.

Once the tooth erupts into the oral cavity, it undergoes a process of "posteruptive maturation." This process increases the mineral content of enamel, since saliva is supersaturated with respect to the enamel mineral. The presence of fluoride accelerates this process. As pointed out by Margolis, Moreno, and Murphy (1986), as little as 0.024 ppm of fluoride can increase the remineralization process from partially saturated buffers. Once formed, enamel has no further biologic activity and events occurring in the oral cavity are controlled by physicochemical conditions; hence the importance of demineralization/remineralization equilibrium and factors that may affect it. Since salivary pH is buffered, it is the plaque fluid pH that becomes acidic and starts the decay process. It is at this point that oral hygiene, fluoride exposure, and the use of sealants becomes increasingly important for the prevention of dental decay. Fluoride may affect many of the complex events occurring during plaque development, metabolism, demineralization, and remineralization. At low concentrations, the most probable mechanisms of action are the inhibition of the enzyme enolase (reduced acid production and sugar transport) and the inhibition of demineralization and enhancement of remineralization in the fluids bathing the tooth. The source of this fluoride may be saliva, enamel, plaque, and/or daily fluoride applications (e.g., water, toothpastes, or rinses).

COMMUNAL WATER FLUORIDATION

The addition of fluoride to communal water supplies is a relatively new method of controlling dental decay. Dr. S. McKay, who practiced in the Rocky Mountain area of the United States, noted that his patients who had intrinsic brown stains (mottling) had less dental decay than those without stain. Dr. H. Trendly Dean conducted investigations in the 1930s linking this brown stain and a lower caries incidence with the presence of fluoride in the drinking water (Newbrun, 1986b). The next step was to compare towns having varying levels of natural fluoride in the water with towns having minimal fluoride to determine what concentration could effectively inhibit decay without enamel mottling. From these results researchers determined the optimum concentration of fluoride, which varies from 0.7 to 1.2 ppm, depending on the climate.

In 1945, Grand Rapids, Michigan, added fluoride to its water supply; the caries incidence over the next several years was compared with that in nearby Muskegon, Michigan, which had a very low fluoride level. Likewise, Newburgh, New York, was fluoridated and compared with its neighbor, Kingston, New York. The results of these "sister city" studies showed a significant reduction in caries as well as unequivocal safety (American Dental Association [ADA] Council, 1984; McClure, 1970; Stallard, 1983; Wei, 1974).

After these initial studies, efforts to fluoridate communities throughout the country were launched. Most major cities are fluoridated; however, there are continuing efforts to fluoridate additional communities and to ward off the efforts of antifluoridationists, who typically cite poten-

tially harmful effects and the issue of mass medication in their efforts to remove fluoride from the public drinking supply. Despite 40 years of safety data that reveal no trends toward increased disease among populations drinking fluoridated water, antifluoridation groups persist in presenting to legislative bodies information that would suggest there are harmful effects. Most dentists and hygienists agree that water fluoridation is desirable, and they are willing to work in community campaigns to ensure that the public votes in favor of adding the ion to their water (Isman, 1984). The most effective way to lobby in favor of this public health measure may be to include a discussion of water fluoridation in one-on-one patient education in the dental office. In this way, people seeking dental care will be educated to the benefits of fluoridation and ready to speak and vote in favor of adding or retaining a fluoridation program in the community.

FLUORIDE FORMULATIONS AVAILABLE FOR CONTROL OF CARIES

If your patients' water supply is not fluoridated, *sodium fluoride* drops should be prescribed for daily use by infants. Lozenges, which are sucked or chewed then swished and swallowed, are prescribed for older children. Table 21-1 shows the recommended doses of daily fluoride tablets or drops (ADA Council, 1984). It is important to coordinate with the child's pediatrician or family physician to ensure that the proper amounts are recommended (Levy, 1986).

A conference on the "Changing Patterns of Fluoride Intake," held in Chapel Hill, North Carolina, in March, 1991, discussed the issues of fluoride usage, ingestion, and fluorosis. One recommendation from the conference concerned the use of fluoride supplements. The use of fluoride tablets has been shown to be a risk factor for dental

Table 21-1. Recommended doses of daily fluoride tablets or drops

| Patient's age | Fluoride concentration of drinking water (ppm) | | | Suggested product |
| | Less than 0.3 | 0.3 to 0.7 | More than 0.7 | |
	Recommended mg of fluoride per day			
Birth to 2 years	0.25	0	0	Drops
2 to 3 years	0.50	0.25	0	Tablets or drops
3 to 13 years	1.00	0.50	0	Tablets

Modified from American Dental Association Council on Dental Therapeutics: *Accepted dental therapeutics,* ed 40, Chicago, 1984, The Association.

fluorosis, as has early use of fluoride toothpaste. It was also stated that from the age of 20 to 30 months the anterior surfaces of the teeth are most sensitive to overexposure to fluoride. This time corresponds to the late secretory and early maturation stage of amelogenesis. Using this information, the scientists at the meeting concluded that a change in the supplement schedule would be appropriate. The change finally adopted is reflected in the patient age category. The suggested ages would be 0 to 3 years, 3 to 5 years, and 5 to 13 years. This change has not been reviewed by the American Dental Association at this time. Recommendations in Table 12-1 may be revised when they consider the topic.

Sodium fluoride was one of the first forms of fluoride to be applied topically to the teeth. The original protocol called for applying a 2.0% solution to clean, dry teeth for 3 to 4 minutes at ages 3, 7, 11, and 13, the ages at which newly erupted teeth are present in the mouth. Four applications are given 1 week apart. Caries reductions of 30% to 40% have been measured among children living in low-fluoride areas. Sodium fluoride is chemically stable, has an acceptable taste, is nonirritating, and causes no tooth discoloration. Its major disadvantage is the need to see the patients weekly for 4 consecutive weeks (Horowitz and Heifetz, 1986).

Sodium fluoride is included in some toothpastes in a 0.22% concentration, which yields a 0.1% fluoride, or 1000 ppm, product. It is stable, provides good remineralization, and is readily taken up into the enamel (Reintsema, Schutof, and Arends, 1985). Sodium fluoride is also the active ingredient in most fluoride oral rinses sold over the counter (0.05% or 0.025%) or by prescription (0.20%). The formulation's stability in solution makes it ideal for delivering fluoride in a ready-made rinse that may be stored for several months. The 0.025% solution is intended for twice-daily use, the 0.05% solution for once-daily use, and the 0.20% prescription solution for once-weekly use. Even a 0.01% sodium fluoride rinse (not currently marketed) used for 60 seconds twice daily was found to produce a layer of acid-resistant mineral at the outer layer of cementum in an in vitro/in vivo study with subjects wearing slabs of demineralized tooth in a prosthetic device while rinsing and during daily activities (Terenaka and Koulourides, 1987).

The famous Three Village Program studies showed that after 7 years of use the 0.2% rinses produced a 47.2% reduction in caries overall and a 78.9% reduction in caries on proximal surfaces (Leske, Ripa, and Sposato, 1984; Leske et al, 1985; Ripa et al, 1983b, 1983c). The Nelson County, Virginia, study showed a 90% reduction in proximal caries after 11 years of weekly rinsing (0.20% rinse) combined with ingesting a 1 mg fluoride tablet daily and using a fluoride dentifrice (Horowitz et al, 1986). Overall, the weekly and daily rinses are considered to decrease caries by 35% (Leske, Ripa, and Sposato, 1984; Horowitz and Heifetz, 1986). In a head-to-head trial, 0.05% and 0.20% rinses were shown to be equivalent (Driscoll et al, 1981). Because they are less costly, most school-based programs use the 0.2% rinses weekly (Horowitz and Heifetz, 1986.)

Rinse container sizes are specified by the U.S. Food and Drug Administration to minimize the possibility of accidentally consuming a toxic or lethal dose. No more than 264 mg of sodium fluoride or 120 mg of fluoride ion should be prescribed at one time (ADA Council, 1984). Fluoride rinses should be stored out of the reach of children, and their use should be supervised by an adult. The rinses must be expectorated after use and not swallowed. Typically children over 5 years of age can manage thorough expectoration, but even they should be evaluated for their ability to control swallowing. Ask the child to swish with a premeasured 10 ml of water and then empty it back into the cup. The amount that is returned should exceed the amount that was premeasured, as the saliva will contribute to its volume. This gauge of ability can help identify subjects who automatically consume whatever is placed in the mouth. Normal rinsing time has been suggested as 1 minute, although this may be reduced in young children.

Stannous fluoride (SnF_2) also can be applied topically. A freshly mixed 8.0% solution is applied to dry teeth for 4 minutes, during which the teeth are continually painted with the solution. The treatment requires a single visit and can result in caries reduction of up to 78%, but usually gives values of 30% (Ripa, 1982). Stannous fluoride is unstable in solution, tastes bad, stains demineralized enamel a yellowish brown color, and can irritate the soft tissues (Ripa, 1982).

Stannous fluoride is now available by prescription in a nonabrasive gel system at a 0.4% concentration, which provides 1000 ppm fluoride. It can be used at home and should be brushed on the teeth twice daily after brushing with a dentifrice and rinsing thoroughly to remove all traces of abrasive from the mouth. As it is brushed on the teeth, the gel quickly becomes a liquid, which is swished among the teeth before expectorating. The stannous fluoride not only aids in the prevention of caries, but also has antihypersensitivity properties (see Chapter 31). Several studies indicate that it has antiplaque and antigingivitis effects as well (Boyd, Leggott, and Robertson, 1988; Hock and Tinanoff, 1979; Mazza, Newman, and Simms, 1981; McDonald, Schemehorn, and Stookey, 1978). The disadvantages are its taste (although the gel preparations are more palatable than the 8.0% solutions), the staining of teeth, and the potential toxicity.

Acidulated phosphate fluoride (APF) was introduced in the early 1960s when it was determined that fluoride uptake is better in an acidic environment (Benediktsson et al, 1982). The fluoride gel is either painted on the teeth or applied in preformed trays on both arches simultaneously. It is applied for 4 minutes, during which uptake is very rapid (Newbrun, 1986). The use of thixotropic gel allows the gel to flow under stress and possibly to penetrate into interproximal areas. When stress is released, the gel becomes highly viscous and therefore tends to adhere to tooth surfaces, and is not easily swallowed (Wefel and Wei, 1979).

Acidulated phosphate fluoride contains 1.23% fluoride ion derived from sodium fluoride and hydrogen fluoride in 0.1 M orthophosphoric acid at a pH of 3.0. Studies show up to 70% reduction in caries, but the average reduction is 28% (Horowitz and Heifetz, 1986). It is available in a variety of flavors and is generally believed to be more acceptable than sodium or stannous fluorides.

At least three manufacturers market a *sequential or combined rinse of APF and SnF$_2$* for professional treatments. These are much higher in total fluoride concentration (0.31% APF and 1.64% SnF$_2$) than normal rinses and, for obvious safety reasons, should not be recommended for home use. Three studies with extracted teeth show that enamel is less soluble after using a sequential rinse (Crall et al, 1983; Shannon, Edmonds, and Madsen, 1974; Shannon, Paoloski, and Wescott, 1974), but most caries researchers agree that a solubility reduction is insufficient to recommend

the use of sequential rinses even under professional supervision. They are easier to use than 4-minute applications of the other agents, but are not supportable as a choice in place of agents proven to be effective in short- and long-term clinical trials (Horowitz and Heifetz, 1986).

Gels for home use on a daily basis can be recommended. They contain 1.1% NaF, approximately half the concentration of the gels used in professional treatment. Applied in custom-made trays, they can be a helpful adjunct for patients with rampant dental decay. Only 5 drops per tray should be used to minimize accidental swallowing. They can be used daily for 3½ weeks; their use then should be reevaluated by a dental professional. School-aged children should be carefully supervised during use; children under age 3 should NEVER be given these products (Horowitz and Heifetz, 1986).

In addition, *sodium monofluorophosphate* (Na$_2$MFP) is used to deliver fluoride in some dentifrices. The average benefit, whether in fluoridated or nonfluoridated communities, is a reduction in caries incidence of 25%, with a range of 15% to 40% (DePaola, 1983). Na$_2$MFP normally requires an enzymatic breakdown of the fluorophosphate bond to liberate free fluoride. These fluoride reactions are slower than those of sodium fluoride (Reintsema, Schutof, and Arends, 1985; White and Faller, 1987). However, Na$_2$MFP seems to produce a more thorough remineralization of the early carious lesion, perhaps because it acts more slowly (Mellberg and Mallon, 1984). These differences may have little clinical relevance when fluoride is available from drinking water, fluoride rinses, and professional treatments.

Fluoride varnishes are available in Europe. They are painted on the teeth and deliver fluoride in a controlled-release system, improving on delivery systems that are quickly washed away by saliva and eating. Presently, fluoride varnishes are not available in the United States. A 2-year study in Finland comparing twice-yearly applications of a varnish with rinsing with 0.20% NaF every 2 weeks showed that the varnishes were significantly better, suggesting that they may be a cost-effective alternative to fortnightly rinsing (Seppa and Pollanen, 1987). Varnishes reduce the incidence of caries by a mean of 48% and show a significantly higher concentration of enamel fluoride at 1 and 5 weeks posttreatment than that achieved with an APF treatment (Clark, 1982).

FLUORIDES AND ROOT CARIES

The effect of fluoride on the prevention of root surface caries has recently received much greater attention than in the past. This is because of the increased awareness that people are retaining more of their teeth, which may become at risk for root as well as coronal caries. A survey by Hand, Hunt, and Beck (1988) has shown a relatively high incidence of root surface caries. Because restoration of carious root surfaces often is unsuccessful, can be quite frustrating, and frequently results in recurrent lesions (Jordan and Summey, 1973), prevention is the ideal way to deal with this and all caries problems. In this regard, several studies have found fluoridated drinking water to be associated with lower prevalence (Brustman, 1986; Burt, Ismail, and Eklund, 1986; Stamm, Banting, and Imrey, 1990) and incidence (Hunt, Eldredge, and Beck, 1989) of root surface caries. Although several laboratories have worked on the effect of topical fluorides on root caries using in vitro model systems (Mellberg and Sanchez, 1986; Wefel, Clarkson, and Heilman, 1987) only one published, placebo-controlled clinical trial designed to test a fluoride agent in the prevention of root caries has reported a statistically significant benefit. Using a fluoridated dentifrice, Jensen and Kohout (1988) reported 67% less root caries over 1 year in the fluoridated groups compared with the placebo control group. Several studies have reported a lower root caries incidence in patients using a 0.05% NaF mouthrinse, although the differences were not statistically significant (Leske et al, 1989; Ripa et al, 1987b).

Thus, although topical fluorides have been shown to be effective in preventing coronal caries, their effectiveness in preventing root surface caries needs further confirmation and elucidation. The development of successful procedures to prevent root surface caries and to arrest and even reverse early lesions is urgently needed. When these preventive approaches are developed, the need for invasive and often unsuccessful restoration of root surface caries will be greatly reduced.

CONTROVERSIES AND CHANGING PROTOCOLS

Historically, dentists and hygienists have delivered fluoride in two primary ways: (1) in dietary sources, such as communal water supplies, and (2) through topical fluoride treatments, in which a high concentration of fluoride is applied directly to the teeth for up to 4 minutes (ASDC Forum, 1984). The former modality is still universally accepted as an important prevention measure. The latter, however, though still widely accepted and practiced, is being re-evaluated.

Professionally applied topical fluorides deliver between 9000 and 19,400 ppm of fluoride to the enamel surface. If the presence of 0.024 ppm fluoride can remineralize tooth structure, as noted previously, the concentration used in professional treatments may be overkill. Fluoride uptake is much greater with an acidic fluoride (APF) than with neutral NaF during the first 4 minutes. Longer treatment times show a diffusion-controlled pattern of uptake. One in vitro study noted that a 6-hour application time was optimal for deep penetration of enamel and the formation of fluorapatite (Arends et al, 1985). This is, of course, not a practice that is easily adopted in dental hygiene care.

In addition, high concentrations of fluoride are not necessarily optimal for deep penetration in enamel. Higher-concentrations form CaF_2 rather than fluorapatite, blocking the diffusion pathways to the deeper enamel and inhibiting ion penetration into the body of a carious lesion (Benediktsson et al, 1982). However, a 1983 study (Bruun, Thylstrup, and Uribe, 1983) showed that carious areas on extracted teeth retained CaF_2 at measurable levels at the surface 8 weeks after treatment with APF, even when subjected to continuous washing. The release of CaF_2 from the enamel over a number of weeks after the concentrated treatment may be of benefit in helping to prevent or remineralize caries (Fejerskov, Thylstrup, and Larsen, 1981) or in affecting accumulation of dental plaque for the short term. In 1988, Lagerlof and colleagues discovered that a coating of pyrophosphate (found in many toothpastes) may enhance the slow release of CaF_2. These findings provide a rationale for the continued use of high-dose, biannual treatments, particularly if patient access to or compliance with use of low-dose fluoride rinses and dentifrices is questionable.

Concentration of fluoride treatment is also a topic of discussion. In vitro tests show that there is no difference in enamel fluoride uptake whether an APF concentration is 1100 ppm, 2300 ppm, 2500 ppm, or 12,300 ppm fluoride ion is used (Dijkman, Tak, and Arends, 1982). A 2-year clinical trial comparing 1.23% with 0.6% APF demonstrated no significant differences between the two concentrations in the control of smooth surface caries, though the higher concentration was more effective on pits and fissures (Hagan, Rozier, and Baseden, 1985). Even drinking fluoridated water has a topical effect on teeth beyond that achieved by the bathing of the unerupted teeth (Mirth et al, 1985). Larsen and Jensen's research (1986) suggests that fluoride activity and pH have a greater impact on CaF_2 than does concentration. Therefore the fluoride concentration in topical treatments may be altered as continued research evaluates fluoride uptake, remineralization, resistance to demineralization, and long-term clinical effects on caries.

The *increased incidence of mild fluorosis* among teenagers compared with the previous decade suggests that children may be exposed to too much total dietary fluoride (Heifetz et al, 1987; Narendran et al, 1987). Fluoride in drinking water, most dentifrices, fluoride rinses, and professionally applied treatments provides cumulative effects. The dental profession has viewed fluoride as incapable of doing harm. However, dental hygienists and dentists are now being urged to assess the levels of fluoride ingested by their patients to minimize the likelihood of fluorosis. Patients should be assessed for all sources of fluoride and the frequency of their ingestion. For instance, children living in a nonfluoridated area may attend a preschool that has fluoridated water. These multiple sources of fluoride must be considered before fluoride supplementation is given.

Children should be supervised when they use fluoride toothpaste to ensure that they do not eat or inadvertently swallow it. Toothpaste should be treated like a drug and placed out of children's reach when not being used under supervision. Consuming large amounts of fluoride toothpaste can cause nausea and vomiting and create a sufficient spike in blood levels of fluoride to cause fluorosis. Even a single elevated systemic dose of fluoride increases the ion concentration in the bone surrounding the developing tooth, where it may be slowly released in sufficient concentrations to cause fluorosis (Angmar-Mansson and Whitford, 1985).

Until 1984, the accepted protocol regarding *preparation of teeth for a topical fluoride treatment* required polishing of all plaque and stain from the teeth to ensure optimal contact of fluoride with enamel. Research results with APF gels

have changed that procedure. A change was first considered when it was discovered that polishing can abrade a thin but significant fluoride-rich layer of outer enamel from the teeth (Vrbic, Brudevold, and McCann, 1967) and further considered when it was discovered that fluoride uptake into enamel was greater when existing plaque remained on the teeth (Bruun and Stoltze, 1976; Klimek, Hellweg, and Ahrens, 1982). However, these combined findings did not immediately translate into an altered protocol.

The first finding occurred when researchers were learning about the importance of the fluoride in the outermost layer of enamel. The second finding was tempered by the discovery that plaque-enhanced uptake resulted from the demineralization the plaque had caused in the underlying enamel; the demineralized structures acquire fluoride more readily than does intact enamel. This latter finding, however, stimulated a series of clinical studies, which established that it makes no difference in uptake or in caries incidence whether plaque is removed with a rubber cup and abrasive, removed with a toothbrush and floss, or simply left on the teeth before topical APF is applied (Bijella et al, 1985; Houpt, Koenigsberg, and Shey, 1983; Leverett and Curzon, 1983; Ripa et al, 1983a; Seppa, 1983; Steele, 1982).

Ripa (1984) recommends the following revised protocol:

Although the prophylaxis/topical fluoride treatment has been a time-honored sequence in clinical dentistry, enough recent laboratory and clinical evidence exists to recommend the elimination of the prior prophylaxis as a routine procedure when professional topical fluoride applications are performed.

This suggested revision and the growing body of information suggesting that polishing has limited therapeutic value make its inclusion as a standard procedure in dental hygiene care questionable (see Chapter 30).

In light of this evidence regarding the necessity of a complete prophylaxis before topical fluoride treatments, dental professionals should begin to investigate other options for patient preparation. Within the dental practice, tooth cleaning is one of the priorities of treatment. Instruction and reinforcement regarding the necessity of effective supramarginal plaque control should be given. In addition, the professional bears the responsibility for removing those soft and hard deposits, both supramarginally and submarginally, which the patient cannot remove. During a preventive appointment, then, scaling, debridment, and selective polishing are important. The clinician can accomplish coronal cleaning in a number of ways other than rubber cup prophylaxis. One alternative might be to have the patient perform supervised brushing and flossing, with or without a fluoride paste. In this way the professional could instruct and reinforce effective behaviors while simultaneously accomplishing the tooth cleaning. If a fluoride paste or gel is used during brushing, the fluoride treatment or application is also accomplished in the same step. If no paste or gel is used, the brushing and flossing can be followed by a topical fluoride treatment if needed.

Another alternative to the traditional prophylaxis is selective polishing of only those teeth with stains that the patient cannot remove. The patient can then brush and floss to remove remaining plaque under professional supervision, and the topical fluoride can be applied. Both of these approaches open up new treatment alternatives that allow the clinician to spend more time instructing patients in home care methods and less time polishing plaque from the coronal surfaces. They also demonstrate to patients that the primary responsibility for supragingival plaque removal lies with them, rather than with the professional.

In addition to using high-concentration professional topical fluoride treatments, clinicians are recommending the use of *daily, low-concentration fluoride rinses* to prevent caries. This pattern is in response to the growing body of information suggesting that frequency of exposure is more critical than concentration. Patients may be asked to rinse daily with 0.05% sodium fluoride rinses or weekly with 0.20% sodium fluoride rinses. Twice-daily rinsing can be recommended with a 0.025% sodium fluoride rinse. The selection should be made primarily with regard to the ability of the patient to expectorate all the rinse from the mouth and to his or her habit. Some people remember to use a rinse if they do so after each brushing; twice daily with 0.025% rinse is best in this case. Others are more likely to comply if the regimen is a weekly one (e.g., every Saturday morning, rinse with the 0.20% solution). School programs often opt for the weekly rinses or institute a program of daily brushing followed by rinsing with the 0.05% solution.

Another controversy concerns the use of *higher-concentration fluoride in dentifrices*. Typically the concentration of fluoride ion in dentifrices has ranged from 800 to 1150 ppm. In 1987, the FDA approved a new drug application for a dentifrice containing 1500 ppm. One toothpaste was immediately introduced with the higher level of fluoride ion; its packaging carries a specific warning regarding the need to supervise children using the product. The debate centers on whether a higher-concentration toothpaste is necessary given the decline in the caries rate and the increased emphasis on limiting ingested fluoride. Clinical trials to demonstrate an incremental benefit from the higher level of fluoride have reported minimal improvement, usually between 10% and 15%, over lower-concentration dentifrices (Stephan et al, 1987) or no difference (Ripa, 1987). This is partly because of the difficulty of securing a test group with a high caries rate. Opponents contend that if little additional benefit is achieved, the risk of ingesting larger quantities of fluoride outweighs the potential good. Proponents contend that certain populations still have a high caries rate and that the dentifrice should be available for them.

FLUORIDE THERAPY PROGRAM

Dental hygienists confronted with persons who have a propensity for caries should design a fluoride therapy program that fits the individual. Adding fluoride to the daily regimen of brushing and flossing requires careful planning and a full assessment of the sources of fluoride already present in the patient's daily activities.

First, assess the family, communal, and school water supply for fluoride. Assay each if necessary. Many sources have natural fluoride; others may not be optimally fluoridated. Determine the need for systemic supplements, following the guidelines in Table 21-1 and those offered by the recent conference in North Carolina (Bowden, 1992). For children, provide the proper prescription for fluoride supplements to the parents, monitor the filling of the prescription (to determine patient compliance), and monitor the use of the supplement by following up with the patient. Remember to adjust the supplement dosage when necessary (as the child ages or as fluoride availability in the drinking supply changes). Following these steps is an important, but frequently ignored, part of the protocol for providing fluoride supplementation (Levy, 1987).

After determining and prescribing the supplement, add a fluoride dentifrice and a fluoride rinse or low-dose home-use gel, giving careful instructions regarding the use of each. In-office topical treatments can be given more frequently than twice yearly, depending on the needs of the patient (Horowitz and Heifetz, 1986). Usually, logic must prevail in how many additional steps can be required of a patient to minimize caries. It will be more effective to add one new source of fluoride that the patient can easily adopt than to add several sources that weigh heavily on his or her time, financial resources, and commitment.

Fluoride gel application

Professional fluoride applications can be delivered by two different methods. The first is the tray technique, which is used to apply fluoride gels to the teeth. The second involves the application of fluoride solution. Fluoride solution cannot be applied in trays because it would spill out into the mouth, and thus it must be "painted" onto the individual tooth surfaces with cotton-tipped applicators. This technique for applying fluoride solution is described later in the chapter.

The widespread use of fluoride gels for professional fluoride applications has significantly increased the ease and simplicity of applying topical fluorides. The gels are inserted into a tray that is designed to fit over all the teeth of one arch, thereby eliminating the need to apply fluoride to individual teeth. The gel is more viscous, or thicker, than the fluoride solutions and is transferred easily into the mouth, where it adheres to the tray and teeth with minimal or no leakage.

Tray selection. A wide variety of fluoride trays are commercially available for use in professional fluoride applications (Fig. 21-1). Although most trays are made of disposable materials, some use disposable liners in a reusable, arch-fitting base (see Fig. 21-1, *top left, bottom middle, left*). The clinician should consider several factors carefully in deciding which type of tray design to purchase. The tray should be available in a variety of sizes to fit primary, mixed, and adult dentitions (Fig. 21-2). The length of the tray should provide complete coverage of all erupted teeth without extending beyond the surfaces of the most distal tooth. The width and depth should provide both effective isolation of teeth and intimate contact of the fluoride gel and the tooth surfaces when it is in place. The ends of the tray should be closed so

that fluoride gel does not spill into the mouth during the procedure. Trays that are custom fitted to the patient's mouth will provide the best fit, because they conform exactly to the teeth and arch (see Fig. 21-1, *top right*). A custom fit improves the amount of contact between the teeth and the fluoride gel and promotes compression of the gel against the teeth and into interproximal areas. Another advantage of custom-fitted trays is that they require less gel to cover all surfaces of the teeth. Larger amounts of gel may be needed in mass-produced trays to ensure that all tooth surfaces are thoroughly coated during the treatment procedure. A technique that minimizes the amount of gel is preferred because it reduces the chances that the patient will swallow excess gel. In addition to vacuum-molded custom-fitted trays, those with foam- or air-filled liners also may enhance the adaptation of the fluoride to the teeth.

When standard, disposable trays are used, no more than 2 g of gel should be dispensed into each tray (about 30% to 40% of tray capacity). Even smaller amounts should be dispensed into trays for small children. When custom-fitted trays are used by patients who require daily or weekly fluoride application with high-concentration gels, only 5 to 10 drops of the product are needed per tray (LeCompte, 1987).

The trays should be made of a material that is comfortable for the patient and will not interfere with the contact of fluoride with the tooth. Use of custom-made wax trays is not recommended, because the waxy material can adhere to tooth surfaces and interfere with fluoride uptake. Trays should be easy to handle and to insert into the mouth when filled. Flexible sponge trays and trays that use paper inserts require slightly more handling than other types of trays, increasing the procedure time (see Fig. 21-1, *top left, bottom far left*). The use of disposable trays reduces the chances of cross-contamination and eliminates the additional time and handling required to sterilize reusable trays. As most reusable fluoride trays are made of heat-sensitive materials, chemical sterilization must be used to decontaminate them.

Application procedure. The same major steps are followed for the application of both fluoride solution and gel. Tray setups for solution and gel application are shown in Figs. 21-3 and 21-4, respectively. The patient should be positioned in an upright position to facilitate evacuation of saliva and fluoride and to reduce the possibility of gag-

(Text continued on p. 466).

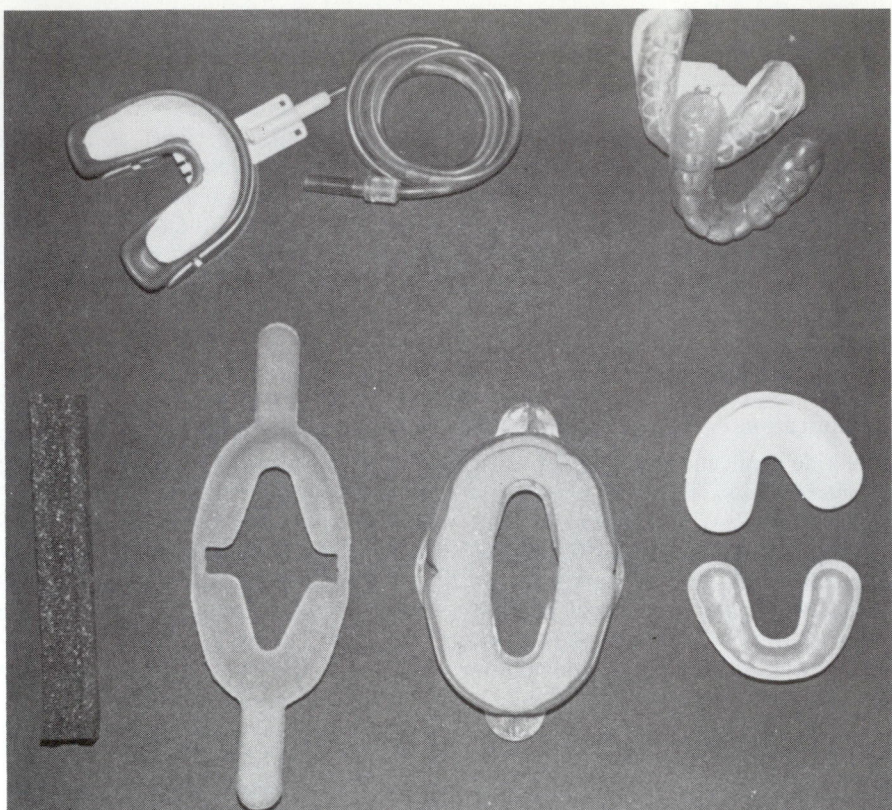

Fig. 21-1. A variety of fluoride trays are available for application of fluoride gels. *Clockwise from upper left:* reusable tray with hard plastic base, rubber membrane liner, and paper inserts (note also saliva ejector attachment on tray); pliable plastic tray made by forming plastic material directly from patient's arch impressions; Styrofoam trays; plastic disposable tray with foam insert; tray in which plastic and foam are fused; foam tray that can be cut and adapted to arch length at time of treatment.

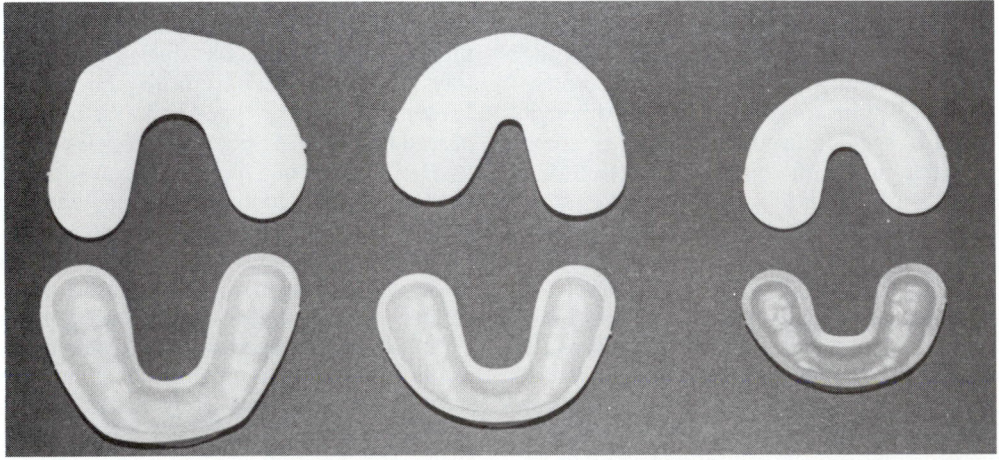

Fig. 21-2. Many disposable fluoride trays come in a selection of arch sizes to ensure optimal fit for each patient.

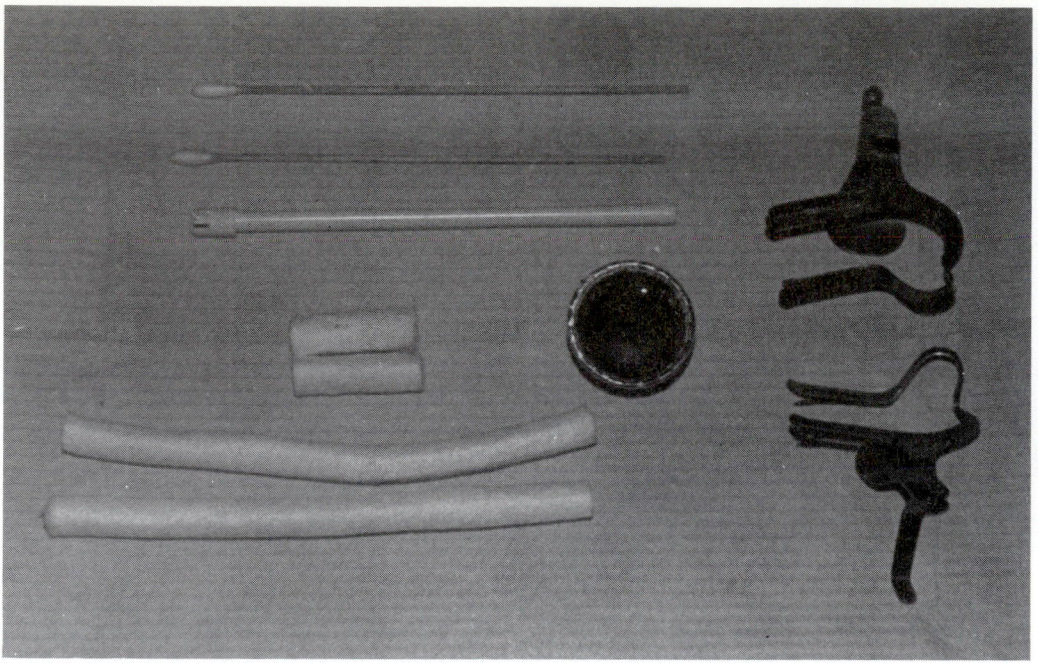

Fig. 21-3. Suggested tray setup for application of fluoride solutions includes cotton roll holders, cotton rolls in two lengths, saliva ejector tip, disposable applicators, and fluoride solution.

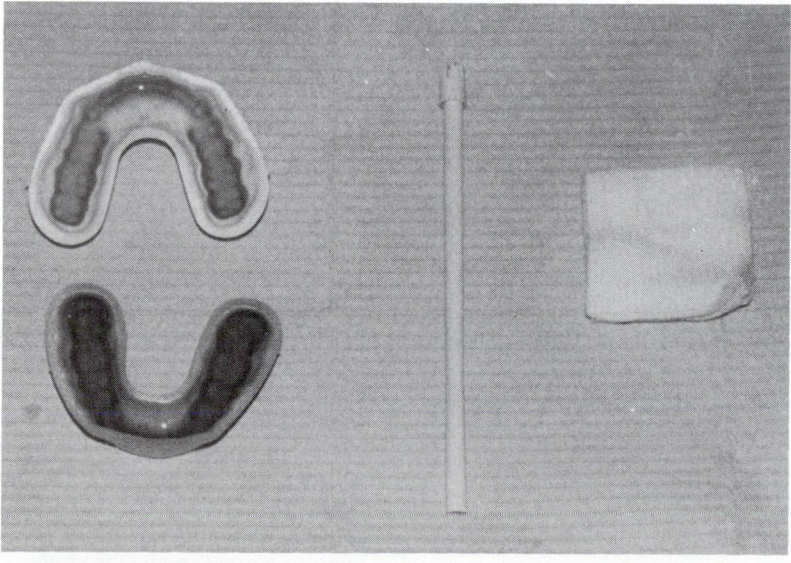

Fig. 21-4. Suggested tray setup for application of fluoride gels.

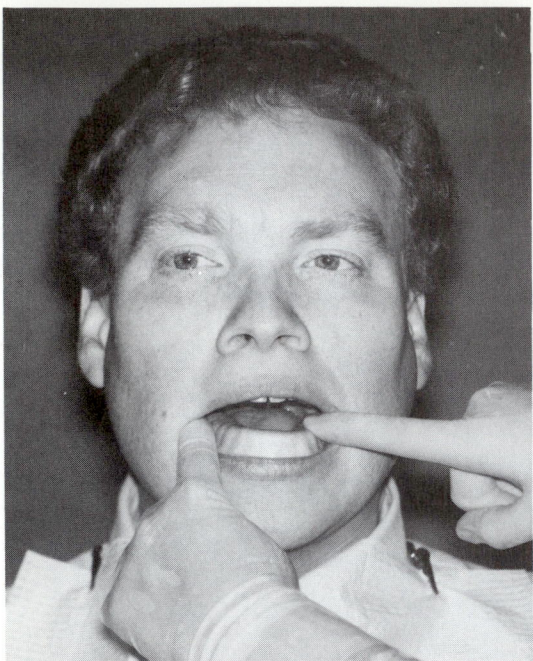

Fig. 21-5. Tray size is selected and tried in patient's mouth to make sure that all teeth will come into contact with fluoride gel.

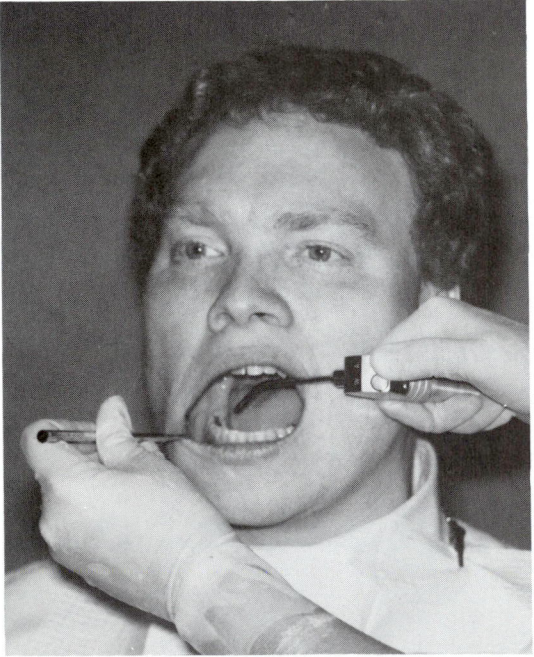

Fig. 21-6. Teeth should be carefully dried and kept as dry as possible until trays are placed. Each arch is dried separately immediately before tray is placed.

ging. All necessary supplies and materials for the procedure should be assembled and the procedure explained to the patient. Patient consent should already have been obtained during the treatment planning stage. It is important to reinforce the patient's knowledge regarding the benefits of the topical fluoride application at this time and to solicit any questions that the patient may have. After the best tray size has been selected for the patient's mouth (Figs. 21-4 and 21-5), both trays should be filled by placing a narrow strip (2 g) of fluoride gel along the bottom of the tray. This amount is sufficient to wet all tooth surfaces thoroughly when the tray is in place but not so much that it overflows the tray boundaries into the mouth where it can be swallowed.

After all materials have been assembled and the patient has been adequately prepared, the first step is to dry all the teeth that will be treated (Fig. 21-6). This should be done slowly and thoroughly to ensure that all tooth surfaces are free of saliva, which might dilute the fluoride concentration and reduce fluoride uptake. The patient should be informed that cooperation is needed to maintain the dry field until the trays are in place. Best results are obtained if the areas least likely to become rewetted are dried first, such as palatal surfaces. Areas near salivary ducts, such as the maxillary buccal and mandibular lingual surfaces, should be dried immediately before the fluoride is applied. Dry the teeth with an air syringe using the following pattern:

Mandibular arch. Dry buccal surfaces; then occlusal surfaces; finish on lingual surfaces.
Maxillary arch. Dry palatal surfaces; then occlusal surfaces; finish on buccal surfaces.

Retract the buccal and labial mucosa away from the dried teeth with either plastic retractors or the fingers of one hand until the tray is placed into position on the teeth with the other hand.

If both arches are to be treated simultaneously, position the mandibular tray first, then place the saliva ejector over the tray, and finally insert the maxillary tray. Ask the patient to close the mouth and to bite gently on the trays. The slight pressure from biting will help force the fluoride gel around and between all the teeth that are being treated. Begin timing the procedure after the tray(s) are in position and all the teeth to be treated are thoroughly wetted with the fluoride. Supervise or monitor the patient for the entire 4 minutes. Place the patient in a fully upright position with the chin tilted down to allow fluids to run to the anterior area of the mouth, where the saliva ejector is placed. All patients, and especially children, should be discouraged from swallowing excess fluoride during the treatment and should be encouraged to rely on the saliva ejector. Patients usually appreciate having disposable tissues on hand to assist in removing excess saliva around the mouth during and after the procedure. These steps are shown in Figs. 21-7 to 21-9.

With some trays, such as the ion-fluoridation tray shown in Fig. 21-1, *top left*, only one tray is put in place at a time. This is because the saliva ejector is attached directly to the tray and because simultaneous use of both trays would be too bulky and uncomfortable for the patient. When using only one tray at a time, dry the arch to be treated. Then place the tray, add the saliva ejector, and ask the patient to close the teeth together gently.

At the end of 4 minutes, remove the trays from the mouth and remove excess fluoride and saliva by means of the saliva ejector or high-speed evacuation. Instruct the patient to expectorate any remaining fluids from the mouth, repeating the process for at least 60 seconds. Expectoration is the most effective way to reduce orally retained fluoride so that it is not swallowed (LeCompte, 1987). Stookey and others (1986) reported evidence that rinsing immediately after fluoride application resulted in less fluoride deposition in incipient caries lesions. Therefore rinsing after a fluoride treatment may reduce the cariostatic potential of the treatment.

The advantages of the tray application methods are as follows:
1. Ease of application.
2. The whole mouth can be treated during a single 4-minute period.
3. Trays are used only once, eliminating sterilization procedures.
4. Improved patient comfort.

The disadvantages of the tray application methods are as follows:
1. Poorly designed or fitted trays may hinder fluoride uptake or allow leakage of gel into the mouth.
2. Cost of disposable supplies.

Controlling gagging. The fluoride treatment may elicit a gag response in some individuals. Mild gagging can usually be controlled through distraction strategies that focus the patient's attention on something other than the fluoride treat-

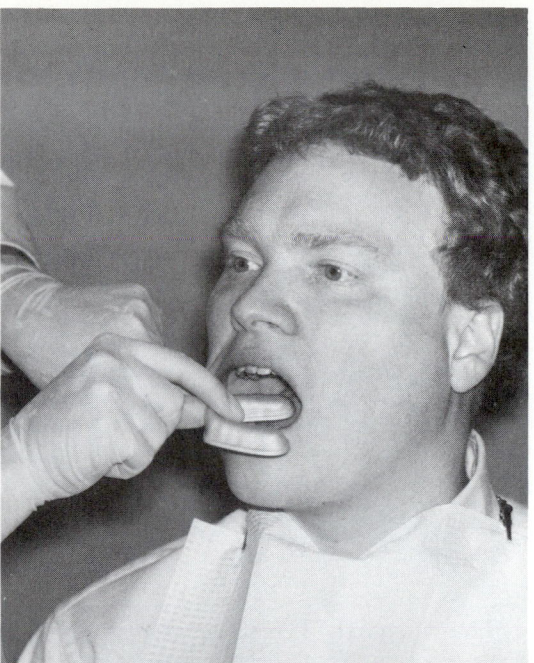

Fig. 21-7. One end of filled mandibular tray is inserted from side of patient's mouth rather than directly from front. This is similar to technique described for insertion of impression trays.

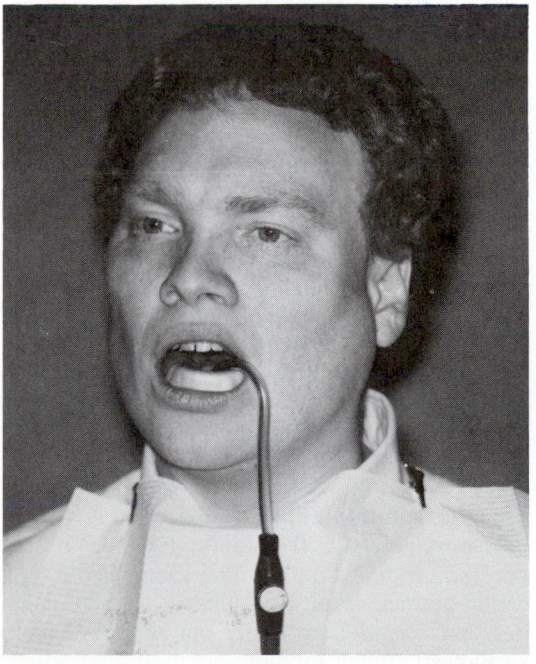

Fig. 21-8. Saliva ejector is inserted *before* maxillary tray is placed.

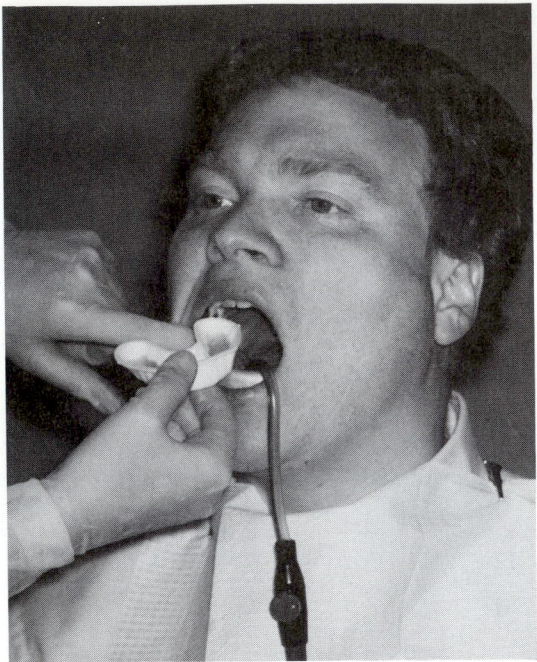

Fig. 21-9. Insertion of maxillary tray.

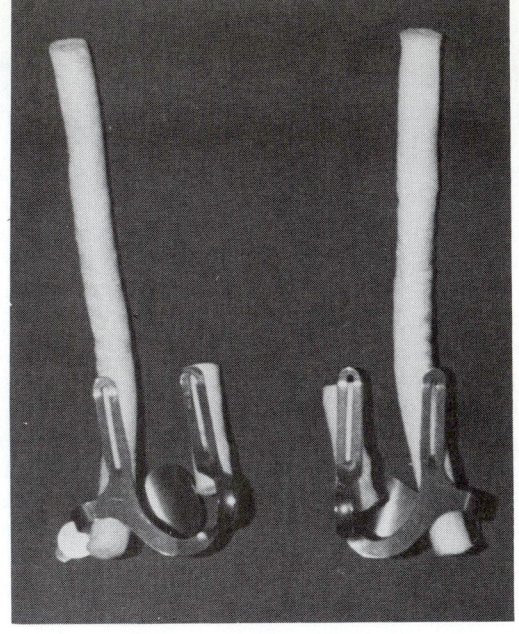

Fig. 21-10. Set of cotton roll holders known as Garmer clamps. Each holder secures two cotton rolls to isolate one half of mouth at a time. Short roll lies against lingual surfaces of mandibular arch, and longer roll isolates buccal surfaces of maxillary and mandibular teeth from mucosa.

ment. Such strategies may include rapidly paced nasal breathing, toe wiggling, or simply talking to the patient about an interesting topic to divert his or her attention.

Patients with more serious gagging problems can be helped by allowing them to practice the procedure in advance (i.e., with empty trays); by giving them some control over the procedure (i.e., holding the saliva ejector); by providing distracting imagery ("imagine walking on the beach in the sunshine"); or by listening to, acknowledging, and discussing their concerns (i.e., about choking, suffocating, and the like) and providing assurance that the procedure poses no risk (Ramsay et al, 1987).

Fluoride solution application

Use of cotton roll holders. Fluoride in solution form requires the painting technique of application because it must be applied in small quantities and would flow easily out of trays and be swallowed. When solutions are used, the teeth are isolated and kept dry by means of cotton rolls.

These rolls are held in place adjacent to the teeth that will be treated so that the tongue, cheeks, and saliva do not touch them during the procedure. Cotton roll holders called Garmer clamps are used to stabilize the cotton rolls in the mouth. Garmer clamps can be obtained in two sizes: adult and child. The cotton rolls are inserted onto metal prongs with a short roll on the lingual side of the clamp and a 6-inch roll on the buccal side (Fig. 21-10). The cotton roll holder is placed gently in the mouth so that the lingual cotton roll isolates the lingual surface of the teeth from the tongue and the lowest half of the buccal roll lies in the mandibular buccal and labial vestibule, with the rest extending out of the mouth (Fig. 21-11). The holder should then be stabilized in the mouth by anchoring the clamp snugly under the patient's chin. The rest of the buccal cotton roll should then be securely positioned so that the free end curves up along the maxillary vestibule and returns labially to the central incisors. Putting a slight twist on the end of the cotton roll before placing the lip over it will hold the anterior end in

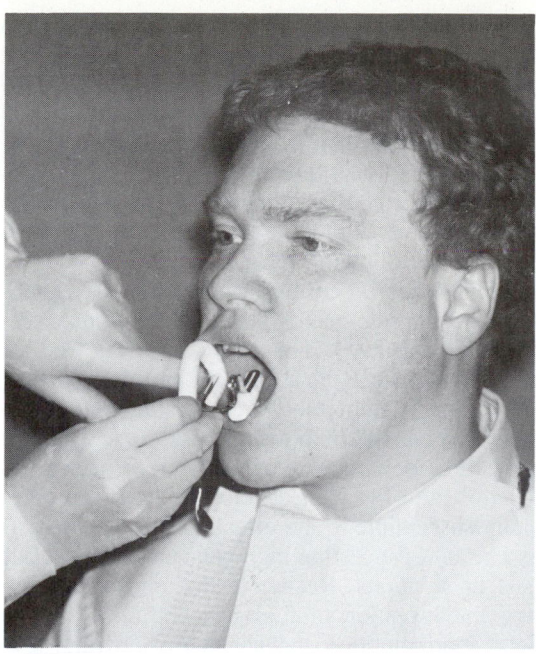

Fig. 21-11. Garmer clamp and cotton rolls are placed with short roll side against lingual surfaces of mandibular teeth and long roll side against buccal surfaces. Note that maxillary extension of buccal cotton roll is folded forward and held until clamps are inserted and stabilized.

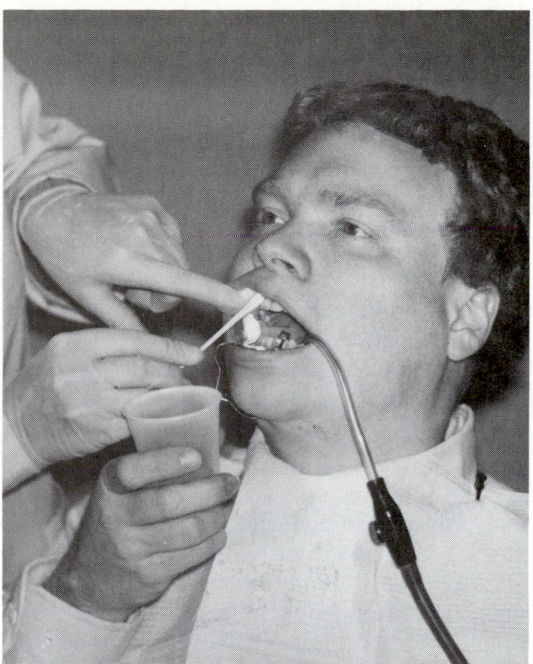

Fig. 21-12. With clamp fastened snugly under the chin and cotton rolls in place, teeth are dried and solution is placed using suggested pattern of application.

place. A final check should be made to ensure that the cotton rolls are effectively isolating the teeth from the cheeks, lips, and tongue but are not touching the tooth surfaces to be treated.

The lingual roll should not extend beyond the distal surface of the last molar, where it might elicit gagging. When the cotton roll holder is in place, the saliva ejector is positioned and the teeth on the side to be treated dried thoroughly following the same pattern as described earlier.

Application procedure. Ask the patient to hold the fluoride solution container close to the mouth, or place it on the bracket table near the mouth (Fig. 21-12). Apply the solution first to the mandibular lingual surfaces, using an application pattern that moves systematically around the quadrant as follows: posterior on the lingual surfaces, anterior on the occlusal surfaces, and posterior on the buccal surfaces. Apply solution to the surfaces of the maxillary arch by starting on the buccal aspect of the molars and moving forward; then wet the occlusal surfaces and finally the lingual or palatal surfaces. Apply the solution

to each tooth liberally with a cotton-tipped applicator, taking care to thoroughly wet all accessible tooth surfaces. After all isolated teeth are covered with solution, begin timing the application. During the application period continue to apply solution to the teeth using the same pattern as before to ensure that they are continuously bathed in fluoride. At the end of the recommended application time, remove the saliva ejector and then the cotton rolls and clamps. Suction all remaining fluoride solution and excess saliva from the mouth, and allow the patient to empty the mouth into a cuspidor or funnel-suction device (depending on the equipment available).

The entire procedure (isolation, drying, application) is then repeated on the opposite side of the mouth.

The advantages of this method of isolation are as follows:

1. It provides effective isolation when fluoride solutions are used.
2. Garmer clamps can be autoclaved and are reusable, reducing the cost of supplies.

The disadvantages of this method of isolation are as follows:

1. The procedure is more time consuming and complicated than tray techniques.
2. Only half the mouth can be treated at one time.
3. Bulkiness of clamps and cotton rolls may be uncomfortable for the patient.

Controlling fluoride ingestion during professional applications

The goal of fluoride therapy is to maximize the benefits of topical or systemic fluoride preparation while minimizing the known risks of using the agent. Fluorides, including the high-concentration gels and solutions used in the dental office, have been proven time and time again to be safe and effective for prevention of decay *when used as recommended*. Recently, however, there has been some concern among members of the professional community that the availability of fluoride from multiple sources—including water, food, diet supplements, school fluoride programs, dentifrices, over-the-counter rinses, and professional applications—might increase the prevalence and severity of dental fluorosis.

A number of investigations have indicated that substantial amounts of fluoride are retained in the mouth after a professional fluoride treatment and subsequently ingested (Ekstrand and Koch, 1980; Ekstrand et al, 1981; LeCompte and Doyle, 1982, 1985; LeCompte and Whitford, 1981, 1982; More et al, 1983; Owen et al, 1979). The large amounts of retained fluoride have been reported to result in elevation of fluoride concentrations in body fluids, including plasma concentrations. There is concern that these elevated levels may result in dental fluorosis when they occur in young children with developing teeth (Ekstrand and Koch, 1980; Ekstrand et al, 1981; LeCompte and Whitford, 1981, 1982). Because fluorosis is most likely to occur in young children, efforts to reduce amounts of ingested fluoride in that group are especially important. Although dental fluorosis does not in itself pose a major public health threat, even this minor side effect can be controlled effectively through proper application technique.

The possibility that a young child might accidentally ingest high doses of fluoride during the professional application procedures is a more serious concern. For this to happen, abuses of accepted fluoride application procedures would have to occur; unfortunately, the death of one child has been reported to result from such abuses (Church, 1976; Horowitz, 1977). Although topical fluoride treatments have consistently been shown to be safe and effective in preventing dental decay, this occurrence emphasizes the need to ensure that the risks, however minor, are minimized. Although each of the following recommendations has been included when describing the technique for application of fluoride gels or solutions, additional emphasis is warranted. They should be followed for all professional applications of fluoride, but they are especially important when treating young children, for whom the potential risks of chronic or acute fluoride overdose are greater. Children under the age of 6 with developing teeth are especially susceptible to the effects of dental fluorosis as a result of ingesting high-concentration fluoride gels or solutions. Recommendations for controlling the ingestion of high-concentration fluoride gels and solutions include the following (LeCompte, 1987).

Patient instruction. Patients should be instructed that the purpose of the procedure is to apply fluoride only to the surfaces of the teeth and that it should not be swallowed. They should be shown how to use the saliva ejector effectively and be placed in a fully upright position with the chin tilted down. It should be explained that maintaining this position will improve the effectiveness of the saliva ejector in removing saliva and excess fluoride.

Tray selection. A tray should be selected that will allow coverage of all teeth in the arch, promote intimate contact of the fluoride to the teeth, and minimize loss of fluoride from the tray and into the mouth. Trays and criteria for their selection were described earlier in this chapter.

Amount of fluoride dispensed. It has been recommended that only about 2 g of fluoride be dispensed into each tray. This is equal to about 40% of the tray capacity. For small children, even smaller amounts should be dispensed. Studies indicate that substantial amounts of fluoride are retained in the mouth or swallowed following all application techniques, both before and after the patient has expectorated (Ekstrand et al, 1981; LeCompte and Doyle, 1982; More et al, 1983). Furthermore, there is wide variation in the amount of fluoride that may be placed in a tray, depending on the discretion of the individual. In studies, the average amount of fluoride gel dispensed per tray, depending on the type of tray system, ranged from 2.0 to 3.6 g (i.e., 14.8 to 44.3 mg of fluoride per tray) (LeCompte, 1987). These amounts are averages, indicating that some individuals were dispensing even greater amounts. Most manufacturers of high-concentration fluoride gels now recommend that only enough gel should be dispensed to fill a third of the tray. The result of over dispensing fluoride gel is that fluoride is ingested unnecessarily by the patient and the product is wasted by the professional.

Use of suction equipment. The use of saliva ejectors and high-speed suction reduces the amount of fluoride that can be ingested during a professional treatment. Saliva ejectors can be used both during and after the procedure, and high-speed suction devices can be used to clear the mouth further after the trays have been removed. Although these devices are effective in removing significant amounts of retained fluoride, data indicate that substantial oral fluoride is retained in both children and adults even when suctioning is used (Eisen and LeCompte, 1985; LeCompte and Doyle, 1985; More et al, 1983).

Expectoration. Instructing patients to empty their mouths repeatedly for 30 to 60 seconds following a fluoride treatment is the single most effective way to reduce orally retained fluoride (LeCompte, 1987). Eisen and LeCompte (1985) reported that suctioning procedures with patient expectoration were more beneficial than suction alone.

Patient monitoring. Patients, especially small children, should be monitored during the entire procedure to ensure that they are following instructions and that they do not swallow the fluoride inadvertently or intentionally. You should never leave the operatory or be in a position from which you cannot see or hear the patient while the fluoride treatment is in progress. Bottles containing fluoride gel or solution should never be kept within reach of young children. Relatively low concentrations of fluoride can cause gastrointestinal irritation. Complaints of nausea, vomiting, or abdominal pain are not uncommon in patients following topical APF gel applications (Whitford et al, 1987). Children who complain of gastrointestinal upset should be given milk and monitored closely for other symptoms. Never give a fluoride treatment to a fasting child; provide a snack before the appointment if the child has not eaten for several hours.

Newer techniques

One way to reduce fluoride ingestion would be to develop a product that produces the same cariostatic effect on tooth surfaces as existing fluoride gels but requires a shorter contact time (i.e., 1 versus 4 minutes). Although 1.23% APF gels have been formulated and marketed with this goal in mind, there has not yet been sufficient evidence generated by independent researchers (i.e., other than the manufacturer) to determine whether these products can be considered as effective as approved APF products applied for 4 minutes (LeCompte, 1987).

Another method of reducing fluoride ingestion may be to use a fluoride "foam" versus the normal gel application. An in vitro study by Wei and Hattab (1988) has shown that fluoride uptake from the foam was comparable to that from gel. A 1990 report by Wei and Chits states that fluoride retention was significantly less with foam than an APF gel. No clinical data are yet available to support a claim of a reduction in dental decay with fluoride foam, but it may be a promising vehicle for professional applications in which ingestion of fluoride is a concern.

Recommended dosages for daily or weekly applications using custom-fitted trays

Certain patients may require frequent use of high-concentration fluoride gel for prevention of rampant caries, especially those who are undergoing cancer therapy or suffering from xerostomia. The recommended application procedures for these patients involve use of a custom-fitted acrylic tray for delivery of the fluoride. Because of the close fit of these trays to the teeth, less fluoride gel is required and excessive amounts of gel are likely to be forced out of the tray when it is placed. Current recommendations are that only 5 to 10 drops (1 to 2 mg) of fluoride preparation should be dispensed into trays used for frequent fluoride application. If patients perform this procedure at home, they should be shown the amount of fluoride to dispense and instructed regarding the importance of expectorating after the treatment is completed.

Awareness of fluoride dosages in professional applications

In addition to complying with recommendations regarding fluoride application technique, the hygienist must always be aware of the amount of fluoride being given to the patient and understand the relation of this quantity (expressed as mg F/ml) to toxic dose levels. Chronic overexposure to fluoride, even at low concentrations, can result in dental fluorosis in children under the age of 6 with developing teeth. Acute overdosage resulting in poisoning or even death can occur if high-concentration gels or solutions are abused. Lyon (1985) stated that "it is the legal as well as moral

Table 21-2. Estimated safe, toxic, and lethal dosage levels of fluoride

Certainly lethal dose (CLD) = an estimated dosage range with the potential for causing death when consumed.
Safely tolerated dose (STD) = an estimated dosage that can be consumed without producing symptoms of serious acute toxicity.
Probably toxic dose (PTD) = the estimated minimum dosage that could cause toxic signs and symptoms.

For a 70-kg adult:

Certainly lethal dose (CLD) = 5-10 gm NaF or 32-64 mg F/kg†
Safely tolerated dose (STD) = (1/4 CLD) 1.25-2.5 gm NaF or 8-16 mg F/kg†
Probably toxic dose (PTD) = 5.0 mg F/kg‡

CLDs, STDs, and PTDs of fluoride for children of selected ages:

Age	Weight (lb)*	CLD (mg)†	STD (mg)†	PTD (mg)‡
2	22	320	80	50
4	29	422	106	66
6	37	538	135	84
8	45	655	164	102
10	53	771	193	120
12	64	931	233	145
14	83	1206	301	189
16	92	1338	334	209
18	95	1382	346	216

*3rd percentile of the normal age-specific weight distribution.
†Modified from Heifetz SB, Horowitz HS: *ASDC J Dent Child* 51:257, 1984.
‡Modified fromWhitford GM: *J Dent Res* 66:1056, 1987.

responsibility of every hygienist to be able to determine how much fluoride is being administered to a patient."

Only trained dental professionals who are legally permitted to apply topical fluoride preparations should perform office fluoride treatments. Each dentist and hygienist must know how much fluoride they are giving to patients and how that quantity compares with the certainly lethal dose (CLD) and the safely tolerated dose (STD) guidelines presented in Table 21-2. Table 21-3 estimates the amount of fluoride that is commonly used in professional fluoride treatments and the associated dosages for each of the three common fluoride preparations. It can be seen that if recommended amounts of fluoride are used according to the suggestions in this chapter, the total fluoride dose is well below the suggested CLD for any age level. It should be noted, however, that if the stated amounts of an 8% SnF_2 solution, for instance, were to be ingested by a 2-year-old child, the dose would exceed the STD for that age/weight level. Close monitoring of the fluoride application procedure and care to ensure that containers of fluoride gel or solution are kept out of the reach of children can prevent accidental ingestion of these products.

If a toxic overdose of fluoride is known or suspected, the hygienist must be able to calculate quickly the total amount of topical fluoride gel or solution that may have been ingested and use that information to recommend appropriate treatment for fluoride overdose. These quantities can be estimated by using the information in Table 21-3, or they can be calculated more exactly using the simple equations in Table 21-4. More detailed explanations of how to calculate the concentration of any type of topical fluoride product are available so that dental professionals can ascertain acceptable dosages of other fluoride products or combinations of products (Bayless and Tinanoff, 1985; Heifetz and Horowitz, 1984; Lyon, 1985).

Table 21-3. Amounts of fluoride in professionally administered topical fluoride treatments

Agent	Frequency	F concentration	Volume	Total amount of F
2% NaF	Series of 4 every 3 yr	0.91%	2.5 ml	22.8 mg
8% SnF_2	1 or 2/yr	1.95%	5 ml	97.5 mg
10% SnF_2	1 or 2/yr	2.44%	5 ml	122 mg
APF	1 or 2/yr	1.23%	5 ml	61.5 mg

Modified from Heifetz SB, Horowitz HS: *ASDC J Dent Child* 51:257, 1984.

Table 21-4. Rapid method of calculating amount of fluoride ingested

Form	Formula
NaF	$(4.5) \times$ (no. ml swallowed) $\times$ (NaF concentration) $=$ mg F^- (e.g., 0.05%, 1.1%)
SnF$_2$	$(2.4) \times$ (no. ml swallowed) $\times$ (SnF$_2$ concentration) $=$ mg F^- (e.g., 0.4%, 8%, 10%)
APF	$(10) \times$ (no. ml swallowed) $\times$ (F^- concentration) $=$ mg F^- (e.g., 1.23%)

Modified from Bayless JM, Tinanoff N: *JADA* 110:209, 1985.

Table 21-5. Emergency treatment for fluoride overdose

Milligram fluoride ion per kilogram body weight*	Treatment
Less than 5.0 mg/kg	1. Give calcium orally (milk) to relieve gastrointestinal symptoms; observe for a few hours 2. Induced vomiting not necessary
More than 5 mg/kg	1. Empty stomach by induced vomiting with emetic; for patients with depressed gag reflex caused by age (<6 months old), Down's syndrome, or severe mental retardation, induced vomiting is contraindicated and endotracheal intubation should be performed before gastric lavage 2. Give orally soluble calcium in any form (e.g., milk, 5% calcium gluconate, or calcium lactate solution) 3. Admit to hospital and observe for a few hours
More than 15 mg/kg	1. Admit to hospital immediately 2. Induce vomiting 3. Begin cardiac monitoring and be prepared for cardiac arrhythmias; observe for peaking T-waves and prolonged Q-T intervals 4. Slowly administer 10 ml of 10% calcium gluconate solution intravenously; additional doses may be given if clinical signs of tetany, or Q-T interval prolongation develops; electrolytes, especially calcium and potassium, should be monitored and corrected as necessary 5. Adequate urine output should be maintained using diuretics if necessary 6. General supportive measures for shock

*Average weight/age: 1-2 years = 10 kg; 2-4 years = 15 kg; 4-6 years = 20 kg; 6-8 years = 23 kg.
Modified from Bayless JM, Tinanoff N: *JADA* 110:209, 1985.

After calculating the amount of the overdose, the hygienist can determine which emergency measures to implement. Table 21-5 suggests emergency treatment measures for acute fluoride overdose based on the quantity of fluoride ingested. Whitford (1987) suggested that an oral dose of 5.0 mg F/kg body weight should be regarded as the "possibly toxic dose" (PTD)—that is, the minimum dose that could cause toxic signs and symptoms. He further recommended that an emergency should be assumed to exist and that immediate emergency treatment and hospitalization should be given if it is even suspected that 5.0 mg F/kg or more has been ingested. This information should be kept where it can be used immediately in case of an emergency. The conversion units listed in Table 21-6 will help the dental professional translate into useful data the information found in labels, advertisements, and research articles describing fluoride concentration levels and dosages.

Table 21-6. Basic conversion factors

1 kilogram (kg)	= 2.2 lbs
1 gram (gm)	= 1000 mgs
1 ounce (oz)	= 30 ml (volume)
1 ounce	= 28.3 gm (weight)
1 gm/100 ml	= 1% (%=parts/hundred)
% × 10,000	= parts/million (ppm)
1 mg/ml or mg/gm	= 1000 ppm

Adapted from Lyon TC: *Dent Hyg* 59:58, 1985.

SELECTING EFFECTIVE FLUORIDE PRODUCTS

As with many other consumer items, a myriad of fluoride products are promoted by dental sales representatives, at professional meetings, in advertisements in both lay and professional publications, by other professionals, and by patients themselves. Proponents of each product indicate that theirs is the best, the cheapest, the most efficient, the safest, or the most popular of its kind on the market. How do dental professionals sort out all of these claims to ensure that they are using or recommending the best product for their patients? A number of suggestions can help professionals make these important choices.

Products that claim to have therapeutic value must have their safety proved to government bodies such as the Food and Drug Administration before they can be marketed for public consumption. Simply knowing that a product is safe, however, is not enough to indicate its choice over other similar products. The professional literature should be consulted regarding research conducted to document its efficacy (ability to produce the desired benefit under controlled conditions), its effectiveness (ability to produce the stated benefit under normal-use conditions), and its comparative efficacy or effectiveness (how it compares with other similar products of an established reputation). A product such as a topical fluoride preparation must go through a number of research stages before it can be recommended safely. First, laboratory studies must be done to determine the properties and effects of the product using models or extracted teeth, and then the product may be used in live animal studies to establish its safety and effectiveness. These studies are followed by controlled use of the substance in vivo; that is, in the mouths of live human beings. Finally, the product must be tested under realistic circumstances of actual use on large population samples. This entire process can take years or even decades to complete, but the final evidence obtained from long-term clinical studies on humans is an important requirement for a product to be professionally recognized as an effective fluoride product.

As a service to the profession and as an aid to practitioners, the American Dental Association has councils (e.g., the Council on Dental Therapeutics and the Council on Dental Materials, Instruments, and Equipment) whose task it is to evaluate the claims of safety and effectiveness of therapeutic and preventive dental products, materials, instruments, and equipment. These councils evaluate data on the safety, efficacy, composition, and quality of products. They review all labels, package inserts, and advertising to ensure the use of scientifically accurate statements. In addition, these councils encourage, establish, and support research on the therapeutic value of agents used in dentistry. The results and discussion of their findings, as well as lists of accepted products, are compiled for easy reference in a publication entitled *Accepted Dental Therapeutics*. In addition, the councils provide more current updates of the status of new products and of newly accepted products in reports published frequently in the *Journal of the American Dental Association*. Dental professionals should consult these reports and recommendations before adopting any new forms of fluoride treatment. Products that have been approved and accepted by these councils can be used and recommended with confidence. For the most current information on the status of new therapeutic agents or products, the professional can also contact the secretaries of these councils by phone at the offices of the American Dental Association.

Dental researchers and faculty members at dental schools may also be consulted for accurate and up-to-date information on new techniques, concepts, or products. Dentists and hygienists should participate in continuing education programs to keep updated in the latest methods and approaches to dental care. Finally, all professionals have a responsibility to keep up to date with professional literature by reading journals published by their professional associations and other related sources. Dental professionals also should be aware of information that is being disseminated to the general public through magazines, newspapers, and television so that they can respond accurately when consulted about claims transmitted by these media. Finally, dental professionals need to review the information supplied by manufacturers of dental materials, instruments, equipment, and products, because many important details can be ascertained from it. Dental professionals also should consider the reputation of a manufacturer within the dental profession when evaluating products. In summary, dental professionals are responsible to their consumers to use accepted and approved methods and products and to be informed regarding the products that are available to the general public. To fulfill this responsibility, they must be assertive in their search for reliable information and develop their skills as critical evaluators of new information and new products.

ACTIVITIES

1. Visit the local pharmacy and grocery store and identify all the products available for oral hygiene that include fluoride. Note the type of fluoride included, the concentration, and the directions for use.
2. Calculate the total fluoride available to a person who consumes four 8-ounce glasses of fluoridated water, rinses with a 0.05% sodium fluoride rinse according to manufacturer's instructions, and brushes three times daily with a 2500 ppm fluoride dentifrice using 1 g of paste at each brushing.
3. Review antifluoridationist literature and prepare a list of their arguments. Locate the sources of their references and review the articles that are available.
4. Review the results of the Grand Rapids/Muskegon and Kingston/Newburgh clinical trials.
5. Conduct a seminar for parents of young children and discuss the ways in which their children use toothpaste.
6. Review the literature for epidemiologic studies that describe trends in the following areas:
   a. Caries incidence
   b. Fluorosis
   c. Water fluoridation
   d. Use of low-concentration fluorides
      Prepare a panel discussion of one or more of these issues, presenting the data and the controversies generated.
7. Survey local family physicians and pediatricians to determine whether they prescribe fluoride drops or lozenges for their patients and in what concentrations.
8. Survey your town or city and surrounding areas for the presence of fluoride in the drinking water. Take a sample of water from the public supply, from several wells, and from neighboring cities to the health department to assess the level of fluoride in the water.
9. Interview local dentists and hygienists regarding the historical efforts to fluoridate the local community.
10. In groups of five, review the literature describing the percentage of caries reductions achieved with (1) each of the topical fluoride agents, including high-concentration professionally applied gels and solutions; (2) home use rinses; (3) dentifrices; (4) home-use gels; and (5) sequential rinses of acidulated phosphate fluoride and stannous fluoride.

Each group should prepare a report describing the research design, the number of subjects, the age of the subjects, the duration of the trial, the agent(s) tested, the method of evaluation, whether the water supply was fluoridated, whether other fluoride sources were available to the study subjects, and the results.

11. Tour a local water plant and find out how community water fluoridation is implemented and monitored.
12. Determine which students come from areas where the water supplies were fluoridated (optimum level) and relate this to each student's number of caries. Can any trend be determined?
13. Plan and discuss setting up a clinical study to investigate a new anticariogenic agent in your (or a hypothetical) town. Would you participate, or would you let your child, brother, sister, or other family member participate if you knew you might receive the placebo product?
14. Invite representatives of dental manufacturing companies to discuss their fluoride products and supplies. Collect a wide variety of fluoride trays and discuss advantages and disadvantages of each tray design.
15. Perform a topical fluoride treatment for a partner in your class (see box on p. 476).
16. Construct scenarios in which the clinician made errors during the topical fluoride application, then have the class critique the procedures and discuss the possible results of the errors.
17. Demonstrate the effectiveness of fluoride by soaking an egg in a high-concentration fluoride solution overnight. Then take the test egg and a control egg and soak them in household vinegar. Compare the results.
18. Select several members of the class and have each dispense fluoride gel into similar or different tray designs. Weigh each set of trays to determine how much gel was dispensed. Compare results and compute the total fluoride dosage that would be delivered to each patient. Are there differences? How much variation is there? Discuss ways to determine how much fluoride gel is actually needed for the topical procedure.
19. Check the most current edition of *Accepted Dental Therapeutics* for a list of fluoride products that have proven effectiveness. Identify products available to the public that are not on the list. Perform a literature search on these items to determine what claims have been made regarding their effectiveness or lack of effectiveness.

Fluoride Application Procedure

Suggested check-off sheet

Mark **S** for satisfactory completion or **U** for unsatisfactory completion of each criterion in the appropriate space.

PERFORMANCE CRITERIA:	FACULTY	STUDENT
1. Assess the need for topical fluoride therapy		
2. Explain the benefits of fluoride, describe the application procedure, and obtain the consent of the patient		
3. Evaluate the teeth for removal of calculus, stain, and plaque		
4. Assemble all necessary supplies		
5. Seat the patient in an upright position		
Tray technique		
6. Select the appropriate-size tray and check the fit in the patient's mouth		
7. Dispense the proper amount of gel into each tray		
8. Dry the mandibular teeth and isolate them		
9. Insert the mandibular tray		
10. Insert the saliva ejector		
11. Dry the maxillary teeth and isolate them		
12. Insert the maxillary tray		
13. Ask the patient to close the mouth and bite the teeth together gently		
14. Begin timing the procedure		
15. Monitor patient comfort		
16. Remove the trays after the full 4 minutes have elapsed		
17. Remove excess fluoride with a saliva ejector or high-speed evacuation		
18. Allow the patient to expectorate for 30 to 60 seconds		
19. Instruct the patient not to eat, rinse, or drink for 30 minutes following the procedure		
Solution technique		
6. Attach cotton rolls to holders properly for maximum effectiveness and patient comfort		
7. Insert cotton roll holders and stabilize them in the mouth		
8. Check the placement of the cotton rolls in relation to the soft and hard tissues		
9. Dry the teeth using the prescribed pattern		
10. Insert a saliva ejector		
11. Apply the solution, using the prescribed pattern, to all tooth surfaces on the isolated side of the mouth		
12. Begin timing the procedure after all surfaces have been covered		
13. Repeat the application pattern throughout the 4-minute period to keep surfaces continuously wet with fluoride		
14. Remove the cotton rolls and holder after the full 4-minute period has elapsed		
15. Evacuate excess saliva and fluoride from the mouth, and allow the patient to expectorate		
16. Repeat steps 6 through 15 for the other side of the mouth		
17. Instruct the patient not to eat, rinse, or drink for 30 minutes following the procedure		

REVIEW QUESTIONS

1. The microorganism most closely associated with dental caries is:
2. True or false:
   a. Fluorapatite is formed in the deep layers of enamel.
   b. Calcium fluoride is formed at the surface of the enamel when exposed to topical fluoride.
   c. Calcium fluoride may serve as a reservoir, releasing fluoride over a number of weeks.
   d. Surface layer fluoride may be more important in preventing dental decay than a high concentration of fluorapatite.
   e. Topical fluoride, even in low concentrations, helps enable calcium and phosphorus to remineralize enamel.
   f. The optimal level of fluoride in communal water supplies is 10 ppm.
3. What is dental fluorosis?
4. What is posteruption maturation?
5. What is the recommended regimen for each of these rinses?
   a. 0.05% NaF.
   b. 0.025% NaF.
   c. 0.20% NaF.
6. Is it necessary to polish the teeth before applying topical fluoride or a fluoride mouthrinse?
7. What was the purpose of the Grand Rapids/Muskegon and Kingston/Newburg caries trials?
8. Describe, in order, the steps involved in performing the following procedures:
   a. A tray application of fluoride gel.
   b. The application of fluoride solution.
9. When should the 4-minute timing of the fluoride application begin?
   a. After the teeth are dried.
   b. As soon as the first tray is in place, or solution has been applied to the first treated teeth.
   c. When all teeth to be treated have been thoroughly wetted with the fluoride gel or solution.
10. State the lethal dose of fluoride for adults; for children. Compare these amounts with those which are normally dispensed in a topical fluoride treatment.
11. Which of the following are effective antidotes for accidental fluoride poisoning?
    a. Milk.
    b. Lime water.
    c. Preparations containing large amounts of magnesium.
    d. All of the above.
12. If a 2-year-old child ingests 10 ml of 8% SnF_2 solution while the dental professional is not watching, how many milligrams of fluoride would he or she ingest?
13. In the case above, would the total fluoride dose be over the CLD for a 2-year-old child?
14. Should hospitalization be recommended for the above child in addition to such measures as giving milk or inducing vomiting?

REFERENCES

American Dental Association Council on Dental Therapeutics: *Accepted dental therapeutics,* ed 40, Chicago, 1984, The Association.

Angmar-Mansson B, Whitford GM: Single fluoride doses and enamel fluorosis in the rat, *Caries Res* 19:145, 1985.

Arends J et al: Time dependence of F uptake in demineralizing enamel from 1000 ppm fluoride, *Caries Res* 19:450, 1985.

ACSD Forum: The topical fluorides—how should they be used? *ACSD J Dent Child* 51:150, 1984.

Bayless JM, Tinanoff N: Diagnosis and treatment of acute fluoride toxicity, *JADA* 110:209, 1985.

Bowden JW, editor: Workshop report, group 3, *J Dent Res* 71:1224, 1992.

Benediktsson S et al: The effect of contact time of acidulated phosphate fluoride on fluoride concentration in human enamel, *Arch Oral Biol* 27:567, 1982.

Bijella MFB et al: Comparison of dental prophylaxis and toothbrushing prior to topical APF applications, *Community Dent Oral Epidemiol* 13:208, 1985.

Boyd RL, Leggott PJ, Robertson PB: Effects on gingivitis of two different 0.4%SnF_2 gels, *J Dent Res* 67:503, 1988.

Brunn C, Stoltze K: In vivo uptake of fluoride by surface enamel of cleaned and plaque-covered teeth, *Scand J Dent Res* 84:268, 1976.

Bruun C, Thylstrup A, Uribe E: Loosely bound fluoride extracted from natural carious lesions after topical application of APF in vitro, *Caries Res* 17:458, 1983.

Brustman B: Impact of exposure to fluoride-adequate water on root surface caries in elderly, *Gerodontics* 2:203, 1986.

Burt BA: The epidemiology of oral diseases. In Striffler DF, Young WO, Burt BA, editors: *Dentistry, dental practice, and the community,* Philadelphia, 1983, WB Saunders.

Burt BA, Eklund SA, Loesche WJ: Dental benefits of limited exposure to fluoridated water in childhood, *J Dent Res* 65:1322, 1986.

Burt BA, Ismail AI, Eklund SA: Root caries in an optimally fluoridated and a high-fluoride community, *J Dent Res* 65:1154, 1986.

Charleton G et al: Associations between dental plaque and fluoride in human surface enamel, *Arch Oral Biol* 19:139, 1974.

Church LE: Fluorides—use with caution, *J Maryland Dent Assoc* 19(Aug):106, 1976.

Clark DC: A review of fluoride varnishes: an alternative topical fluoride treatment, *Community Dent Oral Epidemiol* 10:117, 1982.

Clarkson B et al: Rational use of fluorides in caries prevention and treatment. In Ekstrand J et al, editors: *Fluoride in dentistry,* Copenhagen, 1988, Munksgaard.

Crall JJ et al: SEM and electron microprobe analysis of enamel treated with two-step topical fluorides in vitro, *Caries Res* 17:481, 1983.

DePaola PF: Clinical studies of monofluorophosphate dentifrices, *Caries Res* 17(suppl 1):119, 1983.

Dijkman AG, Tak J, Arends J: Comparison of fluoride uptake by human enamel from acidulated phosphate fluoride gels with different fluoride concentrations, *Caries Res* 16:197, 1982.

Downer MD: Changing patterns of disease in the western world. In Guggenheim B, editor: *Cariology today,* Basel, Switzerland, 1983, Karger.

Driessens FC et al: Posteruptive maturation of the tooth enamel studied with the electron microprobe, *Caries Res* 19:390, 1985.

Driscoll WS et al: Caries preventive effects of daily and weekly fluoride mouth rinsing in an optimally fluoridated community: findings after eighteen months, *Pediatr Dent* 3:316, 1981.

Eisen JJ, LeCompte EJ: A comparison of oral fluoride retention following topical treatments with APF gels of varying viscosities, *Pediatr Dent* 7:175, 1985.

Ekstrand J, Koch G: Systemic fluoride absorption following fluoride gel application, *J Dent Res* 59:1067, 1980.

Ekstrand J et al: Pharmacokinetics of fluoride gels in children and adults, *Caries Res* 15:213, 1981.

Featherstone JDB, ten Cate JM: Physicochemical aspects of fluoride-enamel interactions. In Ekstrand J et al, editors: *Fluoride in dentistry,* Copenhagen, 1988, Munksgaard.

Fejerskov O, Thylstrup A, Larsen MJ: Rational use of fluorides in caries prevention, *Acta Odontol Scand* 39:241, 1981.

Granath L, McHugh WD: Basic prevention for the individual. In Granath L, McHugh WD, editors: *Systematized prevention of oral disease: theory and practice,* Boca Raton, Fla, 1986, CRC.

Hagan PP, Rozier RG, Baseden JW: The caries-preventive effects of full- and half-strength topical acidulated phosphate fluoride, *Pediatr Dent* 7:185, 1985.

Hand JS, Hunt RJ, Beck JD: Coronal and root caries in older Iowans: 36 month incidence, *Gerodontics* 4(3):136-139, 1988.

Harper DS, Loesche WJ: Inhibition of acid production from oral bacteria by fluorapatite derived fluoride, *J Dent Res* 65:30, 1986.

Heifetz SB, Horowitz HS: The amounts of fluoride in current fluoride therapies: safety considerations for children, *ASDC J Dent Child* 51:257, 1984.

Heifetz SB et al: Prevalence of dental caries and fluorosis in four acres of Illinois: a 5-year follow-up survey, *J Dent Res* 66 (abstract):164, 1987.

Hock J, Tinanoff N: Resolution of gingivitis in dogs following topical applications of a 0.40% stannous fluoride and toothbrushing, *J Dent Res* 58:1652, 1979.

Horowitz HS: Abuse use of fluoride, *J Public Health Dent* 37:106, 1977.

Horowitz HS, Heifetz SB: Topically applied fluorides. In Newbrun E, editor: *Fluorides and dental caries,* Springfield, Ill, 1986, CC Thomas.

Horowitz HS et al: Combined fluoride, school-based program in a fluoride-deficient area: results of an 11-year study, *JADA* 112:621, 1986.

Houpt M, Koenigsberg S, Shey Z: The effect of prior toothcleaning on the efficacy of topical fluoride treatment, *Clin Prev Dent* 5(4):8, 1983.

Hunt RJ, Eldredge JB, Beck JD: Effect of residence in a fluoridated community on the incidence of coronal and root caries in an older adult population, *J Public Health Dent* 49:138, 1989.

Iijima Y, Katayama T: Fluoride concentrations in deciduous enamel in high- and low-fluoride areas, *Caries Res* 19:262, 1985.

Isman R: Knowledge and attitudes of dentists about fluoridation, *JADA* 109:924, 1984.

Jensen ME, Kohout FJ: The effect of a fluoridated dentifrice on root and coronal caries in an older adult population, *JADA* 117:829-832, 1988.

Jordan HV, Summey DL: Root surface caries: review of the literature and significance of the problem, *J Periodontol* 44:158, 1973.

Keltjens HMAM et al: Microflora of plaque from sound and carious root surfaces, *Caries Res* 21:193, 1987.

Klimek J, Hellwig E, Ahrens G: Fluoride taken up by plaque, by the underlying enamel and by clean enamel from three fluoride compounds in vitro, *Caries Res* 16:156, 1982.

Lagerlof F et al: Effects of inorganic orthophosphate and pyrophosphate on dissolution of calcium fluoride in water, *J Dent Res* 67:447, 1988.

Larsen MJ, Jensen SJ: On the properties of fluoride solutions used for topical treatment and mouth rinse, *Caries Res* 20:56, 1986.

LeCompte EJ: Clinical application of topical fluoride products—risks, benefits, and recommendations, *J Dent Res* 66:1066, 1987.

LeCompte EJ, Doyle TE: Oral fluoride retention following various topical application techniques in children, *J Dent Res* 61:1397, 1982.

LeCompte EJ, Doyle TE: Effects of suctioning devices on oral fluoride retention, *JADA* 11:357, 1985.

LeCompte EJ, Whitford GM: The biologic availability of fluoride from alginate impressions and APF gel in children, *J Dent Res* 60:776, 1981.

LeCompte EJ, Whitford GM: Pharmacokinetics of fluoride from APF gel and fluoride tablets in children, *J Dent Res* 61:469, 1982.

Leske GS, Ripa LW: Three-year root caries increments: implications for clinical trials, *J Public Health Dent* 49:142, 1989.

Leske GS, Ripa LW, Sposato A: Posttreatment benefits from participation in a school-based fluoride mouthrinsing demonstration program: results after 4 to 6 years of rinsing, *Clin Prev Dent* 6(1):16, 1984.

Leske GS et al: Posttreatment benefits from participation in a school-based fluoride mouthrinsing program: results after up to 7 years of rinsing, *Caries Res* 19:371, 1985.

Leverett DH, Curzon MEJ: Effect of flossing and brushing immediately prior to weekly fluoride mouthrinsing, *Pediatr Dent* 5:187, 1983.

Levy SM: Expansion of the proper use of systemic fluoride supplements, *JADA* 112:30, 1986.

Levy SM: Compliance by health care providers with recommended systemic fluoride supplementation protocol, *Clin Prev Dent* 9(5):19, 1987.

Lyon TC: Topical fluorides: How much are you using? *Dent Hyg* 59:58, 1985.

Manly RS, Harrington DP: Solution rate of tooth enamel in an acetate buffer, *J Dent Res* 38:910, 1959.

Margolis HD, Moreno EC, Murphy BJ: Effect of low levels of fluoride in solution on enamel demineralization in vitro, *J Dent Res* 65:23, 1986.

Mazza JE, Newman MG, Sims TN: Clinical and antimicrobial effect of stannous fluoride on periodontitis, *J Clin Periodontol* 8:203, 1981.

McClure FJ: *Water fluoridation: the search and victory,* Bethesda, Md, 1970, National Institutes of Health.

McDonald JL, Schemehorn BR, Stookey GK: Influence of fluoride upon plaque and gingivitis in the beagle dog, *J Dent Res* 57:889, 1978.

Mellberg JR, Mallon DE: Acceleration of remineralization in vitro by sodium monofluorophosphate and sodium fluoride, *J Dent Res* 63:1130, 1984.

Mellberg JR, Sanchez M: Remineralization by a monofluorophosphate dentifrice in vitro of root dentin softened by artificial caries, *J Dent Res* 65(7):959, 1986.

Mellberg JR et al: The relationship between dental caries and tooth enamel fluoride, *Caries Res* 19:385, 1985.

Mirth DB et al: Comparison of the cariostatic effect of topically and systemically administered controlled-release fluoride in the rat, *Caries Res* 19:466, 1985.

More F et al: Ingestion of fluoride during a topical application, *J Dent Res* 62(abstract):262, 1983.

Nakagaki H et al: Distribution of fluoride across human dental enamel, dentine and cementum, *Arch Oral Biol* 32:651, 1987.

Narendran S et al: Fluorosis in fluoridated and nonfluoridated communities, *J Dent Res* 66(abstract):164, 1987.

Newbrun E: Mechanism of fluoride action in caries prevention. In Newbrun E, editor: *Fluorides and dental caries,* ed 3, Springfield, Ill, 1986a, CC Thomas.

Newbrun E: Water fluoridation and dietary fluoride. In Newbrun E, editor: *Fluorides and dental caries*, ed 3, Springfield, Ill, 1986b, CC Thomas.

Owen D et al: Monitoring ingestion and urinary excretion of topical fluoride, *J Dent Res* 57(abstract):1256, 1979.

Ramsay DS et al: Problematic gagging: principles of treatment, *JADA* 114:178, 1987.

Reintsema H, Schuthof J, Arends J: An in vivo investigation of the fluoride uptake in partially demineralized human enamel from several different dentifrices, *J Dent Res* 64:19, 1985.

Retief DH, Harris BE, Bradley EL: Relationship between enamel fluoride concentration and dental caries experience, *Caries Res* 21:68, 1987.

Ripa LW: Professionally (operator) applied topical fluoride therapy: a critique, *Clin Prevent Dent* 4(3):3, 1982.

Ripa LW: Need for prior toothcleaning when performing a professional topical fluoride application: review and recommendations for change, *JADA* 109:281, 1984.

Ripa LW: Topical fluorides: a discussion of risks and benefits, *J Dent Res* 66:1079, 1987.

Ripa LW et al: Effect of prior toothcleaning on biannual professional APF topical fluoride gel-tray treatments: results after two years, *Clin Prev Dent* 5(4):3, 1983a.

Ripa LW et al: Supervised weekly rinsing with a 0.2% neutral NaF solution: results after 5 years, *Community Dent Oral Epidemiol* 11:1, 1983b.

Ripa LW et al: Supervised weekly rinsing with a 0.2% neutral NaF solution: results of a demonstration program after six school years, *J Public Health Dent* 43:52, 1983c.

Ripa LW et al: Clinical comparison of the caries inhibition of two mixed NaF-Na₂PO₃F dentifrices containing 1000 ppm F: results after two years, *Caries Res* 21:149, 1987a.

Ripa LW et al: Effect of a 0.05% neutral NaF mouthrinse on coronal and root caries in adults, *Gerodontology* 4:131, 1987b.

Schamschula RG et al: Interrelations between the fluoride concentrations in dental plaque and enamel and exposure to fluoride, *Aust Dent J* 27:360, 1982.

Seppa L: Effect of dental plaque on fluoride uptake by enamel from a sodium fluoride varnish in vivo, *Caries Res* 17:71, 1983.

Seppa L, Pollanen L: Caries preventive effect of two fluoride varnishes and a fluoride mouthrinse, *Caries Res* 21:375, 1987.

Shannon IL, Edmonds EJ, Madsen KO: Single, double, and sequential methods for fluoride applications, *ASDC J Dent Child* 41:115, 1974a.

Shannon IL, Paoloski SB, Wescott WB: Dental hygiene students in the fluoride laboratory, *Dent Hyg* 48:87, 1974b.

Stallard RE, editor: *Proceedings, International Conference on Fluorides and Dental Health, Nairobi, Kenya,* New Brunswick, NJ, 1983, S & S Printing Services.

Stamm JW, Banting DW, Imrey PB: Adult root caries survey of two similar communities with contrasting natural water fluoride levels, *JADA* 120:143, 1990.

Steele RC et al: The effect of tooth cleaning procedures on fluoride uptake in enamel, *Pediatr Dent* 4:228, 1982.

Stephan KW, McCall DR, Tullis JI: Caries prevalence in northern Scotland before and after 5 years water defluoridation, *Br Dent J* 163:324, 1987b.

Stephan KW et al: Three-year oral health trial with zinc-containing monofluorophasphaate dentifrices, *J Dent Res* 66(abstract):459, 1987.

Stookey GK et al: The effect of rinsing with water immediately after a professional fluoride gel application on fluoride uptake in demineralized enamel: an in vivo study, *Pediatr Dent* 8:153, 1986.

ten Cate JM, Duijesters PPE: Influence of fluoride in solution on tooth demineralization, *Caries Res* 17:193, 1983.

Teranaka T, Koulourides T: Effect of a 100-ppm fluoride mouth rinse on experimental root caries in humans, *Caries Res* 21:326, 1987.

U.S. Public Health Service, National Institute of Dental Research: *The prevalence of dental caries in United States children, 1979-1980,* NIH publ no 82-2245, Washington, DC, 1981, US Government Printing Office.

Vrbic V, Brudevold F, McCann HG: Acquisition of fluoride by enamel from fluoride pumice pastes, *Helv Odontol Acta* 11:21, 1967.

Wefel JS: Mechanisms of action of fluorides. In Stewart et al, editors: *Pediatric dentistry: scientific foundations and current practices,* St Louis, 1981, CV Mosby.

Wefel JS, Clarkson BH, Heilman JR: Histology of root surface caries. In Thylstrup A, Lesch SA, and Quist V, editors: *Dentine and dentine reactions in the oral cavity,* England, 1987, IRL Press.

Wefel JS, Silverstone LM, Clarkson BH: Remineralization of artificial white spot lesions in human dental enamel. In *Conference on Foods, Nutrition and Dental Health, American Dental Association Health Foundation,* vol 2, Chicago, 1982, American Dental Association.

Wefel JS, Wei SH: In vitro evaluation of fluoride uptake from a thixotiopes gel, *Pediatr Dent* 97:100, 1979.

Wei SH: The potential benefits to be derived from topical fluorides in fluoridated communities. In Forester DJ, Schulz EM, editors: *International Workshop on Fluorides and Dental Caries Reduction,* Baltimore, 1974, University of Maryland School of Dentistry.

Wei SH, Kanelis MJ: Fluoride retention after sodium fluoride mouthrinsing by preschool children, *JADA* 106:626, 1983.

Wei SH, Chits FF: Fluoride retention following topical fluoride foam and gel application, *Pediatr Dent* 12:368, 1990.

Wei SH, Hattab FN: Enamel fluoride uptake from a new APF foam, *Pediatr Dent* 10:111-114, 1988.

White DJ, Faller RV: Fluoride uptake from anticalculus dentifrices in vitro, *Caries Res* 21:40, 1987.

Whitford GM: Fluoride in dental products: safety considerations, *J Dent Res* 66:1056, 1987.

Whitford GM et al: Topical fluorides: effects on physiological and biochemical process, *J Dent Res* 66:1072, 1987.

SUGGESTED READINGS

Aasenden R et al: Effects of daily rinsing and ingestion of fluoride solutions upon dental caries and enamel fluoride, *Arch Oral Biol* 17:1705, 1972.

American Dental Association Council on Dental Therapeutics: A guide to the use of fluorides for the prevention of dental caries, *JADA* 113:506, 1986.

Carlos JP: Topical fluorides: optimizing safety and efficacy—introduction, *J Dent Res* 66:1055, 1987.

Driscoll WS et al: Prevalence of dental caries and dental fluoride in areas with optimal and above-optimal water fluoride concentrations, *JADA* 197:42, 1983.

Duxbury AJ et al: Acute fluoride toxicity, *Br Dent J* 153:64, 1982.

Ekstrand J, Koch G, Petersson LG: Plasma fluoride concentrations in pre-school children after ingestion of fluoride tablets and toothpaste, *Caries Res* 17:379, 1983.

Ellingsen JE, Ekstrand J: Plasma fluoride levels in man following intake of SnF_2 in solution or toothpaste, *J Dent Res* 64:1250, 1985.

Fehr FR von der, Löe H, Theilade E: Experimental caries in man, *Caries Res* 4:131, 1970.

Hattab FN: Diffusion of fluorides in human dental enamel in vitro, *Arch Oral Biol* 31:811, 1986.

Katz S et al: *Preventive dentistry in action,* ed 3, Upper Montclair, NJ, 1979, DCP.

McCall DR et al: Fluoride ingestion following APF gel application, *Br Dent J* 155:333, 1983.

Newbrun E: Topical fluoride therapy: discussion of some aspects of toxicology, safety, and efficacy, *J Dent Res* 66:1084, 1987.

Ripa LW: The roles of prophylaxes and dental prophylaxis pastes in caries prevention. In Wei SH, editor: *Clinical uses of fluoride,* Philadelphia, 1985, Lea & Febiger.

Tinanoff N et al: Effect of a pumice prophylaxis on fluoride uptake in tooth enamel, *JADA* 88:384, 1974.

Tyler JE, Andlaw RJ: Oral retention of fluoride after application of acidulated phosphate fluoride gel in air-cushion trays, *Br Dent J* 162:422, 1987.

Vrbic V, Brudevold F: Fluoride uptake from treatment with different fluoride prophylaxis pastes and from the use of pastes containing a soluble aluminum salt followed by topical application, *Caries Res* 4:158, 1970.

Wefel JS: Critical assessment of professional application of topical fluorides. In Wei SH, editor: *Clinical uses of fluoride,* Philadelphia, 1985, Lea & Febiger.

Wei SH, Kanelis MJ: Fluoride retention after sodium fluoride mouthrinsing by preschool children, *JADA* 106:626, 1983.

22 PIT AND FISSURE SEALANTS

Susan J. Daniel
Bonnie Dafoe

LEARNING OUTCOMES

The dental hygienist will be able to

1. Understand and appreciate the role of dental sealants in the prevention of oral disease.
2. Correctly follow tooth selection criteria for sealant placement.
3. Practice the accepted sequence of steps for sealant placement.
4. Determine by using evaluative criteria the acceptability of a placed sealant.
5. Discuss with a patient or guardian the rationale for sealants.
6. Discuss trends in sealant use.
7. Discuss possible reasons for underuse of sealant techniques in community and private practice settings, given their success as a preventive therapy.

Dental sealants, also referred to as pit and fissure sealants, aid in the prevention of carious lesions by protecting the pits and fissures of teeth from bacterial activity. Although the caries rate among schoolchildren aged 5 to 17 in the general population has declined, the rate of decay in pits and fissures remains high. In 1989 the National Institute of Dental Research reported that approximately 50% of all school-aged children had dental caries and that two-thirds of that decay was located on occlusal surfaces. Further, 15% to 20% of children 5 to 17 years of age are considered to be at high risk for caries (Stamm et al, 1988). In addition, some groups within the population have been categorized as being at high risk for caries. Among Native Americans, the caries rate has been reported to be as high as 80% (Niendorff, 1985). Considering the possible amount of pit and fissure decay, the value of dental sealants as a significant risk reduction procedure can be appreciated. You may have dental sealants in some of your teeth, and as a dental hygienist you will, in most states, be placing dental sealants. After exploring the history of sealant development and the retention rates and success of sealants, this chapter will present the mechanism by which sealants adhere to the tooth; the types of dental sealant materials criteria for selection of teeth to be sealed; application techniques evaluation of sealant placement, and trends in sealant use. Remember as you read this chapter that this is a preventive measure you will regularly perform in your practice.

Methods other than sealants have been used in an attempt to lower the rate of pit and fissure caries. Approaches have included eradication of the occlusal anatomy by reshaping the occlusal grooves (enameloplasty) or placement of conservative occlusal restorations before decay begins (Craig, O'Brien, and Powers, 1983). As both of these methods remove sound tooth structure, neither would seem to be a true preventive measure.

Obturation of pits and fissures on the occlusal surface with materials such as silver nitrate, zinc chloride, potassium ferrocyanide, or red copper cement has also been tried. This procedure has been unsuccessful primarily because of the materials' physical or chemical properties.

Fluoride seemed an obvious answer to the problem of occlusal decay, because it has a systemic effect on the actual quality of the enamel. Though fluorides do reduce the number of caries, studies indicate that proximal and smooth surfaces, not the occlusal surfaces, enjoy the most benefit from systemic fluoride therapy (Ripa, 1973).

Reducing the retentive nature of the occlusal anatomy, therefore, is the key to achieving a significant reduction in pit and fissure caries. A fissure that is less likely to harbor debris and/or bacteria is less likely to decay. The sealants used today are materials that coat the pits and fissures and act as a physical barrier to prevent oral bacteria and nutrients from developing the acidic conditions necessary to destroy tooth structure. The factor that makes today's sealants more successful than other coverage techniques is an acid-conditioning process that alters or enlarges the naturally occurring enamel pores. With the increase in surface area resulting from this technique, the sealant is able to penetrate the enamel better and to achieve a reliable mechanical bond (Gwinnett, 1973). It is important to know the short- and long- term retention rates reported in the literature to assist in presenting sound rationales for sealants as a part of your patients' overall oral disease prevention program.

Retention of properly placed sealants is excellent, as evidenced by two studies in which 87% (Buonocore, 1971) and 97% (Whyte, Leake, Howley, 1987) were fully intact after 2 years. In terms of preventing decay, 99% of the sealant-treated teeth were free of decay, whereas 60% of the nontreated teeth had developed caries (Buonocore, 1971). At 4 years, after a single placement of sealant, full retention was reported to be 50% with an 84% reduction in caries (Going, 1977). After 5 years, one study reported a 39% rate of effectiveness in preventing decay (Horowitz, Heifetz, and Poulsen, 1977). Even after 10 years and a single application of sealant, 84% of occlusal surfaces on permanent first molars were found to be sound (Simonsen, 1987).

When fluorides and sealants are combined, the preventive benefits are enhanced. After 2 years a control group who participated in a weekly mouthrinsing program with 0.2% neutral sodium fluoride solution were 78.4% caries-free. The group who received sealants in addition to the weekly mouthrinses remained 96.4% caries-free (Ripa, 1987). As the aforementioned studies indicate, dental sealants do prevent occlusal decay in pits and fissures. Now, let us see how they work.

THE BONDING MECHANISM

Buonocore (1975) suggested that the occlusal surface of a tooth is similar to an iceberg: much of what exists cannot be seen. In fact, with conventional explorer examination much cannot be determined with tactile sense. The explorer may "catch" in the tooth because of a deep narrow noncarious fissure. Three principal types of pit and fissure configurations have been described: V types, U types, and I types (Figs. 22-1 to 22-3). In addition, miscellaneous shapes exist as small

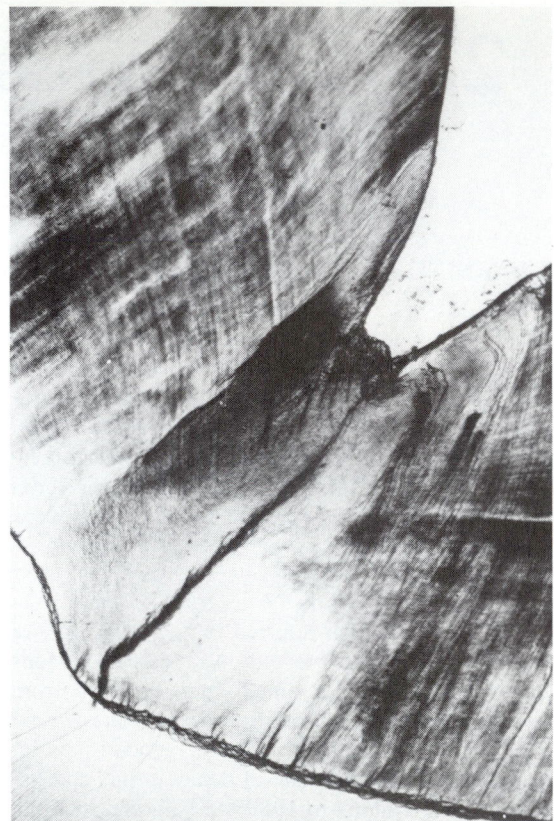

Fig. 22-1. Photomicrograph showing wide V-type fissure. (From Gwinnett AJ: *J Am Soc Prevent Dent* 3:21, 1973.)

round openings, fissures that have pits associated with their bases or walls, or continuous grooves that separate cusps (Fig. 22-4). To protect these anatomic defects from the inevitably high percentage of carious lesions, acid-etch resin sealants are useful. Success depends on using a highly effective bonding technique and a leakage-resistant material.

Mechanical bonding refers to a physical entrapment of material within pores or cavities, whether naturally or artificially created (Gwinnett, 1973). The etching process, also called conditioning, involves applying an acidic gel or a 30% to 50% acidic solution to the pits and fissures to be sealed. The acid removes inorganic material and creates tiny crevices or micropores. This rough and reactive porous surface provides more surface area, as well as tiny pits into which the sealant resin can flow and form a strong mechanical bond.

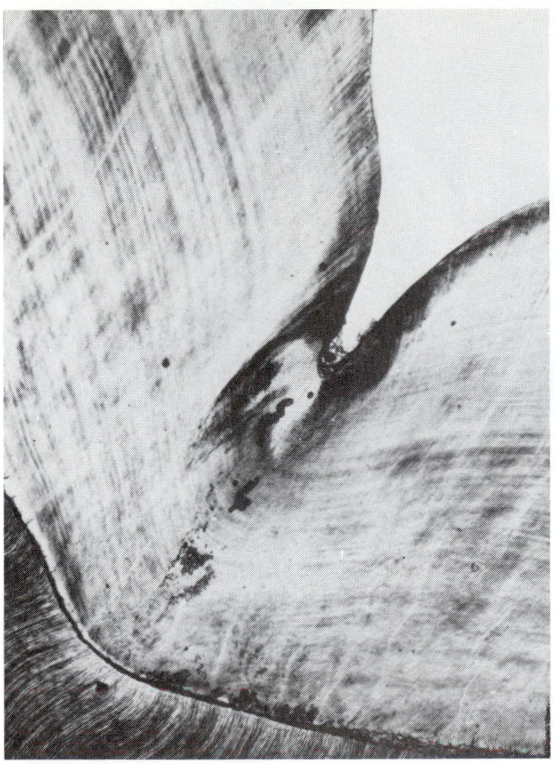

Fig. 22-2. Photomicrograph showing narrow U-type fissure. (From Gwinnett AJ: *J Am Soc Prevent Dent* 3:21, 1973.)

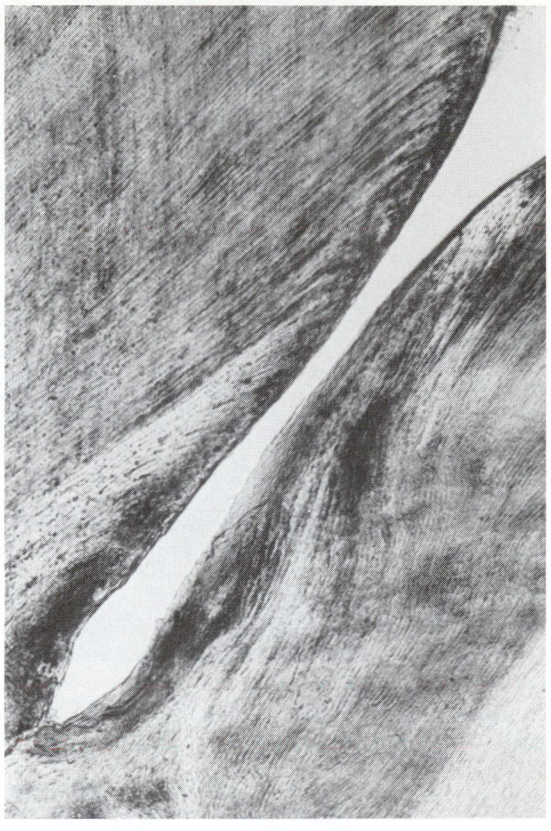

Fig. 22-3. Photomicrograph showing I-type fissure, a narrow constrictive configuration that is somewhat bulbous toward its base.
(From Gwinnett AJ: *J Am Soc Prevent Dent* 3:21, 1973.)

Three basic etching patterns can be observed by scanning electron micrograph. The conditioned enamel surface shows enamel rods that have lost material from the rod cores (Fig. 22-5). The surface may show a preferential loss of rod peripheries, or the enamel surface may show no specific pattern but still be etched satisfactorily. All three types of etching patterns can be observed on a single tooth. Failure of a sealant to properly bond is always a result of this resin-enamel interface (Silverstone, 1987).

As conditioning does remove enamel structure, does it harm the tooth? Most of the conditioned tooth surface is covered by dental sealant; however, if conditioned enamel is left exposed, minerals in the saliva replenish the surface (Silverstone, 1987).

Researchers have reported that decay that is inadvertently sealed in a tooth does not appear to progress when the sealant is firmly bonded (Handelman, 1983; Mertz-Fairhurst, et al, 1979a). The margins of sealed surfaces have been shown to resist leakage of dye and radioisotopes even after being boiled in water. A study of residual carious material under sealed lesions suggested a complete cessation of the carious process. No clinical or radiographic signs were seen to suggest that the health of the sealed tooth had been compromised (Mertz-Fairhurst et al., 1986). When carious or sound surfaces were sealed for the first time, the retention rates for the sealant materials were the same after a 2-year period (Handelman, 1987a).

The results of these studies support the safety of sealing small, incipient caries. The nature of the sealant margin compares favorably with other

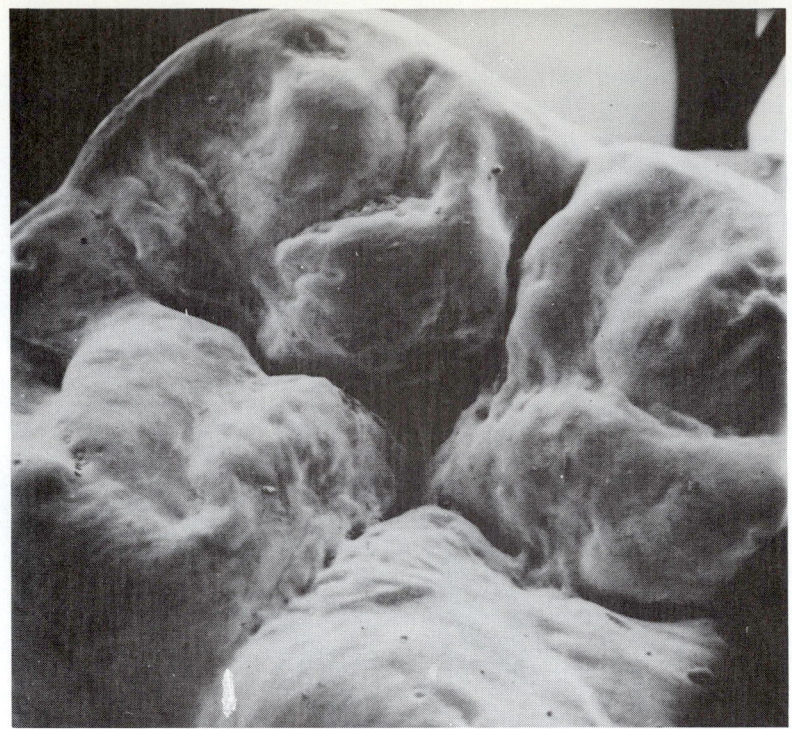

Fig. 22-4. Scanning electron micrograph showing random distribution of pits and fissures on occlusal surface. (From Gwinnett AJ: *J Am Soc Prevent Dent* 3:21, 1973.)

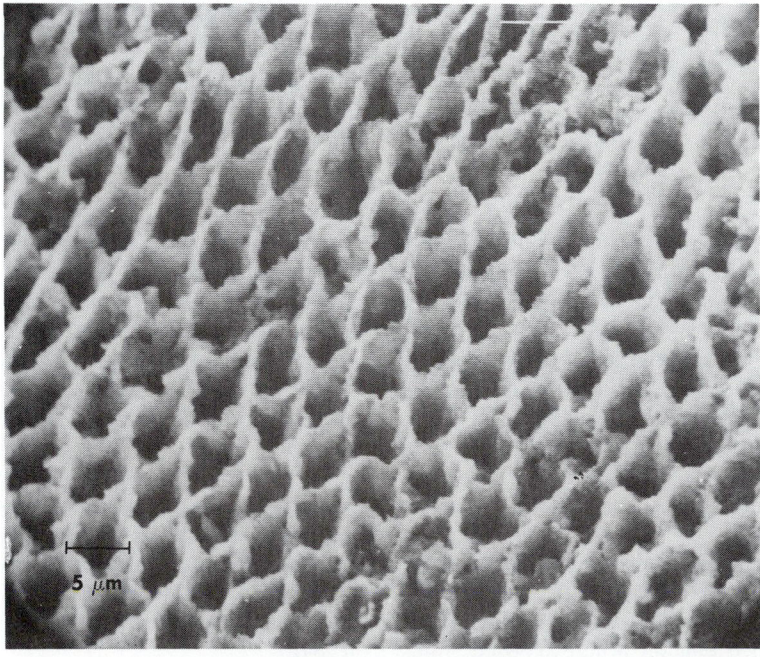

5 μm

Fig. 22-5. Scanning electron micrograph of enamel surface that has been etched (conditioned) with phosphoric acid for 60 seconds. Note loss of enamel prism core, which will encourage sealant retention. (From Silverstone LM: *Preventive dentistry,* Fort Lee, NJ, 1978, Update.)

current restorative material margins that, despite microscopic leakage, arrest the decay process and resist recurrence of caries to a high degree. Dennison and colleagues (1980) compared the margins of amalgam restorations with sealants retained after 18 months. Deterioration around the margin was present in 50% of the amalgam restorations. Sealant margins remained undetectable in 55% of cases. Sealants have proven themselves, therefore, as effective materials for protecting pits and fissures from the caries process.

SEALANT MATERIALS

Dental sealants are made from several types of material. However, most are bisphenol A-glycidyl methacrylate (BIS-GMA) materials, which are polymerized either by an organic amine or by ultraviolet or visible light (Craig, O'Brien, and Powers, 1983). Amine-accelerated materials are supplied as two-component systems and require mixing. Ultraviolet and visible light–polymerized materials require no mixing.

To ensure success with these materials, careful handling is necessary. It is especially important that the sealant material not be exposed to air during storage, since this may cause evaporation. Evaporation in turn would make the material less fluid and thereby reduced penetration into the pits and fissures. Further, visible light-cured materials will begin to polymerize if left exposed to light. Sealant materials should always be fresh, and other sealant equipment such as brushes and light sources should be well maintained and free of extraneous debris.

Mertz-Fairhurst and others (1982) reported a comparative clinical study of two different pit and fissure sealants in which 49% of the teeth remained sealed with one product and 78% remained intact with the other product 6 years after a single application.

In another study, which compared autopolymerized versus light-polymerized fissure sealants, Houpt and coworkers (1987) found no significant difference in their clinical performance and retention after 31 months. Other studies have compared products for their microhardness, bond strength, and abrasion loss (Strang et al, 1986; Dorignac, 1987). Sealants are not as hard as composite resins or metals and, therefore, exhibit greater wear. However, the bond strength is comparable with other bonded composite resins. Hardness, tensile bond strength, and resistance to wear are important properties for sealant materials to possess, given their exposure to conditions in the oral cavity.

Improved sealant materials are being developed. One such material incorporating a slow-release fluoride is promising. A methacryloyl fluoride–methyl methacrylate (MF–MMA) copolymer resin showed after testing that 70% to 80% of the fluoride was tightly bound to the enamel, suggesting that such a sealant could theoretically protect the enamel from caries attack even after detachment (Tanaka et al, 1987).

Glass ionomer cements have also been used to seal pits and fissures; however, reported retention rates are not as good as those with the BIS-GMA formulations. In two studies, retention rates of glass ionomer cements were reported to be 75% at 4 months (Torppa-Saarinen and Seppa, 1990) and 82.5% at 12 months (McKenna and Grundy, 1987).

Varnishes containing fluorides are also being used to seal pits and fissures, because they require less time for placement and may be more suitable for application at an early age (3 to 5 years). Children of this age are less likely to remain still, and salivary contamination of the sealant site frequently occurs (Raadal et al, 1990). Varnishes do not, however, have the longevity of traditional sealants, but they could provide a preliminary preventive measure before dental sealant placement. In addition, the fluoride is continually released, providing an increased uptake in the enamel and dentin for caries prevention (Acuna et al, 1990). Given the possibility of salivary contamination during tooth preparation and sealant placement, one study has investigated a varnish made of a new material (Bayer D520) that relies on humidity to initiate the self-curing chemical reaction process. The initial set requires approximately 60 seconds, and complete hardness is obtained in about 6 hours. At the end of 2 years, 57% of the teeth were found to be either totally or partially covered by the sealant/varnish (Duggan and Midda, 1987).

Another material in the early developmental stages is a polymeric coating that can be painted over all supragingival tooth surfaces to prevent the caries process (Johnston and Bowen, 1991). Once available, this material could be beneficial not only for the prevention of occlusal decay, but also for the prevention of root caries on exposed cementum.

> **Pit and fissure sealant products approved by the Council on Dental Materials, Instruments, and Equipment (January, 1992)**
>
> **Acceptable**
>
> Concise, 3M Dental Products Division.
> Delton, Johnson & Johnson Professional Dental Care, Inc.
> Delton (tinted), Johnson & Johnson Professional Dental Care, Inc.
> Delton (light-cured), Johnson & Johnson Professional Dental Care, Inc.
> Delton (light-cured) Opaque, Johnson & Johnson Professional Dental Care, Inc.
> Delton (self-cured) Opaque, Johnson & Johnson Professional Dental Care, Inc.
> Helioseal, Ivoclar Vivadent.
> Oralin, Mission White Dental Inc.
> Visio-Seal, ESPE GmbH & Co.
> Prisma-Shield (tinted), L D Caulk Co.
> Prisma-Shield, L D Caulk Co.
>
> **Provisionally acceptable**
>
> Sealite, Kerr Manufacturing Co.

Research shows that most sealant materials are comparable and effective. There appear to be no health-related risks to either the patient or dental professionals. No systemic toxicity from the chemical use of sealants has been reported; however, one study found mild to moderately severe foreign body reactions in the subcutaneous tissue when sealant materials were implanted into the backs of guinea pigs (Ranalli et al, 1989). It is recommended that protective glasses be worn when using light-cured materials to prevent possible retinal damage from light sources (NIH, 1984).

Materials approved by the American Dental Association Council on Dental Materials, Instruments, and Equipment can be found in the box above. The Council encourages manufacturers to submit their products for evaluation. These evaluations are based on laboratory tests of mechanical and physical properties and biologic acceptability as well as clinical data on biocompatibility and effectiveness as a caries-preventive material. Clinical studies on retention may also be included. Participation by manufacturers is voluntary.

INDICATIONS FOR SEALANT APPLICATION

Ideally, all pits and fissures should be sealed soon after eruption. However, if this is not financially feasible, the patient's caries susceptibility should be evaluated. You need to consider several factors. One of the best predictors of new caries is the patient's previous and existing caries activity (Disney et al, 1992; Stamm et al, 1988, 1990). Also, pit and fissure morphology has been shown to predict caries susceptibility (Disney et al., 1992). Deep, narrow pits and fissures tend to retain more oral bacteria than teeth with shallow grooves and are less accessible to cleaning methods. In the permanent dentition, molars are more susceptible to caries than are premolars. In the primary dentition, the second molars are more susceptible than the first molars (Ripa, 1973). A thorough review of the patient's dental history could reveal previous caries. The patient's attitude about preventive dentistry may be assessed by investigating home care practices and frequency of care by the dental hygienist. Sealant protection is intended to be used as part of a total preventive program. Regular professional care, fluoride application (systemic and topical), and individual home care are the components of the preventive plan.

The pattern of dental caries differs greatly from tooth to tooth and surface to surface. At least 70% of occlusal surfaces in permanent molars eventually become decayed or filled. The peak of caries in these teeth is reached about 10 years after eruption, between the ages of 16 and 22 years. Walter (1982) reported that 37% of 120 naval recruits aged 17 to 24 years developed new caries within a 5-year period; 90% of these were on occlusal surfaces. Occlusal decay of premolars is less prevalent, with only 30% to 45% becoming carious. Since the peak for caries development in premolars is between the ages of 30 and 40 years, sealing of these teeth in adults may be advantageous.

Sealants can prevent the need for occlusal fillings in 50% of molar teeth. Because the overall caries rate is lower in premolars, sealants will do no better than obviate 10% of the need for occlusal restorations in these teeth (Eklund and Ismail, 1986). In general, when a patient is identified as being caries susceptible, despite other preventive measures, the teeth should be protected as soon after eruption as possible. The Dental Branch of the

Sealant application guidelines for third-party payers

1. Sealants are indicated for previously unrestored, deep, narrow pits and fissures that show no evidence of caries.
2. Presence of interproximal caries should be ruled out before sealant placement.
3. Sealants should be placed as soon as possible after eruption, when the tooth is free of gingival contact and when there is no tissue flap to interfere with application procedures.
4. Consider overall caries status. Seal newly erupted teeth promptly when there is evidence of current carious lesions and/or previous restorations on other teeth, malpositioned teeth, and any other condition promoting decay.
5. Only use sealant products accepted by the Council on Dental Materials, Instruments, and Equipment of the American Dental Association.
6. Sealants should be applied according to the manufacturer's instructions.
7. Fluoride treatment should be applied after sealant application.
8. If needed, one application per tooth may be allowed every 3 to 5 years with one repair allowed (lesser fee) in the intervening time.

From DiLeone CM: *Dent Hyg* 61(1):18, 1987.

Indian Health Service (U.S. Department of Health and Human Services) requires all permanent molars to be sealed within 2 years after eruption.

The Consensus Development Conference on Dental Sealants (NIH, 1984) suggested these priorities for sealant application:

	Priority
General population	1. Permanent first molars (ages 6 to 8)
	2. Permanent second molars (ages 11 to 13)
High caries-susceptible children	1. Permanent first molars
	2. Permanent second molars
	3. Permanent premolars
	4. Primary molars

Teeth should be selected as candidates for sealants after a careful evaluation with an explorer and compressed air. A radiographic examination may also be necessary. Pit and fissure sealants are contraindicated where the proximal surfaces are carious, as the restorative procedure requires a portion of the occlusal table for retention. Occasionally there is a question about a "sticky" fissure. On explorer examination, the instrument tip is retained or "sticks" for a brief instant in the pit or fissure; this causes the patient no discomfort. If there is no evidence of decay penetrating the dentinoenamel junction (DEJ) on a bitewing radiograph (an incipient lesion), placing a sealant is preferable to leaving the tooth in a vulnerable state or preparing it for a prophylactic amalgam restoration (Ball, 1986a and b). This practice may be controversial, but it is rationalized by the fact that sealed incipient carious lesions do not progress (Going, 1978; Mertz-Fairhurst et al., 1979a and b). Sealants represent the most conservative treatment for preventing caries while preserving the most tooth structure.

The box notes guidelines for sealant application suggested for Medicaid as well as other insurance carriers, which may be used as a summary of general considerations.

SEALANT APPLICATION

Although manufacturers' products differ, the basic steps in sealant application are similar. It is essential to note that the quality of the end product is determined to a great extent by the clinician's attention to (1) strict clinical dryness, (2) accurate timing for conditioning and rinsing, (3) fresh sealant material, and (4) adherence to recommended setting (polymerization) procedures.

Application technique

1. Prepare the tooth surface, cleaning it of hard and soft deposits. Using a bristle brush, polish the surface with pumice and water. Use of a polishing paste with fluoride or a fluoride treatment before sealant application is contraindicated, since the fluoride interferes with the etching/conditioning technique (Silverstone, 1978). Rinse the teeth thoroughly with water.
2. Isolate the teeth with cotton rolls held in place by the Garmer clamp or with an absorbent paper triangle such as Dri-Angles (Dental Health Products, Inc, Youngstown, NY) in conjunction with cotton rolls (Figs. 22-6 and 22-7). It is extremely important to keep the working area dry. The rubber dam procedure may be used when the sealant is to be applied to several teeth in the quadrant; however, satisfac-

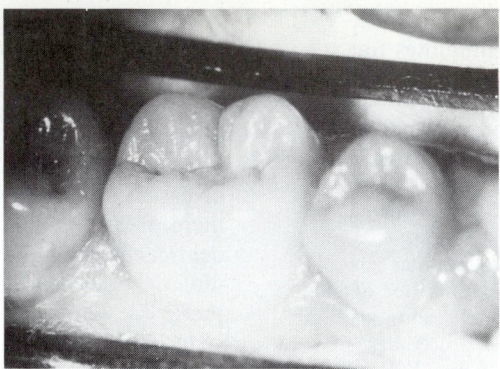

Fig. 22-6. Teeth are isolated with Garmer clamp and cotton rolls.
(Courtesy LD Caulk Co., Milford, Del.)

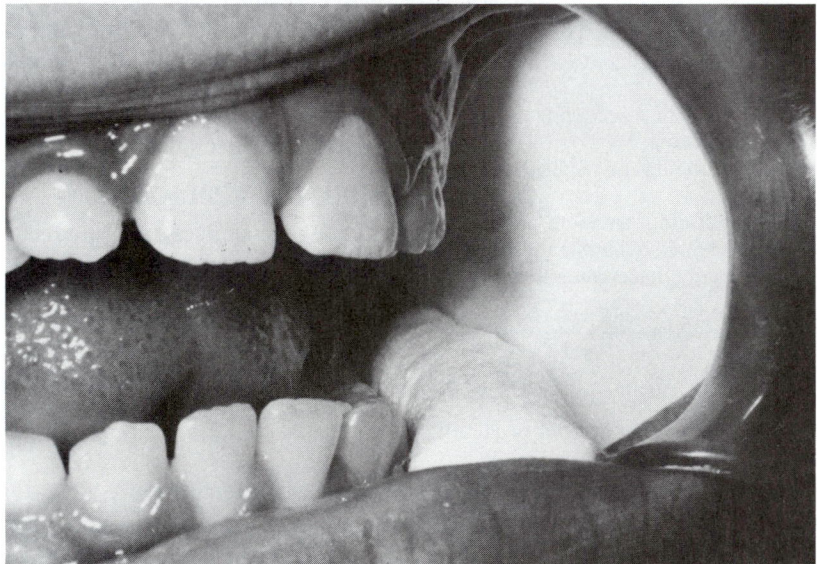

Fig. 22-7. Dri-Angle placed over Stensen's duct for moisture control.

tory results can be obtained with frequent changing of cotton rolls and Dri-Angles. A study comparing rubber dam versus cotton roll isolation found the average 6-month retention rate was 95% regardless with both methods of isolation (Straffon et al, 1985). Another study compared the Vac-Ejector (Whaledent International, New York, NY) (consisting of a bite-block and rubber tongue shield that connect to the high-speed evacuation line) to cotton-roll and Dri-Angle isolation; again, there was no difference in retention rates between the two methods of isolation (Wood, Saravia, Farrington, 1989). Once the teeth are isolated, dry the area with clean, dry compressed air (Fig. 22-8). Maintain suction during the procedure to assist in moisture control.

3. Apply the conditioner for the enamel-etching process following the manufacturer's directions for acid concentration and conditioning time. A brush for painting the conditioner on the occlusal surface is recommended, although

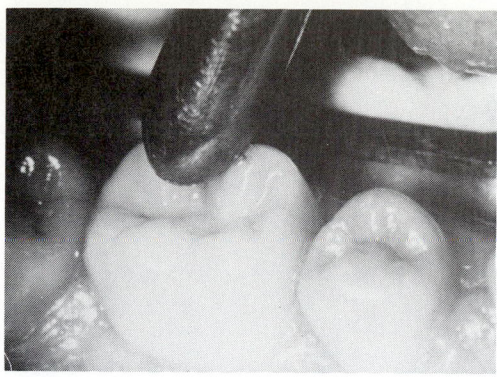

Fig. 22-8. Teeth are dried with compressed air.
(Courtesy LD Caulk Co., Milford, Del.)

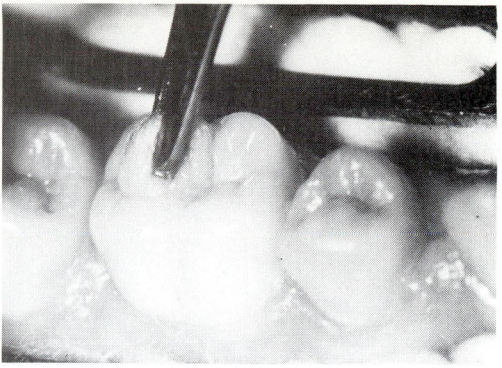

Fig. 22-9. Conditioner is applied according to manufacturer's directions.
(Courtesy LD Caulk Co., Milford, Del.)

a cotton pellet can be used (Fig. 22-9). Fine brushes are more accurate in placing the acid than cotton pellets, since the latter may absorb too much of the solution or cause air to be trapped in the fissure (Silverstone, 1983).

4. After the appropriate conditioning time (usually 60 seconds), rinse the area with water to thoroughly remove the conditioning solution. Suction all remaining fluid. Immediately dry the teeth, taking care not to let saliva come into contact with the conditioned surface, as this interferes with the bonding of the sealant. *This is the most critical period in the sealant application.* Study results show that after an exposure of saliva of 1 second or greater, a tenacious surface coating, which cannot be removed by washing, forms on the etched enamel surface (Fig. 22-10) (Silverstone, 1987). This exposure to saliva may require a 10-second re-etching. Inspect the teeth for a dull, chalky surface (Spohn and Berry, 1979) (Fig. 22-11). If the entire surface to be sealed does not appear chalky or if the teeth have been contaminated with saliva, repeat the conditioning procedure for 10 seconds.

5. Apply the sealant by brushing the liquid on the conditioned tooth surface (Fig. 22-12). Concentrate the sealant in the central pits and fissures (Fig. 22-13) and include the cuspal planes (Fig. 22-14). Remember to include the lingual grooves and buccal pits. Trace the fissures with an explorer to enable air bubbles to rise and the sealant to penetrate.

Sealants with a high coefficient of penetra-

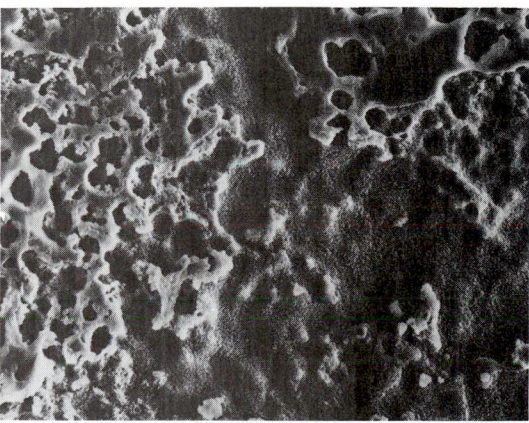

Fig. 22-10. Scanning electron micrograph showing human enamel that was etched for 60 seconds, then contaminated with human saliva for 5 seconds. Shown after rinse with water, the etched surface is completely obscured. Magnification × 1000.
(Courtesy LM Silverstone, Aurora, Colo.)

tion (low viscosity) appear to penetrate the fissures by capillary action, reducing the likelihood of air entrapment. As the viscosity of the material increases, so may the entrapment of air (Powell and Craig, 1978). It is especially difficult to obtain even coverage on maxillary molars because the sealant tends to flow from the mesial to the distal because of patient positioning. Take care not to apply excess of sealant or to let the sealant flow into the contact area.

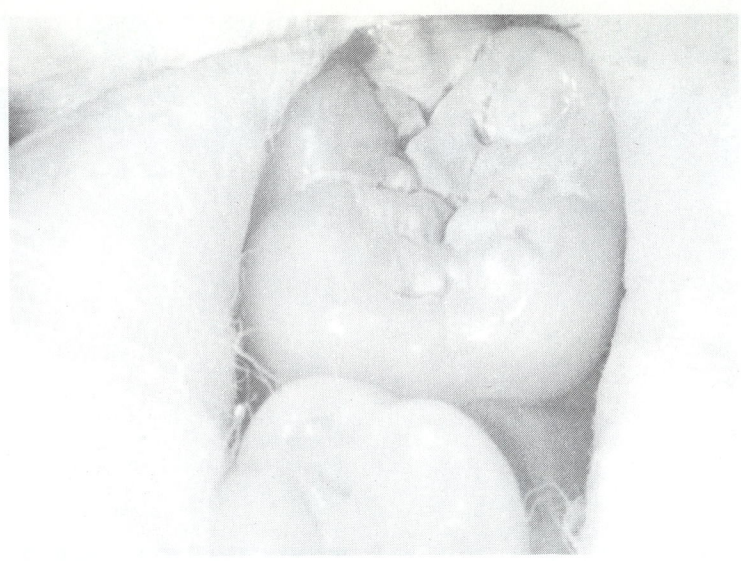

Fig. 22-11. Conditioner is rinsed off, and teeth are dried. Note dull, chalky appearance.
(From Spohn EE, Berry TG: *Pit and fissure sealants.* In Boundy SS, Reynolds NJ, editors: *Current concepts in dental hygiene,* vol 2. St Louis, 1979, CV Mosby.)

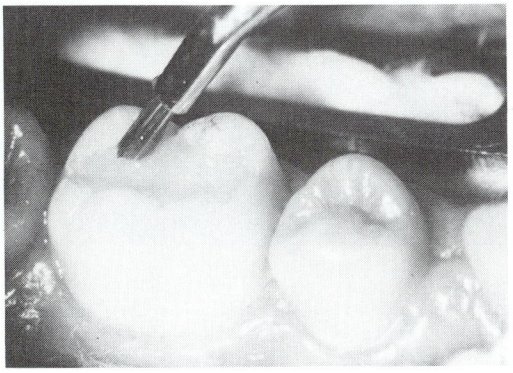

Fig. 22-12. Sealant is brushed on conditioned surface.
(Courtesy LD Caulk Co., Milford, Del.)

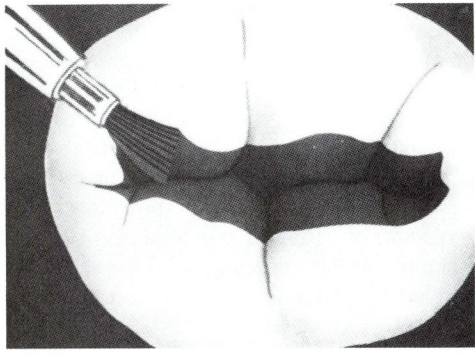

Fig. 22-13. Sealant is concentrated in central pits and fissures.
(Courtesy LD Caulk Co., Milford Del.)

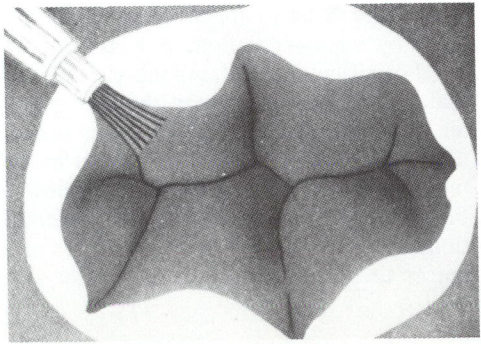

Fig. 22-14. Inclined planes of cusps are covered to complete coverage of occlusal surface.
(Courtesy LD Caulk Co., Milford, Del.)

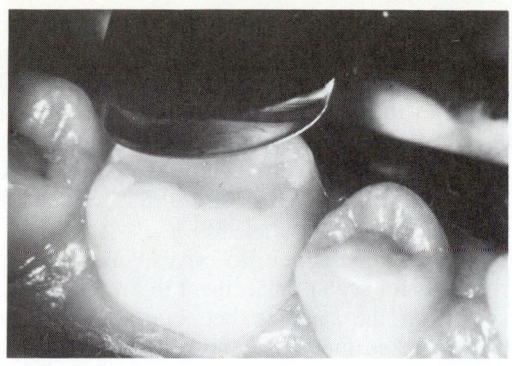

Fig. 22-15. Liquid sealant is polymerized with curing light according to manufacturer's directions.
(Courtesy LD Caulk Co., Milford, Del.)

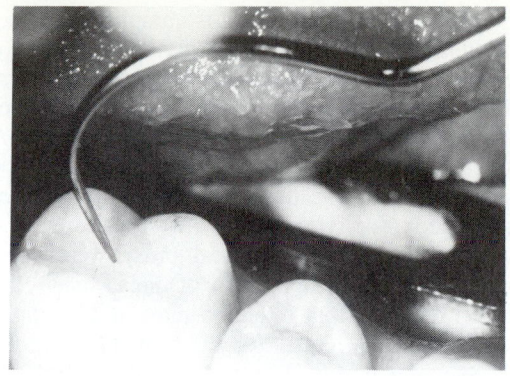

Fig. 22-16. Surface is evaluated with an explorer to check total coverage.
(Courtesy LD Caulk Co., Milford, Del.)

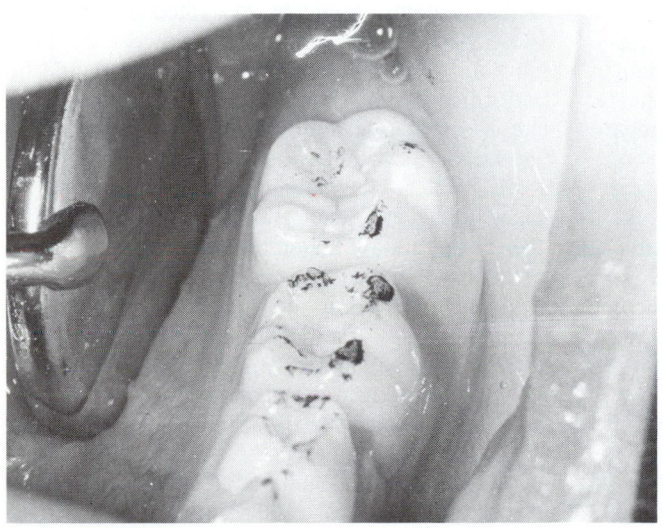

Fig. 22-17. Occlusal relationship is checked. In this case minimal occlusal contact occurs on sealant.
(From Spohn EE, Berry TG: Pit and fissure sealants. In Boundy SS, Reynolds NJ, editors: *Current concepts in dental hygiene,* vol 2, St Louis, 1979, CV Mosby.)

6. If polymerization is to occur chemically, follow the manufacturer's directions for the appropriate period of time (usually 1 minute). If ultraviolet light or visible light is needed for polymerization, follow directions for placement of the light wand and for correct exposure time. Current ultraviolet light sources vary in their output and become less effective over time because of deposits that accumulate on them (Silverstone, 1983). Maintain the light source according to the manufacturer's specifications (Fig. 22-15) and observe the recommended warm-up time (2 to 5 minutes). You can determine the efficiency of the light source by testing a drop of sealant on a glass slab with a 20-second exposure (Craig, O'Brien, Powers, 1983).

7. After polymerization occurs, rinse with water and wipe the occlusal surface. A small cotton pellet can be used to remove sealant that has failed to polymerize. Evaluate the surface carefully with a probe or an explorer to ensure that a smooth, hard surface has been achieved (Fig. 22-16). Check for incomplete coverage and voids. Repeat the entire procedure in areas with voids or incomplete coverage.

8. Check the occlusal relationship with articulating paper (Fig. 22-17). Using floss, make certain that the contact areas are free of sealant.

9. A fluoride treatment may be given after the

entire sealant application is complete.

Alternative methods for preparing the teeth for sealants have been suggested by several authors. (Shapira and Eidelman, 1986; Gerke, 1987; De-Craene et al, 1988; and DeCraene et al, 1989). A pre-etch prophylaxis of the tooth surface to be sealed has been questioned. The retention rates of pre-etched prophylaxis of tooth surfaces with a slurry of pumice and conical brush were compared with no prophylaxis. Donnan and Ball (1988) reported that retention rates at 12 months were essentially equal for the unpumiced group (97.3%) and pumiced groups (96.6%). Mechanical preparation of the tooth has also been investigated. In a study where a #1 round steel burr was run at low speed over the fissure to remove plaque, organic debris, and surface enamel, the retention rate of the sealant was 88%, compared with 65% for the control group, after 6 years (Shapira and Eidleman, 1986). This technique not only removes tooth structure but would, in many states, prohibit the dental hygienist from preparing the tooth for sealant placement. Moreover, other tooth preparation alternatives appear to result in retention rates that are as high or higher.

Some operators advocate going a step further, by using a dentin bonding agent after opening the fissure with a burr. In some fissures, the enamel may be so thin that preparation of the tooth, even scraping with an explorer, may expose parts of the dentin. A very conservative composite restoration, or a glass ionomer cement, could be placed and then the entire surface sealed. The restoration bonds with the cavity wall, resulting in minimal leakage (Henderson, 1985; Simonsen, 1987). Houpt and others (1985) studied the concept of sealing rather than cavity extension for prevention. After 4 years, 156 of 205 occlusal composite restorations showed complete retention of the sealant. Caries appeared in only 13 teeth. Conservative cavity preparation with sealant is successful and preserves valuable tooth structure.

Retention rates have been investigated using less than the standard 60-second etching time. (Fuks et al, 1984; Eidelman et al, 1985; Chosak, 1987; Eidelman et al, 1988). Eidelman, Shapira, and Houpt (1988) reported 91% retention after 3 years with a 20-second etch.

Several studies have investigated the use of the air-powder polisher to prepare teeth for sealants. When this device was used to clean the tooth surface, the bond strength of the sealant to the enamel was greater than with the traditional method—flour of pumice and rubber cup or brush attachment. This greater bond strength can be attributed to the increased wetting surface that results from better cleansing of the enamel micropores (Brockman, Scott, and Eick, 1989, 1990; Garcia-Godoy and Medlock, 1988; Scott and Greer, 1987; Scott et al, 1988).

Researchers continue to investigate efficient techniques for sealant placement that will produce results with the same or better efficacy as currently accepted methods. The results of more invasive preparation techniques are also being studied, but further consensus must be reached before new application recommendations are made.

Follow-up evaluation

Dental sealants should be evaluated periodically. Close visual examination to assess wear, air bubble voids, and partial or complete loss should be performed every 6 months. In many cases if the site was contaminated during placement, the sealant will be lost within 6 to 12 months. When clinically indicated, bitewing radiographs may be taken to determine the tooth's status underneath the sealant and on the proximal surfaces. The failure rate of sealants ranges from 5% to 10% the first year (Mertz-Fairhurst et al, 1984). During a 36-month study, 31% of the treated teeth required at least one retreatment (Straffon et al, 1985).

Like other resin-based materials, dental sealants exhibit wear (Conry, Pintados and Douglas, 1990; Pintado, Conry, and Douglas, 1991). Wear or abrasion of this unfilled resin is a desirable characteristic that can reduce the need for occlusal adjustment when the tooth is slightly overfilled. However, wear may be caused by factors other than normal mastication. The use of the air-powder polisher on dental sealants has been reported to cause wear (Huennekens, Daniel, and Bayne, 1991). Wear was evident after repeated applications of the air-powder polisher to simulate several recall appointments. Although the sealant could not be detected visually or with an explorer, when the teeth were cross-sectioned, sealant remained at the bottom of the fissure. Therefore some protection may exist in teeth even when the sealant cannot be detected clinically.

Assessment of sealants can be complicated. Sealant products differ in appearance, and the patient may have more than one type of sealant placed. Tinted sealants may be easier to examine visually than clear ones. The clinician should review the patient's record and complete a careful visual and explorer examination of all teeth. A decision about the status of each tooth containing sealant should be made and recorded.

Criteria to determine adequate placement and the need for replacement are helpful in the evaluation of sealants. One investigation attempted to identify the evaluation instrument that would provide the highest level of reliability for examiners. Global, checklist, and criterion-referenced instruments were compared. Experienced and inexperienced examiners both achieved a higher reliability when written criteria were used for evaluation (Daniel and Scruggs, 1987). A sample evaluation instrument is found in the following box.

Sealant evaluation form—criterion referenced

Examiner _____Tooth #___
Coverage: Area
___ Sealant covers all occlusal, lingual, and/or buccal pits, fissures, or grooves onto the inclined planes
___ Sealant coverage excludes one pit, fissure, or groove
___ Two or more pits, fissures, or grooves are uncovered
___ Sealant is not apparent on any pits, fissures, or grooves
Coverage: Quantity
___ Sealant is sufficient for all areas covered
___ Sealant is overfilled; appears too bulky
___ Sealant is underfilled; needs more bulk
___ Sealant is not apparent on any pits, fissures, or grooves
Porosity
___ Sealant contains no voids or other defects
___ Sealant contains more than one void or defect
___ Sealant is not apparent on any pits, fissures, or grooves
Retention
___ Entire sealant cannot be removed with the explorer
___ Part of the sealant is removed with the explorer
___ All of the sealant is removed with the explorer
___ Sealant is not apparent on any pits, fissures, or grooves
___ Total points   Comments:

From Daniel ST, Scruggs RR: *J Dent Educ* 51:4, 1987.

Using established criteria will provide some standardization in the way you evaluate your patients' sealants. Make notations in the record about the condition of the sealants at each visit, because this information will assist you in determining the need for sealant replacement.

Replacement procedure

When a sealant is identified as defective and in need of replacement, the tooth should be prepared by cleaning the surfaces as described in the application section, step 1.

Following this, the sealant surface should be roughened up a bit with an explorer or small burr. This prepares the surface for the acid-etching process. Proceed with the customary application steps according to the manufacturer's instructions.

TRENDS IN SEALANT USE

Acceptance of the use of dental sealants in the general practice of dentistry has been slow. A 1985 National Health Interview Survey revealed that whereas the public is generally aware of the importance of a number of factors in the prevention of tooth decay, only 18% had heard of and knew the purpose of dental sealants (Corbin, 1987). It is possible that such a good educational campaign has been done with fluorides and oral hygiene that patients do not understand the added value of sealants for the prevention of occlusal decay (Gift and Frew, 1986).

Sealant usage has increased since 1983, when a Consensus Development Conference of the National Institutes of Health focused on dental sealants in the prevention of decay. In 1983 a survey of hygienists practicing in Minnesota and Wisconsin indicated that sealants were being used in only 54% of the offices in which they worked (Duffy et al, 1986). More recent studies showed that between 70% and 95% of general dentists used sealants to some degree (Bander, 1986; Faine and Dennen, 1986; Rubenstein and Dinius, 1986; Gonzalez et al, 1991). Bander noted that younger dentists who practice with hygienists tend to use sealants more. Possible influences on sealant use include recent exposure to sealants during professional school, the fact that younger dentists tend to have younger patients who may require the service more often, and the fact that the procedure is often performed by hygienists. Rubenstein and Dinius (1986) found that 97% of pediatric dentists in Virginia apply pit and fissure sealants.

The consensus panel recommended that certain populations, including low-income, immigrant, disabled, and institutionalized children, have an urgent need for preventive measures including sealants (National Institutes of Health, 1984). Several community-based sealant programs have published results that support the benefits of sealants. In Iowa, a study found that for low-socio-economic-status children, who display more episodic than regular preventive dental care behavior, sealants were more important than the usual prophylaxis-fluoride regimen (Jones, 1986).

A school-based study in New Mexico compared children who received sealants on their first permanent molars with classmates who did not. After 6 years the sealed group had developed 6% occlusal decayed, missing, or filled teeth, compared with 27% in the unsealed group (Calderone and Davis, 1987).

A Head Start program in Tennessee found that sealants are retained in primary molars after 1 year at a rate comparable to that in permanent molars. The program involved 3- to 4-year-olds and suggests the potential benefits of a sealant program with children who are highly susceptible to caries (Hardison et al, 1987).

After 7 years of a fluoride mouthrinsing program in an elementary school, a 50% reduction in tooth decay was noted. The majority of carious surfaces involved pits and fissures. The investigator followed this study by combining sealants with the mouthrinsing program. After 2 years, the children remained 96% caries free (Ripa, 1985, 1987).

Another school-based program used a fluoride mouthrinse for 10 years and added a sealant program in the eighth year. The researchers reported an additional decrease in decayed, missing, and filled surfaces (DMFS) per child in the two years of sealant use (Sterritt and Frew, 1988; Sterritt et al, 1990).

Success with pit and fissure sealants is well documented, but other issues are related to the low use of sealant techniques. (Romberg et al, 1988; Mitchell and Murray, 1989). Concern over cost-effectiveness and the reluctance of insurance providers to cover sealants has had an effect. Other factors reported to be responsible for low sealant use have included state practice acts and the attitudes of dentists. Now that most state practice acts define sealants as a function of dental hygienists, this should no longer be a factor. As for the attitude of the dentist/employer, several studies have found a relationship between sealant use and the dentist's presentation of sealants as a preventive measure to the patient. When information about sealants and the need for them was presented to the patient, acceptance and placement followed (Cohen and Sheiham, 1988a and b).

A study of costs by Ripa (1985) found that, assuming the cost of a single surface restoration to be twice the cost of a sealant, treating the unsealed group was 1.64 times more expensive than treating the sealed group.

Eklund (1986b) studied a variety of factors to assess the costs to an insurer of amalgam restorations versus sealants. Cost is tied to the level of dental caries in a population. If the potential caries rate is low, the cost of a preventive procedure is less likely to represent a true savings in the long run. Sealants as a covered benefit for molars may not increase insurance premiums if fees and copayments are properly balanced. A substantial decline in caries prevalence could diminish the economic argument for sealants.

Cost-effectiveness can be related to the level of education and scope of practice of the operator. Dental hygienists can place sealants while permitting the dentist to provide other patient services. This can affect income generated in the private setting or reduce the cost of care in community and public health settings. The dental hygiene appointment provides an opportunity to check sealant status, making follow-up and reapplication a logical part of the hygienist's routine. In many cases, the dentist's willingness to delegate this function and the hygienist's desire to provide the service have determined how often sealants are used in practice. Most hygienists have received instruction about sealant application either during training or through approved continuing education courses. The longterm effects of a 1-day course show significant increases in the number of clinicians applying sealants and in the frequency of application (Tilliss, 1986).

Sealant usage has been related to the type of dental supervision required by state practice acts. A state sealant program in New Mexico focused attention on the hygienist's role, eventually bringing revision of the practice act to allow general supervision of hygienists (Siegal and Calderone, 1986).

The issue of cost will continue to be debated. Several state Medicaid programs now offer sealants as a covered benefit, and this trend will undoubtedly grow. For many years, patients have been willing to pay for sealants regardless of insurance coverage because they desire comprehensive preventive dental care for themselves and their children.

The dental profession must be more actively involved in educating the public about sealants: their effectiveness, safety, and the rationale for their use. Encouraging adoption of guidelines for third-party payers in all states and seeking support for federally funded programs are worthwhile activities to increase the public's access to sealants. Educating patients within the practice has also been found to be a factor in the use of sealants, with Lang, Weintraub, and Choi (1988) reporting that most patients learn about sealants from their dentist, not from the media.

Sealant techniques and materials are part of the era of conservative restorations and caries prevention. Continued research, the development of new products, and increased use of these methods will ensure that sealants make an important contribution in the practice of dentistry. Given the content presented in this chapter, you can have an influence on your dentist/employer and patients in regard to the use of sealants in your practice.

ACTIVITIES

1. Practice sealant technique on a typodont or on extracted teeth using various manufacturer's products.
2. Practice techniques for isolation with Garmer clamp with cotton rolls and Dri-Angles with cotton rolls.
3. Practice a four-handed technique for sealant application.
4. Identify an appropriate patient and apply a pit and fissure sealant.
5. Put together an informative brochure or poster about sealants for the patient waiting area.
6. Role-play, with a peer, the presentation of dental sealants as a preventive measure against caries and the need for this preventive agent.

REVIEW QUESTIONS

1. Describe the acid-etching process. What is the significance of this step in the sealant technique?
2. How might the following list of factors be considered in determining whether the sealant application is appropriate for this particular patient?

   Patient age: 12 years old.

   New resident; moved from nonfluoridated area.

   Teeth Nos. 3, 14, 19 and 30 restored.

   Teeth Nos. 18 and 31 erupted recently.

   No current radiographic evidence of interproximal caries.

   Home care and plaque control are good.

   Parents concerned about diet and regular dental care.
3. List the steps to be followed in the sealant application procedure.
4. Sealants have been adopted slowly by dentistry over the past 20 years despite documentation regarding their success as a safe preventive measure. List possible reasons for the slow adoption of sealants.

REFERENCES

Acuna V et al: In vitro fluoride uptake by enamel and dentin—a comparative study of two varnishes, *Acta Ondontol Scand* 48:89, 1990.

Ball IA: An update on fissure sealants. I, *Dent Update* 13:380, 1986a.

Ball IA: An update on sealants. II, *Dent Update* 13:419, 1986b.

Bander VM: Dentist use patterns for pit and fissure sealants and topical fluorides, *J Dent Educ* 50:656, 1986.

Brockman SL, Scott RL, Eick JD: The effect of an airpolishing device on tensile bond strength of a dental sealant, *Quintessence Int* 20:211, 1989.

Brockman SL, Scott RL, Eick JD: A scanning electron microscopic study of the effect of air polishing on the enamel-sealant surface, *Quintessence Int* 21:201, 1990.

Buonocore MG: Caries prevention in pits and fissures sealed with an adhesive resin polymerized by ultra-violet light: a two-year study of a single application, *JADA* 82:1090, 1971.

Buonocore MG: *The use of adhesives in dentistry,* Springfield, Ill, 1975, Charles C Thomas.

Calderone JJ, Davis JM: The New Mexico sealant program: a progress report, *J Public Health Dent* 47:145, 1987.

Chosack A: The parameters influencing time of application of fissure sealants, *Clin Prev Dent* 9:17, 1987.

Cohen L, Sheiham A: The use of pit and fissure sealants in the General Dental Service in Great Britain and Northern Ireland, *Br Dent J* 165:50, 1988a.

Conry JP, Pintado MR, Douglas WH: Quantitative changes in fissure sealant six months after placement, *Pediatr Dent* 12:162, 1990.

Corbin SB: 1985 NHIS findings on public knowledge about oral diseases and preventive measures, *Public Health Rep* 102:53, 1987.

Council on Dental Health and Health Planning and the Council on Dental Materials, Instruments, and Equipment: Pit and fissure sealants, *JADA* 114:671, 1987.

Council on Dental Materials, Instruments, and Equipment: Personal communication, January 1992.

Craig RG, O'Brien WJ, Powers JM: *Dental materials: properties and manipulation,* ed 3, St Louis, 1983, CV Mosby.

Daniel SJ, Scruggs RR: The reliability of three methods for evaluating dental sealants, *J Dent Educ* 51:182, 1987.

DeCraene GP, Martens C, Dermaut R: The invasive pit and fissure sealing technique in pediatric dentistry: an SEM study of a preventive restoration, *J Dent Child* 55:34, 1988.

DeCraene GP et al: A clinical evaluation of a light-cured fissure sealant (Helioseal), *J Dent Child* 56:97, 1989.

Dennison JB et al: A clinical comparison of sealant and amalgam in the treatment of pit and fissures. I: Clinical performance after 18 months, *Pediatr Dent* 2:167, 1980b.

Dennison JB et al: A clinical comparison of sealant and amalgam in the treatment of pits and fissures. II: Clinical application and maintenance during an 18-month period, *Pediatr Dent* 2:176, 1980a.

DiLeone CM: Dental sealants: information and guidelines for insurance carriers, *Dent Hyg* 61:18, 1987.

Disney JA et al: The University of North Carolina Caries Risk Assessment Study: further developments in caries risk prediction, *Community Dent Oral Epidemiol* 20:64, 1992.

Donnan MF, Ball IA: A double-blind clinical trial to determine the importance of pumice prophylaxis on fissure sealant retention, *Br Dent J* 165:283, 1988.

Dorignac GF: Efficacy of highly filled composites in the caries prevention of pits and fissures: two and one-half years of clinical results, *J Pedodont* 11:139, 1987.

Duffy MB et al: Dental hygienists' knowledge, opinions, and use of pit and fissure sealants: a comparison of two states, *J Public Health Dent* 47:121, 1986.

Duggan G, Midda M: Clinical trial of a new fissure sealant, *J Int Assoc Dent Child* 18:17, 1987.

Eidelman E et al: Fissure sealant impression after 20 and 60 seconds etching: a SEM study, *J Dent Res* 64 (special issue): 147, 1985.

Eidelman E, Shapira J, Houpt M: The retention of fissure sealants using twenty-second etching time: three-year follow-up, *J Dent Child* 55:219, 1988.

Eklund SA: Factors affecting the cost of fissure sealants: a dental insurer's perspective, *J Public Health Dent* 46:133, 1986.

Eklund SA, Ismail AI: Time development of occlusal and proximal lesions: implications for fissure sealants, *J Public Health Dent* 46:114, 1986.

Faine RC, Dennen T: A survey of private dental practitioner's utilization of dental sealants in Washington state, *J Dent Child* 53:337, 1986.

Fuks AB, Grajower R, Shapira J: In vitro assessment of marginal leakage of sealants placed in permanent molars with different etching times, *J Dent Child* 51:425, 1984.

Garcia-Godoy F, Medlock JW: An SEM study of the effects of air-polishing on fissure surfaces, *Quintessence Int* 19:465, 1988.

Gerke DC: Modified enameloplasty-fissure sealant technique using an acid-etch resin method, *Quintessence Int* 18:387, 1987.

Gift HC, Frew RA: Sealants: changing patterns, *JADA* 112:391, 1986.

Going RE et al: Four year clinical evaluation of a pit and fissure sealant, *JADA* 95:972, 1977.

Going RE: The viability of microorganisms in carious lesions five years after covering with a fissure sealant, *JADA* 97:455, 1978.

Gonzalez CD, Frazier PJ, Messer LB: Sealant use by general practitioners: a Minnesota survey, *J Dent Child* 58:38, 1991.

Gwinnett AJ: The bonding of sealants to enamel, *J Am Soc Prev Dent* 3:21, 1973.

Handelman SL: Effect of sealant placement on occlusal caries progression, *Clin Prev Dent* 4:11, 1983.

Handelman SL: Clinical radiographic evaluation of sealed carious and sound tooth surfaces, *JADA* 113:751, 1987a.

Handelman SL: Retention of sealants over carious and sound tooth surfaces, *Community Dent Oral Epidemiol* 15:1, 1987b.

Hardison JR et al: Retention of pit and fissure sealant on the primary molars of 3-4 year old children after one year, *JADA* 114:613, 1987.

Henderson HZ: The sealed composite resin restoration, *J Dent Child* 52:300, 1985.

Horowitz HS, Heifetz, Powlsen et al: Retention and effectiveness of a single application of an adhesive sealant in preventing occlusal caries: final report after 5 years study in Kalispell, Montana, *JADA* 95:1133, 1977.

Hicks MJ, Glaitz CM, Call RJ: Comparison of pit and fissure sealant utilization by pediatric and general dentists in Colorado, *J Pedodont* 14:97, 1990.

Houpt M et al: Occlusal composite restorations: 4-year results, *JADA* 110:351, 1985.

Houpt M et al: Autopolymerized versus light-polymerized fissure sealant, *JADA* 115:55, 1987.

Huennekens SC, Daniel SJ, Bayne SC: Effects of air polishing on the abrasion of occlusal sealants, *Quintessence Int* 22:581,1991.

Johnston AD, Bowen RL: Protective coatings for tooth crowns, *JADA* 122:49, 1991.

Jones RB: The effects for recall patients of a comprehensive sealant program in a clinical dental public health setting, *J Public Health Dent* 46:152, 1986.

Lang WP, Weintraub JA, Choi C: Fissure sealant knowledge and characteristics of parents as a function of their child's sealant status, *J Public Health Dent* 48:133, 1988.

McKenna EF, Grundy GE: Glass ionomer cement fissure sealants applied by operative dental auxiliaries—retention rate after one year, *Aust Dent J* 32:200, 1987.

Mertz-Fairhurst EJ et al: Clinical progress of sealed and unsealed caries. I. Depth changes and bacterial counts *J Prosthet Dent* 42:633, 1979a.

Mertz-Fairhurst EJ et al: Clinical progress of unsealed caries. II. Standardized radiographs and clinical observation, *J Prosthet Dent* 42:633, 1979b.

Mertz-Fairhurst EJ et al: Current status of sealant retention and caries prevention, *J Dent Educ* 48(supp):18, 1984.

Mertz-Fairhurst EJ et al: A comparative study of two pit and fissure sealants: six-year results in Augusta, GA, *GADA* 105:237, 1982.

Mertz-Fairhurst EJ et al: Arresting caries by sealant: results of a clinical study, *JADA* 112:194, 1986.

Mitchell L, Murray JJ: Fissure sealants: a critique of their cost-effectiveness, *Community Dent Oral Epidemiol* 17:19, 1989.

National Institutes of Health: Consensus development conference on dental sealants and the prevention of tooth decay, *JADA* 108:233, 1984.

Niendorff W: Findings from the oral health survey, *Indian Health Service Dent Newsl* 26: 47, 1985.

Powell KR, Craig GG: An in vitro investigation of the penetrating efficiency of BIS-GMA resin pit and fissure coatings, *J Dent Res* 57:691, 1978.

Pintado MR, Conry JP, Douglas WH: Fissure sealant wear at 30 months: new evaluation criteria, *J Dent* 19:33, 1991.

Raadal M et al: Evaluation of a routine for prevention and treatment of fissure caries in permanent first molars, *Community Dent Oral Epidemiol* 18:70, 1990.

Ranalli DN et al: Toxicity testing of sealants: a tissue implant study, *J Pedodont* 13:270, 1989.

Ripa LW: Occlusal sealing: rationale of the technique and historical review, *J Am Soc Prev Dent* 3:32, 1973.

Ripa LW: The surface-specific caries pattern of participants in a school based fluoride mouthrinsing program with implications for the use of sealants, *J Public Health Dent* 45:90, 1985.

Ripa LW: Caries prevention in children: the use of fluoride mouthrinses and pit and fissure sealants, *NY State Dent J* 53:16, 1987.

Romberg E, Cohen LA, LaBelle AD: Importance of variables associated with practitioners' estimates of pit and fissure sealant, *J Public Health Dent* 48:138, 1988.

Rubenstein LK, Dinius A: Dental sealant usage in Virginia, *J Public Health Dent* 46:147, 1986.

Scott L, Greer D: The effect of an air polishing device on sealant bond strength, *J Prosthet Dent* 58:384, 1987.

Scott L et al: Retention of dental sealants following the use of airpolishing and traditional cleaning, *Dent Hyg* 62:402, 1988.

Shapira J, Eidelman E: Six-year clinical evaluation of fissure sealant placed after mechanical preparation: a matched pair study, *Pediatr Dent* 8:204, 1986.

Siegal MD, Calderone JJ: Controversy over the supervision of dental hygienists: impact on a community-based sealant program, *J Public Health Dent* 46:156, 1986.

Silverstone LM: *Preventive dentistry,* Fort Lee, NJ, 1978, Update Publishing International.

Silverstone LM: The current status of adhesive sealants, *Dent Hyg* 57:44, 1983.

Silverstone LM: The current state of sealant research, *J Mass Dent Soc* 36:15, 1987.

Simonsen RJ: Retention and effectiveness of a single application of white sealant after 10 years, *JADA* 115:31, 1987.

Spohn E, Berry T: Pit and fissure sealants. In Boundy SS, Reynolds NJ, editors: *Current concepts in dental hygiene,* vol 2, St Louis, 1979, CV Mosby.

Stamm JW et al.: The University of North Carolina Caries Risk Assessment Study. I. Rationale and content, *J Public Health Dent* 48:225, 1988.

Stamm JW et al: The University of North Carolina Caries Risk Assessment Study. II. Baseline caries prevalence, *J Public Health Dent* 50:178, 1990.

Sterritt GR, Frew RA: Evaluation of a clinic-based sealant program, *J Public Health Dent* 48:220, 1988.

Sterritt GR et al: Evaluation of a school-based fluoride mouthrinsing and clinic-based sealant program on a non-fluoridated island, *Community Dent Oral Epidemiol* 18:288, 1990.

Straffon LH et al: Three year evaluation of sealant: effect of isolation on efficacy, *JADA* 110:714, 1985.

Strang R et al: Further abrasion resistance and bond strength studies of fissure sealants, *J Oral Rehabil* 13:257, 1986a.

Strang R et al: Laboratory studies of visible-light cured fissure sealants: setting times and depth of polymerization, *J Oral Rehabil* 13:305, 1986b.

Tanaka M et al: Incorporation into human enamel of fluoride slowly released from a sealant in vivo, *J Dent Res* 66:1591, 1987.

Tilliss TS: Application of pit and fissure sealant: long-term effects of a one-day continuing education course, *Dent Hyg* 60:300, 1986.

Torppa-Saarinen E, Seppa L: Short-term retention of glass ionomer fissure sealants, *Proc Finn Dent Soc,* 86:83, 1990.

U.S. Department of Health and Human Services, Public Health Service, Indian Health Service: *Oral health program guide for the Indian Health Service. Section II. Dental disease prevention and health promotion, 1991.* Rockville, Md, HHS, US Government.

Walter RG: A longitudinal study of caries development in initially caries-free naval recruits, *J Dent Res* 61:1405, 1982.

Whyte RJ, Leake JL, Howley TP: Two-year follow-up of 11,000 dental sealants in first permanent molars in the Saskatchewan health dental plan, *J Public Health Dent* 47:177, 1987.

Wood AJ, Saravia ME, Farrington FH: Cotton roll isolation vs Vac-Ejector isolation, *ASDC J Dent Child* 56:438, 1989.

SUGGESTED READINGS

Chapko MK: A study of the intentional use of pit and fissure sealants over carious lesions, *J Public Health Dent* 47:130, 1987.

Cohen LD: Pit and fissure sealants – an underutilized preventive technology, *Int J Technol Assess Health Care* 6:378, 1990.

Corbin SB et al: Patterns of sealant delivery under variable third party requirements, 50:311, 1990.

Curro FA, Levi M: Extending sealant therapy to the adult population, *NY State Dent J* 53:32, 1987.

Faine RC: The use of dental sealants in the Washington state medical assistance program: a one-year report, *J Dent Child* 54:451, 1987.

Garcia-Godoy F, Gwinnett AJ: An SEM study of fissure surfaces conditioned with a scraping technique, *Clini Prev Dent* 9:9,1987.

Hosoya Y, Goto G: The effects of cleaning, polishing pretreatments and acid etching times on unground primary enamel, *J Pedodont* 14:84, 1990.

Kuthy RA, Ashton JJ: Eruption pattern of permanent molars: implications for school-based dental sealant programs, *J Public Health Dent* 49:7, 1989.

Martens LV, Glasrud PH, Gambucci JR: Changes in sealant use by general practitioners in private practice, *Quintessence Int* 18:53, 1987.

Rock WP et al: A comparative study between a chemically polymerized fissure sealant resin and a light-cured resin, *Br Dent J* 152:232, 1982.

Simonsen RJ: Potential uses of pit and fissure sealant in innovative ways: a review, *J Public Health Dent* 42:305, 1982.

CARE OF REMOVABLE APPLIANCES

Judith C. Berry

LEARNING OUTCOMES

The dental hygienist will be able to

1. List several types of removable appliances and their uses.
2. State a rationale for cleaning dental appliances.
3. Describe the advantages and disadvantages of different cleansing agents and methods of cleansing removable appliances.
4. Discuss important considerations in the care of soft tissues and abutment teeth and/or implant fixtures of patients with removable appliances.
5. Describe an aseptic technique for professional ultrasonic cleaning of removable appliances.
6. State the reasons for denture identification.
7. Describe and compare three basic methods for marking dentures.
8. Discuss the importance of mouth protectors for prevention of oral injuries.
9. Compare the advantages and disadvantages of the three types of mouth protectors discussed.

Although the number of edentulous individuals is declining, there are still nearly 20 million of them in the United States. More than 90% of these people have some form of prosthodontic replacement, and an estimated one third of them need replacement or refitting of their existing dentures. Despite this need, a study done in 1985 by the National Institutes of Health reported that more than half of edentulous people had not visited a dentist in the past 3 years. A number of attitudinal, financial, and other barriers may be implicated in this failure to use dental services (Lebel, 1989). Many people may not be aware of the importance of regular dental care for evaluating soft tissues for disease, for examining existing dental appliances for fit and function, and for preventive education. You can fulfill an important role by informing patients of the importance of oral examinations and preventive and corrective services. You should educate patients regarding hygienic care for all types of removable dental appliances.

An understanding of oral hygiene maintenance and the motivation to apply these concepts are as critical for patients with removable appliances as for those with full dentition. Patients need to be instructed in the proper care and cleaning of appliances, as well as in maintaining the health of

the soft tissues, remaining teeth, and/or implant fixtures. Removable dental appliances to be discussed include complete dentures, partial dentures, overdentures, removable orthodontic appliances and retainers, bite (interocclusal) splints, and mouth protectors.

TYPES OF REMOVABLE APPLIANCES

Removable dental appliances are usually constructed partially, if not entirely, of a type of plastic resin. These plastics are divided into two categories according to their reaction to heat: thermoplastic and thermosetting materials. Thermoplastic material can be softened, hardened, and resoftened by heat. This type is usually used for mouth protectors for sports. The thermoset plastic undergoes a chemical reaction under heat to acquire a hard set. It cannot be softened and then returned to a desired shape. Dentures, for example, are made of the thermoset material. The type of material used dictates the method by which it can be cleaned and/or disinfected. Heat, some chemicals, and the loss of moisture from the plastic can result in dimensional change and/or other adverse effects.

Complete dentures are appliances designed to replace all teeth in an entire arch. The parts of a

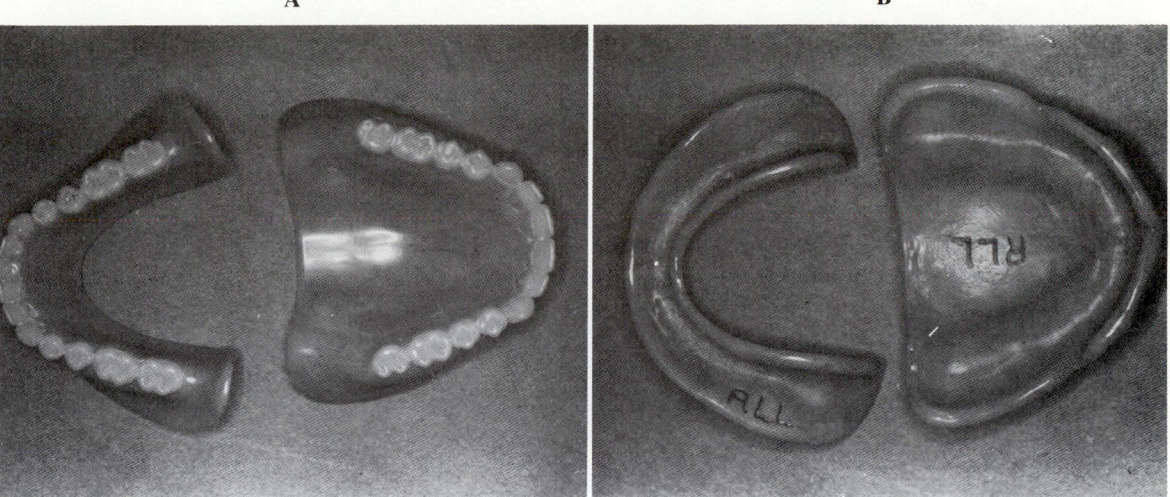

Fig. 23-1. Full dentures. **A,** Polished surfaces and occlusal surfaces. **B,** Tissue or inner surfaces.

complete denture are as follows: the denture base; the tissue surface; and the occlusal surface. The *denture base* is that part which rests on the oral mucosa and to which the denture teeth are attached. It usually is constructed of plastic resin or metal. The surface that is in direct contact with the alveolar ridge is called the *tissue* or *inner surface*. The external surface is called the *polished surface* because of its highly polished appearance. The *occlusal surface* of the denture is formed by the occlusal surfaces of the denture teeth. Denture teeth may be made of either plastic resin or porcelain (Fig. 23-1).

Removable partial dentures replace one or more but not all teeth in a given arch. The denture base is usually made of a metal alloy or plastic resin. Teeth in partial dentures may be made of porcelain, plastic resin, or metal. Partial dentures may also have bars of rigid metal called *major connectors*, which may span the palate in maxillary dentures or the lingual surfaces of the teeth in mandibular dentures. Partial dentures are anchored or supported by natural teeth (abutment teeth) by means of metal clasps and/or occlusal rests (Fig. 23-2).

An *overdenture* is a complete denture supported by both retained natural teeth and/or implant fixtures and the alveolar ridge (Fig. 23-3). The presence of natural teeth and/or implant fixtures offers an advantage over a completely edentulous arch because the teeth or fixtures help to preserve surrounding bone, reduce occlusal stresses on the edentulous ridge, and stabilize and retain the overdenture (Fenton, 1992). The teeth or implant fixtures are reduced in height to allow a denture to fit over them. Overdentures are indicated for situations in which existing teeth can no longer support a removable fixed or partial denture and the additional stability of the denture and preservation of the alveolar ridge are especially desirable. (Wallers, 1990). They are used more frequently for replacement of teeth on the mandibular arch (Johanson and Sivers, 1987). The denture may have special retentive features such as mechanical attachments or magnets built into it, corresponding to features in the abutment tooth or implant, to provide significantly greater retention and stability to the denture (Fig. 23-3).

Removable *orthodontic appliances and retainers* are made of lightweight plastic materials that anchor the wire and clasps used to move teeth or stabilize their position following removal of fixed orthodontic appliances (Fig. 23-4). *Mouth protectors,* or mouth guards, are plastic or vinyl forms that are worn over maxillary teeth to prevent injuries to dentition, the temporomandibular joint, and other oral tissues during contact sports or other recreational activities in which blows to the head, face, or mouth might occur (see Fig. 23-8). Interocclusal splints (bite splints) are plastic resin

(Text continued on p. 502.)

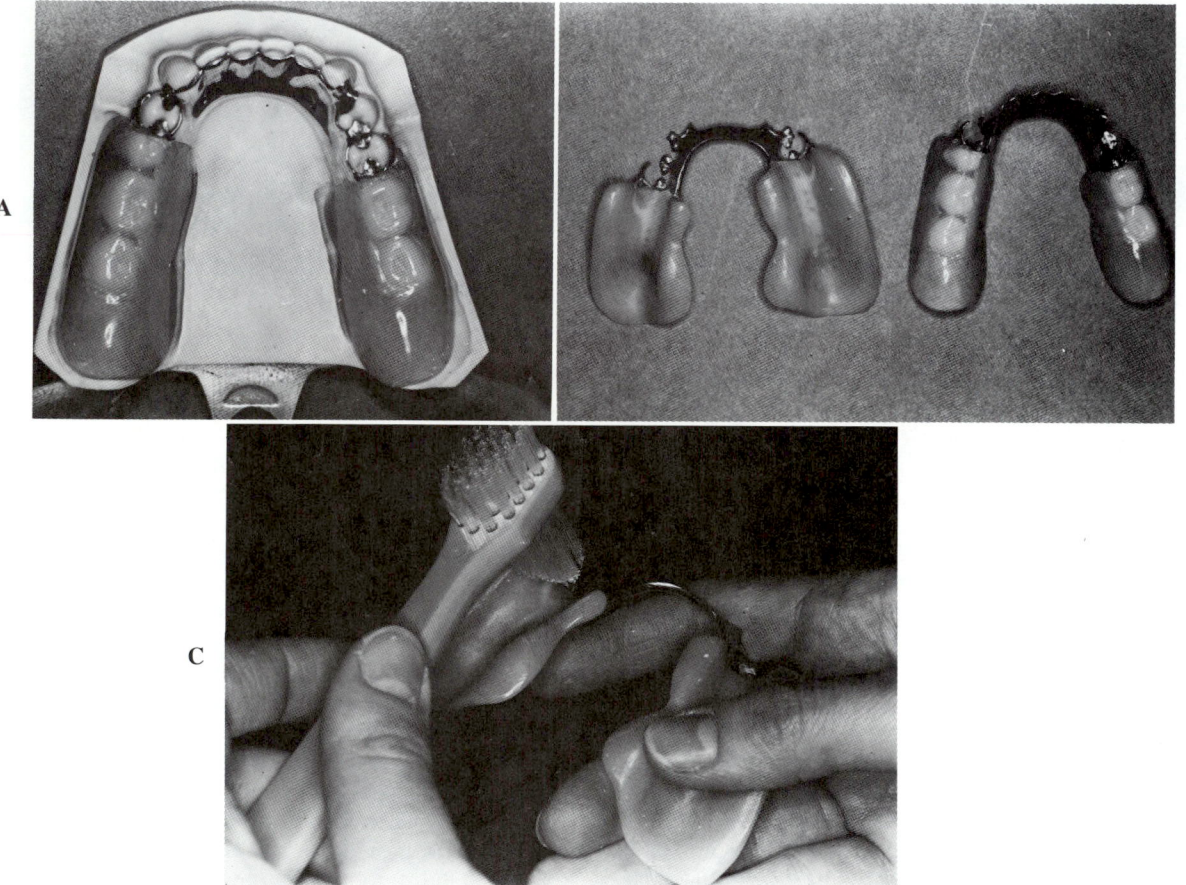

Fig. 23-2. Partial denture. **A,** Partial denture on typodont model. **B,** Partial denture, teeth and soft tissue sides. **C,** Cleaning soft tissue side with a denture brush.

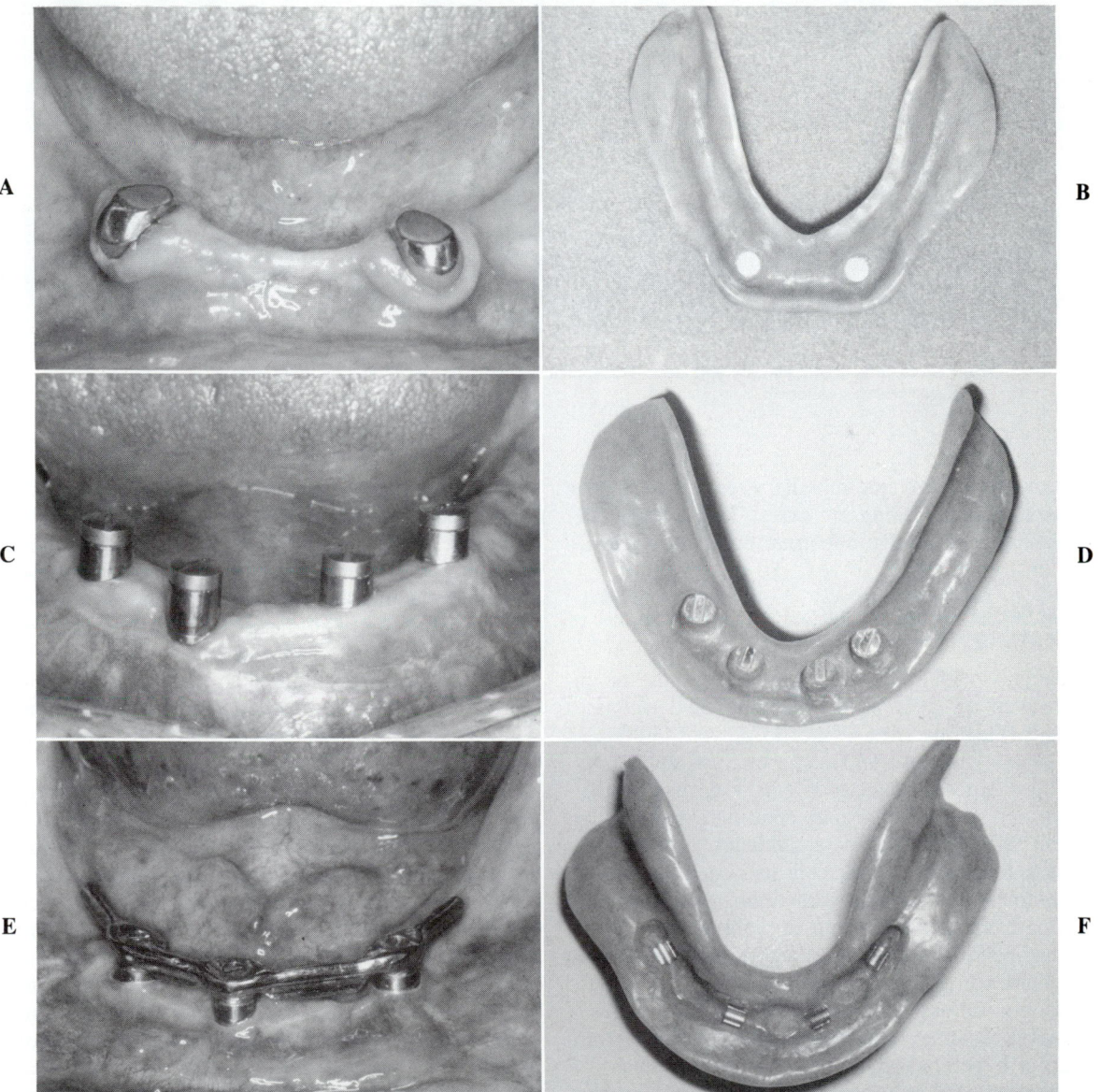

Fig. 23-3. Overdenture and abutments. **A,** Natural teeth with gold alloy cap. **B,** Tissue side of denture with recessed areas for abutments. **C,** Four implant abutments with metal "keepers." **D,** Tissue surface of magnet-containing overdenture. **E,** Bar connector over implant abutment placed to provide additional stability. **F,** Metal clips incorporated into denture to hold to the bar connector.

(Courtesy Dr. James Fowler, Department of Prosthodontics, University of Texas Health Science Center at San Antonio Dental School.)

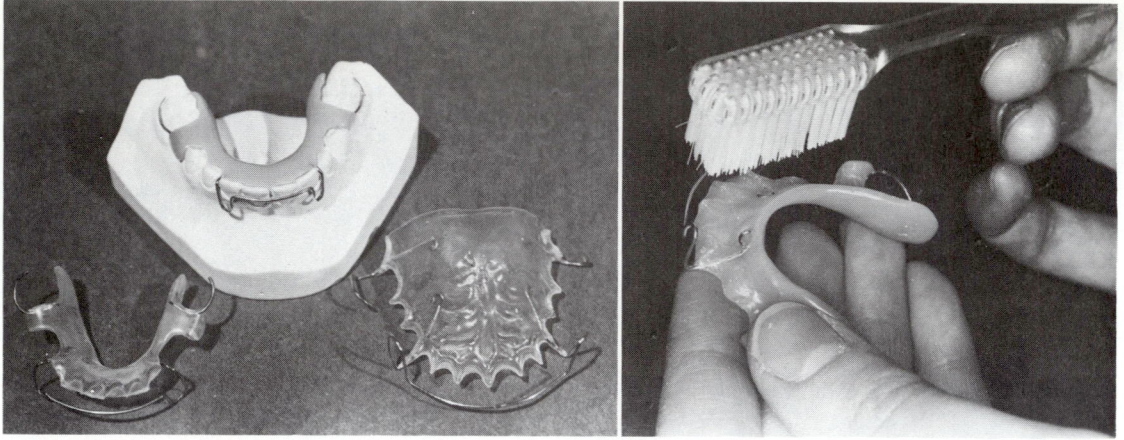

A

B

Fig. 23-4. Orthodontic Hawley appliance. **A,** Appliance placed on model and on table surface. **B,** Brushing appliance with a toothbrush.

forms worn over the maxillary teeth to distribute parafunctional biting pressures. This is especially important to relieve nocturnal bruxism (Attansio, 1991).

IMPORTANCE OF ORAL HYGENE MAINTENANCE

Patients with removable appliances must be instructed on their proper handling and cleaning. Daily cleaning is necessary to prevent buildup of plaque, calculus, and stain on oral appliances. These deposits create problems in terms of esthetics and mouth odor and contribute to irritation and infections, such as candidiasis, gingivitis, or periodontitis in the adjacent mucosa and caries in abutment teeth. *Denture stomatitis* describes pathologic changes that occur in the mucosa of appliance-bearing tissues. Although usually associated with dentures, this condition may occur with orthodontic or other appliances. In its mild forms it may appear as a localized inflammation or pinpoint hyperemia. Less mild forms appear as diffuse, smooth redness in a pattern that correlates directly with the tissue surface of the prosthesis. In its most severe form, denture stomatitis appears as inflammatory papillary hyperplasia (overgrowth) of the soft tissue that lies beneath and adjacent to the denture base (Budtz-Jorgensen, 1978). It is usually a result of poor oral hygiene, ill-fitting appliances, and/or reduced patient resistance to infection (Iacopino and Wathen, 1992).

Irritation of soft tissues underlying prosthetic appliances can be attributed to a number of possible causes. A major etiologic factor is poor oral hygiene. This results in the formation of mature plaque, which contains microorganisms that cause tissue inflammation, along with pathogenic yeast microorganisms, primarily *Candida albicans* (Budtz-Jorgensen, 1983; Catalan et al, 1987). *Candida albicans,* although part of the normal oral flora, can cause an inflammatory condition known as candidiasis in susceptible tissues. This condition can be provoked and/or worsened by constant wearing of the appliance. In a relatively healthy individual, candidiasis can be treated as a localized infection with an antifungal preparation such as clotrimazole (Iacopino and Wathen, 1992) and improved hygiene of dentures and soft tissue surfaces. It may be necessary to soak the denture in an antifungal solution because the continued presence of the organism in the denture may reinfect the patient. However, for patients whose immune response has been suppressed as a result of drug or radiation therapy or through an acquired immunodeficiency (e.g., human immunodeficiency syndrome) resulting in a generally weakened physical condition, the localized infection can become systemic and life-threatening. Optimal control of the pathogens is imperative for these patients, as well as for anyone undergoing prolonged therapy with immunosuppressive drugs, antibiotics, or corticosteroids who may be susceptible to yeast infection (Budtz-Jorgensen, 1978).

Irritation of soft tissues underlying dentures also may be attributed to an uneven distribution of stresses resulting from an improper fit of the denture. The dentist is responsible for evaluating the appliance and adjusting, relining, or replacing it. Patients should be warned against repairing or relining their own dentures to improve retention. Home repairs or relining can cause additional problems in the oral tissues, so patients should be encouraged to seek professional help.

Complete oral hygiene involves procedures to clean both the appliance and the soft tissues and abutment teeth or implants. Procedures for cleaning the removable appliance will be discussed first. The information presented is applicable for partial and complete dentures and other appliances unless otherwise noted.

PROCEDURES AND AGENTS FOR CLEANING APPLIANCES
Brushing with mild abrasive powder, or paste, soap or sodium bicarbonate

Dentures may be cleaned either mechanically with a brush and a mild abrasive substance or by chemical action. Although rinsing with water is helpful after eating and during cleaning procedures to remove food particles and debris, it is not sufficient to remove plaque and other materials adhering to the appliance.

Using a brush or a brush in combination with chemical soaking are effective ways of mechanically removing denture plaque. A study comparing brushing with a dentifrice formulated for denture use and two popular chemical-soak cleansers found brushing with an abrasive to be superior to soaking for removal of accumulated plaque from all denture surfaces (Tarbet et al, 1984). Dentures should be brushed after each meal, if possible, or at least once daily, preferably before bedtime. A soft denture brush is recommended because its two-head design facilitates contact of the bristles with all surfaces of the denture. The longer, rounded tuft of bristles is used to clean the tissue surface of the denture. The flat, rectangular portion should be used to clean the polished and occlusal surfaces (Fig. 23-5). A regular soft toothbrush can be used for cleaning dentures as long as its design permits access to all denture surfaces for thorough scrubbing. Only a soft-bristled brush should be used; hard bristles and/or excessive, prolonged pressure can abrade and damage the denture acrylic. The internal attachments on the tissue side of the overdenture should be cleaned with a soft denture brush or a pipe cleaner. Care must be exercised to avoid damage to the internal attachments incorporated into the overdenture (Jumber, 1981).

Metal clasps on *partial dentures* should be brushed using a small, tapered brush designed specifically for that purpose (available through a dental products supplier). Plaque control is especially important because accumulation around

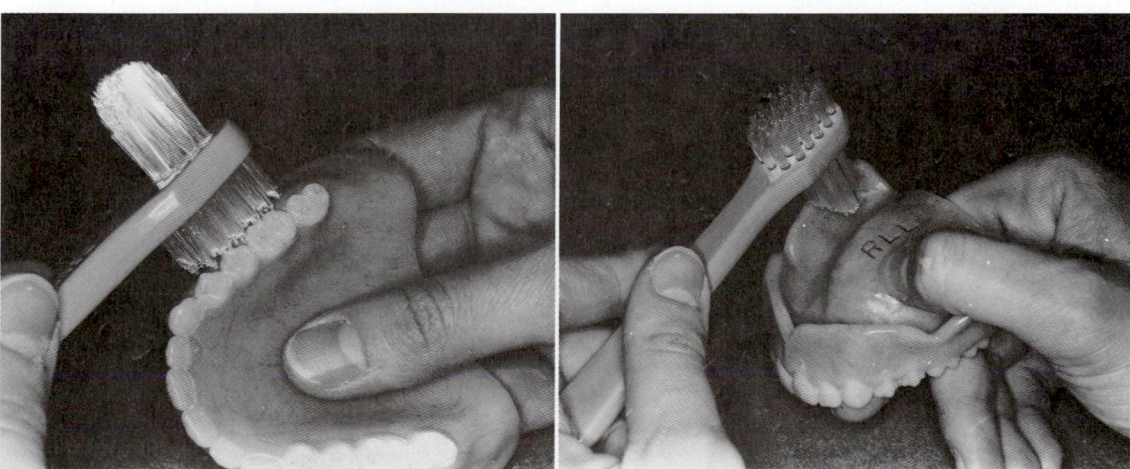

A   B

Fig. 23-5. Mechanical brushing of full denture. **A,** Teeth are brushed with flat, rectangular side of a denture brush, and, **B,** inner surface is brushed with small rounded brush. It is suggested that this be done over a sink partially filled with water to cushion impact if denture is dropped.

abutment teeth and under clasps presents significant potential for damaging the gingival tissues and causing caries. Denture brushes or regular toothbrushes can damage or distort these clasps, affecting their ability to anchor the partial denture properly. The clasps must be handled with special care.

Modifications in the brush may be useful for physically impaired patients. Attach rubber suction cups to the bottom of a soft-bristled fingernail or vegetable-brush so that it will adhere to the inside of the sink. The denture can then be brushed by holding it with both hands and moving all surfaces over the bristles of the brush. Fingernail brushes with plastic handles that curve over and around the side of the hand may also be helpful for individuals who cannot grasp a brush with a regular handle.

A number of powders and dentifrices are commercially available. They contain a mild abrasive (e.g., calcium carbonate), which is less likely to damage acrylic resin than the abrasives in toothpastes. One disadvantage of cream dentifrices is that they are not as easily rinsed off after cleaning. If the patient chooses a commercial powder abrasive or dentifrice, the product should be listed in a current American Dental Association publication of accepted denture cleaners. Appliances can be cleaned satisfactorily and safely with facial soap or sodium bicarbonate and water. Patients should be warned, however, never to use other household cleansers because they are often destructively abrasive and may be toxic if ingested.

The appliances should be rinsed thoroughly under cool running water after cleaning to remove plaque, debris, and the cleaning agent. Brushes should also be rinsed thoroughly and then allowed to air-dry. Patients who have partial dentures or overdentures should have a separate brush for cleaning the abutments. Patients can check the effectiveness of plaque removal from abutments and the appliance with disclosing agents (Ralph and Basker, 1989).

To avoid accidents, patients should be instructed how to handle the appliance during cleaning procedures, because it may be extremely slippery. Hold the appliance firmly but without excessive pressure over a sink filled with water during the cleaning process. You may line the sink with a rubber mat or towel as protection against breakage if the appliance falls. Appliances should never be rinsed or soaked in hot water because

high temperatures can damage the acrylic resin. (Crawford et al, 1986; Robinson et al, 1985). After cleaning at night, store appliances in a container of water or one of the recommended commercial soaking agents unless the dentist has recommended wearing them at night. Rinse appliances well before returning them to the mouth. Containers used to store dental appliances should also be cleaned after each use. To prevent microbial buildup in the container, scrub with soap and water and then rinse with a diluted commercial bleach solution.

Dentures with soft liners should be cleaned carefully to avoid damaging the lining and thereby compromising the fit. A simple rinsing of soft liners and gentle brushing with a soft tooth brush are good interim measures to minimize damage (Zarb, 1990). The manufacturer of the specific soft liner used may offer additional recommendations for the care of its product. Dentures with soft linings should be stored in plain water rather than in a commercial soaking solution and should be placed in the storage container with the occlusal surfaces down so that the weight of the denture will not distort the lining material.

Home (personal) sonic or ultrasonic units

Although thorough brushing of dentures is probably the most effective way of removing denture plaque, some denture wearers may not have the motivation or physical ability required to perform this task regularly and effectively. For these individuals, the use of a sonic or ultrasonic cleaner may be a more acceptable alternative. Both sonic and ultrasonic units are commercially available. Sonic cleaners operate by generating audible electrosonic energy waves; ultrasonic cleaners operate by means of high-frequency sound waves. Most units available to the general public are of the sonic type, which produce less mechanical agitation of solutions than do the ultrasonic units seen in dental offices. The cleaning ability of sonic cleaners has been compared to chemical immersion cleansers (Muenchinger, 1975). Although no ultrasonic cleaner has been shown to remove *all* plaque, ultrasonic cleaning is more efficient than either a commercial chemical immersion cleanser or a sonic cleaner (Palenik and Miller, 1984).

There is disagreement as to the effectiveness of these mechanical cleaners in reducing denture plaque. Abelson (1981) found that an ultrasonic cleaner and water were effective in removing plaque accumulations, more effective than a 15-minute soak in commercial denture solutions. Myers and Krol (1974) stated that sonic cleaners helped remove calculus and stain from dentures. Nicholson et al. (1968) found sonic cleaning with a hypochlorite (bleach) solution was more effective in plaque removal than use of hypochlorite solution alone. Though the cleaning ability of ultrasonic devices may be related more to the chemical solution than to the ultrasonic action, Budtz-Jorgensen (1979) did report that the device enhances the effectiveness of the disinfecting solution.

Chemicals used for immersion

Chemical solutions for soaking appliances are an alternative to mechanical cleansing. These cleansers require less patient effort and compliance, and the solution reaches surfaces on the denture that may be inaccessible to the denture brush. Among the several types of chemical denture cleansers are alkaline hypochlorites, alkaline peroxides, dilute acids, enzymes, and antibacterials.

Alkaline hypochlorites (e.g., household bleach) are effective denture cleansers because they dissolve mucin and other organic substances, thus destroying the plaque matrix so that it can be rinsed or brushed away. These solutions are also bactericidal and fungicidal, making them useful in treating denture stomatitis and disinfecting dentures. Destruction of the plaque matrix also inhibits calculus formation, and the bleaching action of the solution removes stains from denture acrylic. Alkaline hypochlorites are available as commercial products (e.g., Mersene) or as a homemade preparation in which 1 teaspoon of household bleach and 2 teaspoons of sodium salts, such as Calgon, are combined in 4 ounces of warm water. Appliances should be soaked in these solutions for only 10-to-15 minutes for maximum effectiveness (Abelson, 1985). Hypochlorite solutions have an unpleasant taste and odor, so dentures treated by this method should be brushed and thoroughly rinsed afterward. Patients may want to soak dentures in commercial alkaline peroxide rinses after treatment with hypochlorites to minimize taste and odor aftereffects. However, because appliances with metal parts are deleteriously affected by bleach, they should not be placed into a bleach-containing solution. Kastner et al. (1983) also found that a solution of bleach and sodium salts (Calgon) significantly increased the flexibility of the metal clasps of partial den-

tures, resulting in poor retention of appliances.

Alkaline peroxide preparations are commonly available in tablet or powder form. They consist of an alkaline detergent combined with sodium perborate or percarbonate. When dissolved in warm water, they form an alkaline solution of hydrogen peroxide. The release of oxygen by hydrogen peroxide causes a bubbling or effervescent action that produces a mechanical cleaning effect. This action occurs only during the 10- to 15-minute period the solution is bubbling; additional cleaning is not achieved after this period.

Regular use of these agents, followed by brushing and rinsing, helps prevent the formation of stain and calculus. Many of these preparations contain enzymes, which enhance antibacterial action and break down the plaque matrix so it becomes easier to brush or rinse away. These products have been found to be safe and effective for all types of dentures and are the agents of choice for appliances containing metal parts.

Caution is needed in storing alkaline peroxide tablets so that they cannot be ingested by accident. Tablets can be mistaken by elderly or visually impaired persons for antacid tablets and accidentally ingested. These products should also be stored out of the reach of small children.

Dilute acids are also used to clean dental appliances with no metal parts. They include 3% to 5% hydrochloric acids (may include phosphoric acid), white household vinegar, and more concentrated commercial preparations used in ultrasonic units by dental professionals. Acid solutions dissolve the inorganic components formed on the appliance and remove stains that are not removed by regular cleaning methods. These acidic chemicals should be used with care because they corrode metals. An effective stain and calculus removal solution is made by combining 1 to 2 teaspoons of *white* household vinegar in 4 ounces of warm water. When calculus formation is noted, the appliances should be soaked in this solution overnight.

Antibacterial agents such as chlorhexidine gluconate have also been suggested for denture soaking solution. These agents have both antibacterial and antifungal properties, but they may stain the denture teeth after repeated use. They work by adhering to the surface of the appliance and providing continuing presence of the active disinfectant ingredient to the target area (Anderson, Gher, and Powell, 1991).

Appliance-soaking containers and solutions as a potential source of infection. Proper care of appliance soaking containers is especially critical for patients whose immune system is suppressed. Chemical soaking solutions and their containers can serve as growth media for pathogenic microorganisms that form on the appliances, allowing them to act as reservoirs of microorganisms into which clean appliances might be placed. After storage, the appliances can become a source of infection for the patient. Because of the vulnerability to infection of patients with suppressed immune systems, disposable containers should be used and discarded. Appliances should be cleaned with a disinfecting detergent (see Chapter 3) and then rinsed before being reinserted (DePaola and Minah, 1983; DePaola et al, 1984a, 1984b).

COMPARING THE EFFICACY OF DENTURE CLEANSERS

Comparison of the efficacy of the various denture-cleaning products is difficult because of the lack of in vivo studies and the wide variations in materials and methods. Studies documenting both quality and pathogenicity of plaque present after use of denture cleansers are needed. Patients should be instructed in proper denture care, including the advantages and disadvantages of available products, and cautioned about the manufacturers' claims of efficacy. Lists of denture cleansers that have been evaluated and accepted for safety, efficacy, quality, and accuracy in advertising claims are updated annually by the ADA Council on Dental Materials, Instruments, and Equipment and the Council on Dental Therapeutics .

CARE OF EDENTULOUS AREAS, SOFT TISSUES, AND ABUTMENT TEETH/ IMPLANTS

Individuals must be instructed about the need to maintain the health of edentulous areas and the abutment teeth or implants, attachments, and surrounding periodontal tissues. As already stated, unless the patient is instructed otherwise by the dentist, dental appliances should be removed at night and stored in water or in alkaline peroxide cleaning solutions. If not maintained in a liquid, the acrylic resin materials of which appliances are formed can dry, resulting in distortion and compromising the fit of the appliance in the mouth.

Dentures and other removable appliances should be removed for an extended period to give the soft tissues beneath the appliance an opportunity to recover from the constant compression between the appliance and the bone. Failure to provide this recovery period can result in irritation of the soft tissues. Most people prefer to remove their dentures and other prosthetic appliances at night because it is less embarrassing and inconvenient to be without them in the privacy of one's own home. Some individuals feel that being without dentures and other prostheses, even at night, is unacceptable. These patients should be encouraged to find other times to do without the prosthesis. It has been recommended that dentures be left out of the mouth for 6 to 8 hours during each 24-hour period (Boucher and Renner, 1982).

After rinsing and cleaning the denture or prosthesis, the individual should clean the intraoral tissues using a soft toothbrush or a washcloth. This not only removes adherent plaque and debris from the tissues but also massages and stimulates circulation and keratinization of tissues. The tissues may be massaged by applying stimulation with the fingers. Instructions for the care of remaining teeth have been discussed in Chapter 20. The importance of meticulous plaque control for the abutment teeth and implants must be emphasized. These abutments are critical to the retention of the prosthetic appliance and the bony ridge. The patient should be instructed in the care of these abutments and then provided with supervised practice to ensure good home maintenance. The ability of teeth and implants to serve as abutments for partial dentures or overdentures depends on the health of the supporting periodontal tissues.

Use of disclosing solution lets the patient evaluate his or her skills of plaque removal. Implants require the same attention as the natural teeth. The only difference is in the type of oral hygiene aids used for implants. The aids must not be metal (e.g., an interproximal brush must have its metal core covered with plastic) to avoid abrading the titanium implant (McKinney, 1991). The individual abutments (see Fig. 23-3, A and C) are much easier to clean than the abutments supporting a bar attachment (Fig. 23-3, E). The mesial and distal surfaces of a single abutment can be reached by angling the bristles of a soft brush into the sulcus area. The bar requires additional hygiene aids to clean under the bar and around the abutments (e.g., interproximal brush, superfloss, Post-Care floss).

For tooth abutments, the use of fluoride dentifrices as well as topical application of fluoride gels is recommended for caries control. Fluoride may be brushed onto the teeth or placed on the inner surfaces of an overdenture before it is inserted into the mouth (Bergman, 1987; Johnson and Sivers, 1987). If the prosthetic device contains metal, acidulated fluoride should not be used because the acidic component will interact chemically with the metal. A stannous fluoride should be prescribed (Statton and Johnson, 1980).

Topical antimicrobial agents, (see Chapter 20) are intended for use as an adjunct to mechanical plaque removal, not a substitute. These agents have been found to be effective in controlling plaque and gingivitis (McKinney, 1991).

Care of removable orthodontic appliances, splints, and mouth guards involves many of the principles already discussed. Appliances should be worn as directed by the dentist. Generally, they should be removed before meals and rinsed and cleaned with a regular toothbrush and soap or mild abrasive (see Fig. 23-4).

Professional cleaning of prosthetic appliances usually includes immersion of the appliance in a professional denture cleanser combined with ultrasonic cleaning. Protective barrier coverings should be worn while handling and cleaning prosthetic appliances. The clinician should receive the appliance in a sealable plastic bag. The chemical solution should be chosen based on the deposits present and the materials of which the appliance is made. The solution should be placed in the bag, completely covering the prosthetic appliance. Place the bag in a beaker of water in the ultrasonic cleaner (Fig. 23-6). The solution contaminated by the appliance can be discarded after cleaning, leaving the other liquids, containers, and surfaces protected from cross-contamination.

After ultrasonic treatment, the appliance should be rinsed thoroughly and brushed with a sterile or disposable denture brush under running water. The original plastic bag should be rinsed before the appliance is placed into it. The addition of a small amount of mouthwash to the solution will make the prosthetic appliance taste better when it is replaced in the mouth. Stains and deposits not removed by the ultrasonic cleaner and brushing may require the use of hand scaling instruments followed by laboratory polishing. Infection con-

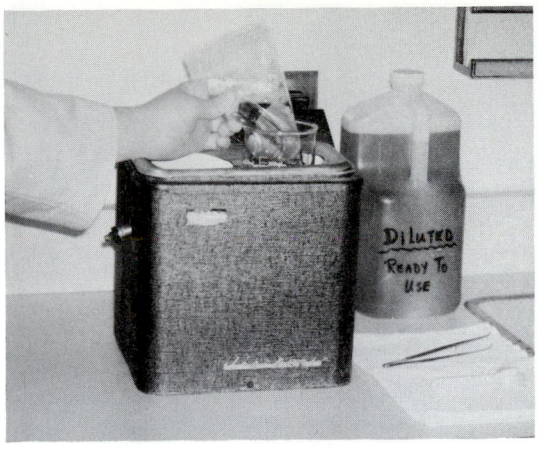

Fig. 23-6. "Zip-lock" sealed plastic bag containing denture and cleaning solution is placed into beaker of water for ultrasonic cleaning.

trol procedures must be observed in the laboratory. Care must be taken when using these methods to avoid scratching or damaging the material, which would make the denture even more susceptible to buildup of plaque, stain, or calculus deposits. Ultrasonic scalers can roughen the surface of acrylic prostheses, so they must be used with caution.

Appliance identification

Dental professionals have recognized the need to mark prostheses for identification. Benefits include postmortem identification; identification of persons who are unconscious or have memory loss; appliance identification in commercial laboratories; identification in institutional situations, such as nursing homes (Seals and Seals, 1985); and facilitation of return of lost appliances.

The ADA guidelines specify that identification must (1) not jeopardize prosthesis strength; (2) be easy, efficient, and inexpensive; (3) be visible and durable; (4) withstand humidity and fire; (5) be cosmetically acceptable to the wearer; and (6) be in the location least likely to be damaged in an accident (Chalian et al, 1986; Johanson and Ekman, 1984; Seals and Seals, 1985).

A variety of techniques has been used for marking prosthetic appliances; including engraving or scribing into the denture surface; surface marking or writing over the denture base; and including paper, plastic, or metal markers in the

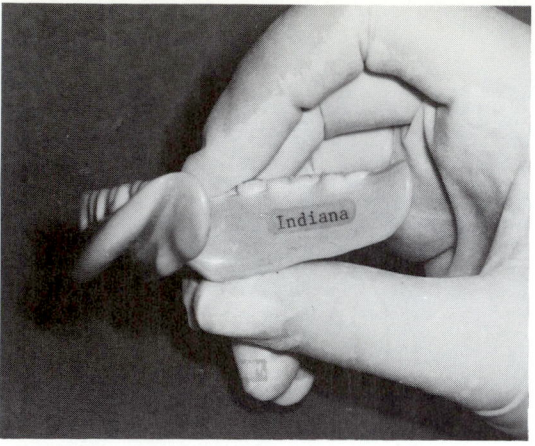

Fig. 23-7. Example of denture marked by inclusion method.

denture's construction (Chalian et al, 1986; Council on Prosthetic Services, 1982; Johanson and Ekman, 1984; Seals and Seals, 1985).

The patient's name or identifying number can be engraved into the prosthesis with an engraving tool. The grooves are then filled with contrasting self-curing acrylic resin or highlighted with a fine-point, alcohol-based felt-tip pen. These markings are then sealed with clear acrylic resin.

The surface marking method involves using an abrasive pad or emery board to roughen a small area, usually at the back of the prosthesis. The identifying name or number is then written over the roughened surface with an alcohol-based felt-tip pen or a hard lead pencil and then covered with clear, self-curing acrylic resin. Surface marking and engraving do not provide truly permanent marks; the prosthesis may therefore need to be marked again after a year or more (Johanson and Ekman, 1984).

The inclusion method provides permanent identification. Strips of paper, plastic, or metal are embedded and sealed into the prosthesis (Fig.23-7). The identifying name or number can be typed on a small strip of thin white paper. A groove the size of the paper strip is created in the prosthesis with a bur. The strip is placed in the groove and covered with clear acrylic resin, and the area is polished (Council on Prosthetic Services, 1982). The name or number can also be placed on a special metal or plastic strip to be embedded into the prosthesis and sealed with clear acrylic resin (Johanson and Ekman, 1984).

Marking dentures for permanent identification is required in several states and in all of the branches of the military service and Veterans Administration. These statutes do not, however, solve the problems of denture identification for individuals with unmarked dentures. Denture identification requires minimal time, materials, and effort. It can be accomplished at a regular dental appointment or through community-based dental health programs (Ames, 1985; Williams et al, 1982). No matter the process used for marking the dentures, standard infection control procedures must be observed.

USE, SELECTION, AND CARE OF MOUTH PROTECTORS

The use of mouth protectors in sports has steadily increased over the past 3 decades. First introduced in boxing and football, mouth protectors are now used widely in any sport where there is a risk of mouth or facial injuries. The introduction of face guards has reduced football injuries involving oral trauma by 50%, and mouth protectors have nearly eliminated the remaining injuries (Seals and Dorrough, 1984). Unfortunately, though oral injuries in a wide variety of physical activities could be prevented with properly fitted mouth protectors, many still occur because of failure to promote the use of protectors for children and adults engaged in activities in which oral or facial injuries are a distinct possibility. (Croll and Castaldi, 1989).

To avoid bulkiness, mouth protectors are usually fitted only over the maxillary teeth, which are the most prone to damage. These devices prevent oral trauma in several ways. They minimize lacerations by holding the soft tissues away from the teeth. They prevent teeth from damage by being hit together when subjected to a blow, and they absorb the impact of a direct blow by spreading its force away from individual teeth. This absorption of impact decreases shock to the temporomandibular joint and mandibular condyle, thus protecting against concussions, neck injuries, and more severe central nervous system damage (Seals and Dorrough, 1984).

Several criteria must be met for mouth protectors to be accepted (Bishop et al, 1985). They must be nontoxic, tasteless, and tissue compatible. They must be comfortable, with a fit that allows retention in the mouth without jaw clenching, and must not interfere significantly with

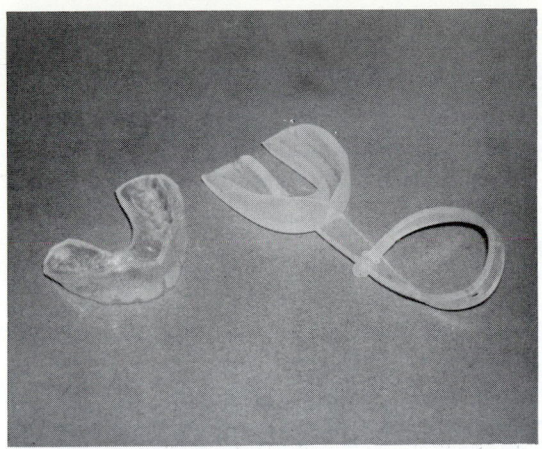

Fig. 23-8. Two types of mouth protectors are shown: custom-fitted *(left),* and thermoplastic mout formed *(right)* types.

speech. Durability and ease of processing and repair are important. Low cost and easy attainability also improve acceptance of mouth protectors.

Four general types of mouth protectors are available for sports (Fig. 23-8): ready-made or stock; mouth-formed (two types), and custom-fitted mouth protectors (Bureau of Health Education, 1984, 1985; Mouth protectors for contact sports, 1983). Although any type of mouth protector will reduce oral injury, the better it is tolerated by the athlete, the more likely it will be worn and injuries prevented. Color-tinted mouthguards have become increasingly more popular because they are easier to locate if dislodged and allow visual recognition that the athlete is wearing a mouthguard (Raymond, 1991).

Although ready-made or stock mouth protectors are available, they are not recommended because they cannot be fitted to the individual. They are uncomfortable to wear, difficult to retain, bulky, and they interfere with talking and breathing.

There are two types of mouth-formed protectors. The shell-liner type consists of a hard outer shell of polyvinyl chloride that provides physical strength. A soft liner made of plasticized acrylic gel or silicone rubber is placed in the mouth, molded to the teeth, and then set by thermal or chemical means. A disadvantage of this type is that repeated biting and exposure to saliva distort the shape and physical properties of the materials. Mouth-formed protectors are not recommended for athletes with fixed orthodontic appliances.

Thermoplastic mouth-formed protectors are made by immersing the preformed plastic shell in boiling water for 10 to 15 seconds, dipping it in cold water for 1 second, and then transferring it immediately to the mouth for adaptation to the teeth. Adaptation can be performed by using finger pressure, tongue pressure, and gentle biting. For best results, however, these protectors should be placed and checked by a dentist. Advantages of this type include comfortable fit, less bulk, reasonable cost, and the ability to re-form the plastic if it becomes loose or distorted. These protectors also can be used safely by individuals with fixed orthodontic appliances if they are fitted by dentists. An added advantage is that many styles include a strap attachment to secure the protector to helmet faceguards, if desired.

Custom-made mouth guards offer optimal fit, comfort, and protection. Importantly, they do not interfere with speech as much as do the noncustom-fit protectors do. Square sheets of a thermoplastic material (e.g., polyvinyl acetate–polyethylene) are custom formed to a cast of the maxillary teeth and tissues and then trimmed for fit and comfort. This procedure should be supervised by a dentist to ensure proper fit and function of the final product. The thermoplastic material is heated and then formed under a vacuum over the maxillary cast for about 2 minutes. The material is then allowed to cool before it is finished. The hardened form is removed from the cast and excess material is trimmed so it does not impinge on frena, muscle, or soft tissue attachments. The protector is then replaced on the cast, and the edges are flamed with an alcohol torch for softening and then smoothed with wet fingers. The protector should be adjusted as needed by the dentist for optimal fit and comfort to the patient. Custom-fitted mouth protectors are usually made to cover all existing teeth in the maxillary arch and palate for most individuals. Variations and modifications can be made for changes in dentition for young athletes, persons who gag easily, patients with Class III jaw relationships, those with orthodontic appliances, edentulous or partially edentulous patients, and other unique situations.

ACTIVITIES

1. Obtain samples of different types of removable appliances, made of different types of materials, from dental offices, laboratories, or dental schools. Discuss the cleaning measures to care for each type of

appliance most effectively, based on its component parts and materials.

2. As a class, plan and implement a community service project. Ideas for projects include providing denture cleaning services, implementing a denture marking service, or making custom-fitted mouth guards for young athletes in conjunction with local dentists. These activities could take place during health fairs or in schools, nursing homes, senior citizen centers, or retirement centers.

3. Survey friends and family members who wear dentures to collect a list of all the methods of cleaning and caring for dentures that they know, including "home remedies"; compile all these into a master list, noting and critiquing the most commonly used techniques.

4. Practice denture-marking methods using old dentures that have been subjected to infection control procedures.

5. Invite a dentist specializing in prosthodontics to address the class about how prosthetic appliances, splints, and mouth guards are made, the importance of proper fit, problems in the patient's adjustment to the prosthesis, and acceptable procedures for relining dentures.

6. Go to a variety of drugstores and grocery stores in the area and compile a list of dental products marketed for use by denture wearers. Compare the list to accepted product lists in *Accepted Dental Therapeutics*. Write manufacturers for more information regarding the uses and effectiveness of these products. Critique the products in terms of safety, efficacy, cost, and acceptability.

7. Visit a dental laboratory and follow the process used to make full and partial dentures.

REVIEW QUESTIONS

1. Which of the following types of cleansers should not be used on prosthetic appliances containing metal parts?
   a. Alkaline peroxide
   b. Dentifrices formulated for denture use
   c. Alkaline hypochlorite solutions
   d. Diluted white vinegar
2. Which method of marking prosthetic appliances is considered to be the most permanent?
   a. Engraving
   b. Surface marking
   c. Inclusion
3. For which arch are mouth protectors usually fitted?
   a. Mandibular
   b. Maxillary
   c. Both arches
4. True or false: Most people with full dentures seek regular dental care.
5. What microorganism seems to be related to denture stomatitis ?

6. What suggestions should be made to patients who complain that calculus forms on their prosthesis?
7. What precautions should the dental professional take to avoid cross-contamination during cleaning procedures for prosthetic appliances?
8. What precautions should individuals take to avoid dropping and breaking their dentures during cleaning?

REFERENCES

Abelson DC: Denture plaque and denture cleansers, *J Prosthet Dent* 45:376, 1981 .

Abelson DC: Denture plaque and denture cleansers: review of the literature, *Gerodontics* 1:202, 1985.

Ames RK: Operation IDENT/nursing home screening project, Broward County, Florida, *Florida Dent J* 56:42, 1985.

Anderson MH, Gher ME, Powell, LV: Paper presented at the meeting of the Academy of Operative Dentistry, Chicago, February 13, 1991.

Attansio, R: Nocturnal bruxism and its clinical management, *Dent Clin North Am* 35:1, 1991.

Bergman B: Periodontal reactions related to removable partial dentures: a literature review, *J Prosthet Dent* 58:454, 1987.

Bishop BM et al: Materials for mouth protectors, *J Prosthet Dent* 53:256, 1985.

Boucher LJ, Renner RP: *Treatment of partially edentulous patients*, St Louis, 1982, CV Mosby.

Budtz-Jorgensen E: Clinical aspects of *Candida* infection in denture wearers, *JADA* 96:474, 1978.

Budtz-Jorgensen E: Materials and methods for cleaning dentures, *J Prosthet Dent* 42:619, 1979.

Budtz-Jorgensen E et al: Quantitative relationship between yeast and bacteria in denture induced stomatitis, *Scand J Dent Res* 91:134, 1983.

Bureau of Health Education and Audiovisual Services and Council on Dental Materials, Instruments, and Equipment: Mouth protectors and sports team dentists, *JADA* 109:84, 1984.

Bureau of Health Education and Audiovisual Services: *Mouth protectors: give your teeth a sporting chance*, Chicago, 1985, American Dental Associations.

Catalan A: Denture plaque and palatal mucosa in *denture stomatitis:* scanning electron microscopic and microbiologic study, *J Prosthet Dent* 57:582, 1987.

Chalian VA et al: Identification of removable dental prosthesis, *J Prosthet Dent* 56:254, 1986.

Council on Prosthetic Services and Dental Laboratory Relations: *Operation IDENT*, Chicago, 1982, American Dental Association.

Crawford CA et al: Denture bleaching: a laboratory simulation of patients' cleaning procedures, *J Dent* 14:258, 1986.

Croll T, Castaldi C: The custom fitted athletic mouthguard for the orthodontic patient and the child with mixed dentition, *Quintessence Int* 20, 1989.

DePaola LG, Minah GE: Isolation of pathogenic microorganisms from dentures and denture-soaking containers of myelosuppressed cancer patients, *J Prosthet Dent* 49:20, 1983.

DePaola LG et al: Evaluation of agents to reduce microbial growth on dental prostheses of myelosuppressed cancer patients, *Clin Prev Dent* 6:9, 1984a.

DePaola LG et al: Growth of potential pathogens in denture-soaking solution of myelosuppressed cancer patients, *J Prosthet Dent* 51:554, 1984b.

Fenton A: The role of dental implants in the future, *JADA*, 123:1, 1992.

Iacopino AM, Wathen WF: Oral candida infection and denture stomatitis: a comprehensive review, *JADA* 123:1, 1992.

Johanson GK, Ekman B: Denture marking, *JADA* 108:347, 1984.

Johanson GK, Sivers JE: Periodontal considerations for over-dentures, *JADA* 114:468, 1987.

Jumber JF: *An atlas of overdentures and attachments*, Chicago, 1981, Quintessence.

Kastner C et al: Effects of chemical denture cleaners on the flexibility of cast clasps, *J Prosthet Dent* 50:473, 1983.

Leble J: Health needs of the elderly, *Dent Clin North Am* 33(1):1, 1989.

McKinney, RV: *Endosteal dental implants*, St. Louis, 1991, CV Mosby.

Mouth protectors for contact sports, *CAL* 47:18, 1983.

Muenchinger FS: Evaluation of an electrosonic denture cleaner, *J Prosthet Dent* 3 3:610, 1975 .

Myers HM, Kroll AJ: Effectiveness of a sonic-action denture cleaning program, *J Prosthet Dent* 32:613, 1974.

National Institutes of Health, *Oral Health of United States Adults,* Pub 87-2868, 1987, Bethesda, MD.

Nicholson RJ et al: Calculus and stain removal from acrylic resin dentures, *J Prosthet Dent* 20:326, 1968 .

Palenik CJ, Miller CH: In vitro testing of three denture-cleaning systems, *J Prosthet Dent* 51:751, 1984.

Ralph JP, Basker RM: The role of overdentures in geriodontics, *Dent Update,* 16:8, 1989.

Raymond KG: Mouthguards, *Dent Hyg* 4:4, 1991.

Robinson JG et al: The whitening of acrylic dentures; the role of denture cleaners, *Br Dent J* 159:247, 1985.

Seals RR, Dorrough BC: Custom mouth protectors: a review of their applications, *J Prosthet Dent* 51:238, 1984.

Seals RR, Seals DJ: The importance of denture identification, *Spec Care Dent* 5(4):164.

Statton RI, Johnson DS: *Fundamentals of removable prosthodontics,* Chicago, 1980, Quintessence.

Tarbet WJ, et al: Denture cleansing: a comparison of two methods, *J Prosthet Dent* 51:322, 1984.

Waller RA: Design, preparation and maintenance of overdenture abutments, *Dent Clinic North Am* 34:4, 1990.

Williams JE et al: A denture identification program for nursing home residents, *Spec Care Dent* 2:76, 1982.

Zarb B et al: *Boucher's prosthodontics treatment for edentulous patients,* St Louis, 1990, CV Mosby.

SUGGESTED READINGS

American Dental Association: *Guide to dental materials and devices,* ed 6, Chicago, 1974, The Association.

Council on Dental Materials, Instruments, and Equipment: Denture cleansers, *JADA* 106:77, 1983.

Council on Dental Materials, Instruments, and Equipment: Accepted dental products, *JADA* 116:249, 1988.

Crawford CA et al: Bleached dentures: misuse of a denture-cleaning agent, *Dent Update* 14(1):29, 1987.

Davenport JC et al: The compatibility of soft lining materials and denture cleansers, *Br Dent J* 161:31, 1986.

Ghalichebaf M et al: The efficacy of denture cleansing agents, *J Prosthet Dent* 48:515, 1982.

Goll G et al: The effect of denture cleansers on temporary soft liners, *J Prosthet Dent* 50:466, 1983.

Harrison A: A simple denture marking system, *Br Dent J* 160:89, 1986.

Hutchins DW, Parker WA: A clinical evaluation of the ability of denturecleaning solutions to remove dental plaque from prosthetic devices, *NY State Dent J* 39:363, 1973.

Kempler D et al: The efficacy of sodium hypochlorite as a denture cleanser, *Spec Care Dent* 2:112, 1982.

Leble J: Health needs of the elderly, *Dent Clin North Am* 33:1989.

McNutt: Oral trauma in adolescent athletics: a study of mouth protectors. *Ped Dent* 11:209, 1989.

Ortman LF: *Patient education and complete denture maintenance*. In Winkler S, editor: *Essentials of complete denture prosthodontics,* ed 2, Littleton, Mass, 1987, PSG.

Rudd RW et al: Sterilization of complete dentures with sodium hypochlorite, *J Prosthet Dent* 51:318, 1984.

Rustogi KN et al: The clinical efficacy of denture cleansers, *Natl Dent Assoc* 37:100, 1979.

Schmidt WF, Smith DE: A six year retrospective study of Molloplast-B lined dentures. Part II. Liner serviceability, *J Prosthet Dent* 50:459, 1983.

Seals RR et al: An evaluation of mouthguard programs in Texas high school football, *JADA* 110:904, 1985.

Shannon IL, Starcke EN: Higher performance denture cleansers, *NY J Dent* 48:246, 1978.

Sharp EW et al: Denture cleansers and in vitro plaque, *J Prosthet Dent* 53:584, 1985.

Waldman HB: The edentulous population: its use and need of dental services, *J Prosthet Dent* 58:643, 1987.

Wright PS: Soft lining materials: their status and prospects, *J Dent* 4:247, 1976.

24 NUTRITIONAL SELF-ASSESSMENT AND MODIFICATIONS

Theresa Levy
Irene Woodall

LEARNING OUTCOMES

The dental hygienist will be able to

1. Describe the role of dietary assessment and planning in dental hygiene care.
2. Briefly describe the ways in which diet and nutrition can affect the overall health of the body and specifically of the oral cavity.
3. Identify the basic role of each of the following nutrients in the health of the patient:
   a. Carbohydrates
   b. Proteins
   c. Lipids
   d. Vitamins
   e. Minerals
   f. Water
4. Describe the usefulness and limitations of the Recommended Dietary Allowances (RDAs) and the four food groups in assessing a person's diet and in recommending modifications.
5. Describe how carbohydrates and plaque promote caries.
6. Explain how diet has been shown to influence cancer formation.
7. Explain strategies for assessing a patient's diet using a 1-day diet review or a 3-day or 7-day diary.
8. Conduct a dietary assessment for a patient, using the self-assessment strategy.
9. Given a variety of completed dietary assessments, assist each patient in determining which components of the diet could be changed, why they should be modified, and how the modification could be accomplished.
10. Identify several environmental factors that affect whether modifications are likely to occur following the self-assessment session.
11. Conduct a follow-up, reinforcement session as part of dental care to evaluate the patient's progress and to assist the patient in identifying alternative approaches to diet modification.

The growing knowledge and awareness of the relationship between good dietary habits and good general health have brought nutritional assessment and dietary counseling into focus as essential components of dental hygiene care. Many of the effects of dietary habits are clearly reflected in the oral cavity, because poor nutrition has negative effects on hard and soft oral tissues as well as on general well-being. Dental hygienists see their patients more frequently and more regularly than do most other health care providers. Thus the hygienist has more opportunity to detect dietary problems and to help the patient adopt changes (Diet, 1984). The hygienist needs to know how to assess a patient's diet, what changes are indicated by the results, and when a patient's nutritional problems require the expertise of a dietitian.

Private dental practices that focus on prevention include nutritional assessment for new patients, with a periodic review at recall intervals for established patients. Other sites, such as hospitals, nursing homes, day care centers, and other community-based settings include nutritional counseling as a significant part of the overall program to improve general and oral health.

Any dental professional who will be assessing patients' diets and helping patients identify changes needs a complete course in nutrition, a good grounding in communication and basic counseling skills, and supervised clinical experience with a range of patients. This can be accomplished as part of the educational preparation with clinic patients. This chapter provides only a survey of basic nutrition and an introduction to the philosophy of nutritional assessment and patient-centered dietary counseling.

For clinicians who understand the basics of proper nutrition, both generally and in oral health particularly, and who include a dietary focus in their everyday clinical care, a dietary assessment for every patient is the best way to ensure that the focus is established and maintained.

The assessment can be a routine component of the overall assessment phase of dental hygiene care. It can provide the means for identifying patients who need simple dietary counseling and those who may need referral to a dietitian or physician. It may also identify those patients whose diets are well within normal limits and who do not need modifications. The critical point, as when any assessment data are gathered, is that the "assumption" of need no longer determines how dietary or nutritional counseling is planned into care. Assessment information can help both the patient and the dental hygienist arrive at a well-informed decision about the need to proceed with further discussions of diet.

IMPORTANCE OF DIET AND NUTRITION IN GENERAL AND ORAL HEALTH

"We are what we eat" is a well-worn, yet appropriate, cliche. Dietary patterns dictate how well the body grows and functions. Failure to consume appropriate amounts of carbohydrates, proteins, lipids, vitamins, minerals, and water can result in general fatigue, dysfunction, and disease.

Carbohydrates, proteins, and lipids are energy-yielding nutrients and provide substrate to build and repair cells. Carbohydrates are the body's major source of fuel. Vitamins and minerals function as regulators in metabolic processes (Hamilton and Whitney, 1991).

Carbon, oxygen, and hydrogen are the three elements that make up *carbohydrates*. The simplest form of a carbohydrate is a *monosaccharide*, such as glucose, fructose, or galactose. *Disaccharides* are double sugars made up of two monosaccharides. Sucrose, lactose, and maltose are disaccharides. The monosaccharides and disaccharides are often referred to as simple carbohydrates or dietary sugars (Hurley, 1992).

Polysaccharides, also known as complex carbohydrates, are long chains of monosaccharide units linked together. Starch, glycogen, and fiber are complex carbohydrates composed of repeating units of glucose molecules. Disaccharides, starch, and glycogen are hydrolyzed to their simplest form (monosaccharide). Energy is ultimately derived from glucose. Glucose is oxidized to carbon dioxide and water, transferring energy in the process to adenosine triphosphate.

Carbohydrates serve other functions in the body. They are an essential component of nerve tissue and can facilitate the oxidation of fats. They contribute to the structural elements of the body, such as collagen. Fiber, which is not digested and absorbed in the human digestive tract, provides a number of healthful benefits (Hurley, 1992). Insoluble fiber, that is, *cellulose, hemicelluloses*, and *lignins*, aids digestion and elimination and is associated with the prevention of colon cancer. Soluble fiber, that is, *pectin, gums,* and *mucilages*, may help lower blood cholesterol and help control diabetes. Because each type of fiber provides distinct benefits, and foods differ in the kinds of fiber they contain, it is important to include a variety of fiber sources in the diet. The National Cancer Institute recommends we consume 20 to 30 g of fiber daily. The current average intake for Americans is 15 g per day (Wardlaw, Insel, and Seyler, 1992). Fiber sources include whole-grain breads and cereals, legumes, fruits and vegetables, nuts, and seeds. Refined grain products are poor fiber sources and should be minimized.

Complex carbohydrates should constitute 50% to 65% of the total diet. Increased complex carbohydrates can replace the less desirable fats, which have been shown to increase the risk of heart disease and cancer (Good news, 1987). Complex carbohydrate intake has declined in the U.S. diet, while that of refined sugars continue to increase. The recommendation is to limit refined sugars to 10% of caloric intake. Currently consumption is at 18% with an average consumption of 130 pounds per person per year, much of it in processed foods (Hurley, 1992). If too much carbohydrate is ingested, the excess is converted to fat and deposited in the body's adipose tissues. Therefore a large intake of carbohydrates can lead to obesity. Frequent ingestion of fermentable carbohydrates promotes tooth decay (Diet, 1984; Firestone, 1982; Nizel and Papas, 1989; Randolph and Dennison, 1981).

Proteins supply energy for the body, but their more critical role is as an essential component of body tissues, enzymes, antibodies, and hormones. Approximately 50% of dry body weight is protein. Proteins are composed of amino acids linked by peptide bonds. The number and arrangement of amino acids determine the type of protein and its function. Twenty-two amino acids are required to build protein structures. The body can synthesize many; however, nine essential amino acids must be obtained in the diet (Nizel and Papas, 1989). The recommended intake for protein is 12% to 15% of calories consumed. The U.S. diet typically provides twice the amount of protein required (Hurley, 1992).

Lipids, a term used for fats and fatlike substances, also have important functions in the body. They are integral components of cells and cell membranes. They are necessary for normal growth and skin health, and they carry the fat-soluble vitamins A, D, E, and K. Stored fats help insulate and cushion the body. Additionally, they lend flavor to food and are digested slowly, thus reducing hunger sensations. Dietary fats are made up predominantly of triglycerides with three fatty acids attached. Saturated fatty acids, found mostly in animal foods, tend to elevate blood cholesterol levels and are implicated in the development of cardiovascular disease. A high-fat intake is also associated with heart disease and several types of cancer as well (Hurley, 1992).

The recommendation is to limit fat intake to 30% of calories consumed and saturated fat to 10%. The average American consumes a diet of 37% fat with 13% to 15% saturated fat (Wardlaw, Insel, and Seyler, 1992). Suggestions for achieving a 30% fat diet include:

Choosing lean meats, fish, poultry, and dry beans as protein sources; using nonfat or lowfat milk and milk products; limiting intake of fats and oils high in saturated fat; trimming fat off meats; broiling, baking or boiling instead of frying and moderating consumption of fat-containing foods, such as breaded or deep-fried foods...and increasing consumption of whole grains, fruits and vegetables (Wardlaw, Insel, and Seyler, 1992).

Caloric intake from carbohydrates, proteins, and lipids should balance with calories expended in daily activities. If intake exceeds energy used, the excess will be converted to and stored as fat deposits, and weight gain will occur. Conversely, if intake is lower than output, weight loss will oc-

cur. Because of the multiple functions that these three nutrients serve, none of them should be strictly eliminated from the diet. Moderation in all three, with the total calories consumed balanced with energy used, is a healthier approach to weight control.

Vitamins, in contrast to carbohydrates, proteins, and fats, do not supply energy. They function as catalysts or coenzymes to regulate metabolism and to assist in forming body tissues. As mentioned earlier, vitamins A, D, E, and K are fat-soluble vitamins. Any excess is stored, and adverse effects can result if this excess reaches critical levels. The other vitamins are water soluble and thus are not readily stored in the body. Excess amounts are largely excreted.

The vitamin B complex consists of 11 different vitamins. All of them are water soluble. All but three (inositol, choline, and paraaminobenzoic acid) are classified as necessary nutrients for human beings. The complete metabolism of carbohydrates depends on the presence of adequate amounts of each of the energy-releasing vitamins: niacin, thiamine, riboflavin, pantothenic acid, and biotin (Nizel and Papas, 1989).

Folacin and vitamin B_{12} play a role in deoxyribonucleic and ribonucleic acid and protein synthesis; thus they are essential in the formation of cells that undergo continued replacement, such as red blood cells. Folacin is poorly absorbed and is easily destroyed in cooking and processing. Thus it is commonly found to be deficient in a high percentage of the population. Oral contraceptives also affect folacin bioavailability (Nizel and Papas, 1989; Pollack and Kravits, 1985). Vitamin B_6 (pyridoxine) serves as a cofactor for enzyme systems involved in amino acid metabolism thus is critical to protein synthesis (Nizel and Papas 1989). Vitamin B_6 was once prescribed to help alleviate premenstrual syndrome symptoms but that practice is presently considered unreliable and dangerously toxic in high doses. (Wardlaw, Insel, and Seyler, 1992)

Because the B-complex vitamins are so interrelated, a discrete deficiency of any one of them probably does not occur; rather there is a deficiency of several. Therefore, for symptoms of Vitamin B deficiency, a supplement that includes the range of B vitamins is indicated. A diet that contains moderate amounts of meats, dairy products, breads and cereals, and green leafy vegetables will supply all of the B vitamins.

Ascorbic acid, or vitamin C, is also a water-soluble vitamin that is found in citrus fruits, red and green peppers, parsley, turnip greens, and other leafy vegetables. Vitamin C plays an essential role in collagen synthesis and is therefore an important component of the organic matrix of teeth and periodontal tissues, including alveolar bone. Its role in collagen formation influences capillary permeability and woundhealing. A person with a vitamin C deficiency often bruises easily because of capillary fragility and may have hemorrhagic tissues. Vitamin C is involved in phagocytosis and acts as a detoxifying agent (Nizel and Papas, 1989). Dietary intake of vitamin C enhances absorption of nonheme iron by 40%, but both must be present in the intestine at the same time to be effective (Olson and Hodges, 1987).

As an antioxidant, vitamin C minimizes cell damage resulting from oxidative substances, such as free radicals. Some sources of free radicals include pollution, tobacco smoke, pesticides, and metabolic end products (Padh, 1991). Research has concluded that smokers require a greater intake of ascorbic acid to achieve the same serum levels as nonsmokers; thus the RDA has been increased from 60 to 100 mg/day (Schectman et al, 1991).

Vitamin C is often mislabeled the "sunshine vitamin," probably because of its association with orange juice and that industry's advertising approaches. However, the real sunshine vitamin is vitamin D, because it forms in the presence of ultraviolet light. It is absorbed through the digestive tract as it is ingested in food and drink. Less dietary vitamin D is required in people with extensive exposure to sunshine. It is commonly added to milk to ensure a dietary source. As vitamin D is best absorbed in the presence of calcium and phosphorus, milk is an ideal medium.

The primary function of vitamin D relates to the absorption and homeostasis of calcium. It distributes calcium and phosphorus ions within the bony matrix. Therefore it is critical to the proper formation of teeth and their supporting bone.

Vitamin D can be extremely toxic if taken in excess. Large amounts can cause intense calcification of bone, formation of renal calculi, and calcification of blood vessels. This is one instance in which megavitamin doses can be extremely harmful (Nizel and Papas, 1989; Randolph and Dennison, 1981).

Vitamin A is another vitamin that can result in severe toxicity if it is ingested in large amounts. Yellow skin and oral mucosa (carotenemia), anorexia, hyperirritability, skin lesions, bone decalcification, and increased intracranial pressures are signs of toxicity.

In its proper dosage, vitamin A is essential for proper vision, control of the differentiation of epithelium in mucus-secreting structures, bone remodeling, normal activity of the reproductive system, and the activity of the body's enzymes. Therefore vitamin A is important to the oral cavity, with its plethora of mucus-secreting structures, and as bone is remodeled to adjust to occlusal patterns and orthodontic treatment. Milk is fortified with vitamin A, and the vitamin is found in many vegetables.

Vitamin K is produced by microorganisms in the intestinal tract. It also occurs in green vegetables, egg yolk, and liver. It is essential for the formation of prothrombin and other clotting factors. Blood will not clot without prothrombin; thus vitamin K is important in health and disease. As it is produced in the intestinal tract, it is not given as a supplement except when pregnancy or an imminent surgical procedure indicates the need.

The last of the four fat-soluble vitamins is vitamin E. Its primary functions relate to reproduction and membrane stability, probably because of its role as an antioxidant in reducing the destruction of lipids carrying other fat-soluble vitamins and necessary fatty acids (Nizel and Papas, 1989).

Several inorganic elements that are essential for health are found in quantifiable amounts in the human body. Calcium, phosphorus, magnesium, sodium, potassium, sulfur, iron, and chlorine all contribute to the growth, development, and function of the body. Trace amounts of elements, including copper, manganese, zinc, iodine, cobalt, molybdenum, selenium, and fluoride, affect the body's biologic systems. Besides these, several other elements found in the body are not considered essential for health or have not been fully studied.

The most critical elements in terms of dietary intake are calcium and phosphorus for the development and health of bones and teeth, iron for hemoglobin formation, iodine for thyroid regulation, and fluoride for decay-resistant teeth. The others are critical as well, but usually are ingested in adequate amounts if the aforementioned specific elements are present in the diet (Nizel and Papas, 1989; Randolph and Dennison, 1982).

Calcium is receiving increased attention because of its link to osteoporosis, a debilitating nutritional disease in which calcium is depleted from the bones, causing skeletal deformities and increasing the likelihood of fractures. This problem is most evident in postmenopausal women, who seem to lose calcium from the system more rapidly. Calcium absorption decreases with age. Impaired renal function, decreased intestinal absorption of vitamin D, and low exposure to sunshine seem to contribute to the problem. Fluoride consumption helps retard the loss of calcium; the concentrations found in community water supplies provide a satisfactory amount. Older adults require 50% to 100% more vitamin D than young adults, and their calcium intake should be 800 to 1200 mg per day. Additional research on the effects of dietary supplementation is needed (Schaafsma et al, 1987).

Calcium deficiency is prevalent and should be checked for as a part of routine nutritional assessment and recommendations. The average woman's intake is 500 mg per day (Fisher, 1990). Persons susceptible to osteoporosis include young, growing people (especially girls) and adults who do not consume dairy products; elderly, sedentary people who live primarily indoors; and patients with anorexia nervosa (Schaafsma et al, 1987). One cup of milk contains approximately 300 mg of calcium; people who cannot or will not consume dairy products can take calcium carbonate supplements. Such a recommendation should be made even for women as young as 20 years of age and certainly for those of 40 or more years (Fahey, Boltri, and Monk, 1987b). Patients should also learn that exercise and vitamin D help bone strength and that cigarette smoking, caffeine, and alcohol appear to be detrimental to calcium balance (Sutnick, 1987).

Water, which serves as the fluid medium for the body's chemical and physical reactions, is probably the most critical dietary component. Without water, all the other nutrients would be incapable of activity. Water carries nutrients and oxygen to all parts of the body through the blood and the lymphatic system. It helps control body temperature and removes metabolic waste in urine and sweat. The average adult consumes and excretes about 2 to 3 quarts of water each day in various forms. People who work in a warm climate and perspire greatly require more. The body needs six to eight 8-ounce glasses of water each day, whether we feel thirsty or not (Getting the most, 1986).

People require different amounts of certain nutrients during times of stress. If an individual is marginally deficient in particular nutrients, stress may make the condition worse. In fact, undernutrition is a form of physical stress (Kipp, 1985). Alcoholics place a special form of stress on the body, frequently have poor diets, and suffer additional nutritional depletion through adverse alcohol-nutrient interactions (Lieber, 1984). Cancer patients have special nutritional needs (Lum and Gallagher-Allred, 1984). Poor nutrition reduces the probability of survival for victims of head and neck cancer. This may result, in part, from compromised immune responses (Brooks, 1985; Homsy, Morrow, and Levy, 1986). Epidemiologic studies have suggested that nutritional deficiencies of vitamin A, riboflavin, and beta-carotene may be linked to tongue cancers in nonusers of tobacco and alcohol (Richie, 1991).

Rapid growth, pregnancy, lactation, and advanced age indicate special nutritional needs (Fahey, Boltri, and Monk, 1987a, 1987b). Athletes require increased levels of certain nutrients and can improve performance by decreasing certain types of food and drink (American Dietetic Association, 1987a; Wilmore and Freund, 1986). Deuster and colleagues (1986) reported that highly trained women athletes consumed diets that exceeded RDA values for some nutrients and were substantially below recommendations for others.

Consuming too much as well as too little of most nutrients can increase the body's propensity for disease. Obesity, scurvy, rickets, and dental caries are prime examples of conditions based largely on deleterious dietary habits. With the mention of dental caries as a nutritional disease, it may become more apparent that nutrition may have a direct effect on oral health as well as on general physical well-being. The oral cavity has been described as a barometer of general health (Randolph, 1977; Randolph and Dennison, 1981). This is particularly true in relation to nutritional problems. The nature of the oral structures allows them to reflect the body's nutritional maladies. The oral mucosa may appear extremely pallid or quite red. The texture of the tissue may indicate edema or friability. Cracks or fissures in the corners of the mouth or a heavily coated tongue may be signs that an individual's general health is less than ideal. The presence of a large number of carious lesions provides information about the patient's consumption of fermentable carbohydrates (Randolph and Dennison, 1981). Another nutritional factor associated with dental health is that tooth loss adversely affects a person's ability to eat correctly. Thus there is a reciprocal relationship between oral health and nutrition (Geissler and Bates, 1984).

TOXICITY

The preceding section mentions the toxic effects of some vitamins taken in large quantities. This is true for the fat-soluble vitamins (A, D, E, and K), for vitamin C, and for pyridoxine (B_6), which recently was found to produce toxic effects including severe sensory nervous system dysfunction and ataxia (Schaumberg, et al, 1983). Minerals such as zinc, fluoride, and iron, essential in prescribed amounts, also produce toxic effects in large doses (Hamilton and Whitney, 1991; Randolph and Dennison, 1981).

In recent years there has been a widespread trend towards taking large doses of vitamin C to prevent or cure infectious diseases and cancer. No well-controlled studies have supported this practice, and several have failed to show significant-differences between vitamin C and placebo. In addition, large doses of vitamin C raise the uric acid level of urine (sometimes triggering gout in susceptible persons); they obscure the results of some medical tests; and they impair the ability of white blood cells to kill bacteria, actually worsening infections. They may cause kidney stones, affect fertility, and induce a deficiency rebound effect in newborns whose mothers routinely took large doses.

Toxic reactions to large doses of vitamins are becoming more of a problem since the awareness of good nutrition has grown among the general public. Some people erroneously assume that more of a good thing is better. Self-prescribed doses may far exceed needed amounts and may be seen as a substitute for eating proper foods. In addition, lay articles advocating the use of megavitamin doses are omnipresent, unwittingly recommending levels of vitamins or minerals that not only exceed what is needed for normal functioning but that actually produce negative effects. In some cases the toxic response is very similar to the deficiency symptoms, which may prompt the person to take even more of the nutrient. It is therefore very important during a nutritional assessment to inquire about what vitamin supplements are being taken, in what doses, and with what frequency (Hamilton and Whitney, 1991).

DENTAL CARIES AND DIET

Much of the research related to the nutritional effect on caries has centered on systemic fluoride's effect on teeth. Teeth with a high fluoride content are less susceptible to caries (Hefferren, Ayer, and Koehler, 1981). Diet-related cariogenic properties include "the chemical composition of the food, the physical form in which it is eaten, the frequency with which it is eaten, the oral clearance time, the concentration of sugars and the organoleptic effect of the food" (Hoffman et al, 1988).

The simple sugars (monosaccharides and disaccharides), both naturally occurring and processed, are highly cariogenic. The cariogenicity of starchy foods is enhanced in the presence of sugar and in cooked form. Cooking changes the nature of the food's starchy base, promoting greater retention and poor oral clearance (Hoffman et al, 1988). Retained complex carbohydrates are reduced by the amylase enzyme in saliva to more simple forms, and they can be fermented by the bacteria in plaque. Retentive, sticky sugars (such as caramels or taffy) that are not quickly diluted by saliva and flushed from the oral cavity promote caries to a greater extent than do liquid sugars (such as soda pop).

Binns (1981) and Newbrun (1982b) have summarized the numerous epidemiologic and clinical studies showing that eating high-sugar diets predicts a high caries rate. People living in countries where sucrose is consumed in large quantities have higher caries rates than people living where sucrose intake is low. Sreebny (1982) confirms that a diet of manufactured or processed food that contains higher levels of sucrose promotes higher levels of caries activity.

Sucrose is used by bacteria in the synthesis of dental plaque (Babcock-Goodman and Suzuki, 1989). The more sugar consumed, especially sucrose, the thicker and more plentiful the plaque (Carlsson and Egelberg, 1965). When oral hygiene is poor, even low quantities of sugar consumption promote caries (Kleemola-Kujala and Räsänen, 1982). Ingested carbohydrates can diffuse into the plaque, where bacteria, especially *Streptococcus mutans,* ferment the simple sugars, producing acid that demineralizes the teeth, initiating a carious lesion (Hefferen, Ayer, and Koehler, 1981).

Plaque is especially important in promoting smooth-surface caries, because it provides the matrix for holding the bacteria and fermenting sugars against a surface that does not otherwise easily retain food. Pit and fissure caries formation relies less on plaque, since the anatomy of the tooth enhances sugar retention and access to acid-forming bacteria.

The longer sucrose is in contact with plaque, the lower the interdental plaque pH (i.e., the greater the acidity of the plaque). Therefore all-day suckers or lollipops, chewing gum, or slowly dissolving hard candies and mints pose a major risk in caries formation. So does a slowly sipped cola or other sugared beverage. The passive, continual availability of sucrose keeps the acidity of the plaque high, enhancing ongoing tooth dissolution (Firestone, 1982; Hoffman et al, 1988; Newbrun, 1982a).

This point is especially evident in cases where babies are put to bed with a bottle of formula, milk, juice, or other substance that contains or is easily converted to simple sugars. The liquid, which stays in the mouth and is periodically replenished as the child sucks during sleep, is chemically reduced and fermented, causing rampant tooth destruction. This is referred to as baby-bottle or nursing caries (Randolph and Dennison, 1981; Ripa, 1988).

Thus a major emphasis in dietary counseling is on reducing the frequency and duration of ingestion of fermentable carbohydrates and eliminating of sticky sweets. Patients who have a high rate of smooth-surface caries (usually on the gingival third of mandibular teeth) are prime candidates for a review of snacking habits. A patient with this clinical finding may keep a box of cookies in the desk drawer at work, eat sugared mints or lozenges, chew gum, or frequently consume sugared drinks such as sweetened coffee or tea, soda pop, or lemonade.

Sreebny (1982) has concluded, based on epidemiologic data, that the "safe" upper limit of daily sugar consumption may be 50 g. For many individuals even this may be too much. Ingesting more than this raises the risk of caries considerably. This amount takes on more significance when the amounts of sugar in typical portions of commonly ingested foods are known: ketchup, 5

g; fruit yogurt, 18 g; canned fruit, 46 g; milk chocolate bar, 26 g; hot chocolate, 12 g; cola, 32 g (Wykeham-Martin, 1981).

Foods with a sugar content of 15% to 20% or higher are poor snack food choices because they are highly cariogenic. Even items that are 10% to 20% sugar should be restricted from between-meal use (Newbrun, 1982a). Sugar, in any form, listed early in the ingredients on a label indicates a highly sweetened product. Several forms of sugar may be added in lesser amounts, but added together contribute significantly to the overall sugar content. Many processed foods today are sweetened with high-fructose corn syrup, which is inexpensive and very sweet (Hurley, 1992).

A number of dietary factors have been found to modify the cariogenicity of carbohydrates. Fiber, some cheeses, fats, phosphates, calcium, calcium lactate, and calcium propionate may have cariostatic properties. Sequence of food intake has been found to be a factor. Studies have shown that ingestion of sugared foods followed by ingestion of nonsugared foods can minimize the pH drop and the cariogenic potential of the diet (Hoffman et al, 1988).

Many sugar substitutes have been introduced to satisfy the public's demand for sweeteners that do not add calories and do not promote tooth decay. Cyclamates came under scrutiny for their links with cancer in laboratory animals and were banned in the United States in 1969. Saccharin-containing products are labeled as hazardous in the United States. Saccharin is banned in Canada, but cyclamates are allowed there. Aspartame is now widely used as a sugar substitute, having been reviewed by the Food and Drug Administration and found to have no adverse effects for most people (American Dietetic Association, 1987b; Babcock-Goodman and Suzuki, 1989; Safety of aspartame, 1986).

In recommending a reduction in sugar intake, the proposed alternatives should be evaluated for their safety in general health as well as for their role in dental health. Every clinician should be aware of what is available, what is "safe," and what foods or snacks it is found in.

PERIODONTAL DISEASE AND NUTRITION

Poor nutrition is not the primary cause of periodontal disease, but it can be considered a contributing factor. "Since all tissue integrity ultimately depends on nutrition and the periodontium is a part of the body, it will be affected by nutrition" (Wilton et al, 1988). Nutritional deficiencies may alter the host's resistance to disease and impair the tissue repair process. Epithelial and connective tissue cells of the periodontium are continually being renewed. The turnover rate of sulcular epithelium is thought to be about 3 to 6 days (Alfano, 1976). This high turnover rate requires a constant supply of nutrients for synthesis of deoxyribonucleic and ribonucleic acid and protein. These tissues are particularly vulnerable, therefore, to deficiencies of nutrients involved in cell formation (Alfano, 1976; Nizel and Papas, 1989). Poor nutrition can thus compromise the integrity of the periodontal tissues, rendering them more susceptible to disease (Alfano, 1976; DePaola et al, 1984; Diet, 1984; Nizel and Papas, 1989). Tissue repair also depends on the nutritional status of the host, and nutrient requirements may, in fact, be elevated (Alfano, 1976). Nutrients that play a major role in the development, maintenance, and resistance of the periodontal tissues include vitamins A and C, folacin, iron, zinc, and calcium (Nizel and Papas, 1989; Pollack and Kravitz, 1985; Randolph and Dennison, 1981).

Recent research suggests that malnourished children are more likely to harbor the bacteria associated with periodontal disease than are well-nourished children (Sawyer et al, 1986). There is growing evidence that nutritional deficiencies may enhance *Candida* infections (Samaranayake, 1986).

Much attention has focused on altered immunity in periodontal disease: the disease becomes active and degenerative when the host is susceptible. It is clear that malnutrition can alter a person's immunity (Homsy, Morrow, and Levy, 1986; Sherman, 1986).

Socransky and Haffejee (1981) point out that "differences in host susceptibility to various infectious diseases have been recognized for decades and periodontal diseases should be no exception." For optimal function, cells of the immune system depend on various nutrients acting as cofactors in metabolic processes. Nutrient deficiencies can affect anatomic development of lymphoid tissue, mucus production, integrity of the skin and mucous membranes, antibody synthesis and response, cell proliferation, chemotactic factors, phagocytic activity, and modulation and regulation of immune processes (Chandra, 1990, 1991; Hamilton & Whitney, 1991; Keusch, 1983; Sherman, 1986). Not only do extreme cases of malnutrition impair the immune response, but mild nutrient deficiencies have an impact as well (Chandra, 1990). Alterations in the immune response can occur early in the development of a nutritional deficiency (Chandra, 1991). Researchers suspect that subclinical nutrient deficiencies may be found in people who "appear healthy," resulting in impaired immunity (Barone, 1988). A number of nutrients are under investigation for their relationship to immunity, including vitamins A, C, B_6, B_{12} and E; pantothenic acid; iron; zinc; copper; beta-carotene; and lipids (Barone, 1988; Chandra, 1990a, 1991b; Hamilton and Whitney, 1991; Sherman, 1986).

Dietary factors such as sugar intake and diets of soft consistency may contribute to bacterial growth and plaque formation (Newman, 1990; Nizel and Papas, 1989). A diet of fibrous, firm foods has a positive influence on the periodontium. Vigorous mastication stimulates salivary flow, increases circulation in the periodontium, strengthens the periodontal ligament, and may increase alveolar bone density (Nizel and Papas, 1989). In light of the relationship between diet, nutrition, and periodontal disease, nutritional assessment and recommendation are an important part of a total periodontal prevention, treatment, and maintenance program.

DIET AND CANCER: NEW FOCUS IN NUTRITIONAL ASSESSMENT

Dental professionals help promote good general health when they help patients replace high-calorie, caries-promoting foods with nutritionally well-balanced choices. This can be accomplished by eliminating or reducing snack foods and high-sugar breakfast choices (doughnuts, sweet rolls, and processed cereals), and for the most part dental professionals limit their nutritional guidance to this sphere. They may emphasize the need for vegetables, fruits, and protein sources, but the diet in general has been a secondary focus for most. New evidence of the importance of diet in relation to cancer in general, however, raises the consideration of how far a dentist or hygienist should extend advice in counseling patients.

The Committee on Diet, Nutrition, and Cancer of the National Academy of Sciences reviewed hundreds of published research findings to identify those pointing conclusively to the influence of dietary habits on cancer formation.* They reviewed epidemiologic studies of population groups with varying dietary patterns and linked the findings of those studies with laboratory and case study results. Based on these findings, the American Institute for Cancer Research (AICR) (1990) devised a set of dietary guidelines, recently revised to reflect the most recent scientific research, for lowering the risk of cancer. These guidelines should be followed in reviewing your own diet as well as the diets of patients:

1. Reduce the intake of total dietary fat from the current average of approximately 37% to a level of 30% of total calories and, in particular, reduce the intake of saturated fat.
2. Increase the consumption of fruits, vegetables, and whole grains.
3. Consume salt-cured, salt-pickled, and smoked foods only in moderation.
4. Drink alcoholic beverages only in moderation, if at all.

The Committee also recommended that carcinogenic and mutagenic contaminants in food be prevented through regulation and continued study of food additives and processing (Palmer and Bakshi, 1983). Though certain chemical additives and pesticides are suspect as potential threats to health, diet and tobacco pose a greater risk, accounting 67% of cancer deaths (Milner, 1989).

Many of the findings relating fat consumption to cancer have come from studies designed to investigate fats and cardiovascular disease. In addition to linking high intake of fats, especially of saturated fats, to heart and blood vessel problems, they have found that diets rich in either saturated or unsaturated fats are highly correlated with cancer of the breast, colon, and prostate gland. Cancers of the testis, uterus, ovary, and pancreas have also been associated with high dietary fat levels (Palmer and Bakshi, 1983).

In these studies persons who had a high fat intake but also consumed large quantities of vegetables had a lower risk of colon cancer. Several other studies have shown that "consumption of vegetables in general, raw vegetables (e.g., lettuce and celery), or cruciferous vegetables in particular (e.g., cabbage, cauliflower, brussels sprouts, and broccoli)" is inversely related to cancer of the alimentary tract (the esophagus, stomach, or colon). It is difficult to determine the mode of their anticarcinogenic activity. Some attribute it to their high fiber content, whereas others cite their vitamin A content or suspect some yet unknown biochemical function (Palmer and Bakshi, 1983). Beta-carotene has recently received much attention as a protective substance. It is found in deep yellow-orange and dark green vegetables and fruits (AICR, 1990).

Fresh fruit consumption or estimated vitamin C intake has also been shown to be inversely related to cancer incidence, especially of the stomach, esophagus, and larynx, and to uterine cervical dysplasia.

Bacon, ham, and other foods preserved with salt, smoke, or salt pickling are now known to be highly carcinogenic, but vitamin C tends to reduce their harmful effect (Palmer and Bakshi, 1983). Vitamin E may also protect against stomach and esophageal cancers associated with eating these types of foods (AICR, 1990).

Numerous studies have shown a correlation between alcohol and cancer of the esophagus, tongue, pharynx, hypopharynx, larynx, lung, lip, glottis, and supraglottic region. Studies also have shown "an interactive role between tobacco and alcohol in tumorigenesis of the oral cavity, larynx, lung, and esophagus" (Palmer and Bakshi, 1983). The incidence of oral cavity cancer among heavy drinkers and smokers is greater than 20 times that of nondrinkers and nonsmokers (Richie, 1991).

Given that dental professionals have the most regular and frequent contact with healthy people, and given the convincing evidence of dietary contributions to cancer, hygienists can assume a role of major importance in reviewing their patient's diets and moving them towards more healthful choices that are likely to reduce the risk of cancer.

CLINICAL ASSESSMENT: INTRAORAL AND EXTRAORAL EXAMINATION

During the complete intraoral and extraoral examination phases, the appearance of the gingivae, teeth, lips, and oral mucosa, as well as the texture of the hair and the skin, may provide some clue

---

*The complete report can be found in National Academy of Sciences: *Diet, nutrition, and cancer,* Washington, DC, 1992, Committee on Diet, Nutrition, and Cancer Assembly of Life Sciences, National Research Council. The Palmer and Bakshi (1983) citation is a summary report of the original 500-page document.

that the patient has nutritional problems that should be carefully assessed (Christakis, 1973). Therefore the dental hygienist is in an ideal position to identify potential nutritional and other general health problems during the complete head and neck examination (Chapter 8).

When a nutrient is not present in the diet, blood and tissue levels are maintained by reserves in specific tissues. No clinical signs are evident until the reserve stores are depleted and biochemical changes occur. Thus a person with obvious clinical symptoms can be assumed to have a relatively long term deficiency rather than a poor diet for a day or two (Chipponi et al, 1982). Similarly, rampant caries reflects nutritional patterns that have existed for more than a few days.

However, the examination procedures are only one step in the nutritional assessment component of care. Just as the patient learns to conduct a self-assessment of oral structures and to observe healthy structures as well as those which have changed in appearance or texture over time, he or she should learn how to self-assess dietary habits. Leading a patient through the self-assessment procedure is a learning procedure in itself. Additionally, it provides key data for making a decision regarding the need for dietary modifications and/or referral.

NUTRITIONAL SELF-ASSESSMENT

One way to include nutritional self-assessment routinely in dental hygiene care is to develop a simple questionnaire that can be used to determine what a "usual" day's diet is like (Nizel and Papas, 1989; Randolph, 1977). This can be done by asking a patient what he or she ate the day before, including at what time of day and the approximate amounts. The questionnaire can be given to the patient to complete, followed by a discussion, or the hygienist can ask the questions in an interview format. Twenty-four hour recalls can provide reliable information if they are completed as interviews (Morgan et al, 1987).

Generally, a patient can be expected to recall with reasonable accuracy the previous day's intake. As with any questionnaire that seeks to gather information but not to place any particular values on behavior, the questions should be phrased in such a way that the patient does not begin to be embarrassed, angry, or puzzled by a failure to comply with the pattern of activities suggested by the questionnaire (Randolph, 1977).

For instance, asking "What did you have for breakfast?" implies that breakfast should have been eaten. An alternative question is, "What was the first thing you ate or drank yesterday?" Then the following question can be, "What time of the day did you eat (drink) that?" and "How much of it did you consume?" A series of such questions can elicit the approximate kinds of foods and beverages consumed, the times of day, and the approximate amounts. Keeping cups, spoons, drinking glasses, and plastic containers handy can help the patient identify more precisely the amounts ingested (Christakis, 1973). It is important to ask about between-meal snacks, glasses of water, and any pills or other medications that were consumed. People often feel that snacks do not count in a dietary assessment and may ignore water or vitamin pills as sources of nutrients.

The question regarding pills and other medications may help expose noncompliance with prescribed dosages of drugs. For instance, if the patient reports during the medical history that a drug to control high blood pressure has been prescribed, the hygienist might assume that the patient takes it. However, if during the dietary assessment the patient fails to report having taken the medication during an entire day, this may be a sign that the patient takes the drug sporadically or not at all, regardless of the fact that it has been prescribed. This is also one way to determine if the patient has adopted any other habits related to prescribed drugs or over-the-counter medications. In any case, just as the other phases of patient assessment can yield valuable clues regarding nutritional problems, the dietary assessment can provide valuable information on the patient's medical status.

Once all the suggested questions have been answered and the dietary form has been completed, the hygienist should ask, "Is this a typical day's eating pattern? Would you normally eat and drink this amount of food at these times of day?" Further questioning should include, "What about on days when you are at work?" (or, "What about on days when you are at home?") A person's eating habits may differ greatly from the weekday to the weekend or from days spent at versus off work (Randolph, 1977; Randolph and Dennison, 1981). If the day described is atypical, the assessment should be repeated at a subsequent visit for a more valid assessment (Christakis, 1973).

According to Randolph (1977), "We tend to

choose food and beverage on the basis of where we are, who we are with, the time of day, the next scheduled activity, the way we feel, the money we have and are willing to spend, and what is available." Current peer group norms (particularly among college students or institutionalized persons and certainly in families) affect dietary choices (Porter, 1987).

A homemaker may have a substantially different pattern of eating when the family is home than when he or she is home alone. A question regarding this may ferret out information about the hoard of chocolate bars in the bed stand or the secret supply of beer hidden in the old refrigerator in the attic. With the right questions, the hygienist can learn a great deal about the patient's dietary habits.

Once a full day's food and beverages have been identified and verified as representing the patient's daily routine, the hygienist should ask the patient to circle in red all those solid foods that he or she knows contain sugar. Most patients can identify a large number of foods that contain sugar (Randolph, 1977; Randolph and Dennison, 1981). An orange pencil should then be used to circle liquids that contain sugar. Dairy foods should be identified by the patient and circled in yellow, meat or meat alternates in blue, vegetables and fruits in green, and bread and cereals in brown. Watching as the patient circles the items according to food group and identifies sugar-containing products allows the hygienist to assess the patient's knowledge of nutrition.

Once the circling is complete, the hygienist should ask the patient if there is anything he or she would like to change about the diet. In most instances, this too will be a strong indicator of what the patient knows but does not necessarily practice. Nutritional behavior (actual food choices) may not correlate well with knowledge about proper nutrition (Shepherd and Stockley, 1987). Hearing the patient say all the right things about what to increase and what to decrease can be quite an awakening. In most instances, the hygienist abandons preplanned lectures on proper diet and nutrition. No doubt there also will be considerable evidence regarding the patient's attitude about changes. For instance, if the patient can identify what should be changed but says, "There's no way I'm going to change it, however," the hygienist may need to be reasonably cautious about offering multiple suggestions for

change. Not all patients want this kind of help; many may resent it. People will not attend to a message unless they have some need to hear what is being said. A person who has no perceived need to change probably will doze through a lecture on what to change in the diet. The hygienist must awaken the need to know; this may not occur until after several encounters or after several decades (Porter, 1987).

Once the patient has had an opportunity to assess what should (or could) be changed in the diet, the hygienist can begin to provide a few insights into the diet of which the patient may not be aware. For instance, most patients are not aware of the vast number of foods that contain refined sugars. Therefore several additional items on the day's menu may need to be circled in red or orange to reflect their actual contents. Keeping common food items in the dental operatory or counseling room can be helpful in showing the patient that ketchup, many canned vegetables, and crackers, for instance, contain sugar. By pointing out how foods are labeled, the patient can learn about concentrations of sugar and salt in the product. In all instances the approach should be "You might be interested to know that. . ." while circling the additional sugared foods.

The foods circled according to food groups should be reviewed for accuracy and to evaluate dietary adequacy. Table 24-1 provides an overview of these food groupings. The "four food groups" have been used as a diet planning and evaluation tool since 1956. In 1991 the U.S. Department of Agriculture (USDA) issued its latest revised plan called the *USDA's Food Guide—A Pattern for Daily Food Choices*. This guide is designed to "represent a total diet, rather than simply a foundation for a diet" (Wardlaw, Insel, and Seyler, 1992). The emphasis is on increasing dietary energy from complex carbohydrates while limiting fat intake. This guide recommends an increase in fruits and vegetable servings from four per day to five to nine per day (including a vitamin C source and a dark green leafy vegetable every day); bread and cereal servings from four per day to six to eleven per day (four or more whole grains); two servings from the milk, yogurt, and cheese group; (lowfat or nonfat choices); and two to three servings from the meat, poultry, fish, dry beans, eggs, and nuts group (5 to 7 ounces total) (USDA, 1990).

National surveys examining food intake have

Table 24-1. The daily food guide

Food group	Suggested servings
Fruits and vegetables	5-9 servings (3-5 vegetables, 2-4 fruits) Count as a serving: 1 c raw leafy greens, ½ c cooked vegetable or diced fruit, 1 medium-size piece of fruit, ¾ c of juice
Breads, cereals, rice, and pasta	6-11 servings (4 or more whole grains) Count as a serving: 1 slice of bread; ½ bun, bagel or English muffin; 1 oz of dry cereal; ½ c of cooked cereal, rice, or pasta
Milk, yogurt, and cheese	2-3 servings (choose nonfat or low-fat products for persons over the age of 2) Count as a serving: 1 c of milk or yogurt or 1½ oz of cheese
Meats, poultry, fish, dry beans and peas, and eggs	2-3 servings (limit to 6 oz daily) Count as a serving: 1-3 oz meat; 3 oz of cooked lean beef or chicken is about the size of a deck of cards; 2 eggs, ½ c cooked beans (eat in place of meat occasionally), 3 oz of tofu

Eat a variety of foods daily, choosing different foods from each group. Most people should have at least the lower number of servings suggested from each food group. Some people may need more because of their body size and activity level. Young children should have a variety of foods but may need small servings (USDA, 1990).

shown that typical U.S. diets are not consistent with these recommendations (Kant et al, 1991a). Only 33% of the U.S. population was found to consume foods from all of the food groups, and only 2.9% consumed at least the recommended number of servings. Foods from the fruit and dairy groups were found to be lacking most often. Servings in the grain and vegetable groups were also likely to be consumed in less than recommended amounts (Kant et al, 1991a). Because certain nutrients are known to be associated with each food group, these dietary intake patterns can be used to identify nutrients that may be lacking in the diet (Kant et al, 1991b).

Two steps that are helpful in determining the effect of the day's diet on the patient's well-being include identifying how long sugar has been active in the oral cavity and how closely the patient's diet adheres to the Recommended Dietary Allowances (RDAs) (Table 24-2) and/or each of the four food groups. The former determination involves counting the number of times sugar was consumed and multiplying by 20. Each time sugar is ingested, it provides 20 minutes of acid production to promote tooth decay and the proliferation of plaque. Therefore calculating the number of minutes (or hours) that acid has been active in the mouth can provide an interesting summary of the effect of the diet on the teeth.

Likewise each of the other items circled in the various colors should be tabulated to determine if their frequency and amounts relate to those suggested by federal standards. The Food and Nutrition Board of the National Research Council of the National Academy of Sciences is responsible for recommending a specific optimum quantity, based on sex and age, for each nutrient. Recommendations are issued every 5 years. The quantities suggested provide a margin of safety and are designed for an average person; therefore they do not address individual differences or the nutritional needs of medically compromised people. As a basic reference, the RDAs provide overall useful guidelines for quantifying a diet. The RDAs are not necessarily a "daily requirement" but should be achieved over a 3-day period (Monsen, 1989).

If specific amounts of nutrients ingested can be identified, they can be compared with RDA standards to determine if intake approximates the optimum levels (Hamilton and Whitney, 1981; Randolph and Dennison, 1981). Many nutrition texts include comprehensive listings of food values that make it possible to perform a detailed analysis of a diet. Nutrient analysis by computer has simplified this process (Randolph and Dennison, 1981). The RDA does not suggest appropriate intakes of fat, carbohydrate, cholesterol, or fiber. It does not describe associations between disease and diet or provide guidance in controlling obesity or in selecting foods (Harper, 1987). Olson (1987) describes the RDA as "a suggested level of intake that prevents signs of deficiency, provides a defined adequate reserve and is fully consistent with

Table 24-2. Food and Nutrition Board, National Academy of Sciences–National Research Council Recommended Dietary Allowances.* Revised 1989. Designed for the maintenance of good nutrition of practically all healthy people in the United States

Category	Age (years) or Condition	Weight† (kg)	Weight† (lb)	Height† (cm)	Height† (in)	Protein (g)	Fat-soluble vitamins Vitamin A (μg RE)‡	Vitamin D (μg)§	Vitamin E (mg α-TE) ‖	Vitamin K (μg)
Infants	0.0-0.5	6	13	60	24	13	375	7.5	3	5
	0.5-1.0	9	20	71	28	14	375	10	4	10
Children	1-3	13	29	90	35	16	400	10	6	15
	4-6	20	44	112	44	24	500	10	7	20
	7-10	28	62	132	52	28	700	10	7	30
Males	11-14	45	99	157	62	45	1,000	10	10	45
	15-18	66	145	176	69	59	1,000	10	10	65
	19-24	72	160	177	70	58	1,000	10	10	70
	25-50	79	174	176	70	63	1,000	5	10	80
	51 +	77	170	173	68	63	1,000	5	10	80
Females	11-14	46	101	157	62	46	800	10	8	45
	15-18	55	120	163	64	44	800	10	8	55
	19-24	58	128	164	65	46	800	10	8	60
	25-50	63	138	163	64	50	800	5	8	65
	51 +	65	143	160	63	50	800	5	8	65
Pregnant						60	800	10	10	65
Lactating	1st 6 months					65	1,300	10	12	65
	2nd 6 months					62	1,200	10	11	65

*The allowances, expressed as average daily intakes over time, are intended to provide for individual variations among most normal persons as they live in the United States under usual environmental stresses. Diets should be based on a variety of common foods in order to provide other nutrients for which human requirements have been less well defined. See original source for detailed discussion of allowances and of nutrients not tabulated.

†Weights and heights of Reference Adults are actual medians for the U.S. population of the designated age, as reported by NHANES II. Thje median weights and heights of those under 19 years of age were taken from Hamill et al. (1979). The use of these figures does not imply that the height-to-weight ratios are ideal.

‡Retinol equivalents. 1 retinol equivalent = 1 μg retinol or 6 μg β-carotene. See original source for calculation of vitamin A activity of diets as retinol equivalents.§

As cholecalciferol. 10 μg cholecalciferol = 400 IU of vitamin D.

‖ α-Tocopherol equivalents. 1 mg d-α tocopherol = 1 α-TE. See original source for variation in allowances and calculation of vitamin E activity of the diet as α-tocopherol equivalents.

¶1 NE (niacin equivalent) is equal to 1 mg of niacin or 60 mg of dietary tryptophan.

the health of most members of a healthy population group."

Publication of the 1985 RDAs (tenth edition) was postponed because of differences of opinion on the proposed changes. The controversy involved a dispute in the interpretation of data concerning certain nutrients. A major issue raised was whether or not the RDAs "apply only to the prevention of deficiency diseases or generally to promotion of growth, maintenance of good health, and the reduction of risk of other diseases" (New FNB, 1986). The nutrients at the center of the debate were vitamins A, C, K, B₁₂, folate, and iron. Some authorities recommended

lowering certain nutrients based on current analytical techniques that allow scientists to estimate levels of nutrient requirements more accurately. However, other scientists supported the concept that certain nutrients are associated with chronic disease prevention, such as cancer, and opposed lowering the RDAs. An increase in vitamin A, for example, is currently advocated by the American Cancer Society and the National Cancer Institute (Nieman, Butterworth, and Nieman, 1992).

The tenth edition of the RDAs was finally published in 1989. Changes were approved "only if substantive new information had become available or to alleviate inconsistencies in the prior

Table 24-2—cont'd. Food and Nutrition Board, National Academy of Sciences–National Research Council Recommended Dietary Allowances.* Revised 1989. Designed for the maintenance of good nutrition of practically all healthy people in the United States

Water-soluble vitamins							Minerals						
Vitamin C (mg)	Thiamin (mg)	Riboflavin (mg)	Niacin (mg NE)	Vitamin B6 (mg)	Folate (µg)	Vitamin B12 (µg)	Calcium (mg)	Phosphorus (mg)	Magnesium (mg)	Iron (mg)	Zinc (mg)	Iodine (µg)	Selenium (µg)
30	0.3	0.4	5	0.3	25	0.3	400	300	40	6	5	40	10
35	0.4	0.5	6	0.6	35	0.5	600	500	60	10	5	50	15
40	0.7	0.8	9	1.0	50	0.7	800	800	80	10	10	70	20
45	0.9	1.1	12	1.1	75	1.0	800	800	120	10	10	90	20
45	1.0	1.2	13	1.4	100	1.4	800	800	170	10	10	120	30
50	1.3	1.5	17	1.7	150	2.0	1,200	1,200	270	12	15	150	40
60	1.5	1.8	20	2.0	200	2.0	1,200	1,200	400	12	15	150	50
60	1.5	1.7	19	2.0	200	2.0	1,200	1,200	350	10	15	150	70
60	1.5	1.7	19	2.0	200	2.0	800	800	350	10	15	150	70
60	1.2	1.4	15	2.0	200	2.0	800	800	350	10	15	150	70
50	1.1	1.3	15	1.4	150	2.0	1,200	1,200	280	15	12	150	45
60	1.1	1.3	15	1.5	180	2.0	1,200	1,200	300	15	12	150	50
60	1.1	1.3	15	1.6	180	2.0	1,200	1,200	280	15	12	150	55
60	1.1	1.3	15	1.6	180	2.0	800	800	280	15	12	150	55
60	1.0	1.2	13	1.6	180	2.0	800	800	280	10	12	150	55
70	1.5	1.6	17	2.2	400	2.2	1,200	1,200	320	30	15	175	65
95	1.6	1.8	20	2.1	280	2.6	1,200	1,200	355	15	19	200	75
90	1.6	1.7	20	2.1	260	2.6	1,200	1,200	340	15	16	200	75

evaluation of data" (Monsen, 1989). A revision in the age/sex groupings extended the 19- to 22-year old group to include 24-year-olds, with a corresponding increase in calcium recommendations from 800 to 1200 mg. It is during this time that building calcium stores is most critical. Recommendations were lowered for iron for most women from 18 mg to 15 mg, assuming that they obtain an adequate diet of meat, poultry, or fish and rich sources of vitamin C. An increase in vitamin C intake for smokers from 60 to 100 mg was recommended (West's Nutrition, 1990). Values for magnesium and folate were lowered dramatically for most groups based on observations concluding that liver stores and folate status were maintained adequately at 50% less intake (Monsen, 1989). The RDAs for vitamin B_6 and B_{12} were also reduced. New RDAs were issued for vitamin K and selenium, both of which were previously in the Estimated Safe and Adequate Daily Dietary Intake (ESADDI) category. The ESADDIs for biotin, copper, and molybdenum were lowered, whereas sodium, chloride, and potassium were given absolute values in the category of Estimated Minimum Requirements. Most significant was the recommendation for sodium set at 500 mg, far below the previous ESADDI of 1100 to 3300 mg range (Monsen, 1989).

For purposes of dietary assessment and most dietary counseling in dental hygiene care, qualitative assessments using the food group guide may be more useful than detailed quantitative analyses. In any case, the patient should be able to determine if his or her food selection is reasonably appropriate. Food choices should be consistent with the Dietary Guidelines for Americans published by the USDA and the U.S. Department of Health and Human Services, revised in 1990. They recommend that individuals over 2 years of age:

1. Eat a variety of foods.
2. Maintain healthy weight.
3. Choose a diet low in fat, saturated fat, and cholesterol.
4. Choose a diet with plenty of vegetables, fruits, and grain products.
5. Use sugars only in moderation.
6. Use salt and sodium only in moderation.
7. If you drink alcoholic beverages, do so in moderation.

These guidelines can be easily incorporated into the USDA Guide for Daily Food Choices (Wardlaw, Insel, and Seyler, 1992).

In addition to these two basic assessments, estimates of caloric intake may be made. The texture of the foods should be identified, as a diet of soft, nonfibrous foods can adhere to the teeth and cause problems with digestion and elimination. The distribution of eating during the day should be identified as well. Encouraging the practice of eating a good breakfast should be viewed as more than "mom's advice." A recent study suggests that persons who eat ready-to-eat cereal regularly for breakfast consume less fat and cholesterol during the day; conversely, those who skip breakfast typically consume a diet that is lacking in essential nutrients during the remainder of the day.

Males who do not eat breakfast tend to eat more during the day than do those who eat breakfast (Morgan, Zabik, and Stampley, 1986). Children who eat breakfast tend to perform better on problem-solving skills in late morning than those who do not (Rapoport and Kruesi, 1984).

Food choices are based on beliefs and attitudes that may be outdated or mistaken. In addition, food choices are a part of daily living and constitute habits that are not easily changed. Research suggests that people select foods and use nutrients based on sensory experiences—some positive and some negative. It may be possible to identify these associations of sensory properties with foods and then use or alter them to improve dietary choices (Mattes, 1987). If habits are changed, changes will affect not only the patients but those around them, most notably their families (Martin, Austin, and Stuart, 1984). Also, the positive results of dietary changes are often delayed, providing little short term reinforcement for continued behavior (Gillespie, 1987). Change must be incremental and directed to those areas in which the patient can identify the need to change and take small, concrete steps to alter behavior.

It is sometimes preferable to draw a line between assessment of need and implementation of dietary counseling. This is especially true if the patient appears to be apprehensive or reluctant to participate. If the assessment shows a need for such counseling, it can be included in a treatment plan and discussed at the case presentation.

Often, the patient may be able to identify at the time of assessment the kinds of modifications that are important for improved health. The patient may say, "I guess I never realized that I ate so few vegetables," or "I knew I was a nibbler, but I would never have said that I was eating at 10 different times during a given day!" If the patient comes to one of these conclusions about the diet, then it may be appropriate to ask, "Would you like some suggestions for modification?" In all likelihood, the patient who has just had a revelation about his or her daily eating patterns will be open to at least a few suggestions for change.

The next question would be, "Where do you think you need guidance?" This question gives the patient the opportunity to say, for example, "Well, I know I can handle adding a few vegetables to my diet, but I really don't know what I'm going to do about all the sugared beverages I drink." This cues the hygienist to ignore the missing vegetables for the moment and turn the patient's attention to substitutes that will make the decrease, and possibly the eventual elimination, of sugared beverages from the diet more tolerable. Once this patient-identified priority is addressed, the hygienist may return to the issue of the vegetables and ask, "What kinds of vegetables do you like? How do you usually prepare them?" Even though the patient may believe he or she can resolve a certain dietary problem, verbally expressing plans for improvement and discussing potential difficulties and different ways to resolve the problem can help clarify the patient's goals and increase the likelihood of change. Another way of bringing the planned change closer to reality is to ask, "What can you do tomorrow to implement the changes you think you need?" The patient may decide to purchase the different foods today to make change possible for tomorrow. In almost all behavior changes, the goals need to be reduced to definable short range steps that the patient can identify and accomplish, one by one. In any case the patient should be given ample opportunity to think and reply.

Merely giving instructions and information without including incremental strategies for behavior change may improve the patient's knowledge and awareness of dietary needs but will have little effect on actual performance (Morasky and Lilly, 1980).

If, after several moments of silence, the patient seems to be at a loss as to how the diet should change, the hygienist can provide missing information. The stock of canned and bottled goods can be brought into view for an assessment of what those foods contain. The hygienist can discuss the retention of food and the frequency of sugar intake in terms of the total amount of time acid is produced in the mouth. Or he or she may point out the vitamins and minerals that are included in the dietary plan, making obvious those which are missing. A brief discussion of how those missing elements affect health and well-being may have an added impact on the patient's perception of the diet. The hygienist may find it appropriate to discuss the effects of an imbalance of caloric intake and use. The patient may decide to expend more calories through exercise as well as decrease intake if obesity seems to be a problem.

In some instances the patient may inquire about what kinds of foods he or she should eat to fulfill a nutritional recommendation. A wise response is to list a number of appropriate foods and ask the patient to specify which ones he or she enjoys and are available. It is important to remember that many food choices may not be available to patients because of financial and/or cultural barriers (Hamilton and Whitney, 1991; Nizel and Papas, 1989; Randolph and Dennison, 1981). Patients may have allergies to certain foods. And, most important, there are some foods a person simply does not like and will not eat.

As mentioned before, it is important for the patient to express what he or she could do the next day to alter the diet in the ways he or she had previously suggested. It is also wise to suggest incremental changes. One small change over a few weeks followed by other small changes may actually result in long term major changes. A crash program to change the entire structure of a person's diet is often short lived, as verified by the numbers of people who have gained and lost and gained back again hundreds of pounds over the years on fad approaches to weight loss. Ideally, the specific changes can be identified in writing for the patient and placed in the record. The date and time of day of each change should be identified as it is implemented, thus tracking whether or not real change has occurred.

Finally, the hygienist should integrate follow-up assessments of progress into each dental hygiene visit. People do not always do everything they say they will do; a supportive, helpful hygienist will remember to identify the areas in which the patient has achieved even minor success and reinforce that change. If recommended changes did not occur, the hygienist might ask, "What seemed to be the biggest roadblock to making the change?" Setting out to remove or diminish each roadblock as it appears can be an effective way to facilitate change over an extended period.

REFERRALS

Even though the dental hygienist has courses in nutrition and feels confident about proper dietary intake, sometimes it is essential to refer the patient to a dietitian or physician for more complete nutritional analysis and counseling (Diet, 1984; Nizel and Papas, 1989; Randolph and Dennison, 1981). In most instances if the patient's health history indicates diabetes, renal disease, food allergies, alcoholism, an obvious chronic nutritional debility, or any other complicated combination of disease and nutritional problems, the hygienist should recommend that the patient see a person more qualified to make recommendations and work with such patients. If an eating disorder such as anorexia or bulimia is suspected, intervention is necessary (Altshuler, 1990). A protocol for these kinds of referrals should be established for the practice site so that coworkers can ensure rapid, safe referral for the patient. Subsequent to such referrals, the hygienist should inquire whether the patient was able to obtain assistance from the dietitian or the physician. Just as medication to control high blood pressure can remain in the bottle, appointments with other health care providers to whom the patient is referred may not always occur. A helpful step is to contact the person to whom the patient was referred to ensure that the patient complied with the recommendation and to determine if the hygienist's findings were accurate. This is one way to establish whether assessment skills in patient observation and history preparation are adequate. A dialogue with other professionals can be beneficial to the dental hygienist as well as to the patient.

SUMMARY

With a solid knowledge of basic nutrition and its relationship to health and disease, the dental hygienist can play a valuable role in helping improve patients' dietary patterns. The use of simple patient self-assessment procedures and the approach of guiding the patient in identifying necessary modifications can result in improvements in health and in patient cooperation in all phases of care. Perhaps the most essential point is for the hygienist to assume a facilitative rather than a directive role. Decisions that the patient makes are most likely to lead to actual behavior change. The hygienist's role is to ensure that the decisions are guided properly and that roadblocks to their fulfillment are identified and reduced.

ACTIVITIES

1. Prepare 1-day, 3-day, and 7-day dietary assessments with a student partner. Use nutritional texts and articles to prepare a comprehensive evaluation of the records to reveal the following:
   a. Caloric intake and expenditure.
   b. Consumption of complex carbohydrates, especially fiber.
   c. Consumption of liquids.
   d. Degree of compliance with the four food groups and the RDAs.
   e. Frequency and form of simple carbohydrates ingested.
   f. Percentage of fat consumed.
2. Compare the percentage of calories from carbohydrate, protein, and fat in your diet with the average American and with the U.S. Dietary Goals.
3. Analyze the fiber content of your diet. Identify foods as excellent, good, and poor fiber sources. List ways to increase fiber in your diet.
4. Videotape the dietary assessment encounter with a student partner to reveal the process of communication, verbal and nonverbal cues, and the approach used by the student dental hygienist.
5. Read Binns NM:*Dent Health* 20(4):5, 1981 on the relationship between caries and carbohydrates.
6. Critique the General Mills advertisement on pp. 142-143 of the January 1981 issue of the *Journal of the American Dental Association*. How are research results manipulated to convince readers that they should counsel patients to eat processed cereals, regardless of their sugar content?
7. In groups of five, visit a grocery store and review labels of products in each of the following categories for the presence of sugar:
   a. Breakfast cereals.
   b. Bread.
   c. Juice.
   d. Canned fruits, vegetables.
   e. Tomato sauce and prepared spaghetti sauces.
8. Compare findings, identifying brand names of products that are high in sugar as well as those that contain little or no sugar.
9. Review the literature regarding nutritional requirements for athletes. Specify which nutrients should be increased or decreased. Refer to: Position of the American Dietetic Association: nutrition for physical fitness and athletic performance for adults, *J Am Diet Assoc* 87:933, 1987, and to more recent citations.
10. Prepare a report on the truth or fiction of one or more of the following popular beliefs:
    a. Honey is more wholesome than sugar.
    b. Fish is brain food.
    c. Eating carrots improves eyesight.
    d. Garlic lowers blood pressure.
    e. Brown eggs are superior to white eggs.
    f. White bread is not as good as whole wheat bread.
    g. Foods are inherently good or bad.
       Refer to the January 1988 issue of the *Tufts University Diet and Nutrition Letter* for information and other topics to research and debate.
11. Learn to estimate food serving sizes in each of the four food groups. At mealtime, measure the amount of a food you would normally consume; then measure out a standard serving and compare.

REVIEW QUESTIONS

1. Identify the three nutrients that provide calories for the body.
2. Which of the three nutrients given in response to Question 1 can cause weight gain if consumed in excess?
3. Match the following nutrients with their important functions in the health of the human body.
   _____ a. Protein
   _____ b. Fat
   _____ c. Carbohydrate
   _____ d. Vitamin B complex
   _____ e. Vitamin D
   _____ f. Vitamin A
   _____ g. Vitamin K
   _____ h. Vitamin E
   _____ i. Iodine
   _____ j. Fluoride
   _____ k. Calcium and phosphorus
   _____ l. Iron
   _____ m. Water

   (1) Contributes to thyroid regulation.
   (2) Serves as fluid medium for the body's chemical and physical reactions.
   (3) Essential for development of healthy bones and teeth.
   (4) Helps teeth become resistant to decay.
   (5) Essential component of nerve tissue.
   (6) Essential component in body tissues, enzymes, and hormones.
   (7) Helps cushion and insulate the body.
   (8) Important in collagen biosynthesis and wound healing.
   (9) Critical for the complete metabolism of carbohydrates and for energy release.
   (10) Formed in the presence of ultraviolet light; important for the absorption and homeostasis of calcium.
   (11) Essential in prothrombin formation.
   (12) Essential in hemoglobin formation.

(13) Primary functions relate to reproduction and membrane stability.

(14) Essential for vision and control of differentiation of epithelium in mucus-secreting structures and in bone remodeling.

4. Why is it a useful strategy to ask the patient to identify the presence or absence of specific foods in his or her diet?

5. What role do the RDAs and the four food groups play in dietary assessment?

6. How does plaque aid caries formation?

7. What role does nutrition play in periodontal disease?

8. Compare the effects of a soft diet with a fibrous diet on periodontal health.

9. What foods have been proved to be highly associated with cancer?

10. What foods tend to reduce the incidence of cancer?

REFERENCES

Alfano MC: Controversies, perspectives, and clinical implications of nutrition in periodontal disease, *Dent Clin North Am* 20:519, 1976.

Altshuler BD: Eating disorder patients: recognition and intervention, *J Dent Hyg* 64:119, 1990.

American Dietetic Association: Nutrition for physical fitness and athletic performance for adults, *J Am Diet Assoc* 87:933, 1987a.

American Dietetic Association: Appropriate use of nutritive and non-nutritive sweeteners, *J Am Diet Assoc* 87:1689, 1987b.

American Institute for Cancer Research: *Dietary guidelines to lower cancer risk,* 1990, Washington, DC, The Institute.

Babcock-Goodman S, Suzuki JB: Dietary control of dental plaque, *J Clin Dent* 1(4):87, 1989.

Barone J: Can diet protect your immune system? *Center for Science in the Public Interest* 15(6):4, 1988.

Binns NM: Caries and carbohydrates—a problem for dentists and nutritionists, *Dent Health* 20(4):5, 1981.

Brooks GB: Nutritional status—a prognostic indicator in head and neck cancer, *Otolaryngol Head Neck Surg* 93:69, 1985.

Carlsson J, Egelberg J: Effect of diet on plaque formation and development of gingivitis in dogs. II. Effect of high carbohydrate versus high protein-fat diets, *Odontol Rev* 16:42, 1965.

Chandra RK: The relationship between immunology, nutrition and disease in elderly people, *Age Aging* 19:S25, 1990.

Chandra, RK: 1990 McCollum Award Lecture. Nutrition and immunity: lessons from the past and new insights into the future, *Am J Clin Nutr* 53:1087, 1991.

Chipponi JX et al: Deficiencies of essential and conditionally essential nutrients, *Am J Clin Nutr* 35(suppl 5):1112, 1982.

Christakis G: Nutritional assessment in health programs, *Am J Public Health* (suppl) 63: 1973.

DePaola DP, Alvares O, Etzel DR: Nutrition and periodontal disease, *TIC* 43(6):5, 1984.

Diet, nutrition, and oral health: a rational approach for the dental practice, *JADA* 109:20, 1984.

Deuster PA et al: Nutritional survey of highly trained women runners, *Am J Clin Nutr* 44:954, 1986.

Fahey PJ, Boltri JM, Monk JS: Key issues in nutrition: from conception through infancy, *Postgrad Med* 81(1):301, 1987.

Fahey PJ, Boltri JM, Monk JS: Key issues in nutrition: supplementation through adulthood and old age, *Postgrad Med* 81(6):123, 1987.

Firestone AR: Effect of increasing contact time on sucrose solution of powdered sucrose on plaque pH in vivo, *J Dent Res* 61:1243, 1982.

Fisher, JG: Osteoporosis in dentistry, *Gen Dent* Nov-Dec, 38:434, 1990.

Geissler CA, Bates JF: The nutritional effects of tooth loss, *Am J Clin Nutr* 39:478, 1984.

Getting the most from the most essential nutrient, *Tufts Univ Diet Nutr Lett* 4(8):3, 1986.

Gillespie AH: Communication theory as a basis for nutrition education, *J Am Diet Assoc* 87(suppl):s44, 1987.

The good news about complex carbohydrates, *Tufts Univ Diet Nutr Lett,* 5(6):3, 1987.

Hamilton EMN, Whitney EN: *Nutrition concepts and controversies,* St Paul, Minn, 1991, West.

Harper AE: Evolution of recommended dietary allowances—new directions? *Ann Rev Nutr* 7:509, 1987.

Hefferren JJ: A look ahead: diet and nutrition research, *JADA* 102:624, 1981.

Hefferren JJ, Ayer WA, Koehler HM, editors: *Foods, nutrition, and dental health,* vols 1-3, Park Forest, Ill, 1981, Pathotox.

Hoffman L et al: Dietary indices of cariogenicity: evolving methodologies, *Clin Nutr* 7:71, 1988.

Homsy J, Morrow WJW, Levy JA: Nutrition and autoimmunity: a review, *Clin Exp Immunol* 65:473, 1986.

Hurley JS: *Nutrition and health,* Guilford, Conn, 1992, Dushkin.

Kant KA et al: Dietary diversity in the U.S. population, NHANES II, 1976-1980, *J Am Diet Assoc* 91:1526, 1991a.

Kant KA et al: Food group intake patterns and associated nutrient profiles of the U.S. population, *J Am Diet Assoc* 91: 1532, 1991b.

Keusch GT: The effects of malnutrition on host response, *Arch Host Defense Mech* 2:275, 1983.

Kipp D: Stress and nutrition, *ASDC J Dent Child* 52:68, 1985.

Kleemola-Kujala E, Rasanen L: Relationship of oral hygiene and sugar consumption to risk of caries in children, *Community Dent Oral Epidemiol* 10:224, 1982.

Lieber CS: Alcohol-nutrition interaction, *ASDC J Dent Child* 51:137, 1984.

Lum LLQ, Gallagher-Allred CR: Nutrition and the cancer patient: a cooperative effort by nursing and dietetics to overcome problems, *Cancer Nurs* 7:469, 1984.

Martin BJ, Austin JB, Stewart JS: Role for the dentist in behavioral intervention: families with poor eating patterns, *Oral Health,* 74(11):11, 1984.

Mattes RD: Sensory influences of food intake and utilization in humans, *Hum Nutr Appl Nutr* 41(2):77, 1987.

Milner I: Food additives offer both risks and benefits, *Environ Nutr* 12(11), 1989.

Monsen ER: The 10th edition of the recommended dietary allowances: what's new in the 1989 RDAs? *J Am Diet Assoc* 89:1748, 1989.

Morasky RL, Lilly KP: Nutrition management for dental health: a behavioral approach, *Clin Prev Dent* 2(4):7, 1980.

Morgan KJ, Zabik ME, Stampley GL: The role of breakfast in diet adequacy in the U.S. adult population, *J Am Coll Nutr* 5:551, 1986.

Morgan KJ et al: Collection of food intake data: an evaluation of methods, *J Am Diet Assoc* 87:888, 1987.

New FNB position paper studied for RDA revision, *CNI Nutr Week* 20:4, Feb 1986.

Newbrun E: Sugar and dental caries, *Clin Prev Dent* 4(3):11, 1982a.

Newbrun E: Sugar and dental caries: a review of human studies, *Science* 217:418, 1982b.

Newman HN: Plaque and chronic inflammatory periodontal disease: a question of ecology, *J Clin Periodontol* 17:533, 1990.

Nieman DC, Butterworth DE, Nieman CN: *Nutrition,* Dubuque, Iowa, 1991, Wm C Brown.

Nizel AE, Papas AS: *Nutrition in preventive dentistry: science and practice,* 1989, Philadelphia, WB Saunders.

Olson JA: Recommended nutrient intakes: guidelines for the prevention of deficiency or prescription for total health, *J Nutr* 116:1581, 1986.

Olson JA, Hodges RE: Recommended dietary intakes (RDI) of vitamin C in humans, *Am J Clin Nutr* 45:693, 1987.

Padh H: Vitamin C: Newer insights into its biochemical functions, *Nutr Rev* 49(3):65, 1991.

Palmer S, Bakshi K: Diet, nutrition, and cancer: interim dietary guidelines, *J Natl Cancer Inst* 70:1151, 1983.

Pollack RL, Kravitz E: *Nutrition in oral health and disease,* 1985, Philadelphia, Lea & Febiger.

Porter SB: Using communication theory: the development of a conceptual framework to map students' thinking about food, *J Am Diet Assoc* 87(suppl):S53, 1987.

Randolph PM: Dietary counseling. In Boundy SS, Reynolds NJ, editors: *Current concepts in dental hygiene,* vol 1, St Louis, 1977, CV Mosby.

Randolph PM, Dennison CI: *Diet, nutrition, and dentistry,* St Louis, 1981, CV Mosby.

Rapoport JD, Kruesi MJP: Behavior and nutrition: a mini review, *ASDC J Dent Child* 51:451, 1984.

Richie JP: Role of nutrition in cancer of the oral cavity, *J Appl Nutr* 43(1):49, 1991.

Ripa LW: Nursing caries: a comprehensive review, *Pediatr Dent* 10:268, 1988.

Safety of aspartame upheld again, *Tufts Univ Diet Nutr Lett* 4(4):2, 1986.

Samaranayake LP: Nutritional factors and oral candidosis, *J Oral Pathol* 15:61, 1986.

Sawyer DR et al: Comparison of oral microflora between well-nourished and malnourished Nigerian children, *ASDC J Dent Child* 53:439, 1986.

Schaafsma G et al: Nutritional aspects of osteoporosis, *World Rev Nutr Diet* 49:121, 1987.

Schaumberg H et al: Sensory neuropathy from pyridoxine abuse, *N Engl J Med* 309:445, 1983.

Schectman G, Byrd JC, Hoffman R: Ascorbic acid requirements for smokers: analysis of a population survey, *Am J Clin Nutr* 53:1466, 1991.

Shepherd R, Stockley L: Nutrition knowledge, attitudes, and fat consumption, *J Am Diet Assoc* 87:615, 1987.

Sherman AR: Alterations in immunity related to nutritional status, *Nutr Today* Jul/Aug, 21:7, 1986.

Socransky SS, Haffejee AD: Microbial mechanisms in the pathogenesis of destructive periodontal diseases: a critical assessment, *J Periodontol Res* 26:195, 1991.

Sreebny LM: Sugar availability, sugar consumption and dental caries, *Community Dent Oral Epidemiol* 10:1, 1982.

Sutnick MR: Nutrition: calcium, cholesterol, and calories, *Med Clin North Am* 71:123, 1987.

US Department of Agriculture, US Department of Health and Human Services: Nutrition and your health: dietary guidelines for Americans, *Home Garden Bull* no. 232, 1990.

Wardlaw GM, Insel PM, Seyler MF: *Contemporary nutrition issues and insights,* St Louis, 1992, Mosby–Year Book.

West's Nutrition Instructor's Network, 1989 RDA, 5:1, 1990.

Wilmore JH, Freund BJ: Nutritional enhancement of athletic performance. In Winick M, editor: *Nutrition and exercise,* New York, 1986, John Wiley & Sons.

Wilton JMA et al: Detection of high-risk groups and individuals for periodontal diseases, *J Clin Periodontol* 15:339, 1988.

Wykeham-Martin J: Hidden sugar, *Dent Health* 20(3):14, 1981.

PART SEVEN

THERAPY

Therapy, or treatment, may run in tandem with educational efforts to help the patient control his or her oral disease, or it may be delayed until the patient is succussful in adopting and maintaining a self-care program. The therapy you provide is based on the dental hygiene diagnosis and treatment plan you have devised; it is modified to account for the dental diagnosis and any treatment that must be integrated into the total plan.

The following chapters introduce you to the treatment procedures encompassed in dental hygiene care. This includes periodontal debridement (and the care of the instruments), application of irrigation and antimicrobial agents, procedures for placing and removing dressings and sutures, cosmetic and therapeutic applications of polishing, treating dentin hypersensitivity, controlling pain, and placing and carving restorations. This part of the text includes an in-depth discussion of many of the fundamental changes affecting dental hygiene practice as a result of research. You may find that the procedures and strategies recommended are quite different from what you experienced as a patient in dental hygiene care or observed in other colleagues' treatment approaches. Therefore you may find it helpful to assimilate the rationale behind these changes so you can discuss the reasons for the altered approach with other dental hygienists, dentists, and your patients. You are learning dental hygiene care at a particularly exciting time for the profession as profound changes in clinical care occur.

25 PERIODONTAL DEBRIDEMENT

Nancy Stutsman Young
Trisha E. O'Hehir
Irene Woodall

Nancy Stutsman Young
Trisha E. O'Hehir
Irene Woodall

LEARNING OUTCOMES

The dental hygienist will be able to

1. Define periodontal debridement and differentiate between the treatment approaches to supragingival debridement, subgingival debridement, and deplaquing.
2. Describe how changing perspectives on the roles of calculus, plaque, and endotoxin in periodontal disease have affected the development of dental hygiene treatment over the past several decades.
3. Identify the beliefs and assumptions that have formed the basis for traditional approaches to root instrumentation.
4. Discuss the scientific basis for periodontal debridement as defined in this chapter.
5. Generate criteria for evaluation of the periodontal debridement process and apply these criteria during and after patient treatment.
6. Compare and contrast the various characteristics of sonic and ultrasonic scaler instruments available to the dental hygienist.
7. Given information about oral conditions and general health status, determine whether or not ultrasonic scaling is an appropriate choice for particular patients.
8. Briefly describe how ultrasonic and sonic scalers remove deposits.
9. Given a patient for whom ultrasonic scaling is indicated, use the proper procedure for ensuring patient confidence, obtaining informed consent, and providing the patient with sufficient information to make an educated choice regarding whether or not to proceed, including:
   a. A patient with large amounts of calculus requiring substantial supragingival and subgingival debridement.
   b. A patient who requires only subgingival debridement as a part of periodontal treatment.
   c. A patient who requires monitoring and coninuing care debridement.
10. Use appropriate measures for managing water flow and evacuation during ultrasonic or sonic instrumentation.
11. Identify the design and usefulness of each of the following tips:
    a. Chisel.
    b. Beaver-tail.
    c. Periodontal probe style.
    d. Universal and right-angle explorer style.
12. Use a sequence and stroking pattern most likely to produce a thoroughly debrided surface (no calculus, endotoxin, or microbial colonies).
13. Contrast ultrasonic and sonic instrumentation principles with those used with hand instruments.
14. Thoroughly debride periodontal and continuing care patients using sonic and ultrasonic instruments and evaluate the success of therapy based on healing response and continued health.
15. Explain to a colleague, employer, and patient how the approach to instrumentation has shifted from an emphasis on mechanical and physical measures of success to one that emphasizes evidence of biological compatability with health.

DEPOSIT REMOVAL—A MEANS OR AN END?

Removal of deposits from the tooth surface is probably the most technically demanding clinical procedure that hygienists master. Development of instrumentation skills has traditionally encompassed a major proportion of time in the dental hygiene curriculum. The emphasis on complete removal of deposits has also been evident from the amount of time devoted to the procedures of scaling, root planing, and polishing during a typical dental hygiene appointment. Hygienists invest so much time and energy in removing deposits that they risk focusing on those procedures more than on the actual goal of all periodontal treatment—the establishment of healthy periodontal tissues. Patients may also associate these procedures with the dental hygiene recall appointment more readily than other vital services such as assessment, diagnosis, dental health education, and health evaluation. The purpose of this chapter is to break away from the traditional emphasis on treatment of the tooth and root surfaces and focus on treatment aimed at establishing and maintaining healthy periodontal tissues.

Current periodontal research findings indicate a need for re-evaluation of many of the assumptions and techniques that have guided the practice of dental hygiene for decades. Practicing dental hygienists and faculty members whose education focused on the "art and science" of calculus removal will find that the research and recommendations presented in this chapter reflect a new perspective on both the objectives of periodontal therapy and the best ways to accomplish treatment objectives. Students will find that, although they will still learn the same basic instrumentation skills as their predecessors, the application of these skills will reflect an understanding of new treatment technologies.

Most importantly, students of the new perspective will participate in defining, practicing, and evaluating both new and old approaches to treatment according to their success in achieving periodontal health. In the context of periodontal health, "success" means stopping the progress of periodontal disease using techniques and approaches that are proven to be the most effective and efficient in achieving that goal and that will result in the least disruption or damage to surrounding tissues and to the patient's general health and well-being.

Definition of debridement

Periodontal debridement refers to the treatment of gingival and periodontal inflammation through mechanical removal of tooth and root surface irritants to the extent that the adjacent soft tissues maintain or return to a healthy, noninflamed state. Periodontal debridement may be accomplished with ultrasonic or hand instruments, depending on operator preference or patient considerations. Bacterial plaque and by-products that are toxic to periodontal tissues (e.g. endotoxins), are the primary foci of periodontal debridement procedures. Removal of calculus is regarded as a secondary concern to the debridement procedure. It contributes to disease because of its plaque-retentive nature. Recognition of the presence, physical nature, and location of these irritants on any given tooth surface is necessary to determine the most effective means of eliminating them through periodontal debridement.

Total debridement may involve any or all of the following three treatment phases:

1. *Supragingival debridement*—removal of all accessible plaque, plaque by-products, and plaque-retentive calculus located on the clinical crown of the tooth, that is, coronal to the gingival margin; its purpose is to support and facilitate the patient's personal plaque control efforts and to support the attainment of healthy gingival tissues.

2. *Subgingival debridement*—removal of accessible plaque, plaque by-products, and plaque-retentive calculus located in inflamed periodontal pockets and apical to the margin of the gingiva; its purpose is to supplement the patient's supragingival plaque control by removing or disrupting bacterial plaque and toxic plaque by-products that are inaccessible to the patient and are promoting inflammation of periodontal tissues; professional subgingival debridement also involves removal of plaque retentive surfaces and deposits, including calculus and poorly contoured restorations, which may promote plaque formation or contribute to plaque retention.

3. *Deplaquing*—removal or disruption of bacterial plaque and its by-products within the gingival sulcus or periodontal pocket as a means of supporting and maintaining periodontal health; it follows the completion of supragingival and subgingival debridement

procedures at re-evaluation and maintenance appointments.

The term *periodontal debridement* will be used throughout this text as a suggested alternative to *scaling* and *root planing,* which are the more traditional terms for treatment of the root surface. However, a general understanding of these two terms will be helpful in comprehending how periodontal instrumentation was previously accomplished in the dental hygiene profession and how it has been described in the periodontal literature. Understanding of these two concepts is also critical to recognizing the differences between their implementation and that of periodontal debridement as explained in this text.

According to the "Glossary of Periodontal Terms" of the American Academy of Periodontology (AAP) (1986), *scaling* is defined as the "instrumentation of the crown and root surfaces of the teeth to remove plaque, calculus, and stains." Typically, scaling procedures focus primarily on removal of visible or easily accessible calculus deposits or heavy stain. Scaling, as it is normally performed, has only limited effect as a means of removing plaque and endotoxins from affected surfaces. This is because scaling strokes are usually applied only to those areas in which calculus or stain is readily detected and because the entire tooth and root surface is not exposed to the type of continuous and overlapping strokes necessary to contact and remove all plaque deposits.

Root planing is defined as "a definitive treatment procedure designed to remove cementum or surface dentin that is rough, impregnated with calculus, or contaminated with toxins or microorganisms" (AAP, 1986). When it is combined with scaling, the result is a more extensive treatment of the root surfaces (see review, O'Leary, 1986). In contrast to scaling, root planing does attempt to adapt the instrument to the entire surface area of the affected root, but it does so at the cost of removing significant amounts of cementum and dentin in an effort to ensure that all contaminants and calculus deposits are removed.

The effectiveness of root planing in the treatment of periodontal disease is well documented, but it carries costs for both patient and operator. Thorough root planing is an intensive treatment in terms of time and professional effort. Depending on the extent of attachment loss and the nature of the deposits and root surface characteristics, root planing can require anywhere from 1 to several

hours per quadrant. Examples of the wide variation in time estimates for accomplishment of thorough root planing have included 2 to 3 hours per quadrant (Chace, 1989), or 30 minutes per tooth (Stambaugh et al, 1981). One study suggested that as many as 30 to 50 strokes per tooth surface *after* removal of detectable calculus were necessary to achieve almost complete removal of cementum (O'Leary & Kafrawy, 1983). Extensive loss of cementum results from this approach to instrumentation.

Dentinal hypersensitivity can occur in some individuals as a consequence of extensive root surface instrumentation. For the clinician the intensive and repetitive hand and wrist motions required to accomplish root planing with hand instruments have been linked to symptoms associated with carpal tunnel syndrome. These may include tingling and numbness in the fingers; night pain in the fingers, wrist, or forearm; and loss of strength or clumsiness in the hand (Conrad et al, 1990; Huntley and Shannon, 1988; MacDonald et al, 1988; Osborn et al, 1990).

The following discussion of the nature of root surface deposits will clarify the belief that this type of extensive root instrumentation may constitute overtreatment and may not be necessary to achieve successful outcomes. Because neither term, *scaling* or *root planing* adequately reflects the nature of root instrumentation described in this chapter, the term *periodontal debridement* is suggested as more appropriate to describe a thorough treatment of the tooth and root surfaces with instrumentation. Although periodontal debridement shares many of the same goals and techniques associated with scaling and root planing, there are significant differences that redirect the clinical approach to root surface instrumentation and its evaluation. These differences will be discussed in this chapter.

The effectiveness of closed debridement

Periodontal debridement may be accomplished as either an "open" or "closed" procedure. "Open" (i.e., surgical) debridement refers to the process of surgically exposing the site for direct visualization and improved access to root surfaces. Using this approach the clinician has the advantage of observing the root surface both for detection of calculus deposits and for easier adaptation of instruments used to debride the root. Because the presence of plaque and endotoxin cannot be reliably detected by visualization of periodontally affected root surfaces, even with the use of disclosing solutions, open debridement offers no advantage to their removal (Eaton et al, 1985). Also, since one cannot discern a difference in the appearance of treated compared with nontreated root surfaces, direct visualization cannot guarantee more thorough or comprehensive treatment. The disadvantages of open debridement include exposing the patient to the additional trauma of surgical manipulation of soft tissues, more postoperative pain, a longer healing period, and greater cost, since most surgical techniques require the expertise of a periodontist.

"Closed" (i.e., "blind" or nonsurgical) debridement is accomplished without surgical exposure of the treatment site. Therefore the soft tissues adjacent to the root surface are left in place so that there is minimal disruption and trauma as a result of treatment. Closed debridement is less painful than surgical therapy and can often be accomplished without anesthesia. With less damage to the soft tissues, healing time is decreased, and the patient experiences less postoperative discomfort than with open debridement.

One disadvantage of closed debridement is that the clinician has almost no visualization of the subgingival root surface and must depend on tactile sensations, combined with knowledge of the pocket and root morphology and root surface characteristics, to guide clinical treatment and decision making. Another disadvantage is that the presence of the adjacent soft tissues restricts the access of instrumentation to the treatment site, especially in deep pockets and furcation areas. The limitation of access complicates closed periodontal debridement procedures, so that the clinician must exhibit a high degree of technical and decision-making skills to achieve successful outcomes.

Closed debridement is sufficient for treatment of most periodontal disease sites and is the most common approach to subgingival debridement used by dental hygienists. This chapter deals primarily with the techniques and decision-making involved with closed debridement. Root debridement is carried out in largely the same way under open conditions, though surgical treatment imposes additional complications. Hygienists employed by periodontists or those with advanced education in the area of periodontics may perform debridement under surgical or open conditions.

Before the 1980s, most clinicians assumed that since instrumentation was more technically demanding within the confines of deep pockets, effective removal of deposits was unlikely under these circumstances. This assumption led to the belief that closed debridement could not be successful in pockets greater than 5 mm and that the only effective treatment for patients with moderate to advanced periodontal disease was through a surgical approach. These assumptions have now proven to be unfounded. Periodontal therapy using closed debridement has been shown to result in treatment outcomes comparable to those produced by open debridement and other surgical approaches.

Several teams of researchers have conducted controlled, long-term, clinical trials to compare the effects of closed debridement (represented as scaling and root planing) and surgical treatment approaches on maintaining attachment levels. Ramfjord and co-workers at the University of Michigan observed 90 participants with moderate to severe periodontal disease for 2 years after being treated. The results indicated that closed debridement was as successful as surgical treatments in maintaining periodontal attachment levels for all levels of disease severity (Hill, 1981; Knowles et al, 1980; Ramfjord et al, 1968, 1982).

Lindhe and co-workers at the University of Gothenburg in Sweden also found that surgical and nonsurgical approaches resulted in equally effective preservation of attachment levels after 2 years (Lindhe et al, 1982a, 1982b, 1984). Pihlstrom and coworkers at the University of Minnesota compared scaling and root planing with modified Widman flap surgery in patients with moderate to advanced periodontitis. Their results also showed no significant differences in the attachment levels obtained by the two treatment approaches at the end of 6½ years (Pihlstrom et al, 1981, 1983).

Researchers at Loma Linda University in California have also examined the effectiveness of nonsurgical therapy for patients with moderate (4 to 7 mm clinical probing depths) and advanced (7 to 12 mm) periodontal disease. Patients received closed debridement performed by hand or ultrasonic instruments in a split-mouth design, that is, one half of the mouth was treated using hand instruments and the other half using ultrasonic instrumentation. Closed debridement effectively reduced bleeding scores and clinical probing depths and achieved clinical attachment gains in both moderate and deep pockets. Results were the same for both hand and ultrasonic treatment approaches (Badersten et al, 1987a, 1987b; Badersten et al, 1981, 1984a, 1984b, 1985).

The results of these studies provide strong evidence that closed debridement can achieve levels of effectiveness comparable to surgical treatment approaches at all levels of severity of periodontal disease. Therefore closed periodontal debridement, which is the more conservative approach and less invasive than surgical therapy, should be the first choice among periodontal therapy options. The success of closed debridement or nonsurgical therapy depends on the degree to which bacterial plaque is removed and/or its composition altered through the combined efforts of the patient and the clinician. Personal and professional plaque control must be achieved at a level compatible with maintaining periodontal health at any given periodontal site (Low and Ciancio, 1990).

Surgical treatment of periodontal disease should be reserved for those sites which do not demonstrate a healing response following closed debridement, plaque control, and appropriate chemotherapeutic therapy. It is the professional's ethical and legal responsibility to evaluate and document site-specific responses to periodontal debridement and determine the need for additional treatment or referral for those sites which do not respond to treatment (Greenwell et al, 1987). Lack of resolution of inflammation in the presence of adequate supragingival plaque control may indicate the need for additional debridement or surgery to gain access to residual plaque deposits. Those sites which fail to show clinical signs of improvement after a reasonable period of following nonsurgical therapy should be re-evaluated for the need for surgical intervention (Kieser, 1990, Ramfjord, 1990).

Claffey (1991) suggested that evidence of persistent bleeding combined with either persistent deep probing depth or increased probing depth, in addition to evidence of probing attachment loss, are the most accurate clinical indicators of progressive periodontitis. These clinical indicators became more accurate predictors as the time interval increased following treatment. He cautioned that clinical changes could be misleading in the early stages of healing (e.g., up to 3 months posttreatment). Longer periods of careful monitoring of these clinical variables against pretreatment and immediate posttreatment baseline data will facilitate more informed decision-making regarding the need for further intervention.

Short-term decision making will be enhanced by the availability of diagnostic tests that sample the pocket microflora of the enzyme levels of the gingival crevicular fluid to determine whether the infection is reduced and if the host response suggests that healing has occurred. Biological markers of healing or persistent tissue destruction will augment our traditional methods of tissue evaluation that inadequately detect persistent disease because debridement triggers a universal clinical appearance of healing (see Chapter 12).

GOALS OF DEBRIDEMENT: PAST AND PRESENT

Our understanding of the nature of periodontal diseases and how to treat them has grown significantly over the last several decades as a result of periodontal research. As more is learned about the exact roles of various etiologic agents in periodontal diseases and about the host's immune response to microbial infection, approaches to treating and preventing periodontal diseases will continue to evolve. In the meantime, outdated and inaccurate assumptions and beliefs that formed the basis for treatment decision making in the past have been replaced by new hypotheses reflecting the most current research knowledge. Several illustrations of how periodontal research about the nature of plaque, plaque by-products, and calculus deposits has enlightened and improved dental hygiene treatment over the past several decades are discussed. Current assumptions about the goals and objectives of periodontal debridement are also examined and evaluated in the context of recent research findings.

Changing perspective on bacterial plaque

In its earliest usage, the term *plaque* referred to a mass of microorganisms and mucinous substances that formed in the absence of adequate oral hygiene. The significance of bacterial plaque to dental caries was established well before its relationship to periodontal disease was known. In the 1950s and early 1960s, the clinical significance of plaque in the context of periodontal disease was thought to be that it produced or attracted stains and provided an organic framework for the attachment of other deposits (e.g., food debris, materia alba, calculus) which were "known" to be irritating to the gingival tissues. At that time, plaque was not regarded as a primary cause of inflammation but a contributing one.

In the 1960s the causal relationship between plaque and disease began to emerge from the periodontal research. The classic study by Löe and others (1965), "Experimental Gingivitis in Man," was instrumental in providing evidence of the direct relationship between plaque and inflammation. From that time on plaque was regarded as the primary etiologic factor in periodontal inflammation.

Early concepts of the role of plaque in the etiology of periodontal diseases included the *nonspecific plaque hypothesis,* which suggested that dental plaque is a homogeneous bacterial mass and that the severity of inflammation is directly related to the overall *quantity* of plaque bacteria in the mouth. Therefore, when plaque accumulation exceeded the host defense capabilities, inflammation was thought to occur (Miller, 1973).

Approaches to patient education based on the nonspecific plaque hypothesis stressed brushing and flossing for the purpose of reducing the quantity of supragingival plaque. Over time, more elaborate plaque control programs, which included use of plaque disclosants, supplemental oral hygiene aids, and behavior modification techniques, became widely recommended. Plaque indices that measured the extent of plaque accumulation were used as indicators of patient success or failure. It was assumed that if the patient could achieve a "low enough" plaque index (although no one was quite sure what numerical value was "low enough"), then the progress of gingivitis and periodontal disease could be halted. Therefore if inflammation was detected at the 6-month recall appointment, it was blamed on improper plaque control on the part of the patient, and home care instructions were repeated. The nonspecific plaque hypothesis could not explain, however, why some patients with seemingly low plaque scores continued to experience periodontal breakdown. An alternative explanation for these cases was needed.

The experimental gingivitis studies of the mid-1960s also contributed to interest in the *specific plaque hypothesis,* first suggested in 1915 (Bass and Johns, 1915). According to this hypothesis, bacterial plaques in nondiseased and healthy sites differ in their compositional quality from those found in diseased sites. These early gingivitis studies demonstrated that as plaque matures its bacterial composition changes and that the pathogenicity of plaque depends more on its maturity than on its quantity (Löe et al, 1965; Theilade et al, 1966).

During the 1970s the nature of plaque bacteria continued to be examined with the aid of phase contrast microscopy and culture studies. Researchers began to identify increasing numbers of bacteria that form the oral flora and to discriminate between the types of organisms associated with health and with disease (Listgarten, 1984; Slots, 1977; 1979). Researchers were also able to differentiate between the nature of supragingival and subgingival plaque.

Fine and others (1978a, 1978b) discriminated between adherent plaque and loosely adherent plaque and compared the two types for their pathologic potential. They found that although the mass of adherent plaque was four to five times greater than that of loosely adherent plaque, the pathogenic potential of the loosely adherent plaque was 2 to 60 times greater. These findings suggested that the threat of plaque could be reduced by alternative methods of plaque removal, such as water irrigation devices. Before this time, these devices had been relegated to a minor supplemental role in treatment because of their inability to remove adherent plaque deposits. The discovery of the greater pathogenic potential of loosely adherent plaque, therefore, increased the professional use of water irrigation devices as well as their recommendation for personal plaque control programs.

With the 1970s and 1980s came an increased emphasis on the specific plaque hypothesis and the suggestion that specific microbes are associated with different forms of periodontal disease (see review: Christerrson et al, 1991). The research interest shifted, therefore, from determining the amount of bacterial plaque associated with disease to identifying the type of bacteria. The advent of anaerobic culturing provided additional information about the nature of bacteria that flourish in the subgingival environment and provided further support for the specific plaque hypothesis. Efforts to discover the pathogenic potential of different bacterial species have led to identification of over 300 types of bacteria in the oral flora. In contrast, students studying dental hygiene in the 1960s might have learned there were only 60 types of bacteria. Only a small number of species, however, are thought to be associated with human periodontal disease (Moore et al, 1983). As researchers zeroed in on the most pathogenic of these bacterial species, interest in the effects of specific antimicrobial agents on these targeted bacteria grew. The advent of antimicrobial therapy promises to provide valuable new approaches to the dental hygiene treatment repertoire.

The specific plaque hypothesis also supported the concept that performing subgingival instrumentation at frequent intervals was an effective means of maintaining periodontal health. Whereas plaque control was regarded as the primary responsibility of the patient in the 1960s and 1970s, "professional plaque control" began to attract interest in the 1980s. It was apparent that supragingival plaque control was effective against gingivitis but that the inaccessibility of subgingival plaque to home care methods allowed periodontitis to persist. Another factor contributing to the interest in professional plaque control was the realization that despite repeated efforts to improve patients' oral health behaviors, gaining widespread patient compliance with rigorous plaque control programs was not only unlikely but also time consuming (see review, Wilson, 1987). Therefore professional interventions aimed at controlling submarginal plaque attracted interest as a treatment approach.

Early studies involving professional plaque control suggested that tooth cleaning (both supramarginal and submarginal) every 2 weeks was effective in maintaining periodontal health (Axelsson and Lindhe, 1974). This treatment regimen, however, is not practical for most individuals. As understanding of the nature of subgingival plaque expanded, it became apparent that a less frequent treatment regimen aimed at removing or disrupting subgingival plaque before it matured to a pathogenic composition could also maintain clinically healthy attachment levels. For most individuals a recall interval of 3 months has been found to be sufficient for preventing periodontal destruction (Axelsson and Lindhe, 1978; 1981). Determination of recall intervals must, however, take into consideration the patient's supragingival plaque control, since it directly affects how rapidly the subgingival plaque will convert to a disease-associated composition. Patients with poor supragingival plaque control will require a recall interval of less than 3 months to control disease.

Several clinical studies have also demonstrated that attachment levels can be maintained even in patients with less-than-perfect personal supragingival plaque control who comply with 3-month recalls for professional subgingival plaque removal (Isidor and Karring, 1986; Isidor et al, 1984; Pihlstrom et al, 1981, 1983; Ramfjord et al, 1982). The success of these studies suggests that thorough instrumentation of the subgingival area removes or disrupts the bacterial composition so that pathogenic flora (motile rods and spirochetes) are converted to flora compatible with health (coccoid cells and straight rods). These findings support the specific plaque hypothesis by demonstrating that, despite the fact that different plaque compositions may be pathogenic for different individuals, it is the disruption of plaque composition that prevents disease rather than the degree of plaque removal (Greenwell, 1990).

Researchers in the mid- to late 1980s began to look beyond the microbial role in disease to consider the interaction between the microbes and the host. This new perspective suggested that periodontal inflammation results from an imbalance in the equilibrium between host and parasite. The imbalance may occur when the quantity or quality of bacteria changes or when the individual's level of immunity is altered or affected by environmental factors (Greenstein, 1990; Listgarten, 1986). The nature of this balance between bacterial challenge and host resistance was described in Chapter 12 and illustrated in Fig. 12-1. Although there is no question that plaque is the cause of chronic periodontal disease, this perspective focuses on the individual's immune response to bacteria—that is, the interaction of the host's defense mechanisms with the plaque microorganisms that trigger inflammation.

Individuals vary in their ability to develop an immune response to a microbial insult. In addition, the microbial composition of plaque is qualitatively different from one individual to another and among different sites within a person's mouth. The response of each site to a specific plaque composition is regulated by the individual's immune system. Therefore individuals with a good immune response may exhibit no evidence of progressive disease despite the presence of extensive mature plaque deposits, while others with less extensive plaque may have generalized or localized evidence of disease.

This perspective has significant clinical implications for how dental hygienists conduct periodontal assessments, make treatment planning decisions, and evaluate the success of their therapeutic interventions. The nature of such a complex interaction suggests the need for both individually based and site-specific assessment and treatment planning, taking into account the wide variation in potential immune responses to the presence of bacteria. The days of approaching all patients with the same treatment regimen (e.g. scaling, root planing, polishing, reviewing brushing and flossing, and assigning a 6-month recall) are gone forever. They have been banished by the realization that each patient's individual characteristics and immune response are critical determinants in designing therapeutic interventions.

Dental hygienists will still work with patients to improve their plaque removal skills, but will also realize that inflammation persists in some individuals or sites despite personal plaque control. In the past, these occurrences were too often blamed on the patient's plaque control behaviors when the situation was actually dictated by the patient's immune response and could not be directly controlled by him or her. Therefore more direct professional interventions to tip the host/microbial balance in favor of the host are being investigated. Examples include professional plaque control (deplaquing) and the growing use of local and systemic antimicrobials.

The focus of the 1990s remains on the nature of the host's immune response. A number of critical questions remain unanswered. For instance, which types or combinations of types of bacteria are most pathogenic, and in what quantity? What individual characteristics or variables are likely to affect the immune response, increasing susceptibility to periodontal disease, and how can these effects be mediated?

A differential host response to periodontal disease has been associated with diabetes mellitus, smoking, and stress, suggesting that these factors affect the immune response. A significant and strong relationship has been reported between diabetes and the prevalence and severity of periodontal disease in a population of Pima Indians in Arizona. This particular group was selected because they were reported to have the world's highest incidence and prevalence of noninsulin dependent type II diabetes mellitus. Diabetes in this population was found to increase the risk of developing destructive periodontal disease about

threefold (Emrich et al, 1991). Although this study suggests that the presence of diabetes affects the host response to periodontal disease, additional studies are needed to verify this result in other population groups.

An association between smoking and progressive bone loss has been established in several Swedish studies using sample populations with high standards of oral hygiene. These results also suggested the linkage of a host response unrelated to plaque-mediated infection (Bergstrom and Eliasson, 1982, 1987; Bergstrom, Eliasson, and Preber, 1991).

The role of environmental factors such as viral diseases and stress on immune functioning is also being studied. Mackinnon and others (1987) reported that mucosal immunity, as measured by a reduction in salivary antibodies (IgA), decreased in athletes after exposure to the physical and mental stresses of intensive training and competition.

The wave of the future appears to be searching for ways to boost the patient's immune response so as to promote and maintain health. If this could be accomplished, then those elements which might normally tip the host/microbe balance in favor of disease (e.g., increase in quantity or virulence of pathogenic bacteria and predisposing conditions such as stress, smoking, diabetes, or genetic immune deficiencies) could be counterbalanced by levels of immune functioning that could withstand the threat. When these possibilities are realized, the role of the dental hygienist will undergo a major shift from that of disease therapist and preventive specialist to that of wellness facilitator. We currently know a lot more about how to prevent and treat disease than we do about how to maintain health and wellness. The future will likely afford new challenges and opportunities for dental hygienists in this area.

Changing perspectives on plaque endotoxins

Gram-negative bacteria exhibit a toxic substance on their outer cell walls known as endotoxin. *Lipopolysaccharide* (LPS) has been suggested as a more accurate term for this substance (Daly et al, 1980), and the terms *endotoxin* and *LPS* are often used interchangeably in the research literature. Lipopolysaccharide is known to be toxic to living tissues. When injected into animals it can cause fever, destruction of bone marrow, changes in white blood cells, shock, and even death (Nowotny, 1969).

The exact nature of the role of LPS in the inflammatory process is still uncertain. Although researchers first thought that LPS was a direct cause of inflammation, more recent research indicates it has a more indirect role in which it "up-regulates," or stimulates the immune system's response to bacterial challenges. Lipopolysaccharide stimulates or activates the body's immune functioning through the production of complement and macrophages which, in turn, lead to accumulation of neutrophils. There is further evidence that production of macrophages stimulated by LPS may lead to tumor necrosis factor (Harmsen, 1988). This factor functions in the immune process by producing necrosis of subcutaneous tumors, but it can also lead to destruction of "innocent bystander" cells. Therefore the presence of LPS can trigger an overly active immune response in the host, which can lead to tissue destruction. It is believed that this mechanism could be at work in periodontal inflammation.

The role of LPS as a possible cause of periodontal disease was suspected as early as 1941 (see review, Daly et al, 1980), and animal studies in the 1960s added to this suspicion. The presence of LPS in dental plaque began to be studied intensively in the 1970s. Shapiro and others (1972) reported a direct correlation between level of inflammation and amounts of LPS present in supragingival plaque at selected sites. Fine and others (1978a, 1978b) compared the concentration of LPS in superficial, loosely adherent plaque and in deeper, adherent plaque. They concluded that subgingival, loosely adherent plaque contained the highest levels of LPS. Because this type of plaque lies adjacent to the soft tissues of the periodontal pocket wall, its proximity promotes toxic breakdown of those tissues.

LPS was first implicated in the cytotoxic nature of diseased root surfaces by Hatfield and Baumhammers (1971). Subsequent studies by Aleo and others (1974, 1975) showed that LPS from periodontally involved cementum caused alterations in live tissue cells, affirming the toxic nature of the cementum resulting from LPS. They also found that cultured human gingival connective tissue cells (fibroblasts) would not attach to a periodontally involved tooth surface unless LPS had been removed. They examined root planing, (i.e. complete removal of cementum), as one way of removing the LPS from diseased root surfaces. Although it had not been established whether the

LPS actually penetrated the cementum or was only associated with the plaque retained on the cemental surface, they referred to the LPS as "cementum bound." This terminology implied that the LPS was actually absorbed by the periodontally involved cementum. This interpretation was used as justification for removal of all or nearly all cementum through extensive root planing as a means of removing all the LPS on periodontally affected roots.

Based on the assumption that removal of cementum was necessary for elimination of LPS on diseased roots, additional studies on root planing were conducted to determine how extensive this treatment should be to ensure complete removal of LPS. Nishimine and O'Leary (1979) treated root surfaces by either hand or ultrasonic instrumentation "until the root surface felt hard and smooth." They concluded that "meticulous" root planing with hand instruments produced LPS values comparable to those of healthy teeth with no periodontal involvement, while treatment with ultrasonic instruments resulted in LPS values almost eight times greater than those reported for teeth treated with hand instruments. Jones and O'Leary (1978) performed "vigorous" root planing of the proximal surfaces of teeth until they felt "hard, velvety smooth and glasslike" so that the teeth had a visibly "dished" appearance. They estimated that this treatment had removed all or nearly all the cementum. Their results demonstrated that root planing to this extent removed nearly all the endotoxin from the diseased root surfaces.

Fine and others (1980) detected additional toxic material on diseased root surfaces after scaling, supporting the assumption that LPS penetrated deeply into the cementum. Daly and others (1982) reported that although LPS penetrated only superficially (within 10 μm of the cementum surface), evidence of microbial deposits could be detected all the way to the cementodentinal junction. They suggested that removal of all cementum was necessary to ensure a surface free of bacterial contamination.

Earlier, Daly and others (1980) had re-examined the assumption that endotoxin penetrated diseased cementum based on the studies of Aleo and others (1974, 1975) and offered a different conclusion. They suggested that some plaque or calculus probably remained in the resorption lacunae on the cemental surfaces of the treated teeth despite the "careful removal of debris" described in the Aleo studies. Because it would have been impossible to discriminate between calculus, plaque, and cementum as the source of the LPS, it was suggested that the term *cementum-associated LPS* would be more appropriate.

A growing body of knowledge emerged during the 1980s to challenge previous ideas about the nature and distribution of endotoxin on periodontally involved root surfaces. Nakib et al (1982) performed an in vitro study to determine the extent of penetration of endotoxin from *Escherichia coli*, a coliform bacterium, into the roots of both periodontally healthy and periodontally diseased teeth. The extracted teeth were washed in distilled water, scaled, and then immersed in differing concentrations of the endotoxin for 2 to 12 weeks. The results indicated that the endotoxin adhered to the tooth surface but did not penetrate the root cementum of either the diseased or healthy teeth. A second part of the study investigated the strength of endotoxin binding to the tooth surface. The teeth were brushed for 1 minute and then re-examined for the presence of endotoxin. They found that brushing removed most of the adherent endotoxin and concluded that a weak bond exists between the endotoxin and the tooth surface.

Hughes and Smales (1986) examined extracted, periodontally involved teeth and also concluded that LPS is present only on the surface of the cementum of periodontally involved teeth and that there was no evidence that LPS penetrated into cementum. In a later study, Hughes and others (1988) reported that most of the LPS that remains on root surfaces after careful scaling is associated with residual plaque and calculus deposits and not with absorption of LPS, or "free" endotoxin, into the surface of the cementum. This study suggested that the presence of retained plaque in resorption lacunae of cementum is more of a therapeutic problem than the removal of cementum-bound endotoxin.

Clinical implications of nature and distribution of LPS. Nyman and others (1986, 1988) investigated the question of whether or not root debridement needed to include the removal of exposed cementum to achieve periodontal health. In the earlier study an animal model was used to test the hypothesis that removal of cementum was a prerequisite for accomplishing optimal healing. Quadrants that were polished subgingivally re-

sponded, as well as those that were treated with meticulous root planing, and in some cases showed superior healing, including the formation of new transseptal fibers.

The second study repeated the method on humans. Patients with moderate to advanced periodontitis were treated using a split-mouth design. Mucoperiosteal flaps were raised in all quadrants, and then the exposed root surfaces of contralateral quadrants were treated by one or the other approach to root debridement. Control quadrants were scaled and root-planed with hand instruments and flame-shaped diamond stones to remove all soft and hard deposits and cementum. The test quadrants were treated with polishing using rubber cups, interdental rubber tips, and polishing paste. Calculus was removed carefully with a curette in the test quadrants to minimize removal of cementum as much as possible.

Following treatment, the surgical flaps were replaced and sutured. Supervised maintenance following treatment included professional tooth cleaning once every 2 weeks for 3 months, followed by recall appointments every 3 months until 24 months after treatment. The results showed that periodontal health was improved by both types of treatment, suggesting that extensive removal of cementum through root planing was not necessary and could not be justified.

Moore and others (1986) investigated the distribution of LPS in periodontally involved root surface–associated materials. They found that washing the root surfaces of periodontally involved extracted teeth removed 39% of the LPS and that brushing the surfaces for 1 minute with a slowly rotating bristle brush removed an additional 60%. Therefore, almost complete debridement (99%) of the LPS on the root surfaces was accomplished by these relatively simple and nontraumatic measures, calling into question the need for traditional methods of treating root surfaces (i.e., root planing with hand instruments). The authors concluded that LPS is only associated with rather than firmly bound to periodontally involved root surfaces. They suggested that polishing the root surface with an abrasive paste would remove LPS during surgical (open) debridement and that passing an ultrasonic instrument lightly over the root surface would remove LPS during nonsurgical debridement.

Cheetham, Wilson, and Kieser (1988) demonstrated that a conservative approach to hand instrumentation was effective in removing most LPS on root surfaces. They executed 15 instrument strokes on each root surface, overlapping the strokes to ensure that the entire root surface was treated. The extent of root smoothness achieved by this procedure was not considered to be important. The small amounts of LPS which remained following this treatment regimen (less than 24 ng) were evaluated as "insignificant," although it should be noted that the soft tissue response to treatment was not determined as part of this in vitro study. Further investigation of the clinical response to this treatment, as well as other conservative approaches to root debridement, is warranted.

The use of ultrasonic instruments has also been proposed as an effective means of accomplishing conservative, yet thorough periodontal debridement. Checci and Pelliccioni (1988) performed an in vitro study in which extracted, periodontally involved teeth were cut in half along the sagittal plane. One half of the tooth was then root-planed with a curette until it felt smooth and glasslike. The other half was treated with an ultrasonic scaler until it exhibited a smooth, calculus-free, and glasslike surface. The teeth were then suspended into dishes containing monkey fibroblasts. Fibroblasts attached to both groups of teeth with no significant differences, demonstrating that both approaches to treatment eliminate root toxicity.

Smart and others (1990) tested the effectiveness of a more conservative treatment approach using ultrasonic instruments. Single-rooted, periodontally involved, extracted teeth with no clinically detectable calculus deposits were debrided. The operator used light pressure and overlapping strokes with a Cavitron TF-10 tip and a medium power setting to accomplish the debridement. Following treatment, LPS levels were reduced to less than 2.5 ng per root surface, a level comparable to that of healthy, noninvolved teeth. These results support the contention that ultrasonic instruments are effective in removing LPS from affected tooth surfaces and in accomplishing deplaquing as part of the periodontal debridement process. A limitation of this study is that it did not consider the potential impact of calculus-associated LPS on root debridement accomplished by an ultrasonic instrument.

Can ultrasonic debridement reduce LPS levels in the presence of calculus deposits? This concern was addressed in a follow-up study by Chiew and others (1991). Lipopolysaccharide levels were measured following use of ultrasonic debridement on periodontally involved teeth that had visually detectable calculus deposits in vitro. A similar technique to the one described previously was utilized in which light pressure and overlapping strokes were applied to treat the entire root surface. Although this technique was intended to extend treatment over the entire root surface, no additional or intentional effort was made to remove calculus deposits during the process. Following this treatment, only small amounts of LPS remained, despite the presence of visually detectable residual calculus deposits. It is interesting that the posttreatment LPS levels were similar to those reported by Smart and others (1990), indicating that the presence of calculus did not affect the outcome. These results suggest that calculus-associated LPS is easily removed by ultrasonic action. This study calls into question the traditional emphasis on subgingival scaling and root planing to remove all calculus and adds to the growing interest in alternative techniques of debridement, which emphasize the removal of subgingival plaque and its products.

In summary, periodontal research conducted in the past several decades has contributed significantly to our knowledge about the existence and nature of LPS and its role in the pathogenesis of periodontal disease. Early assumptions that LPS penetrated into the cementum of periodontally involved roots had significant clinical implications for how root debridement was carried out. More recent investigations, however, have provided evidence that LPS exists only superficially and, in fact, is easily removed by methods other than extensive root planing. These findings should encourage dental hygienists to re-evaluate the justification for traditional methods of scaling and root planing to eliminate LPS and to begin defining and testing alternative approaches to treatment. The next section, on the role of calculus, furthers this perspective.

Changing perspectives on calculus

The association of calculus and periodontal disease has been traced as far back in history as the ancient Sumerians, who lived 5000 years ago (Mandel and Gaffar, 1986). Until the 1960s, calculus was still regarded as a primary cause of periodontal inflammation. Its rough surface was believed to irritate otherwise healthy tissues, causing them to become inflamed. This belief led to a seemingly logical assumption that removal of all calculus was necessary for resolution of the inflammation. Accordingly, dental hygiene education focused on developing and refining instrumentation skills necessary to detect and remove calculus deposits, and treatment expertise came to be measured against calculus removal skills. The goal of treatment was defined clinically as the removal of all calculus, evidenced by a subgingival root surface that felt smooth and a supragingival tooth surface on which no deposits could be seen.

The attainment of root smoothness, although a subjective impression, was used to describe the endpoint of root surface instrumentation. It became equated with surface cleanness and served to indicate that all deposits had been removed. The physical nature of the root surface became a primary criterion for making clinical decisions. Therefore the decision to treat a given site with instrumentation was based on the presence or absence of calculus. The decision to cease instrumentation was based on the physical appearance and feel of the root surface in question. It was assumed that the degree of surface smoothness not only indicated the extent of calculus removal but also provided some level of certainty that new plaque deposits would not be as readily retained in the future.

The interest in calculus removal and root surface smoothness as an indication of treatment success was evident in the periodontal research of the 1950s and 1960s. Researchers examined extracted teeth which had been treated with different types of hand or ultrasonic instruments to determine which approach produced the smoothest surfaces or the least residual calculus deposits. In early studies extracted teeth were scaled or root planed under laboratory conditions (*in vitro*) without the complicating factors of actual intraoral treatment (e.g. saliva, visibility, bleeding, access barriers) (Schaffer, 1956; Barnes and Schaffer, 1960; Jones & O'Leary, 1978; Nishimine & O'Leary, 1979). Later studies examined calculus removal and root surface characteristics following treatment of teeth in the mouth (*in vivo*) (Stende and Shaffer, 1961; Moskow and Bressman, 1964, Jones et al. 1972; Rabbani et al. 1981). These teeth, which had been indicated for extraction due to periodontal disease, were treated with different hand or ultrasonic instruments, and then extracted and examined microscopically. By the early

1970s scanning electron microscopes were being used to study supragingival and subgingival calculus and root surface characteristic at high levels of magnification (Mandel and Gaffar, 1986).

The issue of optimal root smoothness and how best to achieve it has been thoroughly studied in the past four decades (Allen and Rhoads, 1963; Barnes and Schaffer, 1960; Beltin and Spjut, 1964; Ewen, 1966; Ewen and Gwinnett, 1977; Kerry, 1967; Meyer and Lie, 1977; Van Volkinburg et al, 1976; Wilkinson and Maybury, 1973). Most of these studies supported hand instruments, specifically curettes, as the preferred means of subgingival scaling and root planing because they were better than ultrasonic instruments in producing a smooth root surface and removing cementum.

Note that the root surface was the focus of interest in these studies, rather than the periodontal tissues surrounding the treated root. Researchers became so fixated on the nature of the root surface itself that only later, in the mid-1970s and early 1980s did the important question emerge of whether or not a smooth surface made any biologic difference to the adjacent inflamed tissues.

Clinical trials examining the relationship between calculus removal and soft tissue response began to appear in the literature of the late 1970s and early 1980s. Rosenberg and Ash (1974) compared surface roughness after both hand and ultrasonic scaling to an inflammatory index of the adjacent soft tissues. Although hand instruments produced a significantly smoother surface, there was no significant relationship between the two approaches in degree of inflammation after treatment. Khatiblou and Ghodossi (1983) reported that surface roughness played a facilitative role in promoting reattachment of connective tissue to treated root surfaces, casting additional doubt on the biologic rationale for creating hard, glassy-smooth root surfaces.

Despite the mounting evidence in the 1960s and 1970s indicating that bacterial plaque was the primary etiologic agent in periodontal diseases, removal of calculus has maintained its position as a focal point of dental hygiene treatment. Although hygienists intensified their efforts at educating patients to control supragingival plaque, calculus was still the primary focus of subgingival treatment. Treatment planning was based on the need for scaling or root planing. Difficulty levels were determined by the amount and location of deposits, and appointments were planned based on estimates of the time needed to perform scaling and root planing. The endpoint of treatment was defined as the removal of all calculus and stain, and recall intervals were based on how quickly calculus or stains reaccumulated.

Patients have learned to be concerned about calculus from dental professionals. At recall appointments, patients inquire about how much "tartar" or calculus they have accumulated, rather than about the location and extent of bleeding sites or probing depths. Indeed, this focus on calculus as the primary interest of the recall appointment is still promoted in the mass media. In television commercials for calculus-inhibiting dentifrices, patients evaluate their home care success in terms of how much scaling they require.

Dental hygiene students may experience some confusion about how their faculty perceive the importance of calculus in dental hygiene treatment. Though they are exposed to information in textbooks and from faculty about the secondary significance of calculus in periodontal disease, they receive conflicting messages throughout the curriculum which, though unintentional, are still influential. A significant proportion of instructional time is dedicated to learning calculus detection and removal skills because of the belief that motor skills take longer to develop than cognitive learning. In addition, clinical evaluation of students may be disproportionately weighted towards measuring calculus removal as an end product rather than as a process. This may emphasize its achievement over other skills such as patient evaluation or patient education.

These evaluation methods may have been selected because they seemed to be more objective—since calculus deposits can be felt, seen, and measured quantitatively—whereas more qualitative or interpretive evaluation is required for other elements of dental hygiene care. Nonetheless, such systems inadvertently reward students for emphasizing the "smoothness" of the treated root surface rather than the instrumentation process or the soft tissue response to treatment. They encourage students to emphasize their success as calculus removers rather than their ability to motivate patients to perform daily, effective plaque control.

As a result, students may mistakenly perceive that calculus detection and removal is the most critical aspect of patient care. The adage that "ac-tions speak louder than words" applies in this case. An enlightening exercise for faculty and students would be to examine their educational program for consistencies and inconsistencies about what students are told in the classroom, what task they are asked to perform, and how they are evaluated on their performance. This may help to clarify the assumptions underlying these practices.

Much of the professional identity of many practicing hygienists, having been indoctrinated as to the importance of calculus removal, may be centered on perceptions of their scaling and root planing skills. The myth of the "Super Hygienist," who could remove all calculus painlessly in 45 minutes or less regardless of periodontal condition or other complicating factors, has pervaded our professional consciousness over the past several decades. The idea of shifting treatment perspectives away from "cleaning teeth" to treating infected tissues may seem threatening to some clinicians; this is a natural response to change. The excitement which follows, however, when one realizes the close relationship between old and new techniques and the potential for greater treatment success, is well worth the risk of changing perspectives. An even greater degree of professional esteem can be realized when hygienists work together, using their knowledge and skills to redirect and redesign creative approaches to treatment that reflect current knowledge in the field.

Accessibility of calculus to debridement. Current evidence on the significance of calculus to periodontal treatment questions some of the basic assumptions underlying the traditional emphasis on calculus removal. The first assumption is that it is possible to remove *all* calculus deposits which form on the surfaces of the teeth, especially subgingival deposits. After several decades, the abundance of clinical studies focusing on root surface characteristics after scaling and root planing have provided us with an unavoidable conclusion—that removal of *all* calculus deposits from periodontally involved root surfaces rarely, if ever, occurs! The presence of residual calculus (i.e., calculus that was not detected or removed during treatment) has been documented despite the skill or education level of the clinician (hygienist, periodontal resident, or periodontist) (Badersten, 1985; Brayer et al, 1989; Eaton et al, 1985;), the type of instrument used (hand or ultrasonic) (Breininger, O'Leary, and Blumenshine,

1987; Kepic et al, 1990), the type or location of teeth (Buchanan and Robertson, 1987; Kepic et al, 1990; Sherman et al, 1990b), the clinical probing depth (Sherman et al, 1990a, 1990b), or the time alloted for treatment.

Residual calculus has been reported on teeth that had been extensively scaled and root planed, both with open and closed debridement. In fact, it has even been detected on teeth treated with closed debridement followed by a second treatment with open debridement (Kepic et al, 1990). Therefore it cannot be concluded that residual calculus is left behind only because of improper technique, though certainly that may be one explanation. It is apparent that the inaccessibility of calculus within furcations, grooves, and concavities of the root surface and the limitations of current instruments to adapt within these areas are major factors.

Reliability in detecting residual calculus. Another clinical belief that has been disproved by the consistent presence of residual calculus following periodontal treatment is that clinicians can develop sufficient tactile skills to detect all calculus deposits with the aid of a probe or explorer. In each of the studies cited, the operator made a decision that the root surface was clinically smooth with the aid of an explorer or probe. Despite this evaluation, the presence of residual deposits, many of which were reported to be flat and veneer-like, could still be detected microscopically.

One recent study found that trained periodontists evaluated the clinical presence or absence of calculus on treated root surfaces incorrectly more than 50% of the time. In addition, these evaluators were not consistent with each other in their determinations, nor could they reproduce their own findings about root preparation to a high degree (Sherman et al, 1990a). These findings indicate that determination of surface smoothness is not a guarantee of complete calculus removal and that dependence on such a subjective means of evaluating the endpoint of treatment is highly questionable.

The relationship between residual calculus and healing. The clinical significance of the presence of residual calculus depends on its impact on the success or failure of periodontal therapy. It is therefore important to consider the long-held assumption that diseased periodontal tissues would not heal in the presence of calculus deposits. When examined in the light of the many clin-

ical studies that have documented treatment success following closed debridement (i.e., scaling and root planing), it appears that this assumption cannot be substantiated.

Consider the implications of applying the research findings on the prevalence of residual calculus to the assumption that the presence of calculus prohibits periodontal healing. Removal of all calculus from root surfaces is rare if not impossible, even following extensive removal of root surface material. Residual calculus has been observed even when the root surface has been surgically exposed to allow visualization of the treatment area. Even in accessible areas, the presence or absence of residual flat or veneer calculus cannot be determined with the use of explorers. Depending on the type of therapy and the degree of periodontal involvement, treatment success under these circumstances could be predicted to be dismal. Almost half of the nonfurcation sites treated by closed debridement would not respond to therapy. Failure rates of almost 40% in nonfurcation sites treated with open debridement would be expected, with those in furcation areas approaching 100%. Conventional periodontal therapy could be expected to fail in almost 80% of cases of advanced disease if the presence of residual calculus was a valid predictor of treatment failure (Robertson, 1990).

The fact remains, however, that despite the high probability that undetected residual calculus will remain after periodontal treatment, researchers still report high rates of success in achieving resolution of inflammation and maintaining attachment levels following periodontal treatment. If it were true that the presence of residual calculus prohibited healing and periodontal health, then how could such results be explained? An alternative hypothesis, consistent with these proven results, might be that thorough debridement eliminates calculus and associated plaque enough to support healing of periodontal tissues. It might also modify the residual deposits leaving them less plaque retentive and compatible with periodontal health. In other words, each host appears to have a certain "threshold" for calculus tolerance. Reducing calculus below the threshold level allows the host to resolve the inflammation (Robertson, 1990). Many individuals appear able to tolerate the presence of some residual calculus so that periodontal healing can occur.

Sherman and others (1990b) observed both the

extent of residual calculus and the clinical responses to treatment. Patients were treated with scaling and root planing and re-examined after 3 months. Their short-term clinical responses were unrelated to the presence or amount of residual calculus on the treated root surfaces.

Clinical studies in animals and humans have provided further evidence that soft tissues can tolerate calculus in the absence of bacterial plaque. Though plaque-covered calculus deposits will contribute to inflammation, it is the plaque and not the calculus itself which is the source of the inflammation. Individuals who have heavy amounts of supragingival calculus can still maintain gingival health if they practice effective toothbrushing (Gaare et al, 1990).

Blomlöf and others (1987) found that periodontal wound healing in monkeys was not influenced by the presence of small amounts of calculus on the root surfaces. Another study with beagle dogs looked at the degree of inflammation following treatment of calculus-containing root surfaces with either root planing followed by flap surgery or surgery with no root planing (Fujikawa et al, 1988). During the entire 120-day healing period, meticulous daily plaque control was performed on the animals. At the end of the study there was no difference in the degree of inflammation between the two treatment groups.

Chiew and others (1991) found that LPS levels could be reduced significantly when an ultrasonic instrument was used, despite the fact that residual calculus remained over an average surface area of 35% of the root surface. These findings suggest that the pathogenic potential of the treated surfaces could be reduced without removal of all calculus deposits.

Is root planing necessary?

It would be inappropriate to conclude from this discussion that attempting to remove all accessible and detectable calculus during the debridement process is unnecessary. Calculus is plaque retentive, and its presence promotes plaque accumulation and contributes to the chronic nature of periodontal disease. Calculus has been metaphorically described as "a toxic waste dump site" and "a slow release device delivering pathogenic products" within the periodontal environment (Mandel and Gaffar, 1986). In addition, its presence complicates the patient's efforts to manage plaque.

Detection and removal of accessible calculus is an important component of the debridement process. In fact, the approach to periodontal debridement described in this chapter calls on more highly developed instrumentation skills than either scaling or root planing. It is intended to ensure even more comprehensive treatment of all affected tooth and root surfaces through the use of improved instrumentation technologies. This treatment includes removal or disruption of the composition of bacterial plaque and its associated endotoxins as well as elimination of plaque retentive deposits and surfaces over the entire tooth/root surface to promote a healing response. To achieve this goal, hygienists must still become accomplished in techniques of instrumentation (including use of ultrasonic instruments) and be able to navigate complex root morphology. In addition they must be able to work within the confines of the periodontal pocket, apply a working knowledge of the nature of the diseased root surface and adherent deposits, and evaluate the soft tissue response to treatment. One sign of desirable tissue response is attachment gain. Molecular growth factors that enhance reattachment are found in significant quantities in cementum compared with dentin (Somerman, 1987). Therefore planing to remove cementum may be counter-productive as well as unnecessary.

The change in focus toward treating an infection rather than treating the root surface does not imply a less rigorous or less precise approach to treatment by any means. In fact, periodontal debridement probably requires hygienists to be more exacting than traditional approaches do. Consider, for instance, how one would perform instrumentation differently if attempting to remove loose and adherent plaque and endotoxins over the entire root surface area without damaging it instead of trying to remove calculus deposits and the underlying cementum. The implications for instrument selection, stroke patterns, number of strokes, need to overlap strokes, and effective pressure required for a stroke differ significantly. These differences are discussed in detail later in this chapter.

The point to understand is that periodontal debridement, though aimed primarily at removing the threat of pathogenic bacterial plaque, when performed thoroughly will also remove accessible calculus deposits *without* excessive and unnecessary removal of cementum and dentin. Therefore a critical difference between periodontal debridement and root planing is that the former regards calculus removal as a subgoal to achieving periodontal health and cementum removal as unnecessary and undesirable, while the latter regards calculus and cementum removal as a primary goal.

After reviewing current knowledge about the pathogenicity of plaque and endotoxins, the superficial nature of the presence of these pathogens on periodontally diseased root surfaces, the limitations of removing all calculus, and the ability of the periodontal tissues to tolerate small amounts of residual calculus, one must ask two important questions. First, is scaling adequate for treatment of periodontal disease? The answer is a resounding "No!" Scaling is inadequate for total wound debridement. Second, is root planing necessary to achieve periodontal healing? The answer is "Probably not." The rationale for extensive root planing appears to be based on several beliefs and assumptions that cannot be supported by current research findings.

It is possible that root planing, although shown to result in healing, may constitute *overtreatment*. Clinical periodontal treatment has become so caught up in evidence that treatment of the root surface results in improved periodontal health that an illogical assumption has been made that the more extensive the root treatment, the more successful the result. If a little root planing is good, then a lot is even better! It is now necessary to review this assumption and ask how much and what kind of instrumentation is *optimal* for producing successful outcomes for each individual or periodontal site.

The information in this chapter provides a first step toward defining new approaches to treatment that are consistent with our knowledge of the nature of periodontal diseases. Periodontal debridement, as a more conservative and less invasive approach to treatment, would be preferable to traditional root planing techniques if both were shown to be equally effective. Currently, the research on nonsurgical therapy is based on treatment protocols involving traditional scaling and root planing. New research is needed to document and compare the effects of these two approaches to instrumentation. We must expand our knowledge of what approaches are the most effective and efficient in debriding tooth and root surfaces while ensuring an optimal healing response and reducing the risks of treatment for both patient and operator.

THE CHOICE OF HAND OR ULTRASONIC INSTRUMENTS

The first section of this chapter aimed to present critical information about the nature of the diseased root surface and associated deposits and thus enable the dental hygienist to make critical decisions about what needs to be accomplished during periodontal debridement. The next step is to address the choice of how to implement this process—using hand or ultrasonic instruments.

Until very recently, hand instruments, especially curettes, were preferred. This recommendation was influenced by a number of factors. Foremost among these were the previously discussed clinical assumptions, which led to a desire to remove all calculus and most of the cementum to create as smooth a root surface as possible. Early laboratory and clinical studies that relied on profilometer (stylus) tracings of teeth rather than direct evaluation with scanning electron microscopy suggested that curettes produced significantly smoother surfaces than did ultrasonic instruments.

Early generations of ultrasonic instrument tips were also somewhat bulky in comparison to finishing curettes. They did not have the advantage of complex shank designs to permit the same ease of access to navigate subgingival pockets. Therefore ultrasonic instruments were relegated to the role of removing primarily supragingival calculus and stain and easily accessible subgingival calculus. Some practitioners suggested that, with proper technique and experience, ultrasonic instruments could produce results comparable to those of hand instruments during scaling and root planing, but they seemed to represent a minority opinion. Until recently, most clinical textbooks recommended that ultrasonic instruments be used primarily for gross deposit removal, to be followed by the use of hand instruments for definitive fine scaling and root planing.

The shift in perspective towards root debridement as a means of treating an infection rather than treating the root surface itself—combined with greater understanding of the nature of plaque, LPS, and calculus within the periodontal pocket environment—has led to a renewed interest in the use of ultrasonic instruments in the treatment of periodontal disease. Several recent clinical studies have compared the effectiveness of modern ultrasonic instruments to that of hand instruments. The findings add to the general consensus that the two approaches are equally effective in periodontal debridement and support the contention that ultrasonic instruments may be preferable.

Comparisons of hand versus ultrasonic instruments

A number of recent studies have compared the ability of hand and ultrasonic instruments to debride periodontal pockets of bacterial plaque, LPS, and calculus. Breininger, O'Leary, and Blumenshine (1987) found that both methods accomplished effective bacterial debridement of subgingival root surfaces within moderately deep pockets (4 to 7 mm), and that curettes were somewhat more likely to leave apical or calculus-associated plaque than were ultrasonic instruments. Garnick and Dent (1989) also reported that both hand and ultrasonic instruments are effective in plaque debridement. The effects of hand and ultrasonic instruments on the subgingival microflora in deep (6 to 9 mm) periodontal pockets were investigated by Oosterwaal and others (1987). They found the two methods to be equally effective in reducing bleeding and probing depths, and found no differences in the microbial responses to the two methods. Both treatments produced a shift to healthy bacterial composition within the treated sites. Olsen and Socransky (1981) reported that ultrasonic vibrations have a lethal effect on bacteria and that gram-negative pathogens are especially susceptible to sonification. Therefore, in addition to mechanical removal of bacteria, the ultrasonic vibrations provide another means of reducing the bacterial threat.

Treatment of periodontally involved root surfaces with ultrasonic instruments has been shown to reduce the quantity of LPS to nontoxic levels similar to those found on healthy, nonperiodontally involved teeth (Smart et al, 1990). When comparing the effectiveness of hand and ultrasonic instruments in their ability to remove toxic materials from root surfaces, Checci and Pelliccioni (1988) also found both methods to be effective.

A number of studies have documented that ultrasonic instruments are as effective as hand instruments in removing calculus (Johnson and Wilson, 1957; Moskow and Bressman, 1964; Stende and Schaffer, 1961). More recently, Kepic et al. (1990) confirmed that curettes and ultrasonic instruments were equally effective in removing calculus. They also reported that both types of in-

struments left similar amounts of residual calculus and that hand instruments appeared to remove more cementum from proximal surfaces.

Short-term healing effects were examined by Biagini and others (1988). They measured gingival crevicular fluid flow, clinical parameters, and histologic evidence of the healing process of treated sites after both scaling and root planing with hand instruments and ultrasonic debridement. They found no significant differences. Long-term clinical studies comparing the two instrumentation methods have also documented that they are equally effective in treating periodontal disease and maintaining clinical attachment levels (Badersten et al, 1981; 1984a and b; Torfason et al, 1979).

The recent introduction of several brands of sonic scalers has provided an additional instrument choice. Design differences between sonic and ultrasonic instruments, as well as the associated advantages and disadvantages, will be described in the next section. In terms of effectiveness, sonic scalers compare favorably with ultrasonic instruments (Loos et al, 1987). Sonic scalers can be used with or without water coolant because they operate at lower power frequencies and do not generate as much heat as ultrasonic instruments; however, use with water for lavage is recommended.

Walmsley and others (1988) concluded that the presence of the water coolant allowed greater plaque removal from teeth *in vitro* than when water was not used. They concluded that the cavitational activity of the water used during sonic and ultrasonic treatment has an additional effect that supplements the mechanical motion of the tip in debriding the site. Therefore use of a water coolant seems to provide an advantage during debridement.

Gellin and others (1986) compared sonic scalers with curettes in a clinical study of patients with moderate to advanced periodontal disease. They found no consistent differences between the two methods in terms of removal of calculus, nor between the use of the two methods alone or in combination with each other. Loos and others (1987) compared ultrasonic and sonic scalers in patients with moderate to severe periodontal disease. They found no differences in clinical response with either method.

Ritz and others (1991) compared the amount of cementum removed from root surfaces following

12 working strokes with either a curette, a sonic scaler, or an ultrasonic instrument. They found that the ultrasonic instrument removed 12 μm of cementum; the sonic scaler 94 μm; and the curette 109 μm. These results support the use of ultrasonic instruments as the most conservative approach to subgingival debridement.

Advantages of ultrasonic debridement

These studies support the contention that periodontal debridement can be successfully accomplished with either hand or ultrasonic instruments. The choice of instrumentation, therefore, is left to the discretion of the operator and depends on personal preferences as well as patient considerations. A number of advantages to using an ultrasonic instrument should be considered when deciding which approach to select.

Debridement with ultrasonic instruments is less fatiguing to the operator than using hand instruments. The actual work of removing deposits is accomplished by the mechanical action of the ultrasonic instrument rather than by the hand and arm muscles of the operator. Operation of the ultrasonic instrument does not involve the same type of stressful and repetitive finger and wrist motion required by hand instrumentation, which can result in muscle and joint discomfort as well as occupational injuries such as carpal tunnel syndrome.

The use of ultrasonic instruments promotes faster healing of the treated periodontal wound. Ultrasonic instruments do not have the sharp blades of hand instruments, which can lead to inadvertent cuts and tears of soft tissue as a result of improper use or the difficulty of manuevering close to subgingival tissues. By increasing the extent of the periodontal wound, this type of tissue trauma can also delay the speed of healing of the soft tissues. Ultrasonic instrument tips are less capable of inflicting this type of damage and thus decrease healing time. The water irrigation also facilitates cleansing and flushing debris from the treated area as another means of assisting the healing process. New ultrasonic devices are also capable of delivering antimicrobial solutions through the coolant system to further the elimination of plaque bacteria and enhance healing (Nosal et al, 1991; Rosling et al, 1983, 1986, 1989; Taggart et al, 1990). Operator visualization of the treatment area is also improved as a result of the water lavage that constantly clears the site

of blood and debris, which is then carried away by the suction tip.

Newly designed ultrasonic tips are significantly smaller in diameter than most hand instruments to facilitate access into deep pocket areas and beneath tight gingival tissues. More variation in tip design has also improved their adaptability in all areas of the mouth and in areas that are difficult to treat with curettes, such as root concavities and furcations. Another advantage of ultrasonic instrument tips is that their entire surface area is activated so that debridement is accomplished when any portion of the tip contacts the surface to be treated. This makes them much more versatile than hand instruments.

The entire surface of an ultrasonic tip can be used during the procedure. In contrast, only the sharp cutting edge of the curette blade is capable of doing any work. Considering what a small portion of that cutting edge is actually engaged against the tooth surface for any given working stroke, one can appreciate the enormity of the task of treating every square millimeter of root surface with a hand instrument. The cavitational effect of the water coolant, which surrounds the ultrasonic tip as it is working also extends the action of this instrument so that a greater portion of the tooth surface is actually treated than just that area contacted by the tip itself.

Patients often report that debridement by ultrasonic instruments is more comfortable than hand scaling. Not only are the soft tissues not exposed to trauma from sharp cutting edges, but there is also less sensitivity from exposure of dentinal tubules caused by excessive removal of cementum. Smaller ultrasonic tips facilitate more comfortable insertion and adaptation within the pocket, because their reduced diameter requires less distension and manipulation of soft tissues during treatment than larger curette blades. Instrumentation with ultrasonic devices also eliminates the jaw discomfort associated with hand instrumentation, which results from finger rest to stabilize working strokes and the pressure needed to activate working strokes against tenacious deposits.

Ultrasonic debridement requires less treatment time than hand debridement. The time saved can be allocated to other procedures, such as through assessment and monitoring, patient education, or other treatment. The efficiency of ultrasonic instrumentation is also apparent when one considers that the operator can simultaneously accomplish various treatment goals with one procedure, for example removal of calculus, plaque, and LPS; removal of overhangs or excess cement; antimicrobial therapy; soft tissue curettage (removal of inflamed granulation tissue from the pocket wall); and/or subgingival irrigation.

The many advantages of sonic and ultrasonic instruments over hand instruments make it the choice of many clinicians. Therefore the remainder of this chapter will be devoted to explaining how sonic and ultrasonic instruments are used to accomplish periodontal debridement. The use of hand instruments will be described in the following chapter as a supplemental or alternative approach to debridement.

A note of caution is offered for those who might regard the use of an ultrasonic device as a less professionally demanding approach to instrumentation. Despite its many advantages, it would be foolish to think that the use of the ultrasonic scaler requires less training and practice than hand instrumentation. The ultrasonic unit is more complex than hand instruments and requires the control of more variables. Although it is less fatiguing for the operator to use, a great deal of professional skill, understanding, and practice is still required in order to achieve clinical success with this method.

SUPRAGINGIVAL AND SUBGINGIVAL DEBRIDEMENT USING SONIC AND ULTRASONIC INSTRUMENTS
Background

Sonic and ultrasonic instruments use vibrations, similar to sound waves, at power levels best suited to the specific task. Sonic instruments operate at frequencies below 20,000 cycles and ultrasonic instruments at frequencies above this level. These sonic and ultrasonic vibrations are used in medicine and industry as well as dentistry. Ultrasonic visualization is used in medical diagnosis and physical therapy. In industry, ultrasonic applications are used for dispersion of dyes, cutting of hard surfaces, cleaning, welding, soldering, and underwater echo-ranging or sonar. In dentistry, current uses include debridement, amalgam condensation, root canal therapy, and instrument cleaning.

Ultrasonic instrumentation was first used in dentistry in the 1950s. An ultrasonic drill was used to prepare teeth for restorations, but it relied on an abrasive slurry to cut the tooth and there-fore visibility was reduced considerably. About that time, high-speed turbine drills were also developed. As the turbine drill was found to be quite effective, the ultrasonic drill was phased out (Ewen and Glickstein, 1968; Green and Sanderson, 1965).

In 1955, an ultrasonic instrument was introduced for periodontal debridement (Zinner, 1955). This instrument has undergone many changes in design and usefulness since that time. The bulky, complex units are now compact and easy to adjust. The variety of tips has increased, some tips carry the needed water supply through an internal tube, and the size of the tips has changed to provide a finer array. Several manufacturers have developed units, each with unique features (Table 25-1).

Types of instruments

Ultrasonic instruments work by converting high-frequency electrical current into mechanical vibrations. Two types of ultrasonic units are available: magnetostrictive and piezoelectric (Fig. 25-1). Both types have a generator that produces high-frequency electrical current. They vary however, in the way the electrical energy is converted into mechanical vibrations, the pattern of action, and the number of surfaces on the tips that are activated.

The magnetostrictive transducer uses either a stack of flat metal strips (the Cavitron is an example), or a rod of ferromagnetic (capable of being magnetized) material, (the Odontoson M is an example). This magnetostrictive transducer is connected to the working tip to form a handpiece insert. Contained within the handpiece is a coil. When the electrical current is turned on, the coil within the handpiece becomes magnetized. The stack or transducer portion of the handpiece insert reacts to the magnetic field by expanding and contracting in accordance with the alternating current. The rapid expansion and contraction results in vibrations, which are transmitted to the attached working tip. The working motion of the magnetostrictive scaler is generally elliptical.

The first ultrasonic scalers on the market were the manual-tuning, magnetostrictive type. These units were later replaced by automatic frequency tuning machines. The trend is now back toward manual tuning.

The piezoelectric transducer does not require magnetostrictive stacks, and is completely con-

Table 25-1. Sonic and ultrasonic instruments

Manufacturer	Brand name	Frequency cycles/second	Tuning	Lavage choice other than water
Sonic scalers				
Dentsply	Densonic	6,300 Hz	Autotune	No
Kavo	Sonicflex	6,000 Hz	Autotune	Yes
Medidenta Dental Supply	Scalerite	1,500 Hz	Autotune	No
Star	Titan-S	6,000 Hz	Autotune	No
Piezoelectric ultrasonic scalers				
American Medical and Dental Corp.	Neosonic-S	30,000 Hz	Autotune	No
Am dent, AB, Sweden	Am dent 830	25,000 Hz	Autotune	No
Electro Medical Systems	Piezon Master 400	32,000 Hz	Autotune	Yes
Pro-Dentec	PDT Scaler	45,000 Hz	Autotune	No
Spartan USA, Inc.	Spartan Piezoelectric	40,000 Hz	Autotune	No
Young Dental Manufacture	Ultra Scaler	40,000 Hz	Autotune	No
Young Dental Manufacture	Young PS	40,000 Hz	Autotune	No
Magnetorestrictive ultrasonic scalers				
A-Dec	A-Dec (Cavitron)	25,000 Hz	Autotune	No
A/S L. Goof, Denmark	Odontoson M	42,000 Hz	Manual tune	Yes
Dentsply	Cavitron 3000	30,000 Hz	Autotune	No
Dentsply	Cavi-Med 200	25,000 Hz	Autotune	Yes
Dentsply	Bobcat	25,000 Hz	Autotune	No
Dentsply	Cavi-Jet 30	30,000 Hz	Autotune	No
Dentsply	Cavi-Endo 25	25,000 Hz	Autotune	No
JH Maliga Engineering	Microson 101	25,000 Hz	Manual tune	No
Parkell	Le Clean Machine	25,000 Hz	Manual tune	No
Parkell	Perio-Pro	25,000 Hz	Manual tune	Yes
Simplified System, Inc	Sonatron S3X	25,000 Hz	Autotune	No
Ultrasonic Services Inc.	USI-1	25,000 Hz	Manual tune	No

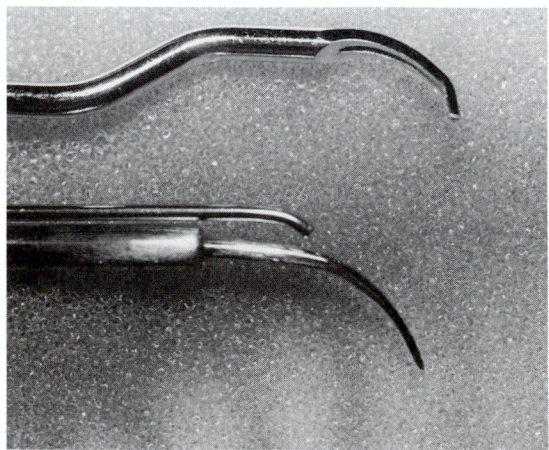

Fig. 25-1. Piezoelectric tip (*top*) functions in a linear direction and has cutting edges to help remove deposits using the two active sides of the tip. Magnetostrictive tip (*bottom*) functions in an orbital pattern and is active on all sides and has no cutting edges. The upper tip has an internal lavage source that necessitates its larger size; the lower tip has an external "trombone" to deliver lavage requiring less bulk for the tip itself.

tained within the handpiece rather than being connected to the working tip insert. Examples are the PDT Scaler by Pro-Dentec. Alternating electrical current is applied to reactive crystals, causing a dimensional change that is then transmitted to the working tip in the form of ultrasonic vibrations. The working tip is small and easily threaded into the handpiece. Separating the tip and the transducer should reduce the cost of the tips and facilitate sterilization and storage. The working motion of the piezoelectric scaler is generally linear. As a result, only two sides of the working tip are activated, limiting its adaptation, especially in deep pockets and furcations.

Sonic instruments also use vibrations of the working tip, but they are mechanical rather than electrical. Vibrations between 2,000 and 6,000 cycles per second are produced by means of air pressure rather than by electrical energy. An example of their mechanics is the Titan-S Sonic Scaler. The handpiece is composed primarily of a hollow rod, a rotor, and several rubber O-rings.

Compressed air is forced through a hollow rod in the handpiece. The rotor is a metal ring 6 mm wide, which encircles the hollow rod above a series of ten scientifically angled holes. As the air passes through the hollow rod, it escapes through the ten holes and causes the rotor to vibrate, causing the entire rod to vibrate in turn. These vibrations are then transferred to the working tip, which is screwed into the hollow rod. The working motion of the sonic scaler is generally elliptical. Through a separate line, water flows through the handpiece and out an opening on the working tip. This line is very narrow within the working tip and must be cleaned with orthodontic wire to prevent deposition of mineral deposits, which would block the water flow.

No superiority in the therapeutic effect of the magnetostrictive, piezoelectric, or sonic scaler has yet been decided by research trials. Because of this fact, several questions of effectiveness have been left unanswered: which of the various frequencies is best, does the linear versus elliptical versus orbital motion of the working tip influence efficiency or healing, and does the amount of fluid lavage (flushing) influence results? Currently, clinicians select equipment based on tip design, ability to sterilize components, and efficiency in debridement.

Tip design

The original Cavitron tips were designed for supragingival debridement and not for subgingival use. In spite of their bulky size, these tips were used in studies comparing hand and ultrasonic instrumentation. Even these bulky tips were as efficient as hand instruments in removing subgingival deposits. A new slimline series is now available from Dentsply, consisting of three "thin-tipped" modified inserts.

The new tips are thinner and are shaped more like exploratory hand instruments (probes and explorers) (Fig. 25-2). This is desirable because the tips can reach even the deepest recesses easily and safely, disrupting the subgingival plaque, removing calculus, and detoxifying the area (Fig. 25-3 and 25-4). Ultrasonic tips can be thin because they do not require the strength necessary to support a cutting edge under pressure. Typically, ultrasonic and sonic tips have no cutting edge. The clinician does not need to apply pressure against the tooth to remove deposits; therefore, the instrument does not require extra bulk to prevent bending and fracturing. The thinner tips require frequent replacement because they wear at a faster rate than thick tips; however, their ability to reach subgingivally and disrupt those areas quickly with minimal clinician fatigue outweighs the reactively minor problem of frequent replacement.

Sonic tips may be smooth and round or have four edges forming a diamond shape. Although the entire tip vibrates, the four edges are more effective than the flat sides for debridement.

The activity of the vibrating tip is enhanced by the cavitation of a fluid lavage that flushes the area. The fluid source is either internal or external. The internal source flows through the tip, carrying the liquid directly to the site. This is preferable, but often the orifice occludes, blocking the liquid. External fluid supply reaches the tip via a "trombone"—a metal tube that aligns with the tip. It is important to select equipment in which this tube is unlikely to become misaligned. The "trombone " should be rigid and not easily bent. Internal tubing is ideal until the orifice occludes, which requires tip replacement (see Fig. 25-1).

Tips are designed singly or in pairs. Single tips possess a universal design, allowing access to areas on both sides of the mouth. Paired tips are designed to complement each other as do the two ends of a cowhorn explorer. Their angles allow each to access half the surfaces. They are usually designated right and left, although the right tip will access the facial surfaces from the right and the lingual surfaces on the left, and vice-versa for the tip designated left.

Curette tip designs have also been adapted to ultrasonic instruments. No research trials using these tips have been reported to date. General limitations of curette tips will hold true for these ultrasonic tips: limited access because of size, and limited application because of a specific cutting edge. These tips may, however, ease the transition from hand to sonic/ultrasonic instrumentation for some practitioners.

Japanese investigators have designed a tip for use in furcation areas. The difference between this tip and the standard ultrasonic tip is a 1 mm ball on the end of the tip. This small ball is designed to give better access to furcation areas and to protect tooth surfaces and tissues. In vitro research found this tip to be more effective than curettes or traditional ultrasonic tips (Oda and Ishikawa, 1989).

Tips are also available for amalgam overhang removal. The first of these was developed for the

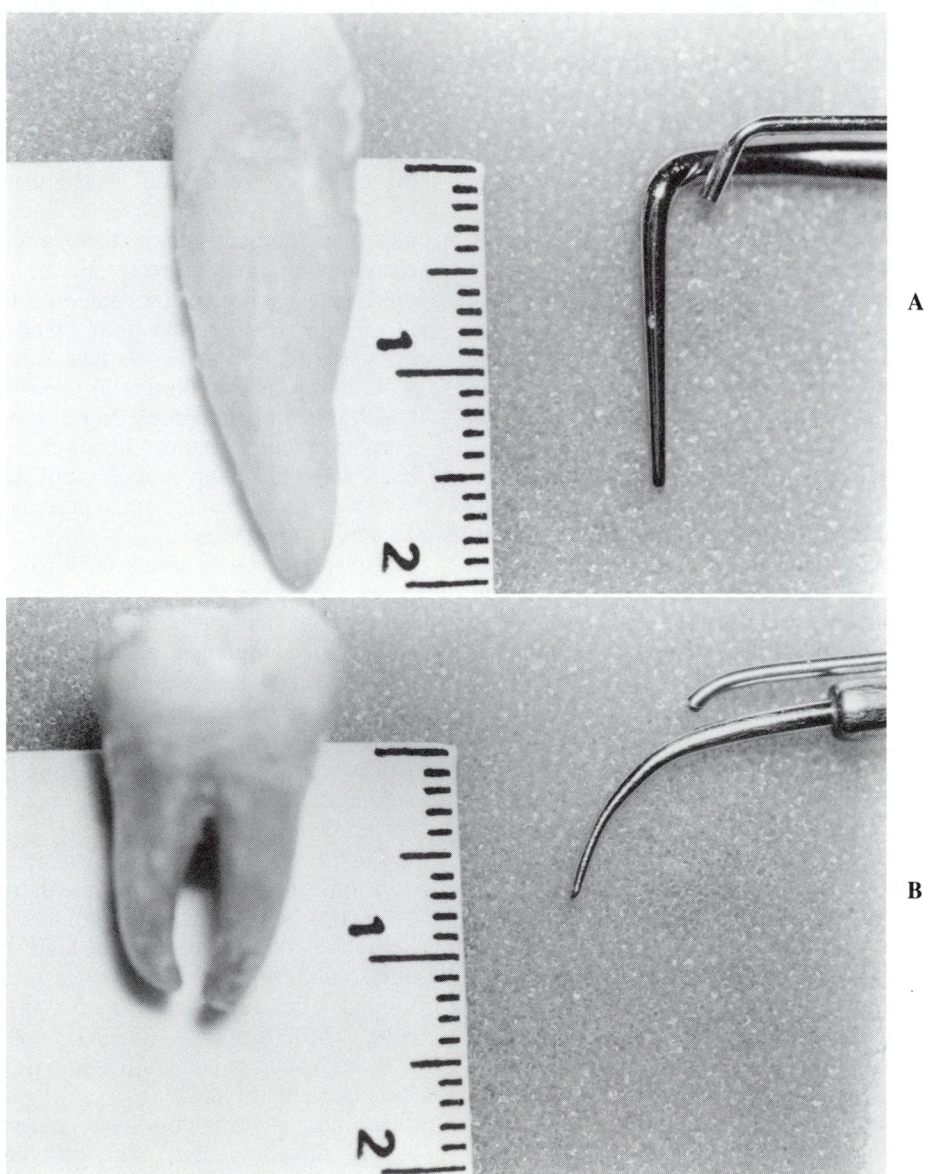

Fig. 25-2. **A**, Newly designed thin tip approximates size of periodontal probe. **B**, Newly designed thin tip approximates size of explorer.

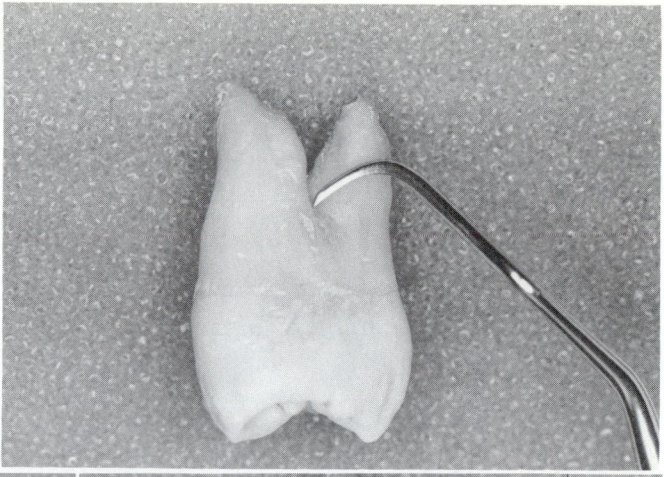

A

Fig. 25-3. **A**, Curette adapted to furcation provides minimal access to root structure; blade must be adapted against tooth to achieve debridement. **B**, Ultrasonic periodontal probe tip can reach all areas accessible to a periodontal probe; all surfaces of magnetostrictive tip are active. **C**, Ultrasonic explorer tip is finer and can reach deep into furcations and areas that are least accessible because of tissue tone or root morphology. Right- and left-angled versions of tip are available.

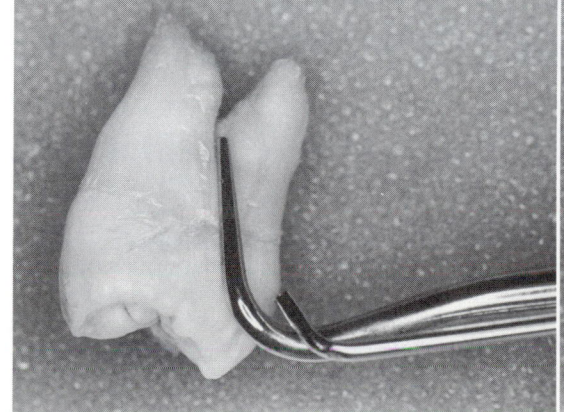

B

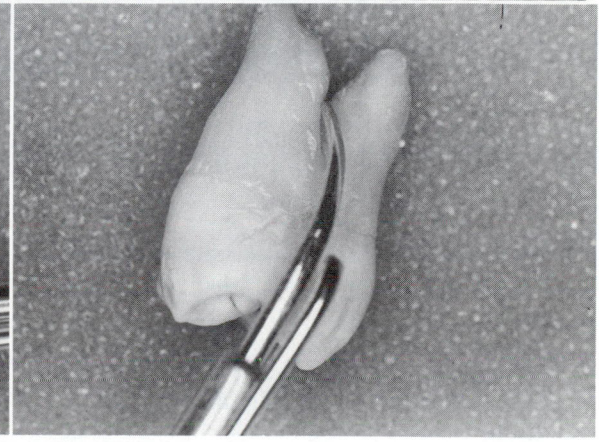

C

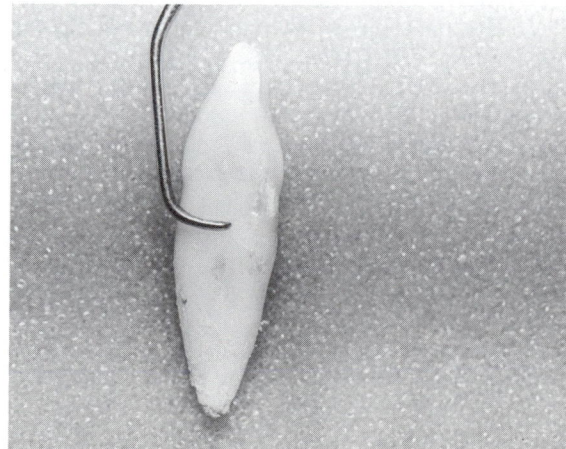

A

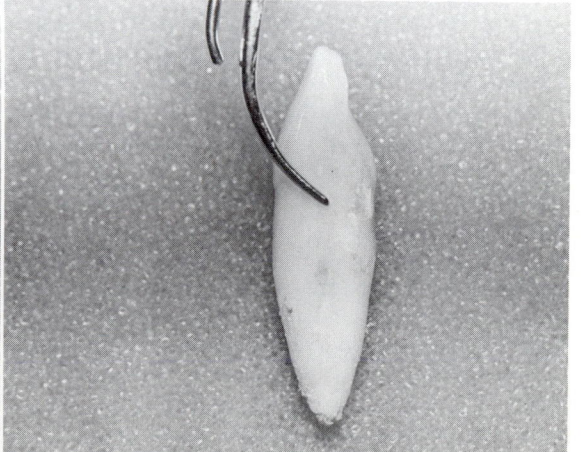

B

Fig. 25-4. **A**, Curette adapted to anterior root structure; adaptation is limited by pocket width of pocket and instrument size. **B**, Ultrasonic explorer tip has access to tight subgingival areas on anterior teeth and can be adapted to reach root concavities and furrows because all surfaces of the magnetostrictive tip are active.

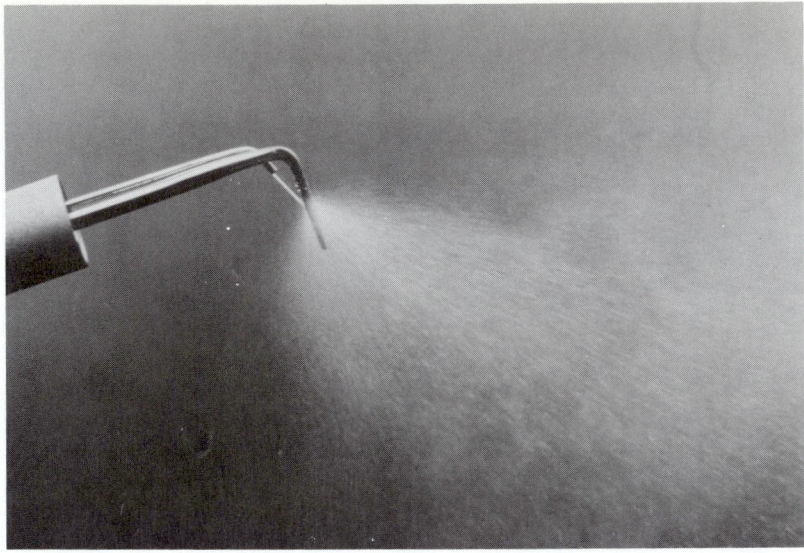

Fig. 25-5. Cavitated spray from tip of activated ultrasonic modulates heat, flushes area of instrumentation, and provides antibacterial activity. Spray of bubbles collapses inward.

Cavitron. Rather than being smooth and round, these paired tips are flat with a file on one side. Check with specific ultrasonic scaler manufacturers regarding tips for overhang removal.

The change of focus from supragingival to subgingival debridement with ultrasonic instruments has led to the design of thinner tips for better access in pocket and sulcus areas. Drs. Tom Holbrook and Sam Low, periodontists in Florida, are credited with the concept of tip modification. They suggest using the original Cavitron tips with external fluid tubing for modification. Newer tips cannot be cut down sufficiently without damaging the internal fluid supply. A large, coarse, fast-cut acrylic stone, mounted in a slow-speed handpiece can be used to reduce the tip (Holbrook and Low, 1989).

Reducing old Cavitron tips this way is no longer necessary because finer tips designed like periodontal probes and curved explorers are available for deep subgingival adaptation.

A sonic tip fitted with a plastic covering can be adapted to implants (Gantes and Nilveus, 1991) and effectively debrides natural teeth.

Lavage

Lavage is important for three reasons: acoustic streaming, which destroys bacterial cell walls; control of heat; and flushing of the area (Fig. 25-5).

As water meets the vibrating tip, it cavitates into a spray of bubbles that collapse inward. This is what causes the halolike appearance of the water at the tip. Ultrasonic instrumentation with a water lavage has an antimicrobial effect. The cavitation activity, heat, and acoustic streaming probably account for the decreased numbers of bacteria at ultrasonically debrided sites. The mechanical effects of cavitation (shock and stress waves) can disrupt and lyse bacterial cell walls (Clarke and Hill, 1970; Crum, 1982; Cunningham, 1982; Rooney. 1972;). One study suggests that the active motile rods typically associated with periodontal disease are the most sensitive to ultrasonics instruments, and that the gram-positive bacteria characteristic of healthy sites are more resistant to sonication (Olson et al, 1981). Bacterial endotoxins are significantly removed by ultrasonic instrumentation, as measured in the lab, (Chiew et al, 1991; Smart et al, 1990). Another study demonstrated that ultrasonically debrided root canals were more often sterilized than hand-instrumented sites (Sjogren and Sundqvist, 1987).

Magnetostrictive ultrasonic devices generate heat within the handpiece and at the working tip. The water serves to cool the handpiece and to protect the tooth surface from excessive heat. Conversely, the warming of the water as it passes through the handpiece provides for patient comfort. If insufficient water is used to reduce heat or if the instrument is held against on an area of a tooth for more than a few seconds, the temperature in the pulp chamber can rise to hazardous levels. The thermal conductivity of restorations and the thickness of tooth structure separating the instrument from the pulp affect the likelihood of a rise in pulp temperature. Usually the patient will feel discomfort and alert the clinician, preventing continued trauma. If the operative site is anesthetized, however, damage could occur (Abrams et al, 1979). Walmsley and colleagues (1986) measured the rise of temperature in the pulp resulting from transference of acoustic energy from the tip through the water coolant to the tooth. The observed increase in temperature suggested that only 3.6% of the energy expended was absorbed by the tooth causing a temperature increase; this suggests that pulp trauma is highly unlikely. However, ultrasonic instruments must be used with water flow and the tip must be kept moving at all times to reduce the possibility of pulp trauma. Sonic instruments do not generate excessive heat and therefore require less water.

Flushing during debridement will clear the area of hard and soft deposits. Calculus, that has been dislodged by the vibrations, attached plaque, and loosely adherent plaque will all be removed by the fluid lavage. This flushing action is also credited with reducing healing time compared with hand instrumentation (Bhaskar, 1972).

Penetration of ultrasonic lavage has been measured using dye instead of water. It was found that the liquid routinely reached the base of the pocket when instrumented with a Cavitron, EWPP tip (Nosal, 1991).

Ultrasonic bactericidal debridement combines the cavitational effects of the instrument with antimicrobial lavage. Traditionally, water has been used as the primary fluid for lavage. The Cavitron and Odontoson M are the first to offer the option of using an antimicrobial solution for irrigation. Previously it was necessary to pressurize a separate container for antimicrobials or sterile water. This technique is still possible with the addition of a pressurized fluid container to which a water valve has been added (Bug Buster, Perio Institute).

More recently, Dentsply introduced a self-contained unit that includes small containers for two antimicrobial solutions. The clinician can select the appropriate irrigant or mix the two for lavage. Tips for the Cavi-Med have an internal fluid tub-

ing that opens at the working end. These tips can be used for ultrasonic debridement, irrigation, or a combination of the two procedures. However, the internal tubing for lavage requires a bulkier tip.

Another option is the Odontoson M, which does not require a pressurized fluid source. Instead, this machine has a 10-inch spear attached to the the fluid tubing. This spear can be placed into a bottle or beaker of antimicrobial solution or a bag of sterile saline, thus expanding the possibilities for fluid lavage. This is the first ultrasonic unit that allows for sterilization of the fluid tubing as well as the handpiece. Thus, the fluid used for lavage can, for the first time, be a sterile solution.

Because the unit does not rely on water pressure from the unit to deliver lavage, it is completely portable for use in special care facilities and for the homebound.

A study using the Odontoson ultrasonic scaler with povidone-iodine instead of water for lavage demonstrated elimination of *Prevotella intermedia* and *Porphyromonous gingivalis* organisms from periodontal pockets, resolution of gingival inflammation, and significant gains in attachment. The attachment level gains were found to be 50% greater than those resulting from surgical access or debridement without antimicrobial lavage (Rosling, 1986). See Genco and Christersson (1990) for procedures used. Also in 1986, Blumenthal and Ewen reported a 7-day trial comparing no treatment, irrigation with water, irrigation with baking soda and hydrogen peroxide, and irrigation with sanguinarine chloride. The latter two treatments were most effective, with sanguinarine producing a 39% improvement in the gingival index compared with 28% with water and 35% with baking soda and hydrogen peroxide (Blumenthal and Ewen, 1986).

Infection control

The fluid spray that accompanies ultrasonic debridement creates an aerosol of water and microorganisms that come into contact with the clinician and settle on adjacent equipment surfaces. For this reason it is essential that, in addition to gloves, the clinician wear protective lenses and a face mask or plastic mask. As with other dental and dental hygiene procedures, the patient should also wear protective lenses and a drape. The dental unit and ultrasonic device should be covered if possible, and the entire area should be disinfected thoroughly after each use. High volume evacuation should be placed immediately adjacent to the working instrument to capture as much aerosol as possible. The air in the operatory should also be continually flushed with a laminar airflow system, which circulates and filters the air of microorganisms (Williams, 1970). When the ultrasonic device is being used, there is a thirty-fold increase of airborne microorganisms, most of which are known to be normal flora of the mouth (Holbrook et al, 1978). Of the airborne contaminants that could infect the clinician or subsequent patients, 97% can be removed with laminar airflow (Williams, 1970). Rinsing with an antimicrobial solution just before instrumentation may significantly reduce this hazard. Preprocedural rinsing with chlorhexidine has demonstrated a significant reduction in salivary bacterial counts immediately after rinsing, as well as during and after a 55 to 70-minute debridement appointment (Veksler et al, 1991). Although the effect has not been studied, using an antimicrobial lavage may also help reduce numbers of suspended viable microorganisms.

Just as instrumentation can contaminate the operating environment, it also can seed bacteria in the surgical site if the lavage is contaminated (Gross et al, 1976). The tubing and water valve connection may also provide an ideal site for bacterial growth. Therefore it has been suggested that sterile lavage solutions be used (Ballinger et al, 1976). Only one ultrasonic unit, the Odontoson M is equipped with sterilizable tubing. For other units, bacterial levels in the tubes can be reduced by flushing with water for 2 minutes prior to use each day and between appointments. Regardless of the fluid source, flushing is important to eliminate backwash of bacteria into the unit and subsequent contamination of the lavage solution.

Another study has shown no statistical differences in postoperative infections between patients treated with ultrasonic debridement using sterile water versus regular tap water (Reinhardt et al, 1982). This result will vary depending on contamination levels in local water supplies and in the equipment.

Preparation of the patient

Perhaps the most important phase of preparation is readying the patient for the procedure. Most patients may never have experienced anything but hand instrumentation. Therefore the first step is to briefly explain to the patient the condition that warrants a debridement procedure, why it should be done, the consequences of not having complete debridement, the likely after effects of the procedure, and the time and cost involved. Included with this explanation should be an introduction to the equipment.

For the person who has never had extensive debridement of any sort and who has large quatities of calculus, this is one way of meeting the criteria for informed consent and introducing the procedure in a helpful fashion:

I would like you to look in the mirror while I show you something. (Patient grasps mirror; clinician retracts lips to expose gingivae and heavy calculus.) These dark, crusty deposits are hard, chalklike pieces of calculus that are firmly attached to the teeth. They usually go hand in hand with disease of the gum tissue (or gingivae) and bone. Their presence makes it difficult for you to perform good oral hygiene, and they typically harbor bacterial plaque on the surface. This is plaque (show deposits on tip of probe from supragingival area and subgingival area), the source of the infection that is affecting your tissues. These deposits and toxins are present on the crowns of your teeth and on the roots. (Answer questions; follow up on patient's nonverbal responses.)

One of the first things we need to do is remove these deposits and toxins. Once they are gone, your tissue should begin to feel better, and it should be easier to keep up your oral hygiene routine. Your teeth and gingivae will look better, too.

Sometimes right after the deposits are removed, your teeth will be sensitive to cold. You've had that crusty insulation for a few years, and once it is gone the teeth will need to generate their own internal insulation. Other than the sensitivity and a couple days of tender gingivae, the procedure should cause no ill effects.

There are two ways we can complete the procedure. One is with hand instruments that are used to scrape or scale the deposits away. (Show the patient a hand scaler; attend to the patient's questions or nonverbals.) The other way is to use the ultrasonic instrument (show the ultrasonic instrument; attend to response). This method takes less time. The instrument generates sound waves that fracture the deposits off your teeth and kills the bacteria in the plaque. A liquid spray on the tip helps disrupt the bacterial clumps and flushes away the toxins. Most patients find that it feels better during and after the treatment if the ultrasonic instrument is used.

Some patients experience some tooth sensitivity during the procedure both with hand and ultrasonic instruments. If you find it uncomfortable, I would like you to tell me. We can try the other procedure or anesthetize the areas so the sensations are not a problem for you.

If we use hand instruments, it make take up to three

or four 1-hour appointments to remove this calculus and disrupt the plaque and toxins on the roots of your teeth. If we use the ultrasonic instruments, the first appointment should result in removal of almost all deposits. (Insert your best estimate of time required based on the difficulty of the case.) The cost per visit, as mentioned earlier, is $. What questions or concerns do you have?

Involving the patient in decision making enhances patient cooperation and reinforces your interpersonal relationship. They become a part of the therapy rather than those served as an object of care.

A thorough discussion of your recommendation of ultrasonic instrumentation is particularly important for long-standing patients accustomed to hand scaling and polishing who will look to you for an explanation. You can modify the basic presentation previously described for those patients:

We're going to be approaching your dental hygiene appointments a little differently now. We've had some major breakthroughs in research recently that suggest we should change some of our methods. For instance, we have always scaled all your teeth with a hand instrument and then polished with an abrasive. Now we know that the most important thing we do when we use an instrument around your teeth is disrupt the colonies of bacteria growing not only on the crowns but down in the spaces between your gingivae and teeth. While the hand instrument can disrupt the colonies, there is a newer approach that uses very thin instruments that can reach easily to the depths of the spaces and deliver an antimicrobial solution at the same time to help flush out the space and medicate the area. The tips vibrate at about 25,000 cycles per second and remove the hard deposits on your teeth while directly dislodging and killing the bacteria that have colonized on your teeth. I simply wipe the tip over your teeth with a few strokes in every area; I won't be pressing it against your teeth, and you won't feel or hear any scraping noise. I think you will find it more comfortable than the hand instruments, and it will take us less time. I can devote the time we gain to thoroughly assessing your periodontal health and making recommendations about areas that need more attention from both of us. How does this sound to you?

If you find this procedure troubling or uncomfortable, let's discuss alternatives. It will be different from what you are accustomed to, but I think you will find it an improvement.

Equipment preparation

The equipment for most ultrasonic units includes a control box, foot or finger control, water con-

nector, and handpiece. Insert tips for the handpieces are separate. Sonic scalers attach directly to the handpiece (compressed air) hosing and require no further set up other than possible pressure adjustment on the dental unit.

For others, the control unit should be moved near the dental chair and plugged into the electrical outlet. Attach and position the foot control; connect the water hose to the dental unit and the handpiece to the unit, being careful to align the prongs with the correct outlet.

When starting the unit after several hours of nonuse, turn the unit on the high setting and activate the foot pedal or finger control, allowing water to flow through the system for at least 2 minutes to clear stagnant water and associated contaminates. (This is not necessary with Odontoson where hosing and handpiece are drained and autoclaved after each use.)

Bleed air from the handpiece so that the liquid flows from the end of the handpiece, allowing air bubbles to rise and dissipate (Fig. 25-6). Attach the tip insert (Fig. 25-7). Select the proper power setting for the tip. Repeat this procedure each time an insert is changed. When you activate the tip, it will automatically tune. When the tip is tuned, the lavage bursts into a halo of fine mist (Fig. 25-8). Adjust the water flow so that it is the proper temperature and so the size of the spray is manageable.

Because of the wide variety of ultrasonic and sonic units, follow the manufacturer's instructions for each unit you encounter.

Instrument sequence

The heaviest instruments are used to remove the heaviest deposits. For a patient who has bridges of calculus, the tip shaped like a chisel can be employed to loosen the bridge in one ro two pieces (Fig. 25-9). The chisel is applied horizontally with a push stroke, flat against the proximal surfaces, and moved from labial to lingual aspects. Once the heavy bridges are removed, the flat-tipped instrument, often referred to as a *beaver-tail* (Figs. 25-10 and 25-11), can be used on all surfaces to remove large deposits, horizontally on the proximal surfaces and vertically on the facial and lingual surfaces. Because of its size and shape, it is not the tip of choice for deep or small deposits.

After using the beaver-tail tip, move to a universal tip that resembles a periodontal probe (see

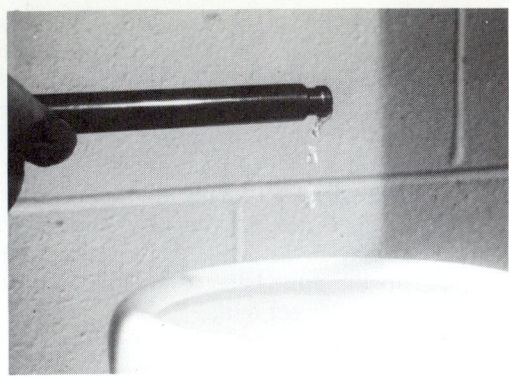

Fig. 25-6. Before placing tip insert, hold activated handpiece upright until water emerges, then turn it to the side and adjust water flow until water trails from edge in steady flow of nearly continuous drips.

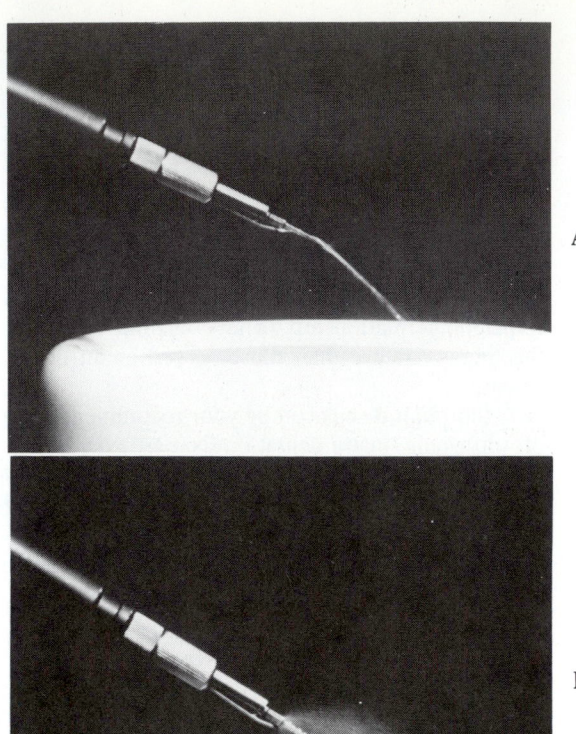

Fig. 25-8. **A**, Before tuning, water runs or sprays off tip in a stream. **B**, When tip is tuned, water sprays around tip in a halo. High-pitched squeal is heard. One or two shakes of handpiece eleminates drop from tip.

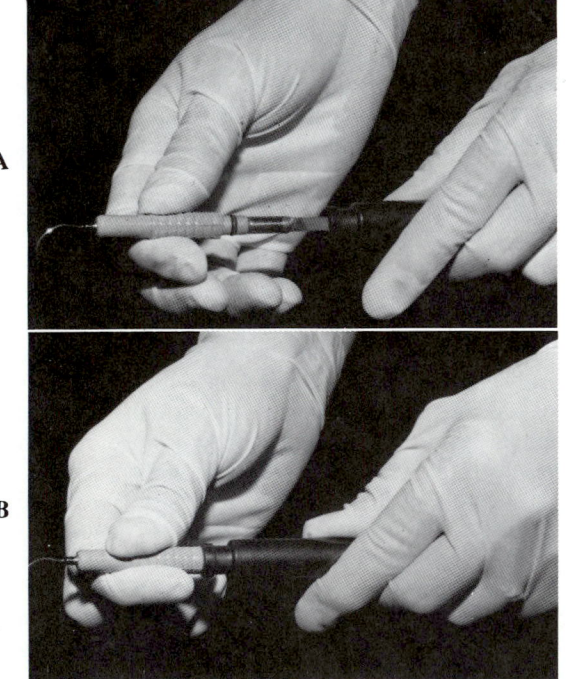

Fig. 25-7. **A**, After water has run freely from handpiece for at least 2 minutes, insert first tip to be used. **B**, Insert is locked firmly in place.

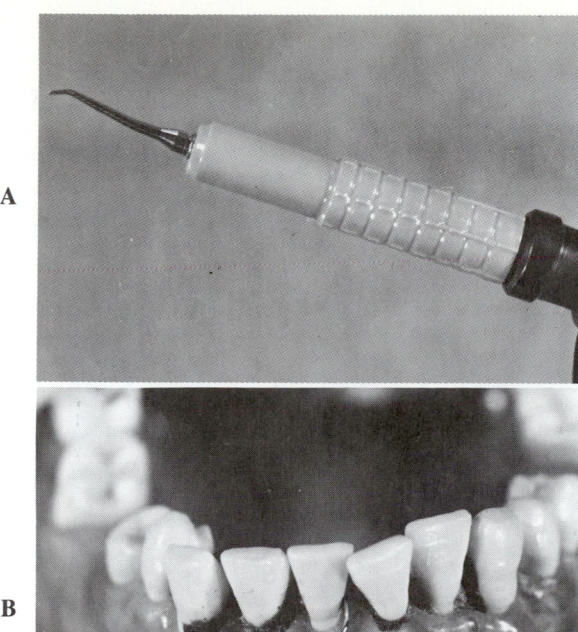

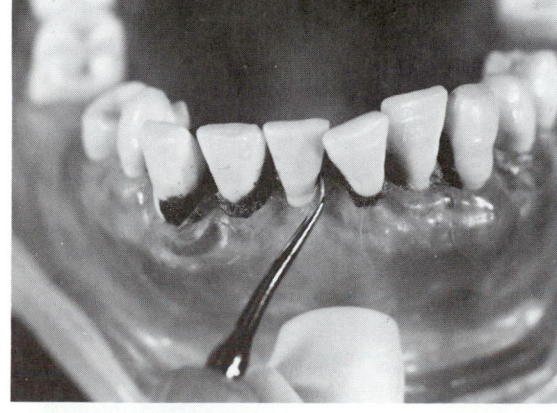

Fig. 25-9. **A,** Chisel-shaped tip is used to loosen and remove lingual bridges of calculus. **B,** Apply "blade" against proximal surfaces from labial aspect with horizontal push stroke. Calculus bridge will loosen and can be lifted out in one or two pieces.

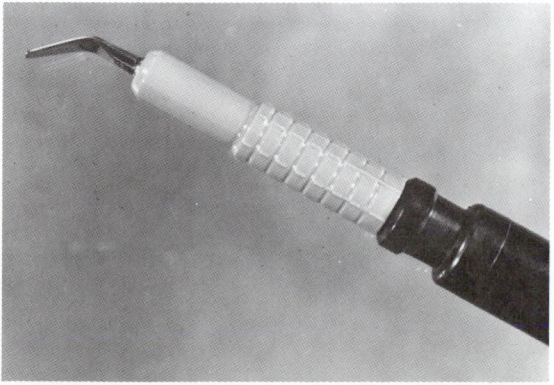

Fig. 25-10. Flat-tipped beaver-tail tip is used to remove large, tenacious deposits throughout mouth.

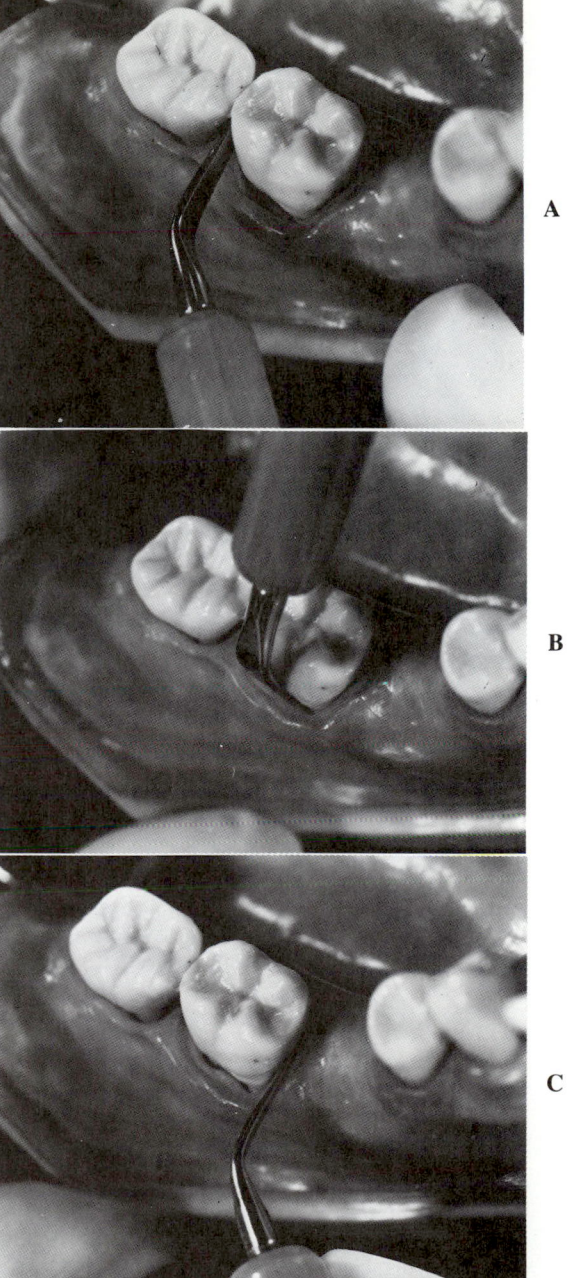

Fig. 25-11. In beginning a pattern of strokes, beaver-tail is used **A,** on distal surfaces from facial and lingual aspects with horizontal stroke, **B,** on facial and lingual surfaces with vertical stroke, and **C,** on mesial surfaces from facial and lingual aspects with horizontal stroke.

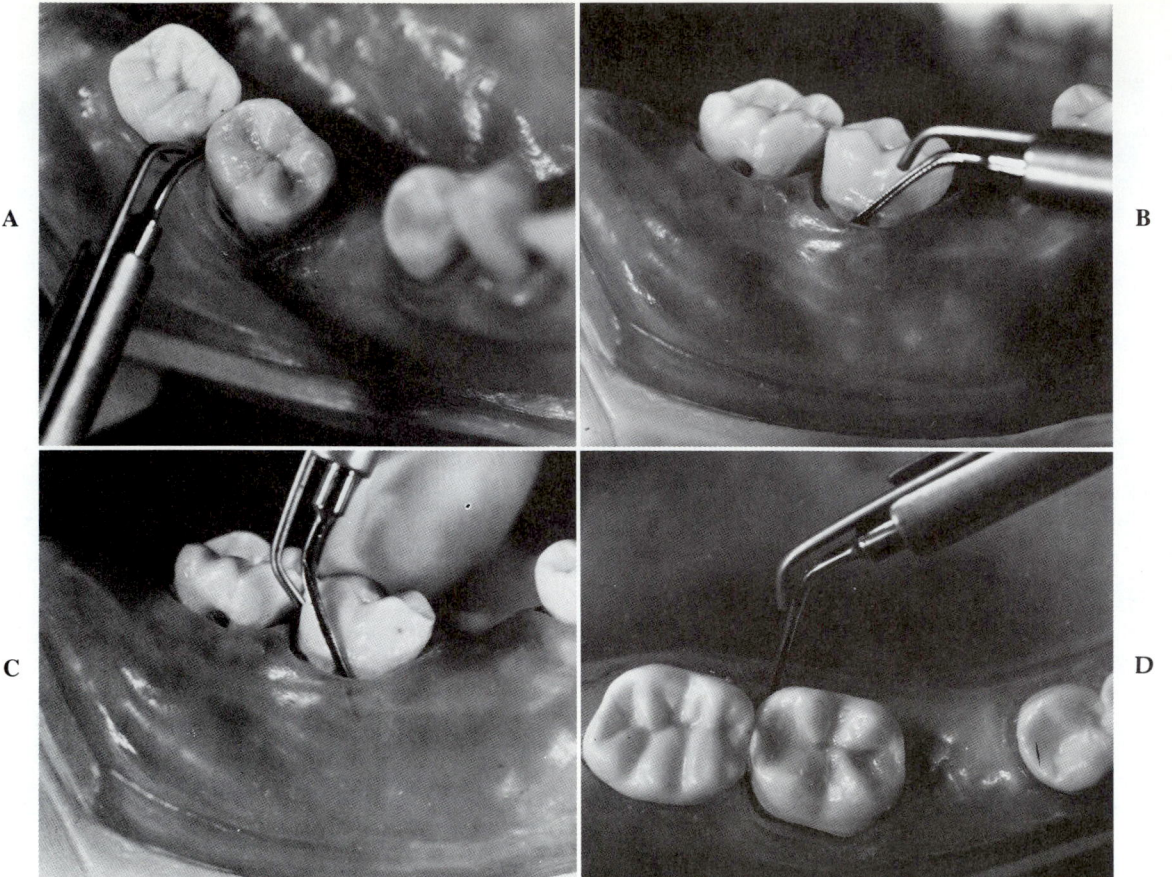

Fig. 25-12. Periodontal probe tip is used **A**, in sweeping motion and in diagonal pattern on facial aspect, **B** and **C**, in cross-hatched diagonal pattern on facial aspect, and **D**, in diagonal pattern from lingual surfaces on distal aspect. Mesial and lingual surfaces are treated similarly.

Fig. 25-2, *A*) or an explorer (see Fig. 25-2, *B*) to remove fine deposits and to debride the root surfaces of microbial colonies and endotoxin. These instruments are applied with a paint-brush motion over all surfaces, using diagonal strokes in a cross-hatch pattern to ensure complete root coverage (Fig. 25-12).

Technique for use

Most textbooks include little about the use of ultrasonic rather than hand instrumentation for subgingival debridement and deplaquing. Although supragingival and subgingival debridement are the objectives of both approaches, the techniques are quite different.

The root surface to be treated should be throroughly evaluated before instrumentation. Detection with an explorer or probe will give the clinician a tactile picture of the surface. Exploring will determine the location and angle of both the cementoenamel junction and the epithelial attachment. It will also provide information on the extent of subgingival deposits and the nature of the root surface, as well as overall root morphology. This information will influence the techniques needed to completely debride the area.

Grasp. A very light pen or modified pen grasp is used for ultrasonic and sonic instruments. The instrument should feel balanced in the hand, with no pull from the cord.

Finger rest. Since a very light touch is used with these instruments, a stable tooth fulcrum is not always needed. An extraoral finger rest is recommended for the maxillary posterior teeth. The position is palm up, with either the back of the fingers resting against the right cheek or the inside of the fingers gently cupped around the angle of the jaw on the left side. Just the opposite would be used by a left-handed operator. Finger rests on the teeth are used for maxillary anterior, as well mandibular areas.

Insertion. The tip of the instrument is directed subgingivally while the instrument is activated. The water lavage will facilitate a comfortable entry into the pocket or sulcus.

Adaptation. Smooth, round magnetostrictive ultrasonic tips are effective 360 degrees around the instrument. The side of the tip is adapted to the tooth surface as the power is concentrated in the last few millimeters of the tip. The tip is adapted to the tooth surface in the same way a periodontal probe is. The side of the tip is held parallel to the tooth surface. The end of the tip should not be adapted at a 90-degree angle to the tooth surface. Unlike curettes, which have a specific cutting edge, most ultrasonic and sonic tips can be activated no matter which side is in contact with the tooth surface. These tips can be adapted on the front, back, or either side. Diamond-shaped sonic tips are more effective on the four-angle edges than on the flat surfaces. As with ultrasonic tips, the power is concentrated in the last few millimeters of the tip. This can be tested by listening to the consistency of the pitch as an explorer is traced over the tip while it is activated. Dead areas will have no sound or low pitch. If a piezoelectric unit is selected, determine which two sides are activated.

Pressure. Extremely light pressure is used with ultrasonic and sonic instruments. With more pressure, ultrasonic instruments may damage the root surface, or sonic instruments will fail to work effectively and the tips will wear down. Some ultrasonic instruments automatically reduce power when excessive pressure is used. This feature prevents trauma to the tooth surface or soft tissues.

Activation. Two motions are used with these instruments: a gentle tapping motion against the side of a specific deposit and a generalized, back-and-forth sweeping motion.

The gentle tapping motion is used to remove calculus deposits. Rather than rubbing the side of the tip over the top of calculus deposits, the side of the tip is held parallel to the tooth surface and the end is used like a periodontal probe to locate and identify the edges of the deposit. The end of the tip is gently tapped against the deposit, and the vibrations from the tip will shatter it. Clinicians who are skilled with hand instruments tend to exert pressure against the deposit, which reduces the effectiveness of the ultrasonic or sonic instrument. The lighter the pressure, the more effective the vibrations will be.

The second motion is a sweeping stroke to remove bacteria from the tooth surface. This motion is similar to an erasing or a coloring motion, in which the side of a lead pencil is used to completely fill in an area. This continuous back-and-forth-motion can be used in different directions on the tooth surface, depending on tip placement. The instrument tip must touch every square millimeter of the surface to remove plaque. To visualize this concept in subgingival areas, use the instrument on supragingival tobacco stain. It will be clear that the instrument tip must touch every aspect of the stain to remove it. Use this information when visualizing instrumentation techniques for subgingival areas. The approach must be methodical and precise. Many overlapping strokes must be used to ensure that the entire surface is covered. These back-and-forth strokes should be made about 6 times per second.

Because of heat buildup in most magnetostrictive-ultrasonic instruments, the movement must be quick but controlled. Sonic instruments build up less heat, and the motions need not be so rapid. A slower, more deliberate motion is recommended for these instruments.

Fluid evacuation

High-speed suction should be used to control the water or antimicrobial lavage accompanying the ultrasonic or sonic instrument. It is advisable to work with a dental hygiene assistant when providing debridement therapy. The quality of high-speed suction will allow for better visibility, a more comfortable experience for the patient, and help reduce the aerosol of microorganisms. When the hygienist must work alone, a saliva ejector will be used for suction. Adaptors are available to accommodate high-volume evacuation to a saliva ejector. One example is the saliva ejector tip adapter made by DCI. The saliva ejector should be placed toward the back of the throat and the patient should be instructed to turn his or her head towards the side where it is placed. As water collects and is not completely removed by the saliva ejector, instrumentation should stop and the patient instructed to close around the saliva ejector like a straw, using his or her tongue to push the remaining water to the tip of the saliva ejector.

Retraction/tissue shielding

The lips and cheeks should be gently pulled out to allow access for the ultrasonic/sonic instrument and to control the spray of water or antimicrobial lavage. This can be done with either the mouth mirror or the fingers. When using the mirror this way, be sure to pull it into the loose tissue rather than resting the mirror head on the alveolar process, which can be very painful.

To control water spray from the maxillary anterior area, be sure that patient is reclined fully and that the water control is turned as low as possible to be effective.

Mirror treatments

Use of the mouth mirror during ultrasonic/sonic debridement procedures can be complicated by the lavage fluid. Many small droplets collect on the face of the mirror and interfere with vision. Defogging solutions, available from dental suppliers, can control this problem. The mouth mirror is dipped into such a solution before use. The water spray from the instrument tip is then directed onto the mirror until it is completely covered. This smooth flow of water over the mirror will allow vision. When defogging solutions are unavailable, wipe the face of the mouth mirror along the inside of the cheek to cover it with mucin. Immediately direct the water flow from the instrument tip onto the mirror. A smooth flow of water will cover the face of the mirror and allow vision.

Power, tuning, and water adjustments

Power and *tuning* are two variables that determine the ability of the instrument to perform properly. Adjusting the power determines the length of the elliptical motion. A "longer stroke" of activity at the tip of the instrument increases its ability to remove tenacious deposits. Gentler actions for plaque debridement are obtained by reducing the power and thus the length of the motion of the tip. Tuning adjusts the frequency of the tip (how fast it is moving). Frequency is expressed in cycles per second or in herz (Hz). Sonic instruments operate at less than 20,000 cycles per second; ultrasonic instruments range from 20,000 cycles to 42,000 cycles per second; you can actually hear when the instrument is in phase or not. It reaches a high-pitched squeak or squeal when it is in phase and a lower, less consistent warbling sound when it is out of phase. This difference is most noticeable when the activated tip is placed against the tooth.

An adequate *water flow* rate is essential for optimum use of the ultrasonic instrument. The ultrasonic, as opposed to the sonic instrument requires water to cool the handpiece. When properly adjusted, the water flow rate should allow for flushing of debris from the pockets and adequate temperature control of the handpiece. There is a general tendency to reduce the flow rate in an attempt to control the spray reaching the patient's face. Contrary to this thinking, reducing the water flow will actually increase the amount of water sprayed outside the mouth. Instead of reaching the end of the instrument tip, the water spray spreads out along the sides of the tip, causing a wider radius of spray with more water reaching the patient's face. The water flow must reach the end of the tip to be most effective.

The three variables of power, tuning, and water are important adjustments to identify and control in meeting the specific needs of different patients and different areas in the mouth.

Treatment options

Fiberoptics. Although widely used in restorative dentistry, fiberoptics have only recently been introduced as an aid for dental hygiene procedures. The fiberoptic light illuminates the area of treatment and transilluminates the tooth surface, enhancing tooth debridement (Reinhardt et al, 1991). Fiberoptics enhance vision in posterior areas, which are difficult to illuminate with the traditional dental light.

Fiberoptics have been internalized in the German sonic scaler by Kavo. The Kavo scaler requires that the unit contain a fiberopic system and that the handpiece hook-ups be wired for fiberoptics.

Add-on fiberoptics have been developed that

can be attached externally to either a sonic or ultrasonic scaler. External attachments consist of a light source (Lumina I, from Zeza, Inc.) and an adapter (Perio Institute) that clamps to the sonic or ultrasonic handpiece (Perio Institute). The adapter has two fiberoptic lights, much like miniature headlights, which illuminate the tip of the instrument.

Papilla reflection. Without adequate subgingival access, procedures where the soft tissue is laid away from the teeth and bone with a surgical flap may be needed for complete debridement. This intermediate procedure provides access yet does not require reflection of the tissue off the bone. Papilla reflection opens up the interproximal area, though it remains a rather conservative procedure. A blade or sharp curette is used to make a diagonal cut through the col area from facial to lingual. The pocket epithelium is removed and the interproximal root surface is visualized. Using this procedure in combination with fiberoptic evaluation, researchers at the University of Nebraska were able to debride root surfaces more effectively than in any other debridement research thus far reported (Reinhardt et al, 1991). A figure-8 or interrupted suture (see Chapter 29) may be used to close the interproximal area. In most cases, closure can be accomplished with a simple fibrin tack, which glues the tissue to the tooth surface with the aid of blood fibrin. A wet gauze is placed over the area and pressure is placed against the facial and lingual papilla in a pinching fashion for 3 minutes. This allows an adhesion to form between the tissue and the tooth surface. In areas where chewing will easily deflect the papilla, a suture is advised.

Approaches to treatment

The various levels of periodontitis will require debridement with increasing levels of competence as pocket depths increase and the complication of furcation invasion occurs (Brayer et al, 1989). The deeper the periodontal pockets, the more difficult and important it is to obtain thorough debridement. The most common approach to debridement is to continue working in an area until it is completed (free of calculus and all surfaces deplaqued). You may opt to complete a sextant, quadrant, half-mouth, or even the full dentition during a given appointment time, depending on the degree of case difficulty, your skill, and the patient's scheduling needs.

Examples of appointment sequencing for the debridement therapy are listed in the following box.

Appointment length can vary, depending on the skill level of the practitioner, from 60 to 120 minutes. It is advisable to allow at least 1 week for healing between appointments. When multiple appointments are planned for debridement, subgingival deplaquing of all areas previously treated should be included at each treatment appointment. Deplaquing is accomplished with light, overlapping strokes with the sonic or ultrasonic instrument. Removal of subgingival plaque, both attached and loosely attached, will enhance the healing process.

Re-evaluation of the periodontal condition and retreatment of nonresponding areas should be scheduled 6 weeks after the last debridement appointment. Bleeding on probing, attachment levels, and tissue tone, color, and contour should be evaluated. This would be the appropriate time to

---

Debridement Therapy Sequencing		
Gingivitis	One appointment	Entire mouth debrided at one appointment
Gingivitis or early periodontitis	Two appointments	Two quadrants at each appointment
Early periodontitis	Three appointments	Two sextants at each appointment
Moderate periodontitis	Four appointments	One quadrant at each appointment
Moderate/advanced periodontitis	Five appointments	Three maxillary sextants and two mandibular quadrants
Advanced periodontitis	Six appointments	One sextant at each appointment

administer the new host response and micribiologic tests to measure the potential for future breakdown (see Chapter 12).

Patient/operator considerations

The noise associated with ultrasonic equipment can be less bothersome to the patient if you provide headphones with music.

In the past, ultrasonic scalers were contraindicated for patients with pacemakers. (Adams et al, 1983) The sound frequencies of the scaler were capable of disrupting the electronic mechanism of the pacemaker. Most newer pacemakers now include a shielding mechanism to prevent interference problems. Sonic scalers use air pressure rather than electrical power and are therefore safe for all pacemakers. Osteomyelitis is another contraindication to the use of ultrasonic scalers (Gross et al, 1976).

ACTIVITIES

1. Review dental hygiene or preventive dentistry textbooks from the 1950s to the present and research what was being taught about plaque and calculus at those times. Discuss or role play how these changing ideas would have been reflected in clinical practice and in patient education dialogues.

2. Critically review television commercials and magazine advertisements in the popular literature for the "hidden messages" and assumptions presented to consumers regarding the objectives of dental hygiene care (e.g., tartar control versus plaque).

3. Examine the clinical evaluation system and share perceptions of the beliefs, assumptions, and values that seem to underly the ways in which dental hygiene care is evaluated. Suggest ways to maximize alignment between evaluation methods and current beliefs, assumptions, and professional values. What are the possible limitations to the suggested evaluation proposals? What might they be? How would these issues relate to self-evaluation or peer review criteria for practicing hygienists?

4. Interview a practicing hygienist to gain an historical perspective of how the profession has changed, especially in terms of treatment approaches. A list of open-ended questions could be formulated by the class, such as: What instruments were you taught to use in school? What were you taught about the relationship of plaque, calculus, and endotoxins and periodontal diseases? In what ways have approaches to instrumentation changed since you graduated?

5. Using extracted teeth, compare the debridement capabilities of various sonic and ultrasonic instruments. Compare various tips, power settings, and strokes. Evaluate ease of use, time involved, water flow, heat buildup, root surface alterations, and operator effects.

6. Compare the effects of hand and sonic or ultrasonic instrumentation on a patient, using the split-mouth method of treatment. Use hand instruments on two contralateral quadrants of the mouth and a sonic or ultrasonic instrument on the other two quadrants. Evaluate root surfaces, gingival tissue, patient perceptions, and operator perceptions immediately after treatment and 7 to 10 days post-treatment.

7. At the next state or local dental convention, visit the exhibitors and collect information on the various sonic and ultrasonic instruments currently available. As a group, compare the advantages and disadvantages of the various instruments, based on this information.

8. Spend several hours assisting a practicing dental hygienist who is proficient with a sonic or ultrasonic instrument. Discuss application techniques.

9. Review Fig. 30-11 and discuss the relative benefits of repeated instrumentation to remove stain, cememtum, and dentin given their effect on tooth morphology. Audit recall files for evidence of patients who exhibit morphological change because of repeated root instrumentation.

10. Using a line drawing of a tooth, use a pencil to trace overlapping vertical strokes over the root area as if debriding the surface. Next use the pencil with horizontal strokes; note how much more surface area is covered by the pencil. Finally, note how diagonal cross-hatchings thoroughly cover the area. This exercise demonstrates that using a single stroking pattern may not adequately debride the surface.

REVIEW QUESTIONS

1. Which of the following reasons describes the limitations of scaling and root planing techniques that are traditionally associated with dental hygiene care?
   a. Dental scaling is likely to remove plaque and endotoxins but is ineffective in removing calculus deposits.
   b. Root planing may remove excessive amounts of cementum in an effort to remove all contaminated material from the root surface.
   c. Scaling and root planing focus clinical attention primarily on root surface characteristics rather than the healing response of soft tissues.

2. Closed debridement has been shown to be an effective treatment approach for which of the following levels of periodontal disease?
   a. Gingivitis.
   b. Early periodontal disease.
   c. Moderate periodontal disease.
   d. Severe periodontal disease.
   e. All of the above.
   f. a and b only.

3. What is the nature of the relationship between LPS and the root cementum of periodontally involved teeth, according to recent research reports?
   a. LPS is found on superficial layers of the cementum.
   b. LPS is found to penetrate deeply into cementum and dentin.
   c. LPS can be removed easily by rinsing, polishing, brushing, and light instrumentation.
   d. LPS can be removed only with extensive removal of root cementum.

4. Among the following choices, the most reliable measure of the success of periodontal debridement is:
   a. removal of plaque as determined by disclosing solution.
   b. removal of calculus as determined by exploration of the tooth surface and use of compressed air.
   c. resolution of clinical signs of periodontal inflammation.
   d. a and b.

5. Which of the following statements comparing hand and ultrasonic instruments is true?
   a. Hand instruments are more effective in removing plaque and associated LPS from subgingival areas than ultrasonic instruments.
   b. Hand and ultrasonic instruments are equally effective means of removing calculus.
   c. Ultrasonic instruments have been shown to remove more cementum during use than hand instruments.
   d. Healing following debridment with hand instruments is superior to that following debridement with ultrasonic instruments.

6. Which of the following is *not* an advantage of ultrasonic instruments when compared to hand instruments?
   a. Decreased inadvertent tissue trauma during debridement.
   b. Newly designed tips allow access to areas that hand instruments cannot reach e.g, furcations, deep pockets, root concavities).
   c. Patients report more comfortable debridement with ultrasonic instruments.
   d. Use of ultrasonic instruments requires increased stress on hand and arm muscles, which could result in occupational injury such as carpal tunnel syndrome.
   e. Treatment time is decreased.
   f. Water lavage or antimicrobial irrigant enhances healing process.

True or False. If the statement is false, correct it to make it accurate.

7. Dental hygienists must remove all calculus deposits from teeth because periodontal healing cannot occur in the presence of calculus.

8. Calculus causes periodontal disease.

REFERENCES

Aleo JA et al: The presence and biologic activity of cementum-bound endotoxin, *J Periodontol* 45:672, 1974.

Aleo JA et al: In vitro attachment of human fibroblasts to root surfaces, *J Periodontol* 46:639, 1975.

Allen EF, Rhoads RH: Effects of high speed periodontal instruments on tooth surface, *J Periodontol* 34:352, 1963.

American Academy of Periodontology: Glossary of periodontal terms, *J Periodontol* 57 (suppl), 1986.

Axelsson P, Lindhe J: The effect of a preventive programme on dental plaque, gingivitis and caries in school children. Results after one and two years, *J Clin Periodontol* 1:126, 1974.

Axelsson P, Lindhe J: Effect of controlled oral hygiene procedures on caries and periodontal disease in adults, *J Clin Periodontol* 5:133, 1978.

Axelsson P, Lindhe J: Effect of controlled oral hygiene procedures on caries and periodontal disease in adults, *J Clin Periodontol* 8:281, 1981.

Badersten A et al: Effect of nonsurgical periodontal therapy. I. Moderately advanced periodontitis, *J Clin Periodontol* 8:45, 1981.

Badersten A et al: Effect of nonsurgical periodontal therapy. IV. Operator variability, *J Clin Periodontol* 12:190, 1985.

Badersten A et al: Effect of nonsurgical periodontal therapy. II. Severely advanced periodontitis, *J Clin Periodontol* 11:63, 1984.

Badersten A et al: Effect of non-surgical periodontal therapy III. Single versus repeated instrumentation, *J Clin Periodontol* 11:114, 1984b.

Badersten A, Nilveus R, Egelberg J: 4-year observations of basic periodontal therapy, *J Clin Periodontol* 14:438, 1987a.

Badersten A, Nilveus R, Egelberg J: Effect of nonsurgical periodontal therapy. VIII. Probing attachment changes related to clinical characteristics, *J Clin Periodontol* 14:425, 1987b.

Bhaskar SN, Grower MF, Cutright DE: Gingival healing after hand and ultrasinic scaling—biochemical and histologic analysis, *J Periodontol* 43:31, 1972.

Barnes JE, Schaffer EM: Subgingival root planing: a comparison using files, hoes and curettes, *J Periodontol* 31:300, 1960.

Bass CC, Johns IM: *Alveolodental pyorrhea*, Philadelphia, 1915, WB Saunders.

Belting CM, Spjut PJ: Effect of high-speed periodontal instruments on the root surface during subgingival calculus removal, *JADA* 69:578, 1964.

Bergstrom J, Eliasson S: Noxious effect of cigarette smoking and age on bone loss in men, *Arch Environ Health* 37:246, 1982.

Bergstrom H, Eliasson S: Cigarette smoking and alveolar bone height in subjects with a high standard of oral hygiene, *J Clin Periodontol* 14:466, 1987.

Bergstrom H, Eliasson S, Preber H: Cigarette smoking and periodontal bone loss, *J Periodontol* 62:242, 1991.

Biagini G et al: Root curettage and gingival repair in periodontitis, *J Periodontol* 59:124, 1988.

Blomlöf L et al: New attachment in monkeys with experimental periodontitis with and without removal of cementum, *J Clin Periodontol* 14:136, 1987.

Blumenthal NM, and Ewen SJ: A short term evaluation of ultrasonically delivered medication in the treatment of moderate periodontal disease, *Ill Dent J* 55(1):12, 1986.

Brayer WK et al: Scaling and root planing effectiveness: the effect of root surface access and operator experience, *J Periodontol* 60:67, 1989.

Breininger DR, O'Leary TJ, Blumenshine RVH: Comparative effectiveness of ultrasonic and hand scaling for the removal of subgingival plaque and calculus, *J Periodontol* 58:9,1987.

Buchanan SA, Robertson PB: Calculus removal by scaling/root planing with and without surgical access, *J Periodontol* 58:159,1987.

Chace R: (letter) *J Peridontol* 60:592, 1989.

Checchi L, Pelliccioni GA: Hand versus ultrasonic instrumentation in the removal of endotoxins from root surfaces in vitro, *J Periodontol* 59:398, 1988.

Cheetham WA, Wilson M, Kieser JB: Root surface debridement—an in vitro assessment, *J Clin Periodontol* 15:288, 1988.

Chiew SYT et al: Assessment of ultrasonic debridement of calculus-associated periodontally-involved root surfaces by the limulus amoebocyte lysate assay, *J Clin Periodontol* 18:240, 1991.

Christersson LA et al: Dental bacterial plaques. Nature and role in periodontal disease, *J Clin Periodontol* 18:44, 1991.

Claffey N: Decision making in periodontal therapy: the re-evaluation, *J Clin Periodontol* 18:384, 1991.

Claffey N et al: The relative effects of therapy and periodontal disease on loss of probing attachment after root debridement, *J Clin Periodontol* 15:163, 1988.

Conrad JC et al: Peripheral nerve dysfunction in practicing dental hygienists, *J Dent Hyg* 64:382, 1990.

Cunningham WT et al: A comparison of antimicrobial effectiveness of endosonic and hand root canal therapy, *Oral Surg* 54:238, 1982.

Daly CG et al: Bacterial endotoxin: a role in chronic inflammatory periodonal disease? *J Oral Pathol* 9:1, 1980.

Daly CG et al: Histological assessment of periodontally involved cementum, *J Clin Periodontol* 9:266, 1982.

Eaton KA et al: The removal of root surface deposits, *J Clin Periodontol* 12:141, 1985.

Emrich L et al: Periodontal disease in non-insulin-dependent diabetes mellitus, *J Periodontol* 62:123, 1991.

Ewen SJ: A photomicrographic study of root scaling, *J Am Soc Periodontol* 4:273, 1966.

Ewen SJ, Gwinnett AJ: A scanning electron microscopic study of teeth following periodontal instrumentation, *J Periodontol* 48:92, 1977.

Ewen SJ, Glickenstein C: *Ultrasonic therapy in periodontics,* Springfield, Ill, 1968, Charles C Thomas.

Fine DH et al: Studies in plaque pathogenicity. I. Plaque collection and limulus lysate screening of adherent and loosely adherent plaque, *J Periodont Res 13:17,* 1978.

Fine DH et al: Studies in plaque pathogenicity. II. A technique for the specific detection of endotoxin in plaque samples using the limulus lysate assay, *J Periodontol Res.* 13:127, 1978.

Fine DH et al: Preliminary characterization of material eluted from the roots of periodontally diseased teeth, *J Periodontol Res* 15:10, 1980.

Fujikawa K et al: The effect of retained subgingival calculus on healing after flap surgery, *J Periodontol* 59:170, 1988.

Gaare D et al: Improvement of gingival health by toothbrushing in individuals with large amounts of calculus, *J Clin Periodontol* 17:38, 1990.

Gantes B et al: The effects of hygiene instruments on dentin surfaces: scanning electron microscopic observations, *J Periodontol* 63:118, 1992.

Gantes BG, Nilveus R: The effects of different hygiene instruments on titanium surfaces. Scanning electron microscopic observation, *Int J Periodontics Rest Dent* 11:225, 1991.

Garnick JJ, Dent J: A scanning electron micrographical study of root surfaces and subgingival bacteria after hand and ultrasonic instrumentation, *J Periodontol* 60:441, 1989.

Gellin RG et al: The effectiveness of the Titan-S sonic scaler versus curettes in the removal of subgingival calculus, *J Periodontol* 57:672, 1986.

Genco RJ, Christersson LA: Antiinfective therapy for gingivitis and periodontics. In Genco RJ, Goldman HM, Cohen DW: *Contemporary periodontics,* St Louis, CV Mosby, 1990.

Greenstein G: Advances in periodontal disease diagnosis, *Int J Periodont Rest Dent* 10:351, 1990.

Greenwell H et al: Periodontics in general practice: perspectives on nonsurgical therapy, *JADA* 115:591, 1987.

Greenwell H et al: Periodontics in general practice: professional plaque control, *JADA* 121:642, 1990.

Gross A et al: Microbial contamination of dental units and ultrasonic scalers, *J Periodontol* 47:670, 1976.

Harmsen AG: Role of alveolar macrophages in lipopolysaccharide-induced neutrophil accumulation, *Infect Immun* 56:1858, 1988.

Hatfield CG, Baumhammers A: Cytotoxic effects of periodontally involved surfaces of human teeth, *Arch Oral Biol* 16:465, 1971.

Hill RW et al: Four types of periodontal treatment compared over two years, *J Periodontol* 52:655, 1981.

Holbrook T, Low S: Power-driven scaling and polishing instruments, *Clin Dent* 3:1, 1989

Hughes FJ, Smales FC: Immunohistochemical investigation of the presence and distribution of cementum-associated lipopolysaccharides in periodontal disease, *J Periodont Res* 21:660, 1986.

Hughes FJ et al: Investigation of the distribution of cementum-associated lipopolysaccharides in periodontal disease by scanning electron microscope immunohistochemistry, *J Periodont Res* 23:100, 1988.

Huntley DE, Shannon SA: Carpal tunnel syndrome. A review of the literature, *Dent Hyg* 62:316, 1988.

Isidor F, Karring T: Long-term effect of surgical and non-surgical periodontal treatment. A 5-year clinical study, *J Periodont Res* 21:462, 1986.

Isidor F et al: The effect of root planing as compared to that of surgical treatment, *J Clin Periodontol* 11:669, 1984.

Jones WA, O'Leary TJ: The effectiveness of in vivo root planing in removing bacterial endotoxin from the roots of periodontally involved teeth, *J Periodontol* 49:337, 1978.

Jones S et al: Tooth surfaces treated in situ with periodontal instruments, *Br Dent J* 132:57, 1972.

Kepic TJ et al: Total calculus removal: An attainable objective? *J Periodontol* 61:16, 1990.

Kerry GJ: Roughness of root surfaces after use of ultrasonic instruments and hand curettes, *J Periodontol* 38:340, 1967.

Khatiblou FA, Ghodossi A: Root surface smoothness or roughness in periodontal treatment. A clinical study, *J Periodontol* 54:365, 1983.

Kieser JB: *Periodontics: a practical approach,* London, 1990, Wright.

Knowles J et al: Comparison of results following three modalities of periodontal therapy related to tooth type and initial pocket depth, *J Clin Periodontol* 7:32, 1980.

Lindhe J et al: Healing following surgical/non-surgical treatment of periodontal disease, *J Clin Periodontol* 9:115, 1982.

Lindhe J et al: Scaling and root planing in shallow pockets, *J Clin Periodontal* 9:415, 1982 .

Lindhe J et al: Long-term effects of surgical/nonsurgical treatment of periodontal disease, *J Clin Periodontol* 11:448, 1984.

Listgarten MA: Subgingival microbiological differences between periodontally healthy sites and diseased sites prior to and after treatment, *Int J Periodont Rest Dent* 4:27, 1984.

Listgarten MA: A perspective on periodontal diagnosis, *J Clin Periodontol* 13:175, 1986.

Löe H et al: Experimental gingivitis in man, *J Periodontol* 49:337, 1965.

Loos B et al: An evaluation of basic periodontal therapy using sonic and ultrasonic scalers, *J Clin Periodontol* 14:29, 1987. Low SB, Ciancio SG: Reviewing nonsurgical periodontal therapy, *JADA* 121:467, 1990.

Macdonald G et al: Carpal tunnel syndrome among California dental hygienists, *Dent Hyg* 62:322, 1988.

Mackinnon LT et al: The effects of exercise on secretory and natural immunity, *Adv Exp Med Biol* 216A:869, 1987.

Mandel ID, Gaffar A: Calculus revisited: a review, *J Clin Periodontol* 13:249, 1986.

Miller WD: *Micro-organisms of the human mouth*, Basel, Switzerland, 1973, S Karger.

Meyer K, Lie T: Root surface roughness in response to periodontal instrumentation by combined use of microroughness measurements and scanning electron microscopy, *J Clin Periodontol* 4:77, 1977.

Moore J et al: The distribution of bacterial lipopolysaccharide (endotoxin) in relation to periodontally involved root surfaces, *J Clin Periodontol* 13:748, 1986.

Moore WEC et al: Bacteriology of moderate (chronic) periodontitis in mature adult humans, *Infect Immun* 42:510, 1983.

Moskow BS, Bressman E: Cemental response to ultrasonic and hand instrumentation, *JADA* 68:698, 1964.

Nakib NM et al: Endotoxin penetration into root cementum of periodontally healthy and diseased human teeth, *J Periodontol* 53:368, 1982.

Nishimine D, O'Leary TJ: Hand instrumentation versus ultrasonics in the removal of endotoxins from root surfaces, *J Periodontol* 50:345, 1979.

Nosal G et al: The penetration of lavage solution into the periodontal pocket during ultrasonic instrumentation, *J Periodontol* 62:554, 1991.

Nowotny A: Molecular aspects of endotoxin reactions, *Bacteriol Rev* 33:72, 1969.

Nyman S et al: Role of "diseased" root cementum in healing following treatment of periodontal disease, an experimental study in the dog, *J Periodont Res* 21:496, 1986.

Nyman S et al: Role of "diseased" root cementum in healing following treatment of periodontal disease: a clinical study, *J Clin Periodontol* 15:464, 1988.

Oda S, Ishikawa I: In vitro effectiveness of a newly-designed ultrasonic scaler tip for furcation areas, *J Periodontol* 60:634, 1989.

O'Leary TJ: The impact of research on scaling and root planing, *J Periodontol* 57:69, 1986.

O'Leary TJ, Kafrawy AD: Total cementum removal: a realistic objective? *J Periodontol* 54:221, 1983.

Olsen I, Socransky SS: Ultrasonic dispersion of pure cultures of plaque bacteria and plaque, *Scand J Dent Res* 89:307, 1981.

Oosterwaal PJ et al: The effect of subgingival debridement with hand and ultrasonic instruments on the subgingival microflora, *J Clin Periodontol* 14:528, 1987.

Osborn JB et al: Carpal tunnel syndrome among Minnesota dental hygienists, *J Dent Hyg* 64:79, 1990.

Pihlstrom BL et al: A randomized four-year study of periodontal therapy, *J Periodontol* 52:227, 1981.

Pihlstrom BL et al: Comparison of surgical and nonsurgical treatment of periodontal disease: a review of current studies and additional results after 6½ years, *J Clin Periodontol* 10:524, 1983.

Rabbani GM et al: The effectiveness of subgingival scaling and root planing in calculus removal, *J Periodontol* 52:119, 1981.

Ramfjord SP et al: Oral hygiene and maintenance of periodontal support, *J Periodontol* 53:26, 1982.

Ramfjord SP et al: Subgingival curettage versus surgical elimination of periodontal pockets, *J Periodontol* 39:167, 1968.

Ramfjord SP: Long-term assessment of periodontal surgery versus curettage or scaling and root planing, *Int J Technol Assess Health Care* 6:392, 1990.

Reinhardt R et al: Clinical effects of closed root planing compared to papilla reflection and fiber optic augmentation, *J Periodontol* 62:317, 1991.

Ritz L et al: An in vitro investigation on the loss of root substance in scaling with various instruments, *J Clin Periodontol* 18:643, 1991.

Robertson PB: The residual calculus paradox, *J Periodontol* 61:65, 1990.

Rosenberg RM, Ash MM: The effect of root roughness on plaque accumulation and gingival inflammation, *J Periodontol* 45:146, 1974.

Rosling BG et al: Microbiological and clinical effects of topical subgingival antimicrobial treatment on human periodontal disease, *J Periodontol* 10:487, 1983.

Rosling BG et al: Topical antimicrobial therapy and diagnosis of subgingival bacteria in the management of management of inflammatory periodontal disease, *J Clin Periodontol* 13:1975, 1986.

Schaffer E: Histological results of root curettage of human teeth, *J Periodontol* 27:296, 1956.

Shapiro L et al: Endotoxin determinations in gingival inflammation, *J Periodontol* 43:591, 1972.

Sherman PR et al: The effectiveness of subgingival scaling and root planing. I. Clinical detection of residual calculus, *J Periodontol* 61:3, 1990.

Sherman PR et al: The effectiveness of subgingival scaling and root planing. II. Clinical responses related to residual calculus, *J Periodontol* 61:9, 1990.

Sjogren U, Sundqvist O: Bacteriologic evaluation of ultrasonic root canal instrumentation, *Oral Surg Oral Med Oral Pathol* 63:366, 1987.

Slots J: Microflora in the healthy gingival sulcus in man, *Scand J Dent Res* 85:247, 1977.

Slots J: The subgingival microflora and periodontal disease, *J Clin Periodontol* 6:351, 1979.

Smart GJ et al: The assessment of ultrasonic root surface debridement by determination of residual endotoxin levels, *J Clin Periodontol* 17:174, 1990.

Somerman MJ et al: In vitro evaluation of extracts of mineralized tissues for their application in attachment of fibrous tissue, *J Periodontol* 58:349, 1987.

Stambaugh RV et al: The limits of subgingival scaling, *Int J Periodont Rest Dent* 1:30, 1981.

Stende GW, Schaffer EM: A comparison of ultrasonic and hand scaling, *J Periodontol* 32:312, 1961.

Taggart JA et al: A clinical and microbiological comparison of the effects of water and 0.02% chlorhexidine as coolants during ultrasonic scaling and root planing, *J Clin Periodontol* 17:32, 1990.

Theilade E et al: Experimental gingivitis in man. II. A longitudinal clinical and bacteriological investigation, *J Periodont Res* 1:1, 1966.

Torfason T et al: Clinical improvement of gingival conditions following ultrasonic versus hand instrumentation or periodontal pockets, *J Clin Periodontol* 6:165, 1979.

Van Volkinburg JW et al: The nature of root surfaces after curette, cavitron and alpha-sonic instrumentation, *J Periodont Res* 11:374, 1976.

Veksler A et al: Reduction of salivary bacteria by pre-procedural rinses with chlorhexidine 0.12%, *J Periodontol* 62:649, 1991.

Walmsley AD et al: Dental plaque removal by cavitational activity during ultrasonic scaling, *J Clin Periodontol* 15:539, 1988.

Wilkinson RF, Maybury JE: Scanning electron microscopy of the root surface following instrumentation, *J Periodontol* 44:559, 1973.

Wilson TG: Compliance: a review of the literature with possible application to periodontics, *J Periodontol* 58:706, 1987.

Zinner DD: Recent ultrasonic dental studies, including periodotia, whthout the use of an abrasive, *J Dent Res* 3-4:748, 1955.

SUGGESTED READINGS

American Acadeny of Periodontology: *Proceedings of the world workshop in clinical periodontics*. Section II. Nonsurgical periodontal treatment, 1989.

Badersten A et al: Effect of nonsurgical periodontal therapy, *J Clin Periodontol* 8:57, 1981.

Ballieux RE: Impact of mental stress on the immune response, *J Clin Periodontol* 18:427,1991.

Bower R: Furcation morphology relative to periodontal treatment. Furcation entrance architecture, *J Periodontol* 50:23, 1979.

Ewen SJ et al: A comparative study of ultrasonic generators and hand instruments, *J Periodontol* 47:82, 1976.

Greenstein G: Periodontal response to mechanical non-surgical therapy: a review, *J Periodontol* 63:118, 1992.

Leon L, Vogel R: A comparison of the effectiveness of hand scaling and ultrasonic debridement on furcations as evaluated by differential darkfield microscopy, *J Periodontal* 58:86, 1987.

Lie T, Meyer K: Calculus removal and loss of tooth substance in response to different periodontal instruments, *J Clin Periodontol* 4:250, 1977.

Pearlman BA: Ultrasonic root planing, *Aust Dent J* 27:109, 1982.

Philstrom BL et al: Molar and nonmolar teeth compared over 6½ years following two methods of periodontal therapy, *J Periodontol* 55:499, 1984.

Schaffer EM: Objectice evaluation of ultrasonic versus hand instrumentation in periodontics, *Dent Clin North Am,* Mar, p 165, 1964.

Thilo B, Baehni P: Effect of ultrasonic instrumentation on dental plaque microflora in vitro, *J Periodontol Res* 22:518, 1987.

Waerhaug J: Effect of rough surfaces upon gingival tissue, *J Dent Res* 35:323, 1956.

Walmsley A et al: Effect of cavitational activity on the root surfaces teeth during ultrasonic cavitational scaling, *J Clin Periodontol* 17:306, 1990.

26 SELECTING AND ADAPTING HAND INSTRUMENTS

Nancy Stutsman Young
Irene Woodall

LEARNING OUTCOMES

The dental hygienist will be able to

1. Consider patient, operator, and logistical factors to determine whether periodontal debridement is best accomplished with hand or ultrasonic instruments.
2. Determine which type of hand instrument and which instrument design is most appropriate to use based on the type and location of deposits.
3. Use a modified pen grasp, finger rest, and hand and wrist motion while implementing both exploratory and working strokes to provide efficient and effective debridement with the following instruments:
   a. Sickle scalers
   b. Universal curettes
   c. Gracey curettes
   d. Hoes
   e. Files
   f. Chisels
4. Adapt the appropriate working and cutting edge of any hand instrument in all areas of the mouth.
5. Demonstrate effective blade angulation for insertion and activation of working strokes with all types of hand instruments.
6. Evaluate the nature of the tooth surface and the type of deposits to be removed and apply appropriate levels of pressure against the surface to accomplish effective working and exploratory strokes while avoiding damage to hard and soft tissues.
7. Provide alternative finger rest, or fulcrum, positioning when needed.
8. Demonstrate time and motion efficiency in selecting and using instruments for debridement and in managing patient-operator position changes.
9. Identify clinical factors that may complicate the debridement process and plan how they may be controlled.
10. Explain the advantages and limitations of methods of evaluating the debridement procedure both during and after treatment.

CHOOSING HAND INSTRUMENTS FOR DEBRIDEMENT

The goals and objectives of periodontal debridement discussed in Chapter 25 can be accomplished with either ultrasonic or hand instrumentation. The advantages of ultrasonic instruments were presented and discussed, and it was recommended that they be considered the preferred method for debridement. Ultimately the decision of whether to use hand or ultrasonic instruments depends on patient and operator preferences and on the availability of both types of instrument. You should be prepared to accomplish periodontal debridement by either approach so that you can work effectively in any type of treatment environment.

Indications for hand instruments are the following:

1. *With patients for whom ultrasonic instrumentation is not recommended.* These include patients with known contagious dis-

eases that could be transmitted through dental aerosols, patients with some types of heart pacemaker devices, and patients with implants requiring debridement with non-metal instruments (see Chapter 25).

2. *In treatment environments where ultrasonic instrumentation is not available.* In the past ultrasonic instruments were recommended primarily for removing gross supragingival deposits, and many dental practices did not consider them a necessary part of the operatory equipment. New recommendations for the use of these instruments in almost all phases of periodontal debridement and new instrument tip designs have greatly expanded their use. However, some dental practices still have older models of ultrasonic devices, which can be fitted only with instrument tips that are too large to gain access to submarginal areas. In such practices the use of hand instruments will still be required to perform definitive submarginal debridement. Hygienists working in public health settings without easy access to electricity or suction evacuation may also be restricted to using hand instruments for debridement.

3. *As valuable supplements to the ultrasonic debridement technique.* The wide variation in hand instrument designs permits clinicians to try different adaptive approaches in difficult-to-reach areas of the mouth. Hand instruments provide more information to the clinician's fingers during debridement, as there are no ultrasonic vibrations to confound the tactile sense. Many hygienists prefer to complete the final phase of subgingival debridement in selected areas with a sharp curette to ensure that the surface has the desired qualities.

4. *For clinicians not trained in the use of ultrasonic instruments and who may feel that they can perform debridement more thoroughly with hand instruments.* Once such clinicians are introduced to the advantages of ultrasonic instruments, however, it is likely that their opinions will change. As with all new instrumentation techniques, practice and experience are necessary to help one gain confidence and expertise in using ultrasonic instruments effectively. During the transition period of learning to use ultrasonic instruments, these hygienists may wish to continue using hand instruments as a supplement until their comfort level with the newer technology is increased.

5. *When patients prefer hand instruments to ultrasonic instruments.* Reasons for this may include discomfort caused by the noise or the feeling of vibration against the tooth surface. Before resorting to the use of hand instruments, however, the clinician should attempt to deal with the source of the discomfort and relieve it if possible. The clinician can make the noise levels less objectionable by providing earphones so the patient can enjoy music during the procedure. Another alternative might be disposable earplugs. Hypersensitivity related to dentin exposure can be treated in advance of debridement by any of the means discussed in Chapter 31. Use of local anesthesia during the procedure also eliminates this type of discomfort. Some patients who have never had treatment with ultrasonic instruments may be slightly uncomfortable with the feeling of the vibrations against their teeth at first but often become accustomed to the feeling after a short time. Explaining to patients how the instrument works, its effectiveness, and its safety may allay their concerns and anxiety. If these measures fail to reduce patient discomfort, the clinician should consider using hand instrumentation.

PRINCIPLES OF INSTRUMENTATION COMMON TO EXPLORING AND DEBRIDEMENT

The basic principles of instrumentation presented in Chapter 9 are essential in learning how to use cutting instruments for deposit removal. The modified pen grasp, finger rest placement, stroke activation, and stroking patterns discussed in relation to detecting deposits and subgingival probing are applicable to all types of hand instruments.

Recall that, in the modified pen grasp, the instrument is held between the thumb and the first *two* fingers, with the first two sections of the index finger flat against the instrument for maximum control. The third finger, or ring finger, is used as a *finger rest,* or *fulcrum,* giving the movements of the instrument control and stability. Usually the finger rest is on the occlusal or incisal surfaces of the teeth, near the operative site.

The *stroke* is produced by pivoting on the finger rest while activating a unified hand and arm motion that rotates the wrist in either a lateral (left to right) or vertical (upward) direction. These movements are modified as the instrument navigates the various surfaces of the tooth so that overlapping and controlled strokes are generated in a prescribed *stroking pattern* to explore or debride each surface. The stroking pattern may be vertical, oblique or diagonal, circumferential, or a combination.

Exploratory strokes require minimum pressure against the tooth and a light grasp so that the nerves in the fingers can detect the slight variations in the texture and morphology of the teeth, which cannot be seen when working beneath the gingival margin but can be felt with a fine explorer or probe.

The *adaptation* of the instrument maintains the terminal portion of the instrument tip against the tooth as it moves around the circumference. Correct adaptation is critical for examining the root surface and for protecting the soft tissues from accidental damage caused by the point of the instrument. All of these principles are important in exploring, probing, and removing deposits.

Debridement with hand instruments is accomplished by scraping, or *scaling*, the tooth surface with a sharp cutting edge. The sharpened blade on hand instruments used in debridement therefore distinguishes them from the probe, explorers, and ultrasonic instruments described in earlier chapters. This same feature requires the mastery of two new principles of instrumentation for safe removal of deposits with hand cutting instruments: *working stroke* and *angulation*. These principles will be discussed after the descriptions of basic instrument design and adaptation of the sickle scaler.

SICKLE SCALER: DESIGN AND USE
Blade design

The basic design of the working end of a sickle scaler is shown in Fig. 26-1. The working end is formed by two cutting edges terminating in a point. Each of the two cutting edges is formed at the junction of the facial surface and a lateral surface. The two lateral surfaces join at the bottom of the instrument to form an unused third edge. Thus there are two hazards for potential trauma

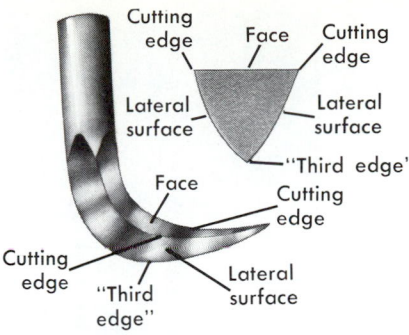

Fig. 26-1. Sickle scaler has two cutting edges. Lateral surfaces join at back of instrument to form a third "edge" that should be dulled to reduce possible tissue trauma. Face (or bevel) of instrument is the surface between the two blades that converges to form a point.
(Adapted from Seibert JS: *Contin Dent Educ* 1:8, 1978.)

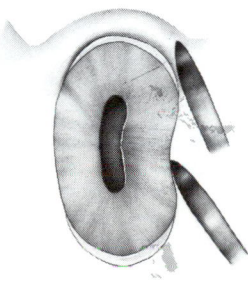

Fig. 26-2. Side of point of sickle scaler must be carefully adapted to tooth to ensure that it does not pierce soft tissue, particularly as it is guided around line angles of tooth.
(Adapted from Seibert JS: *Contin Dent Educ* 1:8, 1978.)

during debridement: the sharp, pointed tip (just as with the point on the explorer), and the sharp edge on the bottom of the instrument. Careful adaptation is necessary to ensure that these features do not lacerate adjacent soft tissues (Fig. 26-2). The "third edge" can be made less of a problem by dulling the underside of the sickle blade with a sharpening stone. A few strokes directly across the bottom of the scaler will reduce the potential for tissue trauma from this edge.

Use

The relatively short shank and straight working end restrict the sickle scaler's usefulness. Generally it is limited to removing supragingival depos-

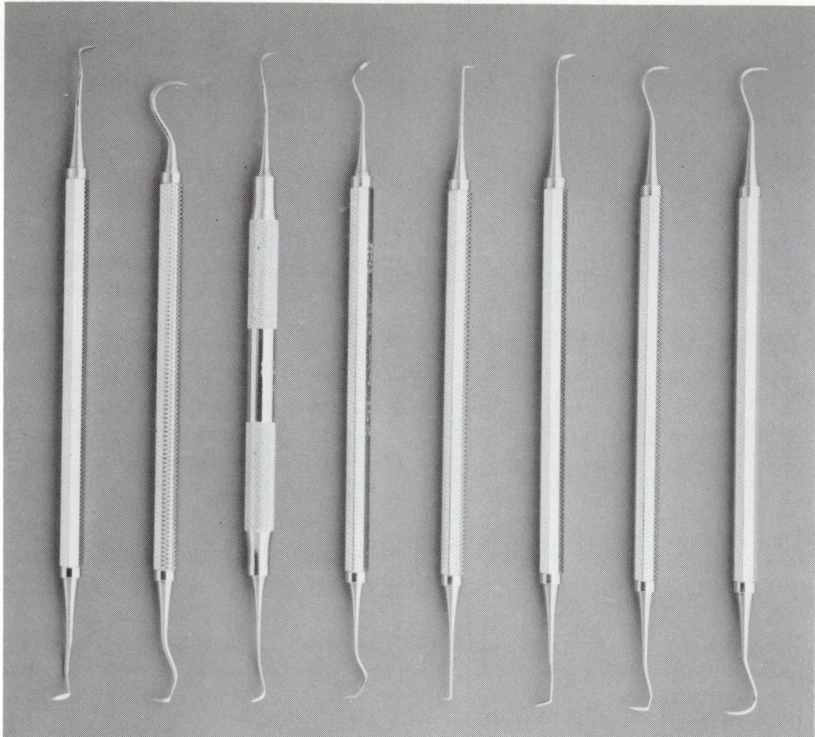

Fig. 26-3. Blade designs of sickle scalers may either be straight or curved. (Courtesy Hu-Friedy Co., Chicago.)

its or those found only 1 to 2 mm beneath the margin of the gingiva. Because it cannot be adapted effectively in deep pockets without damaging adjacent soft tissues, it is not recommended for subgingival debridement. The solid design of the instrument makes it strong enough to remove reasonably heavy deposits as long as it is sharp and used with adequate pressure against the tooth during the working stroke.

The straight blade of some sickle scalers permits only limited contact of the cutting edge with the tooth surface during any given stroke. This design feature makes it less efficient for deplaquing and total debridement of exposed root surfaces than the curved blades of curettes, as far more strokes would be necessary to treat an entire surface area thoroughly. Sickle scalers designed with more curved working ends (similar to the Hartzell explorer design) still have the disadvantages of the sharp point and back, making them more hazardous than curettes for extensive use adjacent to soft tissues.

Anterior designs

Sickle scalers designed for use in anterior regions have a simple, straight shank design. The working ends or blades are perpendicular to the shank and may be either straight or slightly curved (Fig. 26-3). A useful rule to remember when analyzing where an instrument is best adapted is as follows: *The simpler the shank design, the more anterior the intended area of use for the instrument.* Anterior sickle scalers can be adapted on anterior proximal surfaces or on the direct facial and lingual surfaces of teeth with a horizontal or circumferential stroke (Fig. 26-4).

Posterior designs: selecting the correct working end

Sickle scalers designed for access to posterior areas have contraangled shanks (i.e, they have one or more bends in the shank). These double-ended instruments have working ends that are mirror images of each other. Selecting the proper end of a

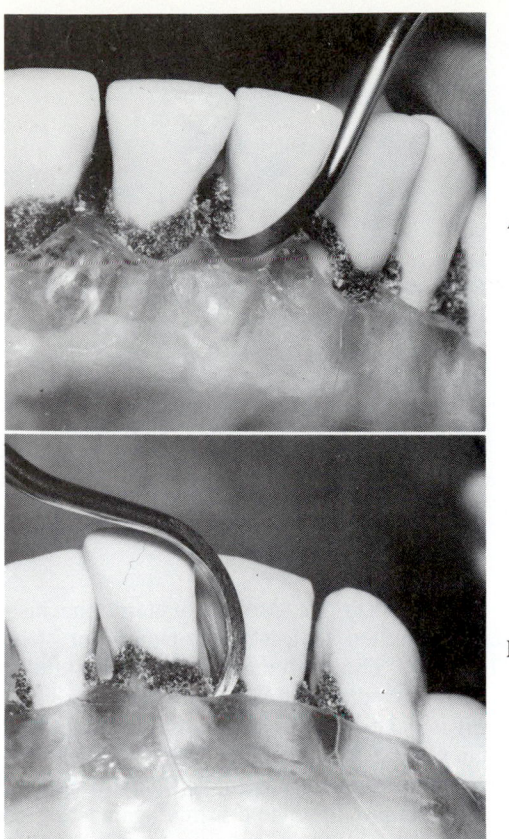

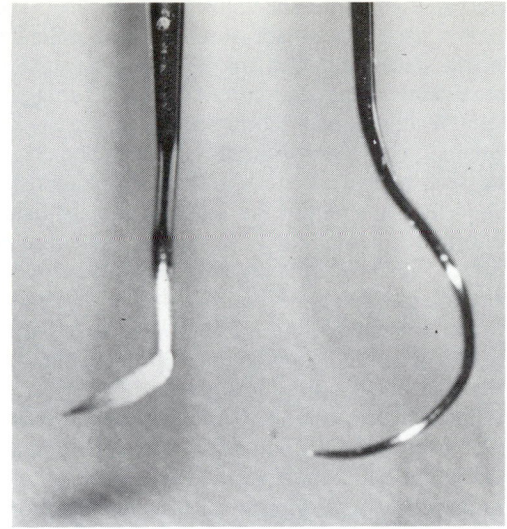

Fig. 26-5. By comparing ends of contraangled (pigtail or cowhorn) explorer and sickle scalers, it is possible to find matching ends that curve in same direction. Sickle scaler can then be selected for use in areas of dentition by following the same principles as for selecting appropriate end of contraangled explorer.

Fig. 26-4. **A,** Anterior sickle scaler with less angular working end in this case is shown adapted to mandibular anterior tooth on proximal surface. Shank is angled in towards midline of tooth to ensure that angle of blade to tooth is less than 90 degrees. Side of tip is carefully adapted to tooth to avoid piercing soft tissue with point of sickle. **B,** Anterior or straight-shanked sickle can be used with circumferential or horizontal stroke on direct facial and lingual surfaces to remove deposits that are otherwise inaccessible. Extreme care is necessary in adapting blade and in ensuring use of short strokes to prevent tissue trauma.

posterior sickle scaler is a reasonably easy task once proper end selection with the cowhorn or pigtail explorer has been mastered (Chapter 9). The best way to determine the proper end is to place the double-ended sickle scaler next to the cowhorn or pigtail and determine which ends match. One end of the cowhorn will curve in the same direction as one end of the sickle scaler (Fig. 26-5). The other ends will likewise match. Careful comparisons will reveal that the terminal

shank of the instrument adjoining the working end matches the terminal shank of the explorer. Therefore the process used to select the proper end of the explorer is also used to select the proper end of the sickle scaler. The end of the explorer used on the mandibular right buccal, for instance, provides a model for the end of the sickle scaler that is appropriate for that area of the mouth.

Alternatively, the clinician can place either end of the sickle scaler against the mesial surface of a tooth in the mandibular right sextant and see which end is aimed across the mesial surface and also has a terminal shank parallel to the long axis of the tooth. Its mate should be usable on the lingual surfaces of the mandibular right sextant, with the shank parallel to the long axis of the tooth.

ADJUNCT INSTRUMENTS

Instruments other than sickle scalers and curettes may be used as adjuncts in the debridement process. These include the periodontal hoe, file, and chisel. In general these instruments are used in patients with heavy calculus deposits, although some clinicians may select them for adaptation to surfaces that require specialized approaches. The chisel is used strictly for supramarginal calculus removal. Hoes and files may be used to supplement sickles scalers and curettes in both supragingival and subgingival debridement.

Studies comparing curettes, files, and hoes have shown that curettes produce the smoothest root surface and inflict the least amount of damage to the cementum and surrounding soft tissues (Kerry, 1967; Wilkinson and Maybury, 1973). Therefore curettes are recommended for use in final debridement of root surfaces. Hoes and files may be used as supplemental instruments for heavy and fine scaling in preparation for root debridement by the curette. Clinicians skilled in the use of hoes and files can adapt them in submarginal areas with good results. The size of the working ends of these instruments has decreased over the years, improving their accessibility to submarginal areas. Although the use of these instruments may speed the debridement process, it should always be followed by the use of a curette. Not only does the curette design facilitate optimum adaptation to the root surface, but the rounded toe and back also protect the soft tissues from trauma during the procedure.

Design and use of hoes

The hoe is usually limited to removal of large ledges of calculus (Seibert, 1978). Calculus that rings the tooth, particularly on the facial, lingual, and distal surfaces of teeth that have no posterior tooth adjacent to them, can be removed relatively easily with a hoe.

Fig. 26-6 shows the design of a hoe. It has one blade. The angle of the shank determines the area of use. Generally the instruments are paired so that one end can be used on the facial surface and its mate can be used on the lingual surface of a given tooth. The companion instrument has one end that can be adapted on the distal surface of a tooth, while its mate can be adapted on the mesial surface of the tooth. The mesial and distal ends are useful when the adjacent tooth is missing. Thus they are especially helpful in removing ledge calculus from the distal surface of the last tooth in the quadrant and on the direct lingual surface of the lower anterior teeth, especially when a large bridge of calculus is present.

The same modified pen grasp, finger rest and wrist motion as used with the previously described instruments are used with hoes. However,

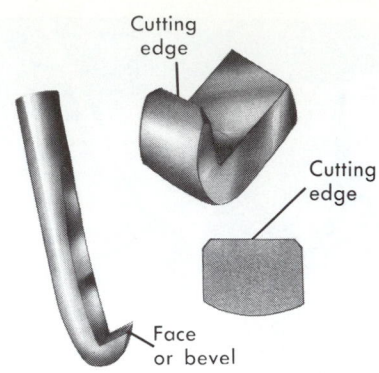

Fig. 26-6. Hoe has one blade and firm shank. When placed beneath a ledge of calculus, a vertical stroke will usually be successful in removing deposits. As shown, corners of blade should be clipped off with sharpening stone.
(Adapted from Seibert JS: *Contin Dent Educ* 1:8, 1978.)

in implementing the stroking pattern, the instrument is limited to a vertical pattern of strokes (Fig. 26-7). The instrument is placed into the sulcus and moved apically past the deposit of calculus. It is not possible or advisable to force the instrument near the attachment because of its bulk. Once the instrument has moved past the ledge of calculus, it should be held firmly against the tooth with the horizontal pressure of a working stroke and moved coronally out of the sulcus. The blade should engage the deposit and remove it in large pieces. The instrument can be used to detect any residual pieces of calculus, but it is not known for fine detection potential. It is a heavy working instrument that generally precedes additional scaling with fine curettes.

A sterile set of hoes may be kept for heavy cases. They are not regular inclusions in a standard tray setup for scaling, however, because of their limited use.

Design and use of chisels

The chisel is another instrument that is usually kept as an adjunct. The Zerfing chisel is illustrated in Fig. 26-8. It is used solely to remove large ledges of calculus from the lingual surfaces of the anterior teeth. It is used with a horizontal push stroke with the blade held against the proximal surfaces of the anterior teeth and entering from the labial aspect (Fig. 26-9). The blade is adapted against the distal surface, then against the mesial surface, and so on with a gentle push

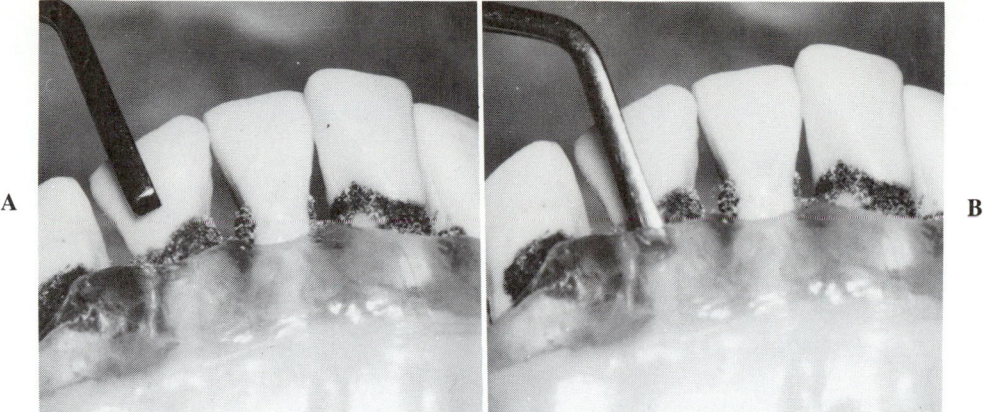

Fig. 26-7. **A,** Hoe with shank parallel to long axis of tooth. **B,** Instrument is moved below edge of calculus with exploratory stroke. Vertical working stroke pattern will engage and remove deposit.

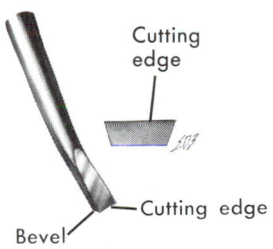

Fig. 26-8. Chisel has single blade and straight shank. Cutting edge is at end of instrument so that when it is pushed against a deposit, leading cutting edge will engage calculus. It is sharpened with flat stone on bevel.

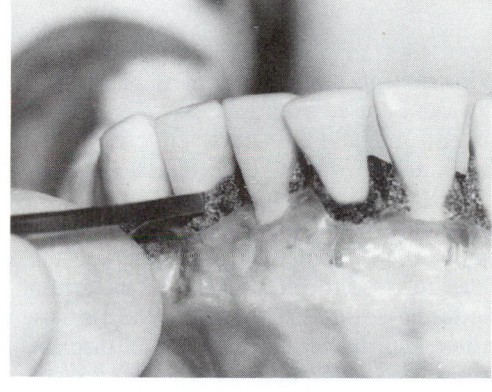

Fig. 26-9. Chisel is used solely to remove lingual calculus on anterior teeth by placing blade against proximal surfaces from labial aspect and pushing toward lingual aspect.

stroke between the teeth until the large bridge of calculus is adequately loosened and can be removed from the lingual aspect of the teeth. It is never to be pushed down into the gingival sulcus, and it is not designed for a pull stroke out of the sulcus. Its sole function is in the anterior areas, where most instruments would crumble the deposit, and more time would be required to remove a bridge formation of heavy calculus.

Design and use of files

When an area of subgingival calculus defies removal with universal curettes, sickles, hoes, and other instruments generally used for universal scaling, a file can be used effectively to crush the deposit and roughen it so that other instruments can remove the fine remnants of calculus (Fig. 26-10). The size of files varies, but generally the small fine files that can be readily adapted subgingivally provide the greatest flexibility and accessibility. In design, files are like several small hoe blades placed in a row on a flat head. They are usually paired to allow access on direct facial and lingual surfaces with one pair of instruments and on mesial and distal surfaces with the other pair of instruments. Thus, in basic design and areas of

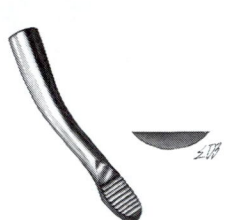

Fig. 26-10. Files are composed of a series of parallel blades on a flat working head. Heavy files have a few large blades, whereas fine files have many small blades.

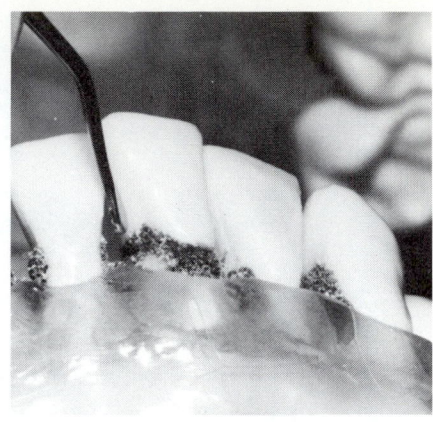

Fig. 26-11. File is adapted to crush calculus and smooth area. Follow-up strokes with a curette are important for removing small fragments and smoothing tooth structure.

access, files are quite similar to hoes. However, the instruments designed for mesial and distal surfaces can be used even in areas where there is an adjacent tooth. Files have a variety of head shapes, ranging from rectangular to oval to oblong.

In addition, the number of cutting edges, or "lips," on each varies. Also varying are the size of the lip closest to the shank and the size of the rake farthest from the shank (the heel); these determine how far the instrument will displace soft tissue when used in pockets. The lip closest to the shank should be 90 degrees to the back of the head of the instrument, and the rake angle between lips should be 55 degrees to the back of the head. Ratcliff files are large, thick, working files with four lips. Others, such as the Rhein 31/32 and UW B46, are best used as finishing files to smooth the roots after calculus has been removed and for finishing restorative margins; such files have 10 or more lips. Hirschfeld files remove calculus in many otherwise inaccessible areas, such as root furrows, deep pockets, and places where the gingival tissues are tight. They have only three rakes and small heads (Hoople, 1985).

Fig. 26-11 illustrates a file approaching the mesial surface of a tooth. The instrument is carefully inserted between the papilla and the tooth, is used to find the tenacious deposit, and is engaged against the deposit with the head of small blades pressed against the deposit and ground into it,

crushing it. Horizontal and vertical strokes can follow this crushing motion. A curette or a finer file can be used to finish the area.

Files are usually considered adjunct instruments and therefore may not be used routinely in general practice or in a recall program. However, in some parts of the country they are used extensively for calculus removal and smoothing root surfaces and are often preferred to curettes for these purposes. They can be extremely valuable in certain clinical situations. The effectiveness of files to debride plaque and plaque by-products from root surfaces has not been established, so they cannot replace curettes for all aspects of the periodontal debridement process.

Plastic instruments for debridement of dental implants

The surfaces of titanium implant abutments can be scratched and damaged by stainless steel or other metal instruments (Fox et al, 1990). Meticulous plaque control is crucial to the long-term success and maintenance of implants. In most cases using home care plaque control devices (e.g, brush, floss, interdental brush, and so on) and polishing the abutment with a rubber cup and polishing paste should be sufficient for removing soft bacterial deposits. When professional debridement for removal of calcified deposits on implant abutments is required it should be accomplished with plastic instruments that will not dam-

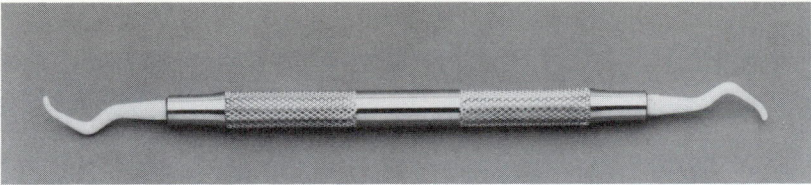

Fig. 26-12. Example of plastic-tipped instrument suitable for debridement of implant abutments. (Courtesy Hu-Friedy Co., Chicago.)

age their surfaces. Plastic-tipped instruments with a variety of blade and shank designs made specifically for this purpose are available. An example is shown in Fig. 26-12.

ALTERNATIVE FINGER REST PLACEMENT

As described in Chapter 9 and earlier in this chapter, the usual location for a fulcrum or finger rest is on the occlusal surfaces of teeth. The tooth surface should be dry so that the clinician's finger is less likely to slip, particularly during a working stroke, when control is absolutely essential. If the finger rest is lost, the instrument may accidentally traumatize the patient's palate, lip, or gingiva or the clinician's hand. The first choice for a finger rest is on a dry, stable tooth. Resting on slippery mucosa or no finger rest at all are unsafe choices.

There are instances when an alternative finger rest is needed: (1) to reach inaccessible areas, (2) when even slight pressure against the lip or stretching of the lips is not easily tolerated, (3) when there are not enough teeth in the sextant to provide a finger rest, or (4) when removing a particularly tenacious calculus deposit demands the greater leverage available from having a more distant finger rest.

Fig. 26-13 shows an alternative rest for the lingual aspect of the maxillary left quadrant for a right-handed clinician. The left index finger is laid across the mandibular arch in the area of the premolars, and the fulcrum finger of the right hand rests stably on it. This is a useful approach for patients with small mouths or when there are few teeth in that sextant to provide a fulcrum.

Fig. 26-14 shows the fulcrum finger placed on the left index finger, which is resting securely in the labial vestibule, retracting the lip. This alternative is useful when using circumferential strokes on the facial surfaces or when there are

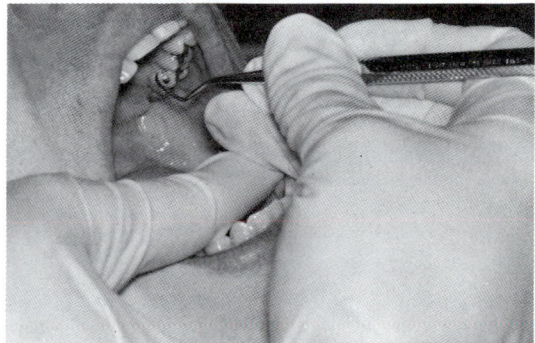

Fig. 26-13. Alternative fulcrum placement for maxillary left lingual sextant uses left index finger resting on mandibular arch.

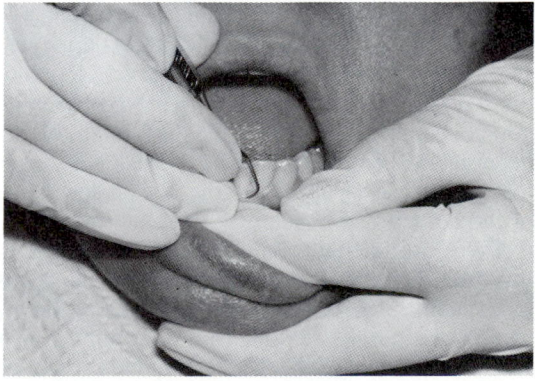

Fig. 26-14. Finger rest on index finger placed in mandibular anterior vestibule.

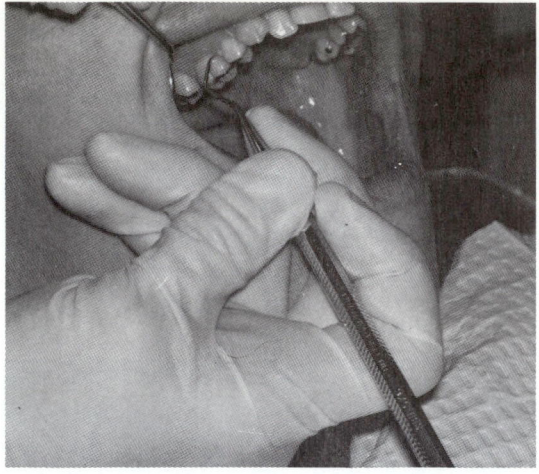

Fig. 26-15. Backs of third and fourth fingers are pressed extraorally against cheek for finger rest for access to maxillary right buccal area.

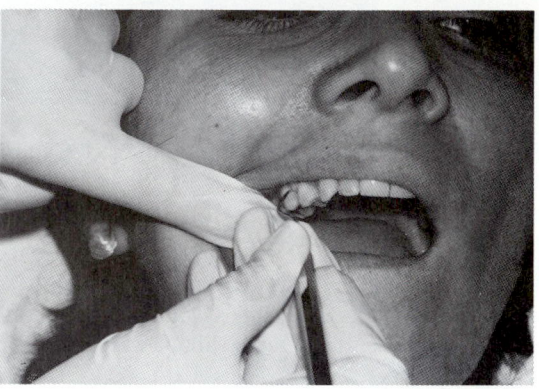

Fig. 26-16. Left index finger retracts cheek; right finger rests on it for access to maxillary right buccal area.

too few teeth to provide a ready finger rest site. It is the fulcrum of choice when using a horizontal, facial-to-lingual push stroke with a chisel.

Chapter 9 contains much information regarding access to the buccal aspect of the maxillary teeth in the sextant closest to the clinician. Two rests are described: one posterior to the operative site and one anterior to it. The two approaches require different wrist motions (see Fig. 9-22 for a right-handed clinician or 9-34 for a left-handed clinician). The finger rest posterior to the operative site is described as using the orbicularis oris muscle at the corner of the mouth to provide much of the stability, particularly for extreme posterior instrumentation sites. When the last tooth in the quadrant is being explored or scaled, all finger rest support is localized on the elastic resistance of the corner of the mouth.

There are two other alternatives for access to this area. Fig. 26-15 shows a rest where the backs of the third and fourth fingers are pressed firmly against the cheek, serving as an extraoral finger rest. Alternatively, the left index finger can be used to retract the cheek, with the right fulcrum finger resting on it (Fig. 26-16).

Although it was once considered heresy to teach many alternative hand placements for establishing a finger rest, experienced clinicians know that creative approaches are necessary to gain access to areas of the mouth that are remote or pro-

vide no ready conventional fulcrum. These approaches include establishing a finger rest on the mandible while treating teeth in the maxilla and on the opposite side of the arch, causing the fulcrum finger and the grasp of the instrument to separate. Virtually any approach to stabilizing the instrument is acceptable as long as a firm grasp and stable finger or hand rest can be established to ensure both safe use of the instrument and sufficient leverage to enable removal of deposits.

PRINCIPLES OF INSTRUMENTATION SPECIFIC TO DEBRIDEMENT
Angulation

While basic principles of end selection, grasp, finger rest, stroke activation, and stroke patterns are applicable to the use of both explorers and instruments used for debridement (e.g, sickle scalers and curettes), *angulation* is a critical difference that is important when using cutting instruments. These instruments have a working end or blade with two cutting edges, one of which is adapted and angled against a given tooth surface. This "working edge" must be angled to the tooth so that it can engage the deposits optimally and so that the edge which is not placed against the tooth surface (i.e, the "opposite cutting edge") does not cut into the soft tissue that lies adjacent to the debrided area.

To ensure that these two needs are met, the

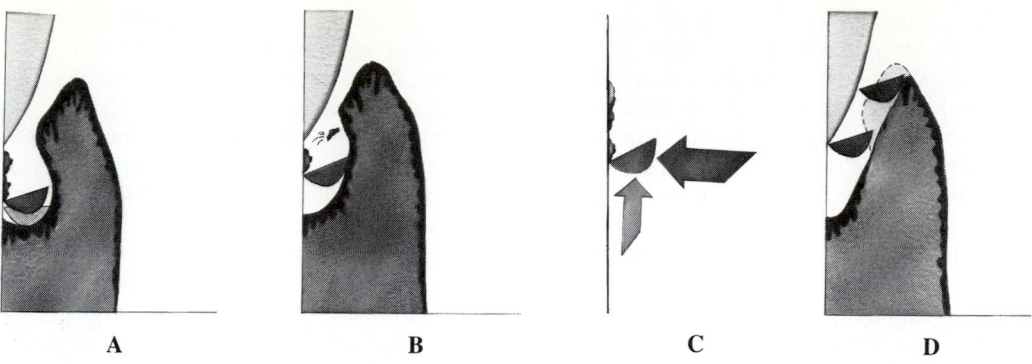

A   B   C   D

Fig. 26-17. **A,** Scaler inserted to base of sulcus and beneath a calculus deposit. **B,** Calculus being removed by properly angulated blade (more than 45 degrees and less than 90 degrees to tooth). Calculus is removed by increased horizontal pressure against tooth as working stroke is activated and, **C,** motion out of sulcus is completed. **D,** Coincidental curettage of sulcus wall occurs in some instances as cutting instrument moves out of sulcus.

(Adapted from Seibert JS: *Contin Dent Educ* 1:8, 1978.)

blade should be angled so that it is less than 90 degrees and more than 45 degrees to the tooth (Fig. 26-17, *B*). If the angle of the blade is less than 45 degrees to the tooth (i.e., "too closed"), the working edge will not be in direct contact with the tooth surface, and the face of the blade will be almost completely in contact with the tooth, resulting in ineffective debridement. If the angle of the blade is at 90 degrees or more to the tooth (i.e., "too open"), the working edge will be tipped too far away from the tooth to treat it effectively, and the opposite cutting edge will scrape or cut into the soft tissues of the sulcus or pocket. This angulation error can result in unnecessary tissue trauma as well as decreased effectiveness in debridement.

When instruments are used for subgingival debridement (primarily curettes), the angulation of the blade is closed to nearly 0 degrees while the instrument is being inserted into the sulcus or pocket to protect the soft tissue wall from trauma posed by the opposite cutting edge. While traveling in an apical direction during the insertion, the working edge is in contact with the tooth surface and provides tactile clues as to the location of calculus deposits and the pocket base. This information is especially useful for locating the boundaries of calculus deposits so that the cutting edge can be placed immediately apical to the deposit for the beginning of the working stroke. Once the

blade is in place for the beginning of the working stroke, the angulation is increased to between 45 and 90 degrees to begin the working stroke.

For strictly supragingival use, the sickle scaler can be maintained at an effective working angulation at all times. Although the sickle scaler is used primarily for supragingival debridement, it can be safely adapted a few millimeters below the gingival margin under certain circumstances, such as in areas beneath tight contacts or when supragingival calculus deposits rest slightly below gingival margins. Under these conditions, care should be taken to insert the sickle using a closed angulation.

Working stroke

One critical difference between probing or exploring and removing deposits is the type of stroke used. Although the same gentle, exploratory stroke is used with a scaler in moving into the sulcus, the actual debridement occurs when the motion out of the sulcus becomes a *working stroke*. A working stroke involves increased pressure laterally against the tooth as the instrument is pulled in a coronal direction.

The lateral pressure needed to create a working stroke is produced by tightening the grasp on the instrument handle and increasing the amount of force applied by the hand and transmitted through the cutting edge to the tooth surface. The amount of lateral pressure is determined by the nature of the work and the purpose of the stroke. For instance, older, subgingival deposits that are firmly attached to the tooth surface require more lateral pressure to accomplish their removal than do recently mineralized or supragingival deposits. Debridement of light, grainy deposits may require moderate lateral pressure during working strokes, whereas deplaquing or careful smoothing of selected cementum surfaces is accomplished with light amounts of pressure against the cutting edge. Exploratory strokes require little or no lateral pressure.

The clinician must assess the nature of the tooth surface and associated deposits and use this information when determining how much pressure to apply to each working stroke. The lateral pressure of each stroke should be sufficient to debride the surface without unnecessary removal of cementum or dentin. Use of too much pressure may cause excessive removal of root cementum, inflict nicks or gouges in root surfaces, and contribute needlessly to fatigue in the clinician's hand and fingers. If too little pressure is applied when removing tenacious calculus deposits, the instrument will skim over the surface of the deposits so that they are smoothed or "burnished" rather than completely removed (Fig. 26-18). The object of calculus removal is not to chip away, shave, wear down, or smooth the deposit but to fracture it cleanly away from the tooth whenever possible. As calculus deposits become burnished they also become harder to detect and to remove.

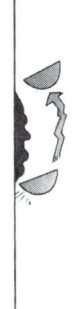

Fig. 26-18. Instrument may merely chatter over or smooth down a calculus deposit if insufficient horizontal pressure is used or if blade is dull.
(Adapted from Seibert JS: *Contin Dent Educ* 1:8, 1978.)

The clinician must continuously reappraise the amount of pressure to be applied for each succeeding stroke as the surface is modified by the cutting edge of the instrument. Since varying amounts of resistance will be encountered during working strokes, depending on the tenacity of the deposits' attachment to the tooth surface, the clinician must apply matching levels of lateral pressure to accomplish thorough debridement while maintaining control of the instrument. When removing a calculus deposit, for example, the amount of force required to dislodge the deposit must be discontinued at the moment the deposit fractures away from the tooth to prevent the instrument from being propelled further in an uncontrolled motion. A constant pressure should be maintained for the duration of each stroke. Controlling the force behind each working stroke and matching the amount of pressure to the nature of the deposits are important skills to develop.

A critical element in ensuring a light-handed approach to instrumentation is to use the least amount of pressure necessary to accomplish the debridement procedure. With a light-handed approach, unnecessary loss of tooth material can be avoided and operator fatigue and patient discomfort reduced. Alternating the use of exploratory strokes with working strokes is important to provide tactile information used in assessing how debridement is progressing and what modifications of adaptation and stroke are needed to complete the task in an efficient and effective manner.

Exploratory and working strokes should generally be maintained subgingivally until debridement at a given site is completed. As with the probe and explorers, the instrument should not exit completely from the sulcus with each stroke. Rather, the instrument should remain in a subgingival position unless removal and reinsertion are necessary to avoid tissue trauma during readaptation of the cutting edge as it moves around the tooth. After completing the working strokes, the clinician can use the instrument to remove loose calculus or other debris and flush the area thoroughly with an irrigant (see Chapter 28).

The sharpness of the cutting edge of hand instruments has a direct impact on stroke effectiveness. A dull cutting edge diminishes the productivity of both exploratory and working strokes. A detailed description of instrument sharpening techniques is provided in Chapter 27.

UNIVERSAL CURETTE: DESIGN AND USE
Blade design

A universal curette is shown in Fig. 26-19. It, too, is a paired instrument. Universal curettes come in a variety of blade sizes and shank lengths for use in all types of debridement. The shape of the working end of curettes allows them to be used safely in subgingival areas. The universal curette has a rounded toe instead of a point and

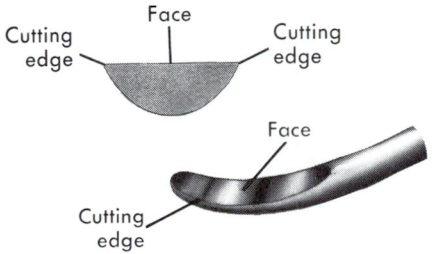

Fig. 26-19. Universal curette has rounded back and rounded toe, which enhance its use in subgingival areas. This back and toe are less likely to cause inadvertent trauma than are sharp-edged back and pointed toe of sickle scaler.

does not have a third edge on the back. It is generally more spoon shaped and less hazardous to surrounding soft tissue than sickle scalers. Yet it is a relatively strong instrument that can be extremely useful in removing heavy, deep deposits. The curved blade (which extends around the toe to form two useful cutting edges) allows it to be more readily adapted to curved root surfaces.

Selecting the correct working end

The same process used in selecting the proper end of the paired explorer and the paired, contraangled sickle scaler is used in selecting the proper end of the universal curette. Placing the universal curette next to the contraangled sickle scaler and explorer allows the clinician to match ends based on direction of curvature and location of the terminal shank. When the universal curette is in place, the terminal shank should be parallel to the long axis of the tooth as the toe of the instrument is aimed across the proximal surface of the tooth to be scaled (Fig. 26-20, *B*). The same principles

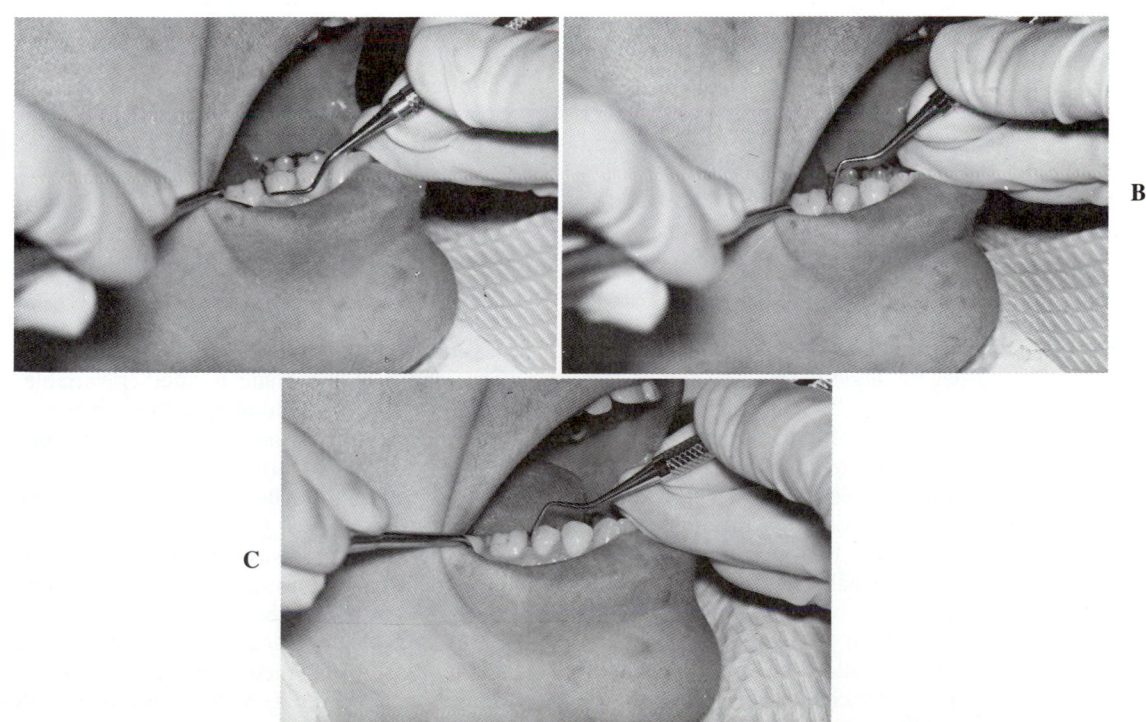

Fig. 26-20. A, Universal curette is adapted with toe directed proximally but with terminal shank perpendicular to long axis of tooth. **B,** Universal curette is adapted with terminal shank parallel to long axis of tooth. **C,** Angulation is closed to less than 90 degrees but more than 45 degrees before beginning working stroke.

of grasp, fulcrum, wrist motion, and stroke are used with this type of instrument.

In general the shank and working end designs of the universal curette allow the instrument to be used more extensively throughout the dentition than the sickle scaler. Just as with the cowhorn explorer and the paired contraangled sickle scaler, the instrument can be used in any given sextant from the facial or lingual surfaces, *with one edge adapting against the mesial aspect and the opposite edge on that same end adapting on the distal aspect*. In other words, the same end of the instrument is used for all proximal surfaces in a given sextant from the buccal aspect. The opposite end is used in that same sextant from the lingual aspect on all proximal surfaces. The two edges on a given end of the instrument make it possible to scale the mesial surface and then the distal surface and so on by merely changing the edge being used and the orientation of the shank in relation to the long axis of the tooth.

With the universal curette it is possible to use the opposite end of the instrument to scale most distal surfaces as well. That is, the end that normally would not be used on a given sextant from a particular aspect can be used on the distal surfaces safely and with the proper angulation. For example, one end can be used on the mandibular right area from the buccal aspect; the other end can be used in that quadrant from the lingual aspect. With the universal curette the end used from the lingual aspect can also be used on distal surfaces from the buccal aspect. The terminal shank, however, will not be parallel to the long axis of the tooth in this case. Fig. 26-20, *A*, shows the position for using the opposite end. By raising the shank to a 45-degree angle to the long axis of the tooth, the instrument can be adapted safely on the distal surface. Generally this particular use of the instrument is an adjunct to regular patterns of instrumentation, largely because it necessitates an additional change of ends of the instrument, which is not necessary if the opposite edge of the same end is used as usual. It is helpful to know that this adaptation can be safely accomplished, as there are times when a slightly different approach to an area will allow the right adaptation to remove a particularly challenging deposit.

When inserting the universal curette for subgingival scaling, the blade should be closed against the tooth to 0 degrees and inserted to the base of the sulcus past the deposit with this same closed angle. At the base of the sulcus the angle is opened to between 45 and 90 degrees and prepared for the working stroke to remove the deposit (Figs. 26-21 and 26-22).

The stroking pattern can be a series of vertical or oblique strokes that overlap (Fig. 26-23) to cover the root or crown surface. This stroke is used for initial scaling around the tooth and is highly successful in removing most deposits. A second kind of stroke is the circumferential or horizontal stroke (Fig. 26-24). The stroking pattern engages the deposits on the sides and allows another approach to calculus that will not come off with a vertical stroke. It is a useful stroke for removing small pieces at the line angles of teeth and for gaining access to the very base of the pocket and to furrows and grooves on root surfaces that may be incompletely treated by vertical strokes (Fig. 26-25).

Selecting a curette: design variations

Many varieties of universal curettes are available; therefore considerable opportunity exists for selecting a specific curette for a particular patient's need. Variations in shank angle, shank strength, and shank length allow for use in remote or more anterior areas of the dentition, for heavy tenacious deposits, or for very deep or relatively shallow pockets. Tissue tightness to the tooth often dictates the size of the shank or blade that may be selected. Extremely tight tissue will not allow a heavy, large instrument adequate access to remove subgingival deposits. Attempts to use instruments that are too large and bulky for existing conditions will also increase the potential for unnecessary tissue trauma and patient discomfort.

The length of the blade is another variable in selecting a universal curette. Longer blades are needed to gain access across the relatively broad proximal surfaces of posterior teeth but may be quite inappropriate for use on the narrow mandibular anterior teeth.

The universal curette is often the instrument of choice for removing moderate or heavy amounts of calculus and when the width and depth of the pocket can accept the heavier shank. In comparison, the design characteristics of area-specific curettes, such as the Gracey series of curettes, make them preferable for use in deep, tight periodontal pockets and for comprehensive root surface debridement after heavy calculus deposits have been removed. The design characteristics

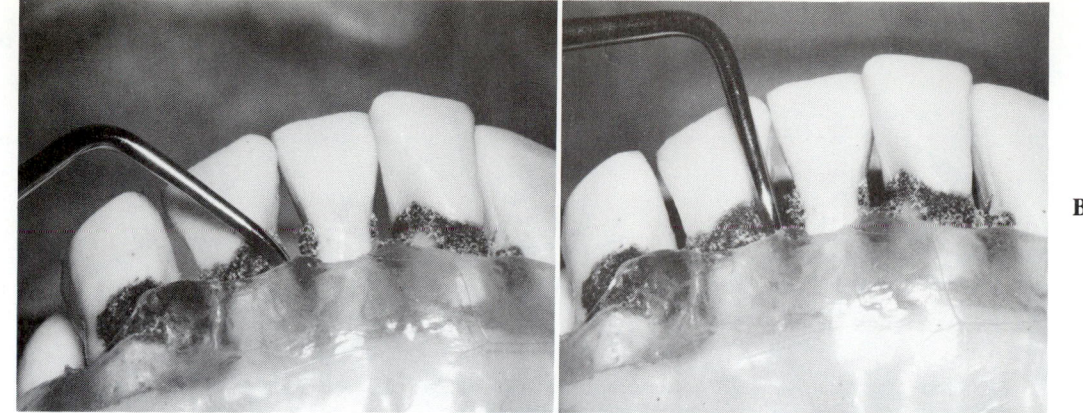

Fig. 26-21. **A,** Curette inserted at 0 degrees and then, **B,** opened to approximately 75 degrees in sulcus.

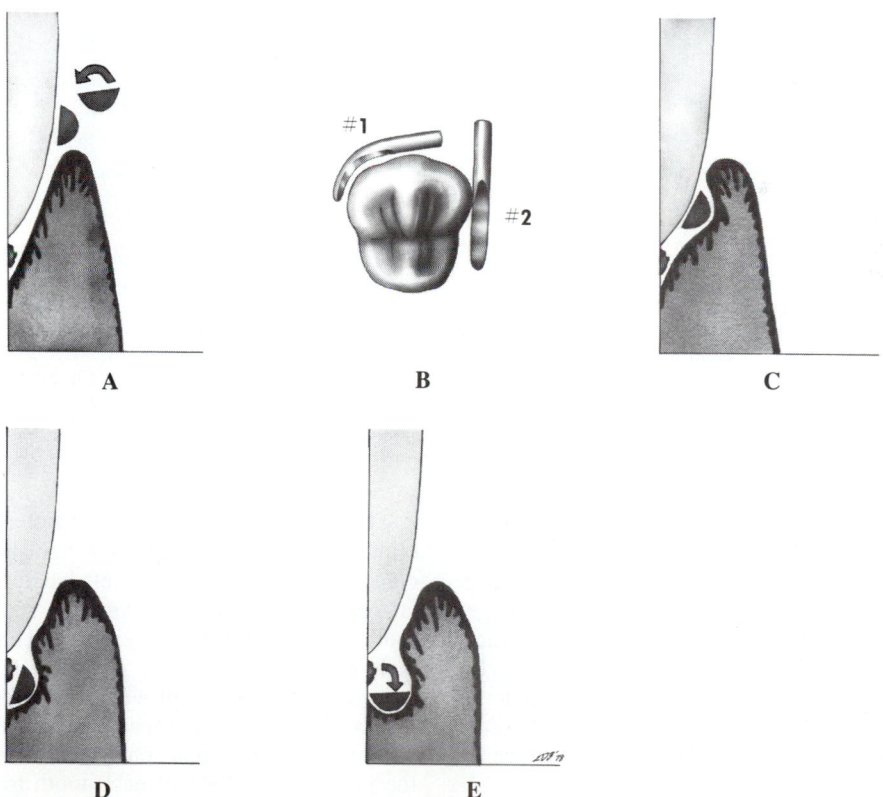

Fig. 26-22. **A,** Curette is inserted into sulcus at 0 degrees angulation so that it resembles curette no. 1 in **B.** Curette is moved into sulcus and past calculus with exploratory stroke, **C** and **D.** At base of sulcus, blade is opened to between 45 and 90 degrees before beginning working stroke, **E.** If 90-degree angle (as shown here) is used, soft tissue will be removed also. Closing it to 75 to 80 degrees minimizes this hazard. (Adapted from Seibert JS: *Contin Dent Educ* 1:8, 1978.)

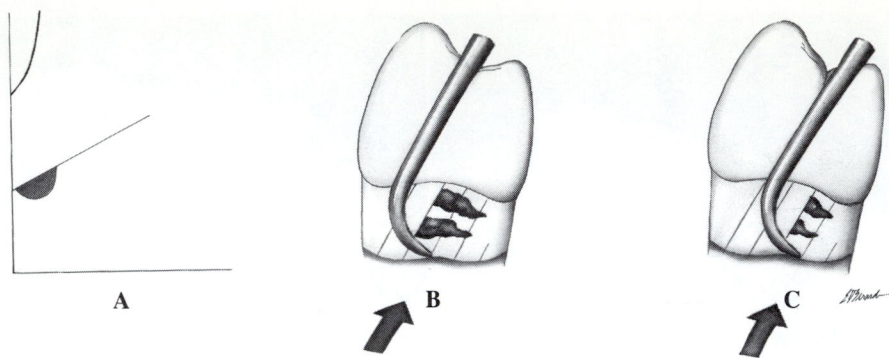

Fig. 26-23. Once blade is engaged at proper angle to tooth, as suggested in **A,** vertical or oblique overlapping working strokes can be used to remove calculus deposits in **B** and **C.**
(Adapted from Seibert JS: *Contin Dent Educ* 1:8, 1978.

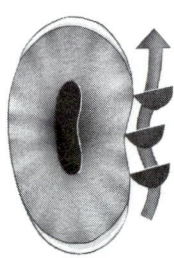

Fig. 26-24. Horizontal or circumferential stroke uses blade with toe aimed more apically so that blade engages lateral side of deposits rather than the most apical aspect of deposit. Horizontal strokes are useful when vertical stokes are not successful and for removing deposits from line angles and from the very base of a pocket. Horizontal stroke also helps obtain adaptation in root furrows and grooves.
(Adapted from Seibert JS: *Contin Dent Educ* 1:8, 1978.)

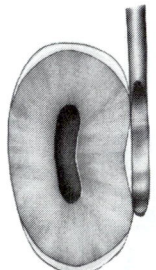

Fig. 26-25. Often a vertical stroke will not be adequate in scaling convoluted roots, especially in furrows and deep grooves. Adaptation is critical, as calculus often forms in these protected areas. Rather than trying to adapt full length of blade to proximal surface as shown, adapt first 2 mm of blade and follow contours of root as shown in Fig. 26-2.
(Adapted from Seibert JS: *Contin Dent Educ* 1:8, 1978.)

and use of these instruments will be discussed in detail later in the chapter.

There are some general guidelines for selecting universal curettes: (1) reserve heavy, large curettes for heavy deposits and finer, smaller curettes for finer deposits or for access to tight subgingival areas; (2) use instruments with long shanks for deep pockets; and (3) select the blade length according to the size of the tooth surface to be scaled.

Sequence of debridement

Whether the universal curette or the sickle scaler is being used for debridement, the same general sequence is followed as described in detail in Chapter 9.

The mandibular posterior sextant closer to the clinician (mandibular right for right-handed clinicians; mandibular left for left-handed clinicians) is treated first, moving from the most posterior tooth through the first premolar. The distal, facial, and mesial surfaces are treated using overlapping exploratory and working strokes as calculus is detected and engaged for removal. The stroking pattern should carry the instrument past the proximal midline of each tooth to ensure that typically elusive deposits are not left.

The clinician then treats the mandibular sextant on the opposite side of the mouth, approaching it from the lingual surfaces. The lingual surfaces on the side of the mouth nearer the clinician are next, and then the buccal aspect of the opposite side of the mouth is treated. At this point all the posterior teeth are treated. If the instrument has reached sufficiently far across the proximal surface under the deposits to engage and remove them with overlapping strokes, few should remain. This can be accomplished with either a posterior sickle scaler or a universal curette with only one position change (moving to the rear position for the buccal surfaces on the side away from the clinician) and with only one instrument change (changing ends when moving from the lingual surfaces of the distant sextant to the lingual surfaces of the near sextant). The anterior teeth can then be treated either from the rear or front position.

Many clinicians stop and explore the mandibular teeth for remaining deposits before moving to the maxilla. If it is determined that debridement is incomplete, time will be needed to return to these locations, perform additional treatment, and recheck.

When debridement is completed on the mandibular teeth, the clinician moves to the buccal aspect of the maxillary sextant closer to the clinician and then to the lingual aspect of the distant posterior maxillary sextant. The clinician changes ends and positions (to a rear position) and treats the lingual surfaces of the nearer maxillary sextant, followed by the buccal aspect of the distant sextant. The anterior teeth are then scaled from the rear position. The maxilla is explored for residual deposits and retreated as needed.

Particularly difficult deposits may require the use of adjunct hand instruments such as the hoe, file, or chisel. Use of these instruments will be discussed later in this chapter. Deposits located in areas defying access by normal means may need to be approached with an unconventional adaptation or fulcrum placement.

GRACEY CURETTES: DESIGN AND USE

Several factors must be considered when selecting a curette for subgingival debridement. The instrument must be adaptable to a wide variety of pocket depths and shapes. It must be versatile enough to be used in any part of the mouth and to reach apically into deep pockets. It must have a blade design that facilitates its use in small, confined areas, such as furcations. The curette must also be designed with maximum ability to transmit minute vibrations from light calculus deposits and rough cementum and yet be rigid enough to

remove all deposits effectively. The presence of deep, narrow, periodontal pockets requires a comparatively narrow blade that can gain access to these areas without traumatizing adjacent soft tissues. The Gracey curette designs meet all of these criteria and are preferred over other types of curettes for subgingival debridement by many clinicians. Examples of the various area-specific Gracey curette designs are shown in Fig. 26-26.

Blade design

There are several differences between the design of a Gracey curette blade and that of a universal curette blade. One major difference is that the two cutting edges are not parallel. Instead, the Gracey curette has offset cutting edges so that one edge appears to be lower than the other (Fig. 26-27). In the universal curette design both cutting edges can be correctly adapted for use on a tooth, but only the *lower cutting edge* of the Gracey curette should be adapted to the tooth for working strokes. The Gracey curette also has a characteristic beveled surface adjacent to one of its cutting edges that universal curettes do not have.

The different blade design of the Gracey curette gives it a *self-angulating* capability. This means that when the Gracey curette is correctly adapted to the tooth so that the terminal shank (i.e, the portion of the shank nearest the blade) is parallel to the long axis of the tooth, the blade is already aligned at the optimum working angulation, and further adjustments are unnecessary.

Area-specific shank designs

Gracey curettes are examples of area-specific curettes. Unlike universal curettes in which one double-ended instrument is adaptable to all tooth surfaces, each Gracey curette has a unique shank configuration that facilitates optimum adaptation and access to a specific area or tooth surface. This design feature means that total debridement requires the use of a combination of instruments. The following list gives the design numbers of the Gracey curettes shown in Fig. 26-26 and the areas for which optimum adaptation can be obtained:

Gracey ½ and ¾: Anterior teeth

Gracey ⁵⁄₆: Anterior and premolar teeth

Gracey ⅞ and ⁹⁄₁₀: Posterior teeth, buccal and lingual surfaces

Gracey ¹¹⁄₁₂ and ¹⁵⁄₁₆: Posterior teeth, mesial surfaces

Gracey ¹³⁄₁₄: Posterior teeth, distal surfaces

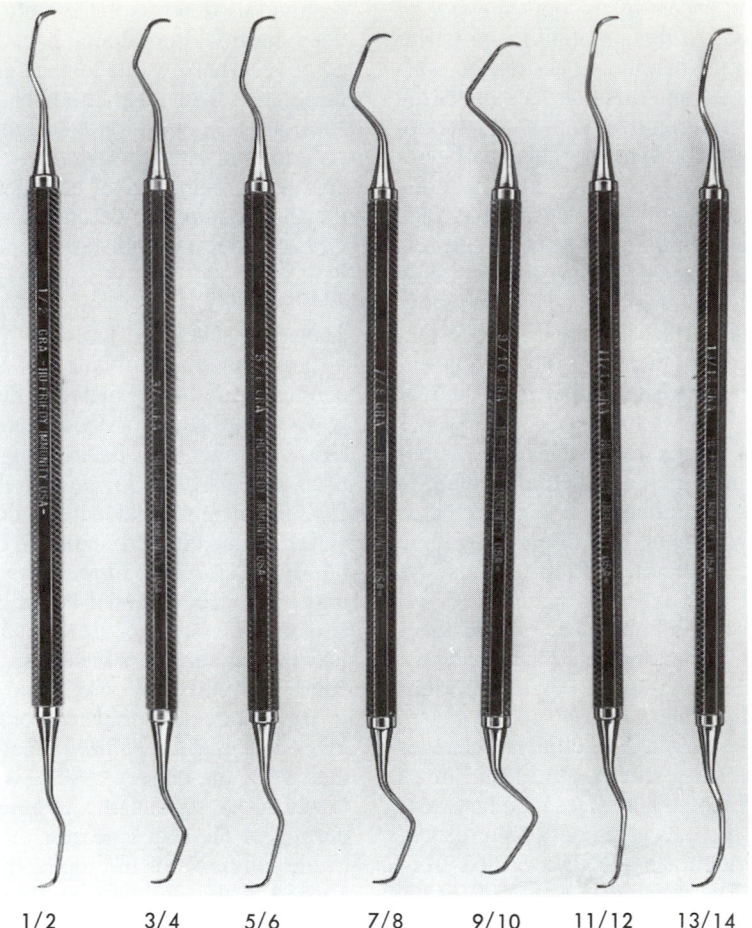

| 1/2 | 3/4 | 5/6 | 7/8 | 9/10 | 11/12 | 13/14 |

Fig. 26-26. Gracey curettes provide a variety of shank designs to facilitate access to all areas of dentition. Working-end design is well suited to removal of fine deposits in subgingival areas. (Courtesy Hu-Friedy Co., Chicago.)

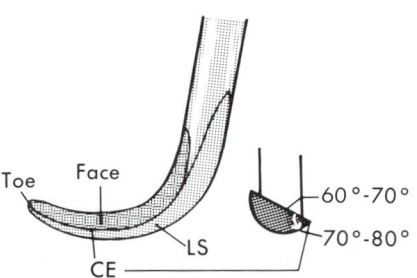

Fig. 26-27. Note offset relationship of cutting edges on this Gracey curette so that one blade appears lower than the other.

(Note: The Gracey curettes used for posterior proximal surfaces may also be combined as $^{11}/_{14}$ and $^{12}/_{13}$ so that one double-ended instrument can be used to treat both mesial and distal surfaces in one buccal or lingual sextant without exchanging instruments.)

A number of modifications of Gracey curettes are also available to improve their adaptability to a variety of clinical situations. Rigid shank designs facilitate removal of moderately heavy or tenacious calculus deposits. Flexible shank designs improve tactile sensitivity during debridement and are effective for removing light and easily dislodged deposits. The "Mini-Five" series of Gracey curettes have shorter, smaller blades to

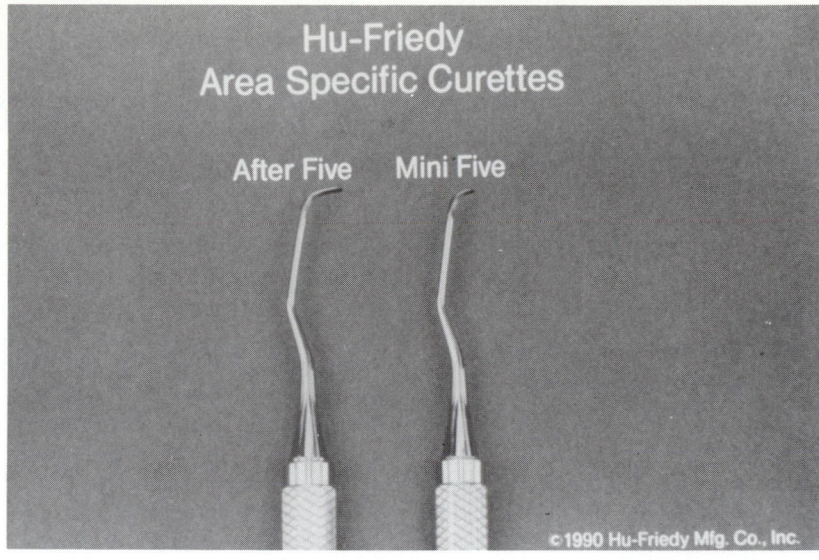

Fig. 26-28. Modifications of Gracey curettes: the "After Five" and "Mini-Five" series. (Courtesy Hu-Friedy Co., Chicago.)

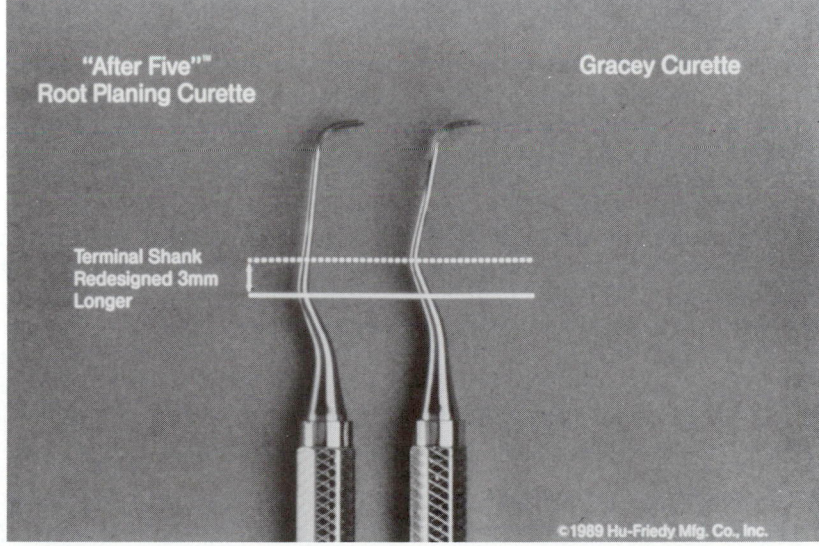

Fig. 26-29. Comparison of a regular Gracey curette and an "After Five" curette demonstrates the longer terminal shank design of the "After Five," which facilitates access to deep periodontal pockets. (Courtesy Hu-Friedy Co., Chicago.)

permit improved access to narrow or confined areas (Fig. 26-28). The "After Five" series is designed with longer than average terminal shanks that allow extension of the blades into deep periodontal pockets (Figs. 26-28 and 26-29).

Gracey curettes designed for use in anterior segments of the mouth have a relatively straight and simple shank design, whereas those designed for harder-to-reach areas in the posterior segments of the mouth have shanks with more complex and convoluted designs. Although each of these curettes is useful in its own way, the efficient clinician will limit the choice of instruments for periodontal debridement to only those designs that are absolutely required to get the job done. Too much time can be wasted hunting for essential instruments among a tray cluttered with extras. Although preferences will vary among clinicians, a good "starter set" of Gracey curettes that provides accessibility to any area of the mouth includes the $\frac{1}{2}$, $\frac{7}{8}$, $\frac{11}{12}$, and $\frac{13}{14}$. Additional instruments can be kept sterilized and stored for immediate availability when they are needed to supplement the basic tray setup.

Selecting and adapting the correct working end

The first step in selecting the appropriate instrument is to associate the shank design and design numbers of each Gracey curette with the area or surfaces for which it is intended to be used. Next, the clinician must determine which working end of the selected instrument adapts to the treatment site. This decision is made by placing the lower cutting edge of the blade against the tooth surface with the toe leading in the direction in which working strokes will be employed. The face of the curette blade should appear partially closed against the tooth surface when the lower cutting edge is correctly adapted. If the correct working end has been chosen, the terminal shank will be oriented parallel to the long axis of the tooth.

The same principles for angulation and activation of working and exploratory strokes that were described earlier for universal curettes also apply to the use of Gracey curettes. The only significant difference is that the offset blade design makes it easier to accomplish effective angulation. Remember that these instruments are designed so that viewing the orientation of the terminal shank assists the clinician in establishing an effective working angulation. When the terminal portion of the shank is parallel to the long axis of the tooth, the angulation is in the optimum range for working strokes.

PERFORMING SUBGINGIVAL DEBRIDEMENT WITH HAND INSTRUMENTS

The instrumentation skills used for supragingival debridement must be highly developed and refined to facilitate effective subgingival debridement. The clinician must have mastered the prin-

ciples of adaptation, insertion, and angulation and must be able to direct working strokes effectively to avoid injuring the inflamed soft tissues. Mastery of instrumentation skills is crucial during subgingival debridement because of the repeated overlapping strokes needed to treat every portion of the root surface during this procedure. The ability of the clinician to control the amount of pressure applied to each working stroke must also be developed so that the root surface is not gouged or over-treated, resulting in unnecessary loss of cementum. In addition, the clinician has to evaluate the progress of the procedure continuously and to determine if adjustments in pressure or angulation are needed either to accelerate or minimize the removal of deposits or cementum, depending on the quality of the surface.

The most important skill required for subgingival debridement is the clinician's ability to receive a wide variety of delicate tactile sensations, to discriminate among them, and to interpret them accurately. The clinician must detect roughness, graininess, or subtle abnormalities of the root surface that may indicate the presence of fine or burnished calculus deposits or ridges and gouges created by earlier instrumentation. Because of the nature of these surface irregularities, they will be less obvious to the tactile sense than were the larger deposits and plaque-retentive surfaces that were encountered during initial debridement. At other times the clinician may be unable to detect any surface roughness at all but must still perform thorough debridement of the surface cementum to remove plaque and its associated endotoxins from the pocket.

The exact type of attachment between endotoxins (also known as lipopolysaccharide [LPS]) or endotoxin-like substances and the cementum surface has not been established. Recent evidence, however, suggests that cementum-associated LPS is relatively superficial and easily removed from the root surface (see Chapter 26). Clinicians should therefore use conservative approaches to debridement that will avoid unnecessary removal of the cementum and must depend primarily on the healing response in each site to determine if the root surface has been made biologically acceptable to the adjacent soft tissues.

Armamentarium

Other instruments or supplies needed for subgingival debridement are a mouth mirror, explorer,

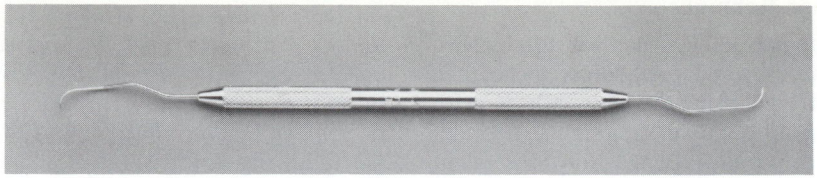

Fig. 26-30. Design of EXD11-12AF periodontal explorer facilitates access to the apical extent of deep periodontal pockets.
(Courtesy Hu-Friedy Co., Chicago.)

probe, sharpening supplies, and anesthesia setup. A fine, long-shanked explorer or periodontal probe should be included because this procedure requires optimum tactile sensitivity for detection of fine deposits and root irregularities. The design of the exploring instrument should allow the clinician access to even the deepest pockets. Curved explorers (such as the pigtail or cowhorn) cannot reach the apical extent of all pockets. The length of the explorer's working end, its ability to be maneuvered in deep pockets, and its ability to transmit subtle vibrations (that is, diameter of the working end) must all be considered. Some explorers that fit these criteria, such as the fine No. 17 or No. 20 design shown in Chapter 9 (see Fig. 9-10), may not adapt easily to the distal surfaces of posterior teeth because of their straight design. For these surfaces the clinician may elect to use a periodontal probe or another instrument for exploration. A periodontal explorer such as the Hu-Friedy EXD11-12AF (designed with a shank similar to the Gracey $11/12$ curette) can facilitate exploration in deep periodontal pockets (Fig. 26-30).

The experienced clinician can also use a sharp curette blade to accomplish much of the detection. There are many advantages to developing tactile sensitivity with the curette blade for definitive exploration. According to basic instrumentation principles, this ability is necessary as a prelude to each working stroke performed with the instrument. The student should take time to practice and develop skill in using the curette for exploration, because it will increase operating efficiency. This skill will facilitate deposit removal, because the clinician will have a more accurate idea of location and type of deposit. Using the curette for exploration also maximizes efficiency, as it eliminates the need for frequent switching between curette and explorer to provide evaluation feedback. Beginning students should depend on an explorer to evaluate the tooth surface until they have developed their tactile sensitivity with the curette. For all clinicians the final check of the debridement process requires use of the explorer (or probe, if preferred) for a definitive tactile evaluation of the treated root surface.

The importance of frequent sharpening of curettes during root planing procedures was clearly demonstrated by a study that evaluated the amount of wear (dulling) that the cutting edges of curettes underwent during prescribed numbers of strokes (Tal et al, 1985). Curettes that had been used for only 15 strokes showed signs of dulling, as evidenced by the presence of a slight bevel (i.e, rounding of the edge) when observed under a scanning electron microscope. Even wider bevels were observed after 45 strokes. Since 15 to 45 working strokes might easily account for the treatment of only one or two teeth, instruments must be resharpened frequently to maximize their effectiveness and efficiency.

The decision to use topical or local anesthesia or nitrous oxide and oxygen conscious sedation during subgingival debridement depends on individual patient needs. Many patients find any kind of instrumentation in inflamed areas somewhat uncomfortable, and because of the exacting requirements of this procedure, it may be necessary and advisable to administer pain control. Since discomfort during debridement therapy is often directly correlated with the presence of inflammation in the gingival tissues, delaying the subgingival debridement until after the patient has developed effective daily plaque control habits is recommended. After marginal gingivitis has been reduced, there is less need for local anesthesia. Pain control should be introduced only for patient comfort when even safe and effective techniques produce symptoms of pain.

Instrumentation technique

Remove supragingival deposits first to improve visibility and access to the periodontal pocket area and to support the patient's early efforts with daily plaque control. Initial subgingival debridement includes removal of the most obvious calculus deposits and plaque retentive surfaces (e.g, amalgam overhangs) that require the use of universal curettes, hoes, or files. The pattern of gross calculus removal in a pocket area should proceed in an apical direction until the entire area has been cleared of easily detected deposits. When deposits are too tenacious or too large to be removed in a single, controlled stroke, remove them in segments. Place the tip of the curette under one edge of the deposit so that each succeeding working stroke reduces the size of the remaining deposit until none remains. Periodontal hoes and files may also be used to supplement the curette for removal of especially heavy or tenacious deposits.

After completion of gross calculus removal, begin the debridement by focusing on methodical coverage of the entire root surface with the cutting edge of the instrument for removal of fine, grainy calculus deposits; root surface irregularities; subgingival plaque; and cementum-associated LPS. Gracey curettes are ideally suited for these purposes. Either a rigid or flexible shank design can be used, depending on the nature of the work to be done. Rigid shanks facilitate removal of deposits requiring moderate to heavy working strokes. The more flexible shank design improves the effectiveness of lighter strokes during final debridement procedures, when maximum tactile information is desired from the working end of the instrument.

Apply the curette blade to all accessible root surfaces while determining the number of strokes, length of strokes, and amount of lateral pressure necessary to treat each surface area. There are no easy formulas to help guide these decisions. Clinical experience is the best teacher. Unfortunately, there is also little guidance provided by the research literature on how to accomplish optimum subgingival debridement with hand instruments. Almost all clinical studies involving closed subgingival debridement with hand instruments have used traditional scaling and root planing approaches to instrumentation. The limitations of these approaches have been thoroughly discussed in Chapter 25.

The task, then, is to *redefine hand instrumentation as a way to render the root surface biologically acceptable to the soft tissue wall of the periodontal pocket without causing unnecessary loss or damage to either hard or soft tissues.* Consider the following objectives that support the goal of achieving resolution of inflammation and periodontal health:

1. Removal of pathogenic bacterial plaque
2. Removal of plaque-associated LPS
3. Removal of plaque or LPS-bearing calculus
4. Elimination of selected plaque retentive surface irregularities
5. Conservation of root surface material
6. Minimal disruption or damage to adjacent soft tissues

Plaque and its associated LPS are present in the pocket as superficially adherent deposits and as loosely adherent deposits. The loosely adherent deposits can be removed from the pocket environment by the "scooping" action of the spoon-shaped curette blade as strokes are generated along the root surface. Loose deposits can also be removed through subgingival irrigation of the pocket area. Use of antimicrobial solutions for this purpose further reduces the bacterial population in the pocket.

Adherent plaque and cementum-associated LPS appear to be easily removed with light pressure during instrumentation (Cheetham et al, 1988; Smart et al, 1990). The clinician's challenge in removing these deposits with a cutting edge is to achieve actual contact with every square millimeter of the root surface to remove bacterial plaque. This task requires careful overlapping of strokes applied in a variety of patterns that will ensure complete adaptation of the cutting edge to all aspects of the root. The difficulty of achieving this goal is discussed further in the section on root morphology.

The lateral pressure applied to working strokes must be varied to match the resistance of the deposit being removed. Well-established subgingival deposits may be difficult to remove because they are usually harder than supragingival deposits and because of how they attach themselves to the root surface. These deposits penetrate into irregularities of the cementum surface (e.g, resorption lacunae, nicks, and grooves resulting from previous instrumentation) and become attached to the root surface by means of a mechanical lock. At the same time, the cementum underlying the deposits is relatively soft and can be easily gouged by a sharp cutting edge. Lateral pressure of the blade against the root surface should be moderate at first until the surface debris is removed. These strokes should be followed by lighter strokes to remove superficial plaque and LPS deposits while care is taken to preserve cementum. Working strokes should be applied with even and controlled amounts of pressure against the tooth. The clinician should be careful not to apply heavy pressure at the onset of the stroke; instead, the same amount of pressure should be applied through the entire stroke. This will prevent ditching of the cementum at those areas where the strokes begin.

Strokes used for initial calculus removal may be shorter than the ones required for the final stages of subgingival debridement. When the purpose of the working stroke is calculus removal, the objective is to fracture the deposit cleanly away from the tooth, and the working stroke can end as soon as the deposit is dislodged. Since subgingival debridement combines the objectives of calculus and plaque removal into one procedure, the initial strokes should be relatively short, overlapping, and controlled, with each morphologic element of the root treated thoroughly. As debridement reaches its final stages and the surface becomes smoother, the strokes can be lengthened to blend the boundaries of each of the treated areas into each other. Short strokes should be used initially because they are somewhat easier to control and adapt when more resistance or irregular surface characteristics are encountered.

The application of different types of stroking patterns over a given surface is likely to produce more complete treatment coverage of the area than the use of only one stroke direction. For instance, if initial debridement for calculus removal is done with vertical strokes, additional strokes to complete the debridement of plaque and superficial deposits and irregularities should include a series of overlapping oblique and horizontal strokes over the same area (Fig. 26-31). Instrument adaptation for vertical and horizontal strokes is shown in Figs. 26-32 and 26-33. This pattern of strokes is similar to the pattern recommended for debridement with ultrasonic instruments described in Chapter 25.

Subgingival debridement using hand instruments requires significantly greater time than does supragingival debridement. Whereas most suprag-

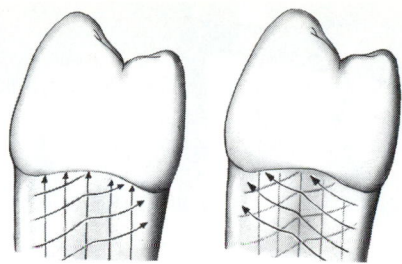

Fig. 26-31. Thorough debridement is achieved through the use of a wide variety of overlapping strokes.

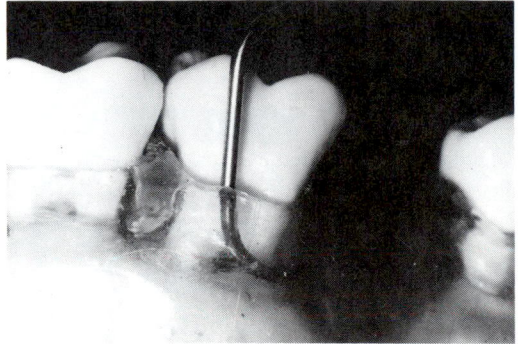

Fig. 26-32. Gracey ⅞ curette is properly adapted for implementation of vertical stroke on mesiobuccal line angle of tooth No. 30. Note that terminal shank is parallel to long axis of tooth for this stroking pattern. This adaptation ensures proper working angulation of lower cutting edge against tooth surface.

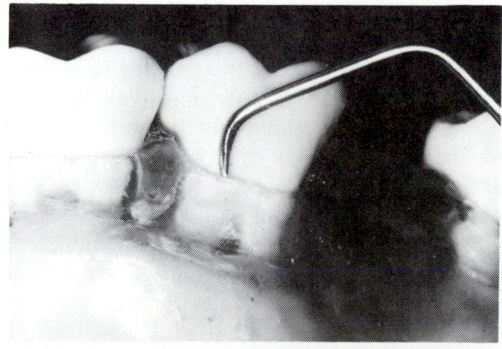

Fig. 26-33. Gracey ⅞ curette is being inserted in preparation for horizontal stroke. Note that toe will be along base of pocket and that terminal shank is not parallel to long axis of tooth.

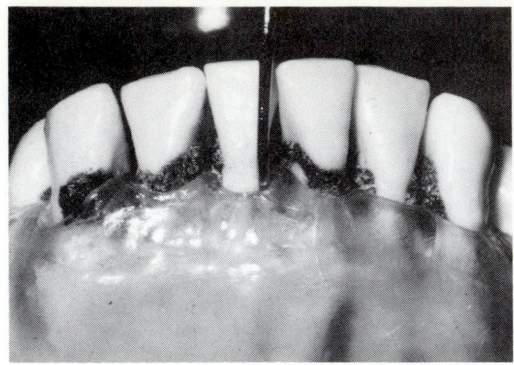

Fig. 26-34. Gracey ½ curette is being adapted to mesial surface of lower right incisor. Again, note that terminal shank is adapted parallel to long axis of tooth. Deviation from this orientation will result in working angulation that is too open or too closed.

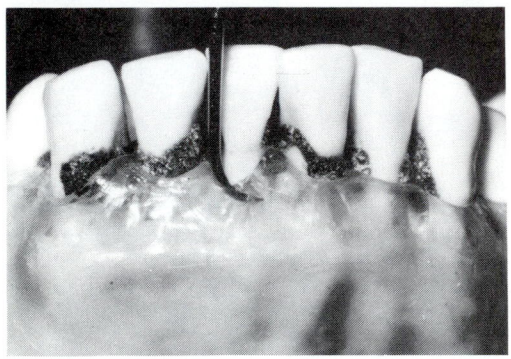

Fig. 26-35. Adaptation of curette blade along narrow labial surface of mandibular incisors is difficult and must be done with a great deal of tactile sensitivity to ensure that toe does not gouge into soft tissues.

ingival plaque can be removed by means other than use of hand cutting instruments (e.g. brushing, flossing, using of other oral hygiene aids, or engine polishing), subgingival debridement can only be accomplished by complete treatment of the entire root surface of the pocket with short, overlapping, continuous, and repeated strokes with the chosen instrument. The amount of time needed to accomplish subgingival debridement depends on the severity of the periodontal disease and other limiting factors, which will be discussed in a later section. However, 5 to 15 minutes *per tooth* is not an uncommon requirement for debridement using hand instruments.

Obviously, subgingival debridement is a much more exacting and definitive process than suprag-

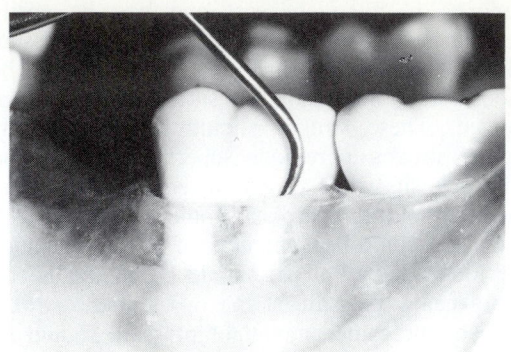

Fig. 26-36. A variety of approaches to debridement of buccal surface of mandibular left molar tooth, in which furcation opening poses additional work. One approach is to use Gracey ⅞ curette on all surfaces except distal surface of mesial root, where it will not adapt. Starting at distal line angle and using vertical and oblique strokes, Gracey ⅞ curette can be used easily in this buccal area.

ingival debridement and requires a great deal of precision. It cannot be mastered after a few experiences, and many clinicians will admit that it is the most difficult treatment procedure to perfect. Students will increase their appreciation of this fact as they perform some of the activities recommended at the end of this chapter. A variety of approaches to subgingival debridement with hand instruments is shown in Figs. 26-34 to 26-39.

Technique considerations

The significance of calculus deposits to subgingival debridement is still somewhat unclear (see Chapters 12 and 25). It is clear that residual calculus is practically inevitable after debridement, no matter how thorough one's technique, and that the presence of small amounts of residual calculus does not have an appreciable effect on healing. Although it is generally agreed that plaque-adherent calculus contributes to inflammation, it also appears that gingival health can be attained in the presence of calculus that does not harbor plaque bacteria. As reviewed earlier, several trials show that healing occurs following subgingival closed flap debridement and after open flap instrumentation when calculus removal is incomplete (veneered deposits and microscipic remnants). Measures of residual LPS levels following ultrasonic debridement that did not focus on calculus removal showed that LPS levels after treatment were significantly reduced in spite of the presence of readily detectable, submarginal, residual calcu-

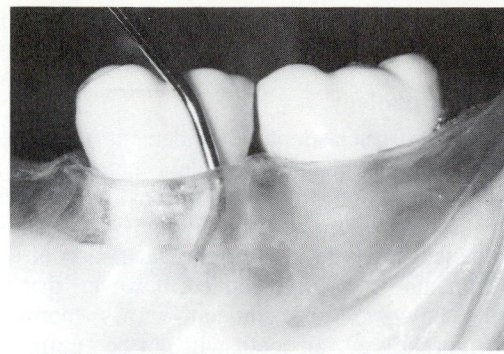

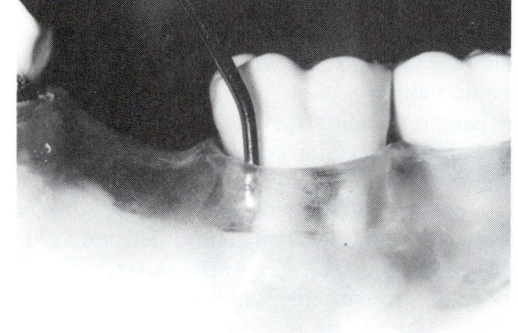

Fig. 26-37. **A,** Gracey ¹¹/₁₂ curette is adapted to mesial surface of distal root and into furcation area. This instrument can also be successfully adapted on buccal surfaces of tooth and root with success. As with Gracey 7/8 curette, this instrument will not adapt to distal surfaces of either root. **B,** Debridement is continued on mesial surface of tooth and mesial root. It is optimally designed to serve this surface. Note that terminal shank is always parallel to long axis of tooth when this instrument is correctly adapted.

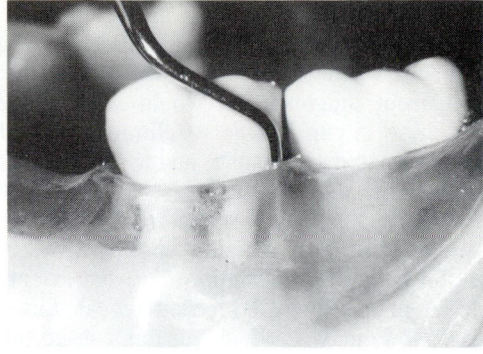

Fig. 26-38. Correct adaptation of Gracey ¹³/₁₄ curette. Again, terminal shank, which is somewhat buried submarginally, is oriented as parallel as possible to long axis of tooth to facilitate adaption and angulation.

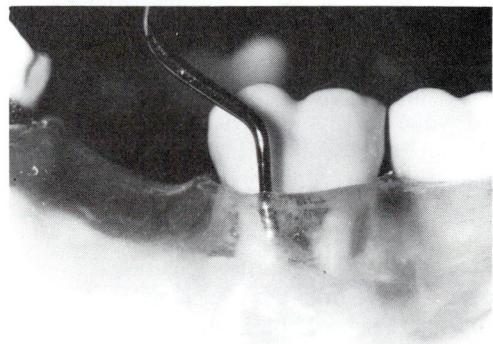

Fig. 26-39. Gracey ¹³/₁₄ curette allows adaptation of blade into furcation area so that distal surface of mesial root can be treated. This is the instrument of choice for this area on tooth.

lus deposits (Smart et al, 1990). Although ultrasonic rather than hand instruments were the mode of treatment in this study, the results suggest that bacterial plaque and associated toxic by products might be superficially located on calculus deposits, much the same as they appear to be located on cementum surfaces. The clinical implications of this are that the instrumentation technique should focus on thorough plaque debridement of the root surface with less concern for residual calculus deposits.

There are a number of reasons why calculus removal is important to the objectives of periodontal therapy:

1. Calculus harbors plaque and LPS, both of which must be removed to resolve inflammation.

2. Calculus removal, especially large ledges and nodules during debridement, also facilitates subgingival plaque control.
3. Calculus removal clears the surface of hard deposits that may prohibit the instrument from coming into close contact with subgingival plaque deposits.
4. Calculus removal facilitates future plaque removal efforts by creating a smoother surface.
5. Calculus removal permits closer adaptation of the soft tissues to the root surface during healing.
6. Calculus removal creates a more uniform root surface quality so that tactile information related to actual root morphology is more readily interpreted.

In many cases instrumentation for removal of adherent plaque requires little modification to accomplish the simultaneous removal of fine calculus and root roughness. It would seem prudent under these circumstances to eliminate calculus that is detectable, accessible, and removable without damage to the root surface.

There are a number of important unanswered questions critical to defining an effective technique for hand instrumentation: To what extent do bacterial plaque and LPS penetrate calculus deposits? How much residual calculus can be tolerated by healthy tissues? How important a role does calculus play in promoting plaque reaccumulation? How does the presence of calculus affect the potential for attachment gain or reattachment? What is the clinical significance to the patient of losing significant amounts of cementum in an effort to remove "all" the calculus from root surfaces? Without answers to these questions, the reasonable approach seems to favor attempting to remove all detectable calculus deposits encountered while attempting to debride the root surface of bacterial plaque. No intentional effort should be made, however, to remove cementum that may harbor residual calculus in irregularities in its surface. After calculus deposits that interfere with further root surface instrumentation have been fractured away from the cementum surface, additional strokes should be applied using a technique sufficient to accomplish plaque debridement as described above.

Periodontal debridement therapy is a central focus of the treatment provided by dental hygienists. Outdated philosophies and approaches to therapy need to be replaced with research-based alternatives. There is an immediate need for dental hygiene researchers and practitioners to design and implement clinical trials to test new approaches to debridement and report much needed answers to questions about debridement techniques. Information leading to design and refinement of optimum approaches to periodontal debridement using both hand and ultrasonic instruments must be openly discussed and distributed among hygienists to facilitate the delivery and implementation of these approaches to actual practice settings.

COMPLICATING FACTORS

A number of factors complicate the subgingival debridement process: limited access to the root surface, bleeding, sensitivity, and root texture. In many situations access to the affected area is difficult if not impossible.

Root morphology

Because most periodontal debridement occurs beneath the gingival margin, unless there has been gingival recession, the clinician must have a reliable mental picture of root morphology to assist tactile sensations in guiding the adaptation of the instruments. It should be added, however, that no matter how well the clinician knows "normal" root morphology, all teeth will not be "normal." Information about the patient's periodontal condition collected as part of the periodontal assessment (see Chapter 12), as well as interpretation of specific tooth morphology and deposits as seen on the patient's radiographs (see Chapter 10), will also facilitate decision making during the debridement process. This awareness of root morphology, coupled with a keenly developed tactile sense, will allow the clinician to detect and navigate the contours of root surfaces, including depressions, grooves, line angles, and furcation entrances. The curette blade and explorer must follow the irregular contour of root surfaces exactly, delivering both exploratory and working strokes that cover every square millimeter of the root surface. In addition, this task must be accomplished without traumatizing the inflamed soft tissues with which the instruments are in close contact.

It is often difficult to achieve effective adaptation of curettes to the proximal surfaces of teeth for complete subgingival debridement because of the presence of concavities that lie within 5 mm apical to the cementoenamel junction on most teeth (Fox and Bosworth, 1987). These concavities are likely to become exposed to the pocket environment after even minimal loss of periodontal tissues and may be too deep to be reached either by a curette or by flossing. As a result, deposits that form in root concavities may remain undetected. Clinicians must be aware of the presence of concavities on proximal surfaces so that instrumentation in those areas will be as thorough as possible (Fig. 26-40). In addition, patients must be taught to use alternative measures to control plaque on these surfaces (such as an interproximal brush, rubbertip stimulator, or Perio-aid), because flossing is more likely to bridge these areas than to clean them.

Exposed *furcation* entrances and the complex anatomy of root surfaces play a significant role in the pathogenesis of periodontal disease and pose a

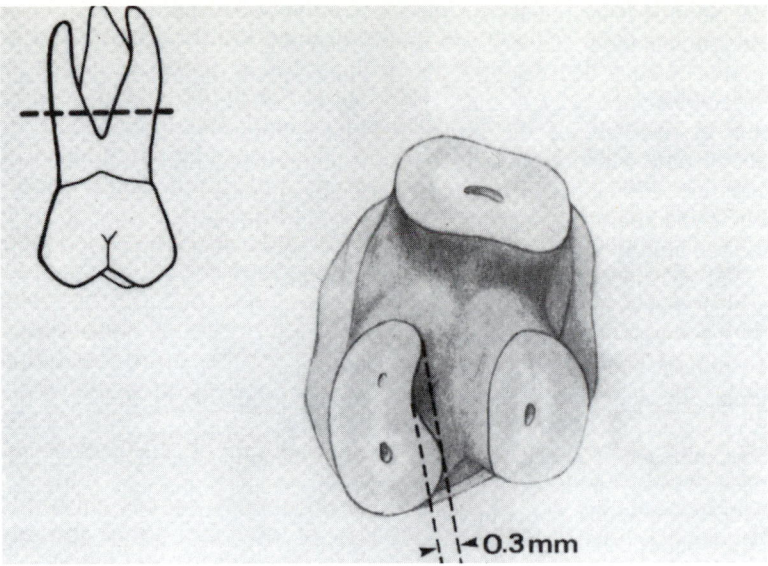

Fig. 26-40. Root morphology, including concavities and furrows, makes instrumentation difficult and requires careful instrument selection and adaptation.

significant challenge (Bower, 1979b; Gher and Vernino, 1980; Goldman et al, 1985; Ramfjord, 1987). Furcation involvements may be large enough to permit the accumulation of plaque and its endotoxins but too small and in too confined an area for access with a curette. Bower (1979a) compared the width of several commonly used curettes and determined that 58% of the furcation entrances studied had entrance widths smaller than the width of most curette blades. He concluded that it was unlikely that curettes would be able to clean the entrance area to furcations in a clinical situation. Access to furcations in maxillary molars and premolars is especially limited. Unlike the buccal and lingual furcations of mandibular teeth, these maxillary teeth have furcation openings on mesial and distal surfaces adjacent to other teeth. In addition, there may be trifurcation involvements rather than bifurcation involvements. Ultrasonic instruments using newly developed fine tips have demonstrated greater success in the treatment of furcations when compared with curettes. Their use is recommended for these areas whenever possible. Certainly, the clinician must be well aware of the root morphologies of these teeth to treat these difficult areas (Fig. 26-41).

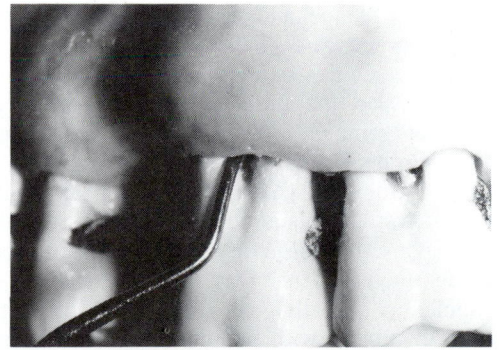

Fig. 26-41. With transparent gingiva removed, it can be seen that access to furcation areas is limited and that there is little room for maneuvering even with narrow blade of Gracey curette. In addition, this area is not normally visible during instrumentation. It is easy to see why these areas complicate subgingival debridement procedures.

Pocket morphology

Another critical area for instrumentation during subgingival debridement is the *apical extent of the pocket.* Waerhaug (1978a) studied the effect of subgingival plaque removal on this area and reported that the proximity of the plaque front to the epithelial junction could be as close as 0.5 mm. Because this plaque results in destruction of the gingival fiber apparatus, it is crucial that it be removed during instrumentation. To ensure the removal of subgingival plaque and calculus, the curette must be inserted all the way to the dentoepithelial junction at the base of the pocket. Since most pockets become narrower at their apical extent, the pressure of the sulcular tissues against the instrument blade as it is inserted may make the clinician prematurely think that the base has been reached. Not only must the curette reach the base of the pocket, but compression of these tissues may also be necessary to locate the cutting edge near the pocket base and below the plaque and calculus that has formed there (Waerhaug, 1978b). This does not mean, however, that instrumentation should be pursued at the base of the pocket without consideration for the soft tissues. Excessive damage to the gingival fibers underlying the junctional epithelium and damage to the deeper periodontal ligament could result in the formation of an even deeper pocket after healing. You must walk the fine line between damaging underlying soft tissues and allowing calculus and plaque deposits to remain subgingivally. The goal is to remove the plaque and calculus with as little soft tissue damage as possible.

Effective plaque and calculus removal at the base of pockets is a challenge, and deposits are often missed in this part of the pocket. Waerhaug (1978b) issued the ultimate challenge when he stated that "removal of 99% of subgingival plaque is likely to be just as bad as no plaque control at all in the long run." Although the clinical significance of residual plaque deposits depends on the host response to the quality and quantity of those deposits, their presence may increase the speed of repopulation of pathogenic bacteria in that site. Again, disruption with fine ultrasonic instruments may be more efficient and less damaging.

An almost certain result of debridement with hand instruments will be some *coincidental curettage*. This is the unintentional removal of soft tissue from the pocket wall adjacent to the treated root surface. It is impossible for the opposite cutting edge of the curette to avoid contact with the pocket wall (see Fig. 26-17, *D*).

Another access problem is posed by the *proximity of roots*, as in the lower anterior areas, making instrumentation in these confined areas difficult. Additional access problems may be experienced in distal pockets of posterior teeth where there is not much room for manipulation of an instrument to gain leverage for working strokes.

Control of bleeding

Bleeding is another complicating factor during subgingival debridement. Bleeding can be expected whenever instrumentation is done in an inflamed area. It serves a useful purpose during subgingival debridement by clearing loosened calculus, plaque, and other debris from the pocket, thereby promoting healing. The disadvantage of bleeding is that it hampers visibility and fulcrum stability. For optimum working conditions the area should be kept as free of blood as possible. This can be accomplished easily with water irrigation and suctioning devices. Slight bleeding can be controlled by blotting and light pressure to the wound site with a sterile gauze sponge. More profuse bleeding can be controlled through the use of frequent irrigation and suctioning during the procedure. A stream of water from the water syringe may be directed at the area, followed by suction evacuation of the fluids. Do not use a forced spray of water and air combined to rinse the area because it increases the production of blood-contaminated aerosols, which then are propelled at the operating team, possibly causing infection from cross-contamination (see discussion of aerosols in Chapter 3). For patients who need anesthesia, the vasoconstrictor in the anesthetic solution will provide some hemostasis or control of bleeding to the area where it is injected. Control of bleeding will make the patient more comfortable and increase tolerance of the procedure. Patients may not realize that bleeding is a normal response to instrumentation in inflamed areas, and they should be assured in advance that it is expected.

Patient sensitivity

Patient sensitivity often accompanies periodontal debridement. This sensitivity may arise from the inflamed soft tissues or from the root surface. Because patient cooperation and comfort are important, this sensitivity should be controlled. Optimum instrumentation skills will minimize the pain and trauma for the patient but often are not sufficient to eliminate it. Nitrous oxide and oxygen conscious sedation and/or a local anesthetic should be available. Tolerance of pain varies greatly among patients; while some may tolerate the procedure well without anesthesia, others may need anesthesia for all aspects of treatment. The use of any type of anesthesia must not be a cover-up for poor instrumentation technique; all treatment should be performed with concern and respect for the soft tissues whether or not anesthesia is used. Damage caused by inappropriate instrumentation will not only hinder wound healing and repair of the gingiva but also discourage patient trust and confidence in the clinician.

As a result of removal of cementum or dentin on the root surface during subgingival debridement, the patient may experience increased root sensitivity to stimuli such as hot or cold temperatures. The patient should be informed of this possible complication and why it may occur. In many cases this is only a temporary discomfort for the patient and can be controlled with the aid of proper desensitization procedures performed in the office and at home (see Chapter 31).

EVALUATION AFTER HEALING

Indicators of the success of therapy are first apparent 10 to 14 days after treatment and again at regular intervals (see Chapter 35). These evaluations determine whether debridement was successful in creating a biologically acceptable area.

Regardless of how clean the area looks, how smooth it feels, and how it sounds when instrumented, the tissues may not react favorably. They may continue to bleed or lose periodontal attachment. A radiographic survey may show continued bone loss. Once the initial treatment is complete, it is your responsibility to evaluate healing and to monitor the patient at regular intervals.

Assessment of the patient's healing response is based on the clinical criteria described in the section on periodontal assessment in Chapter 12. The biologic markers are more important at this point, because they may show that there is continuing destruction deep in the periodontal tissues that may not yet be detectable with a periodontal probe or radiographs.

POSTTREATMENT EVALUATION

If the clinical signs and biologic markers show that the patient is healed and well, the patient should be scheduled for a reevaluation in 2 to 3 months. At that appointment, repeat the full array of assessment procedures and use an ultrasonic or fine hand instruments to disrupt (deplaque) the subgingival areas.

If the markers show continued disease, there are several options:
1. Sample the sites for microbiologic evaluation.
   a. Determine the composition of the flora.
   b. Test for resistance to antibiotics.
   c. Prescribe antibiotics if necessary (prescription written by a dentist.)
   d. Place slow-release antibiotics at sites showing continued destruction.
2. Repeat debridement in areas of poor healing.
3. Refer patient for surgery (in consultation with dentist).
4. Use nonsteroidal anti-inflammatory agents (e.g., ibuprofen, flurbiprofen).

Frequently healing will be good at the posttreatment evaluation, but evidence of disease recurrence may appear at subsequent evaluations. The options outlined above apply in these instances also (see Chapter 35).

Barriers to healing

A *periodontal abscess* can occur when foreign substances, such as calculus or food particles, occlude the pocket opening, preventing drainage of inflammatory exudate. It is not unusual for a periodontal abscess to occur after gross debridement of deep periodontal pockets. After the initial debridement, the superficial tissues heal and the pocket orifice tightens and shrinks so that it becomes more adapted to the tooth. The presence of significant amounts of plaque-embedded calculus or heavy plaque deep in these pockets can contribute to the septic environment that abscesses. A similar result might occur if the patient initiates sudden and vigorous toothbrushing in an area of periodontitis and subgingival calculus. Clinicians should be aware that incomplete debridement, either by intent (e.g., "gross scale") or by omission (e.g., failure to detect and remove calculus), can have this result. Periodontal abscesses are treated by removing the irritant, followed by draining the exudate through a surgical incision or excision of the pocket wall (Kieser, 1990).

Entrapment of calculus, bacteria, and debris in the pocket and adjacent soft tissues following their removal from the root surface will also hinder healing after subgingival debridement with hand instruments. Although bleeding and the curette may bring out much of the debris, the pocket should still be thoroughly irrigated with a stream of water or an antimicrobial irrigant to cleanse the area further (Moskow, 1962). Because water with high bacterial counts could contaminate wound areas, the water supply to the dental unit should be tested. To minimize the risk of infection, all surgical wounds should be irrigated with a sterile normal saline solution or an antimicrobial agent rather than tap water. Southard et al. (1989) suggested that irrigation with chlorhexidine immediately after subgingival debridement and weekly for 4 weeks can significantly reduce pathogens and enhance healing (see Chapter 28 on subgingival irrigation). Oxygenating rinses may also help cleanse and debride these areas.

Healing is further enhanced by the application of gentle compression and readaptation of the tissues to the teeth. This procedure will assist in stopping the bleeding and in forming a thin blood clot against the tissues. Healing is enhanced by the formation of a thin rather than a thick blood clot. Performing these procedures immediately after completion of subgingival debridement will help accelerate tissue healing and achieve an optimum tissue response.

EVALUATION DURING TREATMENT

Evaluation is ongoing during instrumentation. As you use your hand instruments, you continuously attend to visual, tactile, and audio cues that suggest when a site is completed.

Visual indicators

Visual clues are most helpful when evaluating supragingival surfaces. By observing the color and texture of exposed root surfaces, you can identify the presence of residual calculus deposits, extrinsic stain, and other organic material. Drying the tooth surface with a stream of compressed air helps identify white flecks of mineralized deposits. Subgingival deposits that lie close to the gingival margin may also be visualized by deflecting the gingival margin away from the tooth with compressed air. Transillumination of the tooth surface (i.e. directing a bright beam of light through the tooth) may also help detect calculus deposits that appear as shadowed areas. Fiberoptic light sources are especially useful for this purpose. You can disclose the exposed portions and identify those areas that still attract the disclosant because of surface deposits or root irregularities. Organic material and instrumentation debris may also retain the stain immediately after instrumentation, so that not all visibly stained surfaces may represent potential microbial threats to the periodontal tissues (Breininger, 1987).

Audio indicators

The use of audio cues in evaluation is outdated. It has only limited usefulness when applied to newer approaches to debridement that do not stress root smoothness as a criterion for treatment success. Current approaches to debridement no longer regard a "squeaky clean" root surface to be the same as a biologically acceptable one and discourage the excessive removal of cementum associated with a "squeaky" surface. Audio cues are mentioned here only because they provide some additional sensory information that may support other more valid means of evaluation. In general deposits on the root surface produce a scratchy, coarse sound when a sharp curette blade is applied during a working stroke. As the root is debrided of plaque and calculus, the sound of the curette blade against the root begins to diminish or take on a higher pitch. By listening to the sound produced by the curette, you may receive some clues as to the changing nature of the pocket during instrumentation.

Tactile indicators

The most frequently used indicator for evaluating subgingival debridement is tactile. An acute sensitivity to vibrations transmitted through the instruments to the fingers helps identify surface changes as they occur. The tactile sense also guides you carefully around the root morphology during all working and exploring strokes to ensure optimum adaptation and angulation of the instrument against the root surface. It takes a great deal of time and experience to distinguish between the rough, bumpy, irregular, somewhat sticky feel of the diseased root surface embedded with calculus and plaque and a thoroughly treated root surface.

You can develop an acute tactile sense by learning to concentrate on the quality of sensations received through the fingertips and to accurately interpret what they represent. Reception of tactile vibrations is easiest when a light grasp is maintained on the instrument for all exploration of the root surface. Another aid in developing and maximizing the tactile sense is the use of fine (i.e, delicate) instruments; these include explorers with small-diameter working ends, as described in Chapter 9, and curettes with fine blades and thin, light shanks, such as the Gracey finishing curettes. Many clinicians also find that instruments with hollow handles transmit more vibrations than those with solid handles. The fingers can detect more subtle vibrations with a sharp curette than with a dull one. The procedure can be performed much more quickly and easily if the instruments are kept optimally sharp.

Exploring exercises on extracted teeth will help you develop and improve detection skills. One such exercise, described at the end of Chapter 12, is to explore an extracted tooth with the eyes closed, concentrating on the different textures and curves of the root surface. Comparisons also can be made using different instruments and a variety of root surfaces irregularities. After the surface is explored and a mental image of its appearance is formed, look at the tooth and evaluate the accuracy of the impression. Continue to test your tactile sense while working with patients by comparing the feel of different root morphologies, deposits, and restorations and analyzing what makes them feel different from each other. With practice a fine, discriminatory tactile sense will develop.

Clinicians frequently evaluate the effectiveness of subgingival debridement on the basis of tactile information, because this is often the only source of information available during the procedure. In the past a "finished" root surface was described as velvety smooth, glasslike, or hard to an explorer, as these clinical characteristics seemed to accompany the removal of calculus and diseased cementum. The concepts of smoothness and hardness, however, are no longer viewed as valid, reliable indicators that a root surface is biologically acceptable. Both qualities can be measured only subjectively, because they are evaluated according to the tactile skills, clinical experience, and interpretation of each clinician. (These same limitations call into question the validity of the audio cues.)

Differences among the hardness levels of healthy cementum, periodontally involved cementum, and dentin have been found to be insignificant when measured on extracted teeth (Rautiola and Craig, 1961). Under these conditions, it is highly unlikely that one can accurately assess the clinical nature of the root surface material being removed during hand instrumentation on the basis of how "hard" the surface feels to an explorer or curette. Also, it has been clearly demonstrated that root surfaces that feel smooth to an explorer still harbor calculus deposits that can be detected visually. The remaining deposits may be either burnished or simply too small to be detected through the tactile sense.

If a surface that feels smooth can still harbor calculus, then it certainly can harbor plaque and its byproducts. Clinical smoothness of a root surface is not a reliable means of preventing plaque accumulation or gingival inflammation, nor can it or any other clinical cue be relied on as a final test of the effectiveness of the subgingival debridement procedure. It cannot provide any assurance that the root surface is free of plaque or LPS, or that the root is biologically acceptable to the soft tissues. In fact, some research indicates that a rough root surface that is biologically clean may be preferred as a means of gaining clinical attachment (see Chapter 25).

Although clinical indicators or cues provide helpful feedback on the progress of subgingival debridement, the only valid and reliable measure of the success of subgingival debridement is the response of the soft tissues to the treatment when supported by effective mechanical and chemical supragingival plaque control by the patient. Emerging tests of pocket microflora and host enzymes add to our ability to determine response to therapy and to establish a treatment end point.

CONCLUSION

The fields of subgingival debridement with ultrasonic and hand instruments are currently undergoing significant analysis. Research findings have led to a revision of how we perform these procedures in daily practice. While the belief in the importance of achieving a biologically clean surface as the focus of treatment still remains, the issues of *how* that should be achieved and how to determine *when* the task is complete are continually evaluated and evolving.

ACTIVITIES

1. Compare the contraangled sickle scaler and the universal curette with the cowhorn or pigtail explorer. Identify which ends match in terms of the direction of the shanks. Given either end of the contraangled sickle scaler or universal curette, identify all areas in the dentition where that end may be used so that the point aims across the intended proximal surface, the terminal shank is parallel to the long axis of the tooth, and the handle exits the mouth from the front.
2. Use the suggested sequence of positions to adapt the contraangled sickle scaler, straight sickle scaler, and universal curette in each sextant of the dentition. Be certain to do the following:
   a. Use a modified pen grasp.
   b. Establish a stable finger rest.
   c. Use all fingers as a unit to generate a hand and wrist motion while pivoting on the fulcrum finger.

d. Adapt the side of the tip to the tooth to avoid piercing the tissue with the point or toe of the instrument.

e. Angulate the face of the instrument at greater than 45 degrees and less than 90 degrees to the tooth.

f. Execute an exploratory stroke around the tooth with the scaler or curette, using horizontal pressure against the tooth when engaging a deposit (working stroke).

g. Use the *opposite end* of the universal curette on distal surfaces and analyze its usefulness.

3. Adapt the hoe, chisel, and file on a typodont and on calculus-laden teeth set in plaster. Explore apically with the hoe and file to detect calculus and engage horizontal pressure apically to remove it. Use a push stroke from labial to lingual surfaces to loosen a bridge of calculus by engaging the blade of the chisel on the proximal surfaces.

4. Scale a quadrant for a more advanced student's patient. Ask the advanced student to watch the procedure and offer suggestions. Observe as the student uses air, light, explorer, probe, and/or disclosant to evaluate for residual calculus.

5. Role-play ways of responding to hypothetical patients, employers, and peers who describe the dental hygienist as a person who cleans teeth.

6. Develop a role definition of dental hygiene that adequately describes the class's perception of how the oral prophylaxis fits into the scope of practice.

7. Compare the effects of a dull blade and a sharp blade for calculus removal from plaster-mounted, calculus-laden teeth.

8. Compare the shank sizes and shapes and the sizes of the working ends for the following instruments:
   a. Sickle scalers
   b. Universal curettes
   c. Gracey curettes
   d. Hoes
   e. Files

9. Given descriptions of clinical conditions, such as amounts and locations of calculus, sulcus or pocket depth, and gingival tissue conditions, practice selecting appropriate hand instruments for removing the deposits.

10. Review the radiographs that show supragingival and subgingival calculus. Select scalers and/or curettes that would most efficiently remove the deposits.

11. Practice debridement on extracted, sterilized, molar teeth. Simulate deposits on the root surface by coating an area of the root to represent pocket morphology using nail polish, a colored wax crayon or magic marker. Establish a finger rest and begin implementing working strokes over the surface. Note how much of the coating material is removed with each stroke, the extent to which overlapping must occur to "clean" the root surface, the number of strokes required per surface area, and the effect of cross-hatching stroke patterns.

12. Using extracted, sterilized teeth or photos of root morphology from dental anatomy textbooks, summarize the characteristic root morphology found on each permanent tooth. Discuss approaches to adaptation of hand instruments to root surface concavities and furcations. Discuss which teeth would be the hardest to treat because of their root morphology. Note the variability of morphology among examples of the same tooth type.

13. If the facilities and personnel are available, perform subgingival debridement for a patient who will be undergoing periodontal surgery. Observe the surgery to see the effectiveness of your technique when the tissues are lifted away from the tooth.

14. Examine and compare Gracey curettes and their new variations (longer terminal shank, less flex, thinner blade) for ease of use.

15. Analyze the designs of a number of unfamiliar instruments for clues as to how, where, and for what purpose they might be used most effectively.

16. Treat several patients with a split-mouth approach, using hand instruments on one side of the mouth and an ultrasonic instrument on the other side. Evaluate the two approaches for operator and patient perceptions of advantages and disadvantages. Compare the effectiveness of both approaches for deposit removal and healing response.

17. Review the literature on carpal tunnel syndrome and discuss the potential relationship of this problem to hand instrumentation techniques and difficulty level of debridement. How might you prevent this problem and other related occupational injuries to the hands?

REVIEW QUESTIONS

1. Using hand instruments for debridement relies on two major principles not required for exploring and probing. What are they?

2. Are the following statements true or false? (Correct the false statements.)
   a. A chisel is used with a pull stroke.
   b. A chisel is useful for removing ledge calculus that is readily accessible to a heavy instrument.
   c. The file is used to crush calculus.
   d. The universal curette is used primarily for removing deep calculus in periodontal pockets.
   e. The sickle scaler is the most versatile instrument, as it is effective for deep scaling as well as supragingival scaling.
   f. Metal hand instruments should never be used for treatment of titanium metal implant abutments.

3. Which of the following characteristics would you look for in an instrument designed for removal of heavy, submarginal calculus on proximal surfaces of molar teeth? (Identify all that are appropriate.)

a. A relatively straight, linear shank
b. A shank with two or more angles
c. A short blade length
d. A relatively long blade length
e. A light, flexible shank
f. A heavy, rigid shank
g. A relatively short terminal shank
h. A relatively long terminal shank
4. Compare supragingival and subgingival debridement and deplaquing using hand instruments in terms of decision making related to each of the following factors:
a. Instrument selection
b. Number of strokes
c. Direction of strokes
d. Pressure of strokes
5. Compare the following features of the Gracey curettes to universal curettes:
a. Blade size
b. Cutting edges
c. Shank design
6. Write a brief response to each of the following statements, indicating whether or not you agree and your rationale. (There are many ways to respond. Your answers can be judged on the strength and appropriateness of the rationale used to support them. Use these statements as a stimulus for group discussion.
a. When using hand instruments, one should always establish a firm, intraoral finger rest or fulcrum as close to the working area as possible.
b. If a work environment has a modern ultrasonic or sonic instrument with a variety of instrument tips designed for access to all areas of the mouth and all types of pocket configurations, there would be no need for hand instruments for periodontal debridement.
c. If residual calculus remains after periodontal debridement procedures, it doesn't really matter whether or not we remove it during the debridement process.
d. A clear understanding of normal root anatomy is as important as developing good exploration and tactile sensory skills when using hand instruments for periodontal debridement procedures.
e. The use of visual, tactile, and audio cues is sufficient to determine that periodontal debridement is completed.

REFERENCES

Bower RC: Furcation morphology relative to periodontal treatment: furcation entrance architecture, *J Periodontol* 50:23, 1979.

Bower RC: Furcation morphology relative to periodontal treatment: furcation root surface anatomy, *J Periodontol* 50:366, 1979.

Breininger DR et al: Comparative effectiveness of ultrasonic and hand scaling for the removal of subgingival plaque and calculus, *J Periodontol* 58:9, 1987.

Cheetham WA et al: Root surface debridement-an in vitro assessment, *J Clin Periodontol* 15:288, 1988.

Fox SC, Bosworth BL: A morphological survey of proximal root concavities: a consideration in periodontal therapy, *J Periodontol* 57:811, 1987.

Fox SC et al: The effects of scaling a titanium implant surface with metal and plastic instruments: an in vitro study, *J Periodontol* 61:485, 1990.

Gher ME, Vernino AR: Root morphology—clinical significance in pathogenesis and treatment of periodontal disease, *JADA* 101:627, 1980.

Goldman MJ et al: Effect of periodontal therapy on patient maintained for 15 years or longer: a retrospective study, *J Periodontol* 57:347, 1985.

Hoople S: Files provide desirable results in patient treatment procedures, *RDH* 5(10):22, 1985.

Kerry GJ: Roughness of root surfaces after use of ultrasonic instruments and hand curettes, *J Periodontol* 38:340, 1967.

Kieser, JB: *Periodontics: a practical approach,* London, 1990, Wright.

Moskow BS: The response of the gingival sulcus to instrumentation: a histological investigation. I. The scaling procedure, *J Periodontol* 33:282, 1962.

Ramjord SP: Surgical periodontal pocket elimination: still a justifiable objective? *JADA* 114:37, 1987.

Rautiola CA, Craig RG: The microhardness of cementum and underlying dentin of normal teeth and teeth exposed to periodontal disease, *J Periodontol* 32:113, 1961.

Seibert J: Incorporating root planing and gingival curettage into a clinical practice, *Contin Dent Educ* 1:8, 1978.

Smart GJ et al: The assessment of ultrasonic root surface debridement by determination of residual endotoxin levels, *J Clin Periodontol* 17:174, 1990.

Southard S et al: The effect of 2% chlorhexidine digluconate irrigation on clinical parameters and the level of *Bacteroides gingivalis* in periodontal pockets, *J Periodontol* 60:302, 1989.

Tal H et al: Scanning electron microscope evaluation of wear of dental curettes during standardized root planing, *J Periodontol* 56:532, 1985.

Waerhaug J: Healing of the dento-epithelial junction following subgingival plaque control. I. As observed in human biopsy material, *J Periodontol* 49:1, 1978.

Waerhaug J: Healing of the dento-epithelial junction following subgingival plaque control. II. As observed on extracted teeth, *J Periodontol* 49:119, 1978.

Wilkinson RF, Maybury JE: Scanning electron microscopy of the root surface following instrumentation, *J Periodontol* 42:559, 1973.

SUGGESTED READINGS

Abrams H et al: Root anatomy: its effect on periodontal prognosis and treatment. In Clark JW: *Clark's Clin Dent* 3(11):1, 1990.

Nield JF: *Fundamentals of dental hygiene instrumentation,* ed 2, Philadelphia, 1988, Lea & Febiger.

Pattison AM: *Periodontal instrumentation,* ed 2, Norwalk, Conn, 1992, Appleton & Lange.

Perry, DA: *Techniques and theory of periodontal instrumentation,* Philadelphia, 1990, WB Saunders.

27 INSTRUMENT SHARPENING

Laura Mueller Joseph
Nancy Stutsman Young

LEARNING OUTCOMES

The dental hygienist will be able to

1. State the advantages of using sharp periodontal instruments.
2. Determine instrument sharpness, by evaluating three criteria.
   a. Light reflection
   b. Cutting edge under magnification
   c. Ability to "bite" into a testing stick
3. Maintain the design features of universal curettes, Gracey curettes, and sickle scalers during the sharpening procedure.
4. Describe four different techniques for sharpening instruments.
5. State the rationale for sharpening the lateral surfaces of curettes and sickle scalers.
6. Determine the appropriate care of an Arkansas sharpening stone.
7. Describe two techniques for sharpening curettes and sickle scalers using a hand-held sharpening stone.
8. Integrate instrument sharpening into daily clinical practice

A clinician's success in all instrumentation procedures is directly related to the quality of the instruments used. Effective scaling and debridement depend on the use of sharp instruments for their success. There are a number of advantages to using sharp instruments. First, a sharp cutting edge is more effective in removing calculus from tooth surfaces. Dull instruments are more likely to smooth over or burnish calculus deposits than remove them cleanly from the tooth surface. A sharp cutting edge can shear off deposits and plane root surfaces with less effort and fewer strokes. Sharp cutting edges will also deliver more sensitive tactile feedback to the clinician during scaling and root planing when exploratory strokes are used to gain information.

Instruments must be sharp at the beginning of the appointment and should be resharpened frequently during instrumentation. Tal and others (1985) found that cutting edges of curettes had been slightly beveled (dulled) after only 15 strokes on root surfaces of extracted teeth. Wider bevels were seen after 45 strokes. Depending on the condition of the root surfaces, the number of strokes taken before dullness results will vary.

Dental hygienists who work with properly sharpened instruments are more effective and more efficient. When instruments are sharp, fewer strokes are needed to remove calculus deposits from the tooth. A sharp cutting edge allows more effective exploration which saves time by eliminating the need to switch back and forth constantly between an explorer and the scaling instrument. Both patient and clinician will benefit from the time saved during the appointment. An additional benefit to the professional is that instruments that are resharpened frequently require less recontouring than those which are allowed to get extremely dull. Only a small amount of metal must be removed from well-maintained instruments, so less time is required to sharpen them and they tend to last longer.

The use of a sharp instrument can make scaling procedures more pleasant for both the clinician and patient. Less effort is needed for a scaling stroke when sharp instruments are used. The patient will appreciate a light and gentle approach. When dull instruments are used, working strokes must be repeated again and again in the same area until the deposits are finally removed. This repetition can be tiring for the hygienist and unpleasant for the patient. It is easy to understand that the short time it takes to sharpen instruments effectively is justified by the benefits that are gained.

IDENTIFICATION OF SHARP VERSUS DULL INSTRUMENTS

The first step in learning how to sharpen instruments is developing the ability to determine whether or not an instrument is optimally sharp. There are a number of ways to evaluate instrument sharpness. Experienced clinicians can determine when their instruments are getting dull by the increased effort needed to remove calculus deposits. A beginning clinician, however, has not had the opportunity to develop a sense for what a sharp instrument can be expected to accomplish. Several other ways to detect a dull instrument are available that may be easier for the beginning clinician to use.

One of the best ways to test instrument sharpness is by applying the cutting edge to be tested against an acrylic or plastic rod. Special acrylic testing sticks have been designed for this purpose and are available from instrument manufacturers (Fig. 27-1). Place the instrument's cutting edge against the surface of the testing stick at the same angle that would be used to implement a working stroke against the tooth surface. If the edge is sharp, it will "bite" into the plastic surface when light pressure is applied. If the instrument tends to drag, slide, or grate across the surface, it is not sharp. Evaluate the entire length of the cutting edge for dullness. If a commercial testing stick is not available, a plastic disposable cotton-tipped applicator or a disposable evacuation tip can serve the same purpose. Commercial testing sticks are made of materials that can be sterilized and included on each tray setup so that instruments can be tested during treatment procedures.

Another way to detect a dull cutting edge is to examine it under a microscope or a magnifying lens. Hold the instrument so that the cutting edge faces a strong light source. A dull surface reflects light, so that a white area or a bright light line will be visible where the cutting edge should be (Fig. 27-2, *B*). If the cutting edge is truly sharp, there should not be a flat surface (bevel) at the junction of the facial and lateral surfaces. When the instrument is correctly sharpened only a thin, dark line will be visible where these two surfaces meet (Fig. 27-2, *A*). This evaluation method is only useful when a specific time has been set

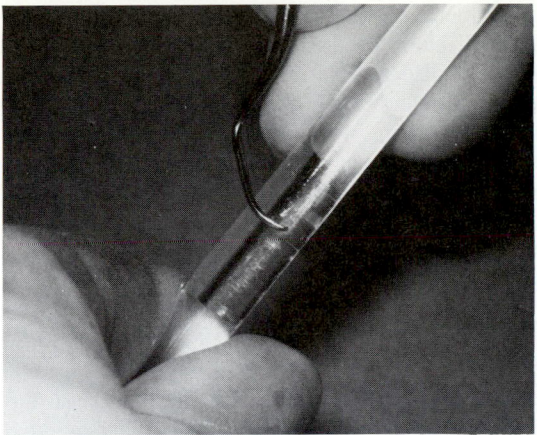

Fig. 27-1. Acrylic testing stick is used by applying light pressure against stick with the instrument at its working angle.

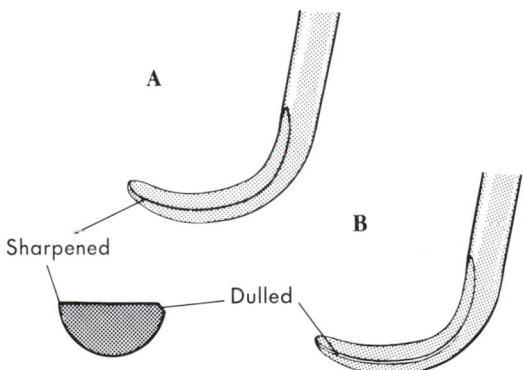

Fig. 27-2. A, A sharp cutting edge will not reflect light. **B**, A dull cutting edge will appear as a bright area at junction of face and lateral surface.

aside to sharpen instruments and a special work area with a good light source and a microscope or magnifying lens is available.

It should be noted that the reliability and validity of the light reflection method has been questioned. Sassie (1987) found that cutting edges that appeared dull using this method were judged to be clinically sharp when examined under much higher magnification using a scanning electron microscope. Therefore instruments might appear to be dull when they are still clinically acceptable.

One method that should *never* be used to test

instrument sharpness is to apply the edge to a fingernail. Not only does this damage the fingernail, but it is also a violation of aseptic technique. Instrument sharpening is often performed at the chairside during a patient appointment. If the clinician were to use this method to test the sharpness of scaling instruments, the instruments would be contaminated and no longer acceptable for patient treatment.

APPLICATION OF INSTRUMENT DESIGN TO SHARPENING TECHNIQUES

Each type of periodontal instrument has specific design characteristics that must be preserved during sharpening. The clinician must understand exactly how these design principles affect the use of each type of instrument so that sharpening techniques are employed that preserve original instrument contours. The two types of instruments used most frequently for scaling and root planing procedures are the sickle scaler and the curette. Design characteristics of both of these instrument types will be discussed.

Sickle scalers

Design features of sickle scalers are shown in Figs. 27-3 and 27-4. There are actually two different blade designs for sickle scalers: straight and curved blades. The straight blade design is shown in Fig. 27-3. The side view shows that the two cutting edges of this sickle form a gentle arc that converges in a sharp tip. Both cutting edges are used so both must be sharpened. The pointed tip of the sickle scaler provides access beneath tight contact areas. A significant design feature of the straight sickle blade is the squared-off back of the blade, which can be seen in the cross-sectional view of Fig. 27-3.

Fig. 27-4 shows the design characteristics of a curved sickle blade. The facial surface of the instrument forms a slight curve as it extends from the shank of the instrument to the pointed tip. The lateral surfaces of this sickle are flat and converge at the pointed back. Differences in the back design can be seen by comparing the cross-sectional views of these two sickle scalers.

For both of these instruments the lateral surfaces and the facial surface form an internal angle of approximately 70 to 80 degrees. When properly applied, the sharpening stone will form a complementary angle of 100 to 110 degrees with the base of the sickle blade.

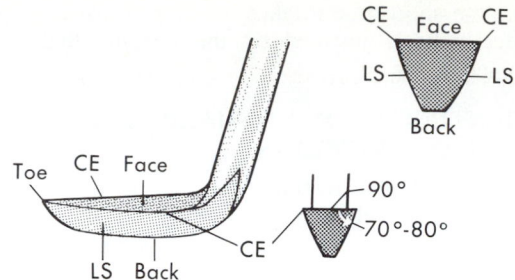

Fig. 27-3. Straight sickle. Face is basically flat; back surface is also flat.

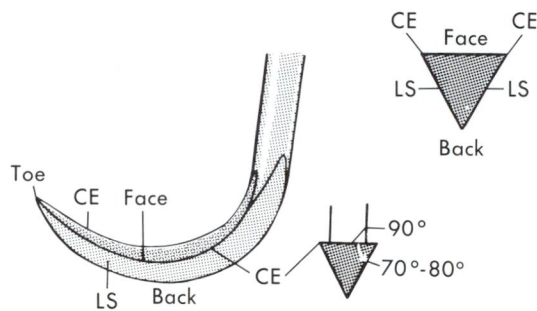

Fig. 27-4. Curved sickle. Note pointed back.

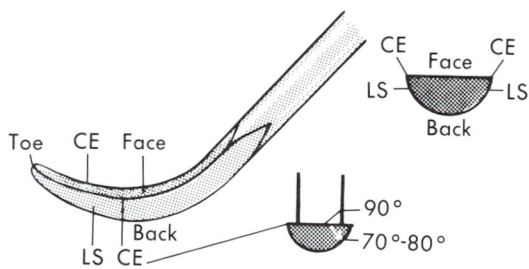

Fig. 27-5. Universal curette. Note that the two cutting edges are parallel. Round back and toe are important design features.

Curettes

Design characteristics of the universal curette are shown in Fig. 27-5. The side view of the universal curette blade shows two parallel cutting edges, both of which are used during scaling and root planing. The two cutting edges converge in a rounded toe. It is important to maintain a rounded toe during the sharpening procedure because this is one of the design features that allows this instrument to be used safely in subgingival areas. Failure to maintain this design could result in trauma to the soft tissues when the curette is inserted below the gingival margin.

Another important characteristic of the curette is that the lateral surfaces are curved, rather than flat, and form a rounded back surface. A cross-sectional view of the universal curette looks like a half circle. This design feature allows the instrument to navigate in tight pockets without damaging the adjacent soft tissues. The rounded back must be preserved during sharpening. The cross-sectional view of the universal curette shows that the facial surface of the blade forms a 90-degree angle with the shank of the instrument. The internal angle of the curette blade is the same as that of the sickle scaler—70 to 80 degrees.

The design features of the Gracey curette (see Fig. 26-27) are the same as those of the universal curette with two notable exceptions. The blade is slightly offset at an angle of about 60 to 70 degrees from the shank of the instrument so that the two cutting edges are not parallel to each other. Instead, one of the cutting edges appears to be lower than the other when the instrument is held so that the last bend in the shank (terminal shank) is perpendicular to the floor, as pictured in Fig. 26-27. Only this "lower" cutting edge is used during periodontal procedures so only one of the cutting edges should be sharpened on a Gracey curette blade. Other design characteristics described earlier for the universal curette (e.g., rounded back, rounded toe, internal angle of 70 to 80 degrees) are also present on a Gracey curette blade.

SHARPENING TECHNIQUES

Techniques for sharpening periodontal instruments vary according to the type of sharpening device used. The most common technique employs hand-held sharpening stones. In other techniques smaller cylindrical or conical stones are mounted on slow-speed handpieces, or flat or rounded stones are mounted on stationary sharpening (or honing) machines. Sharpening may also be accomplished using a rotating abrasive felt wheel (DeNucci and Mader, 1983). Each method has certain advantages and disadvantages.

Instrument sharpening using a hand-held sharpening stone has the advantage that it can be performed anywhere in the dental office where there is adequate light and a good working surface. The use of a hand-held stone also allows the clinician to control the exact speed and pressure with which the instrument is being sharpened so that there is no unnecessary loss of instrument surface as a result of over-sharpening. This technique is recommended for routine sharpening of instruments.

There are two ways in which a hand-held stone can be used for sharpening. One method is to hold the instrument stationary while moving the stone against it; the second method is to stabilize the stone and drag the instrument blade across the surface of the stone. Both techniques are discussed and shown in this chapter so that the clinician can decide which to use. Use of hand-held stones is a very practical approach to instrument sharpening because it can be accomplished easily at the chairside during patient treatment. It requires only commonly available, inexpensive equipment. In addition, hand sharpening techniques are easily mastered by beginning clinicians. After the principles and skills of instrument sharpening have been mastered, the advanced clinician may choose to supplement hand sharpening techniques with mechanical ones.

If hand-held sharpening is not preferred, small cylindrical or conical stones mounted on a slow-speed handpiece may be selected. The clinician must carefully control the speed of metal removal and the proper instrument/stone adaptation with this method. If implemented properly and with concern for preserving the original instrument design, this and other mechanical sharpening methods are time-saving approaches. They are useful for sharpening instruments that require a great deal of sharpening or recontouring. An added advantage of this method is that sterile sharpening stones can be available at the dental unit and readily mounted on a slow-speed handpiece for sharpening instruments during patient treatment. Sharpening equipment can be resterilized after use to prevent cross-contamination. The clinician should always wear protective eye wear when using mechanical sharpening techniques because of the risk of flying metal, abrasive particles, and other debris.

Bench-type sharpening or honing machines are also available for sharpening periodontal instruments (Fig. 27-6). The principles of preserving instrument design that apply to hand-sharpening techniques are also followed when using a sharpening machine. The main difference is that the

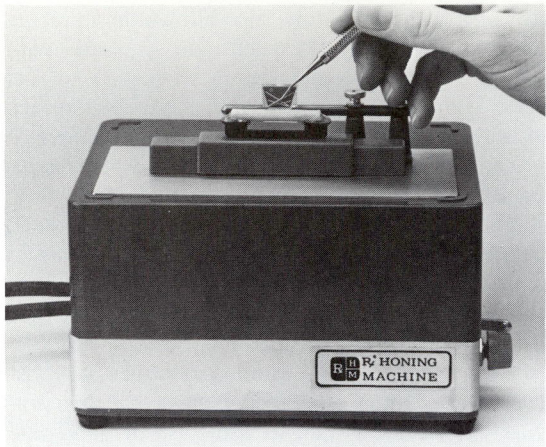

Fig. 27-6. Sharpening/honing machine.
(Courtesy Rx Horning Machine Co., Mishawaka, Ind.)

sharpening stone is mechanically rotated or moved back and forth while the instrument blade is applied to it. The amount of metal that can be removed with this method depends on the amount of pressure applied and the length of time that the blade is in contact with the sharpening stone. These machines can be time-savers if the clinician is skilled in placement of the blade against the stone at the correct angle and if the instrument requires a great deal of contouring. Inexperienced clinicians or those who are unfamiliar with instrument design, however, can ruin instruments much more quickly with this technique than with a manual technique. In addition, the need for special equipment limits the clinician's access to sharpening during patient treatment; this method is more useful when a special time has been alotted specifically for instrument sharpening. The use of honing machines on facial surfaces of instruments may produce an undesirable side effect known as nonfunctional wire edges, which are thin, irregular, metal extensions of the cutting edges (Antonini et al, 1977). Whenever a facial approach to sharpening is employed, instrument blades should be carefully inspected for the presence of nonfunctional wire edges. Their presence could create irregularities in the root surface. A technique for removing wire edges is discussed later in the chapter.

Use of a bench-mounted felt wheel machine has also been described as an effective method for sharpening periodontal instruments (DeNucci and Mader, 1983). In this technique a lateral surface of the instrument blade is held against a rotating felt wheel that has been impregnated with abrasive particles. The disadvantages of this method are the same as those discussed for other mechanical sharpening approaches. Appropriate measures should also be taken to control microbial cross-contamination when using this method.

Sharpening lateral versus facial surfaces

Sharp cutting edges can be created in one of two ways: by grinding the facial surface or by grinding the lateral surfaces. Applying a cylindrical or conical stone to the facial surface of the blade sharpens both sides of the blade simultaneously. Each cutting edge can be sharpened individually by applying a flat stone to each of the two lateral surfaces. Both methods can provide a fine cutting edge when properly implemented. The major advantage of sharpening the facial surface is that it is less time consuming because it sharpens both cutting edges of the blade simultaneously.

A number of authorities recommend not grinding away the facial surface because reducing the depth of the blade decreases the strength of the instrument more quickly than grinding the lateral surfaces (Carranza, 1984; Green, 1972; Paquette and Levin, 1977; Wilkins, 1989). However, evidence against this position was discussed by Murray and others (1984). They found no difference in instrument strength when comparing facial to lateral sharpening. They also noted that both methods result in significant reductions in instrument strength when the size of the instrument blade had been reduced by 20% or more. Clinicians should exercise caution when using instruments that have been sharpened beyond this point because their reduced strength could result in breakage of the tip of the blade if it is applied with much force against heavy or tenacious calculus deposits, restorative materials, or tight contact areas. Removal of broken instrument tips, especially from subgingival areas, can be an arduous task and an unpleasant experience for both the patient and clinician. The clinician can prevent this situation by inspecting instrument blades and exercising good judgment in their use.

Selecting a sharpening stone

Sharpening stones come in a variety of materials and designs (Fig. 27-7). The most popular stone

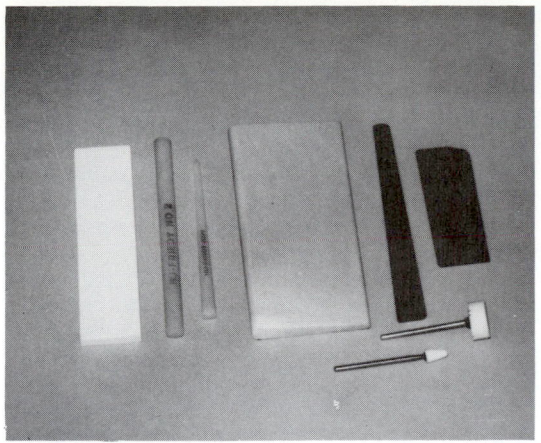

Fig. 27-7. Stones used to sharpen instruments.

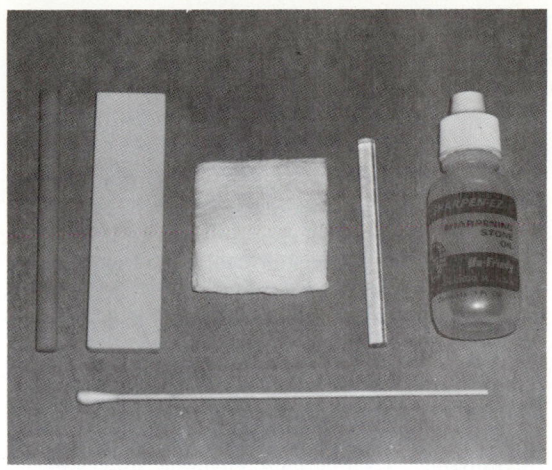

Fig. 27-8. Supplies used for instrument sharpening. *Left to right:* Cylindrical sharpening stone, rectangular Arkansas stone, gauze, testing stick, lubricating oil, and cotton-tipped applicator.

for sharpening periodontal instruments is a natural stone known as Arkansas oilstone. This stone is composed of abrasive crystals that are much finer than those of man-made stones. The quality of a cutting edge is determined by the fineness of the stone with which it is sharpened. An Arkansas oilstone is capable of producing a high-quality cutting edge while not grinding away the metal surface of the instrument as quickly as a coarser stone. Therefore, it is preferred over other sharpening stones for routine sharpening.

Several man-made stones are also available for use in dentistry, including the ruby stone, the India stone, the carborundum stone, and the diamond hone. These stones are impregnated with abrasive crystals such as aluminum oxide, silicon carbide, or diamond particles, all of which are coarser than those of the Arkansas stone. These man-made stones may be useful, however, if a great deal of recontouring is needed, because they grind a surface more quickly than the Arkansas stone.

Sharpening stones are available in rectangular, wedge, or cylindrical shapes. The choice of shape and size depends on the clinician's preference and on how the stone will be used. Small cylindrical or conical stones can be mounted for use in a slow-speed handpiece. Larger or tapered cylinders are used to sharpen the facial surfaces of instruments. Flat or rectangular stones are used to sharpen the lateral surfaces of instruments.

Preparation for sharpening

Have a workbench or countertop reserved for sharpening instruments. This area should provide easy access to all necessary supplies, including an effective light source, a magnifying lens, sharpening oil, applicators, and disinfectant-soaked gauze. If space is not available for this purpose, the methods of sharpening discussed in this chapter can be used wherever an adequate light source and working surface are available.

The supplies needed for instrument sharpening are shown in Fig. 27-8. They include a cylindrical stone (optional), a rectangular or wedge-shaped Arkansas stone, gauze squares, a testing stick, light-grade oil, and a cotton-tipped applicator. Only sterile supplies should be used for instrument sharpening. These supplies must be resterilized after use on contaminated instruments. If all instruments are resharpened at one designated time—either before or after being sterilized—the same sterile stone and testing stick can be used for the entire batch and resterilized for later use. A sterile stone and testing stick should be included on each tray setup if extensive instrumentation is to be performed, because frequent resharpening may be necessary during treatment. A light coating of oil should be applied to the stone with the cotton-tipped applicator. The purpose of the oil is to prevent metal filings from the sharpening procedure from becoming embedded in the surface of the stone. The oil also has a lubricating effect, reducing the heat produced during sharpening and enhancing the ability of the clinician to implement smooth, even strokes over the stone's surface. Other types of sharpening stones may require the use of water as a lubricant or no lubricant at all. Oil is the lubricant of choice for Arkansas stones and India stones. Water is used for ruby, composition, carborundum, and ceramic stones. Manufacturers' instructions should be followed regarding the choice of lubricant. The sterile gauze sponge is used to remove the oil and metal sludge from the sharpening stone and the instruments. To facilitate cleaning and asepsis, the sterile gauze squares may be moistened with an appropriate surface disinfectant solution.

Sharpening with a stationary stone and a moving instrument

Follow the steps outlined here when using this approach to instrument sharpening. Place the Arkansas stone on a flat surface. Coat the surface of the stone with oil using a cotton-tipped applicator. Hold the instrument with a modified pen grasp, as shown in Fig. 27-9, with the third and fourth fingers providing support for the hand on the surface of the table. Grasp and stabilize the stone with the fingers of the other hand as shown. Gloves should be worn during sharpening procedures for maximal asepsis and operator protection. Place the instrument near the top of the stone so that the face forms a 90-degree angle with the stone's surface (Fig. 27-10), then rotate the instrument handle slightly away from yourself until the angle between the face and the stone is 100 to 110 degrees (Fig. 27-11). This is the correct angle for sharpening all curettes and sickle scalers. This angle complements the internal angle of the instrument (70 to 80 degrees) so that the original design of the blade is maintained during sharpening. It is important to maintain this same angle for the entire length of the sharpening stroke. Until you have become experienced at identifying the correct angulation, it may be helpful first to place the instrument so that it forms a 90-degree angle and then open it up slightly another 10 to 20 degrees. Figs. 27-10 and 27-11 show close-up views of the curette blade placed at both 90 and 110 degrees. If you are still uncertain of your angulation, you may use a fixed-stone sharpening guide such as

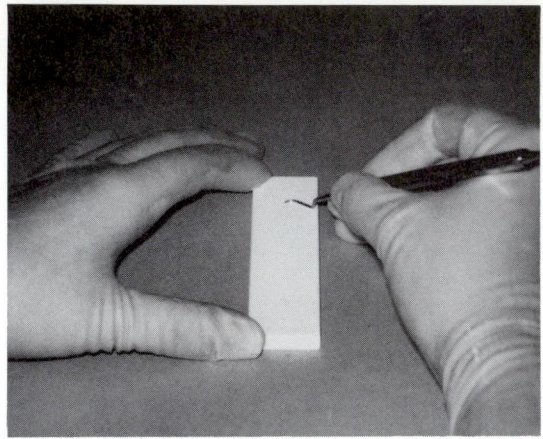

Fig. 27-9. Positioning of stone and instrument for sharpening with stationary stone.

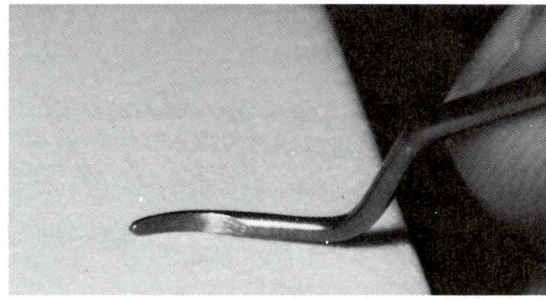

Fig. 27-10. Close-up view of facial surface of curette at 90-degree angle to stationary stone.

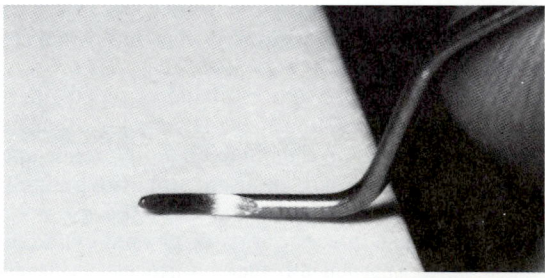

Fig. 27-11. Angle has been opened to 110 degrees before beginning sharpening stroke.

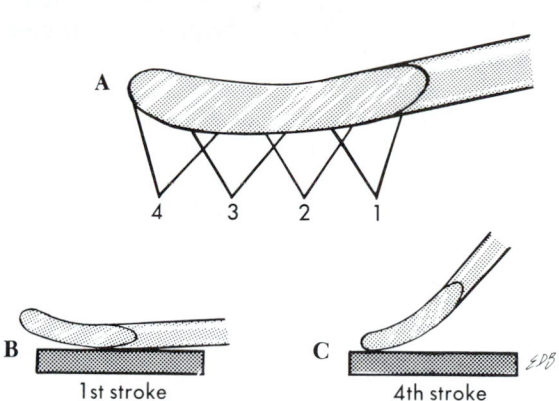

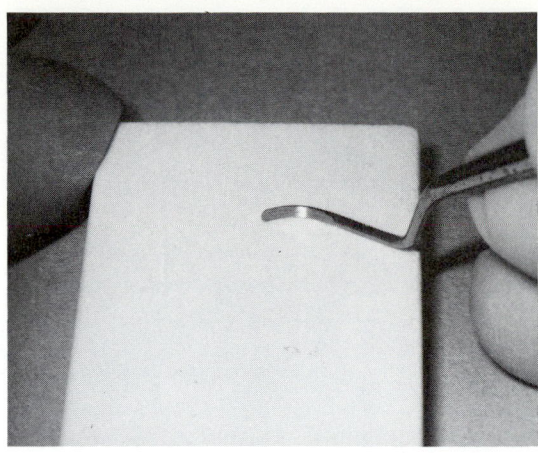

Fig. 27-12. **A,** Four different adaptations of stone are necessary to sharpen entire surface. **B,** First stroke should start at heel of blade. **C,** Last stroke should end at toe.

Fig. 27-13. Stationary stone and moving instrument; stroke begins at top of stone where heel of blade is in contact with stone at an angle of 100 to 110 degrees.

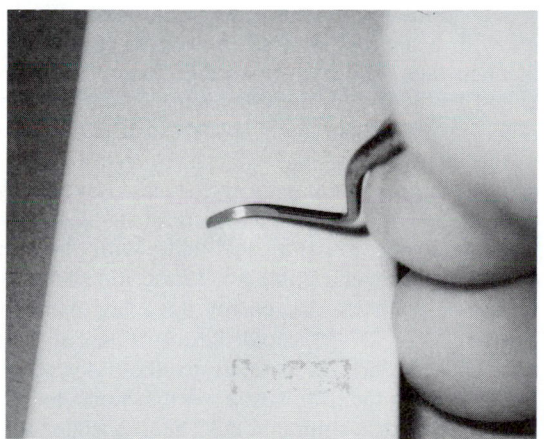

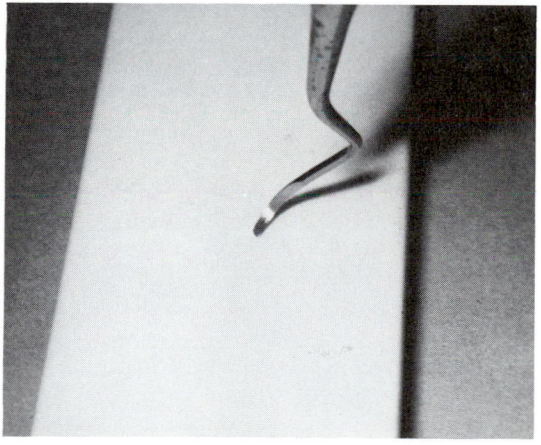

Fig. 27-14. As instrument is pulled forward across stone, blade is slowly rotated toward middle of cutting edge.

Fig. 27-15. As end of stroke approaches, back of cutting edge is lifted so that toe is in contact with stone.

Premier's Disc Sharpener (Norristown, Pa). This aid helps establish the blade-to-stone relationships with a guide that can be rotated to the proper angulation.

After the correct angle has been established, begin the stroke with the heel of the blade adapted to the stone. As you pull the instrument towards you, rotate the instrument blade towards the toe so that the entire blade is sharpened during each complete stroke. Fig. 27-12 shows that four different adaptations of the instrument to the stone may be necessary to ensure that the entire cutting edge has been sharpened. Move the entire hand and arm as a single unit toward you while rotating the wrist. At the end of the stroke, rotate around the entire toe of the blade so that its curvature is maintained. Failure to grind the toe surface evenly may result in a toe that is flattened or pointed instead of curved. The steps involved in a single stroke are shown in Figs. 27-13 to 27-16. Several light strokes may be necessary to sharpen the entire cutting edge completely. After one cut-

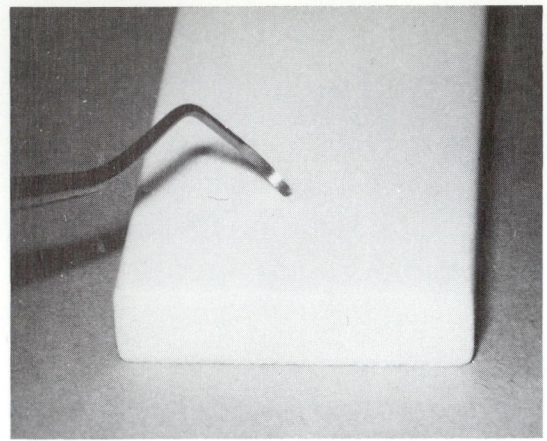

Fig. 27-16. Entire toe should be rounded off at end of stroke so that a sharp point is not created. Less pressure can be used at toe, because it is not a cutting surface.

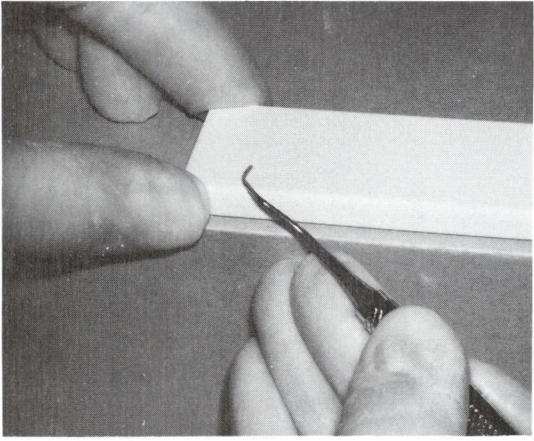

Fig. 27-17. Placement of stone at edge of table to facilitate sharpening of opposite edge of universal curette.

ting edge of the curette has been completely sharpened, sharpen the other edge the same way. You may need to reposition the stone at the edge of the table to facilitate the placement of the opposite cutting edge (Fig. 27-17). After sharpening, inspect the blade carefully to ensure that the original design has been preserved.

Gracey curettes are sharpened in the same way, with few exceptions. Only one cutting edge of the Gracey curette should be sharpened. The clinician must first identify this lower cutting edge. Since the face of the Gracey curette is not perpendicular

to the shank, care should be taken at first to align the facial surface at a 90-degree angle to the stone and then open the angle to the proper sharpening angle of 100 to 110 degrees.

Sickle scalers can be easily sharpened by this method. The same principles of instrument placement and angulation apply. The only major difference is that, because the lateral surfaces of this instrument are flatter and straighter than those of the curette, there is not as much rotation of the blade from heel to toe during each stroke. Stop the stroke at the tip of the instrument to maintain the sharp point. Repeat the sharpening strokes until the cutting edge is sharp then reposition the instrument to sharpen the opposite cutting edge. After sharpening, remove the metal sludge from both the instrument blade and the stone with sterile gauze squares.

Sharpening with a stationary instrument and a moving stone

A second method of sharpening curettes and sickles with a hand-held stone is to hold the instrument in one hand and move the stone across the lateral surfaces with the other hand. The first step is to grasp the instrument to be sharpened firmly in the left hand (if the clinician is right-handed) and brace the hand against the top edge of a counter or table so that the instrument blade extends over the edge of the table with the toe pointing toward the clinician. Grasp the sharpening stone with the fingers of the other hand as shown in Fig. 27-18. Hold the instrument so that its facial surface is parallel to the floor. Fig. 27-18 shows the adaptation of the stone to the cutting edge of a curette at a 90-degree angle. Rotate the top of the stone slightly away from the instrument until the correct angle of 100 to 110 degrees is formed between the stone and the facial surface (Fig. 27-19). Apply short down strokes (½ to 1 inch) to the cutting edge of the blade, being careful to maintain the stone at exactly the same angle during each stroke. Apply pressure against the instrument only during downstrokes to avoid the formation of a wire edge.

Apply sharpening strokes first to the heel of the instrument and then rotate the stone slightly until the entire cutting edge has been sharpened. A separate stroke is needed to maintain the rounded toe. The stone should be adapted to form a 45-degree angle between the bottom half of the stone and the facial surface of the curette (Fig. 27-20).

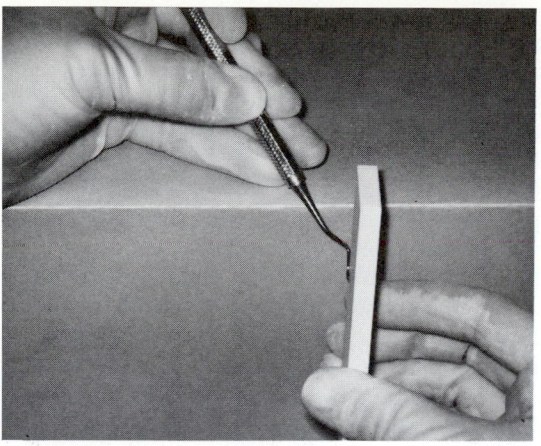

Fig. 27-18. Stationary instrument and moving stone technique. Note position of left hand, which is braced against tabletop. Facial surface of instrument is parallel to floor. Stone is placed at 90-degree angle. Left-handed clinicians hold instrument in right hand and apply stone with left hand.

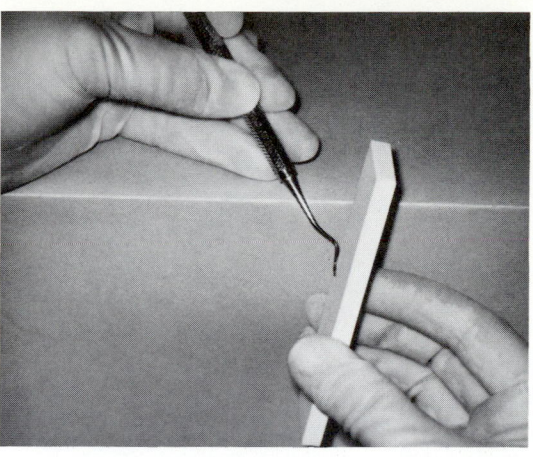

Fig. 27-19. Stone is correctly oriented at an angle of 100 degrees to the facial surface. This exact angle must be maintained for all strokes.

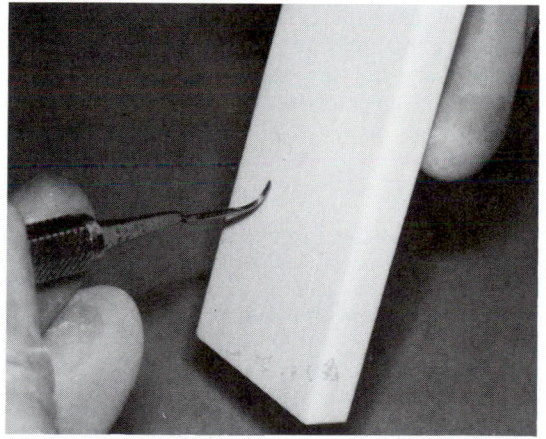

Fig. 27-20. To sharpen toe of curette using moving stone, place stone at 45-degree angle to back of blade.

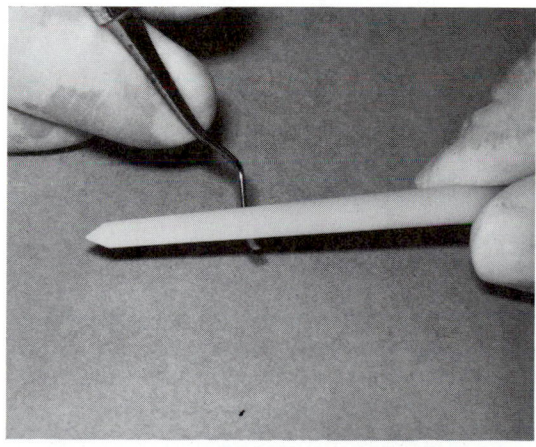

Fig. 27-21. Tapered cylindrical stone is applied to facial surface of curette to assist in removal of wire edges.

Short downstrokes should be applied around the curvature of the toe.

The same technique can be used to sharpen sickle scalers and Gracey curettes. Again, sharpen only the lower cutting edge of a Gracey curette, taking care to position the instrument so that the facial surface is parallel to the floor before positioning the stone to begin the sharpening stroke.

If pressure is applied to both the upstroke and the downstroke using this technique, it may be necessary to smooth the facial surface with a cylindrical stone if wire edges have been created (Antonini et al, 1977). Place the cylindrical or tapered sharpening stone squarely against the facial surface of the curette (Fig. 27-21). Stabilize the instrument and apply light, even pressure to the facial surface while rotating the stone in a counterclockwise direction (i.e., heel to toe). Facial

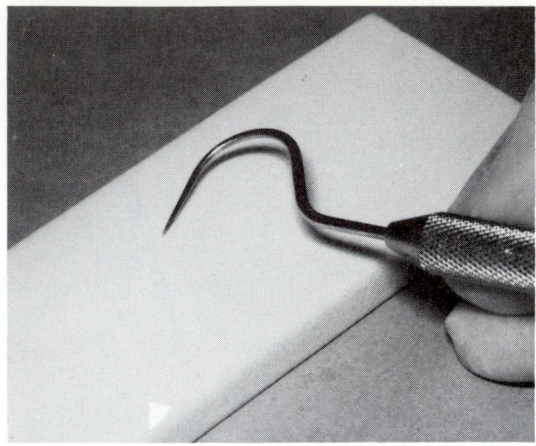

Fig. 27-22. Sharpen explorers by adapting tip to stone at an angle of 15 degrees.

grinding should be done only if wire edges are detected because excessive grinding both here and on lateral surfaces could reduce the instrument size and strength unnecessarily.

Sharpening explorers

Explorers used for detection of decay (e.g., design no. 23 or "shepherd's hook" explorer) should be kept sharp to maximize their effectiveness. Apply the stone to the tip of the explorer at an angle of about 15 to 20 degrees (Fig. 27-22). Use short strokes around the entire point until it becomes sharp. Extremely sharp points are not desirable for explorers that are used primarily for submarginal calculus detection so these instruments do not need to be sharpened unless their tips require recontouring because of damage.

STERILIZATION EFFECTS

Following patient treatment, used instruments should be cleaned ultrasonically or scrubbed by hand before resharpening. Protective gloves should always be worn when sharpening nonsterile instruments to protect against accidental cuts or punctures. Instruments that have been used to treat patients who are known or suspected carriers of serious transmittable diseases should be sterilized before being handled for cleaning or sharpening to protect the clinician from cross-contamination. Once they have been rendered harmless, these instruments can be cleaned, sharpened, and resterilized for use.

Except for these high-risk situations, instruments should be sharpened routinely before being sterilized. If instruments are sharpened after being sterilized and before patient treatment, their sterility may be compromised. Contrary to some beliefs, commonly used sterilization procedures (e.g., steam sterilization at 250° F, chemical vapor at 270° F, dry heat up to 340° F) will not dull the cutting edge of stainless steel instruments (Parkes and Kolstad, 1982; Sassie, 1987). One study found that there was no significant loss of blade sharpness even after 240 sterilization cycles in either the autoclave or the chemical vapor sterilizer (Sassie, 1987). Carbon steel instruments, however, can be dulled slightly by steam or chemical vapor sterilization methods and should be sterilized in a dry heat oven to preserve blade sharpness (Parkes and Kolstad, 1981).

SUMMARY

The clinical judgment to detect when instruments are dull and the technique required to sharpen and recontour instruments properly is a skill that the dental hygienist must develop. The most well-executed scaling and root planing strokes will be ineffective and inefficient if dull instruments are used. Instrument sharpening skills are an indispensible step on the road to becoming an expert clinician.

ACTIVITIES

1. Examine and compare the designs of the following types of instruments under a microscope:
   a. A new instrument.
   b. A well-sharpened instrument.
   c. A missharpened instrument.
   d. A dull instrument.
2. Compare the ease of scaling and root planing on extracted teeth when using an optimally sharpened instrument versus a dull instrument.
3. Observe a demonstration of instrument sharpening using a handpiece-mounted stone or a honing machine and discuss the use of these techniques for routine instrument sharpening in terms of amount of metal removed, ability to control the application of the stone to the instrument, heat generated, contamination control, and access to equipment during patient treatment.

REVIEW QUESTIONS

1. Which of the following methods is not an acceptable way to determine instrument sharpness?
   a. Evaluation of the cutting edge during scaling procedures.

b. Evaluation of light reflection from the cutting edge when observed under magnification.

c. Evaluation of the cutting edge against a plastic testing stick.

d. Evaluation of the cutting edge against the clinician's fingernail.

2. True or false:

a. The Arkansas stone is a man-made, or artificial, sharpening stone.

b. Sterilization by autoclaving will not dull the cutting edges of stainless steel instruments.

c. Both cutting edges of a Gracey curette should be sharpened.

3. What is the internal angle formed by the facial and lateral surfaces of curettes and sickle scalers?

a. 45 degrees.

b. 70 to 80 degrees.

c. 90 degrees.

d. 100 to 110 degrees.

4. Identify two design characteristics of curettes that must be preserved during sharpening.

5. When a stationary instrument is being sharpened with a moving stone, pressure should be applied on the _____.

a. Upstroke only.

b. Downstroke only.

c. Upstroke and downstroke.

REFERENCES

Antonini CJ et al: Scanning electron microscope study of scalers, *J Periodontol* 48:45, 1977.

Carranza FA, editor: *Glickman's clinical periodontology,* ed 6, Philadelphia, 1984, WB Saunders.

DeNucci DJ, Mader CL: Scanning electron microscopic evaluation of several resharpening techniques, *J Periodontol* 54:618, 1983.

Green E, Seyer PC: *Sharpening curettes and sickle scalers,* ed 2, Berkeley, 1972, Praxis.

Murray GH et al: The effects of two sharpening methods on the strength of a periodontal scaling instrument, *J Periodontol* 55:410, 1984.

Paquette DE, Levin MP: The sharpening of scaling instruments. I. An examination of principles, *J Periodontol* 48:163, 1977.

Parkes RB, Kolstad RA: Effects of sterilization on periodontal instruments, *J Periodontol* 53:434, 1982.

Sassie J: Cutting edges of curettes: effects of repeated sterilization, *Dent Hyg* 61:14, 1987.

Tal H et al: Scanning electron microscope evaluation of wear of dental curettes during standardized root planing, *J Periodontol* 56:532, 1985.

Wilkins EM: *Clinical practice of the dental hygienist,* ed 6, Philadelphia, 1989, Lea & Febiger.

28 ORAL IRRIGATION AND ANTIMICROBIAL PLAQUE CONTROL

Laura Mueller Joseph
Barbara Jones

LEARNING OUTCOMES

The dental hygienist will be able to

1. Contrast the views of oral irrigation from the 1970s opposing oral irrigation to those of the present.
2. Determine when it is appropriate to (a) utilize in-office irrigation and/or (b) recommend at-home irrigation for the patients.
3. Instruct patients in the proper method of at-home irrigation using differing irrigation tips.
4. Identify and recommend appropriate antimicrobial plaque control agents for various patient types.

PLAQUE CONTROL: CHEMICAL INHIBITION

Chapter 20 discussed the role of physiotherapeutic aids for plaque control. Toothbrushes, floss, wood wedges, yarn, and other mechanical plaque control methods have been recommended for years as part of the oral health armamentarium. Unfortunately, some patients are unable to control plaque mechanically, even with conscientious effort. Others are unwilling to make the commitment necessary to adequately control plaque using mechanical means. The last two decades have seen the emergence of a new era in plaque control: chemical or antimicrobial inhibition. Antimicrobial agents that reduce plaque and help control resulting gingivitis are now incorporated into dentifrices and oral rinses. Your patients need to understand, that although antimicrobial agents are useful, mechanical plaque control measures remain a necessary part of home care. These products may provide an answer for those patients for whom mechanical methods are not adequate, however.

In addition to antiplaque agents, various anticalculus dentifrices and rinses have emerged on the oral care market. Although these agents contain ingredients that inhibit calculus formation (usually zinc chloride or pyrophosphate), they do not exert an antiplaque effect. Rather, they keep calcium and phosphorus from incorporating into the plaque matrix and thus forming calculus. When recommending these products to your patients, be certain they understand that these products are recommended for calculus inhibition, not plaque control. The patient will still need to practice meticulous mechanical home care to control plaque, or antimicrobial plaque control agents can be incorporated into the home care regimen.

Prescription plaque control agents

Chlorhexidine digluconate has been widely recognized as a powerful antiplaque and antigingivitis agent for over 20 years. Used in Europe at a concentration of 0.2%, chlorhexidine was introduced in the United States as a prescription oral rinse (Peridex, Procter and Gamble). Peridex is a mint-flavored oral rinse (pH 5.5) containing 0.12% chlorhexidine in a base containing 15.0% alcohol.

The research on chlorhexidine is extensive and has unequivocally established its effectiveness against plaque and gingivitis. Patients involved in 6-month studies of chlorhexidine exhibited reductions in plaque of 16% (Lang et al, 1982) and 61% (Grossman et al, 1986) compared with those who used placebo preparations. In addition, gingivitis was reduced by 67% and 39%, respectively. You can confidently recommend chlorhexidine for patients who have serious plaque control and gingivitis problems, as it provides significant benefit with proper use.

However, this benefit is not without adverse side effects (Gjermo, 1989). Your patients may notice alterations in taste sensation, increased calculus formation, tooth staining, and, in some cases, desquamation of the buccal mucosa. Calculus and tooth staining are easily removed with a thorough prophylaxis, and altered taste sensation and mucosal desquamation typically resolve once product use ends. Many dental professionals consider these side effects to be minor given the effectiveness of chlorhexidine.

Chlorhexidine has also been shown to be toxic to red blood cells and to polymorphonuclear cells at concentrations as low as 0.02%. Cells are protected by serum (such as that which flows from the periodontal pocket), but not by saliva (Gabler, Roberts, and Harolds, 1987). Although labeling information for this prescription product does not limit the duration of its use, patients should be closely monitored for adverse effects that may affect compliance. If any adverse response is noted, or if the patient indicates that he or she is unable or unwilling to continue use, you may wish to recommend a different antimicrobial for the purpose of maintaining oral health.

Stannous fluoride is also emerging as an agent that may reduce plaque and gingivitis. The stannous ion makes this agent effective against bacteria because it affects the ability of cells to metabolize polysaccharides. Short-term testing suggests that when administered subgingivally, stannous fluoride reduces bacterial populations, which requires several weeks to return to baseline levels (Mazza, Newman, and Sims, 1981). You can also recommend it for twice-daily home use, instructing the patient to brush a 0.4% stannous fluoride gel onto the teeth, swish the gel around the mouth, and then expectorate. As with any prescription agent, you will want to monitor your patient for adverse responses and compliance with stannous fluoride therapy.

Nonprescription plaque control products

Two nonprescription agents with a strong background of clinical testing are available. One is Listerine, which contains a combination of essential oils (thymol, eucalyptol, menthol, and methyl salicylate) in a 26.8% alcohol base (pH 4.1). Listerine has been on the market for many years as an antiseptic oral rinse and is available without prescription.

Long-term clinical studies of Listerine have shown it to reduce plaque between 14% to 34% (DePaola et al, 1989; Gordon, Lamster, and Sieger, 1985; Lamster et al, 1983). Reductions in gingivitis ranged from 22% to 34%. No serious adverse effects have been observed with regular use of Listerine, although its strong taste (imparted by the active ingredients) may be a major drawback to your patients' compliance. A mint-flavored preparation with 21.6% alcohol partially masks the essential oils taste.

Also available are products containing sanguinaria extract, which is a highly purified extract from the plant *Sanguinaria canadensis*. This extract is comprised of six benzophenanthridine alkaloids, with the principal alkaloid being sanguinarine chloride. Sanguinarine is a cationic molecule that chemically combines with plaque and remains detectable for up to 4 hours at levels capable of inhibiting the growth of pathogenic bacteria. Viadent products (Vipont Pharmaceutical) include toothpaste (with and without sodium monofluorophosphate), which contains 0.075% sanguinaria extract, and oral rinse, which contains 0.03% sanguinaria extract in a 10.0% alcohol base (pH 4.5).

Although short-term testing has demonstrated the effectiveness of the individual products, the greatest effect is achieved when Viadent toothpaste and oral rinse are used together. Longitudinal studies testing the combined use of these products have demonstrated reductions in plaque ranging from 13% to 43% (Hannah et al, 1989; Harper et al, 1990; Kopczyk et al, 1991). Likewise, gingival inflammation was reduced by 17% to 52% and gingival bleeding by 32% to 57%. Testing revealed no emergence of opportunistic organisms or changes in the normal oral flora, nor are adverse responses observed with use of this product.

You can confidently recommend either of these two nonprescription products in the initial phase of plaque or gingivitis reduction or to maintain oral health after use of chlorhexidine.

Other available agents claim antiplaque effects, but long-term studies are either unavailable or inconclusive. Plax is a prebrushing rinse that claims to enable the mechanical action of the brush and floss to remove plaque more readily. However, this claim is based on single-use testing (Emling and Yankell, 1985) and long-term trials have not confirmed the result of the original study (Lobene et al, 1990). Although the active ingredient is not specified, the concentrations of sodium lauryl sulfate and sodium borax suggest that any plaque removal effect may result from surfactant action. The sodium content of this product is high, and thus it may be inappropriate for patients who are on sodium-restricted diets (Wagner et al, 1989).

Hydrogen peroxide and sodium bicarbonate are also suggested to have antimicrobial effects and in fact have been shown to be synergistic (Miyasaki et al, 1986). In spite of the synergistic potential, in vivo clinical testing has been unable to support the plaque inhibitory effect of hydrogen peroxide and sodium bicarbonate beyond that achieved with normal oral hygiene, regardless of delivery method (Cerra and Killoy, 1982; Greenwell et al, 1983 Rosling et al, 1982; West and King, 1983; Wolff et al, 1989). In addition, a study testing hydrogen peroxide and chlorhexidine showed that hydrogen peroxide produced modest reductions in gingivitis and bleeding, but no significant reduction in plaque. In contrast, chlorhexidine produced dramatic, statistically significant reductions in all three parameters (Gusberti et al, 1988).

As you recommend antimicrobial plaque control agents to your patients and see the results in your practice, you will be able to determine which agent works best for specific patient types. Your treatment plans will undoubtedly include use of one or more of the products described here. Your experience in recommending and observing the benefits of these agents will be invaluable in determining what works best for different types of patients.

Antibiotic treatment

In recent years, systemic antibiotics have come to the forefront as an adjunct in the treatment of periodontal disease. Antibiotics are useful for the treatment of refractory periodontal diseases and can be used to selectively suppress proliferating pathogenic bacteria. These antibiotics include tetracycline, amoxicillin, augmentin, metronidazole, doxycycline, and clindamycin. Although systemic delivery is the current method, recent research has demonstrated the effectiveness of both antibiotics and antimicrobial agents when delivered subgingivally or in subgingival slow-release vehicles (for review, see Genco, 1991).

Because the areas of antibiotics and antimicrobials in oral health care are relatively new, re-

searchers will continue to develop and evaluate new products and publish the results. Regular reviews of clinical research literature will prove valuable to you as these findings become available. The increasing number of options will provide a myriad of alternatives to fit patients' oral care needs and preferences.

ORAL IRRIGATION: SUPRAGINGIVAL AND SUBGINGIVAL PLAQUE CONTROL

Nearly all of the devices introduced in Chapter 20 are restricted to supragingival plaque control. Brushing and flossing are effective in the mechanical removal of most supragingival plaque, but are limited in subgingival removal by their physical constraints in conjunction with the gingiva (Plate 1, *I*). Manual brushing approaches between 1.5 to 3.0 mm subgingivally (Waerhaug, 1976), and flossing reaches to a depth of 2 to 3 mm (Reitman et al, 1980). Toothpicks, pipe cleaners, and interdental brushes have minimal effect on subgingival plaque. Even in areas where these devices may be able to move below the margin of the gingiva, their size and shape limit access and usefulness. Thus the dental hygienist must look for adjunctive procedures to assist in the control of periodontal disease.

The combined efforts of periodic professional subgingival debridement and daily at-home self-care can prevent the recurrence of disease by disrupting the subgingival microflora. The tooth root is covered with a highly organized and colonized layer of bacterial plaque that can be compared to a semitropical coastline. For example, when a tropical storm strikes the coastal colonies, the organization and structure, and thus the function, of those colonies is put in disarray. It takes weeks or months for the inhabitants to recover and reorganize; the more thorough the disruption, the longer it takes to rebuild and resume normal activity. The same theory applies to subgingival disruption of colonies. The more regular and thorough the disruption, the more likely the bacteria will be unable to reestablish themselves at levels that can cause tissue destruction.

Oral irrigation is an adjunctive procedure that can disrupt plaque in subgingival areas. The first powered oral irrigation device (Water Pik) was accepted by the American Dental Association in 1968 for its ability to flush food particles and debris from between teeth and under the gingival margin. Although the device was widely recommended, especially for orthodontic and prosthodontic patients, early research found no relationship between debris and periodontal disease and no evidence that irrigation could significantly reduce plaque.

As researchers expanded their understanding of bacterial plaque, however, they discovered that oral irrigation disrupts the subgingival microbiota (Brady, 1973; White et al, 1988). The pulsating action of the water penetrates subgingivally and changes the quality of the plaque, detoxifying it (Cobb, 1988). The introduction of antimicrobial solutions for the chemical control of dental plaque has further expanded the usefulness of the irrigator. Antimicrobial solution can be delivered "site specifically" to the sulcus or pocket by an oral irrigator. These two advances in dental research have made oral irrigation an important procedure in planning preventive care, establishing it as much more than a device to flush away debris.

As described in Chapter 12, plaque is a complex organization of bacteria made up of supragingival and subgingival organisms. The supragingival plaque comprises attached plaque (AP), which clings to the tooth's surface, and an outside layer of loosely attached plaque (LAP), which moves in and out of that attached matrix. Similarly, subgingival plaque includes both an attached layer against the root surface and a loosely attached component floating freely between the root and the epithelial lining of the pocket. The subgingival loosely attached plaque extends beyond the attached component to the epithelial attachment (Plate 1, *I* and *J*).

Gingivitis follows the accumulation of supragingival plaque; regular removal of supragingival plaque will help to prevent gingivitis (Cumming and Löe, 1973). Supragingival plaque influences the establishment and relative proportions of subgingival microorganisms (Kornman, 1986; Loesche and Syed, 1978). However, once mature plaque is established, subgingival plaque cannot be controlled by removal of supragingival plaque alone (Tabita et al, 1981). The loosely attached subgingival plaque that is in direct contact with the sulcular and junctional epithelium is most likely to initiate periodontitis (Carranza, 1984).

The obvious conclusion is that supragingival plaque must be controlled to prevent and treat gingivitis, but subgingival plaque, especially the loosely attached component, must be controlled to prevent and treat periodontitis. Various combinations of professional and home care methods are required for prevention, treatment, and maintenance, depending on the individual patient and his or her disease status.

History of irrigation

Early research on oral irrigation was designed to test its efficacy in removing debris and supragingival plaque. Tempel, Marcil, and Seibert (1975) concluded that water irrigation was significantly more effective than oral rinsing in removing particulate debris and soluble bacterial products, both before and after toothbrushing and flossing. In 1971, Hoover and others found that oral irrigation users had significantly less plaque and calculus accumulation and experienced highly significant reductions in the periodontal index and plaque index in the 3-month test period following prophylaxis.

Lobene (1969) found that oral irrigation, as a supplement to toothbrushing, reduced calculus formation by approximately 50% and effected a 50% reduction in gingivitis. Lobene suggested that the pulsating water jets might have qualitatively altered the composition of the plaque, which in turn accounted for the reduction in gingivitis. A later study by Brady and others (1973) used the electron microscope to verify that the pulsating water of the oral irrigator did remove plaque and produce qualitative changes in the adherent plaque left on the irrigated tooth surfaces.

Eakle, Ford, and Boyd (1985) found that the Water Pik oral irrigtor delivered solution into subgingival pockets of various depths (from 3 to more than 7 mm) and averaged a penetration of approximately half the depth of the pocket.

White and others (1988) verified earlier work of Aday (1982) and West (1982) by evaluating the effect of water irrigation on various bacteria associated with untreated gingivitis and periodontitis at pocket depths up to 6 mm. Irrigated sites improved in both shallow and deep pockets. Results also demonstrated a dramatic reduction of *Bacteroides melaninogenicus* and *Prevotella intermedia* (formerly *Bacteroides intermedius*) organisms, with a statistically significant reduction of spirochetes and motile rods in deep pockets.

An ultrastructural study using oral irrigation and electron microscopic methods (Cobb, Rogers, and Killoy, 1988) evaluated untreated pockets in patients with advanced, chronic adult periodontitis after a single exposure to pulsating oral irrigation with saline solution. They found qualitative differences in microbial morphotypes at various pocket depths with no injury to soft tissues. When compared with rinsing, oral irrigation has proved superior in distribution of antimicrobial agents (Brownstein et al, 1987; Lang and Raber, 1981).

Boyd and others (1985) found that self-administered daily irrigation with 0.02% stannous fluoride resulted in significant improvement in periodontal health when used as an adjunct to brushing and flossing. In 1989, Ciancio and others studied the efficacy of oral irrigation with Listerine as a supplement to normal hygiene. They found that irrigation, with placebo or Listerine, significantly improved probing depths and attachment level measurements. Furthermore irrigation with Listerine significantly reduced plaque and bleeding and was shown to be an effective oral hygiene adjunct, both with and without previous dental prophylaxis. Brownstein and others (1987) showed that irrigation once daily with 0.06% chlorhexidine was superior in reducing the gingival index and bleeding on probing when compared with twice-daily 0.12% chlorhexidine rinsing. Newman and colleagues (1990) reported results of a study confirming the Brownstein work. They demonstrated that irrigation with 0.06% chlorhexidine was significantly better than rinsing twice daily with 0.12% chlorhexidine in reducing gingivitis and bleeding, though without concomitant plaque reduction. In fact, once-daily irrigation with placebo reduced gingival bleeding as well as twice-daily rinsing with chlorhexidine.

Flemmig and others (1990) reported clinical studies which demonstrate the enhanced effect of chlorhexidine on gingivitis when delivered through an oral irrigator. They concluded that irrigation may increase the access of antimicrobial solutions beneath the gingival margin, resulting in improved tissue health. Another study by Jolkovsky and others (1990) evaluated the efficacy of a single in-office irrigation with 0.12% chlorhexidine followed by 3 months of daily home subgingival irrigation with 0.04% chlorhexidine. Results demonstrate significant reductions in gingival inflammation and bleeding compared with standard oral hygiene.

Two other studies evaluated the use of sanguinaria (Viadent) delivered supragingivally. One study evaluated the effects of irrigation and sanguinaria on established plaque and gingivitis (Parsons et al, 1987). The second evaluated their ef-

fects on newly forming plaque and gingivitis (Southard et al, 1987). Both studies used a model in which subjects refrained from brushing for 2 weeks and used only the irrigator, either with water or sanguinaria, or only a manual antimicrobial-loral rinse to control plaque growth. The results showed that irrigation with water or sanguinaria reduced established gingivitis and inhibited the development of gingivitis in healthy subjects. Adding a dilute solution of Viadent (0.00225% sanguinaria) as an irrigant controlled plaque significantly in both studies.

A number of other studies have compared the efficacy of irrigation with that of rinsing and the benefits of irrigating with one chemical agent over another (Aziz-Gandour and Newman, 1986; Derdivanis, Bushmaker, and Dagenais, 1978; Lang and Raber, 1981; Lang and Ramseier-Grossman, 1981; Sanders, Linden, and Newman, 1986). The consistent conclusion appears to be that delivery with oral irrigation enhances the effect of whatever agent is used. Oral irrigation, because of its proven ability to penetrate gently and deeply into periodontal pockets, demonstrates benefit even with dilute concentrations. This can be especially important when prescribing chemical agents that pose problems with taste and staining.

In-office subgingival irrigation

In-office subgingival delivery of antimicrobial agents has been used by many professionals for a number of years. Most of the early research centered on the delivery of chemical agents subgingivally with the use of the hand syringe (Hardy, Newman, and Strahan, 1982; Perry et al, 1984).

In recent years, the powered irrigation device has been fitted with a special handpiece and cannula for subgingival delivery in the operatory (Figs. 28-1 and 28-2). The cannula can be placed into the sulcus or pocket to enable the professional to deliver solutions under extremely low pressure directly into periodontal pockets.

Kelly and others (1985) compared the delivery pressure of the WaterPik powered irrigation device to that of the peristaltic pump and the hand syringe. Delivery force was more consistent and physiologicaly acceptable with the powered irrigator.

Researchers also have examined the use of the powered irrigator with specialized subgingival cannulas in the delivery of antimicrobial solutions. Watts and Newman (1986) found that sub-

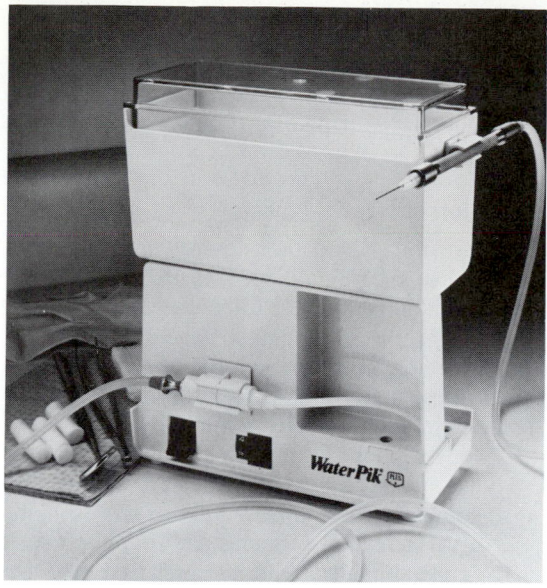

Fig. 28-1. The WaterPik in-office irrigator with a cannula.

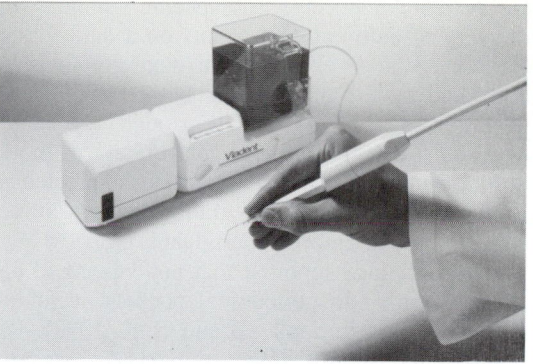

Fig. 28-2. The Viadent Via-Jet irrigator with a cannula and handpiece with heater.

gingival delivery was clinically effective in reducing inflammation and pocket depth but saw no significant difference between results with chlorhexidine versus placebo. Researchers continue to investigate various antimicrobial concentrations and intervals of administration in addition to alternative methods of subgingival delivery. Further research will likely confirm the attributes of powered oral irrigation for site-specific subgingival delivery of chemical agents, at a consistent rate and force, as another adjunctive use of direct irrigation in the dental operatory.

In-office irrigation can be used following routine scaling and root planing to flush away calculus and plaque fragments and to introduce an antimicrobial agent to impede reestablishment of plaque.

Cannulas deliver the irrigant deeper into the pocket than subgingival tips (see Fig. 20-34). The cannula is a blunt needle that attaches to a special office-use handpiece. The cannula has either an end-port with the orifice at the end or a side-port with the orifice on the side. The choice is a matter of professional preference.

The cannula is used much like a periodontal probe. It is gently inserted approximately 3 mm into the pocket or sulcus. The foot pedal is then

activated, starting the gentle stream of liquid into the pocket (Plate 2, *C* and *D*). The liquid should surround the tooth in the moatlike subgingival space and emerge from the pocket (Plate 2, *E*). The cannula is moved around the tooth and on to the next site to be irrigated.

The cannula must be discarded after use. Disassemble the handpiece, autoclave it, and allow liquid to flow through the tubing before and after use.

Placing an antimicrobial solution in the pocket after instrumentation can provide an opportunity to discuss how the patient can incorporate at-home irrigation with an antimicrobial agent appropriate for maintenance therapy.

Patient-applied subgingival irrigation

Understanding and developing a dental health education plan that incorporates patient-administered oral irrigation for the care of periodontal pockets and implants is a major role for the practicing dental hygienist. Researchers are proving that subgingival irrigation provides additional access to hard-to-reach areas. A variety of products and oral irrigation devices are available for dental hygienists to recommend.

As previously mentioned, supragingival plaque control practices are limited in their ability to disrupt subgingival microflora. Because of these limitations, manufacturers have developed devices that can be used by the patient for subgingival delivery (see Figs. 20-32 and 20-33).

Home use of subgingival irrigation allows patients to participate in maintaining bacterial reduction after scaling procedures. It also is beneficial for patients requiring "site-specific" subgingival delivery of antimicrobial agents on a daily basis. However, the level of patient dexterity must be evaluated by the professional before subgingival irrigation is used, as not all patients are candidates for this type of plaque control device. In addition, hands-on educational sessions directed at irrigation use are very important to ensure correct application and enforce compliance.

A recent study reported that patients could deliver solution into periodontal pockets averaging 6.9 to 7.8 mm in depth (Braun et al, 1990). Patients demonstrated safe subgingival irrigation with the PikPocket subgingival irrigation tip. Surprisingly, they irrigated an aqueous solution to approximately 80% of the depth of the periodontal pockets in posterior teeth.

Harper and colleagues (1991) reported the effect of subgingival irrigation with Listerine mouthrinse on the periodontal microflora. This study demonstrated that subgingival irrigation with Listerine promotes significantly greater and more persistent decreases in the pathologic periodontal flora than subgingival water irrigation. The researchers concluded that this treatment may be a useful adjunct to conventional periodontal therapy.

Some patients require site-specific subgingival delivery in their home maintenance regimens for the maintenance of periodontal pockets or implants. Other subgingival irrigation techniques include hand syringes, bulbs, and specialized sulcus tips to assist the patient's home care efficiency. Subgingival delivery tips designed for patient use are currently being evaluated for both efficacy and safety. These tips offer promise for more targeted delivery into deep pockets by patients at home.

As with all oral hygiene procedures, it is important that you *carefully* educate the patient with regard to the proper use of subgingival irrigation devices. Demonstrate the appropriate placement of the subgingival irrigation tip, both for maximum efficiency and for safety.

An additional consideration affecting the recommendation of oral irrigation, with or without an antimicrobial agent, is patient compliance. Dental hygienists need to ask patients "Do you want to do this every day to maintain your dental health?" or "Are you willing to do this?" In a 6-month clinical study, high compliance was reported for patients using oral irrigation, either with water or an antimicrobial solution (Bakdash,

1979). It is vital to remember to meet your patients' needs and wants. If they do not value your suggestion, work with them to find another alternative. Most patients will not comply with home care instructions if they do not value or trust the results.

Irrigation devices

There are many irrigation devices on the market for in-office subgingival delivery. At this point no one technique is superior to another; however, irrigating systems have an advantage over pumps or syringes in terms of the control of pressure. The following systems and devices for subgingival irrigation are commercially available.

1. Jet irrigators have been modified for office use by the Teledyne Water-Pik and Vipont companies and come equipped with subgingival irrigating cannulas and foot controls.
2. A metal canister can be purchased that acts as a reservoir for an ultrasonic unit, thereby permitting solutions to be delivered while roots are being debrided ultrasonically (EZ Enterprises).
3. The Cavi-Med facilitates ultrasonic debridement and irrigation (Dentsply International Inc.).
4. The Odontoson M delivers the antimicrobial of your choice via ultrathin, ultrasonic tips, combining debridement and irrigation.
5. Perio Select facilitates delivering multiple antimicrobial solutions (Sultan Chemists, Inc.).

SUMMARY

Powered oral irrigators are used as adjuncts to preventive dental treatment. They are particularly helpful in patients with plaque control problems and offer a "site-specific" approach to maintenance therapies and antimicrobial solutions. Therefore incorporation of oral irrigation into daily home care practices and in-office treatments may result in improved treatment outcomes.

ACTIVITIES

1. Select a variety of articles about antimicrobial agents from the references or update the list with recent articles. Divide the class into small groups. Ask each group to discuss two or three articles and summarize the findings as compared with information in the chapter.
2. Design a mini-clinical study. Select various nonprescription plaque control preparations. Design a clin-

ical protocol to be used for a period of time. Divide the class into groups, decide what procedures and measurements will be standardized. Carry out the plan, share data, and dicuss the experience.

3. Practice using standard and subgingival oral irrigation tips. Troubleshoot problems that may occur during use. Using nontechnical language, write directions for a patient describing how to use irrigation equipment.

REVIEW QUESTIONS

1. True or false
   a. The oral irrigator's usefulness is limited to flushing away food debris.
   b. The oral irrigator changes the quality if not the quantity of plaque on the teeth.
   c. The irrigator (even with a supragingival standard tip) can deliver liquids approximately halfway into the pocket.
   d. A cannula is a special cone-shaped plastic tip used by the patient at home to carry antimicrobials to the pocket.
   e. Chlorhexidine may alter taste sensation, stain teeth, and irritate the buccal mucosa.
   f. Antibiotics are not useful in supressing proliferating pathologic bacteria.
   g. Periodic professional subgingival debridement and daily home care can prevent the recurrence of disease by disrupting the subgingival microflora, especially if an oral irrigator, used with an antimicrobial agent, is part of the home therapy.

2. List the active agent in each of the following antimicrobials:
   a. Listerine
   b. Viadent
   c. Stannous fluoride
   d. Peridex

REFERENCES

Aday B: *An evaluation of an oral irrigation device's ability to quantitatively reduce the bacterial count of spirochetes, filaments, fusiforms, and motile bacteria from subgingival plaque*, thesis, Kansas City, 1982, University of Missouri.

Aziz-Gandour IA, Newman HN: The effects of a simplified oral hygiene regime plus supragingival irrigation with chlorhexidine or metronidazole on chronic inflammatory periodontal disease, *J Clin Periodontol* 13:228, 1986.

Bakdash MB: Patient motivation and education: a conceptual model, *Clin Prev Dent* 1(2):10, 1979.

Boyd RL et al: Effect of self-administered daily irrigation with 0.02% SnF$_2$ on periodontal disease activity, *J Clin Periodontol* 12:420, 1985.

Brady JM et al: Electron microscopic study of the effect of water jet devices on dental plaque, *J Dent Res* 52:1310, 1973.

Braun RE et al: Periodontal picket depth of delivery with a subgingival irrigating tip, *J Dent Res* 69(abstract 119): 1990.

Brownstein C et al: *Gingival irrigation with chlorhexidine resolves naturally occurring gingivitis*. Paper presented at the annual meeting of the American Academy of Periodontology, 1987, San Antonio, Tex.

Carranza FA, Jr: *Glickman's clinical periodontology*, Philadelphia, 1979, WB Saunders.

Cerra M, Killoy W: The effect of sodium bicarbonate and hydrogen peroxide on the microbial flora of periodontal pockets, *J Periodontol* 53:599, 1982.

Ciancio SG et al: Effect of a chemotherapeutic agent delivered by an oral irrigation device on plaque, gingivitis and subgingival microflora, *J Periodontol* 60:310, 1989.

Cobb CM, Rogers RL, Killoy WJ: Ultrastructure examination of human periodontal pockets following the use of an oral irrigation device in vivo, *J Periodontol* 59:155, 1988.

Cumming BR, Löe H: Optimal dosage and method of delivering chlorhexidine solutions for the inhibition of dental plaque, *J Periodont Res* 8:57, 1973.

DePaola LG et al: Chemotherapeutic inhibition of supragingival dental plaque and gingivitis development, *J Clin Periodontol* 16:311, 1989.

Derdivanis JP, Bushmaker S, Dagenais F: Effects of a mouthwash in an irrigating device on accumulation and maturation of dentalplaque, *J Periodontol* 49:81, 1978.

Eakle WS, Ford C, Boyd RL: Depth of penetration in periodontal pockets with oral irrigation, *J Clin Periodontol* 13:39, 1985.

Emling RC, Yankell SL: First clinical studies of a new prebrushing mouthrinse, *Comp Contin Educ Dent* 9:636, 1985.

Flemmig TF et al: Supragingival irrigation with 0.06% chlorhexidine in naturally occurring gingivitis. I. 6 month clinical observations, *J Periodontol* 61:112, 1990.

Gabler WL, Roberts D, Harold W: The effect of chlorhexidine on blood cells, *J Periodontol Res* 22:150, 1987.

Genco RL: Using antimicrobial agents to manage periodontal diseases, *JADA* 122:31, 1991.

Gjermo P: Chlorhexidine and related compounds, *J Dent Res* 68 (special issue):1602, 1989.

Gordon JM, Lamster IB. Sieger MC: Efficacy of Listerine antiseptic in inhibiting the development of plaque and gingivitis, *J Clin Periodontol* 12:697, 1985.

Greenwell HG et al: Clinical and microbiologic effectiveness of Keyes' method of oral hygiene on human periodontitis treated with and without surgery, *JADA* 106:457, 1983.

Grossman E et al: Six-month study of the effects of a chlorhexidine mouthrinse on gingivitis in adults, *J Periodont Res* 16 (suppl):33, 1986.

Gusberti FA et al: Microbiological and clinical effects of chlorhexidine digluconate and hydrogen peroxide mouthrinses on developing plaque and gingivitis, *J Clin Periodontol* 15:60, 1988.

Hannah J et al: Long-term clinical evaluation of toothpaste and oral rinse containing sanguinaria extract in controlling plaque, gingival inflammation, and sulcular bleeding during orthodontic treatment, *Am J Orthod Dentofac Orthop* 96:199, 1989.

Hardy JH, Newman HN, Strahan JD: Direct irrigation and subgingival plaque, *J Clin Periodontol* 9:57, 1982.

Harper DS et al: Clinical efficacy of a dentifrice and oral rinse containing sanguinaria extract and zinc chloride during six months of use, *J Periodontol* 61:352, 1990.

Harper DS et al: *J Dent Res* 70(special issue): 1991 (abstract 474).

Hoover DR et al: The comparative effectiveness of a pulsating oral irrigator as an adjunct in maintaining oral health, *J Clin Periodontol* 42:37, 1971.

Jolkovsky DL et al: Clinical and microbial effects of subgingival margin irrigation with chlorhexidine, *J Periodontol* 61:663, 1990.

Kelly A et al: Pressures recorded during periodontal pocket irrigation, *J Periodontol* 56:297, 1985.

Kopczyk RA et al: Clinical and microbiological effects of a sanguinaria-containing mouthrinse and dentifrice with and without fluoride during 6 months of use, *J Periodontol* 62:617, 1991.

Kornman KS: The role of supragingival plaque in the etiology and management of periodontal disease, *J Perio Res* (suppl):5, 1986.

Lamster IB et al: The effect of Listerine antiseptic on reduction of existing plaque and gingivitis, *Clin Prev Dent* 5(6):12, 1983.

Lang NP, Raber K: Use of oral irrigators as a vehicle for the application of antimicrobial agents in chemical plaque control, *J Clin Periodontol* 8:177, 1981.

Lang NP, Ramseier-Grossman K: Optimal dosage of chlorhexidine digluconate in chemical plaque control when applied by the oral irrigator, *J Clin Periodontol* 8:189, 1981.

Lang NP et al: Effects of supervised chlorhexidine mouthrinses in children, *J Periodontol Res* 17:100, 1982.

Lobene RR: The effect of a pulsed water pressure cleansing device on oral health, *J Periodontol* 40:667, 1969.

Lobene RR et al: Long-term evaluation of a prebrushing dental rinse for the control of dental plaque and gingivitis, *Clin Prev Dent* 12(2):26, 1990.

Loesche WJ, Syed SA: Bacteriology of human experimental gingivitis—effect on plaque and gingivitis scores, *Infect Immun* 21:830, 1978.

Mazza JW, Newman MG, Sims TN: Clinical and antimicrobial effect of stannous fluoride on periodontitis, *J Clin Periodontol* 8:203, 1981.

Miyasaki TI, Genco RJ, Wilson ME: Antimicrobial properties of hydrogen and sodium bicarbonate individually and in combination against selected oral gram negative facultative bacteria, *J Dent Res* 65:1142, 1986.

Newman MG et al: Irrigation with 0.06% chlorhexidine in naturally occurring gingivitis. II. 6 months microbiological observations, *J Periodontol* 61:427, 1990.

Parsons LG et al: Effect of sanguinaria extract on established plaque and gingivitis when delivered as a manual rinse or under pressure in an oral irrigator, *J Clin Periodontol* 14:381, 1987.

Perry DA et al: Stannous fluoride adjunct to root planing, clinical and antimicrobial effects, *J Dent Res* 63(special issue): 1984 (abstract 702).

Reitman WP et al: Proximal surface cleaning by dental floss, *Clin Prev Dent* 2:7, 1980.

Rosling BG et al: Topical chemical antimicrobial therapy in the management of the subgingival microflora and periodontal disease, *J Periodontol Res* 17:541, 1982.

Sanders PC, Linden GJ, Newman HN: The effects of a simplified mechanical oral hygiene regime plus supragingival irrigation with chlorhexidine or metronidazole on subgingival plaque, *J Clin Periodontol* 13:237, 1986.

Southard GL et al: Effect of sanguinaria extract on development of plaque and gingivitis when supragingivally delivered as a manual rinse or under pressure in an oral irrigator, *J Clin Periodontol* 14:377, 1987.

Tabita P et al: Effectiveness of supragingival plaque control on the development of subgingival plaque and gingival inflammation in patients with moderate pocket depth, *J Clin Periodontol* 52:88, 1981.

Tempel TR, Marcil JFA, Seibert JS: Comparison of water irrigation and oral rinsing on clearance of soluble and particulate materials from the oral cavity, *J Clin Periodontol* 46:391, 1975.

Waerhaug J: The interdental brush and its place in operative and crown and bridge dentistry, *J Oral Rehabil* 33:107, 1976.

Wagner MJ et al: Sodium retention from mouthwashes, *Clin Prev Dent* 11(4):3, 1989.

Watts EA, Newman HN: Clinical effects on chronic periodontitis of a simplified system of oral hygiene including subgingival pulsated jet irrigation with chlorhexidine, *J Clin Periodontol* 13:666, 1986.

West BL: *An evaluation of an oral irrigating device's ability to reduce the microbial count of subgingival plaque at six millimeters in depth*, thesis, Kansas City, 1982, University of Missouri.

West TL, King WJ: Toothbrushing with hydrogen peroxide–sodium bicarbonate compared to toothpowder and water in reducing periodontal pocket suppuration darkfield bacterial counts, *J Periodontol* 54:339, 1983.

White CL et al: The effect of supervised water irrigation on the subgingival microflora of untreated gingivitis and periodontitis, *J Dent Res* 67(special issue): 1988 (abstract 2298).

Wolff LF et al: Four-year investigation of salt and peroxide regimen compared with conventional oral hygiene, *JADA* 118: 65, 1989. Legends

29 PERIODONTAL DRESSINGS AND SUTURING

Trisha E. O'Hehir
Nancy Stutsman Young

LEARNING OUTCOMES

The dental hygienist will be able to

1. List and explain the functions of a periodontal pack.
2. Compare and contrast the properties of a pack that contains eugenol with those of a pack that does not contain eugenol.
3. Describe the placement of a periodontal pack on surgical areas with and without missing teeth.
4. Describe the removal of sutures and of a periodontal pack.
5. Place and remove a periodontal pack on a typodont and/or partner.
6. Place and remove sutures in a simulated situation.
7. Instruct a patient in caring for a periodontal pack.

Dental hygienists are assuming an ever expanding role in the treatment of periodontal disease. More and more dentists and periodontists are using the skills of dental hygienists in the treatment of periodontal disease to provide a team approach that maximizes the training and skills of both types of professionals for the effective and efficient delivery of services to dental care consumers. Among the periodontal treatment procedures that the dental hygienist is qualified to perform are the placement and removal of periodontal dressings after surgical treatment and the removal of sutures following soft tissue healing. In some states, dental hygienists are also licensed to place sutures. This chapter describes both periodontal dressings and suturing.

PURPOSE OF PERIODONTAL DRESSINGS

Periodontal dressings are mixtures of special materials that are initially soft and puttylike in consistency so that they can easily be placed over and adapted to surgically treated oral tissues. After the dressings are properly placed, they harden in the mouth to form a rigid and protective covering for these tissues while they heal. Periodontal dressings have two primary functions: (1) to protect the surgical area and thus promote healing and (2) to increase postsurgical patient comfort. The dressing itself does not contain substances that directly stimulate healing, but it does protect the healing surgical area from irritants such as hot or spicy foods, sharp pieces of food, and mechanical trauma during chewing. Periodontal dressings also protect newly exposed root surfaces from temperature changes, stabilize mobile teeth, protect sutures, help maintain the position of repositioned soft tissues, help control bleeding, and act as a template to prevent formation of excessive granulation tissue (Baer et al, 1969; Blanque, 1962; Carranza and Perry, 1986; Goldman and Cohen, 1980; Grant, Stern, and Everett, 1988; Levin, 1980; Valentine, 1976; Watts and Combe, 1979). Periodontal dressings have been used after most types of periodontal surgery, including flap procedures, gingivectomy, gingivoplasty, mucogingival surgery, and occasionally soft tissue curettage procedures (Carranza, 1984; Goldman and Cohen, 1980; Valentine, 1976; Watts and Combe, 1979).

PRESENT STATUS AND VALUE OF A PERIODONTAL DRESSING

There has been a great deal of debate regarding the value and usefulness of periodontal dressings for routine use following all surgical procedures. Experimental evidence has yet to resolve this controversy. A number of reports have indicated that the routine use of periodontal dressings may not achieve either of the two goals for which they are placed—improved healing and increased patient comfort. Probably the biggest concern is that the presence of a periodontal dressing promotes the accumulation of plaque in and around the wound site. The dressing itself is a plaque-retentive surface that favors the accumulation of plaque. In addition, the presence of the dressing prevents the patient from adequately removing plaque and debris from the area and prevents antibacterial rinses (e.g., chlorhexidine) from reaching the healing surfaces. As a result, inflammation is more likely to occur and healing may be retarded. Studies of the healing process of surgically treated areas found that the tissues healed just as well with or without periodontal dressings (Allen and Caffesse, 1983; Greensmith and Wade, 1974; Jones and Cassingham, 1979; Stahl et al, 1969). Heaney and Appleton (1976) found that the presence of a dressing was associated with increased inflammation and suggested that dressings should be removed within 1 week of surgery. Wampole and colleagues (1978) found a 24% incidence of bacteremia at the time that the postsurgical dressing was changed. They noted that these findings could have serious implications for patients who were already medically compromised and susceptible to systemic infection. Several of these studies asked patients who had experienced surgery both with and without periodontal dressings which approach they preferred. Many patients reported a preference for no dressing and some even said that they experienced more pain as a result of wearing a periodontal dressing (Allen and Caffesse, 1983; Greensmith and Wade, 1974; Jones and Cassingham, 1979). It would seem from these reports that if the surgical procedure is completed in such a way that the flap is well adapted, the flap serves as a sufficient barrier to infection. Open access to the area also allows the individual to cleanse and rinse it thoroughly to keep the area clean. In many cases, depending on the type of surgery, the patient may be more comfortable without a dressing (Sachs et al, 1984).

Although these reports question the need for routine use of periodontal dressings, there will always be circumstances in which a periodontal dressing is indicated. Dressings may be indicated for retention of an apically positioned flap so that it will not be displaced coronally, for additional support to stabilize a free gingival graft, to protect exposed bone from injury during the early stages of healing and thereby reduce patient discomfort, to act as a guide for healing to prevent overgrowth of granulation tissue (Sachs et al, 1984), or to hold slow-release local delivery fibers, gels, or chips in place in the pocket as they dispense medication. The choice of whether to use a dressing depends on the nature of the surgery and the preferences of the dentist or periodontist. The routine use of periodontal dressings following surgery has decreased as a result of better surgical techniques and increased use of antibacterial mouthrinses (Sachs et al, 1984).

TYPES OF PERIODONTAL DRESSINGS

Several different materials are used in the formulation of periodontal dressings. The two most widely used types of dressing materials are zinc oxide–eugenol and zinc oxide–noneugenol dressings. In addition, cyanoacrylates, modified methacrylic gels, and collagen sponges have also been studied for use as periodontal dressings.

The inclusion of eugenol in periodontal dressings is somewhat controversial, and its safety and value as an ingredient in periodontal dressings have been investigated and analyzed by many researchers and clinicians (Baer et al, 1969; Carranza and Perry, 1986; Frisch and Bhaskar, 1967; Goldman and Cohen, 1980; Haugen, 1980; Haugen and Gjermo, 1978; Haugen and Mjor, 1979; Levin, 1980). Eugenol is the main chemical constituent of clove oil, which explains its clovelike odor. It is combined with vegetable oils as the liquid component of zinc oxide–eugenol. As an antiseptic and an anodyne, eugenol is considered to be an *obtundent* material, meaning that it is soothing to living tissues. Some investigators believe that eugenol is an obtundent to all tissues, including bone, and that it should be used in all dressings to promote healing and patient comfort. Other investigators believe that eugenol is irritating to bone and might even stimulate its destruction, and, therefore, that it should not be included in periodontal dressing materials. Reports of animal studies in which zinc oxide–eugenol dressings were placed against exposed bone indicate that there is incomplete healing, or destruction, of the bone as a result of these substances (Carranza and Perry, 1986; Goldman and Cohen, 1980; Haugen and Mjor, 1979; Levin, 1980). Studies done in animals and humans to compare wound healing with zinc oxide–eugenol and zinc oxide–noneugenol dressings have shown no difference in epithelialization and wound healing in spite of the previously mentioned reports of bone destruction (Frisch and Bhaskar, 1967; Haugen, 1980; Haugen and Gjermo, 1978; Levin, 1980). There is no conclusive research to direct the clinician to choose one type over another using the criterion of compatibility with oral tissues, especially bone.

Many clinicians select the type of periodontal dressing on the basis of factors other than the absence or presence of eugenol, such as ease of manipulation, consistency of the dressing, and storage factors. Another important criterion for selection of dressing materials is the potential of patient sensitivity to their ingredients. The dental literature contains several reports of allergic reactions to the eugenol in some dressing materials (Barkin, 1984; Poulson, 1974). In addition, an allergic response to rosin has been described (Lysell, 1976). To decrease the probability that allergic reactions will develop as a result of the presence of periodontal dressings, it is important to assess the patient's history of allergic reactions and relate the allergens to the ingredients in dressing materials.

In general, the antimicrobial qualities of a dressing seem to have only minor effects on wound healing, and the addition of antimicrobial agents to dressings is of questionable merit. The benefits of the antimicrobial substances must be weighed against their potential for causing allergic responses or sensitivity or for altering the normal oral flora (Sachs et al, 1984).

The use of chlorhexidine as an intraoral antibacterial rinse following surgical procedures has shown merit. Although the effect of the rinse is apparently blocked if a dressing is used, it is quite effective in reducing plaque formation and associated inflammation when the surgical site remains exposed to the oral cavity (Addy and Dolby, 1976; Addy et al, 1975; Pluss et al, 1975). The ability of chlorhexidine to inhibit plaque growth makes it a valuable asset in postsurgical care (Sachs et al, 1984).

Zinc oxide–eugenol dressings

Dressings containing eugenol are prepared by mixing a powder and a liquid. The powder is composed of zinc oxide, tannic acid, and rosin. Some powders also contain ingredients such as

Table 29-1. Ingredients and some of the functions of a zinc oxide–eugenol dressing*

Ingredient	Amount	Function
Powder (each 100 g)		
Zinc oxide	40 g	Setting reaction; slightly antiseptic and astringent
Rosin	40 g	Filler to increase strength
Tannic acid	20 g	Slightly hemostatic
Liquid (each 100 ml)		
Eugenol	46.5 ml	Setting reaction; slightly anesthetic; obtundent
Peanut oil	46.5 ml	Regulates setting time
Rosin	7.5 ml	Filler to increase strength

From American Dental Association Council on Dental Therapeutics: *Accepted dental therapeutics,* ed 40, Chicago, 1984, The Association.
*Kirkland Pack, Pulpdent Corp. of America, Brookline, Mass.

kaolin, zinc stearate, or asbestos. Asbestos fibers have been associated with lung disease and are considered a health hazard to dental personnel who prepare the dressings containing asbestos (Bakdash, 1976). Although there is no apparent danger from asbestos to patients after the dressing has been mixed, most products no longer contain asbestos. Tannic acid has also been omitted by some manufacturers because its absorption has been associated with liver disease (American Dental Association [ADA], 1984; Baer et al, 1969; Watts and Combe, 1979). The liquid contains eugenol and an oil such as mineral or peanut oil. Ingredients to modify or improve the color and flavor of the dressing may also be included (ADA, 1984; Carranza and Perry, 1986; Watts and Combe, 1979). Table 29-1 lists the ingredients in one commonly used eugenol dressing and the function of each.

When the components of the zinc oxide–eugenol dressing are mixed, setting (hardening) occurs as a result of the chemical interaction between zinc oxide and eugenol, forming zinc eugenolate. This reaction is a slow one, allowing sufficient time to form, place, adapt, and trim the dressing to fit the wound site before the dressing hardens and becomes brittle. Not all of the eugenol is converted to zinc eugenolate during the reaction, with the result that a certain amount of free, unreacted eugenol is present in the dressing mixture. Because the presence of this free eugenol has been associated with harmful effects on oral tissues in some cases, the use of this type of dressing is controversial.

One reason that clinicians prefer zinc oxide-eugenol dressings is that the material can be mixed in a large quantity, divided into smaller amounts, wrapped tightly, and frozen. After dressing material has been frozen, it must be defrosted to room temperature before it can be used. The ability to mix this material in advance is an advantage because the initial mixing is time consuming. Another advantage of eugenol-containing dressings is that they have a consistency that is firm, heavy, and easy to manipulate. These dressing materials do not stick to the clinician's fingers as readily as the noneugenol materials. A related disadvantage, however, is that the firmness of the material makes it necessary for the clinician to use more pressure to manipulate and adapt the dressing to the soft tissues. Because excessive pressure can displace newly repositioned flaps, a softer dressing material is preferred for these situations.

Zinc oxide–noneugenol dressings

The most common and widely used noneugenol periodontal dressing (Coe-Pack, GC America) is supplied as two pastes or as an automixing system contained within a syringe.

One of the pastes contains zinc oxide, magnesium oxide, and hexachlorophene; the other contains hydrogenated rosin, chlorothymol, and benzyl alcohol (ADA, 1984; Carranza and Perry, 1986; Goldman and Cohen, 1980; Watts and Combe, 1979). Table 29-2 lists the ingredients and functions of each paste. When the two pastes are mixed together, a setting reaction that causes the material to harden occurs between a metallic ion and fatty acids.

The two-paste, noneugenol dressing should be mixed at the time of placement. When first mixed it has a very pliable consistency, making it the ideal choice for placement over a repositioned flap or over other fragile tissues. The noneugenol dressing can be made firmer by adding zinc oxide powder, which is usually mixed with a eugenol liquid; the addition of the powder gives the final dressing material more body and makes it less sticky (Valentine, 1976). Placing a noneugenol dressing in a cup of cold water for several minutes after it is mixed also will have this effect. Noneugenol dressings usually have a more pleasant taste than dressings containing eugenol. Peri-

Table 29-2. Ingredients and some of the functions of a zinc oxide–noneugenol dressing*

Ingredient	Percentage	Function
Paste 1 (pink)		
Zinc oxide	45	Slightly antiseptic and astringent
Magnesium oxide	32	Setting reaction
Peanut oil	11	
Mineral oil	6	Regulate setting time
Rosin oil	3	
Other formulating and bacteriostatic agents	3	Bacteriostatic
Paste 2 (amber)		
Polymerized rosin	53	Increases strength
Coconut fatty acid	30	Setting reaction
Chlorothymol	3	Bacteriostatic
Peruvian balsam	3	Unspecified
Other formulating agents	3	Unspecified

From American Dental Association Council on Dental Therapeutics: *Accepted dental therapeutics,* ed 40, Chicago, 1984, The Association.

odontal dressing products are constantly being improved in terms of strength, setting time, handling characteristics, and patient acceptance.

The automixing system is contained within a syringe. The syringe is made up of two separate cylinders, each containing one of the pastes. As the trigger is pulled, the two pastes mix within the tip of the syringe. The dressing material is then deposited on a mixing pad and within 30 seconds it can be handled and formed into the appropriate shape for placement in the mouth. A slight change in the chemistry of the dressing was necessary to make it thin enough to use in the automixing syringe. This dressing will set slightly harder than the manually mixed system.

Premixed zinc oxide–noneugenol dressings are also available. One such dressing, Peripac (de Trey Frères, S.A., Zurich, Switzerland) contains calcium phosphate, zinc oxide, acrylate, organic solvent, and flavoring and coloring agents (Haugen and Gjermo, 1978). When this material is exposed to air or moisture, it sets by the loss of organic solvent (Watts and Combe, 1979). After it is set, this dressing becomes quite brittle. The Peripac is not as popular as the zinc oxide–noneugenol dressing. Use of these materials has been associated with greater patient pain and swelling than with other dressings (Haugen and Gjermo, 1978). A review of the literature on the physical properties of periodontal dressings indicated that none of the currently used dressings have ideal properties for clinical use and that further research is needed to improve these properties (Sachs et al, 1984).

Collagen dressings

A recent addition to the list of dressings is the collagen sponge. An example of this dressing is CollaCote, (Helitrex, Inc.). This material is type 1 collagen, which is derived from bovine Achilles tendon. It is a completely resorbable dressing that is used to cover and protect palatal graft sites. The sponge is approximately 3 mm thick and can be cut to fit the graft site. It stops bleeding and can absorb 30 to 40 times its weight in fluid, without swelling. In addition to periodontal applications, it is also used following dental extractions.

Cyanoacrylate dressings

A number of researchers have investigated the use of cyanoacrylate as an alternative to suturing and as a surface adhesive and periodontal dressing (Forrest, 1974; Frisch and Bhaskar, 1967; Levin et al, 1975; Ochstein et al, 1969). This material has the unique ability to cement together moist, living tissue surfaces. Cyanoacrylate is either applied in drops or sprayed on the tissue. This method of application is time saving and relatively easy to perform. The characteristics of cyanoacrylate make it a near-ideal periodontal dressing. The material is much less bulky than other dressings. Other advantages include the lack of apparent side effects, easy adherence to living tissues, immediate hemostasis, lack of evidence of systemic toxicity or sensitivity, excellent healing results, precision placement of flaps, decreased suturing time, ease of application, reapplication over existing material, and patient preference over bulky dressings. Cyanoacrylates have been used for surface application only; adhesive that becomes trapped under the soft tissue flap will delay wound healing (Forrest, 1974; Levin, 1980; Levin et al, 1975; McGraw and Caffesse, 1978; Watts and Combe, 1979.) Cyanoacrylate dressings have not yet been approved for other than research use in the United States.

Methacrylic gel dressings

Methacrylic gels are used primarily in dentistry as tissue conditioners or denture liners. They have an elastic-like consistency that is soft and resilient and will flow under pressure, making them ideal for use in dentures. These gels adapt closely to the tissues and are very compatible with the wound site. Tissue conditioners cannot be used alone as dressings because of their poor retention, but they have been used in conjunction with a zinc oxide-noneugenol dressing (Addy et al, 1975; Levin, 1980; Watts and Combe, 1979). Addy and others (1975) reported the application of an antibacterial agent (such as chlorhexidine) by means of a methacrylic gel and zinc oxide-noneugenol dressing. The major advantage of this material is its ability to carry and release medicaments to the soft tissues. Other properties of this material cause it to have less favorable adhesion and retention characteristics than other types of dressings. Methacrylic gel dressings are not widely used.

Addition of antibacterial agents

Antibiotics and other antibacterial agents have been added to periodontal dressings to reduce infection and to promote healing of surgically treated tissues. The effectiveness of adding antibacterial agents to dressings for this purpose, however, has not been proven conclusively (Haugen et al, 1977; O'Neill, 1975). Several concerns exist regarding the addition of antibiotic agents to periodontal dressings. One is that exposure to antibiotics can sensitize a patient to the agent, thereby limiting its application for controlling later infections. A second concern is that the ingredients in the dressing preparations inactivate the antibiotic. Therefore, the risks of antibiotic use may outweigh its intended benefits (Levin, 1980; Watts and Combe, 1979). The addition of chlorhexidine gluconate to methacrylic gel dressings has already been discussed as an effective means of promoting healing (Addy et al, 1975).

MIXING AND APPLICATION OF A PERIODONTAL DRESSING

The materials used for mixing and placing a periodontal dressing are shown in Fig. 29-1. Petroleum jelly is used to lubricate the patient's lips, and the tongue blade is used to mix the dressing components together. The curette and/or cotton pliers are used to adapt the dressing into the inter-

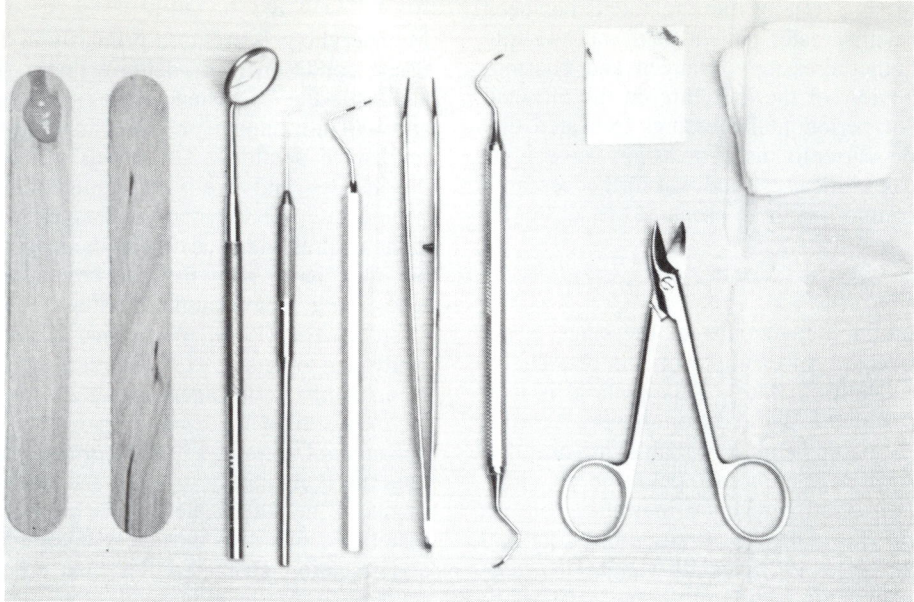

Fig. 29-1. Tray setup for placement of periodontal dressing: petroleum jelly, tongue blade, mirror, explorer, probe, cotton pliers, curette, dry foil, scissors, and gauze.

proximal areas of the wound site. The dry foil may be used to protect the dressing until it hardens.

Preparing the patient

The hygienist should discuss the purpose of the periodontal dressing with the patient and describe how it will be placed, as well as how it will taste, feel, and look in the mouth. When the patient and clinician are ready to begin, the patient's lips should be lubricated with a light coating of petroleum jelly to prevent the moist and sticky dressing material from adhering to the lips while it is being placed. Because noneugenol dressing is commonly used in clinical practice, the technique for mixing and adapting this type of dressing will be discussed first. Later sections will supply additional information on the handling of other types of dressing materials.

Mixing a noneugenol dressing

The following steps are used to prepare a noneugenol dressing. First, mix the dressing according to the manufacturer's directions. For the product shown in the figures, equal lengths of each component paste are expressed from the tubes and mixed until they are well blended and the color is homogeneous (Figs. 29-2 and 29-3). The particular stroke used for mixing is not an important consideration, as it is with some dental materials. Zinc oxide powder may be added to the mix to make the material stronger and less sticky (Figs. 29-4 and 29-5). After the material is mixed, roll it between the palms of the hands (gloves should always be worn) to form it into cylinders about two-thirds the diameter of a pencil (Fig. 29-6). The length of the roll should correspond to the length of the area to be covered by the dressing.

Placing the dressing

Using sterile gauze, gently dry the area to be covered. Bleeding should be controlled before the dressing is placed. Although the dressing will help control bleeding, it should not be considered the primary means of control. If slight bleeding is present, apply pressure to the area with a sterile gauze sponge until it subsides. If this approach does not stop the bleeding, or if profuse bleeding occurs, hemostatic agents or other control measures may be required (Carranza and Perry, 1986). After the bleeding has been controlled and the area has been dried, place the roll of dressing

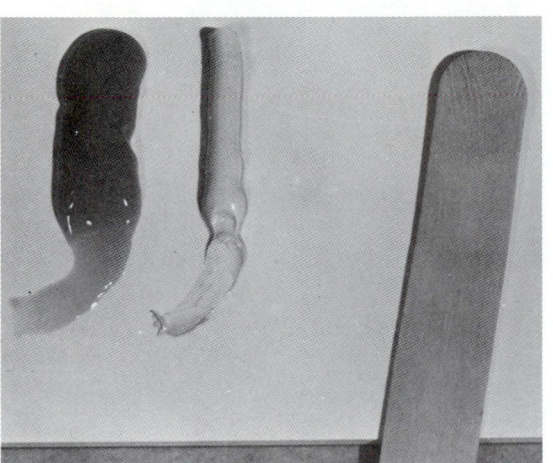

Fig. 29-2. Equal lengths of noneugenol pastes expressed onto pad.

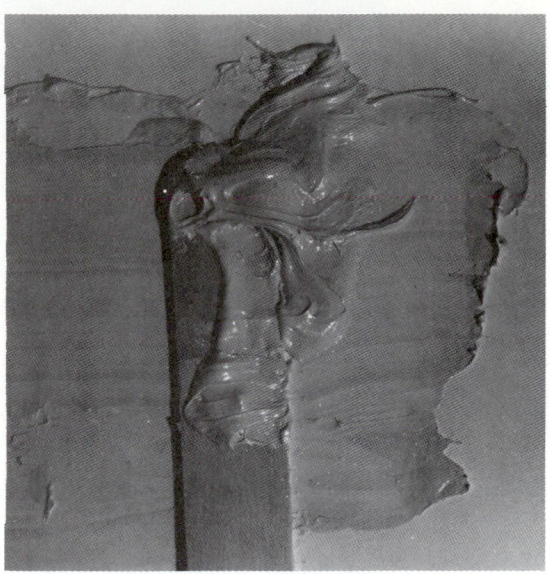

Fig. 29-3. Pastes are mixed until color is homogeneous.

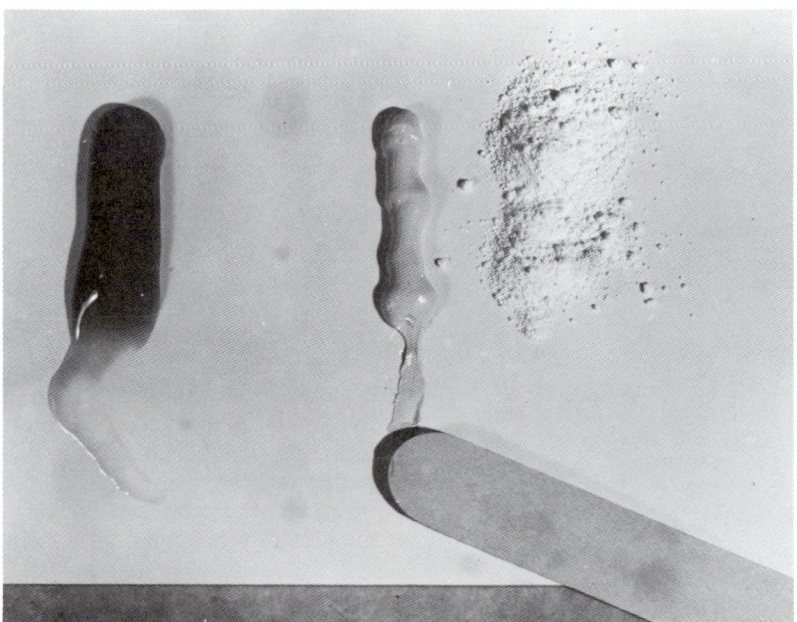

Fig. 29-4. To improve strength and workability, zinc oxide powder is incorporated into paste 1 and then mixed with paste 2.

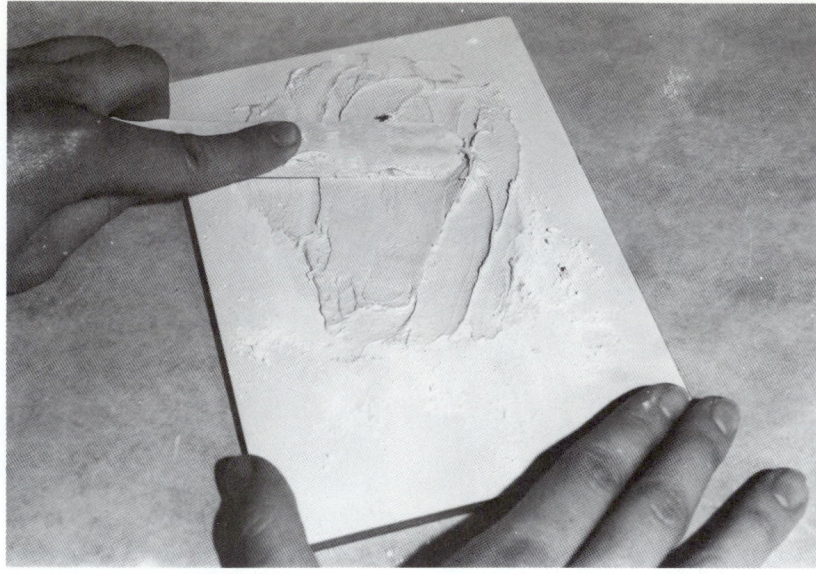

Fig. 29-5. Paste 1, with zinc oxide powder, is being mixed with paste 2 until color is homogeneous.

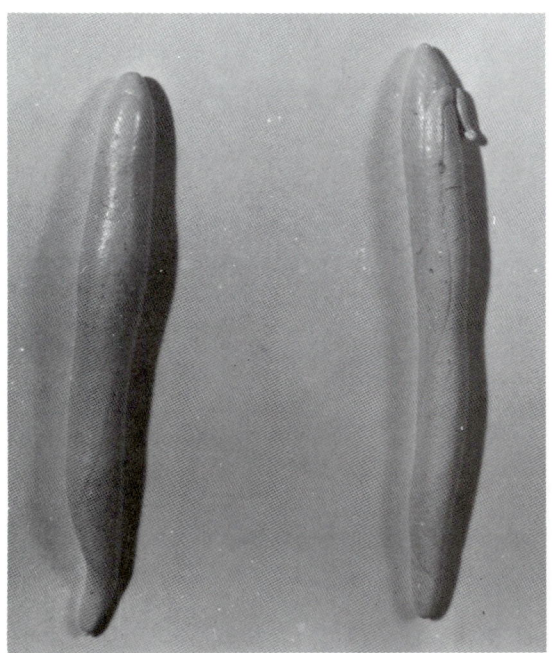

Fig. 29-6. After complete and proper mixing, two rolls, approximating length of wound, are formed.

material so that it wraps around the most distal tooth in the area to be covered. Adapt the dressing to the area by pressing it gently against the wound site and flattening it against the teeth and the soft tissues. The dressing should extend over the entire wound site up to the most anterior tooth involved (Fig. 29-7).

Apply a separate roll of material to the opposite side of the involved area (Fig. 29-8). After placing the rolls of material so that they extend the entire length of the wound site, adapt the material to the teeth and gingiva, using a finger that has been wrapped with damp gauze (Fig. 29-9). Gently compress and flatten the dressing against the teeth and periodontal tissues. Adapt the dressing farther into the interproximal areas using the back of a curette or cotton pliers (Fig. 29-10). Adapt the dressing far enough into the interproximal areas that the facial and lingual surfaces of the dressing are joined together to form a mechanical lock between the dressing and the teeth. If the interproximal spaces are large enough, place small wedges of dressing material in each interproximal area before placing the facial and lingual dressings. As the dressing is adapted, the interproximal

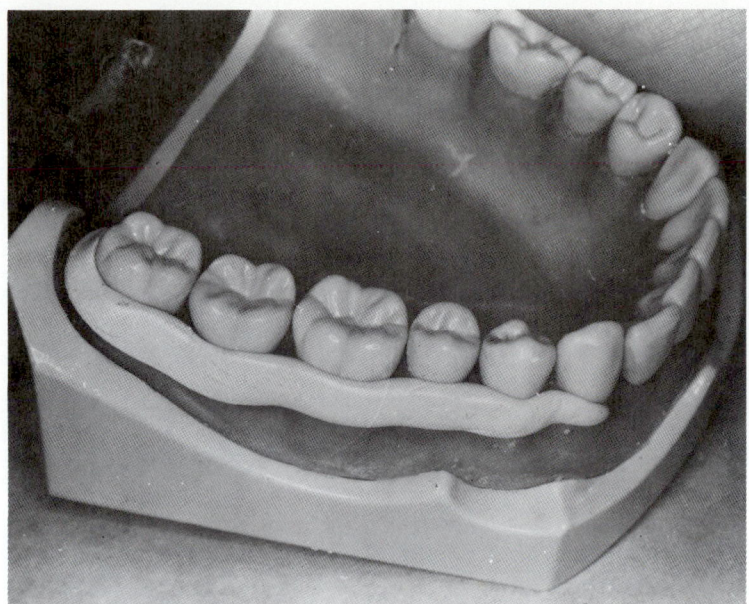

Fig. 29-7. One roll is applied to buccal surface. It is wrapped around distal-most tooth and extends to most anterior tooth.

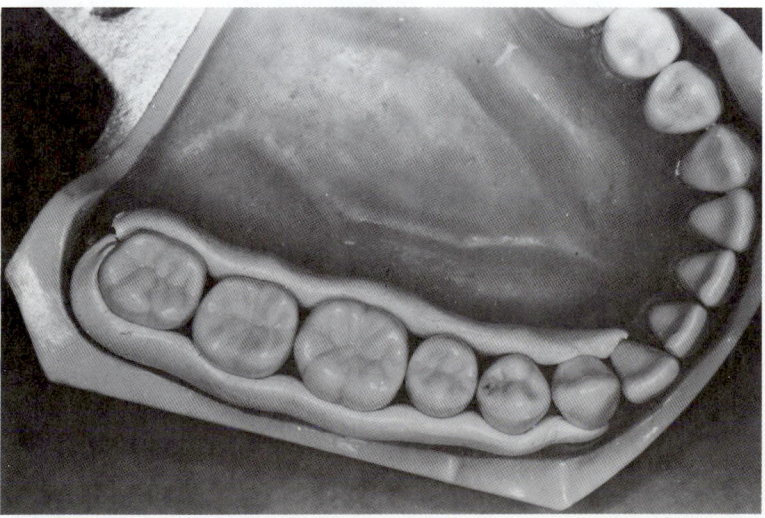

Fig. 29-8. Other roll is applied to lingual surface but is not yet adapted into interproximal areas.

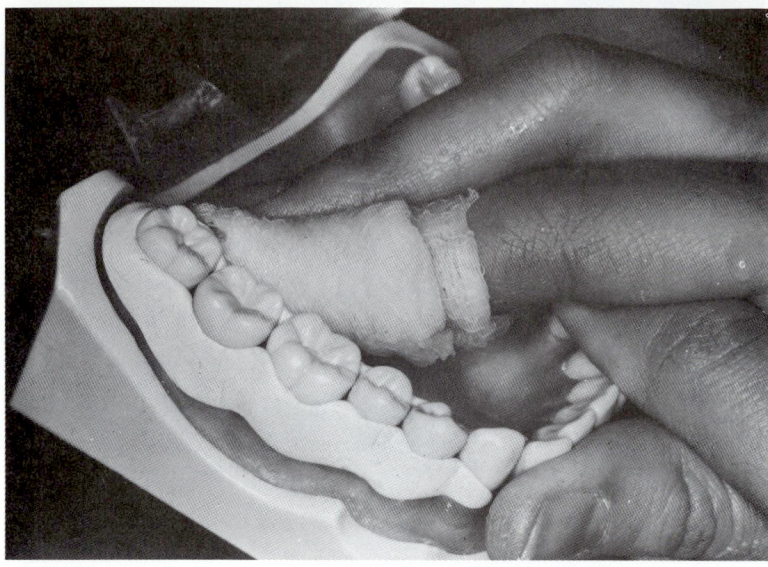

Fig. 29-9. Dressing is adapted with damp gauze wrapped around clinician's finger. (Note: Under normal clinical circumstances gloves should always be worn.)

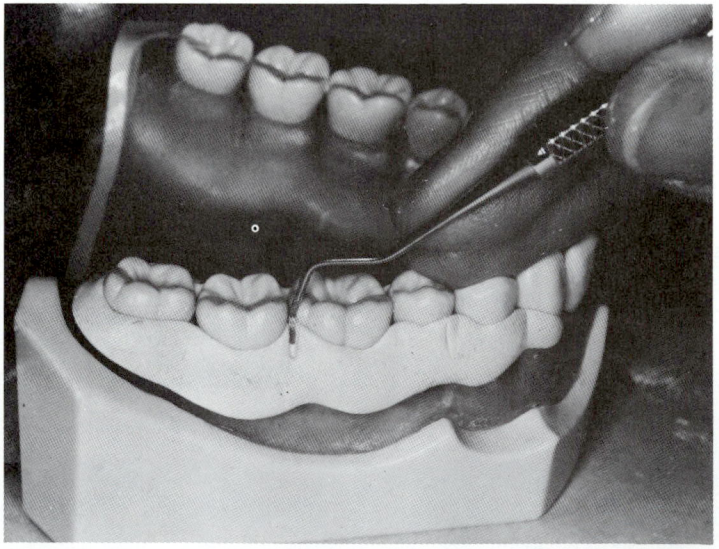

Fig. 29-10. Dressing is pressed into interproximal areas with back of a curette.

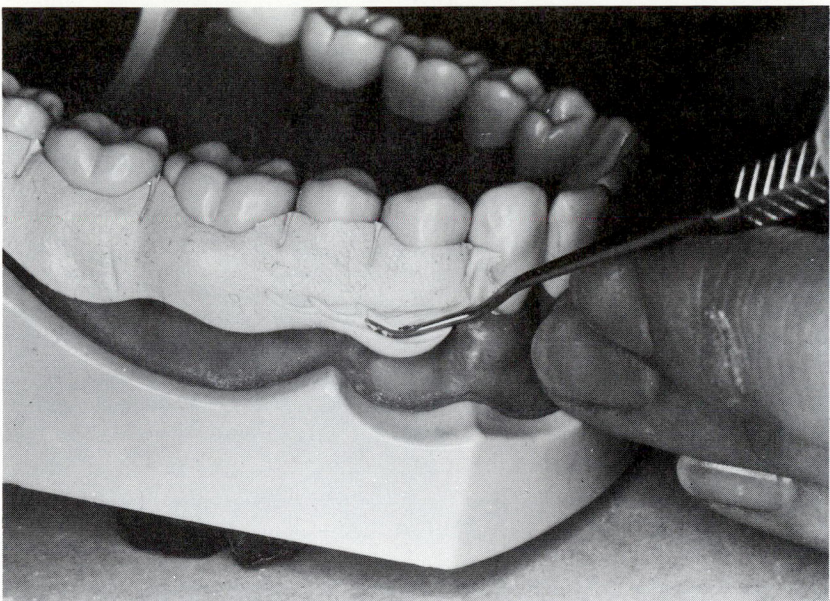

Fig. 29-11. Apical portion of pack is trimmed by gently and firmly pressing curette into material and peeling away excess material.

wedges and the facial and lingual pieces will join together. Even if the facial and lingual dressings do not join, a mechanical lock will still form in the embrasure areas between the teeth. This lock is important for retention of the dressing.

Muscle trimming and removing excess material

Careful molding of the periodontal dressing to the shape of the oral structures will permit the patient to perform normal activities without unnecessary interference or discomfort. After the dressing material has hardened, it should not impinge on the oral musculature. One way of ensuring that this does not occur is to "muscle trim" the dressing. This is done by extending the patient's lips and cheeks over the dressing while it is still soft to identify where it may interfere with muscle attachments. When the tissues are pulled against the apical margins of the dressing, the pressure of the soft tissues will cause the margin to fold occlusally in areas where the dressing interferes with muscle attachments or frenula. The clinician can see where this occurs and trim away the excess material until the interference is eliminated. Curettes can be used to trim excess dressing carefully away from soft tissues. The finished dressing should extend no further occlusally than the

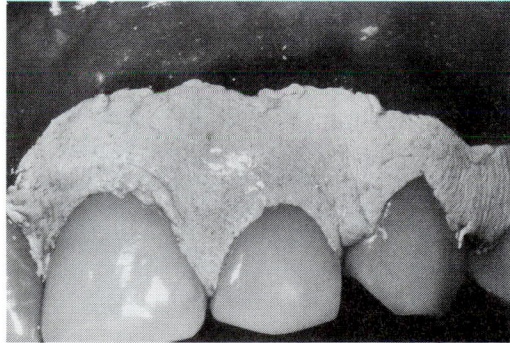

Fig. 29-12. Properly placed, adapted, and smoothed periodontal dressing. It has been muscle molded and trimmed so that none of the material impinges on soft tissue.

middle third of the teeth and should not interfere with normal occlusion. Dressing material that is present on occlusal surfaces or comes into contact with opposing teeth in occlusion must be removed (Fig. 29-11). The clinician must remember that after the dressing hardens it will be very brittle and may irritate soft tissue or break apart if it has not been properly adapted and trimmed. Every effort must be made to provide the patient with a well-contoured, smooth periodontal dressing that is as unobtrusive as possible (Fig. 29-12).

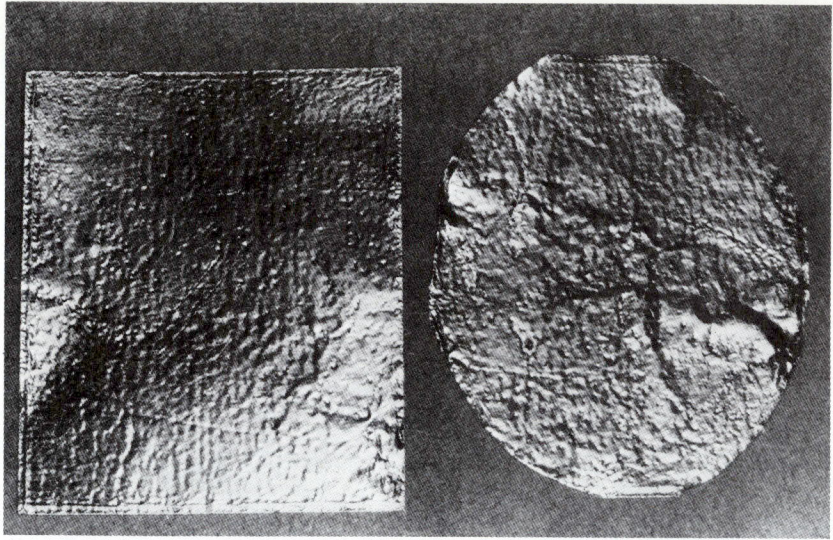

Fig. 29-13. Dry foil on left is as manufacturer supplies it. Foil on right is trimmed and ready to be applied.

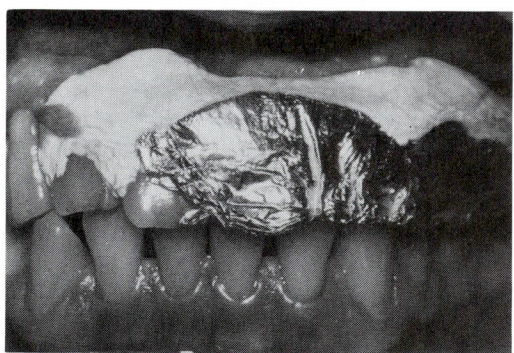

Fig. 29-14. This dry foil had been properly applied; use of foil in anterior is unusual, since it is not esthetically pleasing.

Applying dry foil

Although rarely used anymore, dry foil will be discussed for its historical place in the application of periodontal dressings. Dry foil is a specially treated paper that looks like a small rectangle of aluminum foil (Fig. 29-13). On its nonshiny side, it has an adhesive that can adhere to the periodontal dressing and teeth. Dry foil protects the outer surface of the dressing while it hardens by preventing food and other debris from becoming impregnated into the soft periodontal dressing material, and it helps hold the dressing in place (Fig.

29-14) (Grant, Stern, and Everett, 1988; Nelson et al, 1977; Valentine, 1976). Dry foil also can be placed between composite restorations of teeth and dressings to protect the restorations from deterioration (softening) caused by the components of dressing materials (Watts and Combe, 1981). The dry foil can be removed from the dressing several hours after it has been placed; the clinician can instruct the patient to remove the foil by peeling it away from the hardened dressing. Placing dry foil is not essential or crucial to the success of the periodontal dressing. A dressing will usually harden and remain on the teeth as long as necessary without the application of dry foil.

Evaluating the dressing

Evaluate the placement and adaptation of the dressing according to the criteria presented at the end of this chapter. If any of the criteria are not met, the clinician should modify the dressing appropriately. In most instances there is ample working time to modify or add to the dressing as needed. Some types of dressings, however, set very quickly after being exposed to air and moisture; they must be adapted very quickly before they become hard and brittle. Consult the manufacturer's directions for the exact amount of working time for each type of dressing material.

Date: _____

Dear: _____

    A periodontal dressing has been placed to protect your gums while they heal. The dressing should remain in place until your next appointment. A few instructions are listed below to help you care for your mouth while the dressing is in place.

1. Avoid eating, drinking or rinsing for the next hour. Avoid the following foods until the dressing has hardened completely (next 3 hours): hard foods (e.g., pretzels), sharp foods (e.g., potato chips), sticky foods (e.g., toffee), or spicy foods (e.g., pizza).
2. Avoid rinsing for the rest of the day. After that you may rinse your mouth with warm water or warm saltwater four or more times a day.
3. You may notice some bloodstains in your saliva for 4 to 5 hours. This is not unusual and will correct itself. If there is considerable bleeding, however, it can usually be stopped by applying pressure against both sides of the dressing with a gauze square in the area where the bleeding is originating. Apply firm pressure for 20 minutes. If the bleeding has not stopped after 20 minutes or if it becomes worse, please call the office for instructions. **Do not try to stop the bleeding by rinsing.**
4. Swelling is not unusual and will usually subside in 3 to 4 days. If it does become painful, however, or appears to worsen, please call the office.
5. To keep the dressing clean you can wipe it with moist gauze or cotton or brush it **gently** with a soft toothbrush. The rest of the areas of your mouth can be brushed and flossed as usual. **BE CAREFUL NOT TO DISLODGE THE DRESSING WHILE CLEANING THE MOUTH.**
6. Do not be concerned if pieces of the pack break off. It is not necessary to call us unless sharp edges are left to irritate your tongue or cheeks.
7. If the pack becomes dislodged from the area during the first 2 days after your surgery, please call the office. If it has been more than 2 days, there is probably no need to replace it unless you are experiencing significant discomfort. Simply rinse all fragments of the pack from your mouth and clean the tissues gently until your next appointment. Do not try to replace a dislodged dressing yourself.
8. Avoid smoking. The heat and smoke will irritate your gums and interfere with healing.
9. Be sure to return to the office for your follow-up appointment on _____.
    If you have any questions, please call the office at _____.

Fig. 29-15. Sample patient instruction sheet.

Patient instructions

After placing the dressing, instruct the patient about care of the dressing and oral hygiene procedures. Also provide complete written instructions that can be referred to at home (Fig. 29-15). The patient should be cautioned that the dressing will gradually harden and that care should be taken not to dislodge it within the first few hours. The patient should be advised to avoid eating or drinking within the first hour or until the dressing has hardened. Tart or spicy foods should be avoided immediately after surgery. If the dressing is brushed, it should be done very gently and only with a soft toothbrush. The patient should rinse the mouth thoroughly after eating and can brush and floss the other areas of the mouth. This includes careful brushing of the occlusal surfaces, which are not covered by the dressing.

    Provide the office phone number and tell the patient to call if an emergency arises. There may be some slight oozing of blood from the surgical area. Oozing is considered normal, but profuse bleeding should be reported. The patient should be given an appointment to return to the office in 3 to 5 days to have the dressing removed and the tissue evaluated. In some instances, depending on the type of surgery and the progress of healing, the dressing may be replaced for an additional period.

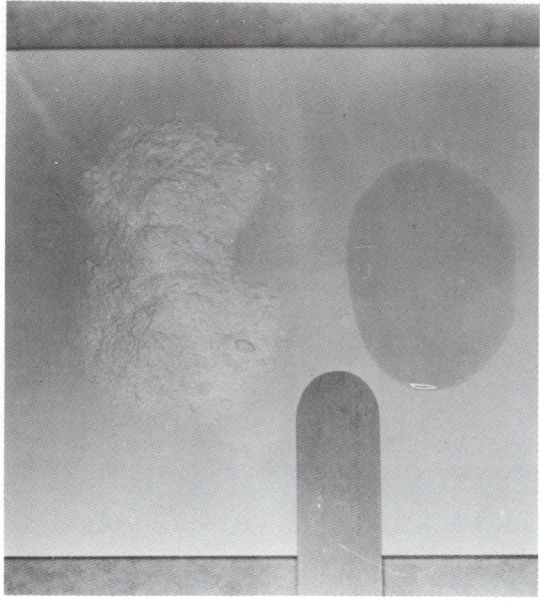

Fig. 29-16. Zinc oxide–eugenol powder and liquid placed on pad before mixing.

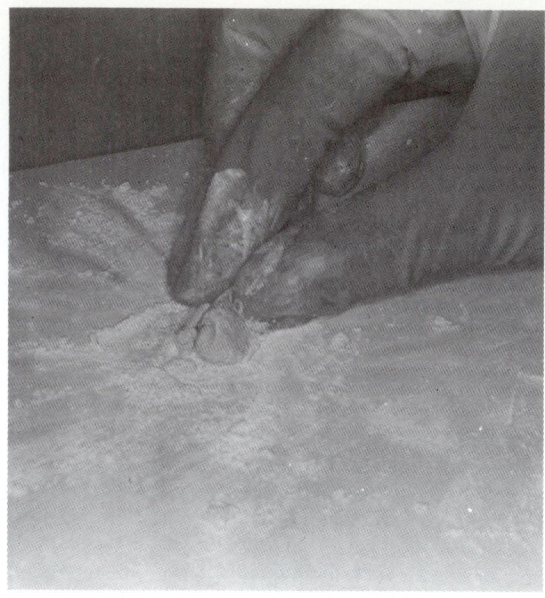

Fig. 29-17. After being mixed with tongue blade, material is kneaded to incorporate more powder.

Alternative dressing procedures

The technique for placing the dressing must be modified for edentulous areas and for isolated or widely separated teeth. If only a few teeth are missing in an area and the dressing cannot be retained there, tie a loop of dental floss around the existing teeth to bridge the open space. The dressing can then be applied against the floss and retained more easily. When a single isolated tooth is present in the arch or groups of teeth are widely separated, place a strip of dressing material around each tooth or group of teeth rather than trying to bridge a wide area with floss. If dressing material will not adhere around an isolated tooth, tie a small strip of gauze around the cervical area of the tooth and then apply the dressing to the area (Carranza and Perry, 1986).

Mixing a zinc oxide–eugenol dressing

The technique for mixing a zinc oxide–eugenol dressing is shown in Figs. 29-16 and 29-17. The material is usually mixed on a waxed pad with a tongue blade, but if a large amount of material is to be mixed, a piece of waxed paper taped to a counter can be used. Follow the manufacturer's directions, which usually require that the powder

be gradually incorporated into the liquid to form a thick paste. The consistency must be very thick; if additional powder is needed, it is added by kneading it into the paste. When the mix has been completed, the dressing is placed as previously described.

Manipulation of a premixed dressing

A premixed dressing should be manipulated according to the manufacturer's directions. Usually, the desired amount of material is removed from the container with a sterile tongue blade and placed on a waxed mixing pad. The material can be formed into two strips of the desired diameter and length and applied as described previously.

REMOVAL OF A PERIODONTAL DRESSING (FIG. 29-18)
Loosening the dressing

If foil is present, loosen and remove it with an explorer (Fig. 29-19). Then, gently loosen the dressing from the soft tissues with a pair of cotton pliers and a curette (Figs. 29-20 and 29-21). After the dressing has been loosened sufficiently, lift it away from the wound site (Fig. 29-22). The dressing often can be removed as one solid strip

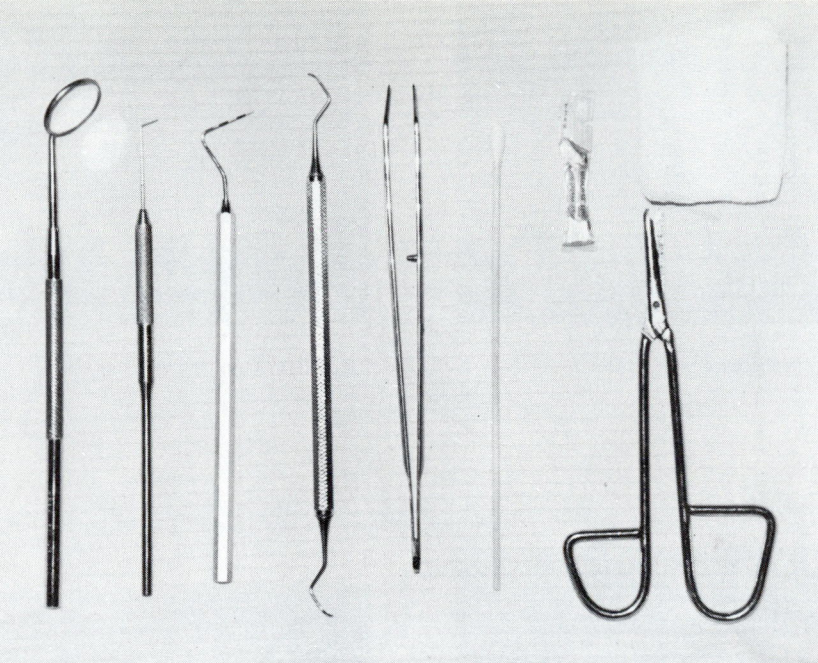

Fig. 29-18. Tray setup for removal of periodontal pack and sutures. Note that suture scissors have a curved blade to reach suture without harming tissue.

(Fig. 29-23). Remove large pieces of excess dressing from the teeth using a curette, being careful not to traumatize tender soft tissues and newly exposed root surfaces (Fig. 29-24). Rinse the area gently with sterile saline or with an oxygenating solution (e.g., Glyoxide, Marian Labs, Inc.) to cleanse it of surface debris (Figs. 29-25 and 29-26). Special care is needed to remove a dressing placed over a sutured area. Instructions for this procedure are discussed in the following section.

After the dressing has been removed, inspect the wound site to evaluate the healing that has taken place. Gently rinse away plaque and other debris that is present so the tissue can be viewed carefully. After 5 to 7 days, the tissues should show evidence of epithelialization and healing. If the tissues appear unusually red or inflamed or if exudate is present, examine and explore the teeth for the presence of plaque and calculus. Remove deposits. Based on the dentist's evaluation, another dressing may be needed until satisfactory

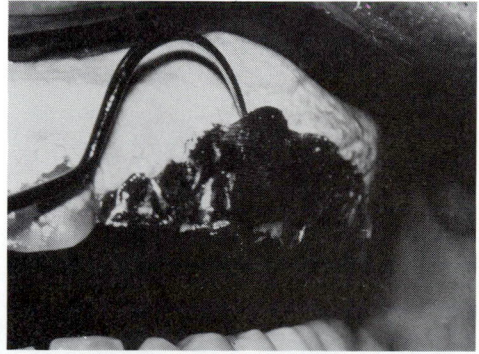

Fig. 29-19. Dry foil is loosened with an explorer and removed.

wound healing has occurred. Root surfaces that have been newly exposed because of shrinkage of soft tissues may be sensitive to tactile or thermal stimuli. Therefore, use compressed air on these surfaces with great care (Carranza and Perry, 1986; Goldman and Cohen, 1980).

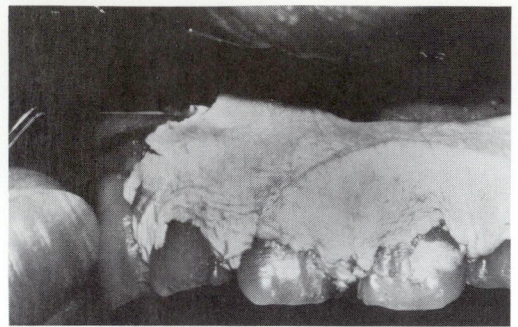

Fig. 29-20. Pack is loosened with a curette.

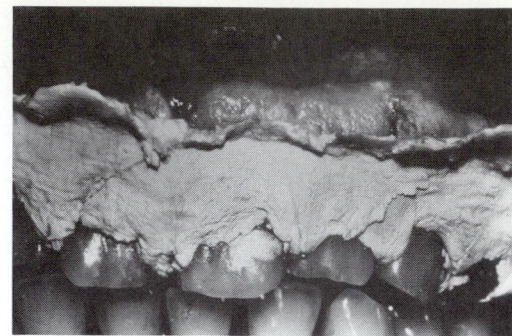

Fig. 29-21. Loosened dressing.

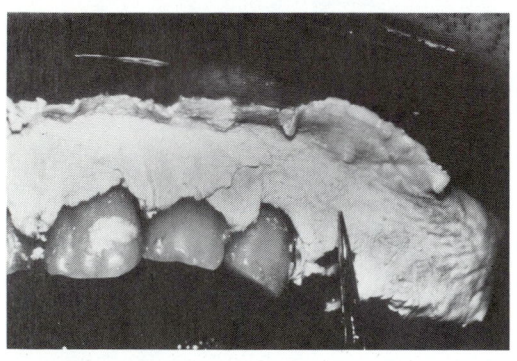

Fig. 29-22. Pack is lifted off wound with cotton pliers.

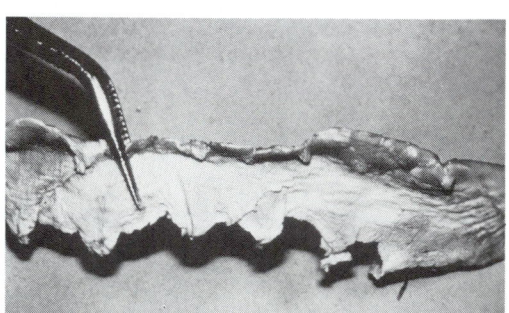

Fig. 29-23. Pack in one piece after removal.

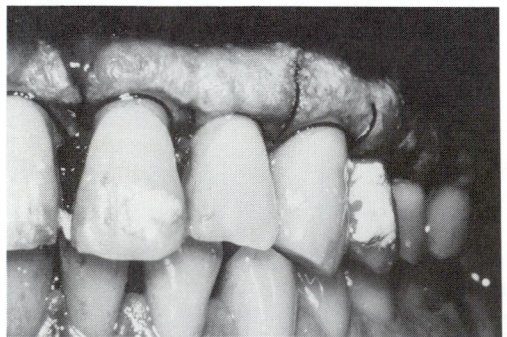

Fig. 29-24. Some large pieces of dressing remain on teeth. Pieces should be removed gently with a curette.

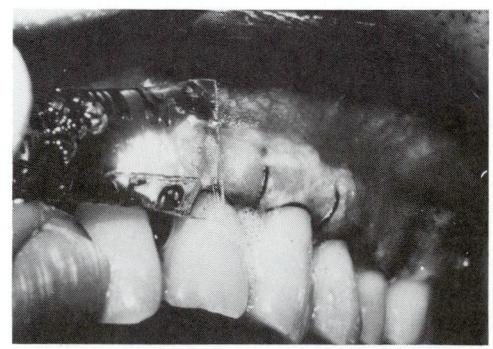

Fig. 29-25. Area is rinsed with oxygenating agent.

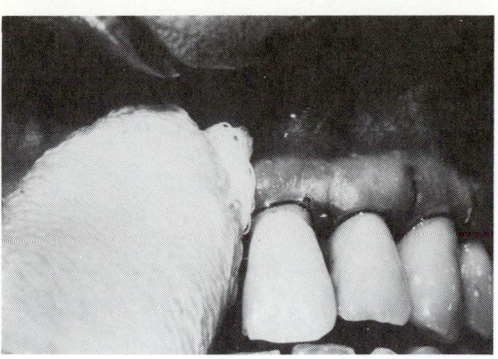

Fig. 29-26. Damp gauze can be used to gently cleanse area of small pieces of dressing and debris.

PLACEMENT AND REMOVAL OF SUTURES

Sutures are used after most surgical procedures to reapproximate (secure together) the soft tissues and to promote healing. Various absorbable and nonabsorbable suture materials are available. The absorbable sutures include surgical gut, collagen, polydioxanone, and polyglactin 910; the nonabsorbable materials are silk, nylon, polypropylene, silver wire, and mersilene (Chung and Weinberg, 1978; Goldman and Cohen, 1980). Black silk suture material is the most popular for periodontal surgery because of its easy manipulation, durability, and strength.

The suture material can be threaded through a needle by the clinician, or it may come already attached (swaged) to the needle by the manufacturer (Fig. 29-27). Swaged needles are more popular among dentists, dental hygienists, and dental specialists. Most of the needles used in dentistry are curved to allow safe, easy manipulation.

Types of sutures

A variety of suture patterns, including interrupted, figure-8, sling, continuous sling, and simple mattress patterns, are used to reapproximate tissues following surgical procedures. The surgeon or dental hygienist licensed to place sutures selects the type of suture based on the type of surgical procedure, healing considerations, and the desired goal of treatment. It is important for the person who is to remove the sutures to know the type of suture placed, the suturing pattern, the number of knots, and the location of the knots.

Thus it is helpful if the clinician who places the sutures indicates this information in the chart. Figs. 29-27 through 29-30 illustrate and describe four types of commonly used sutures: interrupted, figure 8, sling, and continuous sling. Note the pattern of the sutures and the location of the knot.

Dental hygienists licensed to place sutures find the figure-8 suture the most useful for their needs. When the papillae are reflected to gain access for root debridement, the figure-8 suture is used to reposition them. Rather than pushing the papillae apically as the interrupted suture does, the figure-8 suture pulls the papilla together and coronally. To place a figure-8 suture, the needle is inserted into the outer surface of the facial papilla, then drawn through the interproximal area and out to the lingual alongside the lingual papilla. The needle then enters the outer surface of the lingual papilla and is drawn across the interproximal area and out to the facial alongside the facial papilla, where a surgeon's knot is tied. Additional suture patterns are shown in a number of textbooks of periodontology.

Tying a surgeon's knot

To tie a surgeon's knot, a needle holder or hemostat is used. Holding the needle and suture material in one hand and the hemostat in the other, make two loops with the suture material *over* the hemostat beaks. Open the beaks and pick up the one-inch tag end of the suture, and draw the hemostat out of the loops, and set the knot over the papilla. Next make one loop *under* the hemostat beaks and open the beaks again. Pick up the tag end of the suture, draw it through the loop, and tighten the knot. To set the knot, make one more loop *over* the hemostat beaks, as in the first step. The knot should be tight enough to hold the papilla in close apposition to the root surfaces, but not so tight that some tissue swelling will cause discomfort to the patient.

Fibrin tack

An alternative to suture placement is the fibrin tack. This technique is used for isolated interproximal areas in which papilla reflection has been performed. A wet gauze sponge is placed over the interproximal area and pressure is applied for 3 minutes with thumb and index finger from both facial and lingual surfaces. This pressure causes the natural fibrin in the clot to adhere the tissue and tooth together. The fibrin tack has been found

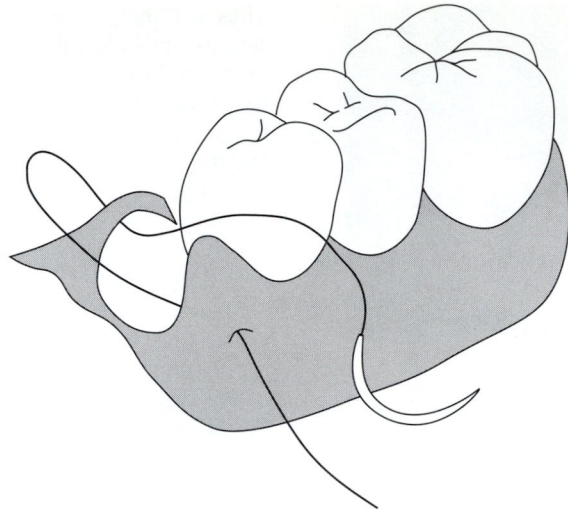

Fig. 29-27. The needle penetrates the outer surface of the first flap. It then passes through the interproximal area and penetrates the outer surface of the opposite flap. The suture is brought back to the first flap.

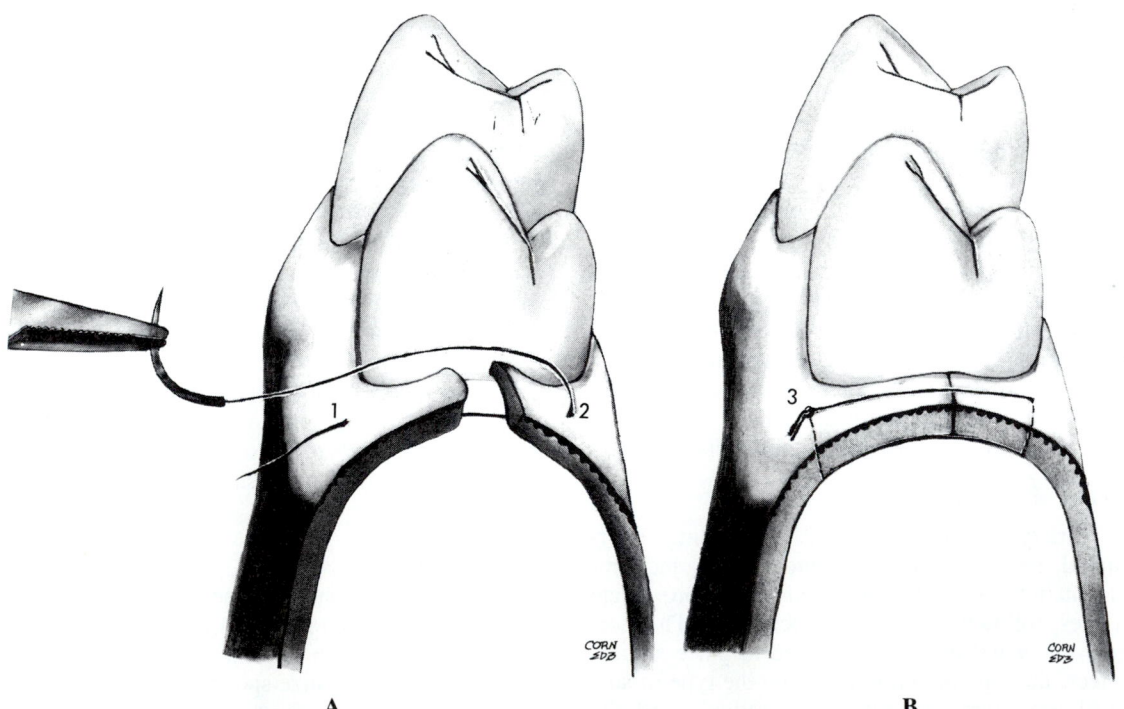

A   **B**

Fig. 29-28. Placement of interrupted suture with a curved, swaged needle, **A,** Suture penetrates *(1)* facial aspect of buccal flap, enters connective tissue of lingual flap, and *(2)* exits lingual flap. **B,** Suture is carried to facial aspect and tied *(3).*
(From Goldman HC, Cohen DW: *Periodontal therapy,* ed 6, St Louis, 1980, CV Mosby.)

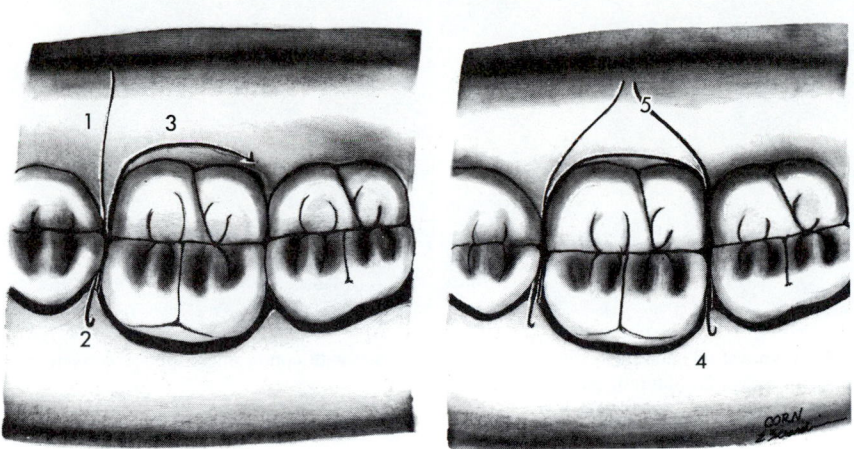

Fig. 29-29. Placement of continuous sling suture to reapproximate buccal tissue. *1,* Needle passes through interdental space from lingual aspect without penetrating tissue and leaves a tail of suture; *2,* buccal tissue is penetrated, and needle passes under contact without entering lingual tissue; *3,* suture is carried around lingual aspect of tooth; *4,* needle penetrates buccal tissue; *5,* suture is knotted on lingual aspect.
(From Goldman HC, Cohen DW: *Periodontal therapy,* ed 6, St Louis, 1980, CV Mosby.)

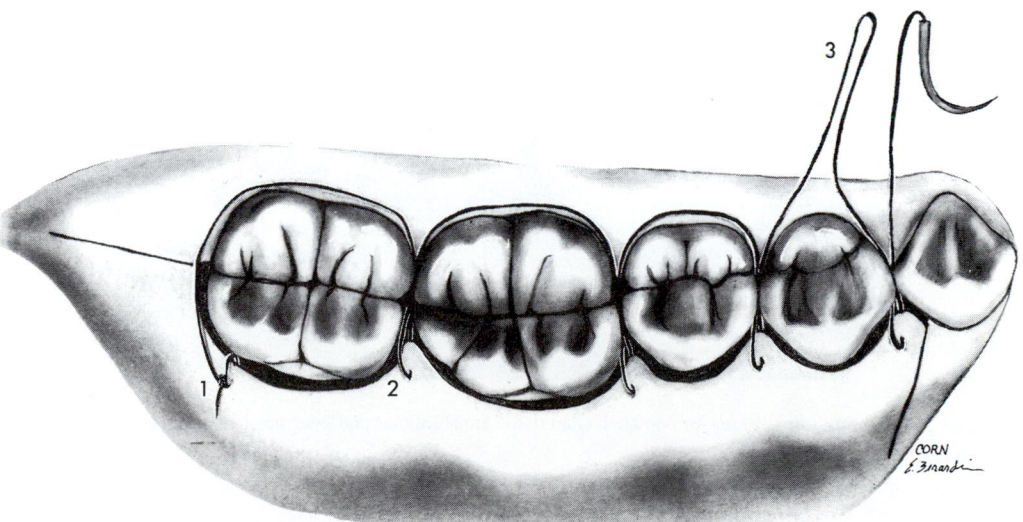

Fig. 29-30. Placement of continuous sling suture to reapproximate lingual tissue. *1,* Loose loop of suture material is tied to ease suture removal; *2,* sling sutures are placed as in Fig. 29-29; *3,* final knot is tied with loop of lingual suture material.
(From Goldman HC, Cohen DW: *Periodontal therapy,* ed 6, St Louis, 1980, CV Mosby.)

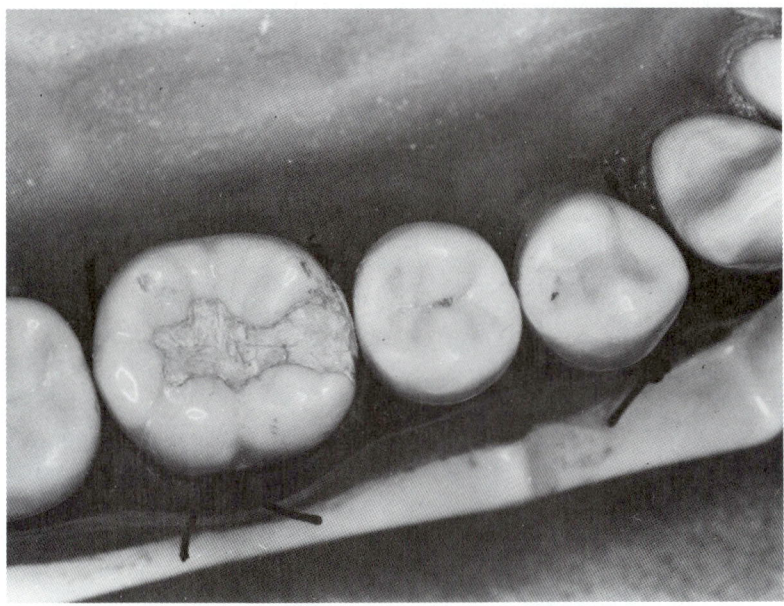

A **B**

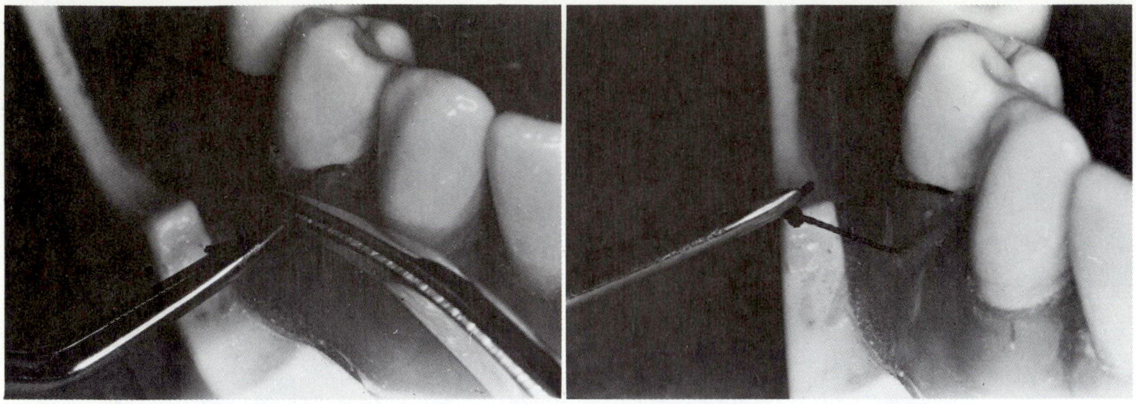

Fig. 29-31. Removal of interrupted suture. **A,** Knot is grasped with cotton pliers, pulled away from tissue, and cut with scissors. **B,** Suture is pulled out of tissue.

Fig. 29-32. Sling suture to reapproximate lingual tissue around molar and interrupted suture mesial to premolar are ready to be removed.

to be as effective as suturing for localized interproximal areas (Reinhardt, Johnson, and Tussing, 1985).

Principles for removing sutures

Removing sutures is a relatively simple procedure, but a few basic principles must be observed. The knot must *never* be pulled through the tissue. Instead, cut the suture so that the knot is pulled *away* from the tissue (Fig. 29-31). When removing the suture, avoid passing through the soft tissues suture material that has been exposed to the oral cavity and may be contaminated by plaque or other oral bacteria and oral debris. Be

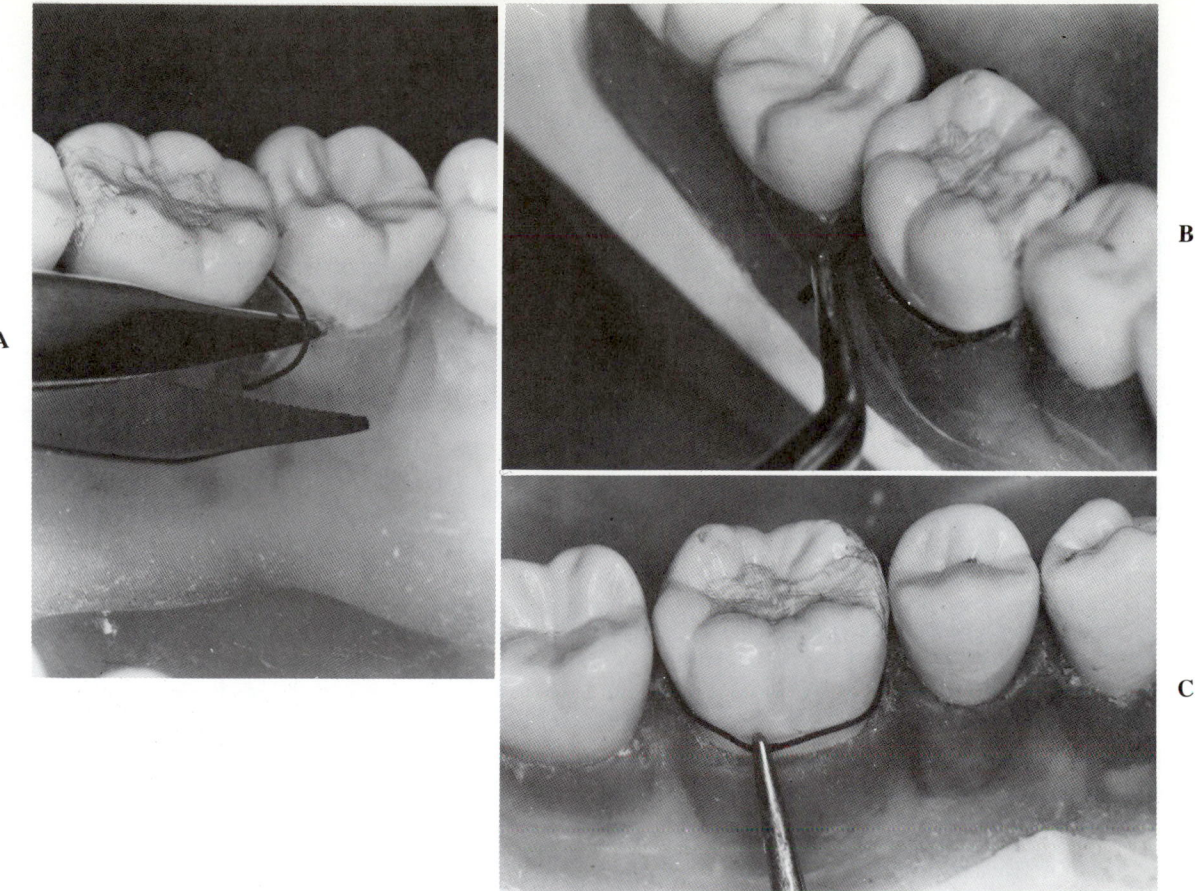

Fig. 29-33. Removal of sling suture. Buccal knot is cut first. **A,** Lingual portions of suture entering tissue are cut. **B,** Loose interproximal suture is removed. **C,** Lingual loop is removed.

certain that all of the suture material and knots are accounted for after the removal procedure. Figs. 29-31 through 29-33 illustrate and describe the correct technique for removal of interrupted and sling sutures.

When removing a dressing that has been placed over sutures, the clinician should be aware of the possibility that the suture material may have become incorporated into the hardened dressing. Under these circumstances, remove the lingual portion of the dressing first. This should be done because sutures are usually knotted on the facial surfaces of the wound site rather than on the lingual surfaces. If the knots have become incorpo-

rated within the hardened dressing, the suture should then be cut from the exposed lingual surfaces, after which the suture material and knots can be removed along with the facial aspect of the pack. After the dressing and sutures are removed, cleanse the area and evaluate the tissue as described previously.

Dental hygienists may be called on to place and remove periodontal dressings or to place or remove sutures. A knowledge of the skills required to perform these functions will help the dental hygienist assume additional responsibilities related to the treatment of periodontal disease (see box on next page).

Placement and Removal of Periodontal Packs

Suggested check-off sheet

Mark **S** for satisfactory completion of **U** for unsatisfactory completion of each criterion in the appropriate space.

PERFORMANCE CRITERIA	FACULTY	STUDENT
1. Assemble the necessary armamentarium		
2. Mix the pack according to the manufacturer's directions		
3. Shape the pack into two rolls, each the length of the site and two-thirds the diameter of a pencil		

Placing the pack

4. Gently adapt the pack to the area with gloved fingers and damp gauze		
5. Adapt the pack interproximally with a curette or cotton pliers		
6. Muscle mold and trim the pack		
7. Smooth the pack		
8. Produce a pack that		
a. Extends to the middle third of the tooth but not onto the occluding surfaces		
b. Extends beyond all margins of the wound		
c. Does not interfere with normal function		

Removing the pack

9. Remove the dry foil if present		
10. Loosen the lingual and buccal packs		
11. Remove the lingual pack		
12. Cut sutures from the lingual portion if necessary		
13. Remove the buccal pack		
14. Cleanse the area with an oxygenating agent		
15. Remove remaining sutures if necessary		
16. Recleanse the area		
17. Gently remove any debris or granulation tissue		
18. Evaluate healing of the wound site		

ACTIVITIES

1. Place and remove a periodontal dressing in one or more of the following situations:
   a. For a partner.
   b. On a typodont with missing teeth.
   c. On a typodont with sutures placed.
2. Conduct a panel discussion with periodontists and/or dentists from your area on the subject of "The need for periodontal dressings."
3. Prepare a table clinic on how to place and remove a periodontal pack.
4. Prepare a review of the literature for any of the types of periodontal dressings.
5. Prepare a presentation about the various suture techniques and the techniques for removing each type of suture.
6. Observe periodontal surgery, suturing, and postsurgical care in a periodontist's office.
7. After having a periodontal dressing placed in your mouth by a fellow student, leave it on until the next day and keep a diary of how it affected your comfort and your ability to eat, talk, and perform oral hygiene procedures.
8. Compile a list of characteristics of an "ideal" periodontal dressing.
9. Place and remove sutures in a piece of fabric held in an embroidery hoop, or in another simulated situation.

REVIEW QUESTIONS

1. List the purposes of periodontal dressings.
2. Which type of periodontal dressing, eugenol or noneugenol, would most likely be placed following a nonsurgical periodontal procedure?
3. After a pack has been placed on a surgical site, the patient asks how to care for it. Briefly outline the directions to be given to the patient.
4. Describe how to remove sutures that have become embedded in the pack.
5. What reasons have been cited for not placing a periodontal dressing as a routine postsurgical procedure?

REFERENCES

American Dental Association Council on Dental Therapeutics: *Accepted dental therapeutics*, ed 40, Chicago, 1984, The Association.

Addy M, Dolby AE: The use of chlorhexidine mouthwash compared with a periodontal dressing following the gingivectomy procedure, *J Clin Periodontol* 3:59, 1976.

Addy M et al: A chlorhexidine-containing methacrylic gel as a periodontal dressing, *J Periodontol* 46:465, 1975.

Allen DR, Caffesse RG: Comparison of results following modified Widman flap surgery with and without surgical dressing, *J Periodontol* 54:470, 1983.

Baer PN et al: Periodontal dressings, *Dent Clin North Am* 13:181, 1969.

Bakdash MB: Asbestos in periodontal dressings, a possible health hazard, *Quintessence Int* 7:61, 1976.

Barkin ME: Acute allergic reaction to eugenol, *Oral Surg* 57:441, 1984.

Blanque RH: Fundamentals and technique of surgical periodontal packing, *J Periodontol* 33:346, 1962.

Carranza FE: *Glickman's clinical periodontology,* ed, 6, Philadelphia, 1984, WB Saunders.

Carranza FE, Perry DA: *Clinical periodontology for the dental hygienist,* Philadelphia, 1986, WB Saunders.

Chung H, Weinberg S: Suture materials in oral surgery: a review, *Oral Health* 68(10):31, 1978.

Forrest JO: The use of cyanoacrylates in periodontal surgery, *J Periodontol* 45:225, 1974.

Frisch L, Bhaskar SN: Tissue response to eugenol-containing periodontal dressings, *J Periodontol* 38:402, 1967.

Goldman HC, Cohen DW: *Periodontal therapy,* ed 6, St Louis, 1980, CV Mosby.

Grant DA, Stern IV, Everett FG: *Periodontics in the tradition of Orban and Gottlieb,* St Louis, 1988, CV Mosby.

Greensmith AL, Wade AB: Dressing after reverse bevel flap procedures, *J Clin Periodontol* 1:97, 1974.

Haugen E: The effect of periodontal dressings on intact mucous membrane and on wound healing, *Acta Odontol Scand* 38:363, 1980.

Haugen E, Gjermo P: Clinical assessment of periodontal dressings, *J Clin Periodontol* 5:50, 1978.

Haugen E, Mjor I: Bone tissue reactions to periodontal dressings, *J Periodont Res* 14:76, 1979.

Haugen E et al: Some antibacterial properties of periodontal dressings, *J Clin Periodontol* 4:62, 1977.

Heaney FG, Appleton J: The effect of periodontal dressings on the healthy periodontium, *J Clin Periodontol* 3:66, 1976.

Jones TM, Cassingham RJ: Comparison of healing following periodontal surgery with and without dressings in humans, *J Periodontol* 50:387, 1979.

Levin MP: Periodontal suture materials and surgical dressings, *Dent Clin North Am* 24:767, 1980.

Levin MP et al: Cyanoacrylate as a periodontal dressing, *J Oral Med* 30:40, 1975.

Lysell L: Contact allergy to rosin in a periodontal dressing, *J Oral Med* 31:24, 1976.

McGraw VA, Caffesse RG: Cyanoacrylates in periodontics, *Periodont Abstr* 26(1):4, 1978.

Nelson EH et al: A comparison of the continuous and interrupted suturing techniques, *J Periodontol* 48:273, 1977.

Ochstein AJ et al: A comparative study of cyanoacrylate and other periodontal dressings on gingival surgical wound healing, *J Periodontol* 40:515, 1969.

O'Hehir T: *Suture technique handout,* Expanded functions in periodontics program, Northern Arizona University, 1988.

O'Neill TC: Antibacterial properties of periodontal dressings, *J Periodontol* 46:469, 1975.

Pluss EM et al: Effect of chlorhexidine on dental plaque formation under periodontal pack, *J Clin Periodontol* 2:136, 1975.

Poulson RC: An anaphylactoid reaction to periodontal surgical dressing: report of case, *JADA* 89:895, 1974.

Reinhardt R et al: Root planing with interdental papilla reflection and fiber optic illumination, *J Periodontol* 56:721, 1985.

Sachs HA et al: Current status of periodontal dressings, *J Periodontol* 55:689, 1984.

Stahl SS et al: The effects of periodontal dressings on gingival repair, *J Periodontol* 40:34, 1969.

Valentine RM: *Expanded duties: a self-determined pace laboratory program,* Philadelphia, 1976, University of Pennsylvania.

Wampole HS et al: The incidence of transient bacteremia during periodontal dressing change, *J Periodontol* 49:462, 1978.

Watts TLP, Combe EC: Periodontal dressing materials, *J Clin Periodontol* 6:3, 1979.

Watts TLP, Combe EC: Effects of noneugenol periodontal dressing materials upon the surface hardness of anterior restorative materials in vitro, *Br Dent J* 151:423, 1981.

SUGGESTED READINGS

Dahlberg WH: Incisions and suturing: some basic considerations about each in periodontal flap surgery, *Dent Clin North Am* 13:149, 1969.

Geiger B et al: Periodontal dressings: rationale and procedures, *Dent Hyg* 55:21, 1981.

Haugen E et al: The sensitizing potential of periodontal dressing, *J Dent Res* 57:950, 1978.

Macht SD, Krizek TJ: Sutures and suturing—current concepts, *J Oral Surg* 36:710, 1978.

Manor A et al: Unusual foreign body reaction to a braided silk suture: a case report, *J Periodontol* 53:868, 1982.

Pihlstrom BL et al: The effect of periodontal dressing on supragingival microorganisms, *J Periodontol* 48:440, 1977.

Stroh C, Chinn SA: *Periodontal dressings,* Seattle, 1976, University of Washington.

30 COSMETIC AND THERAPEUTIC APPLICATIONS OF POLISHING

Susan J. Daniel

LEARNING OUTCOMES

The dental hygienist will be able to

1. Explain to a colleague, a patient, or an employer the relationship of polishing to the therapeutic and cosmetic goals of oral care.
2. Summarize the research findings that suggest the limited therapeutic benefit of coronal polishing and the more relevant therapeutic value of root polishing.
3. Select porte, engine, or air-powder polishing based on the requirements of the patient's oral condition, his or her response to care, and the equipment and time available.
4. Use all of the polishing procedures to remove stain without causing trauma or discomfort.
5. Adopt and implement a successful policy of selective polishing for clinical practice.
6. Explain to a patient the types of tooth-bleaching procedures available and what he or she may expect from treatment.

In the recent past, when you visited a dental hygienist you could expect that the calculus would be scaled and that all of your teeth would be polished. Just as perspectives on scaling and root instrumentation have changed, the principles of polishing have been reviewed and revised as well. The superficial polishing of the crown is now considered as a purely cosmetic procedure with *minimal* therapeutic benefit. Therapeutic polishing, in contrast, refers to polishing root surfaces that are exposed during surgery to reduce endotoxin and the microflora on the cementum. Whether you polish for cosmetic or therapeutic benefit, understanding the polishing process and the resulting effects on the tooth surface is critical to your professional development.

Polishing itself involves smoothing a surface to make it glossy or lustrous; *cleaning* is the act of removing debris, impurities, or extraneous matter. Although the term *polishing* has been used to describe the professional removal of soft deposits and stain from tooth surfaces, in reality this procedure includes both cleaning and polishing. Removal of deposits has usually been achieved by friction created using an abrasive agent and some form of mechanical device. Plaque, stain, and acquired pellicle (which is the acellular bonding apparatus for plaque and stain) are all removed during polishing. Though polishing does remove

plaque and therefore inhibit the occurrence of gingivitis (Huber, Vemino, and Nanca, 1987; Waring et al, 1982), the same benefit can be accomplished with thorough home plaque removal procedures (Waring et al, 1988). Therefore polishing of coronal surfaces has questionable positive effects beyond creating a stain-free smile (Walsh et al, 1985).

Historically, one reason teeth were polished was to remove all soft deposits and stains before the application of topical fluorides to allow for greater fluoride uptake in the enamel (Mallatt and Christen, 1989). However, studies have shown that polishing does not improve the uptake of professionally applied fluoride (Steele et al, 1982; Tinanoff et al, 1974). Dental hygienists formerly considered it their role to polish plaque off the patient's teeth and remove stains. As scientific knowledge has evolved, it has been found that polishing removes part of the fluoride-rich outer layer of enamel (Mellberg, 1977; Retief et al, 1980; Shern et al, 1977). Continuous polishing and hand planing over years of routine care may also cause morphologic changes in the teeth. Essentially, the tooth structure can be abraded away, especially at the cervix of cementum and dentin (Swan, 1979); this has been shown to result from improper angulation of the rubber cup (Christensen and Bangerter, 1987).

As part of clinical assessment, you should identify the types and amount of soft deposits present on patients' teeth to aid in establishing an effective treatment plan. Obviously, stain that cannot be removed by the patient is the primary determinant of the need for cosmetic polishing. Once the type, amount, and distribution of stains have been assessed, the type of abrasive and mechanical device best suited for their removal can be planned.

DENTAL STAINS
Definitions and classifications

Dental stains can be associated with carious enamel, cementum, and dentin; chromogenic bacterial staining of both soft and hard deposits; hemorrhagic staining of soft deposits; exogenous extrinsic staining of the teeth and deposits from food, drink, tobacco, and drugs; and endogenous staining of the teeth by systemic disturbances. Although objectionable because of their appearance, most stains are relatively harmless and do not precipitate disease. Because many patients are more concerned with esthetics than disease, the presence of dental stains may be advantageously used as a motivating factor to improve oral hygiene. In an attempt to achieve whiter and brighter teeth, patients may practice more thorough plaque removal.

Staining or discoloration can occur in three ways: (1) it can adhere directly to tooth surfaces by bonding to the acquired pellicle; (2) it can be contained within calculus and soft deposits; and (3) it can be incorporated in the tooth structure. As you polish the coronal surfaces of the teeth remember that you will be removing not only stain but also soft debris, acquired pellicle, and the outer layer of the enamel. To determine if a type of stain can be removed by polishing, it is important to look at the definitions and classifications of stains.

Discolorations are classified as either endogenous or exogenous (Carranza, 1979; Shaw and Murray 1977; Vogel, 1975; Winter, Murray, and Shaw, 1978). *Endogenous* is the term used for stains that originate within the tooth from systemic disturbances. *Exogenous* stains originate outside the tooth from exposure to environmental agents. Within this classification, exogenous stains are further categorized on the basis of their ability to be removed. *Extrinsic* stains are on the exterior of the tooth and can be removed by the individual or the dental professional. *Intrinsic* stains are of exogenous or endogenous origin and become incorporated into the tooth structure and cannot be removed by the patient or by professional polishing and scaling.

Endogenous stains can be the result of heredity, developmental disturbances, genetic factors, drugs, and trauma (Table 30-1). Both the primary and permanent dentitions may be affected. Medications that the mother or child takes during tooth development can also cause staining. Tetracycline

Table 30-1. Endogenous developmental stains

Type	Appearance	Etiology
Fluorosis	White flecks to brown, pitted enamel (mottled) Focal or generalized depending on severity	Excessive fluoride intake
Tetracycline	Grayish brown rings with or without pits or overall discoloration, depending on duration	Tetracycline ingested during those stages of tooth development
Hypocalcification	White flecks or spots in the enamel, focally or in a linear fashion	Endocrine, metabolic, or unknown causes
Amelogenesis imperfecta	White spots, usually with pitting in a ringlike fashion, or involving the entire enamel Tends to turn brown with age	Genetic
Dentinogenesis imperfecta	Overall bluish translucence to dark tan-brown	Genetic May be seen with osteogenesis imperfecta or as an isolated trait
Dentin dysplasia	Deciduous teeth Looks like dentinogenesis imperfecta	Genetic Permanent teeth appear normal
Porphyria	Dark yellow to brown Enamel, dentin, and cementum are all affected	Genetic disorder of hemoglobin formation

Table 30-2. Endogenous stains of environmental origin

Type	Appearance	Etiology
Incipient caries	White, chalky	Acid-producing bacteria
Active caries	Brown to black	Acid-producing bacteria
Secondary caries	White, gray to brownish black around existing restorations	Marginal leakage of restorations and acid-producing bacteria
Pulpal necrosis	Yellowish black	Trauma

is one example of a medication that is known to cause developmental stains (Rall, 1977). Excessive repeated intake of fluoride during tooth development can cause a range of discoloration, from white flecks to brown pitting of the enamel (mottled enamel). Dental hygienists may be consulted about the effects of these and other compounds on oral tissues.

Environmental endogenous stains can result from pathologic incursions into the tooth, such as dental caries or pulpal necrosis. In addition, metallic stains from dental restorations or prolonged exposure to metals in the air or water may also cause endogenous stains (Table 30-2). Endogenous stains caused by dental procedures (usually from restorative materials, exposure of the dentin to bleeding, and other problems of unknown cause) are termed *iatrogenic* stains. Professional polishing will not remove endogenous stains. Methods for cosmetically improving teeth affected by intrinsic stains include vital and nonvital bleaching (Heringer, 1976); composite restorative materials bonded as overlays, laminate veneers, and less frequently, crowns.

Enamel microabrasion is another option when stain does not permeate the dentinoenamel junction. A thin layer of enamel is removed by burnishing water soluble gel paste containing a mild concentration of HCl and abrasive particles on the tooth (Croll, 1989).

Bleaching involves oxidation, which allows the molecules of discoloration causing the stain to be released. Therefore success depends on how well the bleaching agent can penetrate the tooth structure to the source of discoloration and the necessary length and/or frequency of application (Goldstein and Fineman, 1987).

The standard technique for professional vital bleaching uses 35% peroxide and a heat-generating bleaching light on the enamel surface of the crown. This accepted technique for vital bleaching can successfully remove certain intrinsic stains. However, the process has been found to initiate cervical resorption at the cementoenamel junction if this area is not protected during the bleaching procedure (Lado, Stanley, and Weismann, 1983). Another method of vital bleaching that has gained commercial popularity is the matrix system. This method uses a solution of 10% to 15% carbamide peroxide applied with a plastic matrix or night guard (Goldstein and Fineman, 1987). Because of the lack of long-term studies showing the efficacy and safety of the home-applied matrix technique, these products have been removed from the commercial market.

Bleaching of nonvital teeth uses a similar method for bleaching, but it is applied on the interior of the tooth. A cotton-soaked pellet of 35% hydrogen peroxide is placed into the pulp chamber, and a heat probe is applied at higher temperatures than for vital teeth (Goldstein and Fineman, 1987).

Whether bleaching is performed on vital or nonvital teeth, the application usually must be repeated within 1 to 3 years (Goldstein and Fineman, 1987). Concerns exist about the histologic effects of bleaching and chemical reactions during the application of concentrated peroxides (Cooley, 1976). Effects on the pulp after vital bleaching are unknown, as are potential dehydration effects on the enamel.

Several researchers have used *resin veneers* or *composite materials* in 6- to 12-month evaluations (Cooley, 1976; Spencer, 1972; Stuart, 1975). Results have been encouraging, particularly in matching the color of other teeth in the mouth, in the relatively short time required to do individual teeth (15 to 30 minutes per tooth), and in the excellent patient acceptance after completion of treatments. Difficulties with these materials include flaking or cracking, especially when patients eat fibrous or hard-consistency foods. *Full crowns* are used when major intrinsic staining has occurred; however, this should not be done on a deciduous or young permanent dentition. It is desirable to have complete maturity of the pulp before crowning. A second drawback of this treatment is the expense and time requirements of the procedure. A third difficulty is the creation of an artificial margin between the tooth crown and root, which can be a primary site for plaque adherence. Many dental professionals are reluctant to sacrifice large areas of healthy tooth structure for purely cosmetic purposes.

Environmental exogenous stains result from food, tobacco, tea, coffee, and airborne particles and can be removed. Individuals vary widely in their rate and amount of extrinsic staining. Certain factors are known to predispose a person to the accumulation of both dental deposits and stains; these include enamel roughness, organic salts in saliva, increased or decreased salivary flow, and poor oral hygiene. Extrinsic stains can be identified by color, distribution, and tenacity as well as by age, sex, and home care (Reid, Beeley, and MacDonald, 1977). Most extrinsic stains can be removed with either the rubber cup and polishing agent or air-powder polisher.

Green stain. Green stain occurs primarily on cervical areas of the maxillary anterior teeth and is associated with the primary dental cuticle. It usually is crescent-shaped, close to the gingiva, and colored light green to yellow-green to dark green. Green stains are usually a result of poor oral hygiene and tend to recur after removal. This stain is difficult to remove with polishing agents. If your patient is not allergic to iodine, try a little in the prophylaxis cup to remove the green stain efficiently and effectively.

Gray/green stain. Gray/green stain occurs around the gingival third of teeth in individuals who smoke marijuana. The stain is caused by oils, resin, and pigments found in marijuana.

Black-line stain. Black-line stain usually occurs as a continuous thin band along the gingival margin and follows the crestal contour on lingual or proximal surfaces. It occurs at all ages and is found more often in females. The primary cause of this deposit is iron compounds in saliva or gingival fluid that become embedded in plaque and/or plaque bacteria. This stain is a ferric sulfide compound and can be found in a relatively clean mouth (Reid, Beeley, and MacDonald, 1977).

Orange stain. Orange stain is rare. It occurs at the cervical third of incisor teeth and can be attributed to chromogenic bacteria.

Tobacco stain. Tobacco stains range in appearance from tan to dark brown or black and cover approximately the cervical one-third to one-half of most teeth. It occurs mostly on lingual

Table 30-3. Effect of smoking on extrinsic stain

Number of cigarettes per day	*Percent with moderate to severe stain*
0	18
1 to 10	35
11 to 20	51
>20	78

Modified from Ness L, Rosekrans DdeL, Welford, JF: *Community Dent Oral Epidemiol* 5:55, 1977.

surfaces. It is also commonly found in pits and fissures and other enamel irregularities. Tobacco staining has been found to be directly proportional to the number of cigarettes smoked per day (Ness, Rosekrans, and Welford, 1977) (Table 30-3). Staining can also be found in individuals who smoke pipes or cigars and those who use smokeless tobacco (snuff or chewing tobacco). Tobacco stains may, over time, penetrate the enamel and become intrinsic.

Food stain. Food staining is common in individuals who consume large quantities of coffee and tea. Other categories of food that may contribute to food stains include cola drinks, berries such as raspberries and blueberries, spices, leaves and nuts of the betel plant, and licorice and other candies containing coloring agents. Stains resulting from ingestion of these foods range from tan to dark brown in color and occur over broad tooth surfaces and in pits and fissures.

Metallic stains. Metallic stains vary in color depending on the metal or the metallic salt that is ingested or inhaled. Green or blue-green colors result from copper or brass, whereas brown colors may result from ingestion of materials or dust particles containing iron. The majority of these stains have been attributed to industrial dust, but they may also be found in various foods and water.

Stains caused by drugs and therapeutic agents. Many drugs or therapeutic agents may cause tooth stains; only a few are described here. Surface discolorations and staining have occured after extended topical or systemic antibiotic use and in studies of antibacterial agents with antiplaque activity (Moffit et al, 1974; Solheim, Eriksen, and Nordbo, 1980). These have been attributed to the direct effects of these agents on plaque bacteria. Chlorhexidine, an antimicrobial agent, causes a dark brown stain around the gingival margin within a few weeks to a year with daily

Table 30-4. Extrinsic stains

Stain category	Primary sites	Composition	Associated wtih
Green	Cervical one-third to one-half labial surfaces of maxillary anteriors	Inorganic elements, chromogenic bacteria	Poor oral hygiene; surface irregularities; most common in children
Gray-green	Cervical one-third labial surfaces	Oils, resin, and pigments	Poor oral hygiene; smoking marijuana
Black-line	Thin band along gingival margin on buccal or lingual surfaces	Ferric sulfide	Iron in saliva, gingival fluid; plaque or bacteria; all ages
Orange	Thin line; cervical one-third of incisors	Chromogenic bacteria	Poor oral hygiene; most common in children
Tobacco	Cervical one-third to one-half of lingual surfaces; pits and fissures	Tars, pigments	Smoking, chewing, dipping
Food	Same as with tobacco	Food pigments	Consumption of tea, coffee, cola drinks, berries, spices, betel leaves and nut, candy
Metallic	Cervical one-third; random surfaces	Associated with specific metals	Environmental, food, water
Drug, therapeutic	Cervical one-third, pits and fissures	Plaque bacteria; tin; reactions with food colors	Extended antibiotic use, stannous fluoride, chlorhexidine

use. A brown- to black-pigmented stain in plaque-associated areas has also been reported in several clinical studies and is attributed to dentifrices containing stannous fluoride (Yankell and Emling, 1978). See Table 30-4 for a list of extrinsic stains.

Stains associated with caries. Two discolorations of teeth are associated with primary (initial lesions on unrestored tooth surfaces) and secondary (or recurrent) caries. Initial (incipient) carious lesions will appear slightly whiter, chalky, and dull in comparison with unaffected enamel. These lesions are not typically noted by the patient but should be identified and recorded by the dental hygienist during a thorough dental examination. With increased caries development, the decalcified areas will become stained with food and bacterial debris, and the degree of discoloration will be proportional to the duration of active decay. The second type of discoloration includes those stains which are adjacent to defective restorations (secondary caries). They usually occur because of leakage of saliva and bacteria between the restoration and the tooth. Recurring caries will appear as a gray or brown area adjacent to the margin of a defective restoration. These restorations will need to be replaced.

Stain evaluation

Attempts have been made to develop scoring procedures to evaluate the extent of intrinsic and ex-

Table 30-5. Scoring tooth stains*

Stain characteristic	Score	Description of stain
Intensity	0	None
	1	Light
	2	Moderate
	3	Heavy
Extent	0	None detected
	1	One-third of region
	2	Two-thirds of region
	3	>Two-thirds of region

Modified from Lobene RR: *JADA* 77:844, 1968.
*The facial surfaces of the eight incisors are scored. Each incisor is divided into the gingival and body regions. Each region is scored for both intensity and extent.

trinsic staining. One of the first attempts to evaluate stain clinically was the categorization of both the intensity and severity of the stain and the specific tooth area covered (Lobene, 1968). This scoring system is shown in Table 30-5. It was used to study the effects of dentifrices on tooth stains after controlled brushing times. The products evaluated differed significantly in their ability to remove stains. Another approach to quantification of tooth stain has been by the use of plastic chips of various standardized colors, ranging from white to yellow and brown to black, combined with a tooth-surface-scoring area. This method was used to evaluate new antiplaque materials (Yankell et al, 1982). An index has also been

Table 30-6. Toothpaste composition

Ingredient	Approximate composition (%)	Function
Abrasive(s)	10 to 60	Clean; polish
Water	20 to 50	Provides a vehicle
Humectant(s)	10 to 60	Prevent caking or hardening; retain moisture
Binding agent(s)	1 to 5	Prevent separation; add thickness
Surface active agent(s) detergent(s)	1 to 2	Remove surface deposits, debris; provide foam
Flavor(s), sweetening agent(s)	1 to 3	Add taste
Therapeutic agent(s)	0.01 to 10	Prevent and/or reduce caries, sensitivity, plaque formation, etc.
Miscellaneous	0.1 to 5	Color; preserve; stabilize

Modifed from Yankell S, Emling RC: *Contin Dent Educ* 1:7, 1989.

proposed to detect small changes in staining levels between different groups. In this procedure, stained areas are drawn on a reproduced grid system to determine the area of the tooth covered. No attempt has been made in this system to quantitate the intensity of tooth stain; rather, staining is graded on a stain, no-stain basis (Shaw and Murray, 1977). These measurements are used in research to compare stain development or removal among treatment groups in clinical trials.

Dental abrasives

Toothpastes are formulated to aid in the removal of debris and discoloration from tooth surfaces and to impart a gloss or luster (polish). Toothpastes are composed of many ingredients, each with a specific function (Gershon and Pader, 1972; Goldstein, 1976; Yankell and Emling, 1978) (Table 30-6). Following is a summary of abrasives in toothpastes:

Calcium carbonate ($CaCO_3$ [Macleans, Phillips, Aquafresh]. Precipitated calcium carbonate (chalk) was widely used in dentifrice products until the mid-1950s. This material is decomposed in an acid pH.

Dibasic calcium phosphate ($CaHPO_4$ [Colgate, Viadent regular, Pearl Drops]). The anhydrous or the dihydrate form of dibasic calcium phosphate is used. The anhydrous form is much more abrasive than the dihydrate form. Although dicalcium phosphate dihydrate is not compatible with sodium fluoride or stannous fluoride, sodium monofluorophosphate can be maintained in soluble form in the presence of this agent for relatively long periods.

Calcium pyrophosphate ($Ca_2P_2O_7$ [Gleem]). Calcium pyrophosphate is more abrasive than dicalcium phosphate dihydrate and more compatible

with fluoride compounds because it is one of the most inert calcium phosphate salts.

Tetrasodium pyrophosphate (tartar control toothpastes). Tetrasodium pyrophosphate has abrasive properties and helps prevent precipitation of salivary salts into dental plaque.

Alumina compounds (Ultra-Brite). Hydrated alumina compounds are available in various particle sizes and thus various degrees of abrasiveness. These compounds do not contain calcium and do not appear to react with fluorides.

Hydrated silicas and silicas (Colgate Winterfresh Gel, Viadent fluoride, Sensodyne, Close-up, Crest, Macleans, Aim, Aquafresh). Silica compounds are available in various grades. When coupled with the proper humectant (moisture-retaining agent), silicas can be used to produce translucent or transparent clear gel products.

Effects of toothpastes

With scanning electron microscopy, changes on the tooth surface have been studied after the use of toothpastes that varied considerably in their abrasiveness. After complete tooth cleaning, pellicle was present within 24 hours and increased in thickness with time. Thicker pellicles formed with the use of less abrasive toothpastes. It was concluded that abrasives were necessary to control pellicle thickness and prevent stain buildup. When pellicle was allowed to remain undisturbed, it became more difficult to remove because of changes in its physical properties (Saxton, 1976). This study suggests that dentifrices with mild abrasives should be used properly and on a consistent basis. Because the surface enamel is in a constant state of demineralization and remineralization, a more important reason to use a dentifrice is to ensure regular, low doses of fluoride

ABRASION		POLISHING
Large	Particle size	Small
Irregular	Shape	Regular
High	Concentration	Low
Increased	Hardness	Decreased
Firm	Pressure	Moderate
Rapid	Speed	Slow
Soft (dentin and cementum)	Tooth surface texture	Hard (enamel)

Fig. 30-1. Factors influencing tooth cleaning.

for enamel remineralization. For patients with exposed dentin or cementum, it is imperative to stress proper brushing procedures with a fluoride-containing toothpaste. Because these tooth structures are softer than enamel, they are more susceptible to dental caries and the abrasive action of dentifrices if improperly used. Unfortunately, no standards for the optimal amount of abrasiveness in toothpastes have been established (American Dental Association Council, 1982).

Professional treatment

When cosmetic polishing is warranted, selection of an appropriate abrasive paste is critical. Many hygienists tend to select medium or coarse pastes, typically with pumice as the polishing abrasive (Christensen, 1984). Perhaps the perceived need to remove stains thoroughly and quickly within the allotted appointment time is the best explanation for this choice.

After scaling and root planing, areas of stain may be polished professionally using an abrasive paste. Abrasive agents are incorporated into professional products for the purpose of cleaning and polishing (Fig. 30-1). A dental abrasive changes the surface of the tooth (Russ, 1986) by frictional grinding, rubbing, scraping, and scratching. As this process proceeds from coarse abrasion (cleaning) to polishing, the surface of the tooth passes through various stages; from irregular, to grooved, to finely scratched, with a concomitant increase in smoothness and light reflectance. The last stage is regarded as the polished surface. Although many prophylaxis pastes are available, they vary considerably in their abrasiveness. The abrasives contained in these products essentially are similar to those in dentifrices (Craig, O'Brien, and Powers, 1983; Davis, 1978; O'Brien and Ryge, 1978) the major difference being that the levels of abrasives in professional products are much higher.

Factors determining the abrasiveness and polishing potential of an agent include particle hardness, shape, size, and concentration. Abrasives vary markedly in inherent hardness and shape. For any single abrasive, size is graded from fine to coarse. Compounds with harder, rough-shaped, large particles produce more abrasive action than those with soft, smooth-shaped, small particles. As each of these factors decreases, surface abrasion is lessened and the surface becomes smooth, or polished.

Two abrasive agents used in prophylaxis products or available as chemical compounds are pumice and calcium carbonate. Calcium carbonate can be purchased as chalk or whiting. Pumice is manufactured in a wide variety of particle sizes, and its uses range from abrasive stain-removal to fine polishing of acrylic dentures. Calcium carbonate is also manufactured in several particle shapes and sizes and is less abrasive than pumice. A recent study examining the effects of various cleaning and polishing methods on primary enamel, contraindicated the use of a pumice slurry on primary enamel because of the resulting abrasion (Hosoya and Johnston, 1989). Calcium carbonate produces minimal scratches and results in a smooth polished surface that reflects light.

Although professional products have been categorized as *fine, medium,* or *coarse,* there are no standards to define what these terms mean. One manufacturer's fine prophylaxis paste may be more abrasive than another manufacturer's medium paste. No attempt can be made, therefore, to match one manufacturer's fine abrasive product with another manufacturer's similarly labeled product even if they contain the same abrasive(s). It is, therefore, the responsibility of the dental hygienist to evaluate and select products for patient use based on efficacious results from sound research studies. In published studies, the clinician should look for the composition of the products being compared and for the type of material to

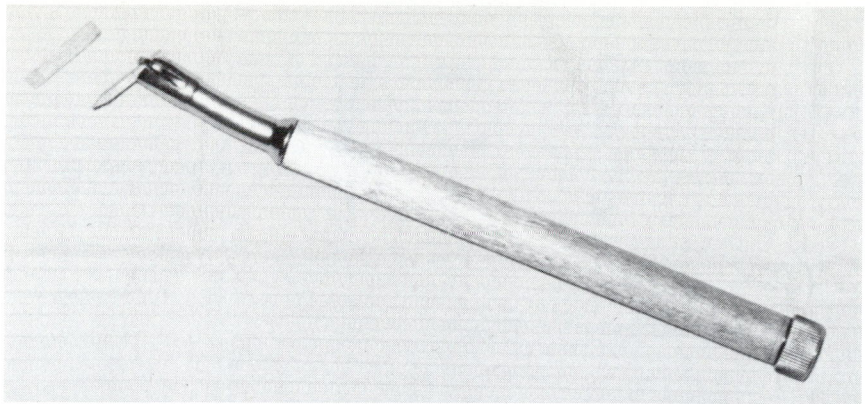

Fig. 30-2. Porte polisher is a hand instrument into which variously shaped orangewood points may be inserted and used to polish teeth with an abrasive.

which the products are being applied. How similar are the products to those used personally, and how similar is the material used to the tooth structure and dental restorative materials? If you cannot find studies of the specific product, ask the manufacturer to supply the information. Further, products can be compared by using them on various materials such as porcelain, copper, or silver, then observing this surface for scratches and luster. However, if the scratches are visible with the naked eye, then the abrasive is not ideal for the tooth or most restorative materials.

Additional factors related to the method(s) of applying the prophylaxis product must be considered in the cleaning and polishing procedure. These include the pressure and speed with which the product is applied and the surface (tooth and/or restorative material) being treated.

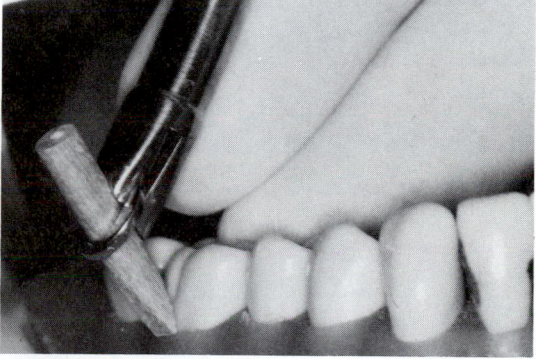

Fig. 30-3. Wooden point is closely adapted to tooth to rub the abrasive against stained areas. Short strokes are used in gingival, middle, and incisal or occlusal thirds of tooth to ensure a clean, well-polished surface.

MECHANICAL DEVICES FOR POLISHING

The simplest device for polishing stains from the teeth is a *porte polisher* (Fig. 30-2). This hand instrument is designed to hold wooden points, which can be adapted to the various aspects of the teeth to rub the abrasive against the tooth surface. Each stroke generated by the wrist motion moves the wedge-shaped, tapered, or pointed wooden point over the tooth surface (Fig. 30-3). This technique requires considerable hand strength and control and is a slow, tedious process. It does, however, offer several advantages: (1) its portability, as it can be used when electricity is not available, at the bedside, or in other settings

where engine-driven equipment cannot be used; (2) the gentle massage provided to the soft tissues with carefully controlled strokes that approximate the gingival margins; (3) easier access to selected tooth surfaces that are obscured by malpositioned teeth; (4) generation of minimal frictional heat; (5) lack of engine noise and thus greater acceptance by patients; (6) minimal bacterial aerosol; and (7) simple procedures for cleaning and sterilizing, as compared with those required for engine-driven handpieces and prophylaxis angles.

In the early days of dental hygiene educatinal programs, porte polishing was one of the first procedures learned because it developed hand

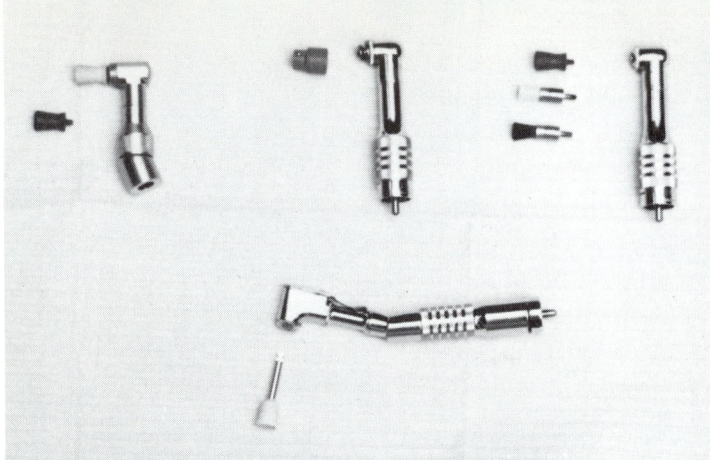

Fig. 30-4. Prophylaxis angles vary in design to accommodate handpiece systems and vary in mechanism used to attach polishing cups or brushes. Attachment may screw in, snap on over a knob, or fit into angle with a mandrel and latching mechanism.

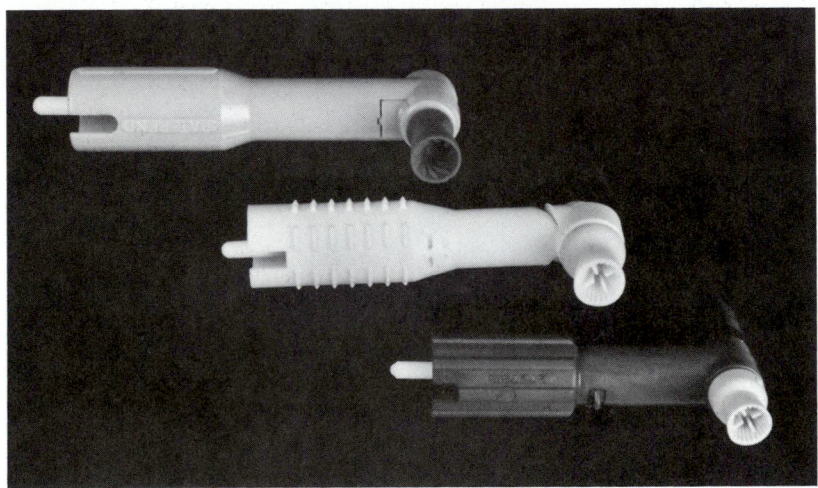

Fig. 30-5. Disposable prophlylaxis angles.

strength, control, and a functional wrist motion. In recent decades, motor-driven polishing has become commonplace, since it requires less time to complete and is usually the method of choice in private clinical practice. It can be used to burnish fluoride or other densensitizing agents into the tooth (see Chapter 31).

Engine-driven polishing is more widely used in clinical practice because it is efficient and requires less effort. The power may be derived from (1) an electric motor, which drives a belt over a series of pulleys to turn the handpiece gears (the old slow-speed "drill"); (2) a small electric motor that attaches to the base of the handpiece and to electric supply hosing; or (3) compressed air supplied by hose to an air-turbine handpiece. Whatever mech-

anism or power source is used in any given clinical setting, it is important for you to be able to operate and maintain the system and to be able to troubleshoot if the polishing instrument fails to function properly. The handpiece and the prophylaxis angle (which holds the rubber cup and brush attachments that polish the teeth) require proper care and maintenance.

The handpiece selected for use should be specifically designed for the system being used; it may screw, snap, lock, or clip onto the power source. Attached to the handpiece is the prophylaxis angle. "Prophy" angles are designed with either straight or contra-angled shanks. They can be reusable after sterilization (Fig. 30-4) or disposable (Fig. 30-5). Cups that attach to prophylaxis angles are designed to have varying degrees of flexibility, and their interior walls can have a ribbed-open, ribbed-webbed or ribbed-turbine configuration. These ribs and webs permit retention of the prophylaxis paste. Cups without webs allow for greater flexibility of the rim. Brushes are designed with different shapes and degrees of flexibility. The cup or brush may attach by means of a metal mandrel that latches into place. The metal mandrel slides through the head of the angle to the latch at the back of the angle head. Other styles of cups and angles enable the rubber cup to screw into the head of the angle. Reverse threads are used so that the rubber cup will not unscrew while running in a clockwise rotation against the tooth. Yet another style allows the cup or brush to snap over a knob on the face of the angle head. The cup and knob must be dry and oil free or the cup will be ineffective. Cups impregnated with fluoride have been shown to increase enamel fluoride content by 400 to 700 ppm and to reduce enamel solubility by 20% to 28% compared with regular rubber cups. They also remove stained pellicle more efficiently and with less abrasion of the enamel than the other cups tested. The cups are made of thermoplastic resins and a 6% mixture of sodium fluoride and stannous fluoride (Stookey and Schemehorn, 1976; Stookey and Stahlman, 1976).

ENGINE POLISHING PROCEDURE

The handpiece and angle must supply adequate torque to maintain the abrasive against the tooth for polishing. The abrasive is carried to the tooth by dipping the rubber cup or brush into the abrasive-filled dappen dish or small prepackaged container. The cup or brush is placed against the tooth, and the rheostat activated so that the applicator rotates, thus polishing the tooth with the abrasive.

The abrasive-filled dappen dish can be held by a finger on the nondominant hand for ready access. Alternatively, a chairside assistant can apply the abrasive directly to the teeth with a plastic syringe, just ahead of the path of the rubber cup or brush. Regardless of how the abrasive is placed on the tooth, it is important that adequate amounts be used. Usually a full rubber cup of abrasive will be sufficient for one or two teeth. A bare or saliva-laden cup void of polishing agent does not polish the teeth and generates heat (Spierings, Peters, and Plasschaert, 1985).

The rubber cup can be adapted to all exposed

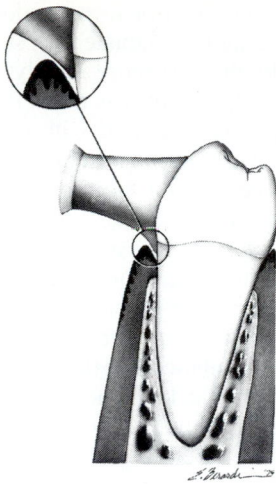

Fig. 30-6. Rubber cup should be adapted so that it slides slightly subgingivally in cervical area.

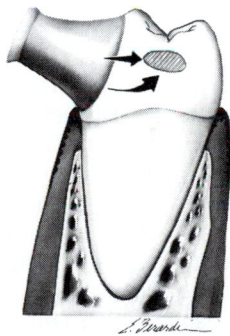

Fig. 30-7. Rubber cup should be adapted so that it has as much access to proximal surface as possible and so that it slides up under contact point.

tooth surfaces. The lip of the cup can be flared and slipped slightly subgingivally to clean the most coronal aspects of the sulcus (Fig. 30-6). It should be applied to proximal surfaces by sliding the lip of the cup as far proximally as possible and slightly under the contact point area (Fig. 30-7). Adapting the lip of the cup into the occlusal grooves will often suffice to remove stains from these difficult areas. When the rubber cup does not remove occlusal stain adequately, a small brush may be used. Brushes *should not* be used on any other tooth surfaces, as they are highly abrasive (Thompson and Way, 1981), difficult to control, and may abrade the soft tissues. Brushes are available with soft or firm bristles. The softer bristles are usually adequate for stain removal, and they hold abrasive more readily.

Whether a cup or brush is used, the attachment and abrasive should be used with *moderate intermittent pressure* (Tilliss and Hicks, 1987). Using intermittent pressure on the tooth allows the heat that is generated to dissipate between each stroke. Constant pressure of the rubber cup or brush on the tooth builds up frictional heat that can cause discomfort, pain, and possible pulp damage. This is especially critical for anterior teeth, which provide minimal insulation for the pulp because they have less dentin and enamel than the posterior teeth. Clinicians should observe the patient's facial expression carefully to detect signs of discomfort from heat. If the patient appears to be in pain, he or she should be asked if there is a sensation of heat. If so, the polishing procedure should be adjusted to reduce heat by lessening the duration of each application and/or the pressure of the cup or brush on the tooth. The speed of the cup is critical in both minimizing frictional heat and in ensuring effective polishing. Operating the cup at high speeds is both harmful and ineffective (Spierings, Peters, and Plasschaert, 1985). As it is rarely possible to determine the exact revolutions per minute (rpm) during operation, it is recommended to use the lowest possible speed that moves the cup or brush against the tooth without stalling. Sound also provides a clue as to whether the cup is rotating too rapidly. A high whine or whistle in the handpiece usually indicates excessive speed. To achieve the lowest possible speed, the rheostat may need to be activated to a high or medium speed and then backed down to a low speed before the tooth is touched with the attachment. Most dental units have a gauge that measures air pressure for each handpiece connector in pounds per square inch (psi). Operating the handpiece at approximately 20 psi seems to be sufficient for stain removal.

Air-powder polishing is a mechanism for polishing the teeth that propels a slurry of water and sodium bicarbonate under air and water pressure. The pounds of pressure per square inch will depend on the type of air polisher being used. In most units the water temperature is warm and thermostatically controlled. The handpiece has a nozzle through which the slurry is propelled when a foot control is activated. The nozzle should be held 3 to 5 mm from the tooth. Holding the nozzle farther from the tooth surface minimizes the

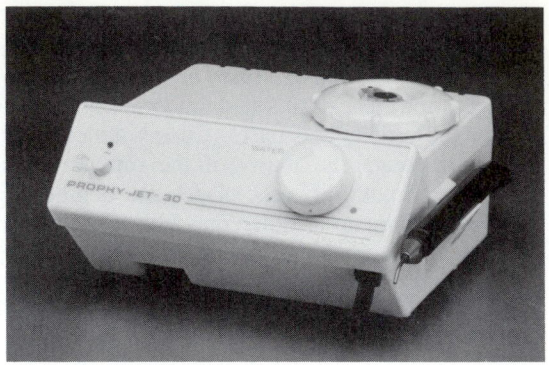

Fig. 30-8. Single unit (Prophy-Jet).

abrasive action (Walmsley,Williams and Laird, 1987). The tip should be angled diagonally towards the tooth and not at right angles to it. The stream should not be aimed at the soft tissue, but towards the occlusal or incisal surfaces. Air-powder polishers are manufactured either as separate units (Fig. 30-8), in combination with an ultrasonic scaler (Fig. 30-9), or to attach directly to the air/water connector on the dental unit (Fig. 30-10). There appears to be little difference in effectiveness of stain removal among the various types of air-powder polishes (Cooley, Braun, and Lubow, 1990). The air-powder polisher removes plaque and stain as well as a rubber cup and in less time (DeSpain and Nobis, 1988; Weaks, 1984). However, it may not prevent plaque reaccumulation as effectively as a rubber cup (Baker, 1988). It has little effect on enamel but can erode cementum and dentin (Boyde, 1984; Kee and Allen, 1988; Galloway and Pashly, 1987; Konturri-Närhi et al, 1990; Peterson et al, 1985).

Some patients require extensive instrumentation on root structure to remove coffee or tobacco stains, particularly at the cementoenamel junction or on areas with extensive recession. If stain is removed with a curette, which is the accepted procedure when a rubber cup or porte polisher cannot adequately reach the areas in question, the root structure will be pared down over the years. This is particularly likely if the patient is on a short recall interval (Fig. 30-11). The air-powder polisher is preferable to the curette in these instances. The air-powder polisher has been shown to remove less root structure than the curette in simulated 3-month recalls for 3 years. In addition, stain was removed more than three times as fast with the air-powder polisher (Berkstein et al, 1987).

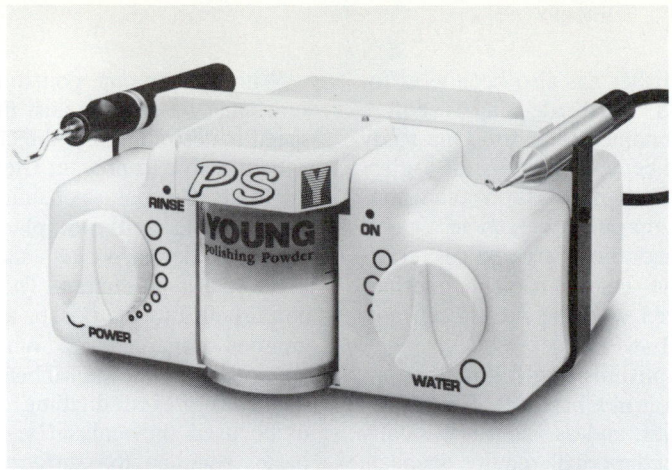

Fig. 30-9. Combination unit (Young's).

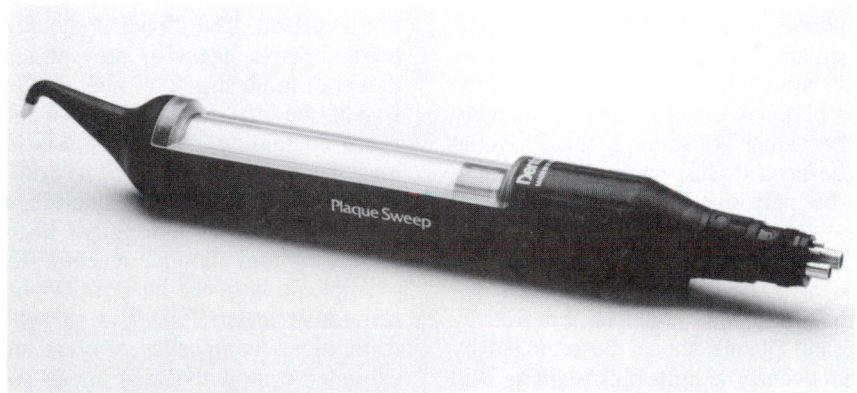

Fig. 30-10. Attach to air/water connector (Plaque Sweep).

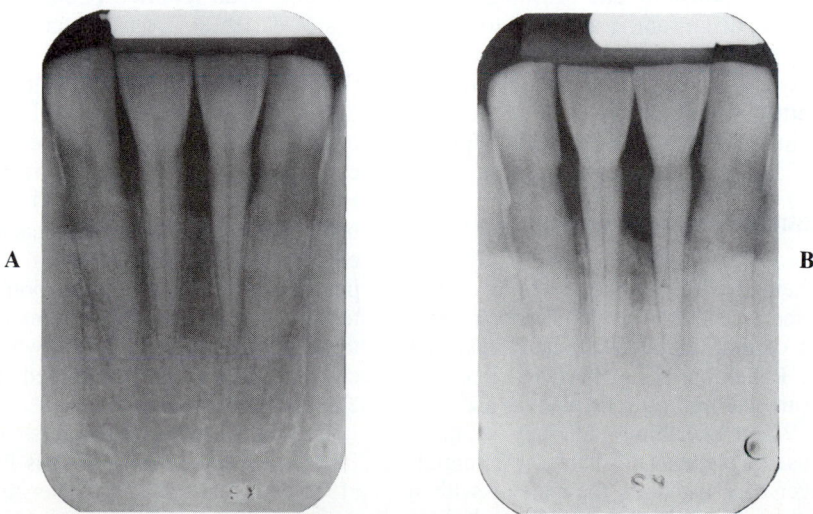

Fig. 30-11. **A,** Radiograph of anterior teeth in 1978. **B,** Radiograph of the same teeth in 1988 after quarterly scaling and polishing, partly to remove tobacco tar from exposed root surfaces. Note the altered root shape.

The air-powder polisher has also been used for debridement of class V abraded areas before placement of glass ionomer cements. One study compared the enamel-cement interface of a glass ionomer cement placed in class V abrasions cleaned by a rubber cup polish versus an air polisher. The air-polished tooth created less microleakage around the enamel-cement interface than the tooth prepared with the rubber cup polisher (Cooley and Lubow 1989).

The sequence of polishing can follow the outline for instrumentation in Chapter 9. Positioning of the patient, clinician, and assistant is basically unchanged. The procedure will require adequate evacuation, as the polishing agent and the mechanical manipulation in the mouth stimulate the salivary glands to secrete more saliva than normal. The trisyringe can be used to flush the areas with a water stream as each arch segment is completed. At the completion of the procedure, the patient should be encouraged to rinse thoroughly to remove all residual polishing agent. Proximal areas should be flossed. Inspection for remaining stain should be performed with good intraoral light, compressed air, and the mouth mirror. Final inspection for plaque should be accomplished with a disclosant as described in previous chapters. Any remaining stain should be removed by the clinician, and plaque should be removed by the patient. Frequently a light pink staining will reappear on the mandibular anterior lingual surfaces with each disclosing and will not disappear despite of repeated polishing and brushing. In almost all cases the disclosant is adherent to a thin sheet of calculus that is not visible unless dried with compressed air. Instrumentation with a scaler or curette is necessary to remove the hard deposit. If stain still exists, the area can be repolished.

Contraindications, precautions, and safety issues

Polishing, whether with a porte, engine, or air-powder polisher, should be approached with knowledge of contraindications, precautions, and safety issues. Polishing is not performed on patients for whom scaling and root planing are contraindicated. When polishing with any of these devices, the use of a stable finger rest is essential. A stable finger rest provides the patient with a sense of confidence in the hygienist's technique and avoids slippage and possible damage to the tissues.

With rubber cup polishing, intermittent pressure must be used against the tooth, slow engine speed is desirable, and the cup must be kept filled with abrasive to prevent frictional heat buildup in the tooth. Cosmetic polishing with the rubber cup after scaling and root planing in patients with deep periodontal pockets should be scheduled for a separate appointment. The polishing agent may be pushed into the pocket and result in increased gingival inflammation. When cemental surfaces are polished with the rubber cup, even pressure is applied to prevent ditching. Brush attachments are to be used on occlusal surfaces *only*. Polishing pastes roughen the surface of composite resins; thus their use should be avoided at those sites (Serio et al, 1988).

Selection of an appropriate abrasive for polishing is critical. The clinician should start with the least abrasive agent to prevent unnecessary removal of tooth structure, moving to the next abrasive if the first fails to remove the stain. If an agent containing fluoride is used, the hygienist must be certain the patient has no history of allergy or toxic reaction to fluoride or prophylaxis pastes. Even with a negative history, a patient may exhibit an allergice reaction (Coyne, 1989).

Application of the air-powder polisher on most restorative materials should be avoided. Esthetic restorations (composites, veneers, porcelain) have exhibited wear with use of the air-powder polisher (Barnes, Hayes, and Leinfelder, 1987; Reel et al, 1984; Eliades et al, 1991). Pitting of porcelain has also been reported (Cooley et al, 1988; Eliades et al, 1991). Even a 5-second exposure results in surface changes in several composite materials (Lubow and Cooley, 1986; Patterson and McLundie, 1984). However it can be safely used near orthodontic brackets (Barnes et al, 1990). Use on cast restorations is also contraindicated (Barnes, Hayes, and Leinfelder, 1987). Air polishing has been shown to wear dental sealants (Huennekens et al, 1991). In the same in vitro study of repeated application of the air polisher, sealant material was not detectable clinically, but was found to be present in the fissures when the teeth were cross-sectioned and examined with a scanning electron microscope.

Use of the air-powder polisher on implant surfaces is controversial. Whereas Parham and others (1989) suggest the air polisher may be used on titanium implants without surface damage, Thompson-Neal, Evans, and Meffert (1989) reported that most professional mechanical cleaning methods cause abrasion to various implant materials. The air-powder polisher has been reported to remove the surface titanium, replacing the oxide layer with sodium bicarbonate particles that may increase surface corrosion (Rapley et al, 1990). One adverse reaction involving pain and submucosal emphysema was reported (Bergendahl et al, 1990). One researcher suggests the use of a 2- X 2-inch gauze square with a fine prophylaxis paste for polishing around nonremovable implant prostheses (Moriarty JD, 1991). In addition, implant surfaces may be polished with a plastic tip, DynaTip (DynaDent, Santa Ana, Calif.), now available to fit over the Titan Sonic Scaler (Gantes and Nilveus, 1991).

The air-powder polisher generates an aerosol of microorganisms that contaminates surfaces several feet from the operative site (Glenwright, Knibbs, and Burdon, 1985; Logothetis, Gross, and Eberhart, 1988). Gloves, mask, protective lenses for the patient, operator, and assistant, and a laminar airflow system to reduce airborne bacteria are important to minimize this problem. Surface areas require thorough disinfection after this procedure.

Systemic concerns exist when the air-powder polisher is used. Blood sample analysis of one patient before and after treatment with an air-powder polisher demonstrated that serum pH rose to a marginally alkaline state, a situation which will normally resolve in a day or two. This may, however, be a potential problem for patients with chronic diarrhea or those who abuse laxatives or use diuretics extensively (Rawson et al, 1985). Snyder et al (1990) found no change in blood chemistry other than an increase in potassium. Another study compared the development of bacteremia in subjects undergoing rubber cup or air-powder polishing. Although the difference was not significant, more subjects receiving rubber cup polishing developed bacteremias than those receiving air-powder polishing. If gingivitis is not present, the likelihood of a patient developing a bacteremia from air-powder polishing is no greater than with rubber cup polishing (Hunter et al, 1989). Small blood clots at the margin of the gingiva have been noted immediately after air-powder polishing, with no signs of abrasion or long-term irritation (Mishkin et al, 1986). Some transient soft tissue abrasion can be expected when the air-powder polisher is used (Konturri-

Närhi et al, 1990). Angling it into a pocket can cause an adverse reaction (Finlayson and Stevens, 1988).

THERAPEUTIC POLISHING

Therapeutic polishing is the removal of toxins from the unexposed root surfaces resulting in a decrease in disease parameters. It is possible to polish root surfaces with the rubber-cup or air-powder polisher; however, the literature cites the use of the air-powder polisher for this purpose (Kozlovsky et al, 1989). The air-powder polisher may be used because of its effectiveness and efficiency, since root surfaces are polished when exposed during a surgical procedure. The air-powder polisher has been found to work well in removing plaque, endotoxins, and stain from root concavities and furcations as an adjunct to periodontal surgery (Horning, Cobb, and Killoy, 1987) and even when a modified flap is laid and calculus is removed without planing the cementum (Nyman et al, 1986, 1988). However, it may offer no measurable benefit over ultrasonic debridement (Krupa et al, 1988). One in vitro study suggests that using an ultrasonic scaler followed by air-powder polishing creates an environment in which fibroblast growth and vitality are greater than using ultrasonic scaling without polishing or leaving the remaining calculus in place (Gilman and Maxey, 1986). Whether used as a follow-up to ultrasonic scaling or on calculus-free root surfaces, the air-powder polisher may play a significant role in the future in the removal of endotoxins on exposed root surfaces during surgery.

When polishing for therapeutic benefits with the air-powder polisher, the hygienist should follow the precautions and considerations presented previously. Most importantly, the clinician should take care to direct the air-powder spray against the root surface, not the exposed soft tissues.

THE ROLE OF POLISHING IN DENTAL HYGIENE CARE

Polishing for cosmetic and therapeutic purposes rather than removing all soft deposits may be a new experience for some patients. Many have learned to consider the professional oral prophylaxis as a full-mouth polish for esthetic reasons or as the key to "healthy gums" (Hunter et al, 1981; Walsh et al, 1985). Accepting some responsibility for this care may be an unfamiliar and perhaps uncomfortable role for some patients. Therefore it is wise to share with the patient the purpose of polishing, the effect of repeated polishing on the teeth, the rate of re-formation of plaque on the teeth after polishing, and the roles all of these play in *prevention* of disease. This explanation may make it easier for the patient to accept the change and reinforce the concomitant plaque control messages offered throughout care. You might try the following approach:

"I know we have polished all your teeth in the past, but we now know that all polishing does is remove stain. The soft debris and plaque can be removed with a toothbrush and dental floss. The plaque can re-form in less than 24 hours; therefore, your work at home is critical to the continued removal of plaque and soft debris, and to the health of supporting tissues. Also, research has shown us that some of the restorations you have in your mouth can be scratched from the use of polishing agents and that a small amount of the tooth structure can be worn away with repeated polishing. Today, I will polish the teeth that have stain and with your help we will remove all the plaque and soft debris with a toothbrush and floss (or other aids as needed)."

Most patients will be receptive to this change if it is presented by a professional who exhibits current knowledge of the profession and care for the patient. If, however, the patient does not accept this change, then it is better to polish the whole mouth with a dentifrice using moderate pressure rather than with a polishing agent (Tilliss and Hicks, 1987).

ACTIVITIES

1. Omit brushing your teeth one morning. Rinse your mouth with grape juice (swallow or spit out), and describe how your mouth feels and the appearance of your teeth and deposits. Which deposits do you think are stained? How do you think this relates to not brushing after meals and eating colored foods? How can you "feel" the grape juice remaining in your mouth? Evaluate the ease of removing the stained deposits.
2. Examine several student partners. If you find intrinsic stains, can you relate them to childhood diseases, medications, fluorides, restorative materials, or other sources? If you find extrinsic stains, can you relate them to tea, coffee, and/or tobacco consumption?
3. Polish stain from a partner's teeth using a porte polisher, engine polisher, and air-powder polisher. Compare the results, the effort and time involved, and your partner's preference.
4. Examine the variety of tips available for use in the porte polisher.

5. Perform routine maintenance on the handpiece and autoclavable prophylaxis angle used for engine polishing in your clinic.
6. Given a nonfunctioning engine polisher, determine why it is not working and correct the problem.
7. Evaluate the effectiveness and quality of disposable prophylaxis angles after clinical application of each.
8. Use the air-powder polisher to polish a quadrant of teeth that are heavily laden with stain. Polish a second quadrant with an engine-driven rubber cup. Compare results in terns of (1) cleanliness of the teeth, (2) time, (3) patient acceptance, and (4) amount of recurrent stain at the recall visit.
9. Role-play an encounter with a patient who wishes to have all of his or her teeth polished regardless of the presence of stain and present a rationale for selective polishing.
10. Take two pennies and draw a line to divide each in half. On one half apply dry pumice with a rubber cup. On the other half apply dry chalk with a second rubber cup. Examine each for scratches. On the second penny, apply a slurry of pumice with a rubber cup to one half and a slurry of chalk with a new rubber cup to the other half. Examine each for differences in smoothness and luster. The same exercise can be performed with any abrasive or polishing method.

REVIEW QUESTIONS

1. Define the following stain classifications:
   a. Exogenous.
   b. Endogenous.
   c. Extrinsic.
   d. Intrinsic.
2. What is the primary importance of the abrasive in toothpaste?
3. Compare abrasives in toothpastes and professional products.
4. What factors affect abrasiveness and polishing?
5. What criteria are used to select a polishing agent?
6. How can frictional heat be minimized during engine polishing?
7. What are the advantages and disadvantages of a porte polisher?
8. What is the primary indication for polishing teeth?
9. How does the air-powder polisher work?
10. What are the indications and contraindications or precautions for use of the air-powder polisher?
11. What effect does polishing of unexposed root surfaces have on disease?
12. What is the difference between cosmetic and therapeutic polishing?

REFERENCES

American Dental Association Council on Dental Therapeutics: *Accepted dental therapeutics,* ed 39, Chicago, 1982, The Association.

Atkinson DR, Cobb CM, Killoy WJ: The effect of an airpowder abrasive system on in vitro root surfaces, *J Periodontol* 55:13, 1984.

Baker DJ: Effects of rubber cup polishing and an air abrasive system on plaque accumulation, *Dent Hyg* 62:55, 1988 (abstract).

Barnes CM, Hayes EF, Leinfelder, KF: Effects of an airabrasive polishing system on restored surfaces, *Gen Dent* 35:186, 1987.

Barnes CM et al: Effects of an air-powder polishing system on orthodontically bracketed and banded teeth, *Am J Orthod Dentofacial Orthop* 97:74, 1990.

Bergendal T et al: The effect of an airbrasive instrument on soft and hard tissues around osseointegrated implants, *Swed Dent J* 14:219, 1990.

Berkstein S et al: Supragingival root surface removal during maintenance procedures utilizing an air-powder abrasive system or hand scaling: an in vitro study, *J Periodontol* 58:327, 1987.

Boyde A: Airpolishing effects on enamel, dentine, cement and bone, *Br Dent J* 156:287, 1984.

Carranza FA Jr: *Glickman's clinical periodontology,* ed 5, Philadelphia, 1979, WB Saunders.

Christensen RP: Brand names and characteristics of polishing products used by dental hygienists in the US: results of a survey, *Dent Hyg* 58:222, 1984.

Christensen RP, Bangerter VW: Determination of rpm, time, and load used in oral prophylaxis polishing in vivo, *J Dent Res* 63:1376, 1984.

Christensen RP, Bangerter VW: Immediate and long-term in vivo effects of polishing on enamel and dentin, *J Prosthet Dent* 57:150, 1987.

Cooley RL, Brown FH, Lubow RM: Evaluation of air-powder abrasive prophylaxis units, *Gen Dent* 38:24, 1990.

Cooley RL, Lubow RM: Effect of air-powder abrasive on glass ionomer microleakeage, *Gen Dent* 37:16, 1989.

Cooley, RL, Lubow RM, Brown FH: Effect of an air-powder abrasive instrument on porcelain, *J Prosthet Dent* 60:440, 1988.

Cooley RL, Lubow RM, Patrissi GA: The effect of an airpowder abrasive instrument on composite resin, *JADA* 112:362, 1986.

Cooley RO: Resin veneer ends discoloration problem, *Dent Stud* 54:28, 1976.

Coyne PJ: Allergic reaction to prophy paste: report of a case, *Northwest Dent* 67:21, 1988.

Craig RG, O'Brien WJ, Powers JM: *Dental materials: properties and manipulation,* ed 3, St Louis, 1983, CV Mosby.

Croll TP: Enamel microabrasion for removal of superficial discoloration, *J Esthetic Dent* 1:14, 1989.

Davis WR: Cleaning, polishing and abrasion of teeth by dental products, *Cosmet Sci* 1:38, 1978.

DeSpain B, Nobis R: Comparison of rubber cup polishing and air polishing on stain, plaque, calculus, and gingiva, *Dent Hyg* 62:55, 1988 (abstract).

Doderich DN, Gulevich TM, Reid A: The effect of rubber cup vs an air-powder abrasive system on root surfaces, *J Probe* 23:135, 1989.

Eliades GC, Tzoutzas JG Voughiouklakis GJ: Surface alterations on dental restorative materials subjected to air powder abrasive instruments, *J Prosthet Dent* 65:27, 1991.

Finlayson RS, Stevens FD: Subcutaneous facial emphysema secondary to use of the Cavi-Jet, *J Periodontol* 59:315, 1988.

Galloway SE, Pashley DH: Rate of removal of root structure by the use of the Prophy-Jet device, *J Periodontol* 58:464, 1987.

Gantes BG, Nilveus R: The effects of different hygiene instruments on titanium surfaces: SEM observations, *Int J Periodont Rest Dent* 11:225, 1991.

Gershon SD, Pader M: Dentifrices. In Balsam MS, Sangarin E, editors: *Cosmetics: sciences and technology,* vol 1, New York, 1972, Wiley-Interscience.

Gilman RS, Maxey BR: The effect of root detoxification on human gingival fibroblasts, *J Periodontol* 57:436, 1986.

Glenwright ND, Knibbs PJ, Burdon DW: Atmospheric contamination during use of an air polisher, *Br Dent J* 159:294, 1985.

Goldstein RE: *Esthetics in dentistry*, Philadelphia, 1976, JB Lippincott.

Goldstein RE, Ronald AF: Bleaching of vital and nonvital teeth. In Cohen S, Burns RC: *Pathways of the pulp*, ed 4, St Louis, 1987, CV Mosby.

Heringer E: Bleaching removes some discoloration, *Dent Stud* 54:31, 1976.

Hosoya Y, Johnston JW: Evaluation of various cleaning and polishing methods on primary enamel, *J Pedodont* 13:253, 1989.

Horning GM, Cobb CM, Killoy WI: Effect of an air-powder abrasive system on root surfaces in periodontal surgery, *J Clin Periodontol* 14:213, 1987.

Huber SJ, Vemino AR, Nanca RS: Professional prophylaxis and its effect on the periodontium of full-banded orthodontic patients, *Am J Orthod Dentofacial Ortho* 91:321, 1987.

Huennekens SC, Daniel SC, Bayne SC: Effects of air polishing on the abrasion of occlusal sealants, *Quintessence Intl* 22:581, 1991.

Hunter EL et al: The prophylaxis polish: a review of the literature, *Dent Hyg* 55(9):36, 1981.

Hunter KM et al: Bacteraemia and tissue damage resulting from air polishing, *Br Dent J* 167:275, 1989.

Kee A, Allen DS: Effects of air and rubber cup polishing on enamel abrasion, *Dent Hyg* 62:55, 1988 (abstract).

Kontturi-Närhi V, Markkanen S, Markkanen H: Effects of airpolishing on dental plaque removal and hard tissues as evaluated by scanning electron microscopy, *J Periodontol* 61:334, 1990.

Kontturi-Närhi V, Markkanen S, Markkanen H: The gingival effects of dental airpolishing as evaluated by scanning electron microscopy, *J Periodontol* 60:19, 1989.

Kozlovsky A, Soldinger M, Sperling I: The effectiveness of the air-powder abrasive device on the tooth and periodontium: an overview, *Clin Prev Dent* 11:7, 1989.

Krupa CM et al: In vitro evaluation of air-powder polishing as an adjunct to ultrasonic scaling on periodontally involved root surfaces, *Dent Hyg* 62:55, 1988 (abstract)

Lado EA, Stanley HR, Weismann MI: Cervical resorption in bleached teeth, *Oral Surg* 55:78, 1983.

Lobene RR: Effect of dentifrices on tooth stains with controlled brushing, *JADA* 77:849, 1968.

Logothetis R, Gross K, Eberhart A: Bacterial aerosol contamination using an air polishing device, *Dent Hyg* 62:55, 1988 (abstract).

Lubow RM, Cooley RL: Effect of air-powder abrasive instrument on restorative materials, *J Prosthet Dent* 55:462, 1986.

Mallatt ME, Christen A: Is a prophylaxis really necessary prior to topical fluoride therapy? *J Indiana Dent Assoc* 68:33, 1989.

Mellberg JR: Enamel fluoride and its anti-caries effects, *J Prev Dent* 4:8, 1977.

Mishkin DJ et al: A clinical comparison of the effect on the gingiva of the Prophy-Jet and the rubber cup and paste techniques, *J Periodontol* 53:151, 1986.

Moffitt JM et al: Prediction of tetracycline-induced tooth discoloration, *JADA* 88:547, 1974.

Moriarty JD: Personal communication, 1991.

Ness L, Rosekrans DL, Welford JF: An epidemiologic study of factors affecting extrinsic staining of teeth in an English population, *Community Dent Oral Epidemiol* 5:55, 1977.

Nyman S et al: Role of "diseased" root cementum in healing following treatment of periodontal desease, an experimental study in the dog, *J Periodont Res* 21:496, 1986.

Nyman S et al: Role of "diseased" cementum in healing following treatment of periodontal disease: a clinical study, *J Clin Periodontol* 15:464, 1988.

O'Brien W, Ryge G: *An outline of dental materials and their selection*, Philadelphia, 1978, WB Saunders.

Parham PL et al: Effects of an air-powder abrasive system on plasma-sprayed titanium implant surfaces: an in vitro evaluation, *J Oral Implantol* 15:78, 1989.

Patterson CJW, McLundie AC: A comparison of the effects of two different prophylaxis regimes in vitro on some restorative dental materials, *Br Dent J* 157:166, 1984.

Peterson LG et al: The effect of a jet abrasive instrument (Prophy-Jet) on root surfaces, *Swed Dent J* 9:193, 1985.

Rall DP: From the NIH: research findings of potential value to the practitioner, *JAMA* 217:635, 1977.

Rapley JW et al: The surface characteristics produced by various oral hygiene instruments and materials on titanium implant abutments, *Int J Oral & Maxillofac Implants* 11:47, 1990.

Rawson RD et al: Alkalosis as a potential complication of air polishing systems, *Dent Hyg* 59:500, 1985.

Reel DC et al: Effect of a hydraulic jet prophylaxis system on composites *J Prosthet Dent* 61:441, 1989.

Reid JS, Beeley JA, MacDonald DG: Investigation into black extrinsic tooth stain, *J Dent Res* 56:895, 1977.

Retief DH et al: In vitro fluoride uptake distribution and retention by human enamel after 1- and 24-hour application of various topical fluoride agents, *J Dent Res* 59:573, 1980.

Russ JC et al: SEM low magnification stereoscopic technique for mapping out surface contours: application to measurement of volume differences in human teeth due to polishing, *J Microscopy* 144:339, 1986.

Saxton CA: The effects of dentifrices on the appearance of the tooth surface observed with the scanning electron microscope, *J Periodont Res* 11:74, 1976.

Serio FG et al: The effect of polishing pastes on composite resin surfaces: a SEM study, *J Periodontol,* 59:837, 1988.

Shaw L, Murray JJ: A new index for measuring extrinsic stain in clinical trials, *Community Dent Oral Epidemiol* 5:1 16, 1977.

Shern RJ et al: Enamel biopsy results of children receiving fluoride tablets, *JADA* 95:310, 1977.

Solheim H, Eriksen HM, Nordbo H: Chemical plaque control and extrinsic discoloration of teeth, *Acta Odontol Scand* 38:303, 1980.

Snyder JA et al: The effect of air abrasive polishing on blood pH and electrolyte concentrations in healthy mongrel dogs, *J Periodontol,* 61:81, 1990.

Spencer DE: A conversative method of treating tetracycline stained teeth, *J Dent Child* 39:443, 1972.

Spierings TAM, Peters MCRB, Plasschaert AJM: Thermal trauma to teeth, *Endodont Dent Traumatol* 1:123, 1985.

Steele RC et al: The effect of tooth cleaning procedures on fluoride uptake in enamel, *Pediatr Dent* 4:228, 1982.

Stookey GK, Scbemehorn BR: Studies evaluating a fluoride-containing prophylactic cup, *Dent Hyg* 50:253, 1976.

Stookey GK, Stahlman DB: Enhanced fluoride uptake in enamel with a fluoride-impregnated prophylactic cup, *J Dent Res* 55:333, 1976.

Stuart R: Treatment of anterior teeth for esthetic problems, *Quintessence Intl* 6:31, 1975.

Swan RW: Dimensional changes in a tooth root incident to various polishing and root planing procedures, *Dent Hyg* 53:17, 1979.

Thomson-Neal D, Evans GH, Meffert RM: Effects of various prophylactic treatments on titanium, sapphire, and hydroxyapatite-coated implants: an SEM study, *Int J Periodont Restor Dent* 9:301, 1989.

Thompson RE, Way DC: Enamel loss due to prophylaxis and multiple bonding debonding of orthodontic attachments, *Am J Orthod* 79:282, 1981.

Tilliss TS, Hicks MJ: Enamel surface morphology comparison: polishing with a toothpaste and a prophylaxis paste, *Dent Hyg* 61:112, 1987.

Tinanoff N et al: Effect of a pumice prophylaxis on fluoride uptake in tooth enamel, *JADA* 88:384. 1974.

Vogel RJ: Intrinsic and extrinsic discoloration of the dentition: (a literature review) *J Oral Med,* 30(4):99, 1975.

Walmsley AD, Williams AR, Laird WRE: The air-powder dental abrasive unit—an evaluation using a model system, *J Oral Rehabil* 14:43, 1987.

Walsh MM, Heckman BH, Moreau-Diettinger R: Polished and unpolished teeth: patient responses after an oral prophylaxis, *Dent Hyg* 59:306, 1985.

Walsh MM et al: Effect of a rubber cup polish after scaling, *Dent Hyg* 59:484, 1985.

Waring MB et al: A comparison of engine polishing and toothbrushing in minimizing dental plaque reaccumulation, *Dent Hyg* 56(12):25, 1982.

Waring MB et al: Plaque reaccumulation following engine polishing or toothbrushing-a 90-day clinical trial, *Dent Hyg* 62:282, 1988.

Weaks LM et al: Clinical evaluation of the Prophy-Jet as an instrument for routine removal of tooth stain and plaque, *J Periodontol* 55:486, 1984.

Winter GB, Murray JJ, Shaw L: Cosmetics and dental history, *Cosmet Sci* 1:1 1978.

Yankell S, Emling RC: Understanding dental products: what you should know and what your patient should know, *Contin Dent Educ* 1:7, 1978.

Yankell SL et al: Effects of chlorhexidine and four antimicrobial compounds on plaque, gingivitis and staining in beagle dogs, *J Dent Res* 61:1089, 1982.

SUGGESTED READINGS

Cross GN, and Carr EH: Patients' acceptance of selective polishing, *Dent Hyg* 57(12):20, 1983.

Manly RS: A structureless recurrent deposit on teeth, *J Dent Res* 22:479, 1943.

Orton GS: Clinical use of an air-powder abrasive system, *J Dent Hyg* 61(11): 513, 1987.

Primosch RE: Rubber cup prophylaxis: a reevaluation of its use in pediatric dental patients, *Dent Hyg* 54:525, 1980.

Rohleder PV, Slim LH: Alternatives to rubber cup polishing, *Dent Hyg* 55(9):16, 1981.

31 CONTROL OF DENTIN HYPERSENSITIVITY

Susan Daniel

LEARNING OUTCOMES

The dental hygienist will be able to

1. Understand the hydrodynamic theory of pain conduction.
2. Describe the three general categories of stimuli that elicit pain response and give examples of each.
3. Discuss the role of plaque in the prognosis of hypersensitivity treatment.
4. Describe antihypersensitive products available for home care.
5. Select office procedures for treating sensitivity based on patient needs and response to agents.
6. Determine if adjustments need to be made in a patient's plaque removal and dietary habits to assist in reducing dentin hypersensitivity.
7. Comment on the current American Dental Association and Food and Drug Administration policies for desensitizing products.

Do you have or do you know someone who has sensitive teeth? If the answer is yes, then you will have a true appreciation for the content of this chapter. If, however, your answer is no, you can still benefit from the content as you encounter patients in your practice who exhibit dentinal hypersensitivity. It has been reported that approximately 40 million adults in the United States have dentinal hypersensitivity at one time or another and that more than 10 million have chronic hypersensitivity (Kanapka, 1982). Hypersensitive dentin is most common among patients aged 20 to 40 years, peaking during the 30s (Flynn, Galloway, and Orchardson, 1985; Graf and Galasse, 1977). The condition has been reported to occur slightly more often in females than males; however, this finding has not been statistically significant (Addy, 1990; Flynn, Galloway, and Orchardson, 1985; Orchardson and Collins, 1987).

What is dentinal hypersensitivity? It can be defined as an adverse reaction or pain in one or more teeth resulting from a thermal, chemical, or mechanical stimulus (Clark, 1985). Microscopic examination of clinically hypersensitive surfaces has shown areas of dentin exposed by gingival recession, abrasion, erosion, periodontal therapy, defective restorations, or caries. The tubules in these areas are also shown microscopically to be wider and more numerous than in nonsensitive areas (Absi, Adams, and Addy, 1986; Absi, Addy, and Adams, 1987; Yoshiyama et al, 1989). Hypersensitive dentin is found almost exclusively on the facial surfaces of teeth at the cervical margins (Graf and Galasse, 1977). The relative frequency of sensitivity of different teeth has been reported as follows: premolars, 38%; incisors, 26%; canines, 24%; and molars, 12% (Orchardson and Collins, 1987).

Now, let's look at how the sensation of pain is transmitted from the exposed dentinal surface to the terminal nerve endings.

HYDRODYNAMIC THEORY

Historically, there have been several theories to explain the mechanism of pain transmission from the dentin to the pulp (Tronstad, 1982; Krauser, 1986a). Frank and colleagues (1972), using SEM, invalidated previous theories when they reported that nerves entering the dentinal tubules extend only to the inner one-third of the dentin from the pulp. As early as the midnineteenth century the work of Dr. Neill of Philadelphia was reviewed and published by Blandy (1850–51). Dr. Neill postulated that:

Dentin consists of hollow tubules, filled with fluid secreted by the pulp, and pressure applied without, by compressing the enamel and the fluid of the tubules, affects the nervous pulp within, by subjecting the latter to a species of hydrostatic pressure, the amount of which can be measured. Whatever reduces the thickness of the enamel or uncovers any portion of the dentine, increases the painful impression caused by external pressure.

Approximately 100 years later, Kramer proposed the "hydrodynamic" theory, which was later expounded on by Alfred Gysi; however, it wasn't until the late 1950s with the work of Martin Brannstrom that the theory was accepted by the dental profession (Rosenthal, 1990). Brannstrom (1966) conducted a series of experiments asking the following questions: How could an area of tooth that has no obvious signs of decay sometimes be so sensitive to the slightest stimulus? Why would exposure to a mere blast of air elicit a pain response? Why would exposure to sugar or salty foods cause pain when many chemical agents known to stimulate nerve fibers do not produce a response when applied to exposed dentin?

The hydrodynamic theory is based on the observation that fluid within the dentinal tubules can flow either outward or inward depending on the pressure variations in the surrounding tissues. The rapid movement of fluid in the open dentinal tubules may subsequently deform the odontoblast or its process, eliciting the transmission of a pain-causing stimulus (Brannstrom and Astrom, 1964). The theory of hydrodynamics clarifies how so many different stimuli can elicit the same pain response.

ETIOLOGY OF HYPERSENSITIVITY

The etiology of dentinal hypersensitivity is multifactorial. Stimuli that may elicit a pain response have been categorized as mechanical, thermal, chemical, or osmotic (Addy, 1990). Dental procedures can contribute to or initiate the onset or progression of hypersensitivity. The clearest example of the hydrodynamic theory and a mechanical stimulus is the dehydration of dentin (i.e., by an air blast). The air causes dehydration, which causes the dentinal fluid to move in an outward direction by capillary action. This, in turn, pulls the odontoblastic process farther into the tubule, stimulating sensory pulpal nerves (Brannstrom and Astrom, 1964). Direct mechanical stimulation can occur during dental instrumentation (e.g., during exploratory procedures or scaling). Mechanical trauma can result from brushing, especially when toothbrushes with firm bristles are used. It has been reported that incorrect brushing

can cause gingival recession and root surface abrasion; this may account for the high incidence of hypersensitive dentin on vestibular surfaces, particularly in teeth at the corners of the arch, in a region that is perhaps most susceptible to toothbrush trauma (Orchardson and Collins, 1987). Patients who chronically clench and grind their teeth often complain of tooth sensitivity. Enamel loss through occlusal wear caused by bruxing can expose dentinal tubules and cause pain (Knight, 1969).

The second type of stimulus that elicits tooth sensation is thermal. Responses can occur when hot and cold foods or liquids are consumed or when cold air reaches the exposed dentinal areas. Heat applied to the dentin results in an expansion of the fluid, putting pressure on the odontoblast, which again stimulates a pain response (Brannstrom and Astrom, 1964).

Sweet, sour, or highly acidic foods, fluids of high osmolarity (salty or sugar solutions), and plaque induce pain by chemical stimuli. Pain produced when sugar or salted solutions are placed in contact with exposed dentin can also be explained by tubular fluid movements. Fluids of a low osmolarity (i.e., the dentinal tubule fluid) have a tendency to flow toward solutions of a higher osmolarity (i.e., salty or sugar solutions) (Berman, 1984). This outward flow of fluid elicits a pain response. Some highly acidic foods (e.g., lemons) can chemically dissolve the enamel, exposing underlying dentin. Hypersensitivity also has been reported in individuals with bulimia because of the repeated exposure of the enamel to highly acidic gastric juices (Miles, 1985). Chemically induced pain has also been attributed to production of lactic acid by bacteria present in plaque. Conversely, other reports have found that the presence of plaque is associated with reduced tooth sensitivity. Addy and Mostafa (1989) reported greater sensitivity in an area of the mouth with the least plaque. In this study, the subjects who were right-handed had less plaque but greater sensitivity on the left side than the right side. It is believed that this negative association may result from the patients' vigorous brushing at the cervical margin, resulting in less plaque but greater abrasion of the exposed dentin.

Some dental procedures result in mechanical and thermal stimuli. More specifically, certain periodontal procedures have been found to result in dentinal hypersensitivity (Wong et al, 1989).

Periodontal therapy may create or increase the exposure of root surfaces, and it is recommended that concepts of hypersensitivity be explained to the patient when such procedures as scaling and root planing in the gingival margin area are to be performed. The root surface is covered with cementum, which is softer than calculus and often is removed by hand or ultrasonic instruments exposing the dentinal surface. Anatomically, the cementum and enamel may not meet at the cementoenamel junction during the developmental process, resulting in a naturally occurring area of exposed dentin (Moss-Salentin and Hendricks-Klyvert, 1990).

It has been reported that root planing can increase root sensitivity (Fischer et al, 1991; Haugen and Johansen, 1988; Hirsch and Clarke, 1989). Conversely, one study reported that root planing produced partially occluded dentinal tubules and a smear layer comprising microcrystals of cementum and dentin. Therefore this partial occlusion may decrease the conduction of a painful stimulus through the dentinal tubule (Addy, Absi, and Adams, 1987). More often, a painful stimulus results from the exposure of root surfaces following periodontal surgery than from root planing (Wallace and Bissada, 1990). What makes one type of dentin exposure respond to painful stimuli more than the other? The difference is analogous to the difference between an acute and chronic wound. That is to say that dentin, once it has been exposed and traumatized, will develop a reparative dentin over time. The tooth will become less susceptible to the root planing stimulus. However, following periodontal surgery, which results in apically positioned gingival tissues in conjunction with root planing, dentin is newly exposed and the root will become acutely sensitive to stimuli until reparative dentin can form.

One study investigated the differences in root sensitivity produced by the air-powder polisher and the rubber cup polisher. The dentinal tubules remained open with the air-powder polisher whereas the rubber cup polish left a smear layer that partially occluded them. Therefore an increase in sensitivity was reported among the group receiving the air-powder polishing (Dederich, Gulevich, and Reid, 1989).

Cavities or crown preparations by the dentist may also elicit sensitivity. For example, sensitivity may result if temporary filling materials are in contact with the dentin for too long a time after a cavity preparation has been performed. This postoperative sensitivity can be avoided if a varnish and base material are placed beneath restorations and crown preparations (Brannstrom, 1986).

NATURAL DEFENSE MECHANISMS

The pulp has several natural defenses to protect itself from irritating stimuli. One of these, reparative dentin, was discussed in the previous section. The tooth can also produce secondary dentin in response to calcification in the pulp chamber from stimuli (Krauser, 1986a). Dentinal sclerosis, if not caused by caries or attrition, can be associated with the aging process affecting the cervical region of the tooth late in life. This process is evidenced by mineralization in the peritubular dentin that can partially or completely block the patent tubule and prevent the passage of painful impulses (Berman, 1984). Yoshiyama and associates (1989, 1990) reported the presence of rhomboidal shaped crystals in dentinal tubules from naturally desensitized dentin.

TREATMENT OF HYPERSENSITIVITY

The majority of treatments for dentinal hypersensitivity attempt in some way to block fluid flow in the tubules. The following section describes some of the common agents as well as the difficulty of assessing their effects.

Although many products are available for use either by the patient or in a professional office, no one accepted modality gives maximum or consistent benefit (Chasens, 1974; Everett, Hall, and Phatak, 1966; Goldman, 1982; Grant, Stern, and Everett, 1979; Peden, 1977; Wycoff, 1982; Yankell, 1982). Many agents have been tested for treating hypersensitive teeth. The essential criteria used to select agents to be tested have not changed since they were developed by Grossman (1935). They are as follows:

1. Easy to use and apply.
2. Nonirritating.
3. Minimum number of dental appointments required (applications).
4. Painless.
5. Minimum application time.
6. Will not discolor teeth.
7. No danger to teeth or soft tissues.
8. Minimum expense.

These criteria apply to both professional and over-the-counter products.

Clinical studies to determine the effectiveness of agents or products for desensitization have been difficult to conduct because of the following:

1. Use of subjective evaluations.
2. Lack of proper controls.
3. Lack of objective measurements.
4. Strong placebo effect in control groups.

Historically, many evaluations have been based on subjective reactions. In these studies, the person's reaction to the products being tested has been based on his or her impressions of whether there was poor, fair, good, or excellent improvement. In addition, several studies have been based on the patient's evaluation under unsupervised use and without a placebo or control product (i.e., a product containing no known effective agent).

In 1986, the American Dental Association Council on Dental Therapeutics established guidelines for evaluating the efficacy of agents used to reduce hypersensitivity:

1. The test data should be quantifiable and reproducible.
2. Critical evaluation must be made of all subjective responses; threshold of response should be established, preferably quantified, and correlated to a clinically definable intensity; it is also recognized that the threshold is a range and not a point.
3. The relationship between the experimental stimulus and the defined area of hypersensitivity must be established by controlled clinical research.
4. There should be no commitment to a specific form of stimulus; if more than one stimulus is used, then these stimuli should be reproducible and interference between them must be minimized.
5. Appropriate statistics should be used, and these should be justified according to the experimental design.

To measure pain accurately, the investigations must assess the subjective pain as well as the characteristics of the stimulus producing it. Pain associated with dentin hypersensitivity has been difficult to assess, and research has not identified a physiologic index that is unequivocally related to changes in pain sensation and not simply related to stimulus intensity.

The criteria for accurate and objective pain measurement are as follows (Ad Hoc Advisory Committee on Dentinal Hypersensitivity, American Dental Association Council on Dental Therapeutics, 1986):

1. Reliability. The procedure yields consistent results with time; reliability across subjects and between test sessions should be determined.
2. Validity. The procedure measures unequivocally a specific dimension of pain.
3. Bias-free. The procedure is independent of method bias or patient or investigator response bias.
4. Versatility. The procedure is applicable for both laboratory and clinical uses.

Two types of instruments have been developed that can be applied to the tooth surface to produce specified temperatures at the probe site (Kanapka, 1982; Smith and Ash, 1964a, 1964b; Tarbet et al, 1982). This equipment has been used to evaluate agents with desensitizing potential and has resulted in acceptance of two products by the American Dental Association (Chasens, 1974; Kanapka, 1982).

A major problem with testing desensitizing agents or products can be the high degree of reduction in sensitivity that occurs in groups treated with control products. This may be the result of a general decline over time (often observed with sensitivity problems) or of improved cleaning by patients who are seen routinely by the dental professional.

Home care procedures should be emphasized as a primary factor in the treatment of sensitivity. It is important to have adequate plaque control procedures well developed by the patient before professional treatments are started (Chasens, 1974; Grant, Stern, and Everett, 1979; Green, Green, and McFall, 1977; Peden, 1977) to enhance the long-term benefits (Wycoff, 1982). In addition to proper brushing and flossing procedures, the use of other topical and interdental aids to remove plaque should be initiated. It is also important to discuss diet with the patient and, if necessary, to eliminate foods that are acidic or sour, and those which are fermentable carbohydrates, which can produce acids in plaque (Addy, Absi, and Adams, 1987; Clark et al, 1990). It is also important to evaluate the patient's toothbrush and dentifrice. Patients should use soft or ultrasoft toothbrushes with minimally abrasive dentifrices. There is no uniformity among toothbrush manufacturers as to the texture of the toothbrush bristles, and one manufacturer's soft bristles may be firmer than another manufacturer's medium bristles (Yankell and Emling, 1978). Toothpaste abrasiveness is another factor that is also difficult to monitor clinically, and it is up to the dental professional to individualize the dentifrice used by each patient. Regardless of treatment, tooth sensitivity can improve with a change in oral hygiene procedures (Gedalia et al, 1978; Hiatt and Johansen, 1972).

COMMERCIALLY AVAILABLE PRODUCTS
Over-the-counter products

Desensitizing toothpastes are widely promoted to both the dental profession and the public. Three of these toothpastes, Denquel Sensitive Teeth Toothpaste (Procter & Gamble Co., Cincinnati, Ohio) and Sensodyne Toothpaste for Sensitive Teeth and Mint Sensodyne (Block Drug Co., Jersey City, NJ), contain potassium nitrate as the active ingredient and have been found to be effective in clinical studies (Council on Dental Therapeutics, 1992). The exact mechanism of action is unknown. Some postulate that potassium nitrate, like most other ingredients, reduces dentin permeability by partially occluding the tubule. Others believe it has a desensitizing action on the fine nerve fibers at the dentinal-pulpal junction.

Another product, Protect (J.O. Butler), contains dibasic sodium citrate in a pluronic gel. The action of this product is thought to be derived from the ability of the polyglycoid to precipitate dentinal or salivary proteins. All of these agents have received "Accepted" status from the ADA and the Council on Dental Therapeutics for their effectiveness in reducing dentin hypersensitivity (American Dental Association Council on Dental Therapeutics, 1992).

Prescription products

One stable stannous fluoride 0.4% gel (Gel-Kam, Canton, MA) has recently received "Accepted" status from the ADA as a desensitizing agent. This product also carries the ADA seal for caries control and remineralization. It is a prescription home-applied gel that has been reported to produce satisfactory results when used for at least 2 weeks (Miller et al, 1969). Stannous fluoride works by occluding the dentinal tubules with tin and fluoride particles. (Blong et al, 1985; Ellingsen and Rolla, 1987; Snyder, Beck, and Horton, 1985; Thrash, 1992; Ellingsen and Rolla, 1987).

Stability of the stannous ion is the essential factor directly influencing the ability of this product to relieve hypersensitivity.

PROFESSIONAL PRODUCTS

Over 100 different agents for reducing dentin hypersensitivity have been reported in the literature (see box). Many of these agents were detrimental to the pulp or discolored the tooth surface. Most modern products used by dental professionals and their method(s) of application have not changed significantly since they were comprehensively reviewed by Everett, Hall, and Phatak in 1966. They have since been described in many textbooks and review articles (Chasens, 1974; Grant, Stern, and Everett, 1979; Peden, 1977). None of these products has been classified as effective for reducing dentin hypersensitivity by the ADA Council on Dental Therapeutics (ADA Council, 1992) or the Food and Drug Administration (see box).

TECHNIQUES

Treatment of hypersensitive teeth should be targeted at reducing the size of the tubules to limit fluid movement. To accomplish this goal one of the following strategies may be taken (Trowbridge and Silver, 1990):

1. Form a smear layer by burnishing the exposed root surface.
2. Apply topical agents that produce insoluble precipitates in the tubules.
3. Place plastic resin within the tubules to occlude the openings.
4. Apply bonding agents to seal the tubules.

Initial preparation of the teeth must be done before any desensitizing agent is professionally applied. Teeth must be free of all hard and soft deposits. In addition, 3% hydrogen peroxide can be applied to the teeth with a cotton pellet for further cleansing. The teeth are then rinsed with warm water, dried, and isolated before treatment. Care should be taken to use air lightly or to dry the sensitive areas with cotton rolls. Rather than specific products, only the ingredient(s) that are claimed to be active are discussed here. As you read about each, notice that most desensitizing agents are applied with a burnishing action. (See Chapter 30 for the discussion of porte polisher with orangewood tips.) One study reported that the action of burnishing with an orangewood stick alone was as effective as burnishing with sodium

Agents Reported in the Literature to Reduce Dentinal Hypersensitivity

Aconite and aconitine, albargine, aluminum salts, ammoniacal silver nitrate, Anderson's remineralizing powder, anesthetic agents (general, anodyne cement, arsenic and arsenious acid, asbestos, atropia

Benzyl alcohol, Buckley's desensitizing paste

Calcium hydroxide, calcium lactate, calcium orthophosphate complex, calcium sucrose phosphate, Campho-Phenique, carbolic acid, carbolized potash, cataphoresis apparatus, caustic agents, cavity varnish, chloral hydrate, chloro-carboline, chloroform, chromic acid, chromium sesquichloride, cocaine phenate, collodion, composite resins, corticosteroids, creosote, cyanoacrylates

Dr. Dowsley's dental obtundent

Electrical osmosis, erythrophicin, ether, ethyl chloride, Eucain, eucalyptus, Eugenol

Fluoride iontophoresis, Formalin, Fowler's solution

Gold, Gottlieb's solution

Hartmann's desensitizer (alcohol, thymol, sulfuric ether), hemicrania, hot water, hydrochlorate of cocaine

Iodine, Kreosotum, lactophosphate of lime

Magnesium hydroxide, menthol, methyl chloride, morphine, Myer's obtundent

Nervocidine, Novocaine, oleate of cocaine, Orthoform, oxide of lime

Paraform, Phenol, phosphoric acid, potassium carbonate-sodium carbonate, potassium nitrate, potassium oxalate, Potassocaine, Prednisolone

Quinine sulfate, Robinson's Remedy

Siloxane ethers, silver iodine, silver nitrate, small dentine obtundent, sodium dioxide, sodium fluoride, sodium monofluorophosphate, sodium silicofluoride, stannous fluoride, Stenocarpin, strontium chloride, strontium sequestrant salts, style obtunding device, sulfuric acid, syrup of the phosphates

Tar water, the Herbst obtunder, the Rahinator, Thymol, trichloroacetic acid

Unslaked lime, Van Wyck obtundent, Vapocain, varnishes and cements, Veratra

Weaver obtundent, Wilcox obtundent, zinc chloride, zinc oxychloride

Modified from Trowbridge HO, Silver DR: *Dent Clin North Am* 34:561, 1990.

Professional Products Used in Treating Dentinal Hypersensitivity

Products or agents that act by partially occluding the dentinal tubules
  Burnishing
  Calcium hydroxide
  Dibasic calcium phosphate
  Iontophoresis
  Fluoride compounds
    Sodium fluoride
    Sodium silicofluoride
    Stannous fluoride
  Formalin
  Potassium oxalate
  Silver nitrate
  Strontium chloride
  Zinc chloride-potassium ferrocyanide
Surface sealing agents
  Bonding agents
  Cements
  Resins
  Varnishes

Modified from Rosenthall MW: *Dent Clin North Am* 34:403, 1990.

fluoride (Pashley, Leibach, and Horner, 1987). Another study found that the action of burnishing with water reduced dentinal sensitivity (Cooley and Sandoval, 1989). The reduction in sensitivity can be attributed to partial occlusion of the dentinal tubules by a smear layer that results from burnishing. However, a smear layer can be dissolved in an acidic environment. Another thing to keep in mind as you read about some of these agents is that optimum results are seldom obtained with one application.

It is claimed that *formalin*, in a concentration of 40%, reduces sensitivity when applied to a sensitive area using a cotton pellet and burnished with a porte polisher. Greenhill and Pashley (1981) reported that a 10% formalin solution was ineffective in decreasing hydraulic conductance. (Remember, hydraulic conductance refers to the ability of a substance or stimuli to produce fluid movement in the tubules.) This agent should not come into contact with the mucosa, as a reaction (precipitation of protein) with the tissues will occur and result in soft tissue irritation.

A solution of basic or ammoniated *silver ni-*

trate is alleged to decrease dentinal sensitivity. This solution is applied directly to the sensitive area and then precipitated with a reducing agent such as eugenol. Its action is to partially occlude the tubules and thereby decrease hydraulic conductance. This preparation may be irritating to soft dental tissue and cause tooth discoloration.

Calcium hydroxide is another agent that decreases dentin permeability by producing a precipitate inside the dentinal tubule (Pashley et al, 1986; Levin et al, 1973). The effectiveness of this precipitate is negatively influenced by an acidic environment. Acids will dissolve the calcium hydroxide crystals within the tubules.

Another product found to be effective in decreasing sensitivity is *dibasic calcium phosphate*. It is burnished into the dentinal surface, depositing minerals into the tubules. It thereby reduces the opening and subsequently the effects of painful stimuli.

Solutions of 40% *zinc chloride* and 20% *potassium ferrocyanide* are used in a two-step process. The solution of zinc chloride is applied with a moist cotton pellet or porte polisher and rubbed vigorously into the tooth surface. Excess solution is removed from the gingival margin. While the teeth are still moist, the second solution of potassium ferrocyanide is applied. This solution is rubbed vigorously until an orange, curdy precipitate forms. One minute is allowed for the reaction to occur, and then the excess is removed from the gingival margin. Scanning electron microscopy revealed a crystalline deposit on the dentinal surface; however, most of the crystals appeared to be too large to enter the tubule. Therefore the reduction in sensitivity with the use of this technique may be attributed to the burnishing action (Greenhill and Pashley, 1981).

Professional products consisting of *fluoride gels and solutions* for caries treatment are used to treat hypersensitivity. The teeth should be free of deposits before fluoride treatment. With generalized sensitivity or many areas of gingival recession, tray or painting procedures are used. If specific teeth are sensitive, fluoride can be burnished into the area with a porte polisher. Also available are fluoride products with claimed desensitization properties. The first contains equal amounts of sodium fluoride, kaolin, and glycerin. This product is rubbed into the dried and isolated sensitive area with a porte polisher for 1 to 5 minutes. The mechanism of action is attributed to the deposi-

tion of insoluble salts. Two products are available that contain *sodium silicofluoride*. The first of these is a saturated solution containing 0.7% in cold water or 0.9% in hot water. This preparation is rubbed into sensitive areas for 5 minutes. A calcium gel forms, which is claimed to be an improved insulating barrier. Sodium silicofluoride is also used with calcium hydroxide in a two-step procedure. Initially, the sodium silicofluoride is applied and allowed to react for 1 to 2 minutes. Then the area is painted with 5% calcium hydroxide and allowed to stand for 1 minute. This combination treatment is claimed to reduce the tubule opening.

Stannous fluoride, in various percentages and forms (solution or gel), has been found to provide relief from dentinal hypersensitivity. Studies have shown reductions in sensitivity with solutions of varying concentrations (Blank and Carbeneau, 1986; Thrash, Dorman, and Smith, 1983). A 0.717% solution is available as a chairside treatment for immediate relief of hypersensitivity. Applied with a sponge applicator, in an individual dose, this product can be helpful when instrumentation of a hypersensitive area is necessary.

Oxalate solutions have shown a reduction in sensitivity and can be applied without the need for burnishing, which is often painful to the patient. Pashley and others (1987) reported a 96% decrease in dentin permeability with the use of a 3% solution of oxalic acid. The dentinal tubules were occluded and the surface covered with an acid-resistant layer of calcium oxalate crystals. This could provide a less painful method of achieving desensitization.

Iontophoresis is another method of treating dental hypersensitivity. The purpose of this procedure is to enhance movement of ions by electric current. With this system, a negative ion, such as fluoride, would be repelled from a negatively charged applicator on the dentin surface, thus increasing the fluoride ion penetration into dentin. An older theory claimed that iontophoresis resulted in the formation of secondary dentin and thus a decrease in sensitivity.

Several clinical studies have reported on the use of iontophoresis, mainly with neutral 2% sodium fluoride as the active agent but sometimes using other ions. Although iontophoresis alone was claimed to be effective against hypersensitivity, modern research indicates that the procedure provides effective therapy when coupled with the active agent, fluoride ion (Kern et al, 1989; Gangarosa et al, 1989; Lutkins et al, 1984).

These double-blind clinical studies that proved effective were performed with the Dentelect ElectroApplicator System (EAS), which is no longer available. The successor to this unit is the Life-Tech Dentaphor II (Life-Tech, Inc.) The Dentaphor II, with its new features, may be considered a third generation system (Gangarosa and Jeske, 1992). The EAS is considered a second generation system, while most first generation systems (Chayes-Siemon, Lemonstron, Desensitron, and 3M's Ionator) were underpowered, had other disadvantages, and are no longer available. Two upgrades of first generation systems are (1) Hampton's Iontophoresis Instrument (Hampton Research), a modification of Chayes-Siemon, and (2) Parkell's Desensitron II (Parkell).

The ideal technique provides immediate, painless relief with a 2- minute application in a high percentage of patients. The treatment may need to be repeated once or twice at weekly intervals, but once desensitization occurs, it is permanent (Gangarosa et al, 1989; Carlo et al, 1982). This technique is easy to use and avoids the major disadvantages of topical medication (i.e., the medication or reaction products are quickly dissolved after any topical application). (For further information on iontophoresis, see Gangarosa and Jeske, 1992.)

The barrel-shaped Lemonstron apparatus has a sable brush at one end. The clinician moistens the brush with a 2% sodium fluoride solution and applies it to the sensitive tooth area. The circuit is completed by the clinician touching the patient. The brush is allowed to contact the sensitive area for 1 minute. Because this unit operates with two penlight batteries and there is no ammeter, the clinician is unsure how much current is being dispensed.

Surface sealing agents such as varnishes, resins, and cyanoacrylate are useful in treating hypersensitivity when other agents are ineffective. Great success has been found using *fluoride varnishes* and *unfilled resins* to cover the outside of the patent tubules (Clark, 1985). More recently, *acid etching and bonding* have been employed to reduce areas of cervical sensitivity (Fusayama, 1988). Another clinician recommends the use of *glass ionomer cements followed by bonding* as an alternative treatment for dentinal sensitivity (Buccinarelli, 1990). A promising product called *cya-*

noacrylate has been shown in clinical studies to have an immediate and long-lasting effect on hypersensitive dentin. Data indicate that this treatment is 33% more effective than sodium fluoride (Bahram, 1987; Javid et al, 1987).

Corticosteroid products also are available for dentin hypersensitivity. These products are used primarily for sensitivity resulting from cavity preparations but are also used for dentin hypersensitivity. Usually the agent is administered by being rubbed into the sensitive site. The mode of action is considered to be that of decreasing pulpal inflammation, implying that hypersensitivity is linked to pulpal inflammation. More research is needed to investigate the existence of this relationship.

Research in the use of *lasers* to reduce hypersensitivity is underway with mixed results. One study reported no significant difference in the reduction of sensitivity with the use of lasers compared with conventional methods (Wilder-Smith, 1988). Earlier studies reported success with the use of lasers in desensitization, however (Matsumoto et al, 1985; Senda et al, 1985). As the search for effective treatments for dentinal hypersensitivity continues, more efficient and effective products will be introduced to both the general public and dental professionals.

As you reflect on the cause of dentin hypersensitivity, you will appreciate the important role of the dental hygienist in the treatment and education of patients with this condition. As discussed in Chapters 25 and 26, instrumentation should stop short of purposeful cementum removal, which often causes hypersensitivity. Because root planing to expose and smooth dentin was the norm in clinical practice during the 1970s and 1980s, you may see many patients who acquired sensitivity this way.

Given that dentin is exposed most frequently on buccal surfaces of premolars, canines, and incisors and that abrasion of these areas contributes to an increase in sensitivity, your educational role is most apparent. You need to thoroughly investigate the patient's home care practices. Ask about and have the patient demonstrate plaque removal techniques. Determine what type of brush, oral physiotherapy aids, and dentifrice are being used. How often does the patient brush and with what degree of pressure? Also, be cognizant of the patient's dominant hand for brushing. Right-handed individuals will apply more pressure to the left side than the right (Addy, Mostafa, and New-combe, 1987). This continuous increase in pressure causes more abrasion to the tooth surface, which can result in exposed dentin and produce sensitivity. If you apply a desensitizing agent or recommend the use of a product at home, by all means investigate the patient's diet. The objective is to occlude the dentinal tubules by introducing a precipitate into the opening in combination with a smear layer on the dentinal surface; foods and beverages that are high in acid will undermine this process. Bacteria found in plaque may also produce an acidic environment; therefore, removal of plaque is important. The techniques for mechanical plaque removal and the degree of pressure applied during this process should be observed by the dental hygienist to facilitate reduction of dentinal hypersensitivity by the patient.

ACTIVITIES

1. Determine whether members of the class have areas of gingival recession or tooth sensitivity. Test both areas with the following: ice, a blast of air, cold water, hot water, and a sharp probe. What is the most severe reaction in terms of speed of response and pain? Do areas of recession and sensitivity differ? Why? What parameters do you think would be best for testing a new antihypersensitivity agent?
2. Review two publications on desensitizing products from before and after 1980. Comment on the occurrence of a placebo effect and on the measurements used.

REVIEW QUESTIONS

1. What are the primary areas where tooth sensitivity occurs?
2. What professional procedures contribute to tooth sensitivity?
3. What stimuli elicit hypersensitivity?
4. What is the primary mechanism of action of desensitizing agents?
5. True or false:
   a. The tooth area closest to the cementoenamel junction is the most sensitive.
   b. The placebo effect often occurs in treating sensitivity.
   c. Regardless of treatment, improved oral hygiene can reduce sensitivity.
6. Describe how the fluoride treatment for caries is:
   a. Different from the fluoride treatment for sensitivity.
   b. Similar to the fluoride treatment for sensitivity.
7. Explain how fluid movement in dentinal tubules can cause a pain response.

REFERENCES

Absi EG, Adams D, Addy M: The patency of dentinal tubules in hypersensitive and non-sensitive dentine, *Br Soc Dent Res*, 1986, (abstract 89).

Absi EG, Addy M, Adams D: Dentine hypersensitivity: a study of the patency of dentinal tubules in sensitive and non-sensitive cervical dentine, *J Clin Periodontol* 14:280, 1987.

Ad Hoc Advisory Committee on Dentinal Hypersensitivity: *JADA* 112: 709, 1986.

Addy M: Etiology and clinical implication of dentine hypersensitivity, *Dent Clin North Am* 34:503, 1990.

Addy M, Absi EG, Adams D: Dentine hypersensitivity: the effects in vitro of acids and dietary substances on root-planted and burred dentine, *J Clin Periodontol* 14:274, 1987.

Addy M, Mostafa P: Dentine hypersensitivity. II. Effects produced by the uptake in vitro of toothpastes onto dentine, *J Oral Rehabil* 16:35, 1989.

Addy M, Mostafa P, Newcombe RG: Dentine hypersensitivity: the distribution of recession, sensitivity and plaque, *J Dent* 15:242, 1987.

Addy M, Mostafa P, Newcombe RG: Effect on plaque of five toothpastes used in the treatment of dentin hypersensitivity, *Clin Prevent Dent* 12:28, 1990.

American Dental Association Council on Dental Therapeutics: *Accepted products categorical listing*, The Association, January 27, 1992.

Ash MM: Quantification of stimuli, *Endodont Dent Traumatol* 2: 153, 1986.

Bahram J: Cyanoacrylate—a new treatment for hypersensitive dentin and cementum, *JADA* 114:216, 1987.

Berman L: Dentinal sensation and hypersensitivity, *J Periodontol* 56: 216, 1984.

Blandy AA: On the sensibility of teeth, *Am J Dent Sci* 1:22, 1850–1851.

Blank LW, Charbeneau GT: Urgent treatment in operative dentistry, *Dent Clin North Am* 30:489, 1986.

Blong MA et al: Effects of a gel containing 0.4 percent stannous fluoride on dentinal hypersensitivity, *Dent Hyg* 59:489, 1985.

Brannstrom M: The hydrodynamic theory of dentinal pain: sensation in the preparations, caries, and the dentinal crack syndrome, *J Endodont* 12:453, 1986.

Brannstrom M: Sensitivity of dentine, *Oral Surg* 21:517, 1966.

Brannstrom M, Astrom A: A study of the mechanism of pain elicited from the dentine, *J Dent Res* 43:619, 1964.

Bucciarelli A: Preventing root sensitivity, *JADA* 120:652, 1990.

Carlo GT, Ciancio SG, Seyrek SK: An evaluation of iontophoretic application of fluoride for tooth desensitization, *JADA* 105:452, 1982.

Chasens AI: The management of tooth pain and sensitivity. In Chasens AI, Kaslick RS, editors: *Mechanisms of pain and sensitivity in the teeth and supporting tissues*, Rutherford, NJ, 1974, Fairleigh Dickinson University.

Clark DC: The effectiveness of a fluoride varnish and a desensitizing toothpaste in treating dentinal hypersensitivity, *J Periodont Res* 20:212, 1985.

Clark DC et al: The influence of frequent ingestion of acids in the diet on treatment for dentin sensitivity, *Can Dent Assoc J* 56:1101, 1990.

Clark DC, Al-Joburi W, Chan ECS: The efficacy of a new dentifrice in treating dentin sensitivity: effects of sodium citrate and sodium fluoride as active ingredients, *J Periodont Res* 22:89, 1987.

Cooley RL, Sandoval VA: Effectiveness of potassium oxalate treatment on dentin hypersensitivity, *Gen Dent* 37:316, 1989.

Council on Dental Therapeutics: Acceptance of Promise with fluoride and Sensodyne—toothpastes for sensitive teeth, *JADA* 113:673, 1986.

Dederich DN, Gulevich T, Reid A: The effect of rubber cup vs an air-powder abrasive system on root surfaces, *Can Dent Hyg/Probe* 23:135, 1989.

Ellingsen JE, Rolla G: Treatment of dentin with stannous fluoride—SEM and electron microprobe study, *Scand J Dent Res* 95:281, 1987.

Everett FG, Hall WB, Phatak NM: Treatment of hypersensitive dentin, *J Oral Ther Pharmacol* 2:300, 1966.

Fischer C, et al: Clinical evaluation of pulp and dentine sensitivity after supragingival and subgingival scaling, *Endodont Dent Traumatol* 7:259, 1991.

Flynn J, Galloway R, Orchardson R: The incidence of hypersensitive teeth in the West of Scotland, *J Dent* 13:230, 1985.

Frank RM, Sauvage C, Frank P: Morphological basis of dental sensitivity, *Int Dent J* 22:1, 1972.

Fusayama T: Etiology and treatment of sensitive teeth, *Quintessence Int* 19:921, 1988.

Gangarosa LP Sr, Jeske AH: Iontophresis: a system for solving some difficult dental problems. In Hardin JF, editor: *Clark's clinical dentistry*, Philadelphia, JB Lippincott, in press.

Gangarosa LP et al: Double-blind evaluation of duration of dentin sensitivity reduction by fluoride iontophoresis, *Gen Dent* 37:316, 1989.

Gedalia I et al: The effect of fluoride and strontium application on dentin: in vivo and in vitro studies, *J Periodontol* 49:269, 1978.

Goldman HM: Dental sensitivity: a periodontist's perspective, *Compend Contin Educ Dent* 3(suppl):S110, 1982.

Graf H, Galasse R: Morbidity, prevalence, and intraoral distribution of the hypersensitive teeth, *J Dent Res* 56(special issue A):A162, 1977 (abstract).

Grant DA, Stern IB, Everett FG: *Periodontics: in the tradition of Orban and Gottlieb*, ed 5, St Louis, 1979, CV Mosby.

Green BL, Green ML, McFall WT Jr: Calcium hydroxide and potassium nitrate as desensitizing agents for hypersensitive root surfaces, *J Periodontol* 48:667, 1977.

Greenhill JD, Pashley D: The effects of desensitizing agents on the hydraulic conductance of dentin in vitro, *J Dent Res* 60:686, 1981.

Grossman LI: A systematic method for the treatment of hypersensitive dentin, *JADA* 22:592, 1935.

Haugen E, Johansen JR: Tooth hypersensitivity after periodontal treatment: a case report including SEM studies, *Clin Periodontol* 15:399, 1988.

Hiatt WH, Johansen E: Root preparation. I: Obturation of dentinal tubules in treatment of root hypersensitivity, *J Periodontol* 43:373, 1972.

Hirsch WR, Clarke NG: Endodontic effects of root planing in humans, *Endo Dent Traumatol* 5:193, 1989.

Javid B, Barkhordar RA, Bhinda SV: Cyanoacrylate—a new treatment for hypersensitive dentin and cementum, *JADA* 114:486, 1987.

Kanapka JA: Clinical evaluation of dentinal hypersensitivity: a comparison of methods, *Endo Den Traumatol* 2:157, 1986.

Kanapka JA: A new agent, *Compend Contin Educ Dent* 3(suppl):S118, 1982.

Kanapka JA: Over-the-counter dentrifices in the treatment of tooth hypersensitivity, *Dent Clin North Am* 34:545, 1990.

Kern DA et al: Effectiveness of sodium fluoride on tooth hypersensitivity with and without iontophoresis, *J Periodontol* 60:386, 1989.

Knight T: Erosion, abrasion, *J Dent Assoc S Afr* 24:130, 1969.

Krauser JT: Hypersensitive teeth. II. Treatment, *J Prosthet Dent* 56:307, 1986.

Krauser JT: Hypersensitive teeth. I. Etiology, *J Prosthet Dent* 2:153, 1956.

Levin MP, Yearwood LL, Carpenter WN: The desensitizing effect of calcium hydroxide and magnesium hydroxide on hypersensitive dentin, *Oral Surg* 35:741, 1973.

Lutins ND, Greco GW, McFall WT Jr: Effectiveness of sodium fluoride on tooth hypersensitivity with and without iontophoresis, *J Periodontol* 55:285, 1984.

Matsumoto K et al: Study of the treatment of hypersensitive dentine by GaAlAs laser diode, *Jpn J Cons Dent* 28:54, 1985.

Miles DA: Dental management and reported cases of bulimic erosion, *Can Dent Assoc J* 51:757, 1985.

Miller JT et al: Use of a water-free stannous fluoride-containing gel in the control of dental hypersensitivity, *J Periodontol* 40:490, 1969.

Moss-Salentijn L, Hendricks-Klyvert M: Pulp and dentin. In Moss Salentijn L, Hendricks-Klyvert M, editors: *Dental and oral tissues, an introduction*, ed 3, Philadelphia, 1990, Lea & Febiger.

Orchardson R, Collins WJN: Clinical features of hypersensitive teeth, *Br Dent J* 162:253, 1987.

Pashley DH, Kalathoor S, Burnham D: The effects of calcium hydroxide on dentin permability, *J Dent Res* 65:417, 1986.

Pashley DH, Leibach JG, Horner JA: The effects of burnishing NaF/kaolin/glycerin paste on dentin permeability, *J Periodontol* 58:19, 1987.

Peden JW: Dental hypersensitivity, *J West Soc Periodontol* 25:75, 1977.

Rosenthal MW: Historic review of the management of tooth hypersensitivity, *Dent Clin North Am* 34:403, 1990.

Smith BA, Ash MM Jr: Evaluation of a desensitizing dentifrice, *JADA* 68:639, 1964a.

Smith BA, Ash MM Jr: A study of a desensitizing dentifrice and cervical hypersensitivity, *J Periodontol* 35:222, 1964b.

Snyder RA, Beck FM, Horton JE: The efficacy of a 0.4% SnF$_2$ solution on root surface hypersensitivity, *J Dent Res* 64(abstract 237), 1985.

Tarbet WJ et al: Home treatment for dentinal hypersensitivity: a comparative study, *JADA* 105:227, 1982.

Thrash WJ: *Long term effects of a gel containing 0.4% stannous fluoride on dentinal hypersensitivity as compared to placebo and no treatment control,* unpublished manuscript, 1992.

Thrash W, Dorman HI, Smith FD: A method to measure pain associated with hypersensitive dentin, *J Periodontol* 54:160, 1983.

Tronstad L: The anatomic and physiologic basis for dentinal sensitivity, *Compend Contin Educ Dent* 3(suppl):S99, 1982.

Trowbridge HO, Silver DR: A review of current approaches to in-office management of tooth hypersensitivity, *Dent Clin North Am* 34:561, 1990.

Wallace JA, Bissada NF: Pulpal and root sensitivity rated to periodontal therapy, *Oral Surg Oral Med Oral Pathol* 69:743, 1990.

Wilder-Smith P: The soft laser: therapeutic tool or popular placebo? *Oral Surg* 66:654, 1988.

Wong R, Hirsch RD: Endodontic effects of root planing in humans, *Endodont Dent Traumatol* 5:193, 1989.

Wycoff SJ: Current treatment for dentinal hypersensitivity: in-office treatment, *Compend Contin Educ Dent* 3(suppl):S113, 1982.

Yankell SL: At home treatment, *Compend Contin Educ Dent* 3(suppl):S115, 1982.

Yankell S, Emling RC: Understanding dental products: what you should know and what your patient should know, *Contin Dent Educ* 1:7, 1978.

Yoshiyama M et al: Scanning electron microscopic characterization of sensitive vs insensitive human radicular dentin, *J Dent Res* 68:1498, 1989.

Yoshiyama M et al: Transmission electron microscopic characterization of hypersensitive human radicular dentin, *J Dent Res* 69:1293, 1990.

SUGGESTED READINGS

Addy M, Mostafa P, Newcombe RG: Effect on plaque of five toothpastes used in the treatment of dentin hypersensitivity, *Clin Prev Dent* 12:28, 1990.

Avery JK: Anatomic considerations in the mechanisms of pain and sensitivity in the teeth and supporting tissues. In Chasens AI, Kaslick RS, editors: *Mechanisms of pain and sensitivity in the teeth and supporting tissues,* Rutherford, NJ, 1974, Fairleigh Dickinson University.

Irvine JH: Root surface sensitivity: a review of aetiology and management, *J NZ Soc Periodontol* 66:15, 1988.

Kanapka JA: Clinical evaluation of dentinal hypersensitivity: a comparison of methods, *Endo Dent Traumatol* 2:157, 1986.

Minkoff S, Axelrod S: Efficacy of strontium chloride in dental hypersensitivity, *J Periodontol* 58:470, 1987.

Parr OD, Brokaw WC: Economical iontophoresis for dentistry, *Quintessence Int* 20:841, 1989.

Pashley DH: Mechanisms of dentin sensitivity, *Dent Clin North Am* 34:449, 1990.

Reinhart TC et al: The effectiveness of a patient-applied tooth desensitizing gel: a pilot study, *J Clin Periodontol* 17:123, 1990.

Sena FJ: Dentinal permeability in assessing therapeutic agents, *Dent Clin North Am* 34:475, 1990.

Sessle BJ: The neurobiology of facial and dental pain: present knowledge, future directions, *J Dent Res* 66:962, 1987.

Stanley HR: Dentin permeability and sensitivity. In Chasens AL, Kaslick RS, editors: *Mechanisms of pain and sensitivity in the teeth and supporting tissues,* Rutherford, JN, 1974, Fairleigh Dickinson University.

Susi FR: Sensory receptor morphology in the teeth and their supporting tissues, *Dent Clin North Am* 22:3, 1978.

32 PAIN AND PAIN CONTROL: TOPICAL AND LOCAL ANESTHESIA

Donna Stach

LEARNING OUTCOMES

The dental hygienist will be able to

1. Explain the uses and limitations of psychosomatic, topical, and local anesthesia in dental hygiene practice.
2. Understand pain, pain perception, pain reaction, and factors that result in variations among individuals.
3. Develop an approach that will minimize pain and assist patients to cope with the anxiety that may be associated with dental treatment.
4. Trace or locate the nerve branches supplying the maxilla and mandible and identify the tissues innervated by each.
5. Select the appropriate injections that will achieve the desired anesthesia, then identify the injection site.
6. Prepare both the patient and the armamentarium for common dental injections.
7. Describe the safety value of each of the following:
   a. Comprehensive assessment of the patient's medical status
   b. Use of anesthetic containing a vasoconstrictor
   c. Aspiration before injection
   d. Slow injection and careful technique
   e. Remaining with the patient after the injection
8. Be prepared to recognize and assist in the management of any emergency or complications that may result from the use of anesthetic agents.
9. Properly apply a topical anesthetic when indicated.

Pain and dental care go hand in hand for many people, as shown by the many cartoons and comedy routines about dental pain. The fear of being hurt prevents some people from seeking routine dental care. Dental personnel use various methods to alleviate patients' pain, such as verbal reassurance, topical anesthetics, local anesthetics, conscious sedation, acupuncture, sedative premedication, general anesthesia, and hypnosis. Two simultaneous movements—patients' increased awareness that dental care need not cause discomfort and more exacting instrumentation and therapy for periodontally involved patients—have led to an increase in the perceived need and use of topical anesthetics, local anesthetics, and nitrous oxide and oxygen conscious sedation. The need to control pain in dental hygiene procedures is diffi-

cult to quantify, but two studies on estimated perceived need—one from a state where local anesthesia is legal for dental hygienists and one from a state where it is not—give us some insights. In California local anesthesia use by dental hygienists was estimated at 10.6% in general practice and 50.2% in periodontal practice (Rich and Smorang, 1984). In a recent study in Iowa, 29% of the patients of dental hygienists received anesthesia, but 70% were perceived by their hygienists as needing pain control measures (Sisty-LePeau et al, 1992). Many states' laws permit dental hygienists to provide anesthesia for their patients. Currently hygienists are allowed to administer local anesthesia in Alaska, Arizona, California, Colorado, Hawaii, Idaho, Missouri, Montana, Nevada, New Mexico, Oklahoma, Oregon, South

Dakota, Utah, Washington, and Wyoming (ADHA, 1992).

Another interesting perspective on the role of local anesthesia in dental hygiene practice comes from dentists in Colorado. Responding to a survey on the impact of a hands-on local anesthesia course taken by dental hygienists, 80% of the dentists felt that anesthesia was administered more regularly to patients who needed it, 75% said patients were more satisfied and comfortable with hygiene procedures, and 82% believed that the hygienist was able to perform a more definitive instrumentation because of improved patient comfort (Cross-Poline et al, 1992).

PAIN

Everyone has experienced pain at some time. Pain has two different components—perception and reaction. *Pain perception* is the physical aspect, the process by which the pain is received and transmitted through the nervous system. The pain perceptors are the nerve end organs that sense the painful stimulus. The message is stimulus transmitted through the peripheral nervous system to the central nervous system, where it is interpreted as pain. Pain perception is the same for most healthy persons, unless the nervous system has been damaged by injury or disease (Bennett, 1984). *Pain reaction* is the interpretation given to the pain perceived plus the response it elicits. Pain reaction varies among people and over time in the same person. It is influenced by conscious and unconscious thinking as well as emotional, cultural, and ethnic factors (Burstein et al, 1979; Christensen, 1980; Foreman, 1979; Spear, 1977). The pain reaction threshold is also markedly affected by a number of drugs (analgesics) that act on the nervous system (McCarthy, 1979). Persons who react minimally to pain are said to have low pain reaction and high *pain reaction thresholds;* the pain reaction threshold is inversely related to pain reaction (Bennett, 1984).

PAIN CONTROL

There are a variety of pain control methods used in dentistry today. Bennett (1984) divided these into five categories:

1. Remove the painful stimulus.
2. Block the pathway of the pain message.
3. Prevent pain reaction by raising the pain reaction threshold.
4. Depress the central nervous system.

5. Use psychosomatic methods.

The first two affect pain perception, the second two affect pain reactions, and the last can influence both pain perception and reaction.

Removal of a potentially painful stimulus is the method used by many patients when they avoid dental care. They reason, usually unconsciously, that if they don't go to the dentist they will not experience the pain or the fear of pain that the treatment might cause. In another example, if pain is caused by the instrumentation technique (e.g., by an overly wide angle or poor adaptation of a curette), its correction will remove the painful stimulus. A third example is resolution of a painful gingivitis either by plaque control methods or medicaments before a course of instrumentation is begun.

Blocking the pathway of the painful impulse is the method being used when either topical anesthetic or local anesthetic drugs are used. The painful stimulus is present, but because the nerve pathways are temporarily shut down, the message never gets to the brain for interpretation.

Conscious sedation, including nitrous oxide and oxygen analgesia, involves raising the pain reaction threshold (discussed in more detail in Chapter 33). Many drugs have analgesic effects and are used in dentistry; included are ibuprofen, acetylsalicylic acid (aspirin), meperidine hydrochloride (Demerol), other narcotics, barbiturates, and psychosedatives.

Central nervous system depression is used in general anesthesia. It prevents any conscious reaction to a painful stimulus.

Psychosomatic methods of pain management can be highly effective alone or in combination with other techniques. Because these methods are nonpharmacologic, they do not have potential for adverse drug reactions. Psychosomatic techniques affect how the mind influences the body and therefore influence both pain perception and pain reaction. They involve basic interpersonal skills, such as being honest, keeping the patient informed and empowered, and using specific relaxation and distraction techniques.

This chapter presents an introduction to the use of psychosomatic methods, topical anesthetic agents, and local anesthetic agents. Although this chapter, along with those on anatomy, pharmacology, medical assessment, and emergency management, provides a solid background for local anesthetic administration, it is not intended as complete instruction for this serious undertaking. All dental personnel—dentists and dental hygienists—should participate in a more in-depth local anesthesia course that includes supervised practice in administering local anesthetics. The administration of local anesthetics is a serious responsibility. When any chemical substance is put in a person's body, it may produce undesired effects as well as desired ones. The practitioner must be able to evaluate both types of effects and initiate the appropriate care. A properly educated dental hygienist is capable of assuming the added responsibilities associated with the administration of local anesthetics, but *proper formal education is essential* (American Association of Dental Schools, 1980). Studies by Lobene (1979) and Sisty-LePeau and others (1986) describe the success of dental hygiene students in administering local anesthesia. After a specific course, the overall adequacy of anesthesia achieved for all procedures was 95%, indicating that dental hygienists can provide local anesthesia with a high degree of accuracy. Malamed (1990) further notes that patients frequently comment on the lack of discomfort when the injection is given by a hygienist.

This chapter provides a general overview of local anesthesia and how to determine when a local anesthetic is needed and which injections will provide the desired effect. The technique of administering an injection is not presented in detail. The ability to determine which injection is needed allows the hygienist to provide or request the appropriate one, to prepare the necessary armamentarium, and to prepare the patient, in addition to applying the topical anesthetic. An understanding of the uses and limitations of topical and local anesthetics will provide the dental hygienist with a realistic understanding of the capabilities of each agent for pain control and enhancement of patient care.

INFLUENCES ON PAIN REACTION

As previously mentioned, pain reaction varies from person to person and may even vary over time for the same person, depending on his or her mental and physical condition. Factors that influence a person's interpretation of the pain resulting from an event can be divided into three categories: cognitive, emotional, and symbolic (Wepman, 1978).

Cognitive factors are those that influence how persons think about pain or when they interpret a sensation as being painful. There is evidence that what the clinician says can modify how patients think and react to painful stimuli. For example, Steblay and Beaman (1982) showed that telling patients that some of their physiologic sensations, such as temporarily increased heart rates, were due to the local anesthetic allowed the patients to properly associate the feelings with the anesthetic. This in turn seemed to allow the patients to be less fearful and experience less pain.

Wepman (1978) has reported an experiment in which patients were told that they would experience less pain if they listened to music through earphones during treatment. The patients seemed to develop ways to cope with the pain by using the music to distract themselves, by tapping a foot, tapping their fingers, or humming. These patients reported feeling less pain.

The above example helps illustrate the concept that people are less susceptible to pain, fear, or anxiety when they feel they have some control over the situation. Patients are more likely to cope with pain if they believe they have some control. Conversely, when patients feel helpless or not in control, they are likely to experience greater pain. Thus allowing patients to have some control over their situation is a good pain management technique (Wepman, 1978).

Emotional factors such as anxiety greatly influence patients' tolerance for pain. In general, increased anxiety is associated with decreased tolerance for pain (a high pain reaction) (Bennett, 1984). For example, a patient, nervous about a scaling procedure, who jumps when the clinician establishes a fulcrum has a high pain reaction and a low pain reaction threshold. Increased anxiety is often exacerbated by patients' feelings of helplessness and vulnerability. To help relieve anxiety, the clinician should strive to create an atmosphere in which the patient feels accepted and able to express his or her concerns, thus giving the patient the feeling of confidence and trust.

Events in patients' lives, such as recent marriage, the birth of a child, change in a job, loss of a job, divorce, or the death of a loved one, may also affect their ability to cope with pain. Because such events create stress and its associated anxiety, it is likely that patients may have a decreased pain reaction threshold. Fatigue affects many people as stress does, and may also lower the pain reaction threshold. Careful listening, as described in Chapter 5, will help the clinician discern if life events are affecting a particular patient and perhaps his or her pain reaction.

The *symbolic factors* affecting pain are unique to each person, but universally pain symbolizes an attack, damage, or a threat. All persons have unconscious symbols and feelings of which they are unaware and which they usually are unable to explain. These unconscious feelings about and symbols of pain affect patients' pain reactions (Wepman, 1978). The dental health professional can recognize that all persons react to pain and are affected by their unconscious feelings. It is not the role of the dental health professional to analyze why a patient reacts to pain in a certain manner. Rather, the role of the professional is to listen and observe so as to discern when patients are in pain and to take steps to alleviate the pain associated with dental treatment.

A variety of other factors, such as fatigue, sex, race, and ethnicity, may affect persons' pain reactions. When people are tired or fatigued, their pain reaction thresholds are decreased (Bennett, 1984). Various authors have indicated that pain reaction may be influenced by sex and race or ethnicity (Bennett, 1984; Christensen, 1980; Spear, 1977; Wepman, 1978). For example, men have a higher pain reaction threshold than women; Latin Americans and Southern Europeans have a lower pain reaction threshold than North Americans or Northern Europeans. As different groups have different cultures that regard expression of emotions and pain in a variety of ways, it is not surprising that pain reactions may vary. While these generalizations may be true for the majority of persons from a particular group, there are many exceptions. Every patient must be treated as an individual with his or her own individual reactions to pain (Wepman, 1978).

PSYCHOSOMATIC METHODS OF PAIN CONTROL

Anxiety and fear of dentistry are interwoven with dental pain. Pain during dental procedures often results in fear (generally of short duration and more cause specific) and dental anxiety (generally more nebulous). Fear and anxiety increase the pain experience, primarily by lowering the pain reaction threshold. Psychosomatic methods of pain control are nondrug methods of helping patients cope with or reduce their dental anxiety and pain. Another closely related term is *iatrosedation*—the reduction of anxiety through the behav-

ior of the health care provider (Malamed, 1989).

Perhaps the most important aspect of psychosomatic pain management is the development of helping relationships with patients (see Chapter 5). Patients will both perceive less pain and react less if they trust the health care provider and believe that they are really cared about as a person. This is more than establishing rapport, such as asking the obligatory "How are you?" (Malamed, 1989; Wepman, 1978). Rather, it is offering a relationship in which the provider genuinely cares about patients' well-being, especially their dental health. The health care provider must be truthful and honest with patients about procedures that are uncomfortable. It is highly inappropriate for the health care provider to tell patients that procedures will not hurt or will only hurt for a second if it is not true. The health care provider should take seriously patients' reports of pain and try to alleviate it. Patients' feelings of pain are sometimes expressed verbally, but often they are communicated nonverbally by knitted eyebrows, rolling eyes, or white knuckles clinging to the chair arms. The astute clinician will be attuned to such communications and ask the patient about the source of the pain.

In addition to developing a helping relationship and being honest with the patient about pain associated with treatment, the health care provider must develop skills to alleviate pain. Some psychosomatic approaches include telling the patient about sensations associated with medication or treatment. Use of a soothing, not singsong, voice can help to relax the patient. The patient can be instructed to take a few deep breaths to help relax and ease tension and to continue breathing normally during treatment. If the clinician is familiar with relaxation techniques, such as tensing and relaxing muscle groups, these may be helpful for some patients (Atterbury, 1978; Foreman, 1979). The use of these techniques in a trusting, helping relationship may allow the patient to feel at ease with the clinician and more in control, thus increasing the patient's pain reaction threshold. Other methods that require further training, such as hypnosis, biofeedback, or progressive relaxation, also can be used.

The patient's dental anxiety will be reduced by a positive relationship with the health care provider. The use of psychosomatic methods has been presented because they are an important but often overlooked component of a pain management program. These methods can potentiate other pain control measures, such as topical or local anesthesia, nitrous oxide and oxygen conscious sedation, and general anesthesia. Psychosomatic methods alone are rarely enough to control the pain associated with dental treatment. The health care provider should use other pain control measures as necessary but always in conjunction with good psychosomatic techniques.

LOCAL ANESTHESIA

Local anesthesia is the primary means of pain control in modern dentistry. It is estimated that 4 million local anesthetic injections are administered annually in the United States alone (Wong and Jacobsen, 1992). An overview of local anesthetic agents, patient considerations, injection sites and technique, and potential complications are presented here.

Local anesthetic agents

Local anesthetics are chemical agents that produce transient and completely reversible loss of sensation in a specific area. Other desirable properties include the following (Bennett, 1984; Malamed, 1990):

1. The agent is sterile.
2. It is stable in solution but will readily undergo biotransformation or metabolism in the body.
3. It is nonirritating to the tissues.
4. It will not cause permanent damage to nerve structure.
5. It has a low systemic toxicity.
6. It has a low potential for producing allergic reactions.
7. It has adequate potency without use of harmful concentrations.
8. There is a rapid onset of the anesthetic effect.
9. Duration of anesthesia is long enough to permit completion of the dental procedure, yet not so long as to require an extended recovery.

Local anesthetic agents are water-soluble hydrochloride salt solutions. The chemical structure is made up of three portions—the lipophilic portion, intermediate chain portion, and hydrophilic portion (Fig. 32-1). The agent is classified by the intermediate chain linkage, which is either an ester or an amide. The hydrophilic portion is responsible for the water solubility of the agent.

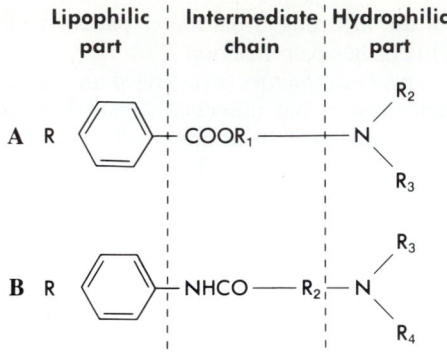

Fig. 32-1. Typical chemical structure for a local anesthetic agent. **A,** Ester type. **B,** Amide type. (From Malamed SF: *Handbook of local anesthesia,* ed 3, St. Louis, 1990, CV Mosby.)

This ensures solubility in the dental cartridge and carries the solution through the interstitial fluid in the tissue to the nerve. The lipophilic group, composed of the aromatic ring structure, enables the agent to penetrate the lipid-rich nerve sheath and membrane where impulse conduction can be blocked (Hersh et al, 1987).

To understand how anesthetic agents work, a brief explanation of how an impulse or message travels along the nerve to the brain is necessary. The message travels by changes in electrical charges that result from the movement of charged ions across a permeable nerve membrane. An inactive nerve has a resting potential from a negative charge on the inside of the nerve membrane. Sodium ions are concentrated on the outside of the membrane and potassium ions on the inside. When a stimulus such as pain produces activity of the nerve fiber, the ion balance changes. This phase is called depolarization. Sodium ions move across the nerve membrane to the inside, and the potassium ions move from the inside to the outside of the nerve membrane. After the impulse has passed along the nerve, repolarization occurs, with the ions moving back to their original concentrations on each side of the nerve membrane. This entire exchange process takes place in 1 millisecond. In this way an impulse wave is transmitted rapidly along the nerve fiber to the brain.

When a local anesthetic is injected in the area of a nerve fiber, the membrane becomes stabilized. Transfer of ions across the membrane is prevented, and the resultant blockage of conduction prevents the patient from feeling any sensation.

Procaine (Novocaine), an ester type of local anesthetic, was the first local anesthetic agent widely used in dentistry. The major disadvantage of ester anesthetics is that they produce allergic reactions in some patients.

Amide anesthetics, developed after the esters, are now used almost exclusively because they do not produce allergic responses. The most commonly used amides include lidocaine (Xylocaine), mepivacaine (Carbocaine), and prilocaine (Citanest). Documented cases of allergic reactions to any of the *pure* amides have been reported as rare (Malamed, 1990) to nonexistent (Bennett, 1984; Giovannitti and Bennett, 1979; Larson, 1977). Allergic reactions have been caused by other contents of the anesthetic cartridge. Preservatives methylparaben and sodium metabisulfite have been documented as causing allergic reactions (Malamed, 1990). Since 1984, use of methylparaben has been discontinued in all single-use local anesthetic cartridges manufactured in the United States. However, methylparaben is still found in multidose vials and topical anesthetic (Malamed, 1990). Sodium metabisulfite is found only in anesthetics that contain a vasoconstrictor.

Vasoconstrictors are added to most local anesthetics to decrease the rate at which they are absorbed from the injection site. This makes the drugs safer by lowering the circulating systemic dose and increases both their effectiveness and duration. This permits the administration of smaller total amounts of the drug and again increases the margin of safety. Commonly used vasoconstrictors include epinephrine, norepinephrine, and levonordefrin (American Dental Association, 1982; Bennett, 1984).

Potency, toxicity, concentration, and maximum safe dose. All drugs have both a desired effect(s) and undesired or side effect(s). In a local anesthetic agent *potency* is the amount necessary to produce the desired effect. *Toxicity* refers to the amount of local anesthetic or vasoconstrictor necessary to produce a toxic overdose (Bennett, 1984). Toxic overdose is the most common potential serious adverse drug reaction to local anesthetics. A toxic overdose occurs when the blood level of drug is too high either as a result of an absolute or relative overadministration of the drug (Malamed, 1990). A relative overdose occurs when the amount of drug administered causes a reaction and is too much for that individual but would have been tolerated by a "normal" person. This is most likely to occur in the presence of some medical conditions (Malamed, 1990). The signs, symptoms, and treatment of a local anesthetic or vasoconstrictor toxic overdose are discussed in Chapter 7. Fortunately toxic overdose can be avoided with excellent anesthetic technique and careful evaluation of the patient's medical status. The blood plasma level of a local anesthetic or vasoconstrictive agent can become too high if (1) too much is given, (2) it is injected intravascularly, (3) it is injected or absorbed rapidly, (4) it is biotransformed (metabolized) slowly, or (5) it is excreted slowly. Thus a toxic overdose can occur if the clinician's technique is faulty (1, 2, and 3) or if the patient is medically compromised (3, 4, and 5). All of these can be avoided or anticipated and compensated for.

One technique that makes local anesthesia injections safer is aspiration. It would be undesirable to inject the anesthetic into a blood vessel, both because it would put a lot of drug into circulation quickly, therefore creating the potential for a drug overdose, and because the drug would be quickly carried away from the site where its action was needed. Because blood vessels are often located near nerves, a method is needed to determine if the tip or open end of the needle is in a vein or artery. The technique used to prevent intravascular injection is called *aspiration*. It is done by pulling back on the thumb ring of the syringe, which puts negative pressure on the anesthetic cartridge. If the needle tip is in a blood vessel, blood will be drawn back into the cartridge. If this occurs, the needle should be withdrawn, and a fresh cartridge placed in the syringe. The needle is then reinserted and aspiration is completed again before depositing the solution.

Local anesthetic and vasoconstrictive agents are available in various *concentrations* (Table 32-1) according to their potency. A weakly potent agent would be produced in a higher concentration to achieve the desired anesthetic or vasoconstrictive effect.

Each local anesthetic and vasoconstrictive agent has a *maximum safe dose* (MSD). This is an estimate of the greatest amount that can be given safely to a healthy 150-pound person (Bennett, 1984; Dafoe, 1982; Malamed, 1979; Rogo, 1982). Table 32-1 lists the MSDs for some com-

Table 32-1. Duration and maximal safe doses

Local anesthetic solution	Duration (min)		Anesthetic dose per cartridge (mg)	Vasoconstrictor dose per cartridge (mg)	Maximal safe dose of anesthetic		Maximal safe dose of vasoconstrictor (mg)	
	Pulpal	Soft tissue			mg/lb of body weight	Maximum (mg)	Healthy individual	Medically compromised individual
2% procaine	0-5	60-90	36		2.7/lb	400		
2% lidocaine	5-10	60-120	36		2.0/lb	300		
4% prilocaine	10-60	90-240	72		2.7/lb	400		
3% mepivacaine	20-40	120-180	54		2.0/lb	300		
0.4% propoxycaine, 2% procaine, and 1:20,000 levonordefrin	30-60	120-180	43.2	0.09	3.0/lb	400	0.5	0.50
2% mepivacaine and 1:200,000 epinephrine	45-60	120-240	36	0.0090	2.0/lb	300	0.2	0.04
2% lidocaine and 1:100,000 epinephrine	60-90	180-240	36	0.018	2.0/lb	300	0.2	0.04
2% lidocaine and 1:50,000 epinephrine	60-90	180-240	36	0.036	2.0/lb	300	0.2	0.04
2% mepivacaine and 1:20,000 levonordefrin	60-90	180-240	36	0.09	2.0/lb	300	0.5	0.50
4% prilocaine and 1:200,000 epinephrine	60-90	120-240	72	0.0090	2.7/lb	400	0.2	0.04
1.5% etidocaine and 1:200,000 epinephrine	90-180	240-540	27	0.0090	3.6/lb	400	0.2	0.04
0.5% bupivacaine and 1:200,000 epinephrine	90-180	240-540	9	0.0090	.9/lb	200	0.2	0.04

Modified from Malamed SF: *Handbook of local anesthesia*, ed 3, St Louis, 1990, CV Mosby; Hersh EV: *Compend Contin Educ Dent* 8:374, 1987.

mon local anesthetic and vasoconstrictive agents. This information is also on the product information sheet in the package of anesthetic cartridges.

It should be noted that the MSDs are expressed in milligrams and that the anesthetic and vasoconstrictive agents are expressed in milligrams per milliliters. Whenever local anesthetic or vasoconstrictive agents are administered, the clinician should calculate the amount of each agent given to ensure that the MSD is not exceeded and record the amount in the patient's record. A standard cartridge contains 1.8 ml. A 1% solution contains 10 mg/ml, so a cartridge of 1% solution is equivalent to 18 mg of anesthetic agent. One cartridge of 2% solution is equivalent to 36 mg of anesthetic agent. Thus if a patient were given two cartridges of a 2% local anesthetic agent, the patient would have received 72 mg of the agent (Bennett, 1984; Dafoe, 1982).

The amount of vasoconstrictor administered should also be calculated and the MSDs observed. Epinephrine, the most commonly used vasoconstrictor, has an MSD of 0.2 mg for a healthy person and 0.04 mg for a person with a cardiac condition (Malamed, 1990). Again, the concentration of the agent must be considered to calculate the amount of drug administered. If one cartridge of solution containing epinephrine 1:100,000 is given, the patient will receive 0.018 mg of epinephrine. Table 32-2 presents the formulas and information necessary to calculate the amounts of local anesthetic and vasoconstrictive agents administered.

When local anesthetic and vasoconstrictive agents are used together, one of the two agents will determine the MSD. For example, the MSD for epinephrine may be reached before the MSD for the local anesthetic in some medically compromised patients, and no more can be given.

The MSD should also be adjusted downward for persons weighing less than 150 pounds (Bennett, 1984; Malamed, 1990). By weight, the MSD for prilocaine (Citanest) is 2.7 mg per pound up to a maximum of 400 mg. Therefore a healthy person weighing 120 pounds can be given 324 mg, or 4 ½ cartridges of prilocaine. A 60-pound child could receive 162 mg of prilocaine or 2 ¼ cartridges of the anesthetic agent. Calculating the MSD according to the patient's weight is the preferred method for small people, particularly children (Bennett, 1984; Malamed, 1990; Rood, 1981).

Table 32-2. Computation of amounts of agents administered

Local anesthetic agents

FORMULA:
1.8 ml per cartridge × Number of cartridges × Concentration of solution = mg adminstered
  1% = 10 ml
  2% = 20 ml
  3% = 30 ml
  4% = 40 ml
EXAMPLE: 2 cartridges of lidocaine 2%
1.8 × 2 × 20 = 72 mg

Vasoconstrictive agents

FORMULA:
1.8 ml per cartridge × Number of cartridges × Concentration of agent = mg administered
  Epinephrine
  1:50,000   = 0.02 mg
  1:100,000 = 0.01 mg
  1:200,000 = 0.005 mg
  Norepinephrine
  1:30,000   = 0.03 mg
  Nordefrin
  1:10,000   = 0.1 mg
  Levonordefrin
  1:20,000   = 0.05 mg
EXAMPLE: 2 cartridges containing epinephrine 1:100,000
1.8 × 2 × 0.01 = 0.036 mg

Medical considerations

A complete and thorough review of the patient's medical history and vital signs is essential before a local anesthetic is administered. Some patients' conditions may contraindicate a local anesthetic agent and/or vasoconstrictor. Most often contraindications are relative and require evaluation of the severity of the patient's condition, modification in the amount of anesthetic, and perhaps type of agent used. An example is a patient with liver dysfunction. A healthy liver is important because it removes amide anesthetics from circulation and biotransforms them. The question becomes one of degree. Ambulatory patients who can walk into a dental office and seek care do have some liver function. Consultation with the patient's physician may be appropriate. Extending treatment over more appointments would result in fewer injections given at each session. Selecting an ester anesthetic, which is metabolized primarily in the blood plasma, is another option.

The following is a list of common medical conditions that need special consideration before local anesthetic injections are given (adapted from

Bennett, 1984; Malamed, 1990):

1. For patients with ischemic heart disease, hypertension, or cardiac arrhythmias, the vasoconstrictor should be kept to a minimum.
2. Kidney and liver disease may slow the elimination of anesthetic agents from the body.
3. History of a stroke is an indication to use the minimum effective doses of anesthetic with vasoconstrictor.
4. When controlled or corrected, thyroid disease does not indicate any need for modification. Clinically hyperthyroid patients are sensitive to vasoconstrictors.
5. Reports of excessive bleeding, bruising, or hemophilia must be investigated. Injections in highly vascular areas, such as the posterior superior alveolar, inferior alveolar, and mental areas, should be avoided.
6. For allergy patients, allergy-producing agents should be avoided. A true allergic reaction can be life-threatening. In patients with many allergies, even if anesthetics are not listed, consider avoiding all esters, including topical.
7. Malignant hyperthermia is an exaggerated, life-threatening response to general anesthetics and possibly amide anesthetics.
8. Atypical plasma cholinesterase is an indication to avoid ester type anesthetics.
9. Methemoglobinemia is a condition in which the blood hemoglobin has reduced capacity to carry oxygen. Two anesthetics, prilocaine and articaine, exacerbate this condition.

Drugs and medications should be investigated in the *Physician's Desk Reference* or similar source for possible interactions with the local anesthetic agents themselves or the catecholamines used as vasoconstrictors.

Because the general population is aging, more elderly people will be requiring routine dental care. Bomberg (1986) points out that about 85% of the population over age 65 have one or more chronic disease conditions and that these patients often take between 3 and 12 medications simultaneously. It is important to establish the current physical state and medication regimen. Age-related changes in the liver, decreased liver mass and blood flow, and decreased renal function suggest that local anesthetic dosage must be revised downward for the medically compromised or frail elderly patient.

Allergic reactions to local anesthetics are mentioned in Chapter 7. Once the agent has been administered, the patient should be observed for at least 3 to 5 minutes, as most reactions occur within that time. If any untoward reaction occurs, the dentist should be informed, proper treatment provided, and the incident recorded in the patient's chart.

Armamentarium

The armamentarium necessary for an injection is illustrated in Fig. 32-2. The syringe is an aspirating syringe, because the clinician can create negative pressure in the anesthetic cartridge by pulling back on the thumb ring. The tray also includes a topical anesthetic; an antiseptic; cotton-tipped applicators; gauze to retract, dry, and hold movable tissues; and the assembled syringe. Fig. 32-3 shows the proper assembly of the syringe, cartridge, and needle. Needles are either short (approximately 1 inch, or 25 mm) or long (approximately 1 5/8 inches, or 40 mm) and come in a variety of gauges (Malamed, 1990). The short needle is used for all common dental injections except the inferior alveolar, Gow-Gates, and infraorbital, which require a longer needle.

The gauge of the needle refers to the diameter of the lumen. The most common gauges used in dentistry are 25, 27, and 30. Of these, the 25-gauge needle has the largest lumen and is recommended for dental injections that pose a risk of positive aspiration, such as the inferior alveolar, posterior superior alveolar, mental, or incisive nerve blocks. Aspiration is easier through a larger needle lumen. The 27-gauge needles are useful for supraperiosteal and local infiltrations, and the 30-gauge needle for localized hemostasis (Malamed, 1990). The small lumen size of the 30-gauge needle does not permit adequate aspiration, so its use is limited to papillary and periodontal ligament injections.

Another delivery system for anesthesia is the jet injector. This instrument is capable of delivering 0.05 to 0.2 ml of anesthetic solution at a pressure of 2000 pounds per square inch. This technique is used primarily to produce topical anesthesia (Bennett, 1984; Malamed, 1990). The actual force of the injection may be disturbing to the patient. Although no needles are required, this type of injection does not produce adequate pulpal anesthesia, which limits its usefulness.

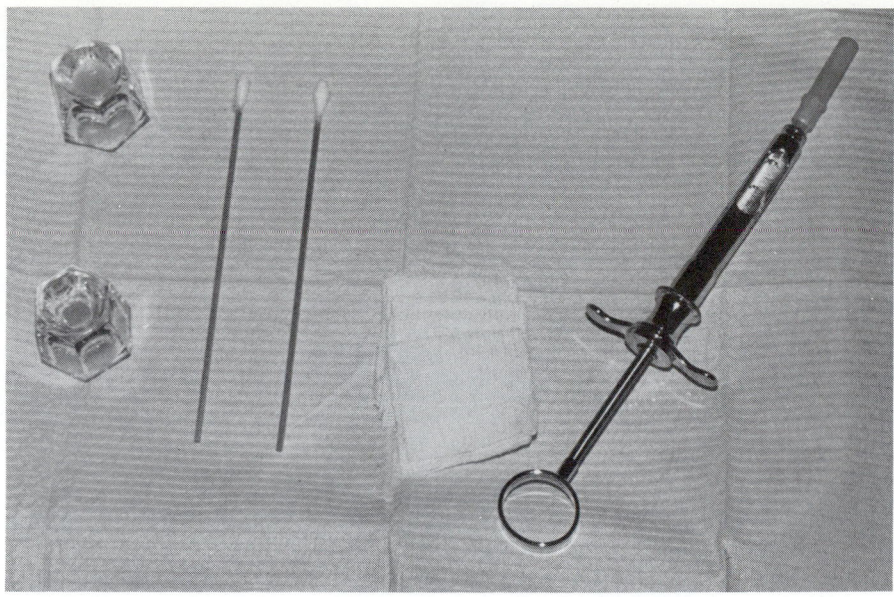

Fig. 32-2. Tray setup for administration of local anesthesia: topical anesthetic, antiseptic, cotton-tipped applicators, gauze, and assembled syringe.

Administration

An understanding of the anatomy of the nervous, vascular, osseous, and muscular structures of the head and oral area is necessary to determine which injections should be given and which technique should be used for administration. Fig. 32-4 illustrates the innervation of the teeth and associated structures of importance in local anesthesia. The nerves supplying the oral structures pictured in Fig. 32-4 are branches of the fifth cranial nerve, the trigeminal nerve. Specific injections and injection techniques have been developed to anesthetize the nerve trunks and nerve branches. When a nerve is anesthetized along the nerve trunk before it branches, *block anesthesia* occurs. When a branch of a nerve trunk is anesthetized by depositing solution in the area of the nerve branch so that the solution filters through the underlying bone to reach the nerve, *infiltration* or *field block anesthesia* occurs (Haglund and Evers, 1972; Sicher and DeBrul, 1975). Infiltration anesthesia depends on the solution filtering through the tissues and bone to reach the nerve. Its effectiveness depends in large part on the thickness of the bone and the distance of the nerve from the deposition site of the anesthetic.

Table 32-3 lists the various injections along with the nerves and tissues anesthetized by each injection. Figs. 32-5 to 32-14 illustrate the injection sites. This can help the clinician determine which injections could be given to achieve anesthesia in a given area. It is important to determine if soft or hard tissue anesthesia is necessary. Not all of the injections provide both; for example, the long buccal injection anesthetizes only the soft tissues over the mandibular molars. If both the teeth and the soft tissue must be anesthetized, an inferior alveolar block plus the long buccal must also be given. In some instances more than one combination of injections may be administered to achieve the desired anesthesia. In those instances the clinician decides which injections to give based on factors such as which combination requires the fewest penetrations, which requires the least amount of solution, the desired duration, the patient's medical condition, and other relevant factors.

A local anesthetic may be required when the patient is experiencing pain in the gingiva and/or teeth. If verbal reassurance does not alleviate the pain, the clinician can consider nitrous oxide and oxygen conscious sedation and/or local anesthe-

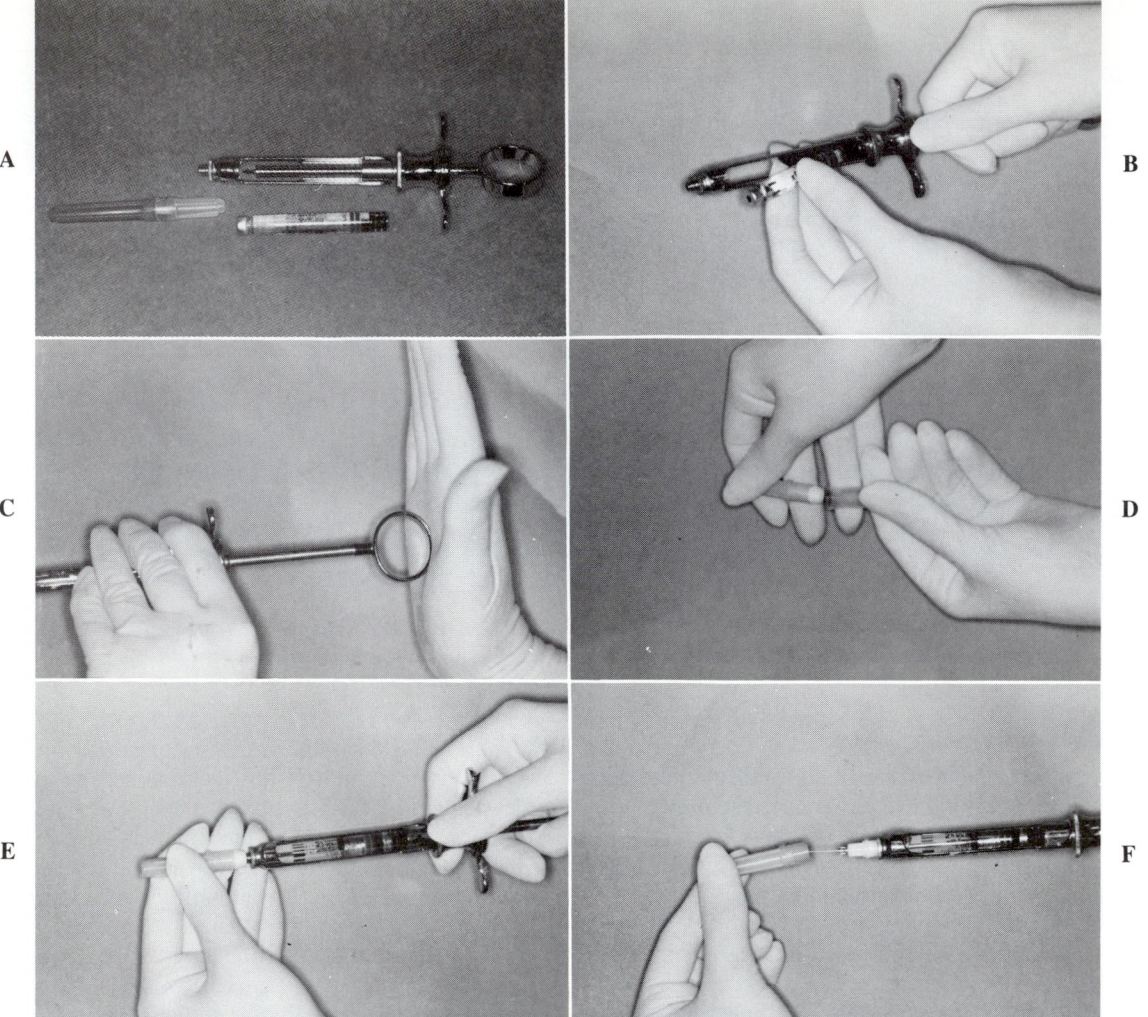

Fig. 32-3. **A,** Syringe, cartridge, and needle. **B,** Aspirator assembly is drawn back, and cartridge is inserted. **C,** Aspirating tip is engaged into plunger with several firm taps against ring. **D,** End of needle to be inserted into cartridge is uncovered. **E,** Needle penetrates diaphragm of cartridge and is screwed into syringe. **F,** Needle is exposed.

sia. Local anesthesia will provide complete anesthesia for a localized area from a single tooth to a quadrant or half of the mouth. It is rare that a patient is subjected to local anesthesia in all four quadrants simultaneously, as it is uncomfortable to have all areas of the mouth, tongue, and lips numb at the same time. Also, the maximum safe dose would be approached. Most clinicians anesthetize a sextant, a quadrant, or the right or left half of the mouth to perform dental hygiene or periodontal procedures.

The clinician is concerned with the osseous, vascular, and muscular anatomy during an injection (Bennett, 1984; Haglund and Evers, 1972; Reed and Sheppard, 1976). The osseous structures are the most reliable landmarks, as they are constant in shape and location. The musculature is important because penetration and trauma to the muscles must be kept to a minimum to avoid muscle trismus or soreness after the injection. A knowledge of the probable location of the blood vessels is important, because rupturing a vessel

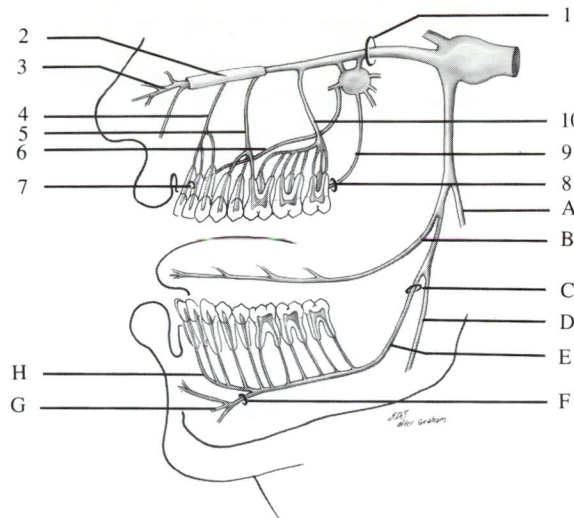

Fig. 32-4. Trigeminal nerve. Maxillary division: (1) foramen rotundum; (2) infraorbital canal; (3) infraorbital nerve; (4) anterior superior alveolar nerve; (5) middle superior alveolar nerve; (6) nasopalatine nerve; (7) incisive foramen (located on palate); (8) greater palatine foramen; (9) greater palatine nerve; (10) posterior superior alveolar nerve. Mandibular division: (A) auriculotemporal nerve; (B) lingual nerve; (C) mandibular foramen; (D) mylohyoid nerve; (E) inferior alveolar nerve; (F) mental foramen; (G) mental nerve; (H) incisive nerve.
(From Graham KB: *Local anesthesia and pain control: a modular approach*, Kansas City, Mo, 1979, Biomedical Communication Services, University of Missouri—Kansas City School of Dentistry.)

can cause internal bleeding and a hematoma and because depositing solution intravascularly can result in an overdose. The clinician must *always aspirate*—pull back the plunger—to create a negative pressure in the cartridge, which will draw blood into the cartridge if the tip of the needle is in a vessel. Blood vessels are associated with each of the nerves. Aspiration will help the clinician avoid injecting into the major blood vessels and decrease the chances of toxic overdose.

Steps for administration

1. Once you have selected the injection to be given, all the anatomic landmarks should be located to identify the penetration site.
2. Dry the penetration site with a gauze square.
3. Apply the topical anesthetic to the area for the appropriate amount of time, then rinse and suction it away or wipe with a gauze square.
4. Retract the movable tissue so you have a clear view of the needle penetration site.
5. Apply the antiseptic solution to the site just before the needle penetrates the tissue. Aseptic technique must be observed to protect the patient from a bacteremia or infection. The needle should touch nothing except the patient's tissues. The cap should remain on the needle unless the setup is being tested or the syringe is being used. Bennett (1984) has advocated the use of an antiseptic solution on the penetration site to lessen the chance of carrying bacteria and debris from the oral

cavity into the tissue. Some clinicians do not use antiseptic solution before injection; others apply it before the topical anesthetic. These preferences in technique do not affect the result of the injection. The rationale used here is that the antiseptic should be the last agent on the tissue before the needle is inserted.

6. If possible, you should establish a fulcrum against which to rest the syringe so you can hold it steady during needle insertion, aspiration, and administration of the solution.
7. Before and during the injection, talk with the patient to provide reassurance.
8. Insert the needle to the proper depth.
9. Complete the aspiration technique.
10. Inject the solution slowly to increase patient comfort and reduce the chance of a toxic reaction.
11. When the desired amount of solution has been administered, remove the needle and syringe.
12. Give special attention to the used anesthetic needle. The risk of needle stick injury is a serious concern because of the potential for transmission of hepatitis and HIV. During the recapping of a used needle, there is increased risk of unintentional needle stick injury. Current Occupational Safety and Health Administration (OSHA) regulations (1991) suggest that there are two options for the management of used anesthetic needles. One is to not recap them, the other is to use a mechanical device or a one-handed technique for re-

Table 32-3. Branches of the trigeminal nerve related to dental local anesthesia

Nerve	Tissues innervated/anesthetized	Injected
Maxillary division		
Greater palatine	Hard tissue: none Soft tissue: palatal tissue from teeth to midline from distal of third molar to cuspid	Greater palatine
Nasopalatine	Hard tissue: none Soft tissue: palatal tissues from left cuspid to right cuspid	Nasopalatine
Posterior superior alveolar (PSA)	Hard tissue: second and third molars; first molar excluding mesiobuccal root; associated supporting structures Soft tissue: overlying buccal tissues	Posterior superior alveolar (PSA)
Middle superior alveolar (MSA) branch of infraorbital	Hard tissue: first and second premolars, mesiobuccal root of first molar, and associated supporting structures Soft tissue: overlying buccal tissues and cheek or lip	Middle superior alveolar (MSA)
Anterior superior alveolar (ASA) branch of infraorbital	Hard tissue: cuspid and incisors and associated supporting structures Soft tissue: overlying facial tissues and lip	Anterior superior alveolar (ASA)
Infraorbital (includes both MSA and ASA)	Hard tissue: premolars, cuspid, incisors, and associated supporting structures Soft tissue: overlying facial tissue, cheek, and lip	Infraorbital
Individual terminal branches of MSA or ASA	Hard tissue: individual premolars, cuspid, incisors, and associated supporting structures Soft tissue: facial tissue and lip overlying individual teeth	Maxillary infiltration
Free nerve endings	Hard tissue: none Soft tissue: individual papillae	Interpapillary
Mandibular division		
Buccal (long buccal)	Hard tissue: none Soft tissue: buccal tissue of molars	Long buccal
Lingual	Hard tissue: none Soft tissue: lingual tissue from molar to midline, including anterior two-thirds of tongue	Lingual
Inferior alveolar (includes dental, mental, and incisive branches)	Hard tissue: molars, premolars, cuspid, and incisors to midline, as well as associated supporting structures Soft tissue: facial tissue anterior to mental foramen, including lip	Inferior alveolar or mandibular block
Mental branch of inferior alveolar	Hard tissue: none Soft tissue: facial tissue and lip anterior to mental foramen	Mental
Incisive and mental branches of inferior alveolar	Hard tissue: premolars, cuspid, incisors, and associated supporting structures Soft tissue: facial tissue and lip anterior to mental foramen	Incisive and mental
Individual terminal branches of mental and incisive	Hard tissue: individual cuspids, incisors, and sometimes premolars Soft tissue: facial tissue and lip overlying individual teeth	Mandibular facial infiltration
Anterior portion of lingual nerve	Hard tissue: none Soft tissue: lingual tissue in area of injection	Mandibular lingual infiltration
Third division nerve block (includes inferior alveolar, mental, incisive, lingual, mylohyoid, auriculotemporal, buccal nerves)	Hard tissue: mandibular teeth to midline; body of mandible; inferior portion of ramus Soft tissue: buccal and lingual tissue; anterior two-thirds of tongue and floor of mouth; skin over the zygoma; posterior portion of the cheek and temporal regions	Gow-Gates technique
Free nerve endings	Hard tissue: none Soft tissue; individual papillae	Interpapillary

Data from Bennett, 1984; Reed and Sheppard, 1976; Sicher and DeBrul, 1975; and Malamed, 1990.

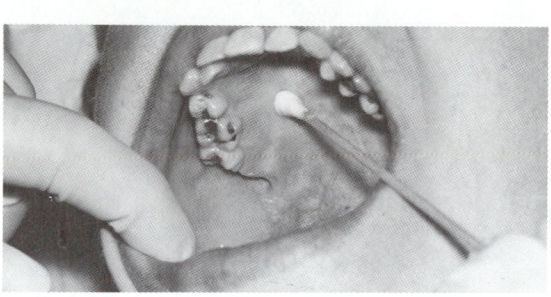

Fig. 32-5. Placement for greater palatine injection is just anterior to the foramen which is typically at the height of hard palate between first and second molars.

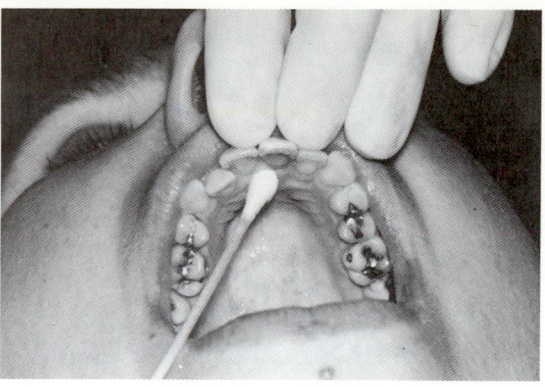

Fig. 32-6. Placement for nasopalatine injection is incisive papilla.

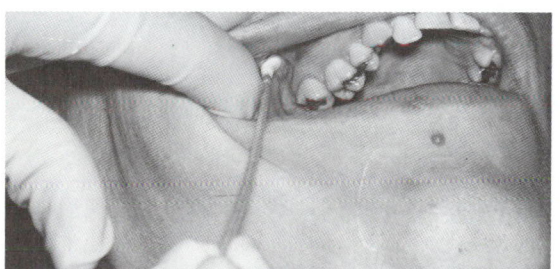

Fig. 32-8. Placement for middle superior alveolar injection is at height of mucobuccal fold between premolars.

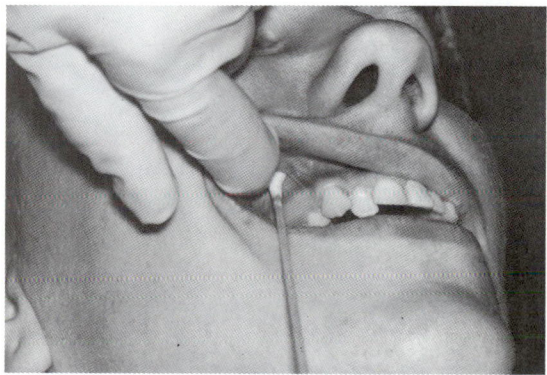

Fig. 32-7. Placement for posterior superior alveolar injection is at height of mucobuccal fold, usually over the second molar.

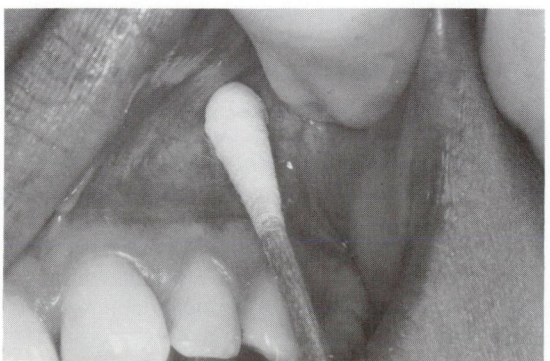

Fig. 32-9. Placement for anterior superior alveolar injection is at height of mucobuccal fold just anterior to the canine.

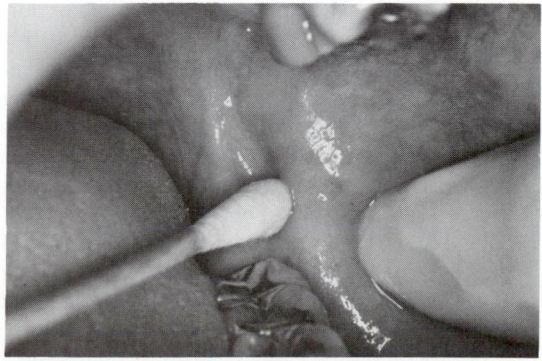

Fig. 32-10. Placement for inferior alveolar and lingual injection is in the pterygomandibular triangle. Approach from across the arch.

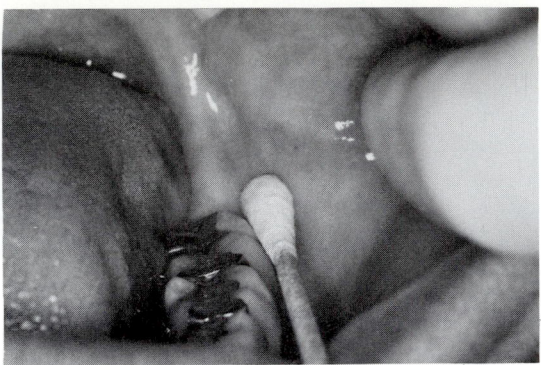

Fig. 32-11. Placement for long buccal injection is buccal to ramus and at height of molar.

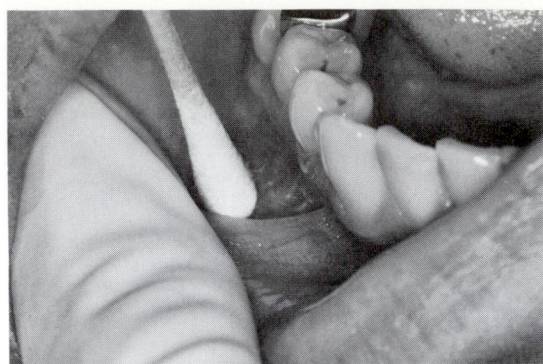

Fig. 32-12. Placement for mental or incisive nerve injection is in mucobuccal fold, over the mental foramen, usually between the premolars.

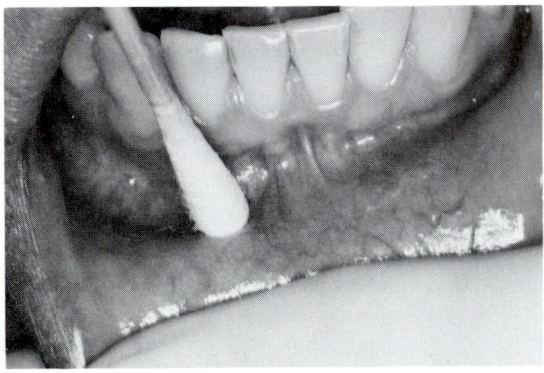

Fig. 32-13. Placement for mandibular facial infiltration is at depth of mucobuccal fold at desired tooth.

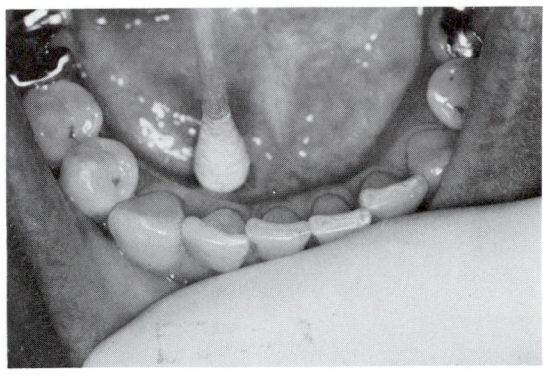

Fig. 32-14. Placement for mandibular lingual infiltration is at depth of mouth adjacent to tooth.

capping. A number of available devices serve as a shield or holder for the needle cap so that operators cannot inadvertently stick themselves while holding the needle cap during a recapping procedure. A sample of this type of device is shown in Fig. 32-15. Another successful one-handed recapping method is called the "scoop" technique. No special device is needed for this. The cap is placed horizontally on the tray, and the needle is inserted or scooped into the cap (Fig. 32-16). Once inside the cap, the syringe is tipped up vertically so the needle can be pushed in completely and the cap snapped into place at the hub. All of this is done without touching the cap. At all times, handling a syringe with a used needle and disposing of needles deserve extreme care.

13. To dispose of needles and other sharps, use a special container that is closable, puncture resistant, and leak proof. It must also be color coded and labeled for hazardous waste (OSHA, 1991). These containers should be located near the area of use. They have an adaptor that allows the needle to be detached and dropped into the container without unscrewing it by hand (Fig. 32-17).

The clinician or another properly trained person should remain with the patient after the injection has been given. Adverse reactions are most likely to occur within the first 3 to 5 minutes after the injection is completed. Systemic reactions associated with local anesthetics and vasoconstrictors include syncope, allergy, toxic overdose, and idiosyncrasy. For more information, refer to the section on local anesthetic reactions in Chapter 7.

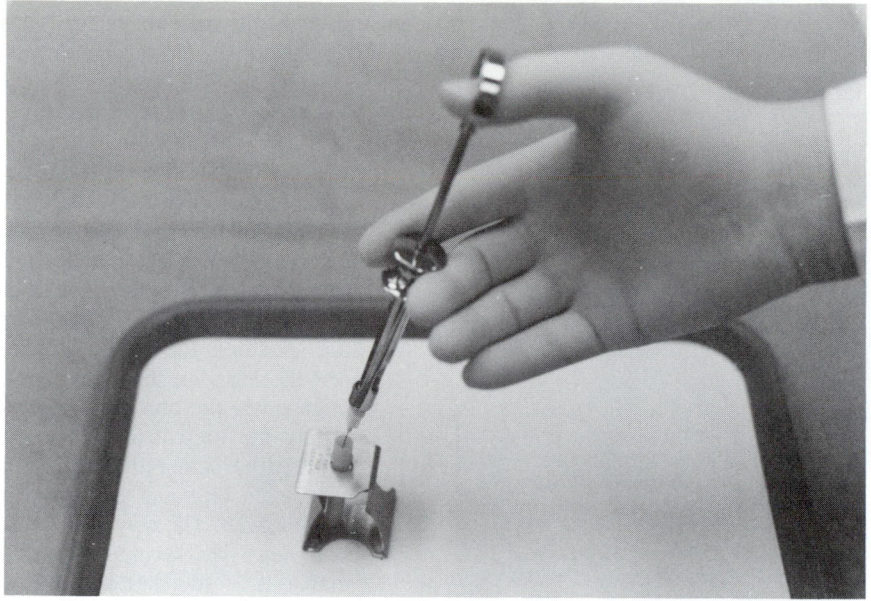

Fig. 32-15. A device for holding the cap of the anesthetic needle so that one-handed recapping can be easily accomplished.

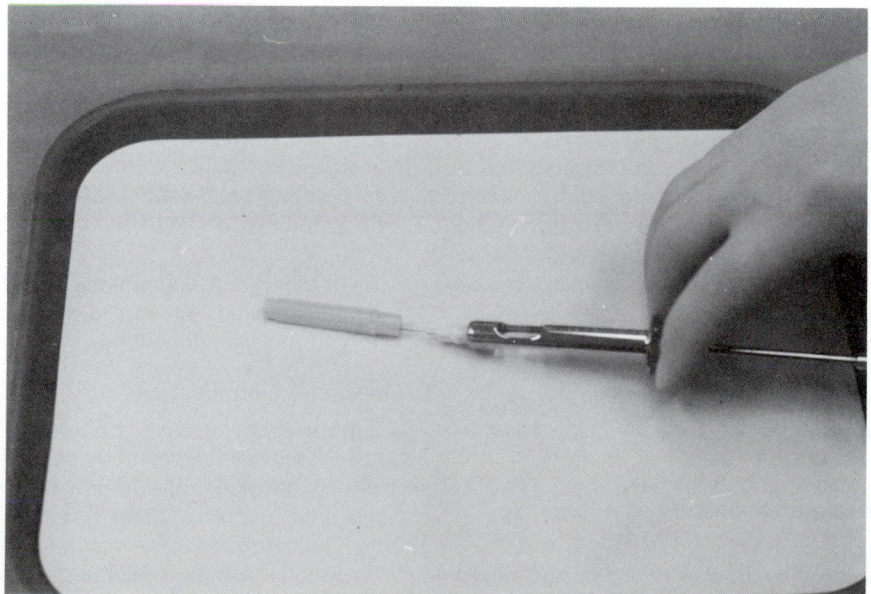

Fig. 32-16. The "scoop" technique for one-handed recapping of the anesthetic needle.

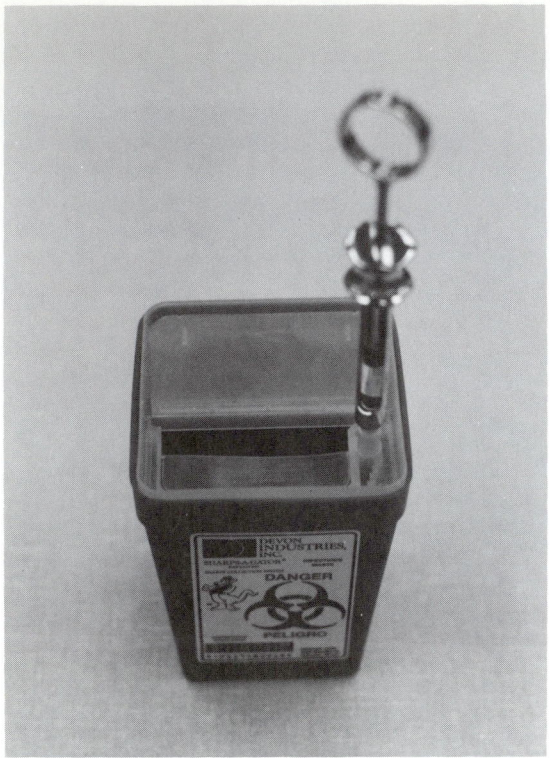

Fig. 32-17. A typical sharps disposal container. The needle is shown in place for removal. The syringe is removed and the used needle drops into the container.

After several minutes, the clinician may test the tissue and teeth to determine if anesthesia has been achieved. At the end of the appointment the patient should be reminded not to chew or bite the soft tissues that are numb. The patient should be instructed to call the office if any unusual sensations or rashes are experienced.

Some modifications in technique are necessary during the administration of local anesthesia to children. Malamed (1990) and Rood (1981) should be consulted if anesthesia is being given to children.

Assisting with administration of a local anesthetic

With an increased awareness of the hazard posed by used needles, it has become usual practice for the syringe and often all of the anesthetic setup to be on the operator's cart rather than on the assistant's cart. Syringes are usually uncapped and re-capped by the person giving the injection, so that the potentially hazardous step of transferring an uncapped needle does not occur.

When assisting another person with the administration of a local anesthetic, follow these steps after the review of the health history and the recording of the patient's vital signs:

1. Prepare the syringe with the appropriate anesthetic agent and a needle of the correct length (see Fig. 32-3). The setup may be tested by removing the cap and squeezing a few drops of solution onto a gauze square. This allows the assistant to examine the needle, position the bevel of the needle, and test the harpoon to make sure it is securely engaged in the plunger of the cartridge.
2. Apply the topical anesthetic for the appropriate time. Rinse the area.
3. When the clinician is ready, pass the antiseptic swab. (If a syringe is passed, it occurs here. The syringe is passed to the clinician out of the patient's view. Each clinician has a preference for this transfer, but in general the assistant must hold the syringe in such a way that the operator can grasp it easily and securely. The assistant should not remove his or her hand until the clinician is in full control of the syringe. As the syringe is moved away from the assistant, the cap is removed and the needle should be positioned so the bevel of the needle is facing the tissue when the injection is performed.)
4. Stand by to reassure the patient.
5. Rinse the patient's mouth. (Meanwhile, the operator recaps the needle.)
6. Remain with the patient, unless the clinician is doing so.
7. In the patient's treatment record, record the amount and type of anesthetic agents used and the injections give (Fig. 32-18).

Anesthetic complications

Local anesthetics have a remarkably safe record. Considering that conservative estimates place use at an excess of 6 million cartridges per week in the United States (Malamed, 1990), we hear of very few serious adverse reactions.

Potentially serious systemic reactions to anesthetic drugs are toxic overdose, allergy, and idiosyncrasy. With careful technique and a thorough evaluation of the patient's medical status, overdose reactions should be avoidable. If one should

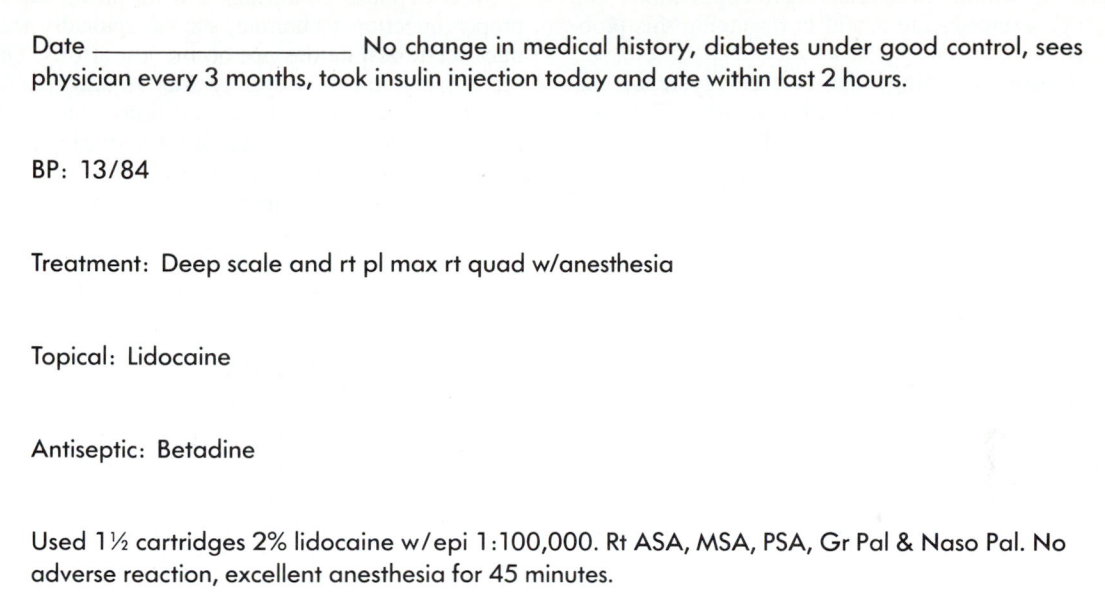

Date _____ No change in medical history, diabetes under good control, sees physician every 3 months, took insulin injection today and ate within last 2 hours.

BP: 13/84

Treatment: Deep scale and rt pl max rt quad w/anesthesia

Topical: Lidocaine

Antiseptic: Betadine

Used 1½ cartridges 2% lidocaine w/epi 1:100,000. Rt ASA, MSA, PSA, Gr Pal & Naso Pal. No adverse reaction, excellent anesthesia for 45 minutes.

Fig. 32-18. Sample chart entry for the administration of a local anesthetic.

occur, prompt recognition and effective CPR should be able to maintain the patient until emergency help arrives. This is the most common of all true adverse drug reactions (Malamed, 1990).

Allergic reactions range from dermatitis and hives to a life-threatening anaphylaxis. While they can be caused by anesthetic agents, they are rare since amides became the standard drug for dental care.

An *idiosyncratic reaction* is an adverse reaction to a normal amount of local anesthetic that is unexplainable on a pharmacologic or biochemical basis. Treatment will vary according to symptoms and usually will be the same as for allergic or toxic reactions (Laskin, 1984). These adverse drug reactions have also been discussed elsewhere in this chapter and in Chapter 7.

There are also a number of localized reactions that can result from the use of local anesthetics. A list of these typically includes hematoma, trismus, tissue sloughing, cheek or lip bites, transient facial nerve paralysis, intraoral lesions, and localized infection (Bennett, 1984; Malamed, 1990).

Hematoma. Hematoma can occur on injection into a highly vascular area or a region where a large blood vessel is located. During the injec-

tion, if the blood vessel is damaged or nicked, bleeding occurs into the tissue. A small amount of blood can accumulate if a vein has been nicked, but a large hematoma can occur very rapidly if an artery has been affected. Usually the bleeding is self-limiting because of pressure that builds up in the tissues. When a hematoma is recognized, pressure should be applied to the area immediately. An ice pack may also be used. Dental treatment should be discontinued. After 24 hours, moist heat is applied to the area to speed up the resolution. Swelling and discoloration will gradually disappear over 7 to 14 days.

Careful technique and attention to anatomic detail will greatly reduce the occurrence of hematomas. However, they can still occur because blood vessels are often associated with the path of the nerve and because of variation in human anatomy that cannot be seen without "x-ray vision."

Trismus. *Trismus* is difficulty opening the mouth because of spasm of the muscles of mastication or a motor disturbance of the trigeminal nerve. Needle insertion, especially multiple injections, rough tissue manipulation, overly large volume of anesthetic solution, or too rapid deposition can cause this. Usually the condition is much improved within 48 hours. Heat applications and gentle exercises are useful in managing this problem.

Tissue sloughing. The surface layers of epithelium are lost because of irritation. This may occur as a reaction to a topical anesthetic or excessive rubbing of the tissue. Following the recommendations for limiting the amount of topical anesthetic used and the time it is in place, as well as gentle treatment of the mucosa, will usually prevent this.

Lip and cheek biting. This occurs when the patient traumatizes the tissue while anesthesia is still present. It is seen most often in children. The trauma can create a significant wound. The best prevention is to use an anesthetic agent that has a duration appropriate to the length of the dental appointment. The patient should be told not to eat, drink, or test the anesthetized area by biting until normal sensation has returned. For children, a sticker can be placed on the forehead or the shirt as a reminder to the patient and the parent to be careful.

Facial paralysis. Facial paralysis is a weakening sensation of the muscles on the side of the face where the injection was given. The most notable findings are inability to close the eyelid, obliteration of the nasolabial fold, and drooping of the corner of the mouth (Laskin, 1984). This is the result of anesthetic solution inadvertently deposited in the parotid gland, affecting the facial nerve, during an inferior alveolar nerve block. The condition is temporary, but the patient will require reassurance. This complication can be completely avoided with the use of proper technique.

Intraoral lesions. Some patients susceptible to recurrent aphthous ulcers or recurrent hepatic lesions will experience intraoral lesions in the area of an injection. These cannot always be avoided, but keeping trauma to a minimum during needle insertion, placement of topical anesthetic and antiseptic, and tissue drying may help. The clinician should treat the symptoms, especially pain, and reassure the patient.

Localized infection. This is sometimes called needle tract infection and may be visible as a red line following the path of the needle in the tissue. It can best be prevented by use of impeccable asepsis, gentle wiping of the tissue surface to remove microorganisms, and use of antiseptic in the area of needle penetration.

Most of these conditions can be prevented by proper injection technique, but occasionally they may occur despite the operator's best efforts. Observe the patient very closely after an injection for anesthetic reactions and complications. Inform the patient and provide instruction for managing these uncomfortable conditions should they occur. Always record the patient reaction in detail in the chart. It is a good idea to periodically review the recognition and management of anesthetic complications or emergencies so that you feel confident and prepared.

TOPICAL ANESTHESIA

Topical anesthesia is achieved by direct application of an anesthetic agent onto the mucous membrane surface (Bennett, 1984). Once placed on the mucous membrane, the agent is absorbed by the free nerve endings in the area, creating an anesthetic effect. Only the free nerve endings in the soft tissue are affected. Topical anesthetic does not anesthetize teeth or root surfaces, as neither the nerve trunk nor its branches entering the teeth are affected.

Topical anesthetic agents

Chemically, topical anesthetics are similar to local anesthetics. There are two groups of topical anesthetics: amides and esters. The amide used as a topical anesthetic is lidocaine (Xylocaine), and the main two esters used as topical anesthetics are tetracaine (Pontocaine) and ethyl aminobenzoate (benzocaine). Benzyl alcohol is also used as a topical anesthetic. For these agents to be effective, they are used in greater concentrations than local anesthetics. For example, lidocaine is used in a 5% or 10% concentration; tetracaine in a 2% concentration; and benzocaine in 10%, 15%, and 20% concentrations (Bennett, 1984; Rogo, 1982). The topical anesthetic is absorbed by the blood vessels in the affected area, making a toxic reaction possible, especially because topical anesthetics are supplied in much higher concentrations (Bennett, 1984; Rogo, 1982).

Topical anesthetics are often liberally swabbed on the tissue. This technique can lead to overapplication and makes the dose control difficult. Many practitioners regard topical anesthetics as relatively harmless agents, but nothing could be further from the truth, thus this emphasis on the chance of toxic overdose.

Topical anesthetics are available in three forms:

gel, liquid, and spray. The gels and liquids are recommended for use before local anesthesia or during scaling procedures for superficial soft tissue anesthesia. Some practitioners also use topical anesthetics during radiographic series or impression taking to lessen patients' gag reflexes. Use of a topical anesthetic in these last two instances must be done judiciously to ensure that the patient maintains some of the necessary protective gag reflex. The use of topical anesthetic sprays should be limited to those with dose-controlled dispensers. Inhaling the agent is not recommended for either the patient or clinician.

The precautions observed for medically compromised patients when selecting a local anesthetic also apply to topical anesthetics. This is particularly true for patients with allergies. Esters, which cause the most allergy problems, are the most commonly used topical agents. If a patient has a history of allergy to ester anesthetics, then lidocaine topical anesthetic should be used. However, methylparaben, an esterlike substance, is used with most amide topical anesthetics, as they are all sold in multidose packages. The clinician should check the package insert accompanying the product to see if methylparaben is used. If allergy is suspected, the safest course of action is to avoid the use of the topical agent, as it is not essential. Topical anesthetics do not contain vasoconstrictors, so the medical conditions affected by vasoconstrictors do not apply to topical anesthetics.

A potential complication of topical anesthetics is tissue irritation. Because a topical anesthetic is applied directly to the mucous membrane, it has the potential to irritate or damage the tissue. This is of particular concern with benzocaine topical anesthetics, because they are produced in very high concentrations. Topical anesthetics are most likely to cause tissue sloughing if left in contact with the tissue too long or if rubbed into the surface. The surface tissue should always be treated gently.

Application

The use of a topical anesthetic before the injection of a local anesthetic and during a scaling procedure is presented in this section. Topical anesthetics are effective only on the soft tissue and are most effective on nonkeratinized soft tissue, where they are more readily absorbed.

Before an injection, a topical anesthetic can be

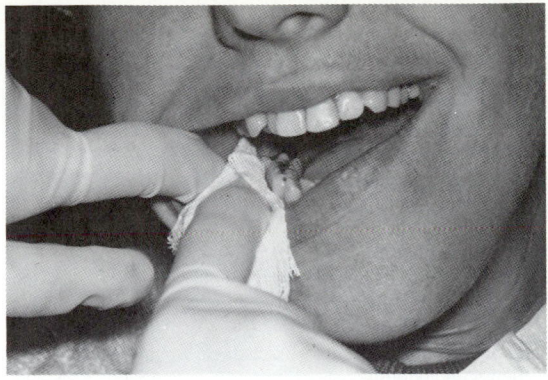

Fig. 32-19. Drying tissue with gauze prior to application of topical anesthetic.

applied to the injection site. Figs. 32-5 to 32-14 illustrate the application of a topical anesthetic to some of the injection sites listed in Table 32-3. Before the topical anesthetic is applied, the area should be dried with either a gauze square or a stream of air (Fig. 32-19). A gauze square has the benefit of removing debris and moisture before the injection. Drying the tissue helps keep the agent in the desired area, and it also ensures that the desired amount is being applied. If there is saliva in the area, the topical anesthetic will be carried away, lessening the amount applied and producing undesired anesthesia in other areas of the mouth. The topical anesthetic should be applied with a cotton-tipped applicator that has been dipped into the agent. To maintain asepsis, the topical anesthetic should be removed from the container and placed into a dappen dish so that the container is not contaminated. The multidose container should not be placed on the patient's treatment tray. The topical anesthetic on the cotton-tipped applicator (Fig. 32-20) is held in place for the appropriate amount of time. The length of application depends on the agent used and is determined by reading the manufacturer's directions accompanying the product. The highly concentrated benzocaine agents usually have very short application times of about 15 seconds; the less concentrated agents, such as lidocaine and tetracaine, may have longer application times of 30 to 120 seconds. The manufacturer's directions should be observed to obtain the desired effect and avoid tissue irritation.

Once the length of application is complete, the

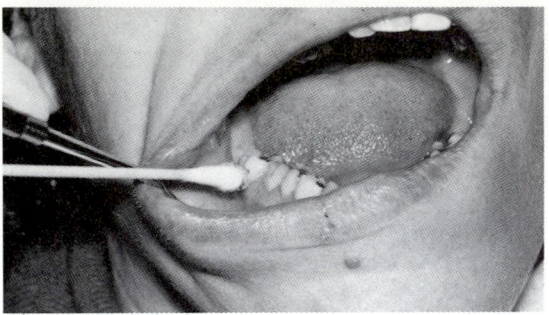

Fig. 32-20. Applying topical anesthetic for interpapillary injection with cotton-tipped applicator.

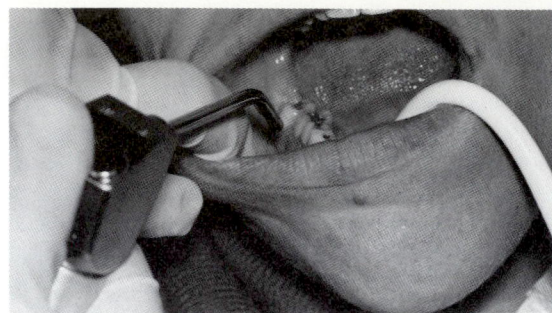

Fig. 32-21. Rinsing area at end of topical application time.

cotton-tipped applicator should be removed and the area thoroughly rinsed to remove the agent (Fig. 32-21). Ideally, the area should be suctioned as it is rinsed. The patient should not swallow the rinse water. Another option is to gently wipe off the excess with a gauze square. After the topical agent is removed, an antiseptic, if one is used, is applied to the injection site, and the injection is given.

The *application of a topical anesthetic during a scaling procedure* requires some modifications to the previous technique. It is still important to dry the area with either a stream of air or a gauze square, but the topical anesthetic can be applied in one of two ways: with a cotton-tipped applicator or a curette. Application with a cotton-tipped applicator will allow the topical anesthetic to reach the outer surface of the papilla and marginal gingiva but not the sulcus. Because the most sensitive tissue is likely to be the lining of the sulcus, it is recommended that the clinician dip the curette into the topical anesthetic and carry it into the sulcus in this manner. Liquid topical anesthetic is most easily carried into the sulcus on a curette. The application time must still be observed and the area thoroughly rinsed.

During a scaling procedure, the topical anesthetic of choice would provide a relatively long anesthetic effect and have a low toxicity. The MSDs of the agents must be observed. Benzocaine has a longer anesthetic effect and a lower toxicity than lidocaine or tetracaine. Benzocaine's longer effect and lower toxicity are due to its low water solubility, which results in slow absorption. But it must be remembered that benzocaine is an ester and that tissue sloughing is more likely. If the patient is not allergic to ester drugs and the clinician observes the application time, benzocaine can provide adequate topical anesthesia. Lidocaine and tetracaine also provide adequate anesthesia and are less likely to produce an allergic reaction and tissue sloughing. As with many agents, the clinician should use several and develop his or her own preferences, to be modified by the patient's medical history.

In general, the least possible amount of topical anesthetic necessary to produce the desired effect should be used. Also, the use of a topical anesthetic in highly vascular areas, such as the floor of the mouth, should be done with care. Observing application times and thorough rinsing are essential.

SUMMARY

Some psychosomatic, topical anesthetic, and local anesthetic approaches to pain control have been presented in this chapter. As the practitioner develops helping relationships with patients and uses the appropriate methods of pain control, his or her patients should have very little or no pain associated with dental treatment.

ACTIVITIES

1. Role-play a fearful patient and use psychosomatic technique to reduce dental anxiety and a potentially exaggerated pain reaction. Discuss how each role felt.
2. Make up a sample of dental hygiene procedures that may require local anesthesia and decide which injections could be given. (Refer to Table 32-3.) Incorporate these into a treatment plan so that care is provided effectively.
3. Using role-playing, practice presenting a treatment

plan that includes local anesthetic so that the patient understands the reasons for its use and accepts it as part of the total care plan.

4. The innervation of the maxilla and mandible described in Table 32-3 is for the permanent dentition. Look up the innervation of the primary and mixed dentitions, and compare and contrast the innervations.

5. Obtain a copy of the laws that govern the practice of dental hygiene in your state. Is administration of local anesthetic permitted? If not, does the class think it should or should not be permitted? What can or cannot be done about the practice act in the state?

6. Participate in a formal local anesthesia course open to dental hygienists to learn how to administer local anesthetics.

7. Referring to Table 32-1, figure out the number of cartridges of each agent that could be given before reaching the maximum safe dose in healthy and medically compromised patients. In which cases was the MSD of the vasoconstrictor reached first?

8. Practice the management of potential complications of local anesthetics. Include a review of CPR.

REVIEW QUESTIONS

1. Draw and label the following nerves:
   a. Posterior alveolar, superior alveolar, middle superior alveolar, and anterior superior alveolar
   b. Lingual, buccal, and inferior alveolar

2. Name the hard and soft tissues innervated by each of the following nerves:
   a. Posterior superior alveolar
   b. Greater palatine
   c. Buccal (long buccal)
   d. Inferior alveolar and lingual combined

3. Name the injections that should be given for each of the following procedures:
   a. Open flap periodontal debridement on the facial and lingual aspects of the mandibular right quadrant
   b. Periodontal debridement on a maxillary left first molar with deep pockets and some furcation involvement
   c. Debridement of the mandibular central incisors with sensitive roots but shallow pockets.

REFERENCES

American Association of Dental Schools: Special report: curricular guidelines for comprehensive control of pain and anxiety in dentistry, *J Dent Educ* 44:279, 1980.

American Dental Association Council on Dental Therapeutics: *Accepted dental therapeutics*, Chicago, 1982, The Association.

American Dental Hygienists' Association. Personal communication, 1992.

Atterbury R: Relaxation by vocal pre-sedation in dentistry, *CAL* 43:18, 1978.

Bennett RC: *Monheim's local anesthesia and pain control in dental practice,* ed 7, St Louis, 1984, CV Mosby.

Bomberg TJ: Local anesthetics and the elderly patient, *Gerodontics* 2:157, 1986.

Burstein A et al: Injection pain: memory, expectation, and experienced pain, *NY J Dent* 49:183, 1979.

Christensen LV: Cultural, clinical, and physiological aspects of pain: a review, *J Oral Rehabil* 7:413, 1980.

Cross-Poline GN et al: The effectiveness of a continuing education course in local anesthesia for dental hygienists, *J Dent Hyg* 66:130, 1992.

Dafoe BR: Providing pain control: local anesthesia, *RDH* 2:46, 1982.

Foreman PA: Behavioral considerations in patient management, *Anesth Prog* 26:161, 1979.

Giovannitti JA, Bennett RC: Assessment of allergy to local anesthetics, *JADA* 98:701, 1979.

Haglund J, Evers H: *Local anaesthesia in dentistry,* London, 1972, Astra Läkemedel.

Hersh EV et al: Local anesthetics: a review of their pharmacology and clinical use, *Compend Contin Educ Dent* 8:374, 1987.

Larson CE: Methylparaben, and overlooked cause of local anesthesia hypersensitivity, *Anesth Prog* 24:72, 1977.

Laskin DM: Diagnosis and treatment of complications associated with local anesthesia, *Int Dent J* 34:232, 1984.

Lobene RR: *The Forsyth experiment: an alternative system for dental care*, Cambridge, 1979, Harvard University Press.

Malamed SF: An update on pain and anxiety control in pediatric dentistry. II. Inhalation sedation and local anesthesia, *Alpha Omegan* 72:29, 1979.

Malamed SF: *Sedation—a guide to patient management,* St Louis, 1989, CV Mosby.

Malamed SF: *Handbook of local anesthesia,* ed 3, St. Louis, 1990, CV Mosby.

McCarthy FM: *Emergencies in dental practice, prevention and treatment,* ed 3, Philadelphia, 1979, WB Saunders.

Melzack R: *The puzzle of pain,* New York, 1973, Basic Books.

Occupational Safety and Health Administration: Rules and regulations, *Fed Reg* 56:64175, 1991.

Reed GM, Sheppard VF: *Basic structures of the head and neck,* Philadelphia, 1976, WB Saunders.

Rich SK, Smorang J: Survey of 1980 California dental hygiene graduates to determine expanded-functions utilization, *J Public Health Dent* 44:22, 1984.

Rogo ES: Providing safe comfortable pain control, *RDH* 1:12, 1982.

Rood JP: Notes on local anesthesia for the child patient, *Dent Update* 8:377, 1981.

Sicher H, DeBrul EL: *Oral anatomy,* ed 6, St Louis, 1975, CV Mosby.

Sisty-LePeau N et al: The administration of local anesthesia by dental hygiene students, *Dent Hyg* 60:28, 1986.

Sisty-LePeau N et al: Use, need, and desire for pain control procedures by Iowa hygienists, *J Dent Hyg* 66:137, 1992.

Spear FC: Cultural factors in clinical pain assessment, *Int Dent J* 27:284, 1977.

Steblay NM, Beaman AL: Reduction of fear during dental treatment through reattribution technique, *JADA* 105:1006, 1982.

Wepman BJ: Psychological components of pain perception, *Dent Clin North Am* 22:101, 1978.

Wong MKS, Jacobsen PL: Reasons for local anesthesia failures, *JADA* 123:69, 1992.

SUGGESTED READINGS

American Dental Association Council on Dental Materials, Instruments, and Equipment: Status report: the periodontal ligament injection, *JADA* 106:222, 1983.

Adriani J, Campbell D: Fatalities following topical application of local anesthetics to mucous membranes, *JAMA* 162:1527, 1956.

Aldrete TA, O'Higgins TW: Evaluation of patients with a history of allergy to local anesthetics, *South Med J* 64:115, 1971.

Bateman PM: Multiple allergy to local anesthetic including prilocaine, *Med J Aust* 2:449, 1974.

Bay N, Connon TM: Management of the fearful patient: role of the dental hygienist, *JDH* 64:188, 1990.

Blackmore JW: Local anesthetics: a review, *Oral Health* 77:11, 1987.

Dietz ER: The dental assistant's role in preparing the anesthetic syringe, *Dent Assist* 56(3):26, 1987.

Fry BW et al: Concentration of vasoconstrictors in local anesthesia change during storage in cartridge heaters, *J Dent Res* 59:1163, 1980.

Gangarosa LP Sr: Newer local anesthetics and techniques for administration, *J Dent Res* 60:1471, 1981.

Gill GJ, Orr DH: A double-blind crossover comparison of topical anesthetics, *JADA* 98:213, 1979.

Graham KB: *Local anesthesia and pain control: a modular approach,* Kansas City, 1979, Biomedical Communication Services, University of Missouri—Kansas City School of Dentistry.

Jastak JT et al: Vasoconstrictors and local anesthesia: a review and rationale for use, *JADA* 107:623, 1983.

Johnson WT et al: Hypersensitivity to procaine, tetracaine, mepivacaine and methylparaben: a report of a case, *JADA* 106:53, 1983.

Kaufman E et al: Difficulties in achieving local anesthesia, *JADA* 108:205, 1984.

Malamed SF: The periodontal ligament (PDL) injection: an alternative to inferior alveolar nerve block, *Oral Surg* 53:117, 1982.

Milgrom P et al: Student differences in achieving local anesthesia, *J Dent Educ* 48:168, 1984.

Milgrom P et al: Local anesthesia: adverse effects and other emergency problems, *Int Dent J* 36(2):71, 1986.

Miller S: Hypnosis—relaxation for you and your patient, *NY State Dent J* 45:221, 1979.

Mollen AJ et al: Needles—25 gauge vs 27 gauge—can patients really tell? *Gen Dent* 29:417, 1981.

Mumma RD Jr et al: Survey of administration of infiltration anesthesia, *Dent Hyg* 51:159, 1977.

Pashley DH: Systemic effects of intraligamental injections, *J Endodont* 12:501, 1986.

Peterson DS et al: Pain sensation related to local anesthetics injected at varying temperatures, *Anesth Prog* 25:164, 1981.

Prensky HD: Current concepts in pain control, *Clin Prevent Dent* 3(1):8, 1981.

Rich SK, Smorang J: Survey of 1980 California dental hygiene graduates to determine expanded-functions utilization, *J Public Health Dent* 44:22, 1984.

Sharp J: Should dental hygiene students be taught to administer local anesthesia? *NM Dent J* 30:8, 1979.

Sheilds PW: Local anesthesia and applied anatomy, *Aust Dent J* 31:319, 1986.

Siskin L: Anaphylaxis due to local anesthesia hypersensitivity: report of case, *JADA* 96:841, 1978.

Walsh MM et al: Mental imagery and local anesthesia, *J Dent Educ* 48:653, 1984.

Yaacob HB et al: The pharmacological effect of Xylocaine topical anesthetics—a comparison with a placebo, *Singapore Dent J* 6:55, 1981.

Yoeman CM: Hypersensitivity to prilocaine, *Br Dent J* 153:69, 1982.

33 NITROUS OXIDE AND OXYGEN CONSCIOUS SEDATION

Donna Stach
Bonnie Dafoe

LEARNING OUTCOMES

The dental hygienist will be able to

1. Define the term *conscious* as used in the philosophy of conscious sedation.
2. Assess a patient's medical, physical and mental status to determine need for anxiety control and appropriateness of nitrous oxide oxygen sedation.
3. Describe the chemical nature of nitrous oxide.
4. Describe the pharmacologic interactions that nitrous oxide with oxygen has on the body.
5. List the indications and contraindications for use of nitrous oxide with oxygen.
6. Describe the sequence of sensations that a patient may experience as the concentration of nitrous oxide is increased from 10% to 50%.
7. Outline safety features of nitrous oxide with oxygen for both equipment and technique.
8. Calculate the percentage of nitrous oxide and the total volume of gas being delivered to a patient.
9. Describe and use the technique for nitrous oxide and oxygen conscious sedation including:
   a. Preparation of equipment.
   b. Induction and titration.
   c. Monitoring of patients.
   d. Conclusion of use.

For many patients, visiting the dental office is an anxiety-producing situation. Because of past experiences or current discomfort, the patient worries that further discomfort is inevitable. Modern dentistry offers excellent pain control techniques, and such measures are necessary for most periodontal and restorative dentistry procedures. Local anesthetics are effective in blocking pain perception but the injection itself may produce anxiety. Before some patients are receptive to local anesthetic techniques, sedation techniques are helpful. Nitrous oxide and oxygen conscious sedation is a conscious inhalation sedation method that is used in about 40% of the dental offices and clinics in the United States today (Malamed, 1989).

The hygienist performs procedures that may cause the patient discomfort. Patients who rely on nitrous oxide and oxygen conscious sedation for other restorative dental procedures may require it for deep subgingival debridement, and placement of temporary restorations or crowns.

Administration of nitrous oxide includes assessing the health and anxiety status of the patient, in-ducing the proper level of sedation, monitoring the patient during analgesia, and oxygenating the patient at the completion of treatment. The terms *assist* or *monitor* in reference to the administration of nitrous oxide are interpreted by state practice acts as induction of the patient to the proper level by the dentist followed by monitoring and oxygenation of the patient following sedation by the hygienist. In 1992, 32 states allowed hygienists to assist, monitor or administer nitrous oxide (American Dental Hygienists' Association, 1992).

Nitrous oxide has been used in dentistry for more than 100 years. Horace Wells, a dentist, first demonstrated its effectiveness during a surgical procedure in 1844 (Langa, 1976). Since that time, the properties and effects of nitrous oxide used with oxygen have been studied and documented.

Nitrous oxide and oxygen conscious sedation is most beneficial in dentistry because it comforts and relaxes the patient. Nitrous oxide alters pain reaction, which is a very individualized interpretation of actual pain perception. When the patient's pain reaction threshold is raised, he or she is able better to relax and cooperate during dental procedures. A study designed to provide statistical estimates of the effects of nitrous oxide on pain and anxiety associated with tooth pulp shock demonstrated that it significantly raises levels of absolute sensation, pain threshold, and pain tolerance. Anxiety levels were reduced to a statistically significant degree (Dworkin, 1983). Additionally, nitrous oxide and oxygen conscious sedation alters the patient's perception of time, so dental appointments seem to pass more quickly. It may also have some amnesia effect, so the patient will not remember the appointment clearly. With a relaxed, conscious, and cooperative patient the appointment can be handled efficiently and comfortably. This results in less stress for both the patient and the clinician.

The basis of understanding nitrous oxide and oxygen conscious sedation is an appreciation of the conscious state. At no time during the administration of this form of inhalation sedation should the patient lose consciousness. The American Dental Society of Anesthesiology defines *conscious* in this way: "A patient is said to be conscious if he/she is capable of rational response to command and has all protective reflexes intact, including the ability to clear and maintain his/her airway in a patent state" (Bennett, 1978). All parts of this definition must be observed. Rational response to command will be especially important in monitoring the patient's conscious state. Retaining the ability to breathe automatically and to cough so that aspiration is avoided enables inhalation sedation to be administered without sophisticated technical support personnel and equipment. With nitrous oxide and oxygen inhalation sedation, vital signs and the function of cardiovascular and respiratory systems will remain within normal limits (Bennett, 1978; Roberts et al, 1982). Often there is a slight decrease in heart rate and cardiac output with a slight increase in total peripheral resistance, which is most likely the result of breathing a high concentration of oxygen (Giovannitti, 1984).

Nitrous oxide affects the central nervous system by depressing the cerebral cortex, thalamus, hypothalamus, and reticular activating system. This results in nervous impulses either not being relayed to the cortex or being interpreted differently (Swepston, 1980). The patient will experience an alteration of mood, and his or her pain reaction threshold will increase. The patient will be in a relaxed and very suggestible state.

A 20% concentration of nitrous oxide has been compared to 15 mg of morphine administered subcutaneously (Chapman et al, 1943). In fact, a 35% concentration has been shown effectively to relieve the pain associated with myocardial infarction (Thompson, 1976). As an important note, nitrous oxide sedation may be helpful in an emergency situation involving a myocardial infarction. It can provide pain control as well as supplemental oxygen for the patient until further emergency help arrives.

Nitrous oxide is a mildly potent anesthetic. *Potency* refers to the amount of medication necessary to achieve a desired effect. A clinical measure of relative potency has been experimentally determined. This is called the *mean alveolar concentration (MAC)*. The MAC is defined as the concentration of anesthetic agent required to prevent movement (reflex reaction to pain) at the time of surgical incision in 50% of patients (DeMartina and Garber, 1979). A very potent medication such as halothane, a general anesthetic, has an MAC of 0.77%. Nitrous oxide has an MAC of 101% (Fordham, 1974). Because it is impossible to deliver a 101% concentration of pure nitrous oxide gas because of atmospheric conditions, it cannot be relied on to relieve response to frank pain perception. In a dental procedure where hard or soft tissue pain will be significant for the patient, nitrous oxide and oxygen conscious sedation must be accompanied by local anesthesia. Heft and others (1984) found that 33% nitrous oxide analgesia reduced the intensity but not the unpleasantness of painful tooth pulp sensations.

Increasing the concentration of nitrous oxide will not significantly reduce true pain perception. A patient responding to pain while under nitrous oxide and oxygen conscious sedation will not be comfortable or cooperative for long.

Nitrous oxide is a colorless, nonexplosive, and sweet-smelling inorganic agent that will support combustion (Malamed, 1989). Commercially, nitrous oxide is supplied in blue pressurized cylinders, in which it is present in both a liquid and a gas state.

Nitrous oxide is nonallergenic and does not react with body tissues. It diffuses across tissue membranes much more rapidly than oxygen. When inhaled, nitrous oxide diffuses across the alveolar membrane in the alveoli of the lungs, entering the bloodstream. With a very low blood gas solubility (0.47) the nitrous oxide molecule travels unchanged in the blood. Nitrogen molecules are usually displaced in the bloodstream by nitrous oxide molecules. Nitrous oxide reaches equilibrium in the bloodstream rapidly and exerts its analgesic effect within minutes (Giovannitti, 1984). As long as the patient continues to breathe the flow of nitrous oxide and oxygen, a concentration of nitrous oxide that will affect the central nervous system will be maintained in the bloodstream. By controlling the external concentration of nitrous oxide and oxygen as it comes from the sedation equipment, the clinician can control the patient's pulmonary alveolar concentration (De-Martina and Garber, 1979).

Nitrous oxide concentration is usually expressed as a percentage of the gas volume being administered. On some nitrous oxide with oxygen delivery systems this percentage can be read directly. On others, the gas delivered is recorded in liters per minute and the percentage must be calculated. In either case it is important to know the total amount of gas, in liters per minute, and the percentage of each gas (N_2O and O_2) being administered to the patient to have an accurate understanding of the drug (N_2O) dose. Below is the equation for calculating percentage of nitrous oxide administered and 2 sample problems:

$$\frac{\text{Liters of } N_2O/\text{minute}}{\text{Total flow of } N_2O + O_2 \text{ in liter/minute}} \times 100 = \% \text{ of } N_2O$$

Example 1: $\dfrac{2 \text{ L of } N_2O}{2 \text{ L of } N_2O + 8 \text{ L of } O_2} = \dfrac{2}{10} \times 100 = 20\%$

Example 2: $\dfrac{3 \text{ L of } N_2O}{3 \text{ L of } N_2O + 6 \text{ L of } O_2} = \dfrac{3}{9} \times 100 = 33 1/3\%$

The alveolar concentration, or percentage, of nitrous oxide delivered, determines the central nervous system sedative effect that the patient will experience. Table 33-1 summarizes the range of responses possible at given concentrations (Bennett, 1978).

The sedation (depression) of the central nervous system resembles the state one experiences just before falling asleep. At concentrations higher than necessary for dental procedures, sleep indeed occurs. To maintain the definition of consciousness, the patient must remain awake and re-

Table 33-1. Signs and symptoms in response to nitrous oxide and oxygen conscious sedation

Concentration N_2O	Response
10% to 20%	Body warmth
	Tingling of hands and feet
20% to 30%	Circumoral numbness
	Numbness of thighs
20% to 40%	Numbness of tongue
	Numbness of hands and feet
	Droning sounds present
	Hearing distinct but distant
	Dissociation begins and reaches peak
	Mild sleepiness
	Analgesia (maximum at 30%)
	Euphoria
	Feeling of heaviness or lightness of body
30% o 50%	Sweating
	Nausea
	Amnesia
	Increased sleepiness
40% to 60%	Dreaming, laughing, giddiness
	Further increased sleepiness, tending toward unconsciousness
	Increased nausea and vomiting
50% and over	Unconsciousness and light general anesthesia

From Bennett CR: *Conscious sedation in dental practice,* ed 2, St Louis, 1978, CV Mosby.

sponsive to verbal commands at all times. If the patient is unable to keep the mouth open or is falling asleep, the amount of nitrous oxide being delivered should be reduced.

In addition to being relaxed and having time perception altered, the patient may experience dissociation (DeMartina and Garber, 1979; Minnis, 1979). This refers to an effect on the patient's ability to maintain his or her spatial orientation. The patient may describe floating or sinking into the chair. The clinician's voice and sounds in the operatory may seem distant. Most people enjoy a slight bit of "escape" from the dentistry at hand. Other patients may interpret dissociation as a feeling of losing control of themselves or the situation. This in itself may be alarming to the patient, thereby reducing the comfort that he or she expects to feel.

Patient reactions at any given concentration of nitrous oxide vary a great deal. The clinician must be sensitive to the physiologic and psychologic personality of the patient. Observing the patient's responses constantly ensures that a comfortable level of sedation is maintained at all times.

A few parameters are noteworthy. When nitrous oxide is administered above a 40% concentration, the patient generally becomes increasingly sleepy and responds sluggishly to commands (Bennett, 1978; Hamburg, 1980). The patient may begin to perspire, look uncomfortable, move in an uncoordinated manner, and complain of nausea. Any of these signs indicates that the inhaled concentration is too high. Although vomiting is rare at recommended levels, it is potentially dangerous and unpleasant for everyone concerned.

A concentration of 30% to 35% is the usual range for nitrous oxide in conscious sedation (Bennett, 1978). Many patients are comfortable at lower concentrations. An administration technique in which the concentration is preset is unacceptable. Sedation is induced with small amounts of nitrous oxide and a constant flow of at least 6 L of oxygen per minute. After a minute or 2 at each increment of nitrous oxide, the concentration is increased until a comfortable state is achieved. This technique is called *titration*. It is possible because of the rapid onset of nitrous oxide's effect and it is one of the advantages of this drug for sedation (Malamed, 1989).

From one appointment to another the same patient may achieve the desired sedation at different concentrations. The time of day, level of fatigue, general mood of the patient, dental procedures being performed, and a variety of other factors all have an influence. In any case, delivering an excess of medication is, at worst, capable of producing a bad experience for the patient and, at best, unnecessary and wasteful.

As a general rule in dentistry, nitrous oxide sedation should never be administered in concentrations greater than 50%. If a patient requires more pain control, another anesthetic modality should be employed.

PATIENT SELECTION

As with all drug interventions, careful patient assessment and selection are critical. When considering patients for nitrous oxide with oxygen seda-

tion, both the physical and psychological status of the patient must be considered. Patients in poor physical condition generally benefit from conscious sedation (Bennett, 1978), both because they do not tolerate stress well and because of the oxygen enrichment (McCarthy, 1989). From the psychologic perspective, patients who are mildly to moderately anxious of dental treatment benefit most. Severely distressed or phobic patients generally need intervention with a more potent drug (Bennett, 1978) or an approach that combines several treatment modalities including, perhaps, progressive desensitization.

Indications

Indications are from Bennett, 1978; Langa, 1976; Malamed, 1989; McCarthy, 1989.

1. The primary indication for the use of conscious sedation with nitrous oxide is for the management of dental fear or anxiety.
2. The other major indication is for the medically compromised patient. The combination of stress with many systemic diseases places the patient at greater risk for a medical emergency or other undesirable reaction. All forms of stress reduction, including nitrous oxide with oxygen, should be used as to make these patients more comfortable.

   Another major advantage for many patients is the oxygen enrichment afforded from use of nitrous oxide with oxygen. A number of high-risk diseases share the complication of *ischemia* (lack or reduction of blood or oxygen to an organ or body part). A patient receiving 35% N_2O is getting 65% O_2, and even at a concentration of 50/50, the 50% O_2 is better than the 20.9% O_2 available in room air.

   Patients with cardiovascular and cerebrovascular diseases are excellent candidates for nitrous oxide with oxygen sedation. Neither hypertension nor cardiac arrhythmias pose any specific contraindication to its use.

   Patients with respiratory diseases require careful evaluation before nitrous oxide is used. It can be used successfully in patients with bronchial asthma, especially if the attacks are stress related. Unlike many other anesthetic gases, nitrous oxide is nonirritating to the bronchial mucosa. In general, it is recommended if the patient would benefit from an oxygen-enriched air supply. It is generally not recommended for patients with chronic obstructive pulmonary disease, nasal obstruction, or infections that could contaminate the equipment.

Key considerations of liver and kidney disease are the breakdown and elimination of a drug or drug by-products by these body systems. Because nitrous oxide is not biotransformed anywhere in the body and enters and exits unchanged almost entirely through the lungs, its use is not contraindicated by dysfunction of these organs.

There are no known allergies to nitrous oxide.

Neither diabetes nor seizure disorders are contraindications for the use of nitrous oxide. It might be especially beneficial if these diseases make patients more fragile to stress.

3. Analgesia is one of the benefits of nitrous oxide with oxygen sedation. Analgesia is defined as the diminution or elimination of pain in the conscious patient (Third Pain Control Conference, 1971). Nitrous oxide does not block all pain perception and must be used in combination with local anesthesia for most procedures. It is most effective in blocking pain perception in the soft tissues and may be sufficient by itself to eliminate mild to moderate discomfort during periodontal instrumentation. In fact, this may be one of the most beneficial uses of nitrous oxide with oxygen sedation (Jastak, 1989; Malamed, 1989).

4. Nitrous oxide with oxygen sedation will diminish the gag reflex. In patients whose overactive gag response makes radiography and impression taking difficult, this type of conscious sedation will make these procedures more comfortable for all concerned.

Contraindications

Contraindications are from Bennett, 1978; Duncan and Moore, 1984; Langa, 1976; Malamed, 1989.

There do not appear to be any absolute contraindications to the use of nitrous oxide and oxygen sedation as long as a sufficient volume of oxygen is always provided and good technique is used. However, it may be relatively contraindicated and is not a good choice for some patients. As always, the key is a clear understanding of the actions of the drugs and the patient's condition.

1. The ability to communicate and cooperate are essential for success with conscious sedation. This may eliminate its use in a young or very disruptive child or handicapped patient who cannot or will not breathe through the nose or leave the nasal hood in place. It may also eliminate patients who cannot understand directions or communicate what they are feeling.

2. Patients with chronic obstructive pulmonary disease (i.e., emphysema, chronic bronchitis) depend on a lowered blood oxygen level to stimulate respiration. Because use of nitrous oxide with oxygen raises the oxygen saturation of the blood, this stimulus is removed and apnea may result. Nitrous oxide with oxygen may be appropriate for patients with mild to moderate disease, but if used for patients with severe conditions it should only be administered by an experienced practitioner (McCarthy, Pallasch, and Gates, 1989).

3. Chronic conditions or acute upper respiratory tract infectious conditions may pose one of several contraindications in inhalation sedation techniques. Blocked nasal passages (i.e, common cold, allergies) or chronic mouth breathing prevent effective use of this drug system. Also any infectious respiratory condition (i.e., common cold or cough, tuberculosis, infectious bronchitis) will contaminate the tubing and breathing apparatus. Although many newer units allow for regular sterilization of this part of the equipment, it still poses an infection control problem in many offices.

4. Several conditions that involve confined air spaces may be adversely affected by use of nitrous oxide. One characteristic of this anesthetic is that it diffuses into any air-containing body cavity, generally replacing nitrogen. Because nitrous oxide diffuses into an air space faster than nitrogen moves out, there is a temporary increase in either the size of the air space or the pressure in the space, depending on the rigidity of the walls. The middle ear is particularly affected by the pressure increase caused by this phenomenon. Nitrous oxide use may be contraindicated for patients with a history of middle ear or tympanic membrane problems or blockage of the eustachian tubes, even if caused by a head cold.

Along the same lines, sinus congestion or blockage, either acute or chronic, may subject a patient to more pressure and discomfort.

Gastrointestinal distention is another possibility. This may be a factor in patients who vomit when higher concentrations of nitrous oxide are administered. It may be contraindicated for a patient with a bowel obstruction. The degree to which this phenomenon will occur is influenced by the concentration of nitrous oxide, the duration of its use, and the vascularity of the air space. The first two of these are under the control of the clinician (Duncan and Moore, 1984).

5. Claustrophobic patients may find the confinement of the nasal hood to be unacceptable.

6. Patients with some types of personality disorders have a tenuous grasp on reality. Because the effect of conscious sedation is to let go of a focus on the present, this may not be a desirable adjunctive treatment. With some recovered drug abusers it may also be prudent to avoid the use of nitrous oxide. Careful patient evaluation and consultation are important.

7. Patients with compulsive personalities who do not like the feeling of "losing control" are more likely to perceive nitrous oxide with oxygen sedation as an unpleasant experience. The level of sedation may also be reduced as the patient resists the effects of the drug in an attempt to remain in control. Careful patient preparation or selection of another management technique are important for a satisfying appointment with these patients.

8. If a patient simply does not want nitrous oxide oxygen sedation, it should not be forced on him or her.

9. Pregnancy might be legitimately included in both the contraindicated and the indicated lists for nitrous oxide use. In general, it is desirable to avoid all unnecessary drugs during pregnancy, especially in the first trimester. In fact, avoidance of optional dental treatment may also be recommended, especially early and late in the pregnancy. However, if anxiety management or mild pain control are needed nitrous oxide with oxygen is "the safest and most highly recom-

mended" (Malamed, 1989). Nitrous oxide is not metabolized in the body, it has little or no effect on most organ systems, and is rapidly eliminated from the body once administration is discontinued. Nitrous oxide does cross the placental barrier and thus affects the fetus. Adequate oxygen levels must be maintained. Consultation with the patient's obstetrician would be prudent.

The question that must be answered in each case is, which has the most potential for harm: the nitrous oxide with oxygen, another drug that might be chosen in its place, the stress produced by providing the treatment without adequate pain and anxiety control, or postponing treatment until after the birth?

There is evidence that chronic exposure to nitrous oxide may result in a higher rate of spontaneous abortions and congenital deformities (American Dental Association, 1977, 1980; Corbett et al, 1973; Duncan and Moore, 1984). This does not appear to be true of occasional use by patients during treatment.

The clinician's discretion and consultation with the patient's physician may be necessary for any patient for whom there is a question about the appropriateness of nitrous oxide–oxygen sedation. In general, no procedure should be performed unless the office personnel would be able to support the patient should an emergency or life-threatening situation occur (DeMartina and Garber, 1979).

EQUIPMENT

Nitrous oxide and oxygen conscious sedation equipment is available as a portable or central system.

A portable unit is shown in Fig. 33-1. The small tanks of oxygen and nitrous oxide permit mobility of the unit throughout the office or clinic. If inhalation sedation is used often, frequent changing of the small tanks may create a problem. The "E" size cylinder of oxygen contains about 66 L, while the "E" size nitrous oxide cylinder contains 1590 L of compressed gas. These figures equate to a 2-hour duration for an oxygen cylinder (at a flow of 5 L per minute) and a more than 5-hour duration for a nitrous oxide cylinder at the same flow rate (American Dental Association, 1983).

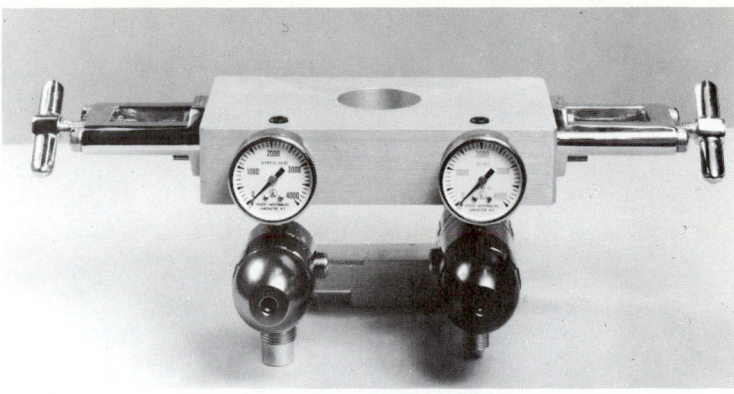

Fig. 33-2. Nitrous oxide and oxygen regulators that affix to portable analgesia machine. Pressure gauges indicate pressure of gas contained in cylinders.
(From Bennett CR: *Conscious sedation in dental practice,* ed 2, St Louis, 1978, CV Mosby. Courtesy Fraser Sweatman, Inc.)

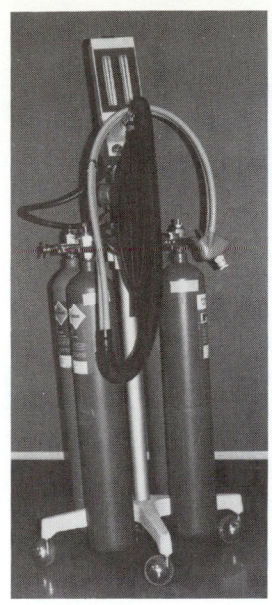

Fig. 33-1. Portable nitrous oxide and oxygen conscious sedation equipment.

Fig. 33-2 illustrates the regulators that attach to the portable unit tanks. These gauges indicate the pressure of the gas in the cylinder. Oxygen is supplied at a pressure of 2100 pounds per square inch (psi). As the oxygen is used, the pressure of the gas falls in direct proportion to this amount. Therefore if one half of the tank has been used, the regulator gauge will read 1050 psi.

Nitrous oxide is present as both a liquid and a gas and is supplied in cylinders at a pressure of 750 psi. The pressure remains the same in the tank until all the liquid is converted into gas. A nitrous oxide tank that is half empty will still read 750 psi; once all the liquid is converted, the pressure will drop quickly until the tank is empty. A tag should be placed on the tank to keep track of the nitrous oxide used, with the date a full tank was opened and the dates and lengths of subsequent appointments at which nitrous oxide was administered.

Central systems run from a bank of several large nitrous oxide and oxygen cylinders. These are called "H" and "G" tanks, respectively. With a central system, lines run to several wall hookups to which the flow meter and mask unit are attached (Fig. 33-3). In addition to showing the

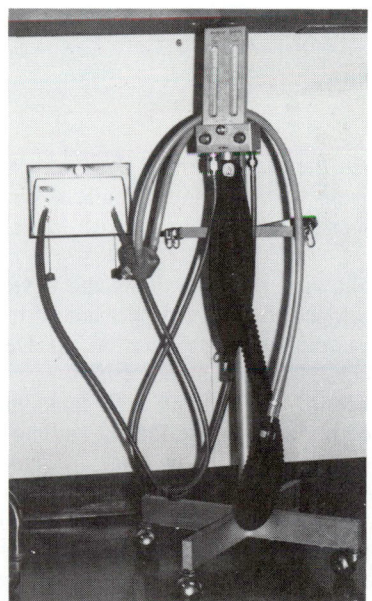

Fig. 33-3. Wall hookup for centralized nitrous oxide and oxygen conscious sedation system.

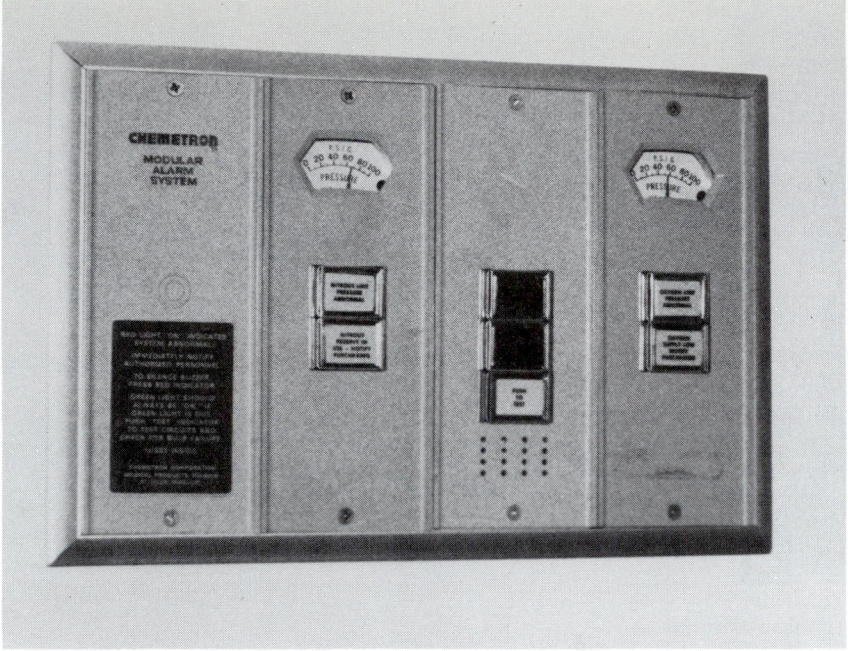

Fig. 33-4. Wall alarm system for centralized system.

pressure in the tanks, central systems usually include a wall- or desk-mounted alarm system that lights up or sounds if supplies are low (Fig. 33-4).

The following safety systems and devices have been developed to ensure proper use of inhalation sedation equipment (Bennett, 1978; DeMartina and Garber, 1979; Malamed, 1989):

- *Universal color coding.* The tanks and associated parts of the equipment (tubing, regulator gauge mount, flow controls) are colored *green* for oxygen and *blue* for nitrous oxide.
- *Pin index or diametric index system.* The connection for the tanks and hoses for nitrous oxide will not adapt to the oxygen hookups. This prevents a person from mistakenly interchanging the gas systems.
- *Minimum oxygen flow.* A preset flow of oxygen is provided at all times when the unit is on. This prevents the administration of pure nitrous oxide.
- *Fail-safe system.* If for some reason the oxygen supply runs below the minimum level, the nitrous oxide automatically shuts off and begins to whistle.

- *Flow meter.* This is a visual indicator of liters per minute flow of both nitrous oxide and oxygen. The flow control valve (dial or lever) is color coded and labeled for each gas (Fig. 33-5). Automatic flow meters are available in which the concentration of nitrous oxide is dialed. The machine adjusts to higher or lower concentrations automatically when the dial is changed.
- *Nonrebreathing system.* Expired gases are not recirculated.
- *Nasal hood and scavenging system.* Two types of nasal hood, the rubber or silicone device that fits over the patient's nose, are available. The traditional nasal hood usually has two tubes that deliver the fresh nitrous oxide and oxygen mixture from the analgesia machine to the mask. Exhaled gas are delivered directly into the dental operatory through a valve at the top of the nasal mask. This has the disadvantage of raising the nitrous oxide levels in the ambient air breathed by the dental personnel. Because of increased concern over chronic exposure, a scavenging system has been built into newer hoods.

- Scavenging nasal hoods are really a hood within a hood (Fig. 33-6 and Fig. 33-7). A fresh mixture of gas enters the internal hood from the tube(s) connected to the machine. When the patient exhales, the expired gases enter the second or outer mask and are drawn away through tubing by the high-speed evacuation system. A quick-connect coupling attaches the exhaust tube of the analgesia machine to the evacuation system. The evacuation system is usually turned on to a moderate level, depending on the volume of gas being delivered to the patient. The high-speed evacuation system should be vented outside the building, away from the windows and air intake vents.
- *Reservoir bag.* The reservoir bag is filled by fresh gas and is large enough to accommodate the volume of the patient's greatest inspiration.
- *Flush valve.* By activating this valve, the clinician is able to deliver 100% oxygen at a high flow rate very quickly. This also enables the machine to be used in manual resuscitation if a full face mask is used.

Attention to nitrous oxide and oxygen conscious sedation equipment is essential. The installation of such equipment should be completed by qualified professionals. After installation, the equipment must be maintained and checked regu-

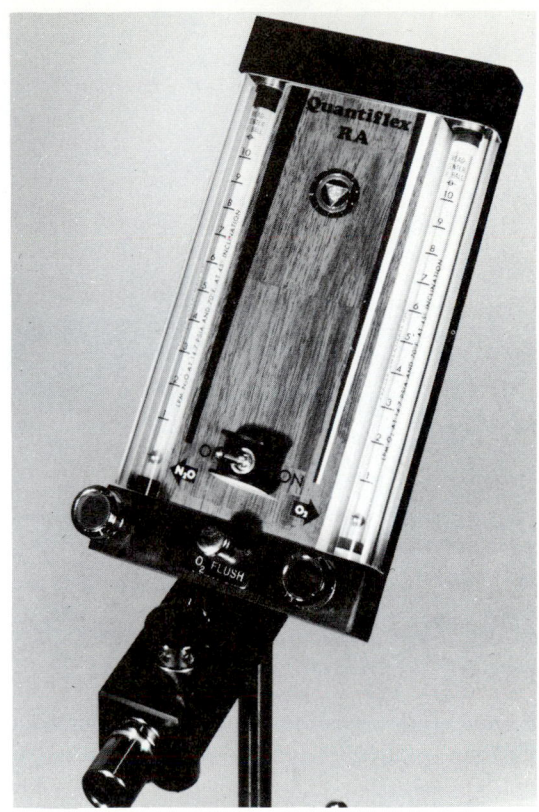

Fig. 33-5. Fraser Sweatman analgesia machine with dials to regulate gas flow.
(From Bennett CR: *Conscious sedation in dental practice,* ed 2, St Louis, 1978, CV Mosby. Courtesy Fraser Sweatman, Inc.)

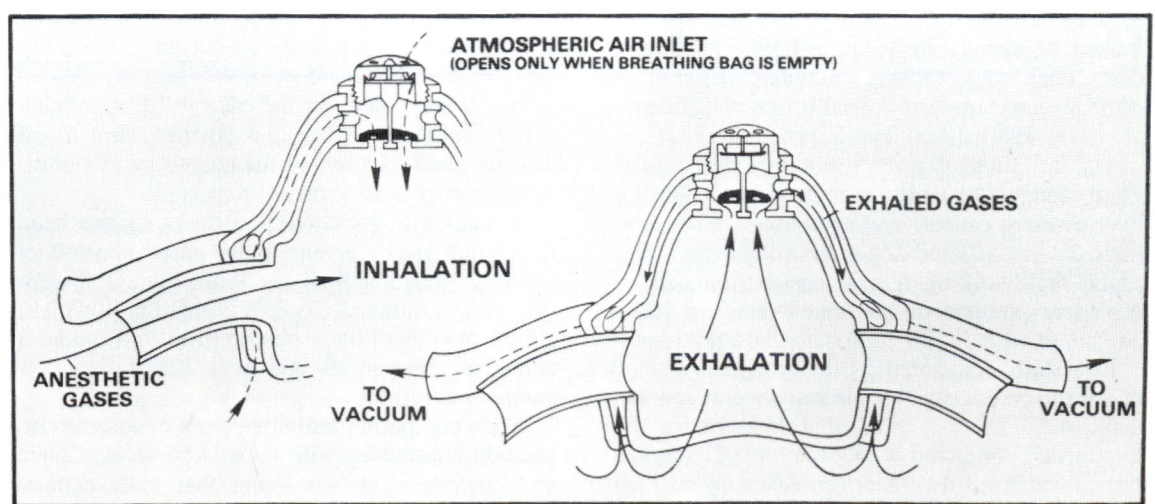

Fig. 33-6. Diagramatic cross-section of a scavenging nasal hood. Note the hood within a hood design.
(From Malamed S: *Sedation, a guide to patient management,* ed 2, St Louis, 1989, Mosby–Year Book.)

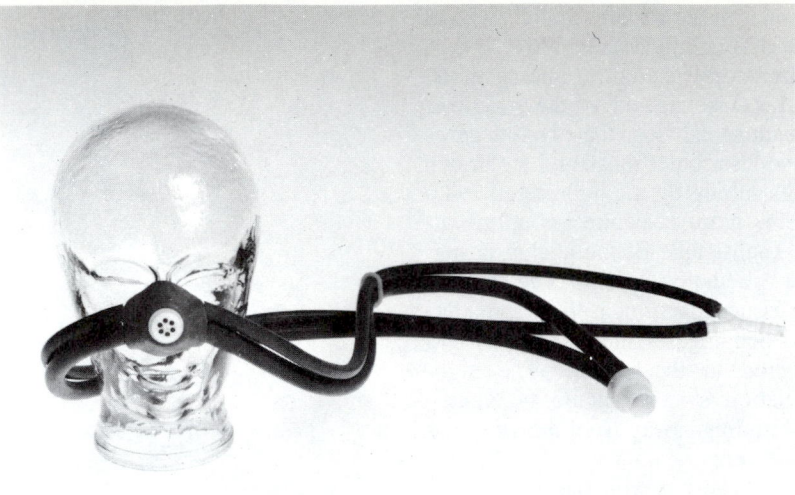

Fig. 33-7. Scavenging nasal mask. (From Bennett CR: *Conscious sedation in dental practice,* ed 2, St Louis, 1978, CV Mosby. Courtesy Narco McKesson.)

larly to ensure proper functioning. The equipment must not be altered in any way, and the manufacturer's guidelines for safe handling must be followed.

CONCERN ABOUT ENVIRONMENTAL CONTAMINATION

In the last several years there has been increased interest in the possible effects of chronic exposure to anesthetic gases. Although few studies have looked at nitrous oxide as a single agent, evidence does suggest that trace contamination of anesthetic gases may be a health hazard (Cohen et al, 1975, 1980; Jastak and Greenfield, 1977).

Major topics of study have included miscarriage, congenital malformation, reduced fertility, liver disease, cancer, and neurologic and psychologic disorders. Knill-Jones and colleagues (1972) found that working female anesthesiologists reported a spontaneous abortion rate of 18.2% as compared with 14.7% in nonanesthesiologists.

In a study sponsored by the American Society of Anesthesiologists, female respondents reported a rate of 1.25 congenital abnormalities per 100 live births, compared with a rate of 0.21 reported by women from the American Academy of Pediatrics. The rates of the wives of men responding in the two associations were 1.56 and 0.90, respectively (Cohen et al, 1974).

A recent retrospective study of female dental assistants concluded that occupational exposure to high levels of nitrous oxide may adversely affect the ability to become pregnant. Those exposed to 5 to 9 hours per week of unscavenged nitrous oxide were only 41% as likely to conceive in each menstrual cycles as unexposed women. Each hour of exposure to unscavenged $N20$ corresponded to a 6% reduction in probability of conception. For those working with nitrous oxide that had a functioning scavenging system, no decrease in fertility was detected (Rowland et al, 1992).

In a 20-year study of the cause of death among anesthesiologists, Bruce and others (1968) found that the rate of lymphoid malignancy was significantly higher than normally expected.

In studies of psychologic effects, it has been found that traces of anesthetic gases may affect memory, reaction time, or temperament. Swepston (1980) outlined a case presentation in which, after 3 months of daily misuse of nitrous oxide, a clinician experienced and was hospitalized for paranoid delusions.

When comparing individuals not exposed to inhalation anesthetics with those who were, Cohen and coworkers (1980) found that male dentists had a 1.7-fold increase in liver disease, a 1.2-fold increase in kidney disease, and a 1.9-fold increase in neurologic disease.

The morphologic characteristics of the bone marrow of 21 dentists who habitually used nitrous oxide was investigated. The study provided direct evidence that exposure to nitrous oxide may cause depression of vitamin B_{12} activity, resulting in measurable changes in bone marrow secondary to impaired synthesis of deoxyribonucleic acid (Sweeney, 1985). Studies conducted with laboratory rats subjected to prolonged nitrous oxide exposure show impaired bone marrow function, damaged spermatogenic cells with decreased testicular function, and increased fetal death in pregnant animals (Corbett et al, 1973; Kripke et al, 1976, 1977).

When humans abuse nitrous oxide for periods ranging from 3 months to 5 years, neurologic symptoms appear. These include paresthesia of the extremities, loss of dexterity and balance, muscle weakness with gait ataxia, impotence, incontinence, and an electric shock sensation traveling upward from the feet to the neck after flexion of the neck. In most cases these symptoms are reversible after discontinuation of the drug abuse (Giovannitti, 1984).

Swenson (1976) studied the mean concentration of halothane and nitrous oxide, measured 15 inches in front of the nasal mask. In a nonrebreathing system in which partial recirculation of exhaust occurs, 1955 parts per million (ppm) of nitrous oxide were found. In a system without recirculation of exhaust, 172 ppm of nitrous oxide were found. Scavenging devices and well-ventilated operatories help reduce the amount of exposure to nitrous oxide for dental personnel.

Investigators will continue to define the hazards and determine the safety standards for nitrous oxide use in dental practice. The National Institute for Occupational Safety and Health (Control of Occupational Exposure to N_2O in the Dental Operatory, 1977) has recommended 50 parts per million as the maximum exposure to nitrous oxide waste gas in the breathing zone of the worker. In a study with pediatric patients, Badger and others (1982) noted that higher than recommended levels persist in operatories in spite of scavenging equipment. Christiansen and others (1985) found that there are significant differences in the effectiveness of scavenging devices, and that neither rubber dam placement nor the patient's talking significantly affected levels of scavenged nitrous oxide. This suggests that better methods for eliminating waste gases and monitoring trace gases in

the dental environment must be developed. Current guidelines for nitrous oxide scavenging and waste gas monitoring equipment are published by the American Dental Association Council on Dental Materials and Devices (American Dental Association, 1990).

To reduce nitrous oxide levels in the dental operatory, the following recommendations can be implemented:

1. Use an approved nitrous oxide scavenging device.
2. Fit the nasal mask to the patient as well as possible.
3. Minimize patient conversation and mouth breathing.
4. Vent the exhaled gases and the patient suction machine to a safe disposal site outside the building.
5. Use a fan to direct exhaled nitrous oxide away from the breathing zone of the operating personnel.
6. Improve circulation in the operatory by opening a window or using a nonrecycling air conditioning system.
7. Use a monitoring system; air sampling equipment is available and relatively inexpensive; a badge can be worn on the lapel to detect nitrous oxide levels in the operator's breathing zone.
8. Maintain equipment; inspect the connectors and test for leakage at frequent regular intervals.
9. Set conservative limits on the duration of nitrous oxide exposure for each patient.
10. Shut off and secure the equipment after each day's use.

There is no convincing evidence that trace concentrations found in dental operatories have any acute effect on the mental or motor functions of the dental personnel while the patient is sedated and treatment is underway. The threshold for psychomotor impairment is in the range of 10% to 20% concentration (Moore, 1983). This cannot be obtained through leakage in the breathing zone if the proper administration guidelines and safety practices are followed. The concern for dental professionals is from chronic low-dose exposure over time.

Concerning professional liability, employers should be aware of the potential dangers of working with nitrous oxide and must inform their employees of the harmful effects. Besides providing information to employees, employers must show that they have followed the recommended and reasonable steps to eliminate danger in the workplace to both employees and patients (Troyer, 1983). If safe conditions do not exist, employees cannot be penalized for activities to preserve and pursue health and safety. If an employer refuses to acknowledge or correct potential nitrous oxide hazards, a formal complaint should be made to the regional Occupational Safety and Health Act office (Rogo, 1986).

ADMINISTRATION

Once the patient is identified as a candidate for nitrous oxide and oxygen conscious sedation, preparation for the experience is in order.

Often an initial experience is helpful for the patient. This is done at a time when no dentistry is to be performed. The patient is familiarized with the sedation equipment and experiences the relaxation effects. In this way the patient looks forward to a comfortable dental appointment. This step may in itself create an important change in the patient's attitude.

Dworkin and others (1984) found that providing information to people receiving a drug for pain relief yields higher sensation thresholds, pain thresholds, and tolerance of pain. This indicates that influencing thought processes in combination with giving analgesia can increase the depth of the analgesia.

Occasionally the patient may have heard about nitrous oxide, or "laughing gas," and may be afraid he or she will do something embarrassing. The clinician should explain that this will not occur. The level of sedation will produce pleasant relaxation, but the patient will be aware of and in control of all actions. The patient is able to control the level of sedation by breathing deeply through the nose (increase effect) or by breathing through the mouth (decrease effect). These maneuvers affect the external concentration, thereby increasing or reducing alveolar concentration. Since mouth breathing will also affect the waste of gas in the dental operatory it is desirable to keep it at a minimum. Watch for mouth breathing or check with the patient periodically about his or her comfort level and reduce the nitrous oxide concentration as needed.

The clinician maintains a professional attitude. The patient's comments are listened to, and positive reassurance is offered. This encourages con-

fidence in the clinician. During sedation, it will be important that the patient trust the clinician's suggestions.

In general, conversation should be kept to a minimum during nitrous oxide–oxygen sedation. Patient conversation, like mouth breathing, lightens the level of sedation and raises operatory nitrous oxide levels. Operator conversation forces the patient to stay focused on the dental setting and the procedures being performed, which, for many patients, counteracts the effect of the nitrous oxide that helps them drift into other more pleasant thoughts.

Other suggestions before the dental appointment include attention to diet and dress. The patient does not need to restrict diet altogether before nitrous oxide and oxygen conscious sedation. A light meal 1 hour or so before the appointment is recommended. For patient comfort, neither an empty stomach nor a full stomach is suggested.

Comfortable, loose clothing is ideal. If desired, clothing at the neck can be loosened. If the patient is wearing contact lenses, they should be removed before inhalation sedation. Gas leaks around the bridge of the nose may produce drying of the eyes with potential irritation to the patient (Malamed, 1989).

Technique

Following are the steps for administering nitrous oxide and oxygen conscious sedation:

1. Review the patient's medical history. Take vital signs.
2. Discuss the procedure with the patient.
3. Prepare the sedation equipment. Use a nasal mask that has been sterilized, a personal mask (inexpensive, often scented masks are available that may be used multiple times but only for one patient), or a disposable paper nose cone that fits inside a conventionally disinfected mask. Check to ensure that the supply of oxygen and nitrous oxide is sufficient to complete the procedure. Attach the nitrous oxide scavenger hose to the high-speed evacuation system. Once the patient is seated in the operatory, show him or her the sedation equipment. Never force sedation on a patient. The patient should agree to try the experience. Reaffirm the comfortable feelings the patient will experience.
4. Turn the oxygen on to a flow of 6 to 8 L

per minute. This flow will be maintained throughout the procedure. The patient can hold the mask and feel the flow of oxygen. If the system does not include a scavenging mask, check the exhalation valve to be sure it is set at *open* and the air dilution valve to be sure it is set at *closed*.

5. Fill the reservoir bag by activating the flush valve. The patient seats the nasal mask himself or herself and adjusts it to a comfortable position. A gauze square placed under the edges of the mask on sensitive areas of the face may be helpful. This pads the mask against the face and closes any leaks around the mask if a perfect fit is not possible. It is especially important to have the oxygen flowing and the reservoir bag filled so that the patient may take a comfortable first breath of pure oxygen.

6. Allow the patient a few minutes to breathe the oxygen. Have the patient practice breathing through the mouth to show how he or she has control of the inhalation technique.

7. Inform the patient that he or she may smell a sweet odor as the nitrous oxide is started at 0.5 to 1.0 L per minute. Reassure the patient that the procedure is going well. Ask the patient to take a few deep breaths while relaxing the arms, hands, and legs. Suggest that he or she rest back in the dental chair for a comfortable and enjoyable dental appointment. The patient may begin to show signs of less tension: relaxed facial expression, relaxed hands, and less movement of the eyes around the room. A patient who feels uncomfortable usually will say so or look distressed.

If a patient comments that nothing has changed, increase the nitrous oxide level another ½ or 1 L per minute. Suggest the reactions that the patient will generally feel at that particular nitrous oxide concentration, such as, "You may be feeling warm or notice tingling in your hands and feet. Everyone responds a bit differently, but a feeling of floating comfortably or relaxing into the chair is common. These feelings are part of the relaxation technique."

Do not be too specific about what sensations the patient will feel. There is a great

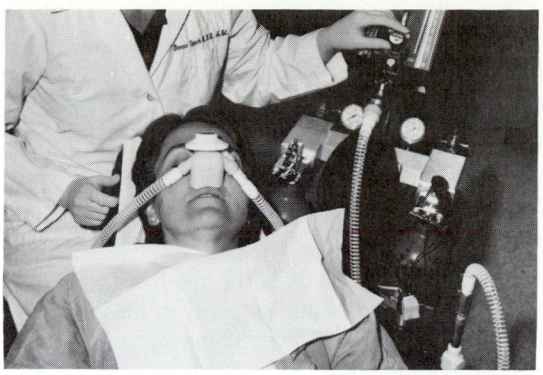

Fig. 33-8. Monitor patient at all times for consciousness, comfort, and cooperation.

deal of individual variation, and some patients will worry if the sensations they experience are not the ones you described.

Once sedation has started, the patient should never be left alone. The operatory and supplies should be fully arranged before the sedation procedure is begun. Constant monitoring must be maintained (Fig. 33-8). One can arrange instruments, write notes, or begin examination procedures while observing the patient. Extremely close monitoring of the patient's every feeling may be anxiety producing if the patient senses he or she is not feeling what has been suggested.

Careful observation of the patient will determine whether the nitrous oxide should be increased to the next step. When the patient is comfortable, he or she may sigh, readjust the body to a more relaxed position, become quiet, and smile slightly. Voices and other operatory noises may be exaggerated or muffled. The middle ear is an air space that is sensitive to pressure changes during nitrous oxide inhalation. Patients may report transient auditory changes (Duncan and Moore, 1984). Speak in a quiet voice, at a slower rate, and in a calming manner. Limit extraneous conversations with a third person in the operatory to create a more calm and quiet environment.

Minnis (1979) has noted that a person under nitrous oxide and oxygen conscious sedation is in a very suggestible state. The effect of the clinician's verbal and nonverbal communication is crucial; how things are said and done is very important. Experimental and control studies confirm the powerful role of mental processes in mediating pain experience (Dworkin, 1983). Be supportive and reinforce how well treatment is going. Comment on how comfortable the patient appears. Ask the patient to let you know if he or she feels otherwise. The softness and sincerity of the clinician's voice may be one of the best instruments for relaxing and reassuring the patient. Weinstein and others (1986) found that the behavior of the clinician is a major influence on the fear-related behaviors of children, even when nitrous oxide is used. Certain verbal directions intended to distract the child's attention from the procedure at hand appear to be especially effective.

The comfort range for each patient varies with the individual. The optimum concentration of nitrous oxide will not generally exceed 35%. Use the formula mentioned earlier to compute the percentage.

8. Once a comfortable level of sedation has been achieved, a local anesthetic can be administered. (Some operators choose to reduce the nitrous oxide concentration after the injection.)

9. Proceed with the appointment plan.

10. Monitor the patient constantly for consciousness, comfort, and cooperation. If the patient is becoming very lethargic, closing his or her mouth often and tending towards sleep, reduce the percentage of nitrous oxide 1/2 to 1 L per minute to lighten the level of sedation. Restlessness may also be a sign that the concentration of nitrous oxide is too high and the patient is no longer comfortable.

11. Near the end of the appointment, reduce the nitrous oxide concentration. The patient will usually maintain satisfactory relaxation if simple procedures are performed, such as polishing, flossing, carving amalgam, or checking occlusion. Place sensible limits on the duration of sedation in the individual case.

About 5 minutes before the end of the appointment, turn the nitrous oxide off completely but leave the oxygen on.

12. Allow the patient to breathe 6 to 8 L of pure oxygen per minute for at least 5 minutes. This step is necessary to avoid diffusion hypoxia, which may precipitate syncope.

Because nitrous oxide diffuses more rapidly than oxygen, the concentration of nitrous oxide in the bloodstream begins to diffuse into the alveolar spaces rapidly when the nitrous oxide is shut off. A temporary state of hypoxia (lack of oxygen) may occur if adequate oxygen is unable to diffuse from the lungs into the bloodstream during the phase of exhaling the nitrous oxide concentration. A lack of adequate oxygen or an increase in carbon dioxide levels in the bloodstream may produce syncope or other adverse cardiac and respiratory effects. When the patient is given oxygen for several minutes after termination of the nitrous oxide flow, diffusion occurs gradually and a hypoxic state is avoided.

Generally, under short-term conditions such as those used in outpatient dental treatment, the patient should be fully recovered after a 5-minute exposure to 100% oxygen at the conclusion of the appointment. However, further benefit is apparently gained from a somewhat longer recuperation before the patient engages in any activity requiring exacting psychomotor skills (McKercher et al, 1980).

13. Remove the nasal mask.

14. Slowly bring the patient back to an upright position. Following the 5 minutes of breathing 100% oxygen, breathing room air for 10 to 15 minutes before dismissal is appropriate. In most cases this much time is necessary to complete appointment procedures. The patient remains in the chair until all sedation effects are gone. The patient should feel normal and be pleased with the dental appointment.

15. Disconnect the portable equipment and prepare the mask for sterilization or other appropriate treatment. Shut the entire system off after each administration if sedation is used infrequently or at the end of the day if the system is used frequently.

Because of the rapid euphoric effects nitrous oxide is capable of creating, there is potential for abuse of this medication. In fact, one or two deaths occur each year because of misuse of nitrous oxide (Swepston, 1980). Lock portable equipment and secure the central system to discourage any such unfortunate occurrences.

16. Record the experience in the patient's chart. Note vital signs before nitrous oxide administration, concentrations of nitrous oxide and oxygen administered, and length of time for inhalation sedation. Also record the length of time the patient received oxygen after the procedure and include any specific postoperative instructions given to the patient. A summary of the patient's reactions will be helpful for future reference.

Conditions during sedation

If a patient becomes uncomfortable or anxious and tries to remove the nasal mask, gently prevent this, as it predisposes the patient to diffusion hypoxia. Immediately flush the system with 100% oxygen while at the same time verbally reassuring the patient that you understand what is occurring and realize that he or she feels uncomfortable (DeMartina and Garber, 1979). Ask the patient to breathe deeply as the pure oxygen is delivered. Within a few moments the patient will begin to feel better. Reassure the patient that everything is fine. He or she is safe and will be feeling better with each breath of oxygen.

When the patient achieves a relaxed state again, complete the dental procedure. Do not let the patient have a bad experience with sedation. At the end of the appointment compliment the patient on his or her cooperation and the successful dental appointment.

An occasional patient may become nauseated and vomit. This usually does not happen when sedation is maintained at a nitrous oxide concentration below 50%. If the patient felt well and ate lightly before the dental appointment, this situation probably will not occur.

If vomiting does occur, help the patient to a position that will prevent aspiration. Hold the head over the cuspidor or use suction to assist evacuation (Swepston, 1980). Again, maintain the mask and flush the system so that the patient is breathing 100% oxygen. Supply the patient with a cool, wet towel to clean up. Refresh the operatory as quickly as possible. The patient probably will be embarrassed. Handle the situation promptly, comfort the patient, and finish the dental procedure. Prevention is possible by maintaining comfort at a lower level of nitrous oxide and observing the early signs of patient distress.

Nausea and vomiting are the most common, unpleasant side effects of nitrous oxide and oxygen sedation (Duncan and Moore, 1984). Instances of dysphoria, claustrophobia, apprehension, and hallucination have also been described. Several cases of sexual phenomena have been reported that involved complaints to law enforcement agencies and required hearings before state dental boards. Usually these incidents have occurred when nitrous oxide was administered in concentrations greater than 50% and when the patient was sedated without an assistant in the room (Jastak et al, 1984). An additional person should be present in the operatory when a patient of the opposite gender is treated. In general, this seems to be a wise safety policy in case of emergency.

Conditions following sedation

In general, an episode of nitrous oxide sedation has no residual effects. The medication is inhaled, it influences the central nervous system while it circulates in the bloodstream, and it is exhaled unchanged. Depending on the nature of the patient and the length of sedation, the patient may retain a relaxed feeling. Often the dental procedure is itself tiring, and the patient may feel a bit fatigued. The age of the patient does not seem to be a significant factor in determining the response to nitrous oxide sedation (Norton, 1984; O'Reilly et al, 1983) but the length of time the patient breathed 100% oxygen does seem to affect recovery for some (Malamed, 1989).

Normal functioning or driving is not contraindicated specifically because of nitrous oxide and oxygen conscious sedation, but the dentist or hygienist may recommend precautions according to the procedures performed or the patient's health status.

Patients whose occupations require operating heavy machinery, using highly skilled motor coordination, or making critical decisions may need to use discretion in returning to these functions. Conventional methods of assessing recovery from nitrous oxide may be inadequate. Somatosensory evoked potentials testing may be useful in accurately describing recovery for specific tasks. Further studies are indicated, but early evidence shows recovery may take longer than 25 to 30 minutes in some instances (Herwig et al, 1984). In general, full recovery occurs within 15 minutes, with the patient feeling fine and able to perform as normal.

CONCLUSION

Nitrous oxide and oxygen conscious sedation is a safe and effective means of providing comfortable dentistry to patients who require minor pain control and who are apprehensive about dental treatment. As the anxious patient gains confidence in the clinician and experiences several successful appointments, he or she may be weaned from nitrous oxide. One may find that increasing positive suggestion and decreasing nitrous oxide concentration produce the desired sedation. The patient is usually pleased with the realization of this new behavior. Seeing such a patient approach and accept dental care without fear is possibly the greatest benefit of nitrous oxide and oxygen conscious sedation.

ACTIVITIES

1. Given patient profiles, discuss the indication for nitrous oxide and oxygen conscious sedation.
2. Watch a demonstration of administration technique. Observe the experience of a clinic patient or classmate with nitrous oxide and oxygen conscious sedation.
3. Simulate administration of or actually administer nitrous oxide and oxygen conscious sedation to a laboratory partner. If actually administering sedation, share the variety of responses that were noted in the group.
4. Administer nitrous oxide and oxygen conscious sedation to an appropriate clinic patient.
5. Investigate the statutes in your state regarding the legality of dental hygienists administering, monitoring, or assisting in the administration of nitrous oxide with oxygen conscious sedation.

REVIEW QUESTIONS

1. Nitrous oxide and oxygen sedation is a form of conscious sedation. What does this mean? (Include a definition of "conscious" in your answer.)
2. Consider each of the following pairs. Check the characteristic that best describes nitrous oxide.
   a. Organic inhalation agent, odorless, and flammable.
   a'. Inorganic inhalation agent, sweet smelling, and nonflammable.
   b. Has a high blood gas solubility as compared with oxygen.
   b'. Has a low blood gas solubility compared with oxygen.
   c. Eliminated unchanged from the lungs.
   c'. Eliminated from the lungs as nitrogen.
   d. An extremely potent anesthetic when administered with oxygen.
   d'. A mildly potent anesthetic when administered with oxygen.
   e. Affects the body's physiologic reaction to pain perception.
   e'. Affects the person's psychologic reaction to pain perception.
3. Explain why nitrous oxide and oxygen conscious sedation is contraindicated for persons with the following conditions:
   a. Emphysema.
   b. Upper respiratory tract infection.
4. Calculate the percentage of nitrous oxide being delivered to a patient at the flow of 4 L per minute of nitrous oxide and 6 L per minute of oxygen. How does this percentage relate to the level recommended for optimal sedation? If this patient were having a tooth extracted, would local anesthesia be indicated?
5. Identify three signs that indicate that the inhaled concentration of nitrous oxide is too great.

REFERENCES

American Dental Association: *Dentist's desk reference: materials, instruments, and equipment,* ed 2, Chicago, 1983, The Association.

American Dental Association Council on Dental Materials and Devices: Expansion of the acceptable program, nitrous oxide scavenging equipment and nitrous oxide trace gas monitoring equipment, *JADA* 95:791, 1977.

American Dental Association Council on Dental Materials, Instruments, and Equipment: Council position on nitrous oxide scavenging and monitoring devices, *JADA* 101:62, 1980.

American Dental Association Monograph Series on Dental Materials and Therapeutics: *Safety and infection control in the dental office,* ed 1, Chicago, 1990, The Association.

American Dental Hygienists' Association: Personal communication, 1992.

Badger G et al: Nitrous oxide waste gas in the pediatric operatory, *JADA* 104:480, 1982.

Bennett CR: *Conscious sedation in dental practice,* ed 2, St Louis, 1978, CV Mosby.

Bruce DL et al: Causes of death among anesthesiologists: a 20 year survey, *Anesthesiology* 29:565, 1968.

Chapman WR et al: The analgesic effects of low concentration nitrous oxide compared in man with morphine sulfate, *J Clin Invest* 22:871, 1943.

Christiansen JR et al: Measurement of scavenged nitrous oxide in the dental operatory, *Pediatr Dent* 7:192, 1985.

Cohen EN et al: Occupational disease among operating room personnel: a national study, *Anesthesiology* 41:321, 1974.

Cohen EN et al: A survey of anesthetic health hazards among dentists, *JADA* 90:1291, 1975.

Cohen EN et al: Occupational disease in dentistry and chronic exposure to trace anesthetic gases, *JADA* 101:21, 1980.

Control of occupational exposure to N_2O in the dental operatory, HEW pub no (NIOSH) 77-171. Cincinnati, 1977, US Department of Health, Education and Welfare, Public Health Service Center for Disease Control, National Institute for Occupational Safety and Health.

Corbett TH et al: Effects of low concentrations of nitrous oxide in rat pregnancy, *Anesthesiology* 39:299, 1973.

DeMartina BK, Garber JG: Analgesia in dental practice, *Contin Dent Educ* 2:5, 1979.

Duncan GH, Moore PA: Nitrous oxide and the dental patient: a review of adverse reactions, *JADA* 108:213, 1984.

Dworkin SF et al: Analgesic effects of nitrous oxide with controlled painful stimuli, *JADA* 107:581, 1983.

Dworkin SF et al: Cognitive modification of pain: information in combination with nitrous oxide, *Pain* 19:339, 1984.

Fordham KC: *Analgesia (medicated air)*. Booklet accepted for course credit by the Academy of General Dentistry, 1974, Radnor, Pa.

Giovannitti JA: Nitrous oxide and oral premedication, *Anesth Prog* 31(2):56, 1984.

Hamburg HL: Establishing a standard technique for nitrous oxide/oxygen sedation, *Dent Surv* 56(3):28, 1980.

Heft MW et al: Nitrous oxide analgesia: a psychological evaluation using verbal descriptor scaling, *J Dent Res* 63(2):129, 1984.

Herwig LD et al: Time course of recovery following nitrous oxide administration, *Anesth Prog* 31(3):133, 1984.

Jastak JT, Greenfield W: Trace contamination of anesthetic gases: a brief review, *JADA* 95:758, 1977.

Jastak JT: Nitrous oxide in dental practice, *Int Anesthesiol Clin* 27:92, 1989.

Jastak JT et al: Nitrous oxide and sexual phenomena, *Dent Anaesth Sedat* 13(2):56, 1984.

Knill-Jones RP et al: Controlled survey of women anesthetists in the United Kingdom, *Lancet* 1:1326, 1972.

Kripke BJ et al: Testicular reaction to prolonged exposure to nitrous oxide, *Anesthesiology* 44:104, 1976.

Kripke BJ et al: Hematological reaction to prolonged exposure to nitrous oxide, *Anesthesiology* 47:342, 1977.

Langa H: *Relative analgesia in dental practice, inhalation analgesia and sedation with nitrous oxide*, ed 2, Philadelphia, 1976, WB Saunders.

Malamed SF: *Sedation: a guide to patient management*, ed 2, St Louis, 1989, CV Mosby.

McCarthy FM: *Essentials of safe dentistry for the medically compromised patient*, Philadelphia, 1989, WB Saunders.

McCarthy FM, Pallasch TJ, Gates R: Documenting safe treatment of the medical risk patient, *JADA* 119:383, 1989.

McKercher TC et al: Recovery and enhancement of reflex reaction time after nitrous oxide analgesia, *JADA* 101:785, 1980.

Minnis R: Psychological effects of conscious sedation, *Anesth Prog* 26:150, 1979.

Moore PA: Psychomotor impairment due to nitrous oxide exposure, *Anesth Prog* 30:72, 1983.

Norton JC et al: The effect of nitrous oxide and age on psychological and psychomotor performance, *Anesth Prog* 31:64, 1984.

O'Reilly JE et al: The effects of nitrous oxide in the healthy elderly: nitrous oxide elimination and alveolar carbon dioxide, *Anesth Prog* 30:187, 1983.

Roberts GJ et al: Physiological changes during relative analgesia—a clinical study, *J Dent* 10:55, 1982.

Rogo EJ et al: Nitrous oxide: an occupational hazard for dental professionals, *Dent Hyg* 60:508, 1985.

Rowland AS et al: Reduced fertility among women employed as dental assistants exposed to high levels of nitrous oxide, *N Engl J Med* 327:993, 1992.

Sweeney B et al: Toxicity of bone marrow in dentists exposed to nitrous oxide, *Br Med J* 291:567, 1985.

Swenson RD: 1976. Scavenging of dental anesthetic gases, *J Oral Surg* 34:207, 1976.

Swepston B: Dental phobia becomes euphoria: advantages of nitrous oxide, parts 1 and 2, *Dent Pract* 1(5):60, 1(6):42, 1980.

Third Pain Control Conference: *American Dental Association, American Society of Anesthesiology, American Association of Dental Schools, guidelines for teaching the comprehensive control of pain and anxiety in dentistry*, Chicago, 1971.

Thompson PL: Nitrous oxide as an analgesic in acute myocardial infarction, *JAMA* 235:924, 1976.

Troyer GT: Liability: important issue regarding nitrous oxide exposure, *Dent Stud* 62:16, 1983.

Weinstein P et al: The use of nitrous oxide in the treatment of children: results of a controlled study, *JADA* 112(3):325, 1986.

SUGGESTED READINGS

Allen WA: Nitrous oxide in the surgery: pollution and scavenging. Some clinical experiences, *Br Dent J* 159:222, 1985.

Brown JP: Efficiency of three nitrous oxide relative analgesia scavenging systems, *Dent Anaesth Sedat* 13:5, 1984.

Bruce DL et al: Trace anesthetic effects on perceptual, cognitive and motor skills, *Anesthesiology* 40:453, 1974.

Dionne RA: The pharmacological basis of pain control in dental practice: N_2O_2, *Compend Contin Educ Dent* 2:271, 1981.

Dworkin SF et al: Cognitive reversal of expected nitrous oxide analgesia for acute pain, *Anesth Analg* 62:1073, 1983.

Dworkin SF et al: Psychological preparation influences nitrous oxide analgesia, replication of laboratory findings in a clinical setting, *Oral Surg Oral Med Oral Pathol* 61:108, 1986.

Hammond NI: Nitrous oxide and children's perception of pain, *Pediatr Dent* 6(4):238, 1984.

Kaufman E et al: Nitrous oxide analgesia in selected dental patients, *Anesth Prog* 29:78, 1982.

Kucey SP: Nitrous oxide contamination in dentistry, *Ont Dent* 61(7):21, 1984.

Littner MM et al: Occupational hazards in the dental office and their control. IV. Measures for controlling contamination of anesthetic gas, nitrous oxide, *Quintessence Int* 14:461, 1983.

Riklin BM: Nitrous oxide—oxygen sedation for the geriatric patient, *J Am Soc Geriatr Dent* 13:8, 1978.

Ship JA: A survey of nitrous oxide levels in dental offices, *Arch Environ Health* 42:3010, 1987.

Sweeney B: Nitrous oxide: panacea or poison? *SAAD Dig* 6:82, 1985.

Wald C: Nitrous oxide—are there any real contraindications? *Quintessence Int* 14:213, 1983.

Yagiela JA et al: Disinfection of nitrous oxide inhalation equipment, *JADA* 98:191, 1979.

34 RESTORATIVE PROCEDURES

Thomas G. Berry
Eric Spohn
Wendy Halowski

The dental hygienist will be able to

1. Classification and nomenclature of cavity preparation
   a. Identify the walls, cavosurfaces, line angles, and point angles of Class I, II, III, IV, and V cavity preparations.
2. Isolation of the teeth
   a. Explain the advantages, disadvantages, and rationale of rubber dam isolation.
   b. List the armamentarium needed to place and remove a rubber dam.
   c. Given a specific tooth, identify the clamps that can be used.
   d. Explain the procedure in terms understood by a patient.
   e. Place and remove a rubber dam.
   f. Evaluate a placed rubber dam to determine if it is clinically acceptable.
   g. Explain the importance of removing all fragments of the rubber dam.
3. Bases and liners
   a. Define bases and liners.
   b. Explain the purposes of bases and/or liners under amalgam and composite resin restorations.
   c. Describe the rationale and contraindications for use and the clinical situations that require a specific base or liner.
   d. Place bases and liners in cavity preparations for amalgam and composite resin restorations.
4. Principles and general procedures for amalgam placement in Class V and Class I amalgam restorations
   a. List the ingredients of dental amalgam and the purpose of each.
   b. Discuss the indications for placement of an amalgam restoration.
   c. Discuss and follow accepted mercury hygiene precautions for both office personnel and patients.
   d. Explain the general procedure for placing an amalgam restoration.
   e. List and discuss the criteria for the placement of a successful class I, class II, and class V amalgam restoration—both process and product.
   f. Place and carve a Class V and a Class I amalgam restoration on typodonts or extracted teeth.
   g. After laboratory proficiency has been achieved, successfully place amalgam as dictated by the patient's needs.
5. Matrix for the conservative Class II amalgam restoration
   a. Describe the functions of a matrix band, retainer, and wedge.
   b. Select correct matrix retainer, band, and wedge for a given clinical situation.
   c. Assemble matrix band and retainer.
   d. Place assembled retainer, matrix band, and wedge on prepared tooth on a typodont.
   e. Evaluate the placed retainer, matrix band, and wedge according to criteria provided.
6. Restoration of the conservative Class II amalgam preparation
   a. Place, condense, carve, and smooth amalgam in a conservative class II cavity preparation.

   b. Remove Tofflemire retainer and matrix band using criteria provided.
   c. Evaluate and adjust occlusal contacts on the restoration.
   d. Evaluate the surface, anatomic form, marginal integrity, occlusal contacts, and proximal contours and contact using criteria provided.
7. Recontouring and finishing amalgam restorations
   a. Explain the rationale for recontouring and finishing.
   b. Differentiate between and describe the indications and contraindications for recontouring and finishing.
   c. Identify the armamentarium necessary for amalgam recontouring and finishing.
   d. Explain how overhang removal is a part of the recontouring procedure and how to use hand instruments to achieve it.
   e. Recontour and finish an amalgam restoration.
   f. Evaluate amalgam restorations to determine if they are acceptable according to the process and product criteria.
8. Properties of composite resin, acid-etching enamel: the Class V and Class III composite resin restoration
   a. Explain the basic formulation of resin and its filler particles, including the purposes of each.
   b. Discuss the indications for a composite resin restoration.
   c. Discuss the basic rationale for acid conditioning of enamel, the procedure involved, and the precautions necessary.
9. Rationale for dentin bonding and the procedure
   a. Describe the difference between light-activated and chemically activated composite resins; list the advantages of each.
   b. Explain the general procedure for placing a composite resin.
   c. List and discuss the criteria for a successful Class III and Class V restoration—both process and product.
   d. Place and contour a Class III and a Class V composite resin restoration on a typodont or extracted tooth.
   e. After laboratory proficiency has been achieved, place a composite resin as dictated by the patient's needs.

Though dental hygiene care focuses on prevention with an emphasis on preventive periodontics, it also involves the prevention and treatment of dental caries. Some licensing jurisdictions have provisions for hygienists to place and carve restorations (see Table 1-1), and hygienists in those states often practice a full range of care that encompasses periodontal and restorative care. In other regions, hygienists will recontour amalgams and correct defects. In all parts of the country, hygienists must properly identify and chart restorations (see Chapter 11) and talk intelligently with patients and dentists about restorative care. Therefore a knowledge of restorative care is an important component of competent clinical practice. This chapter explains the terminology and procedures needed for achieving competence.

CLASSIFICATION AND NOMENCLATURE OF CAVITY PREPARATIONS

The pattern of carious destruction has many variations, and each preparation is therefore unique (see Chapter 11, Fig. 11-6). However, the basic principles of cavity design produce a similarity of cavity outline within each class of preparation.

The following basic components are common to all classes of cavity preparations:

Wall. A vertical or horizontal surface within the cavity preparation named according to closest external tooth surface (e.g., facial, mesial, and lingual walls), for the structure it approximates (e.g., pulpal wall), or for its relationship to long axis of tooth (e.g., axial wall).

Cavosurface. The uncut tooth tissue adjacent to cavity preparation.

Line angle. Line formed along junction of two walls or of one wall and the cavosurface (referred to as cavosurface margin) and named according to walls and surfaces involved.

Point angle. A point formed by the junction of three walls within a cavity preparation and named according to the walls involved.

Class I cavity preparations

A class I preparation on a molar is used to illustrate the derivation of the nomenclature (Fig. 34-1).

Walls. A Class I molar preparation normally has curving walls along the facial and lingual sides that blend with the mesial and distal walls. These vertical walls end at a horizontal wall, called the pulpal wall. The preparation is illustrated as a "box" to aid in learning the nomenclature (Fig. 34-2).

Line angles. The three sets of line angles in the occlusal Class I preparation are named according to the walls involved (Figs. 34-3, 34-4, and 34-5).

Rule number 1: When developing the name of a line angle or a point angle, drop the "al" and substitute "o" at the end of all words in the name except the last one (e.g., line angle formed by the facial wall intersecting with pulpal wall is the faciopulpal line angle or pulpofacial line angle). The remaining line angles formed by the pulpal wall are shown in Fig. 34-3. These line angles are not actually straight but follow the outline form of the preparation. The line angles formed by the intersection of one vertical wall with another are illustrated in Fig. 34-4. In the actual cavity preparation, these are not sharp corners but curves. The names represent hypothetical places along the curves. Fig. 34-5 illustrates the four line angles formed by the intersection of the vertical walls with the cavosurface.

Rule number 2: When cavosurface is one of the words used in developing a term, place it last (e.g., the intersection of the facial wall with the cavosurface is the faciocavosurface line angle). The other three cavosurface line angles are named in a similar manner.

Point angles. The four internal point angles of a Class I occlusal preparation are illustrated in Fig. 34-6. The name of each is derived by combining the names of the involved walls using Rule number 1.

Class II cavity preparations

The Class II cavity preparation removes the proximal surface (Fig. 34-7). The occlusal portion is prepared like a Class I preparation but the marginal ridge is involved to allow access to the

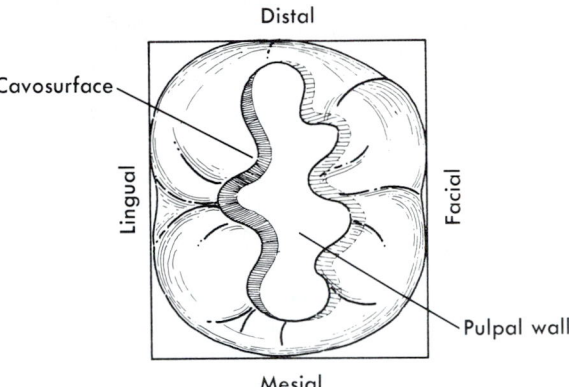

Fig. 34-1. Outline of a Class I cavity preparation. The outer surfaces of tooth are designated mesial, lingual, distal, and facial. The wall at the bottom of the cavity is the pulpal wall. The unprepared external surface of the tooth adjacent to the preparation is the cavosurface.

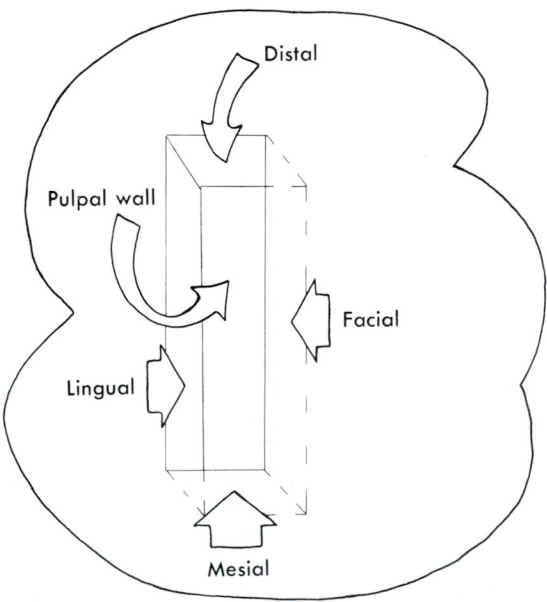

Fig. 34-2. Compare with Fig. 34-1. Preparation is a box with four walls and a bottom. The walls of the preparation are named for the external surfaces to which they are adjacent; the bottom is named pulpal wall because of its proximity to the pulp.

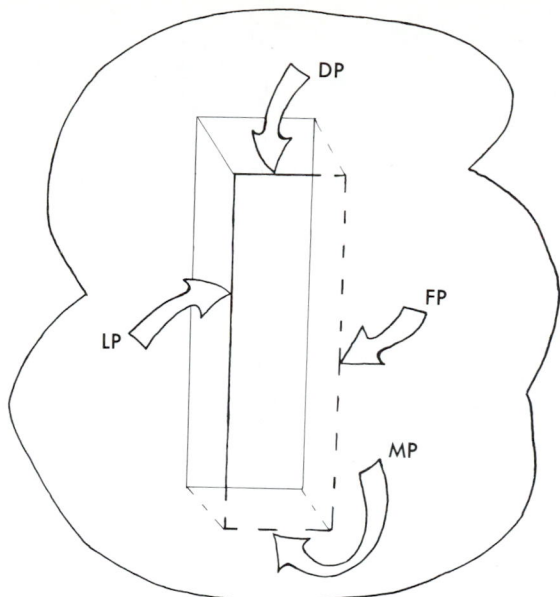

Fig. 34-3. The four line angles formed at the intersections of the vertical walls with the pulpal wall: the mesiopulpal *(MP)*, linguopulpal *(LP)*, distopulpal *(DP)*, and faciopulpal *(FP)* line angles.

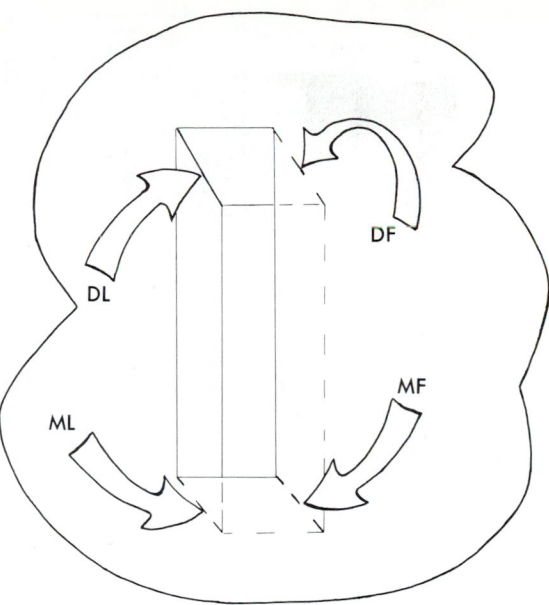

Fig. 34-4. The four line angles formed where the vertical walls intersect one another: the mesiolingual *(ML)*, distolingual *(DL)*, distofacial *(DF)*, and mesiofacial *(MF)* line angles.

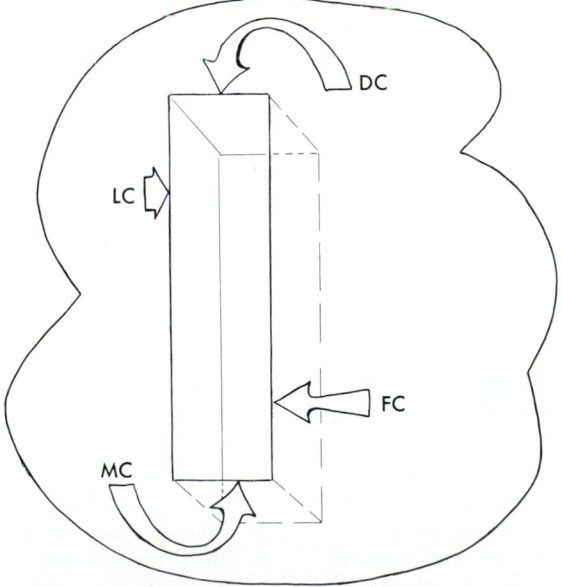

Fig. 34-5. The four line angles formed where the vertical walls intersect the uncut tooth surface (cavosurface): the mesial *(MC)*, lingual *(LC)*, distal *(DC)*, and facial *(FC)* cavosurface line angles.

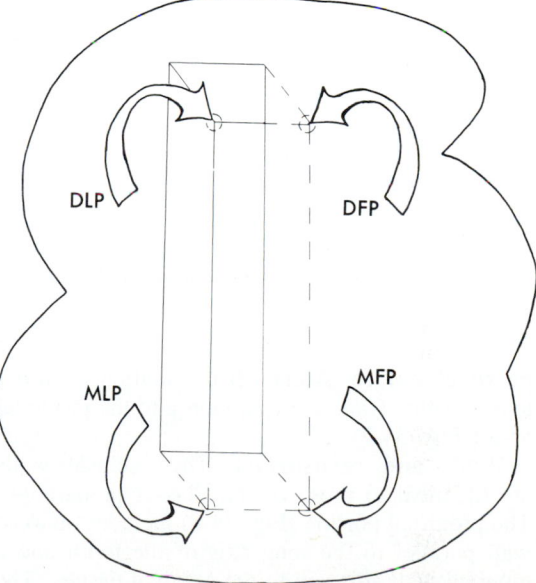

Fig. 34-6. The four point angles formed at the intersection of three internal walls. For example, the intersection of the three walls in the lower left is the mesiolinguopulpal *(MLP)* point angle.

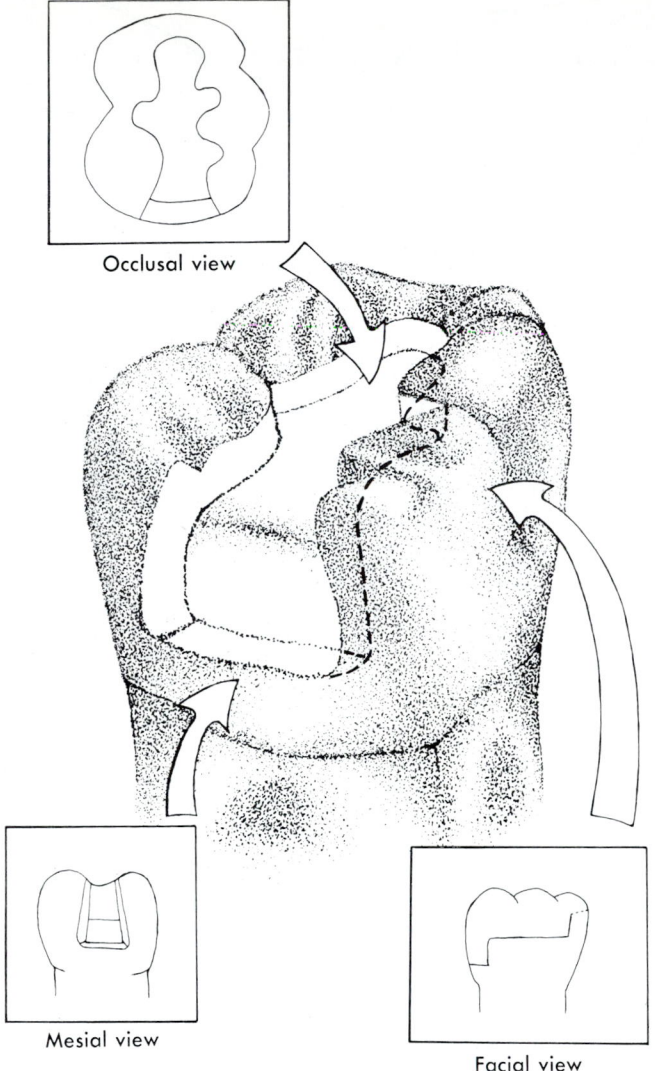

Occlusal view

Mesial view

Facial view

Fig. 34-7. Class II mesioocclusal cavity preparation on tooth No. 19. Compare with the occlusal view in Fig. 34-1.

proximal surface. A class II preparation is an extension of the Class I preparation into the proximal area (Fig. 34-7).

Walls and cavosurface. The occlusal walls are identical to those of the Class I preparation. The proximal portion (Fig. 34-8) includes an axial wall parallel to the long axis of the tooth and a gingival wall adjacent to the gingival tissues. The lingual and facial walls of the proximal portion are termed the *linguoproximal wall* and the *facioproximal wall*, respectively.

Line angles. In the proximal portion the internal and external line angles are:

Internal line angles (Fig. 34-9)

1. Axiopulpal
2. Axiogingival
3. Axiolinguoproximal
4. Axiofacioproximal
5. Gingivolinguoproximal
6. Gingivofacioproximal

External line angles (Fig. 34-10)

1. Linguoproximal cavosurface
2. Facioproximal cavosurface
3. Gingival cavosurface

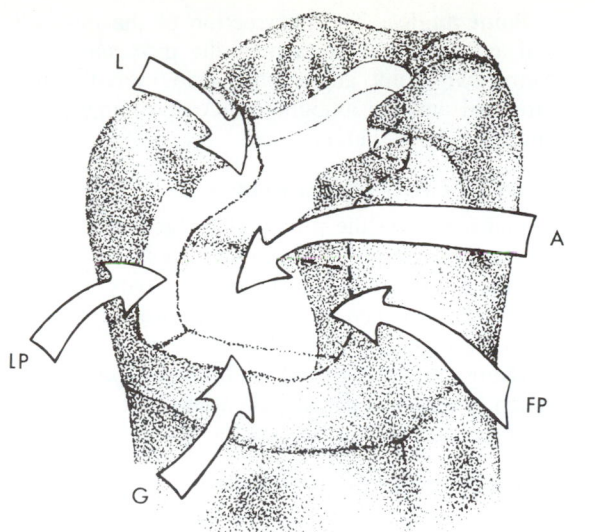

Fig. 34-8. The walls of the proximal portion of this preparation are the gingival *(G)*, linguoproximal *(LP)*, axial *(A)*, and facioproximal *(FP)* walls.

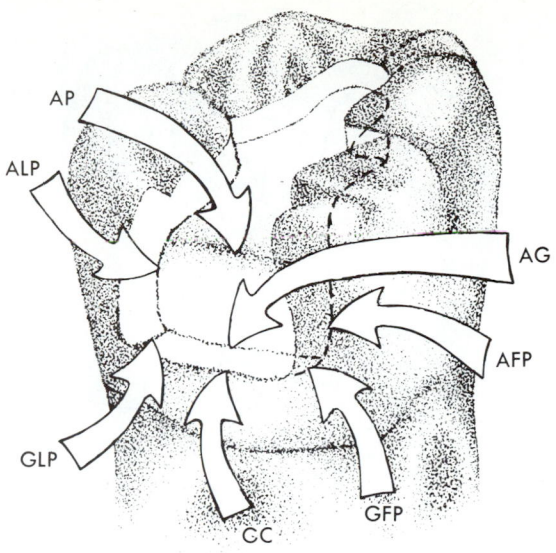

Fig. 34-9. The line angles of the proximal portion of a Class II mesioocclusal preparation: the gingivolinguoproximal *(GLP)*, axiolinguoproximal *(ALP)*, axiopulpal *(AP)* axiogingival *(AG)*, axiofacioproximal *(AFP)*, and gingivofacioproximal *(GFP)* line angles.

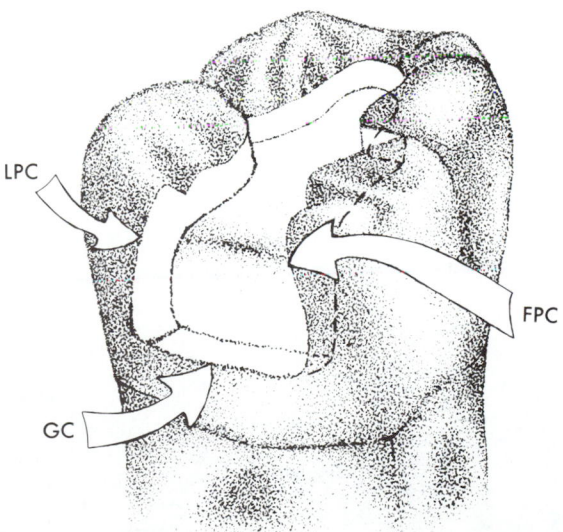

Fig. 34-10. The cavosurface line angles of the proximal portion of the class II preparation: the gingival *(GC)*, linguoproximal *(LPC)*, and facioproximal *(FPC)* cavosurface line angles.

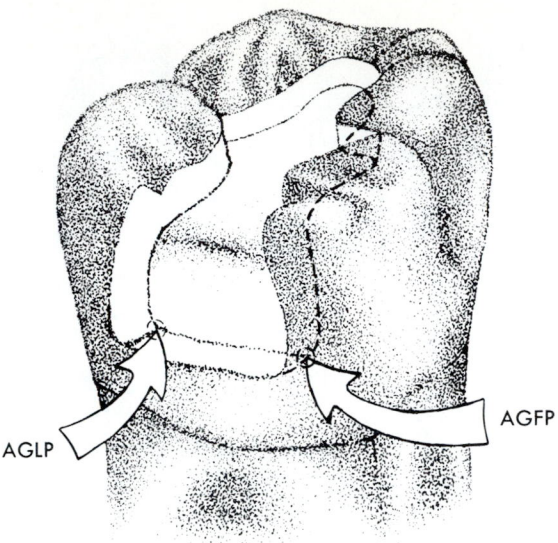

Fig. 34-11. The internal point angles of the mesioproximal portion of the Class II mesio-occlusal preparation: the axiogingivolinguoproximal *(AGLP)* and axiogingivofacioproximal *(AGFP)* point angles.

Point angles. The intersection of the gingival and axial walls with each of the proximal walls forms two point angles: the axiogingivolinguoproximal and the axiogingivofacioproximal point angles (Fig. 34-11).

Class III cavity preparations

Dental caries on the proximal surface of anterior teeth may be removed by either a facial or lingual approach. Fig. 34-12 illustrates the cavity outlines resulting from each approach. The walls resulting from the preparations are also shown.

Using the rules and definitions previously stated, the line angles and point angles for each of the preparations can be identified.

Class IV cavity preparations

An illustration is included for one form of a class IV restoration to develop the nomenclature for this preparation. Fig. 34-13 is a proximal view of the class IV preparation.

Class V cavity preparations

This preparation is similar to a class I preparation except for its location in the gingival one third of the facial or lingual surface. It also may be thought of as a "box" with four sides and a bottom (Fig. 34-14). On an anterior tooth, the occlusal wall is called the incisal wall.

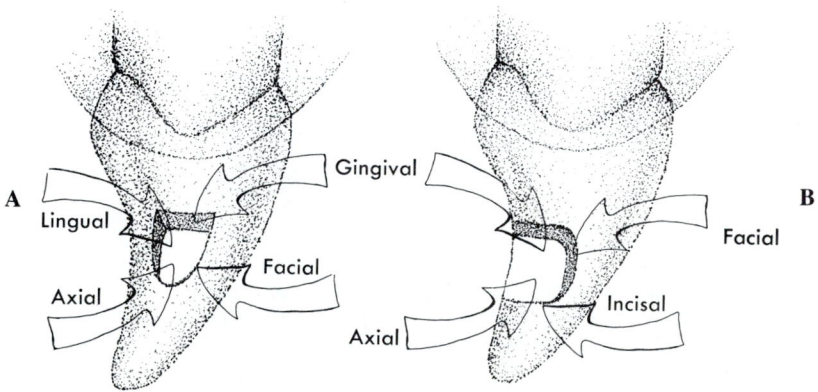

Fig. 34-12. Walls of the Class III cavity preparation: **A,** labial access; **B,** lingual-slot access.

ISOLATION OF THE TEETH

A proper operating field is necessary to perform operative procedures with optimal results. Isolating the field prevents moisture contamination, retracts and controls the soft tissues, protects the patient against aspiration of instruments and materials, and provides optimal visibility of the operating site. This should be accomplished without interfering with the operator's visual or mechanical access to the operating site, injuring soft or hard tissues, or causing discomfort.

The type of isolation required depends on the duration of the procedure and the degree of dryness necessary. For some procedures, cotton roll isolation can be used in conjunction with a saliva ejector and high-volume oral evacuation system. Cotton roll holders can be used in the mandibular arch. Absorbent triangles, placed over the parotid duct, can be used in conjunction with cotton rolls for increased moisture control. Cotton roll isolation offers ease and speed of application. However, there is risk of contamination of the operating field, limited retraction of soft tissues, and no protection against the patient aspirating debris or objects.

The rubber dam meets the criteria listed for isolation. Disadvantages are that the clamp can irritate the gingiva, placement of the dam can be time consuming for the beginning clinician, and some patients are sensitive to the rubber dam. Overall, however, the advantages of using a rubber dam outweigh the disadvantages.

Armamentarium

The necessary armamentarium for rubber dam placement is illustrated in Fig. 34-15. There are several types of rubber dam holders (Fig. 34-16). One of the most commonly used is the Young's frame. It is a metal U-shaped frame, which holds the dam away from the patient's face. The Woodbury holder is an elastic band that fits around the back of the patient's head and is attached to the sides of the dam with three clips on each side. It provides excellent lip and cheek retraction.

The rubber dam clamp (Fig. 34-17) anchors the dam to the tooth. Therefore, this tooth is referred to as the anchor tooth. Clamps may be winged or wingless. The jaws of the winged clamp have small projections that allow the clamp to be mounted on the dam before it is placed on the teeth. The chart in Fig. 34-18 will be helpful in determining which clamps are most likely to fit particular teeth.

The dam material is available in several

Text continued on page 726.

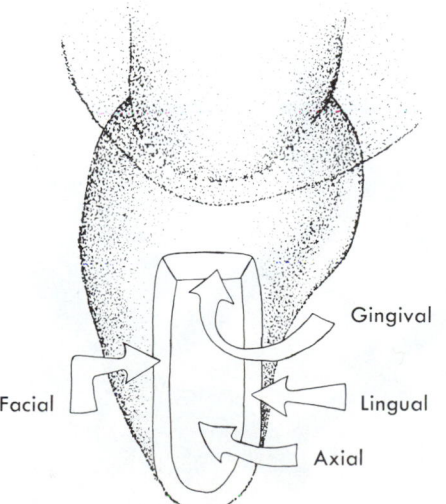

Fig. 34-13. Proximal view of the walls of the Class IV cavity preparation.

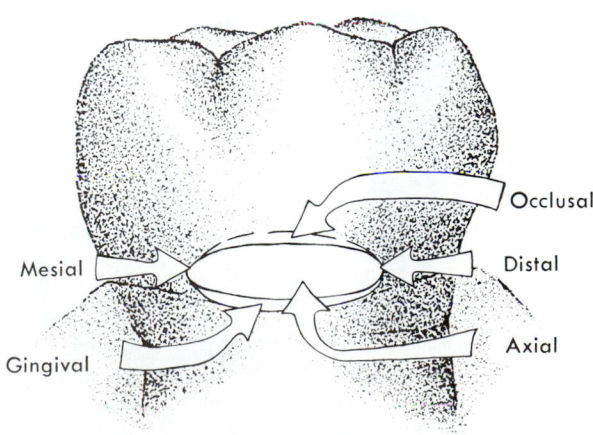

Fig. 34-14. Walls of the class V cavity preparation on a posterior tooth.

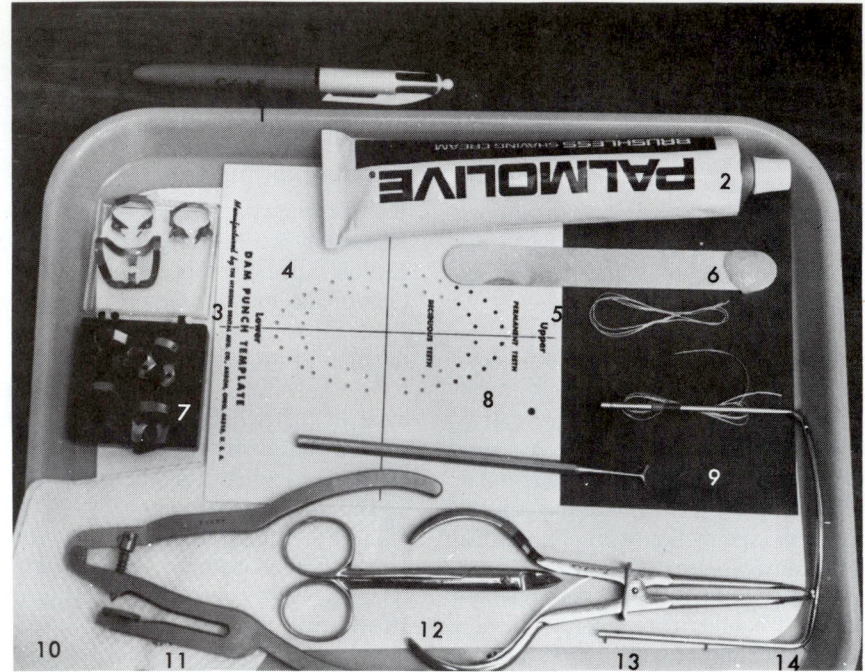

Fig. 34-15. Tray setup for rubber dam application includes: *1*, ball-point pen; *2*, lubricant for rubber dam; *3*, gingival retractors; *4*, rubber dam template; *5*, waxed dental floss; *6*, lubricant on tongue blade; *7*, assorted rubber dam clamps; *8*, T-ball burnisher; *9*, rubber dam material; *10*, rubber dam napkin; *11*, rubber dam punch; *12*, scissors; *13*, rubber dam clamp forceps; *14*, rubber dam holder.

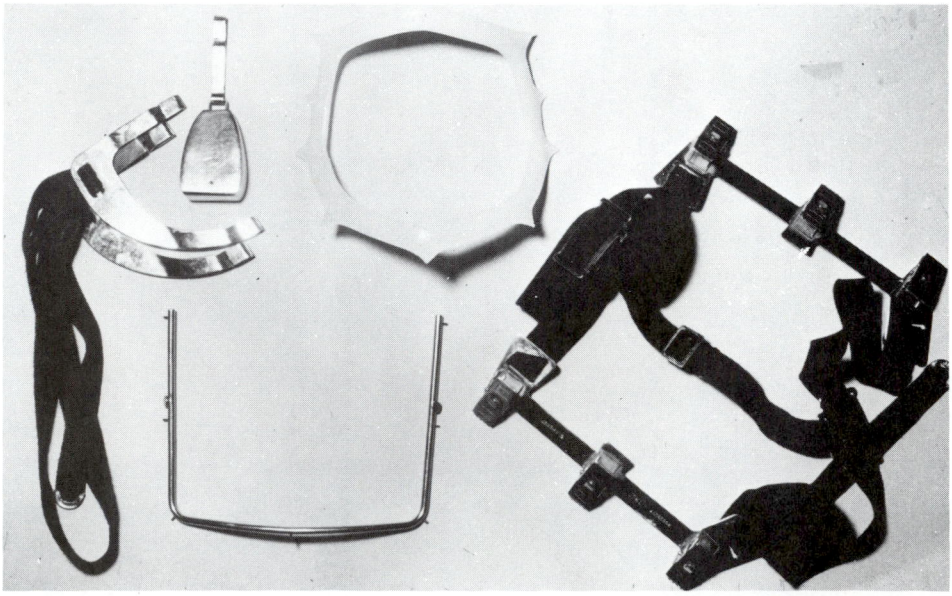

Fig. 34-16. Some examples of rubber dam holders. *Clockwise from upper left:* Wizard holder, weight, plastic frame, Woodbury holder, and Young's frame.
(From Gilmore WH et al: *Operative dentistry,* ed 4, St Louis, 1982, CV Mosby.)

Bow
Forceps hole
A
Jaws
Bow
Forceps hole
B
Wings
Jaws

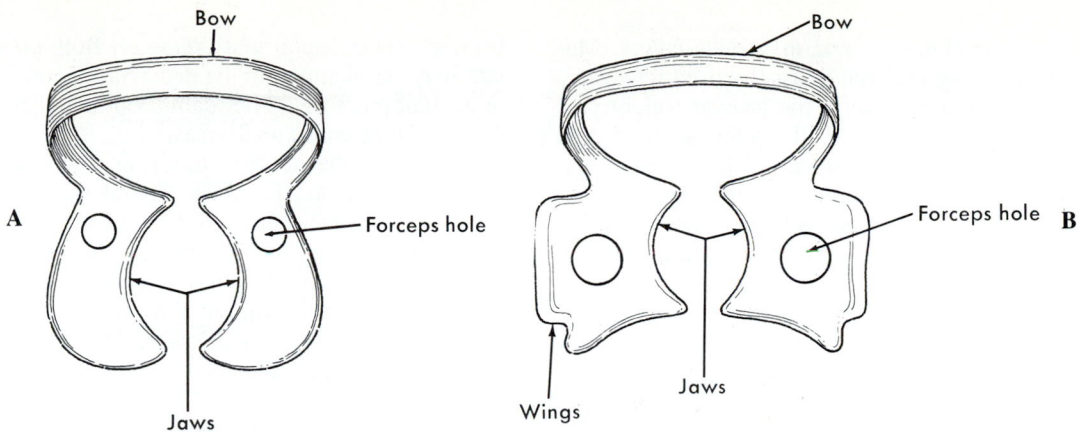

Fig. 34-17. Rubber dam clamps: **A,** wingless; **B**, winged.

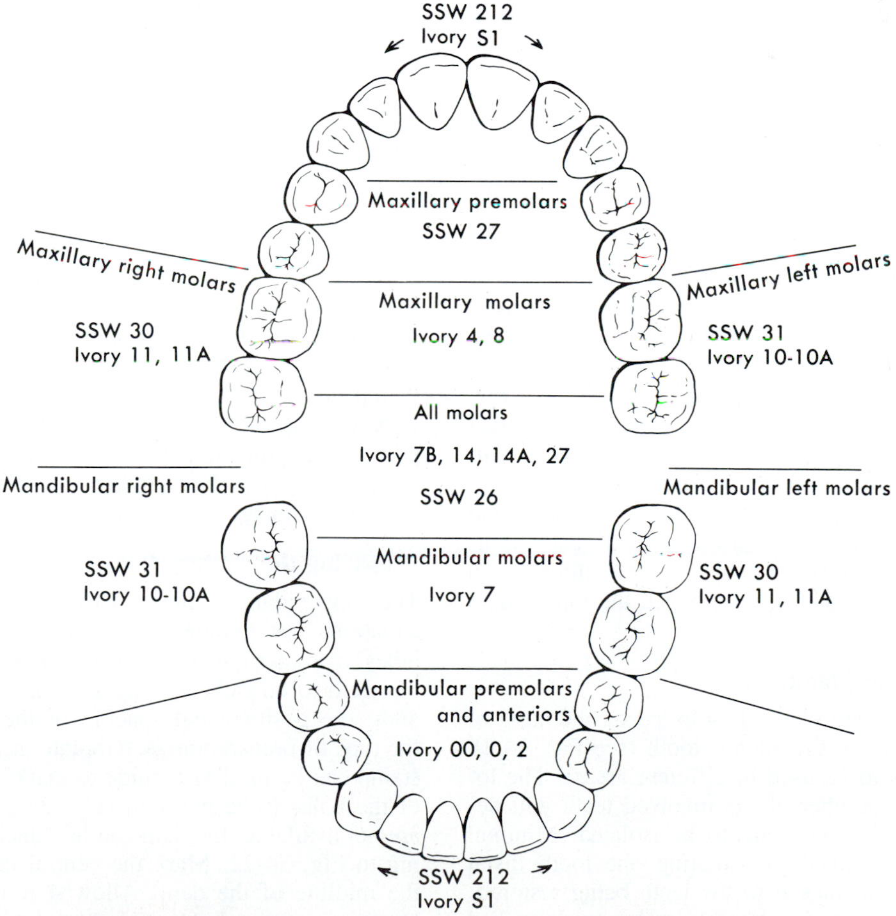

SSW 212
Ivory S1
Maxillary premolars
SSW 27
Maxillary right molars
Maxillary left molars
Maxillary molars
Ivory 4, 8
SSW 30
Ivory 11, 11A
SSW 31
Ivory 10-10A
All molars
Ivory 7B, 14, 14A, 27
SSW 26
Mandibular right molars
Mandibular left molars
Mandibular molars
Ivory 7
SSW 31
Ivory 10-10A
SSW 30
Ivory 11, 11A
Mandibular premolars
and anteriors
Ivory 00, 0, 2
SSW 212
Ivory S1

Gingival retraction
SSW 212 Ivory S3
30 4(maxillary molars)
31 16 (molars)

Deciduous molars
SSW 1A Ivory 8A
2A

Fig. 34-18. Chart of suggested clamps to be used in various areas of mouth.
(From Howard WW, Moller RC: *Atlas of operative dentistry,* ed 3, St Louis, 1981, CV Mosby.)

weights (thicknesses) and in various colors. Medium or heavy material is usually used for restorative procedures because the heavier weight provides better retraction of the gingivae, lips, and cheeks and does not tear easily. Lightweight material is used more often during endodontic procedures because only one tooth is isolated, tearing is less of a problem, and the lighter material is easier to manipulate.

Preparing the patient

If the patient has never experienced placement of a rubber dam, explain the benefits, such as eliminating debris in the mouth and preventing contamination of the restoration site. Briefly explain the procedure so that the patient knows what to expect. As the patient will not be able to talk with the dam in place, suggest signals to be used in case the patient needs to communicate.

Examining the mouth

Examine the site where the dam is to be placed. Floss the teeth to determine if there will be difficulty in passing the dam between any of the teeth. If floss cannot be passed through the contact, determine why. Calculus, restoration overhangs, or rough proximal surfaces should be removed. Teeth with very tight contacts may need to be wedged apart before dam placement. If needed, place a wooden wedge into the involved proximal space for 1 to 2 minutes, then check the contact again with dental floss. Check the patient's occlusion to determine if any unusual anatomy may interfere with the restoration. Note the shape and size of the arch, position of the teeth, edentulous spaces, and fixed prostheses. This information will be needed to correctly punch the rubber dam holes.

Selecting the clamp

The rubber dam clamp is selected on the basis of the anatomy of the anchor tooth (see Fig. 34-18 for clamps to be used in different areas). The location and number of the involved teeth will determine which teeth are to be isolated. Minimal access is obtained by isolating one tooth distal and two teeth mesial to the teeth being restored. Clamp the most distal tooth in the quadrant and extend isolation to the opposite lateral incisor to achieve greater access; maximum retraction of the lips, cheeks, and tongue; and increased number of teeth available for a finger rest. If only the anterior teeth are involved, isolate the first premolar from the contralateral first premolar. Both premolars may be clamped or ligated with dental floss or a small piece of rubber dam used to wedge the dam in the interproximal areas.

Determine the anchor tooth and select the appropriate clamp. Tie floss around the bow of the clamp to permit retrieval if the clamp slips off the tooth. Place the clamp in the forceps. Squeeze the handles together to open the jaws of the clamp. With the tips of the forceps upward, the locking ring will slide towards the handle of the forceps holding the jaws of the clamp open (Fig. 34-19).

Position the clamp over the tooth. Rotate it lingually to seat the lingual jaw first because vision is more restricted in this area. Rotate the clamp facially to seat the facial jaw. Be certain that the jaws do not drag across the tooth, scarring the cementum. Squeeze the handles of the forceps to release the locking ring and allow the jaws of the clamp to engage the tooth. When properly placed, all four prongs should contact the tooth cervical to the height of contour (Fig. 34-20). The clamp should be stable when rocked gently from side to side with light finger pressure and should not impinge on the soft tissue. If these criteria are not met, reposition the clamp or, if needed, select another clamp. If the clamp rotates or slides off the tooth or rests on the papilla, it is too big. If the clamp does not fit over the height of contour or pops off the tooth, it is too small. Because the prongs are pointed and can cut the gingiva or gouge the root surface, forceps should always be used to disengage or reposition the clamp.

Preparing the rubber dam

The rubber dam is punched to suit each clinical situation. The number, size, and location of the holes are determined by the location and size of the teeth to be isolated, the shape and size of the arch, the position and spacing of the teeth, and the type of preparation. A template or rubber dam stamp can be used as a guide to mark the location of the holes to be punched (Fig. 34-21). If these are not available, the dam can be punched according to Fig. 34-22. Mark the central incisors near the midline of the dam. Allow 4 mm of rubber between anterior holes and 5 mm of rubber between posterior holes. Mark the holes for Class V restorations 1 mm to the facial side. Allow an additional 1 mm of rubber between adjacent teeth for the gingival retraction needed for access to the Class V lesion.

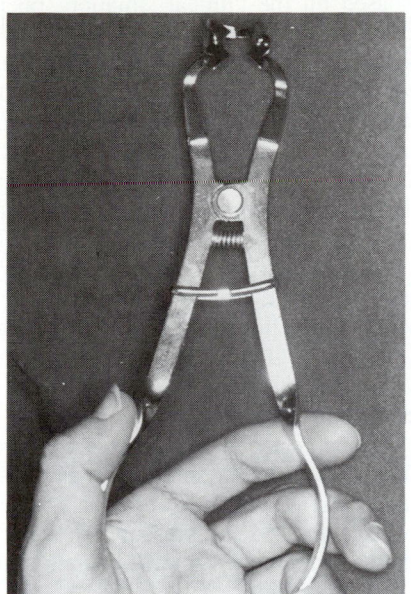

Fig. 34-19. Engage locking ring by pointing forceps upward, then squeeze and release.

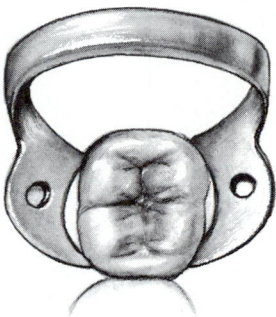

Fig. 34-20. All four prongs of clamp should be in contact with tooth.
(From Howard WW, Moller RC: *Atlas of operative dentistry*, ed 3, St Louis, 1981, CV Mosby.)

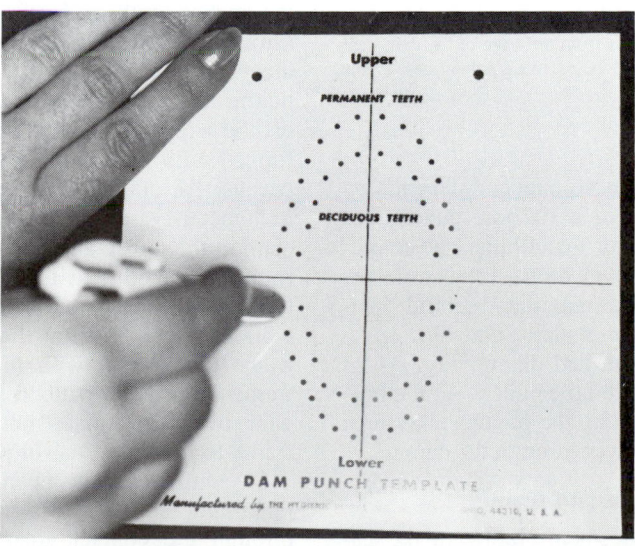

Fig. 34-21. Rubber dam template and a ball-point pen are used to mark the dam.

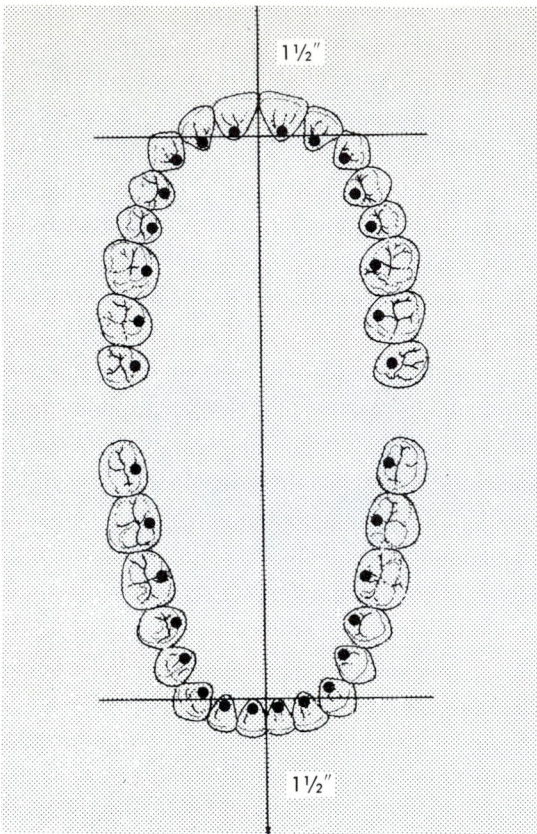

1½"

Fig. 34-22. For the average-sized arch, punch the central incisors approximately 1 1/2 inches from the edge of the dam near the midline. Punch additional holes using guidelines in the text.

The size of the hole to be punched depends on the size of the tooth. For a six-hole punch, use the smaller size 2 hole for mandibular and maxillary lateral incisors; the medium-size 3 hole for premolars, canines, and maxillary central incisors; the size 5 hole for molars; and the size 6 hole for the anchor tooth and clamp. Fig. 34-23 illustrates the use of a five-hole punch. As the hole is punched, pull the dam up the punch spike to be certain it has cut completely through the dam.

Placing the rubber dam and frame

Before rubber dam placement, lubricate the patient's lips with petroleum jelly to protect them against dryness and irritation from the dam. Place the powdered side of the dam facing the clinician to reduce light reflection.

There are two alternative methods of placing the clamp and dam on the tooth. The method chosen is based on the clinical situation, operator's preference, and availability of clamps. If a wingless clamp is used, place the clamp on the tooth and recheck its stability. Orient the rubber dam and place the index finger of each hand on opposing sides of the hole to be placed over the clamped tooth. Stretch the dam to enlarge the hole and slide it over the bow and under each of the jaws, one at a time. When the tooth and clamp are fully exposed with the rubber dam against the gingiva, use a T-ball burnisher blade to pull the floss tied to the clamp through the hole.

The dam may also be placed on the bow of the wingless clamp before placement on the tooth, which may be easier for the inexperienced operator. This allows maximum access and visibility while applying the clamp. Care must be exercised to avoid placing excess pressure on the clamp, thus traumatizing the tooth or surrounding gingiva as the dam is seated.

To use a winged clamp, orient it to the correct hole in the dam. Engage the clamp onto the forceps. Slide one wing into the hole and then stretch the dam towards and over the opposite wing (Fig. 34-24). The dam may be placed on the frame at this stage if desired. Place the clamp on the anchor tooth as described previously, looking through the opening and under the dam to check the position of the clamp relative to the gingiva before releasing the forceps. Pull the rubber dam off the wings and under the clamp. Vision is more limited with this method, but placement is faster because the clamp, dam, and frame are placed simultaneously. After the dam is placed over the clamp, the most anterior tooth is isolated. The frame is placed next to hold the dam away from the patient's face and to provide access to the working area. Position the base of the U-shaped frame downward, with the concave side of the frame toward the patient. Gently pull the rubber dam over the small metal protrusions on the frame to hold the dam in place.

Stretch the dam to open the holes over the the remaining teeth one at a time. Next pass the dam through the contact areas. This is more easily done with the help of an assistant, who stretches the dam over each contact area. Push the rubber through the contact areas holding waxed floss or tape first against one proximal surface and then

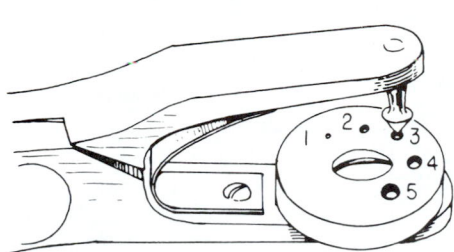

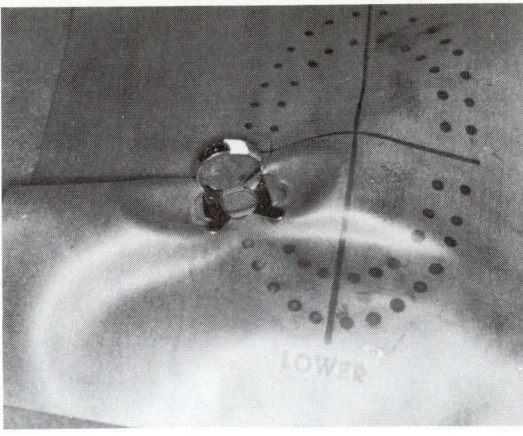

Fig. 34-23. Suggested sizes of holes to be punched in dam for various teeth.
(Modified from Howard WW, Moller RC: *Atlas of operative dentistry,* ed 3, St Louis, 1981, CV Mosby.)

Fig. 34-24. Winged clamp being held by the dam before placement on the tooth.

the other (Fig. 34-25). Do not try to force the whole width of the septum through at once; this is difficult to accomplish and may result in tearing of the dam. If the dam is not fully through the contact areas, it will be difficult to tuck it into the facial and lingual sulci. Repeat the flossing procedure if needed.

After the dam is through the contact areas, the frame is readjusted to hold the dam more tightly. Center it to avoid endangering the patient (i.e., the ends of the frame should be away from the patient's eyes). Tie the floss attached to the clamp to the frame so it is out of the operating field.

Tuck (invert) the dam into the sulcus around each tooth to prevent seepage of sulcular fluid and saliva. Starting at the distal, position the blade of a plastic instrument or T-ball burnisher parallel to the distofacial line angle of the tooth, directed slightly into the sulcus. Slide it to the mesial line angle using the edge of the blade to push the rubber into the gingival sulcus (Fig. 34-26). Simultaneously, direct a stream of air into the sulcus to dry the tooth, rubber dam, and soft tissue to prevent the rubber dam from sliding back out of the sulcus. Repeat this step for each tooth on both the facial and lingual surfaces.

Stabilize the rubber dam by ligating a piece of dental floss around the most anterior tooth (Fig. 34-27) or by wedging a small piece of rubber dam

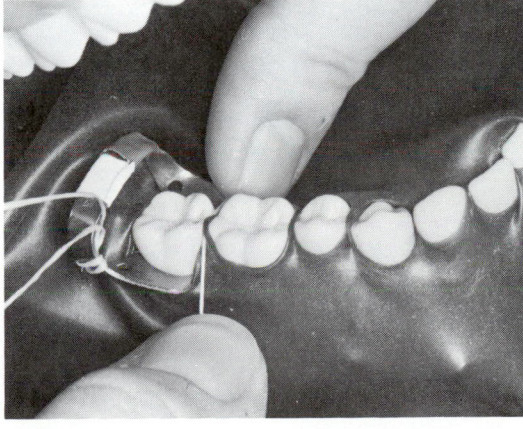

Fig. 34-25. When necessary, push the interseptal rubber through the contacts with dental floss.

into the embrasure between the last exposed tooth and the rubber dam (Fig. 34-28). For dam applications isolating the teeth from first premolar to first premolar, the ligature or rubber dam wedge method of stabilization may be used instead of clamps. After the dam is correctly placed, insert a saliva ejector under the rubber dam onto the floor of the mouth.

A properly applied rubber dam should (1) isolate the working area with no moisture present; (2) expose the teeth to be treated and provide sufficient visual access and finger rests for the clini-

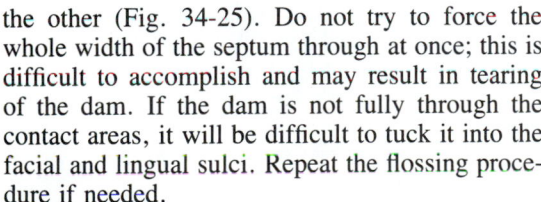

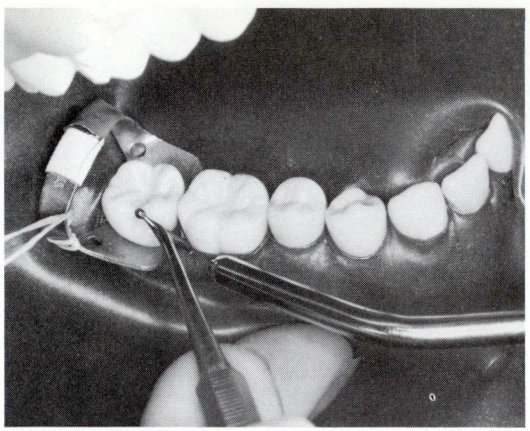

Fig. 34-26. Invert the dam into the sulcus using a thin (not sharp) blade. Air helps to dry the tooth and dam and creates a seal.

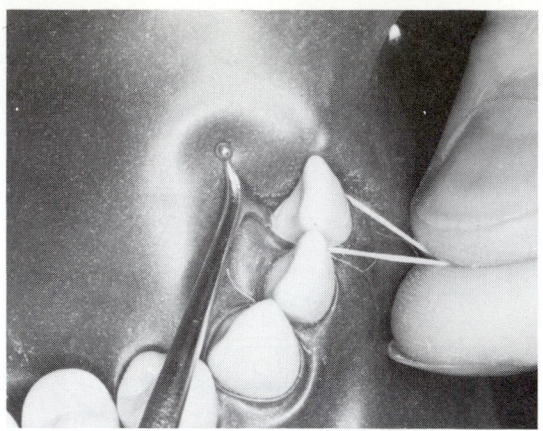

Fig. 34-27. Push the loop of ligature below the cingulum with the blade while pulling the ends in an apical direction.

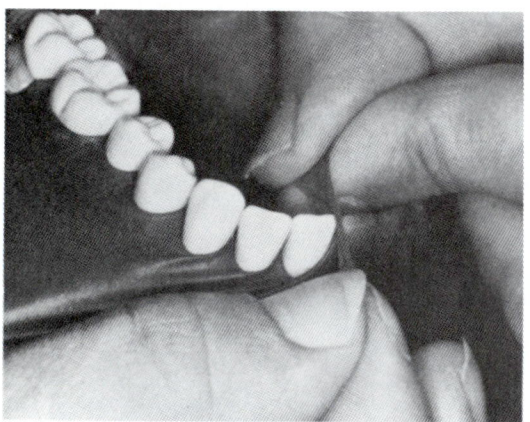

Fig. 34-28. Stretch the piece of rubber dam and push it into the contact area.

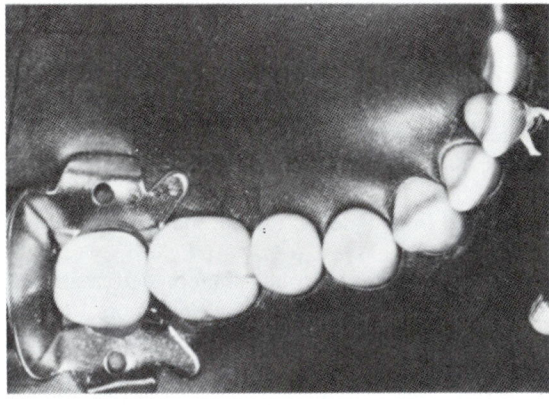

Fig. 34-29. Isolation achieved through a properly mounted rubber dam.

cian; (3) be stable and secure with no potential damage to the hard and soft tissues; (4) be inverted into the gingival sulcus; and (5) be comfortable (Fig. 34-29).

Applying the gingival retractor

The gingival retractor pushes the gingival tissue and rubber dam material away from the site of the Class V preparation. This retractor has two jaws, with prongs, two bows, and notches for the clamp forceps with specific lingual and facial sides (Fig. 34-30). When it is oriented to the tooth, the flat portion of the bow will be to the facial side of the tooth.

Insert the forceps into the notches and expand the jaws of the retractor. For greater access and visibility, seat the lingual jaw first. Slide it gently against the lingual surface until it is apical to the height of contour and flush with, but not impinging on, the gingival tissue. Use the opposite hand to stabilize the lingual jaw. At the same time rotate the forceps to move the facial jaw apically along the facial surface until the facial jaw is apical to the height of contour and contacts the dam overlying the gingiva. Using the jaws of the clamp, gently retract the gingiva and dam to expose the gingival extent of the carious lesion.

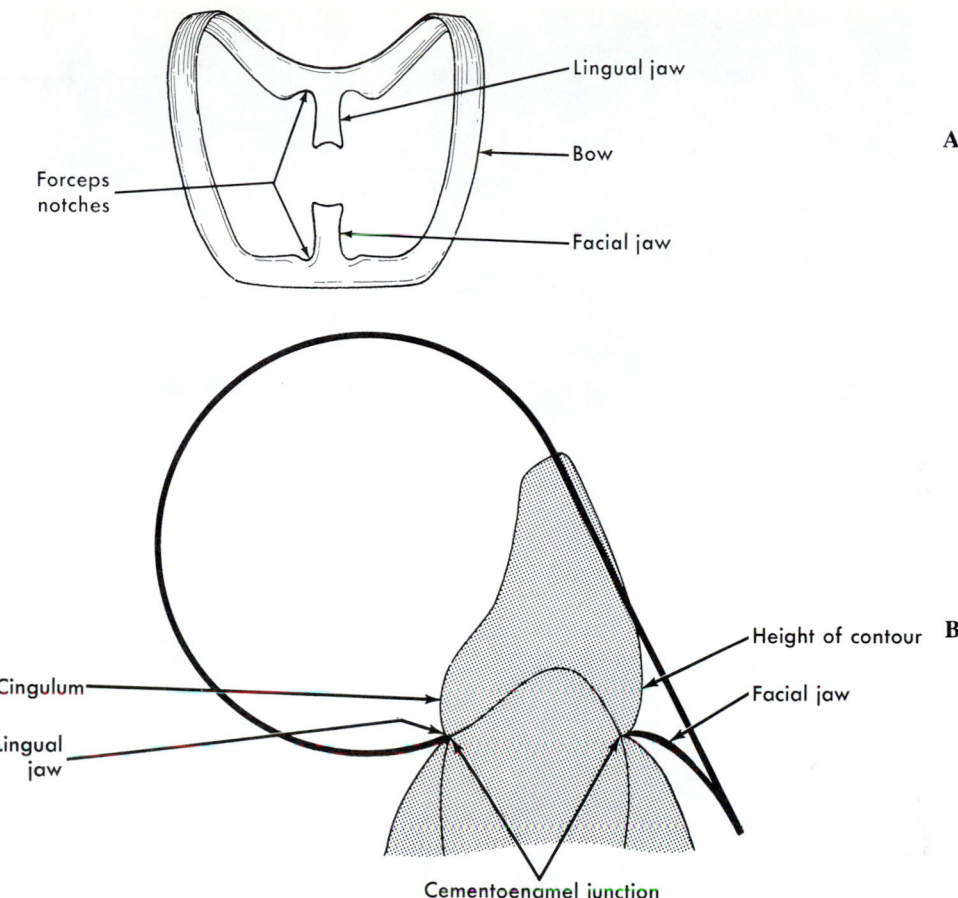

Fig. 34-30. A, Parts of a gingival retractor. **B,** Relationship of the jaws of the gingival retractor to landmarks on an anterior tooth.

Spread the jaws wide enough to avoid scraping against the tooth as the jaws are seated. This would scar the tooth, making it more susceptible to plaque accumulation and caries. If possible, retract the gingiva until it is at least 0.5 to 1.0 mm apical to the gingival margin of the lesion. The bows of the clamp should be parallel to the tooth's occlusal plane to ensure even retraction of the gingiva. Remove the forceps from the retractor while continuing to support the lingual and facial aspects of the retractor with the other hand. Continue the support until dental compound has been placed (Fig. 34-31).

Dental compound stabilizes the gingival retractor to avoid slippage during the procedure. Trauma to the tooth structure and the preparation or restorative material may occur if the clamp

slips. Warm the compound stick over a flame until the end begins to sag. Then temper it in warm water until the material is warm and malleable but not hot. Mold the compound over the top of one retractor bow and the occlusal (incisal) surface. Continue molding the compound until it fills the space between the bow and the tooth. Repeat procedure for the other bow (Fig. 34-32).

Check the retractor to make sure that it resists movement and that it evenly retracts the gingiva and rubber dam. Check the stability with light finger pressure.

Removing the rubber dam

Before removing the dam, use high-volume evacuation to remove all debris from the operative field. If a gingival retractor has been used, re-

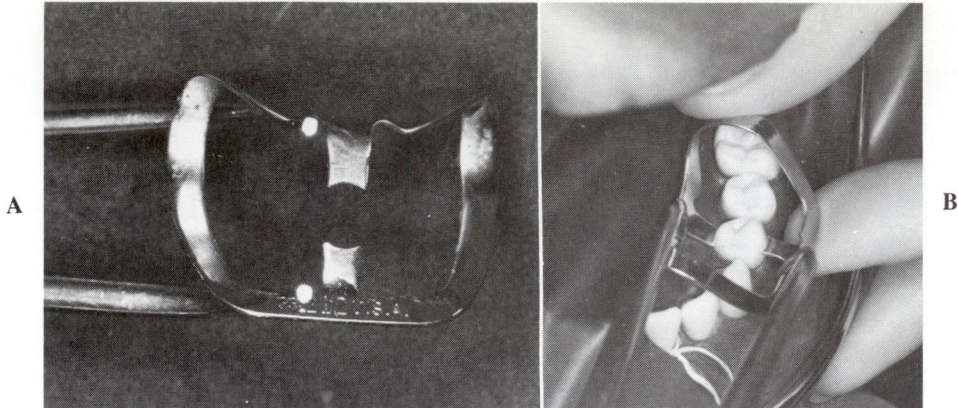

Fig. 34-31. Mounting gingival retractor. **A,** Position of gingival retractor in forceps for mounting in the maxillary left or mandibular right arches. **B,** Placement of retractor in mandibular left arch. (Notice that retractor is positioned in the other pair of notches and turned 180 degrees when compared with **A.**) Seat the lingual jaw first.

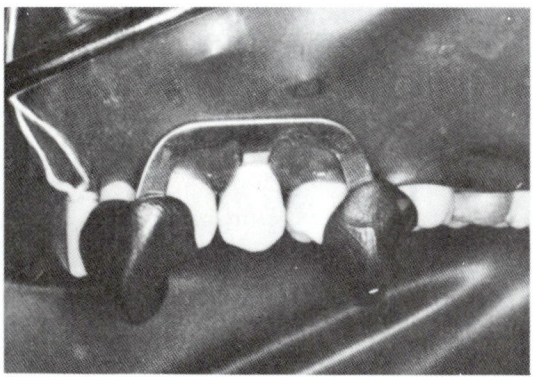

Fig. 34-32. Properly mounted gingival retractor with dental compound stabilizing it.

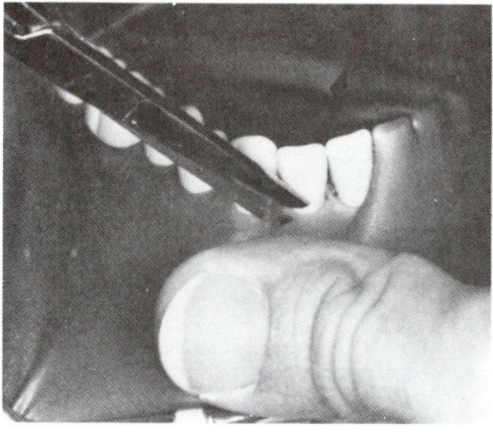

Fig. 34-33. Note that the tip of the lower scissors blade extends well beyond the rubber to ensure complete cutting of the septum each time.

move it first. Apply the forceps in an occlusolingual direction to break the compound off the teeth. Remove the retractor carefully in an occlusal direction without letting it touch the newly placed restoration or the tooth surface. Remove any remaining compound with a sharp instrument. Remove the ligature or rubber dam wedge from the most anterior tooth. Stretch the dam to the facial, away from the teeth. Place one finger under the stretched dam (to protect the patient's lips and cheeks) while cutting the interdental areas of the dam (Fig. 34-33). Cut the entire septum with one stroke from the facial aspect. Pull the dam in a lingual direction.

Pulling an uncut dam up through the contacts or snipping the interproximal areas in stages may cause thin pieces of dam to tear or remain around the tooth. If a ring of rubber dam material remained around the tooth, it would tend to migrate apically because the apex is the most constricted area of the tooth. It could cause a gingival abscess, bone destruction, or even loss of the tooth (Abrams, 1978).

The clamp, dam, and frame are removed at the

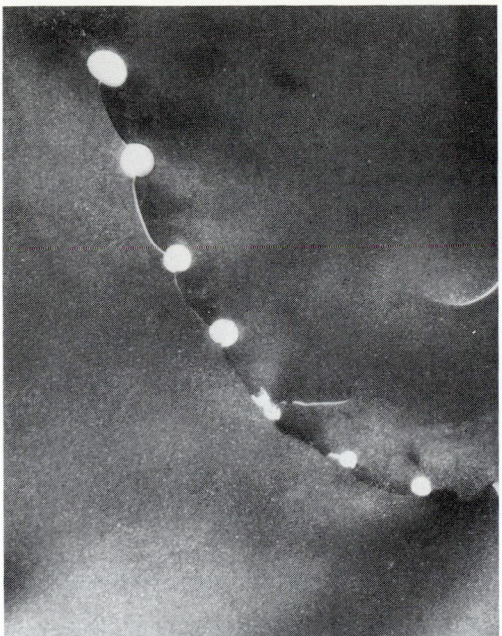

Fig. 34-34. Note that a piece of rubber dam is missing next to the fourth hole from the bottom.

same time. The dam is laid on a light-coloured surface and checked to ensure that there are no small pieces of dam missing, which may remained in the patient's mouth. Except for the severed interdental pieces, the dam should appear as it did before placement (Fig. 34-34). Remove any piece that is left in the mouth with dental floss or an explorer.

Rinse and evacuate the oral cavity. Examine the soft tissue for any trauma. Inform the patient that he or she may experience some discomfort after the anesthetic wears off.

Evaluation criteria
Application of rubber dam
1. Isolated area is clean and dry.
2. Number of teeth exposed provides visual access and finger rests.
3. Clamp is stable and secure and does not impinge on gingiva.
4. Ligature or wedges hold dam securely in place.
5. Dam inverted into the gingival sulcus.
6. Patient is comfortable.
7. Gingival retractor (if used) is stable and retracts the gingiva and dam.

Removal of rubber dam
1. All rubber dam material, ligatures, and other debris have been removed.
2. No significant soft tissue injury is present.

PROBLEMS IN RESTORING TEETH

Pulpitis (inflammation of the pulp) is a concern before, during, and after operative procedures. It can occur from the cavity preparation or the restorative materials. The physical cutting of enamel and dentin, heat generated by rotary instruments, and drying of dentinal tubules by the use of air during cavity preparation can be irritating to the pulp (Langeland, 1972; Stanley, 1961, 1971). Microleakage of various fluids containing microorganisms has been shown to produce considerable irritation to the pulp (Browne et al, 1983). Because most of the materials used in restoring teeth do not truly seal the interface between the cavity wall and the restorative material, microleakage and the entry of microorganisms is a constant potential danger.

Materials expand and contract under the influence of heat and cold. This rate of expansion and contraction differs from that of enamel and dentin. The material undergoing contraction pulls away from the cavity wall. This increases the rate of microleakage. Agents that minimize microleakage are beneficial for both patient comfort and the future health of the tooth. Generally, a dentin thickness of 2 mm or more between the pulp and the cavity wall is enough to insulate the pulp from thermal, chemical, and even bacterial irritation (Cohen and Burns, 1980).

Some materials used in operative dentistry are potentially irritating to the pulp. Chemical irritation can result from molecules from the chemicals seeping into the dentinal tubules. Metal materials such as amalgam readily conduct heat, which may irritate the pulp. Temperature conducted through the materials is a potential source of irritation to the tooth. The greatest source of irritation would appear to be bacterial invasion via microleakage of the restorative materials. All of these problems, however, could be prevented or solved by the materials used under the basic restorative materials.

PROBLEM SOLVERS
Bases and liners

Bases and liners are dental materials used to help the pulp recover from trauma that may have ex-

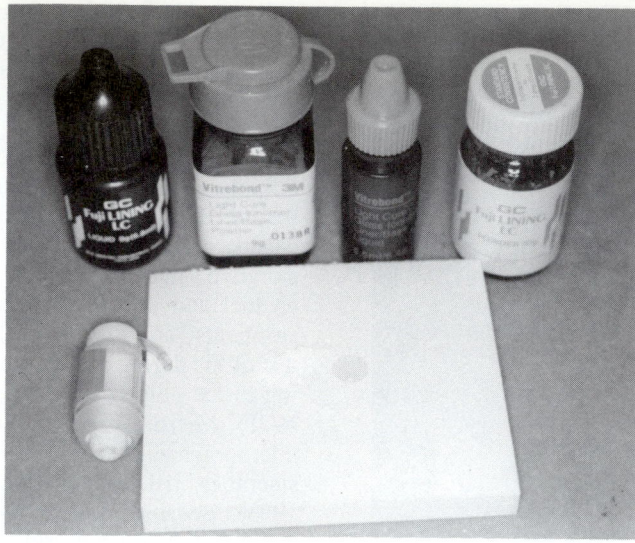

Fig. 34-35. Pictured are some commercially available glass ionomer cements. The mixing pad with the powder and liquid dispensed is shown.

isted before the cavity preparation and to protect it from trauma occurring during or after the restorative procedures. Bases are applied to the pulpal floor or axial walls in relatively thick layers (greater than 0.5 mm). Liners are applied as thin coatings (less than 0.5 mm) to the walls and floor of the cavity preparation. The specific indications for these materials depends on the health of the pulp, the amount of carious invasion, the depth of the preparation, and the restorative material being used.

The most common products used as liners have been varnishes and glass ionomer cements. Varnishes are natural or synthetic resins, such as copal or nitrated cellulose, dissolved in an organic volatile solvent (ether, acetone, or chloroform). Clinically they are used under amalgam restorations to seal the cavity preparation in two ways. Varnish protects the pulp by reducing the ingress of chemical and bacterial irritants into the dentinal tubules. They also decrease the mercury or tin corrosion products from amalgam restorations from entering the tubules and causing discoloration of the tooth. Copal varnish is not recommended for use under composite resin because it interferes with the setting of the resin. A varnish-type dentin sealer composed of methylcellulose is compatible with resin and has been shown to be

effective in reducing dentin permeability against the resin monomer (Tjan et al, 1987). The sealer also helps to seal the microscopic space between the wall of the cavity preparation and the restoration thus reducing leakage of fluids around the amalgam restoration (Murray et al, 1982; Yates et al, 1980). Because it is soluble in oral fluids, the varnish dissolves in time. However, as the amalgam corrodes the resultant corrosion products fill the space once occupied by the varnish to maintain some of the seal originally provided at the interface between the amalgam and the tooth.

Glass ionomer cement is gaining popularity as a base and liner (Klausner et al, 1989) — particularly for use under composite resin (Hosoda et al, 1991) (Fig. 34-35). Glass ionomer is derived by mixing a silicate glass powder with polyacrylic acid and water, which gives a material that can adhere to dentin and that releases a caries, preventing fluoride. Glass ionomer is relatively insoluble and exhibits little microleakage. Other desirable characteristics include radiopacity, pulpal compatibility, good insulating properties, and thermal expansion similar to that of the tooth. Glass ionomers are marketed in several forms. Some are sold as a bulk powder and liquid system, and others are premeasured and encapsulated (Fig. 34-36). Both chemically and light-activated

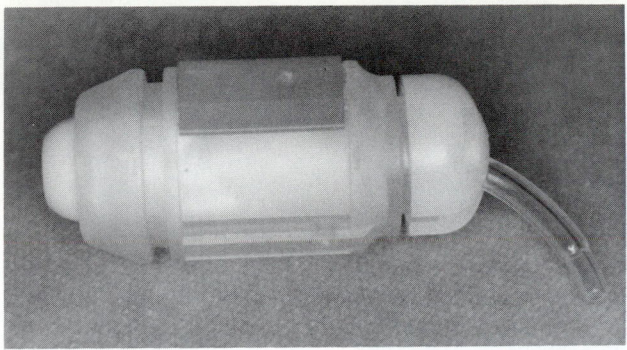

Fig. 34-36. The mixing capsule has a premeasured amount of polyacrylic acid and silicate glass powder enclosed. The spout allows dispensation directly into the cavity preparation.

products are available. The basic difference between the glass ionomer liner and base is the powder-liquid ratio, which makes the liner more fluid and thinner but does not give as strong a material.

A calcium hydroxide base is used in very deep cavity preparations that extend near the pulp when a pulp exposure is possible. Calcium hydroxide stimulates the pulpal tissue to form secondary dentin to protect the pulp from further irritation. In addition to pulpal stimulation, calcium hydroxide has some sealing ability to protect the pulp. Peters and Augsberger (1981) found that a layer of calcium hydroxide provides short-term thermal protection. Its radiopacity makes it visible on radiographs. Both chemically and light-activated materials are available. Calcium hydroxide does not provide a strong base, however. Varnish or a glass ionomer liner can be placed over calcium hydroxide to provide a seal between the calcium hydroxide and the amalgam.

Zinc oxide–eugenol is called an "obtundent" because it reduces the irritability of pulpal tissue and decreases pain. The eugenol gives the familiar oil-of-cloves aroma to the dental office. Although this material has been used as a base in the past, today it is used chiefly as an intermediate or temporary restoration when the prognosis of a tooth is questionable. It is not typically used under amalgam and is contraindicated under composite resin restorations (Millstein and Nathanson, 1983). Caution must be exercised for patients with hypersensitivity to eugenol, exhibited as ulcers or sloughing of the gingival tissues.

PROCEDURES
Armamentarium

The armamentarium for the placement of varnishes includes varnish, cotton pellets, and cotton pliers. Calcium hydroxide is either mixed as two pastes on a mixing pad, or with light-activated products, applied directly. The armamentarium for placement of glass ionomer liners and bases depends on the system used. The bulk powder and liquid systems require a mixing pad and spatula, application instrument (plastic or Dycal instruments for liner), and syringe (for base application). Encapsulated products are dispensed and applied from the capsule thereby negating the need for a syringe. A water-soluble lubricant such as K-Y Jelly or a composite bonding agent for application to the external surface of the restoration prevents dessication of the glass ionomer liner or base. The mixing pad and instruments may be eliminated for the light-activated glass ionomer.

Procedural steps

The sequence of steps and specific products used for a base depends on the type of restoration to be placed, the depth of the cavity preparation, and the condition of the pulp (see box on p. 736).

Amalgam restorations

Minimal depth. Minimal-depth preparations extend about 0.5 to 1.5 mm into the dentin. The remaining dentin is thick enough to provide both insulation and protection during cavity preparation. However, a sealer is needed to seal the dentinal tubules and fill the space between the amal-

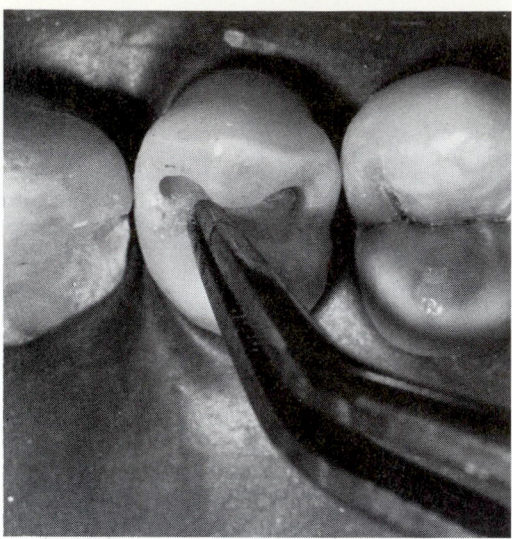

Fig. 34-37. Varnish is applied in all areas of the preparation, including over the cavosurface margin. A small cotton pellet helps control placement of the varnish.

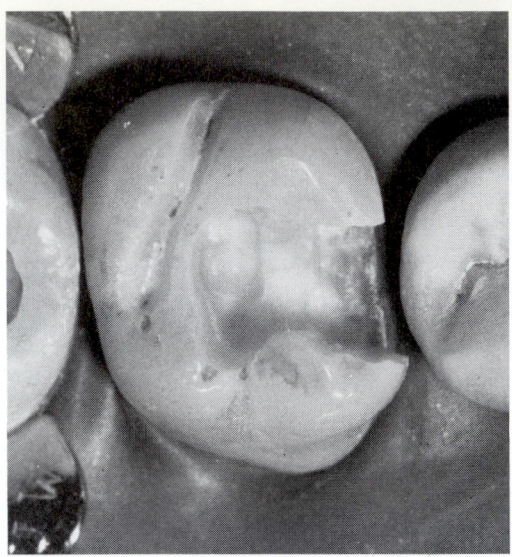

Fig. 34-40. Near pulpal exposures can occur on both the pulpal and axial walls.

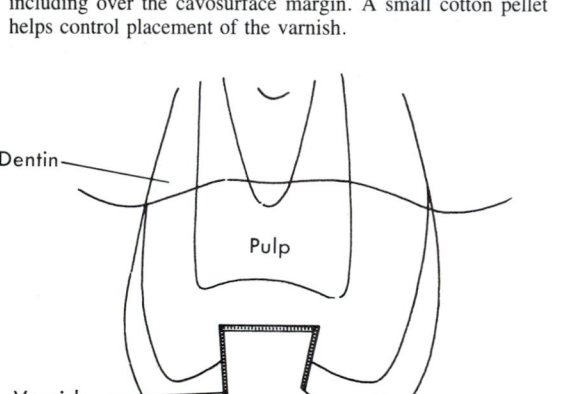

Fig. 34-38. Minimal-depth restorations have a sufficient bulk of dentin remaining to provide thermal insulation. Two coats of varnish are placed before placing the amalgam.

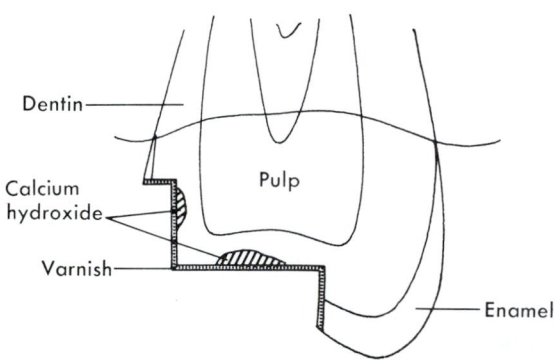

Fig. 34-39. Subaxial and subpulpal extensions in a Class II preparation. Calcium hydroxide or glass ionomer cement is placed in the extensions before the layer of varnish is applied.

Review of Pulpal Protection

Minimal depth

Minimal-depth preparations extend only 0.5 to 1.5 mm into the dentin so sufficient thickness of dentin remains to protect the pulp from potential chemical irritation. The composite resin is placed directly onto the cavity preparation.

Subaxial or subpulpal extension

A thin layer (0.5 mm) of calcium hydroxide is placed in the deepest portion of the cavity preparation. The calcium hydroxide should not be placed into the retentive grooves or along the enamel. Several applications of the material are easier to control than one large amount, particularly in preparations with minimal access.

Near pulpal exposure

Calcium hydroxide is placed in a thin layer (0.5 mm) over the deeper portions of the cavity preparation to provide protection from chemical irritation and stimulate secondary dentin.

Pulpal exposure

The exposure site, along with the surrounding dentin, is covered with a layer of calcium hydroxide, then a temporary zinc oxide–eugenol restoration is placed to allow time for observation of the tooth.

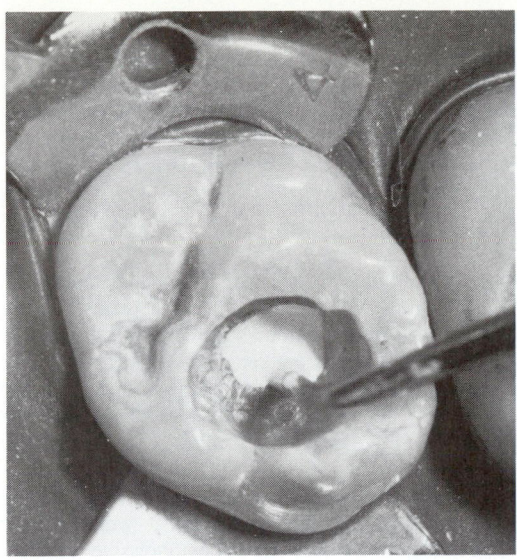

Fig. 34-41. Calcium hydroxide is placed in a thin, continuous layer on the deepest areas of the pulpal or axial wall.

gam and tooth surface. Regardless of their depth, all cavity preparations to be restored with amalgam require a sealer. Varnish is applied over the entire preparation, including both dentin and enamel, with a cotton pellet held with cotton pliers (Fig. 34-37). Two applications are needed to completely coat the tooth surface. The first layer of varnish is dried with a gentle stream of air before the second coat is applied. Strong blasts of air form ridges of varnish that may not dry before amalgam placement. Use a new cotton pellet to apply the second thin coat allowing it to dry before placing the amalgam (Fig. 34-38). Some varnishes come with their own applicator. The solvent in the varnish is highly volatile, so tightly cap the bottle immediately after use.

Subaxial or subpulpal extension. A subaxial or subpulpal extension is an area on the axial or pulpal wall that extends deeper than the rest of the wall (Fig. 34-39). This places the amalgam closer to the pulp, leaving less dentin to protect it. If there is a possibility that the pulpal tissue may be exposed microscopically, calcium hydroxide should be applied in an even layer of 0.5 to 1.0 mm thick. Apply varnish if this is not a concern. A glass ionomer base or liner may be placed over the calcium hydroxide if desired for extra protection. Varnish is the final coating.

Near pulpal exposure. Cavity preparations very close to the pulp require special care (Fig.

34-40). The pulp is already irritated by the caries, and the depth of the preparation adds a further insult. Knowledge of pulpal anatomy, history of the tooth's involvement, radiographic evidence, and experience will aid in determining the approximate nearness to the pulp. If the pink color of the pulp can be seen through the dentin, the dentin is very thin. In these situations, apply calcium hydroxide over the deepest portion of the preparation (Fig. 34-41). Newer and stronger calcium hydroxide materials can be applied in thicker layers to provide some thermal protection as well as protection from chemical or bacterial irritation (Farah et al, 1981; Peters and Augsberger, 1981).

If using a two-paste system, dispense small, equal amounts of base and catalyst pastes on a mixing pad. The placement instrument can be used to mix the material to a homogeneous color. Wipe the instrument clean and pick up a small amount of material. Place the material onto the desired area, spreading an even layer (0.5 to 1.0 mm) on dentin only. Calcium hydroxide placed on enamel must be removed. It will quickly dissolve when exposed to oral fluids, leaving a space at the margin and making the restoration more susceptible to microleakage and recurrent decay. To prevent interference with the retention of the restorative material, avoid placing the calcium hydroxide in any retentive grooves. Calcium hydroxide can be removed using an explorer once the material has set. It tends to smear if removed before it sets. Two coats of varnish are applied over the entire preparation before the amalgam is placed.

Pulpal exposure. Pulpal exposures can occur from either carious or mechanical causes. Depending on the severity and extent of the exposure, it may be decided to treat the tooth endodontically. If, however, the decision is made to observe the tooth for a time to allow recovery, a temporary restoration may be placed. Generally, zinc oxide−eugenol is used as a temporary material because of its relative ease of placement and removal and its palliative effect on the pulp. Calcium hydroxide is first placed over the exposure site and surrounding dentin to stimulate secondary dentin formation and then the zinc oxide−eugenol restoration is placed.

Composite resin restorations

Because the thermal conductivity of composite resin material is similar to that of dentin, thermal irritation is not a problem. The major potential problem is chemical irritation from the monomer in the composite resin. The decision of which material to place is based on the depth of the preparation and the availability of the protective materials compatible with composite resin materials. Copal varnishes and zinc oxide–eugenol are contraindicated because they interfere with the setting of the material (Eliasson, 1979).

The pulp must be protected from the acid used to etch enamel and from the irritating effects of the composite resin materials. Calcium hydroxide is placed in a thin layer in the area closest to the pulp. A glass ionomer base and/or liner can be placed over the calcium hydroxide and over all dentin surfaces for additional protection. A glass ionomer base is used if additional structural support is needed to protect the pulp.

PRINCIPLES AND GENERAL PROCEDURES FOR AMALGAM PLACEMENT: THE CLASS V AND CLASS I RESTORATIONS

Dental amalgam is the most commonly used restorative material, accounting for almost three fourths of the restorations placed (Gilmore et al, 1982). It is adaptable to many situations, offers good durability, and restores function to the tooth. It is easy to mix, adapt into the preparation, and contour. Research on the long-term clinical performance of alloys has indicated that they last for decades, release less mercury than previously thought and do not require resurfacing or replacement as would composite resins (Laswell et al, 1989; Lemmens et al, 1986; Osborne, Norman, and Gale, 1991). Amalgam is a long-lasting, safe, and inexpensive material that is tolerant of operator errors.

Amalgam is composed of several metals. Any combination of metals is referred to as an alloy. If an alloy is mixed with mercury, the result is an amalgam. The mixing process is known as trituration. Dental amalgam is often called silver amalgam because silver is its chief ingredient. Alloy composition varies among manufacturers; the ranges are shown below:

Percentage	Element	Function
40% to 69%	Silver	Combines easily with mercury
11% to 27%	Copper	Adds strength to the alloy, decreases corrosion and tarnish
15% to 30%	Tin	Aids in combining mercury with the alloy
0% to 1%	Zinc	Prevents alloy oxidation during the manufacturing process

All dental amalgams share the following physical properties:

1. Dimensional change. All amalgams undergo dimensional change. The amount depends on many factors. Greater amounts of mercury cause greater expansion and a weaker restoration. Longer mixing time decreases expansion or increases contraction (not a factor within reasonable trituration times). Increased condensation pressure decreases expansion.
2. Variance in strength. Force applied directly to the thicker parts of the restoration is well tolerated. Amalgam exhibits good compressive strength. Force applied to a thin area such as an edge (margin) is not well tolerated. Amalgam's tensile strength is only about one-fifth its compressive strength (Charbeneau et al, 1981).
3. Strength is adversely affected by many factors. Inadequate trituration results in a drier mass, which in turn results in a mass that contains voids (porosity). Excessive mercury produces a weaker restoration that is more subject to corrosion and tarnish (Craig et al, 1989). The correct ratio of mercury to amalgam is specified by the manufacturer. It is usually about 1 to 1 or less. Amalgam has relatively little strength early in its setting reaction. It requires careful protection immediately after placement to avoid fracture of any unsupported portion.

Other characteristics that affect the amalgam are:

1. Moisture can cause undesirable expansion of an amalgam restoration (Craig, 1980). It also interferes with the blending of one carrier load of amalgam with the preceding one. It increases corrosion and thus decreases strength.
2. Amalgam begins the setting (hardening) process as soon as it is mixed. After 2½ to 3 minutes, the working stage of the material has passed. Although it can be loaded into an amalgam carrier and packed into the preparation with some difficulty, it will not become a part of the mass already condensed and will likely fracture or flake away. After 2½ to 3 minutes, mix a new batch of material to add to the already condensed amalgam.
3. When first placed, amalgam is relatively soft. Only the gross excess should be removed. Final

carving should be done when the amalgam offers slight resistance to the instrument.

4. Because amalgam is initially very weak and can be fractured easily, carving strokes should not be directed toward unsupported amalgam; they should be directed from the tooth structure towards the amalgam. If possible, use repeated, short, gentle carving strokes.

Product packaging

Alloy is packaged in powder or pellet form. The mercury may be packaged separately. The powder or pellets and the mercury may be loaded into separate dispensers so correct proportions can be dispensed into the mixing capsule. This method may cause mercury contamination through spills and aerosol production during trituration. Amalgam residue may contaminate future batches. Only sealed prepackaged capsules containing correct proportions of the alloy and the mercury should be used.

The capsules are designed as "one-spill," "two-spill," or "three-spill" capsules. Small preparations may require only a one-spill capsule; large preparations will need one or more two- or three-spill capsules.

Dental mercury hygiene

All personnel who handle mercury should observe good mercury hygiene practices. Although it is extremely rare, some individuals may develop a mercury sensitivity or allergy. Symptoms may vary from local dermatitis to a generalized erythema over the entire body. Symptoms of mercury toxicity include tremor, which is observable in fine voluntary muscular movements (e.g., handwriting), eventually progressing to convulsions; loss of appetite; nausea and diarrhea; depression, fatigue, increased irritability, or moodiness; pneumonitis; nephritis; nervous excitability; insomnia; headache; swollen glands and tongue; ulceration of oral mucosa; and dark pigmentation of marginal gingiva and loosening of teeth. Excessive exposure to mercury or its vapor can cause toxicity, though this is very rare.

The work area should be a well-ventilated space with fresh air exchange and outside air exhaust. The office should be monitored yearly for mercury contamination (more often if contamination is suspected). Periodic urinalysis for mercury should be done for all personnel. Observe the following additional precautions:

- Use precapsulated alloy to minimize mercury spills.

- Avoid direct contact with or handling of mercury, amalgam, or other mercury-containing materials.
- Never heat mercury or amalgam.
- Do not use mercury disinfecting solutions.
- Prohibit eating, drinking, or smoking in the dental operatory.
- Use recommended procedures for cleaning mercury spills and dispose of mercury-contaminated items properly.
- Check clothing and shoes for mercury and amalgam to avoid contamination of nondental areas.

Mixing the amalgam (trituration)

Trituration must wet all of the alloy particles with mercury within the appropriate time. Mixing is done with a motor-driven mechanical device called an amalgamator, which shakes the capsule rapidly back and forth to allow the alloy and mercury to mix (Fig. 34-42). Some capsule designs require a barrier to be broken before the capsule is placed in the amalgamator. Some have a barrier that breaks during mixing, allowing the alloy and mercury to mix. Refer to the manufacturer's directions. Recommended design of the amalgamator includes a covering over the amalgamator arms to prevent spraying of any loose mercury into the operatory environment.

Set the capsule firmly into the identations in the amalgamator arms. A capsule that is not held firmly in place may be flung loose. Set the timer to the number of seconds recommended by the manufacturer for the particular amalgamator being used (this varies from 2 to 25 seconds for a two-spill capsule). The more alloy and mercury used, the greater the mixing time required. When the timer has been set and the covering moved into place, push the button to begin the mixing.

When trituration is completed, remove the capsule. Do not touch the amalgam directly with the fingers to avoid moisture contamination and a mercury hazard. Drop the pellet directly from the capsule into an amalgam well or dappen dish. Reassemble the capsule parts to decrease the possibility of contamination.

The amalgam should be a solid mass with a dull shine and no dry or grainy areas (Fig. 34-43). If it meets these criteria, it is ready to load into the amalgam carrier. If it appears dry and crumbles when pressure is applied, it cannot be well adapted against the walls and into the retentive features. It will not become one solid

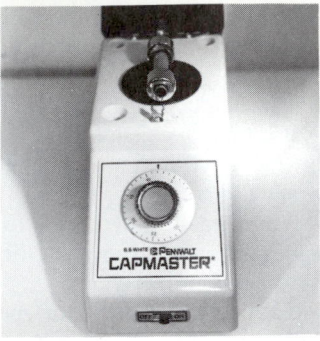

Fig. 34-42. Place the capsule securely in the rocker arms to prevent dislodgement. Close the cover before activating the amalgamator.

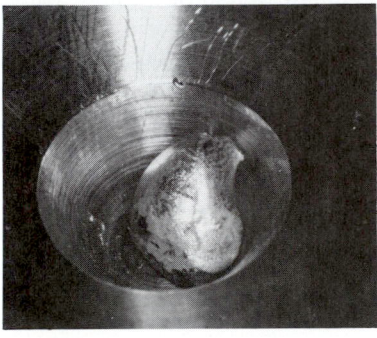

Fig. 34-43. The amalgam should be a single mass, not crumbly, and should have a dull shine.

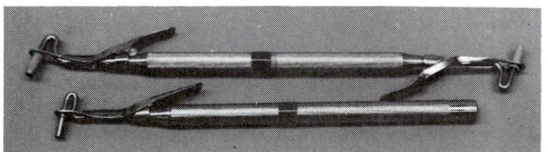

Fig. 34-44. Either single- or double-ended amalgam carrier may be used. Double-ended carrier offers a choice of a large or small end to correspond to the size of the preparation.

mass. Amalgam that is too wet with mercury will be very shiny and quite soft; it will set slowly, will be difficult to carve, and will have significantly less strength than a correctly proportioned mix (Craig, 1989).

Condensing amalgam

The amalgam carrier is used to transfer the amalgam into the preparation. The carriers shown in Fig. 34-44 are the most commonly selected. The end of the carrier is a hollow tube containing a plunger to extrude the amalgam when the lever is depressed. The ends are two different sizes; select the one that fits the preparation. To load the carrier, place a finger under the lever and then insert the end of the carrier into the amalgam mass to force amalgam into the tube. The finger under the lever holds the plunger position, allowing amalgam to enter the tube. Wipe away any excess by dragging the end of the tube against the side of the amalgam well or dappen dish.

Place the first increment of amalgam into the most inaccessible portion of the preparation. In this way, the first increments of amalgam do not hinder placement of later segments. Place a partial load in a small or medium-sized preparation. Too much amalgam obscures the view, hinders the condensation strokes, and makes it difficult to determine if the amalgam is being well condensed. Only large preparations can accommodate placement of a full increment without risk of undercondensation.

Condensation forces the amalgam into all the areas of preparation so each particle of amalgam is attached or melded with previously placed particles to become one solid mass. This creates a tighter fit to decrease leakage of fluids between the amalgam and the tooth structure and also provides retention for the restoration. Amalgam does not bond or adhere to the tooth structure.

Knowledge of the size and shape of the preparation and its retentive areas is important for proper condensation. Retentive areas usually consist of grooves cut into the walls that meet the axial or pulpal wall at a perpendicular angle. These grooves make the interior portion of the preparation larger than the external, thus providing an "undercut" that locks the material into the preparation. Amalgam is condensed into these areas first.

The condenser end (nib) should fit into all areas of the preparation. Before mixing the amalgam, insert the nib into the preparation to ensure that it will fit. A too-large nib will not force the amalgam into the retentive areas. A too-small nib will simply push through the mass of amalgam without condensing it effectively.

Apply condensation pressure toward both internal line angles and the walls themselves. Use a smaller condenser nib to condense into groove extensions and line angles. Even smaller condenser cannot be inserted into all areas. Use side of the instrument to push amalgam laterally into the area. Condensing strokes are primarily directed perpendicularly toward the axial or pulpal wall.

When condensing, each stroke must overlap the previous one. Well-condensed amalgam has two characteristics: (1) overlapping indentations made by the condenser nib and (2) shiny surface because condensing pressure has forced the mercury within the amalgam to the surface.

Each segment must be completely condensed. All loads are manipulated just as was the first segment. This makes the restoration a homogeneous mass rather than several "layers" that will not hold together.

When the preparation is filled, switch to the next larger condenser nib size. This size will help adapt the amalgam to the cavosurface margins as the preparation is overfilled by approximately 1 mm. Overfilling allows for removal of the mercury-rich layer on the surface and ensures sufficient material to carve the desired contours of the restoration. Direct the final condensation strokes toward the cavosurface margins at a 45-degree angle to ensure complete adaptation at the margins. Avoid at the margin could be fatal to the success of the restoration.

At this stage the amalgam should cover all margins, overfill the preparation, have a shiny surface without voids, and exhibit overlapping condensation strokes.

Burnishing amalgam

Burnishing rubs the surface, making it shiny or lustrous. Burnishing an amalgam restoration after condensation provides additional adaptation and compaction of the material over its surface and marginal areas, reduces marginal leakage, and leaves a smoother surface (Charbeneau, 1965; Kanai, 1966; Kato et al, 1968; Svare and Chan, 1972).

With gentle pressure, move a smooth-ended instrument from the fresh amalgam towards and over the cavosurface margin to adapt the amalgam against the margin. This action also removes excess amalgam. Do not to use too much pressure.

The amalgam is burnished immediately after condensation to smooth the surface and better adapt the amalgam. Burnishing after carving when the amalgam has begun initial set allows a final smoothing of the surface.

Carving amalgam

Timing is important in carving. If started too late, the amalgam will be hard and difficult to carve. If started too soon, the amalgam may be too soft, resulting in overcarving as the instrument sinks into the surface. Test the hardness by pulling the carving instrument through an area of excess amalgam. Do not try definitive carving until the amalgam offers some resistance. Remove the gross excess from the margins early.

Carving is a series of shaving strokes that remove only the surface layer. Removing too much at one time results in overcarving or fracture of the restoration. The stroke is controlled by resting the instrument on the tooth structure around the preparation. Adapting the instrument this way guides it in shaping the anatomy and prevents slippage and overcarving. Move the instrument from tooth onto the amalgam rather than from amalgam toward the margins to avoid removing too much at the margin ("ditching") and leaving a ledge of enamel above the restoration.

Carving is much easier if the clinician has a good mental image of the tooth's anatomy. The adjacent and contralateral teeth provide good reference for the anatomy of the tooth being restored. Grooves in the enamel surrounding the preparation must be carved into the adjacent amalgam. If this is not done, a ledge of amalgam will be left at the junction of the enamel groove and the amalgam. This ledge can be detected by drawing an explorer tip along the groove onto the amalgam surface. Amalgam extending over the cavosurface margin ("flash") must be removed. The restoration should not have a jagged outline at the margins with abrupt changes in contour. Jagged contours usually indicate the presence of flash.

The restoration must reproduce the original contours of the tooth. Resting the instrument on the surrounding enamel, with its blade angle corresponding to the angulation of the surrounding enamel, will reproduce the contours desired. No matter the type or location of the restoration being carved, these principles remain the same.

The following sections discuss specific procedures involved in placement of the classes of restorations. Each calls for unique variations and adaptations.

Armamentarium

The armamentarium suggested for amalgam restorations is shown in Fig. 34-45. Specific situations may require other instruments.

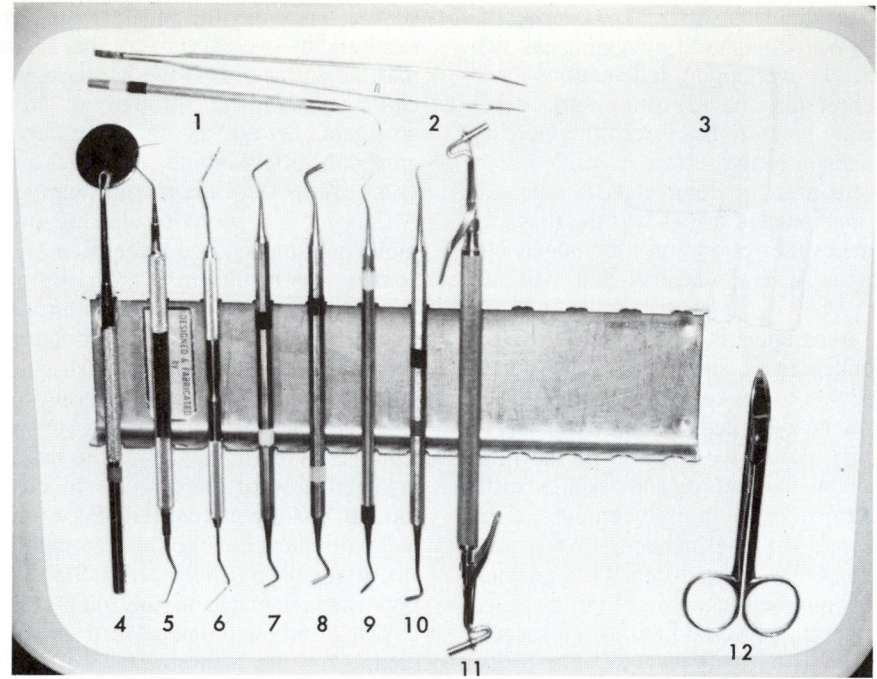

Fig. 34-45. Tray setup for Class V cavity restoration includes: *1,* calcium hydroxide placement instrument; *2,* cotton pliers; *3,* gauze and cotton pellets and rolls; *4,* mouth mirror; *5,* explorer; *6,* probe; *7* and *8,* amalgam condensers; *9,* No. ½ Hollenback carver; *10,* plastic placement instrument; *11,* amalgam carrier; and *12,* crown and bridge scissors.

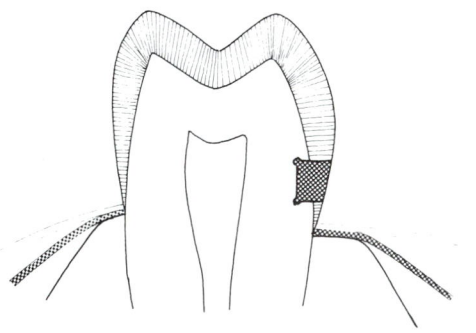

Fig. 34-46. Retentive grooves located in the gingivoaxial and occlusoaxial line angles.

CLASS V AMALGAM RESTORATION

The class V restoration is located in the gingival one third of the facial or lingual surface of anterior and posterior teeth (Fig. 34-46). Esthetic concerns contraindicate placement of amalgam in anterior teeth. This restoration is usually the least complex and easiest to place. Its basic shape is rectangular, although the walls are slightly curved. The preparation is essentially a "box." The axial wall meets the occlusal, gingival, mesial, and distal walls at nearly a right angle. Retention is provided by grooves placed at the occlusoaxial and gingivoaxial line angles. The cavosurface margins are usually even without undulations. Recognition of this outline aids in visualizing the exact margin to which to carve the restoration.

If indicated, place a base according to the criteria previously discussed. Before mixing the amalgam, use the explorer tip (Figs. 34-46 and 34-47)

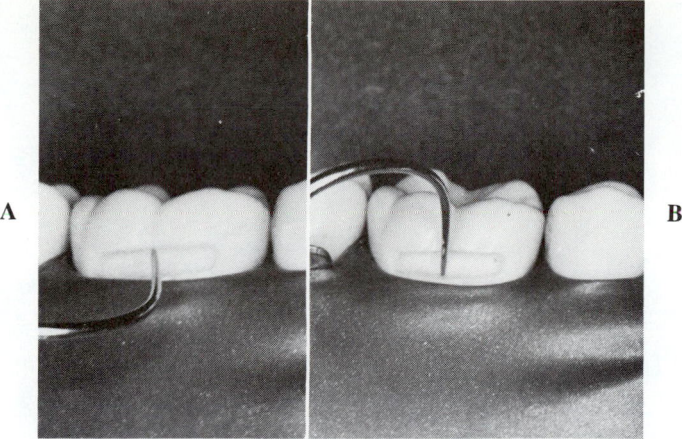

Fig. 34-47. Check retentive grooves with the tine of the explorer. A slight catch will be felt along the occlusoaxial (**A**) and gingivoaxial (**B**) line angles.

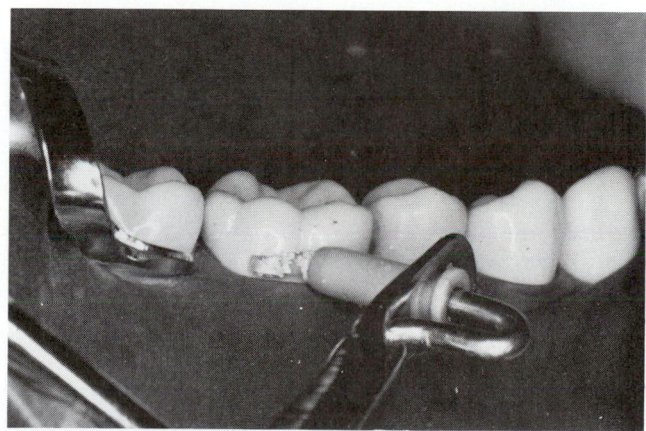

Fig. 34-48. First increment of amalgam being spread along the axial wall.

to remove any base material left in the retentive grooves. Material left in the grooves prevents amalgam from being condensed into the area, reducing or eliminating retention of the restoration.

After the base is set, cover the entire cavity preparation with two coats of varnish.

Placement and condensation

Place one half of the first carrier load of amalgam against the axial wall (Fig. 34-48). Direct the first condensing strokes at a 45-degree angle towards the gingivoaxial line angle to adapt the amalgam against the walls and along the whole length of the retentive grooves (Fig. 34-49, *A*). Continue condensation across the occlusoaxial line angle to the mesioaxial line angle (Fig. 34-49, *B*). Apply condensation pressure at 45 degrees to ensure good condensation into these line angles and retentive grooves.

Compact the remaining amalgam against the axial wall. Use overlapping strokes with enough pressure to produce slight indentations and to make the surface slightly shiny (Fig. 34-50). When the first carrier load is thoroughly condensed, add the second. Continue to condense until the whole axial wall is covered. Most of these condensation strokes are at a 90-degree angle toward the axial wall. Some, however, should be as

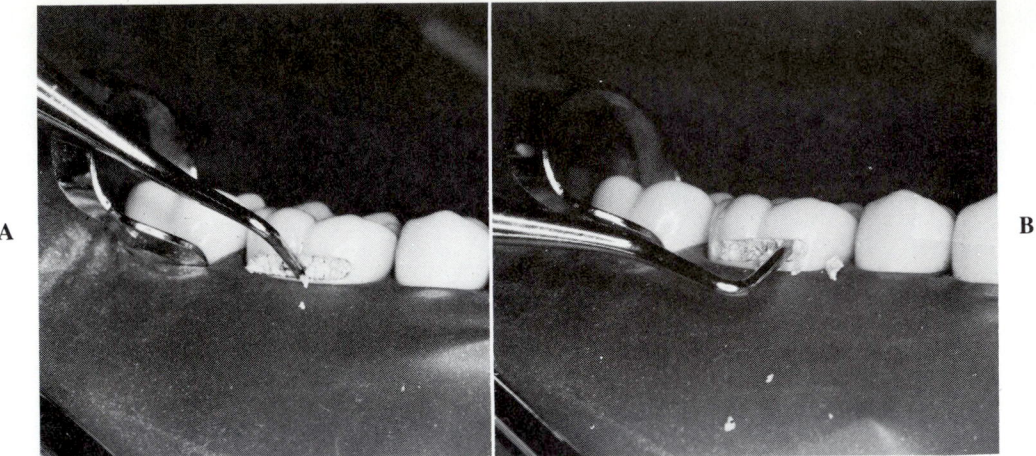

Fig. 34-49. **A,** Angle of condenser nib when condensing into the gingivoaxial retentive groove. **B,** Angling nib of condenser towards the occlusoaxial retentive groove.

nearly perpendicular as possible to the occlusal, gingival, mesial, and distal walls (Figs. 34-51 to 34-54). Adapt the amalgam against those walls to increase retention and decrease leakage along the interface.

As the mass reaches the cavosurface, switch to the next larger condenser nib (Fig. 34-55) to better adapt the final layer over the margins.

Overfill the preparation by 0.5 to 1.0 mm (Fig. 34-56). The outer layer will be removed to eliminate mercury-rich amalgam. The last condensing strokes should be at approximately 45 degrees against the margins. Condense out over the margins slightly. Do not grossly overfill the preparation to avoid a time-consuming and difficult carving process.

At this point, evaluate the restoration carefully according to the following criteria:

1. All margins are covered with amalgam.
2. The preparation is overfilled by 0.5 to 1.0 mm.
3. The amalgam surface is shiny, without voids or grainy areas.
4. Overlapping condensing strokes are clearly visible.

If these criteria are met, the restoration is ready for burnishing.

Initial burnishing

Choose a relatively flat-bladed instrument, such as a beavertail burnisher, for the rather flat Class

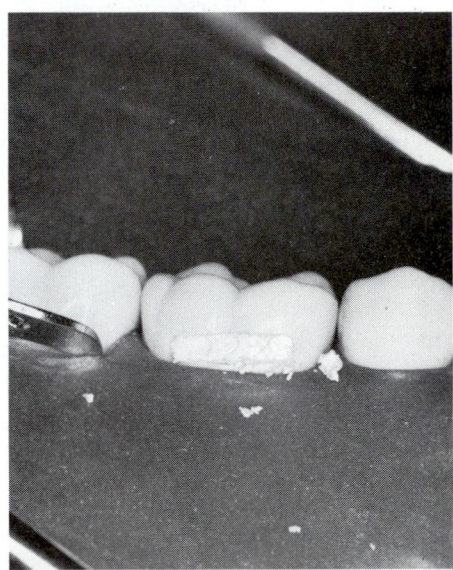

Fig. 34-50. Well-condensed amalgam has a slightly shiny surface with clearly visible overlapping condensing strokes.

V restoration. Rest the instrument tip gingival to the margin, with the side of the instrument contacting the gingival one-third of the restoration on its distal aspect. Pull the instrument along the gingival margin towards and over the mesial margin, then back along the gingival margin across the distal margin. This smooths the material along the margins and better adapts it to the preparation wall (Fig. 34-57).

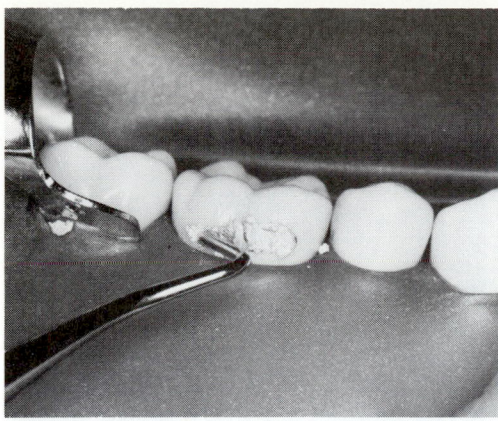

Fig. 34-51. Angle of condenser nib when directed toward the distal wall.

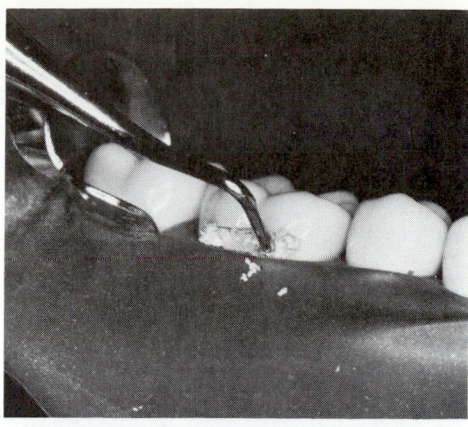

Fig. 34-52. Force of condensation directed toward the gingival wall.

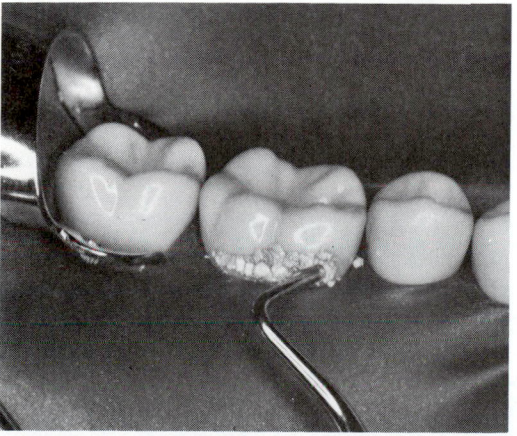

Fig. 34-53. Angle of condenser nib when directed toward the mesial wall.

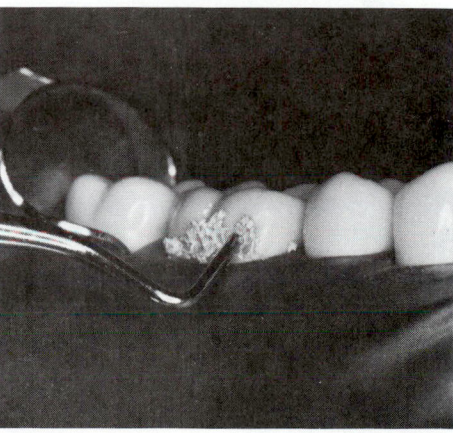

Fig. 34-54. The condenser nib is angled as nearly perpendicular to the occlusal wall as the preparation permits.

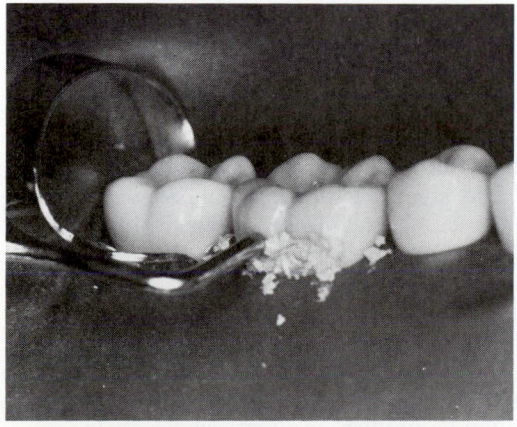

Fig. 34-55. The larger condenser nib is directed at and beyond the cavosurface margins.

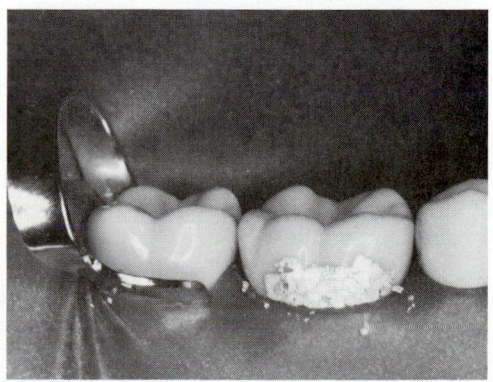

Fig. 34-56. The final increment of amalgam slightly overfills the preparation. Note the overlapping condensing strokes.

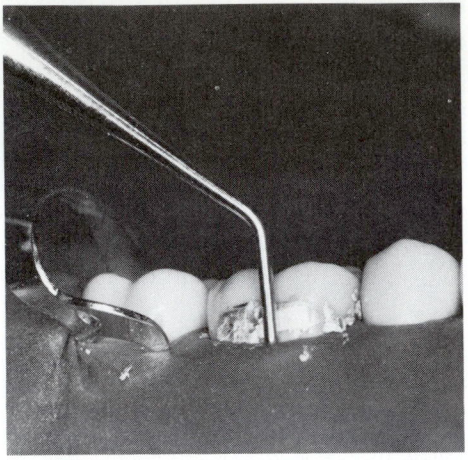

Fig. 34-57. Burnish amalgam with the side of a condenser. A blade-shaped burnisher can also be used.

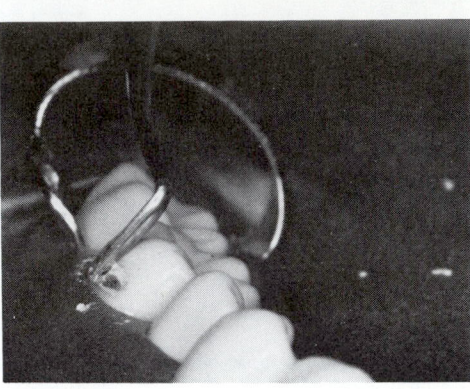

Fig. 34-58. Carving the occlusal margin. The tip of the instrument is not contacting the central portion of the restoration.

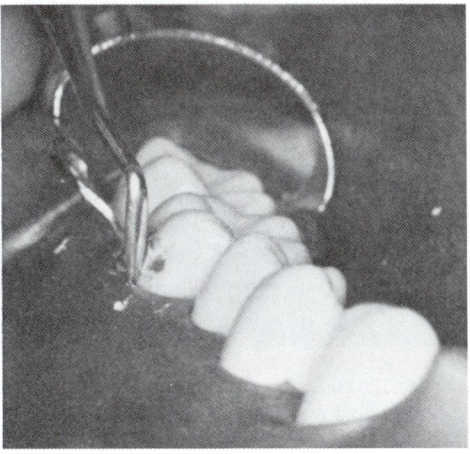

Fig. 34-59. The side of the bladed carver is adapted against both tooth structure and amalgam. The heel of the instrument is not contacting the central portion of the restoration.

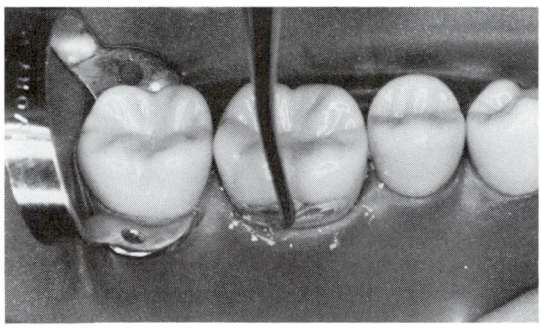

Fig. 34-60. Adaptation of the instrument when carving the distal margin.

With the side of the instrument on the tooth occlusal to the restoration and the instrument tip on the amalgam, repeat the same steps done for the gingival margin. Avoid digging into or gouging the amalgam with the tip.

Burnish the center portion of the restoration by rubbing the instrument lightly over its entire surface from the distal margin to the mesial margin. Use only enough pressure to smooth the surface and better adapt amalgam to the margins. Excessive pressure may gouge the amalgam, resulting in ditching or inadequate contours.

The amalgam surface should be smooth, shiny, and well adapted to the margins. Most of the excess amalgam originally placed should have been pushed away from the margins and eliminated. The restoration is ready for carving.

Carving the amalgam

Visualize the size and form of the original preparation before the amalgam was inserted.

Remove the excess material with the ½ Hollen-

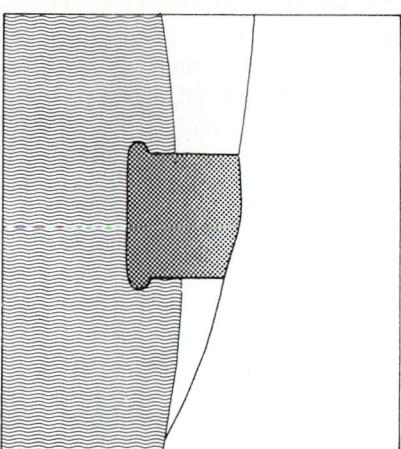

Fig. 34-61. Illustration of an overcontoured Class V restoration. The margins are flush at the cavosurface; however, the center of the restoration is too bulky.

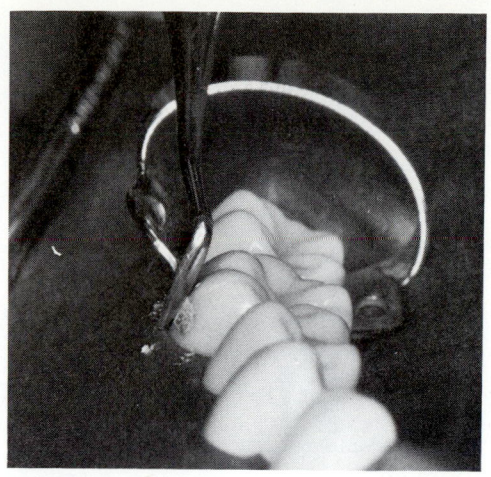

Fig. 34-62. Carving the central portion of the restoration "freehand." The side of the instrument is adapted to excess amalgam only.

back carver. The end with the blade whose a face is perpendicular to the shank of the instrument is adapted to the amalgam. With the blade resting on the tooth structure occlusal to the margin, pull the instrument through the excess amalgam (Fig. 34-58). Do not place the tip on the amalgam surface itself because it may gouge that surface. This procedure is similar to that performed with the burnishing instrument except that the blade will carve away amalgam.

Repeat the procedure along the gingival margin, resting the tip of the instrument on the tooth gingival to the restoration, pulling it from the distal to the mesial, and pushing it back toward the distal (Fig. 34-59). The distal margin is carved with the carver tip resting on tooth structure distal to the restoration and moving occlusogingivally and then back again (Fig. 34-60). The same procedure is performed on the mesial margin.

In all these strokes, only the area immediately adjacent to the margin is shaped. The intent is to remove obvious excess and to begin to form the outer borders of the restoration.

Observe the occlusogingival contour from a mesial view (Fig. 34-61). Because the carving has concentrated on the marginal areas, the middle third will be overcontoured.

To contour the middle third, position the instrument on the distal cavosurface margin and bring it mesially past the mesial margin (Fig. 34-62). This is the first carving movement in which the blade

is not supported by tooth structure. Do not remove all the excess with the first stroke. Overaggressive removal may result in an undercontoured restoration. After the movement is made, re-examine the contours from the mesial to determine if additional reduction is needed. Remove amalgam until the contour is correct. Blend all the segments so the contour is smooth and continuous.

Using very light pressure and the side of an explorer, check all the margins carefully. If flash is detected, adapt the side of the 1/2 Hollenback carver along the marginal area, as previously described. Shave away excess amalgam and then re-examine. An open margin (space between the body of the amalgam and the enamel wall) usually requires replacement of the restoration (Fig. 34-63). A submarginal area (an area where the amalgam does not reach the level of the cavosurface margin) may be corrected (Fig. 34-64) if it is less than 0.2 mm (barely detectable with an explorer). It can be corrected by reducing the adjacent enamel during the finishing and polishing procedure. A difference of more than 0.2 mm usually requires replacement of the restoration.

Check the restoration for the following criteria:

1. Margins are flush with no open margins, submarginal areas, or flash.
2. The anatomic contours are reproduced.
3. The surface has been wiped with a damp cotton roll to help smooth it and wipe away debris.

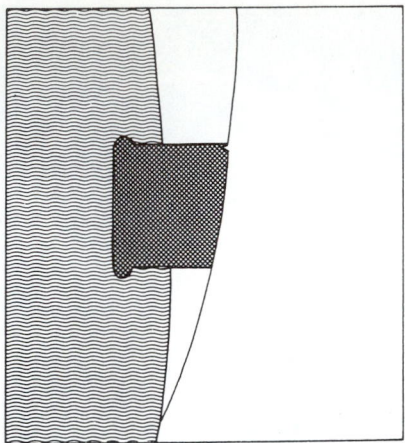

Fig. 34-63. An open margin may be the result of poor condensation at the cavosurface.

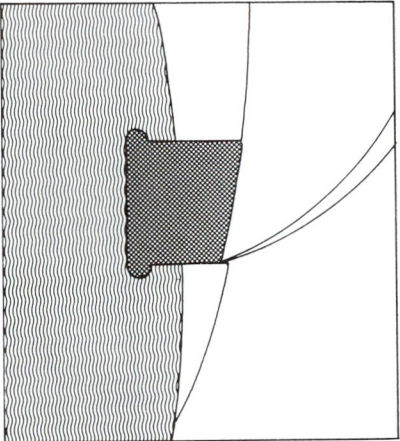

Fig. 34-64. Submarginal areas are detected as the explorer is moved from the restoration to the tooth surface.

Final burnishing

If the amalgam has set and is hard enough to resist alteration of contour, it may be burnished. Adapt the beavertail or ball burnisher as described previously. Use a back-and-forth rubbing motion with enough pressure to produce a smooth shiny surface over the whole restoration, including the margins. Re-examine the restoration to ensure that it meets all of the evaluation criteria listed in the check-off sheet at the end of the chapter.

CLASS I AMALGAM RESTORATIONS

The Class I restoration is more difficult to place because of the grooves and pits of the occlusal surface and the ridges surrounding them, which must be reproduced. Carefully examine the preparation's size and extensions into the grooves (Fig. 34-65). The outline form follows the extension of the carious lesion, but the cavosurface margins should be smoothly rounded with no sharp corners. The walls are parallel or slightly converging toward the occlusal. Apply base, if it is indicated, and two coats of cavity varnish.

Condensation

Deposit only one half carrier load into the distal portion of the preparation (Fig. 34-66). Push the carrier towards the pulpal wall and move it mesially as the amalgam is extruded, wedging the mass into the preparation.

Direct the first condensing strokes toward the distal and pulpal walls, using light pressure to further wedge the mass (Fig. 34-67). Begin condensing at the distal aspect and across the pulpal wall to the mesial wall. Direct the nib toward the internal line angles (Fig. 34-68). Begin with the distopulpal line angle and move the nib to include the faciopulpal, mesiopulpal, and linguopulpal line angles.

Add the next amalgam increment and condense it into the smaller grooves. Although most of the condensation will be accomplished with the nib end moving perpendicular to the pulpal floor, the side of the nib may be used to push amalgam sideways into groove extensions (Fig. 34-69).

Add and condense the amalgam until the preparation is slightly overfilled (Figs. 34-70 and 34-71). Change to a larger condenser nib and direct the final condensing strokes at a 45-degree angle against the margins to adapt the amalgam in these critical areas (Fig. 34-72). Evaluate the restoration after condensation is completed. It should exhibit the previously listed criteria for newly condensed amalgam.

Initial burnishing

The grooves and fossae or pits of a class I restoration require a football-shaped, egg-shaped, or ball burnisher (Fig. 34-73). Place the more pointed end in the center of the tooth with the side resting on both tooth and amalgam. Beginning at the most distal aspect of the facial margin, move the burnisher to the mesial using relatively

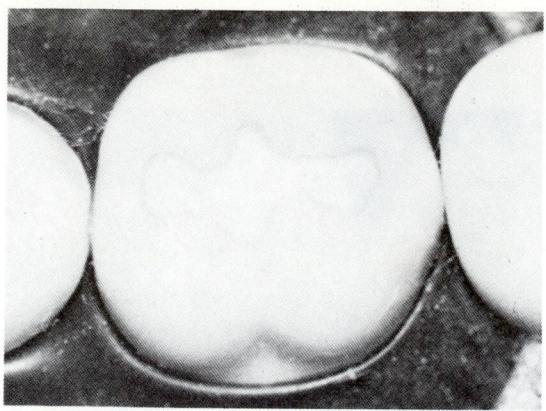

Fig. 34-65. Outline of a Class I cavity preparation.

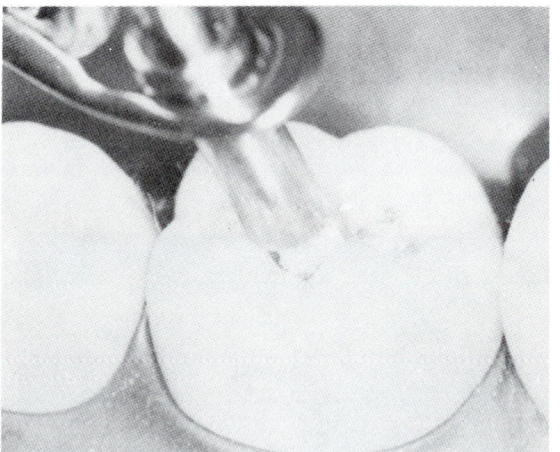

Fig. 34-66. Placement of the first increment of amalgam.

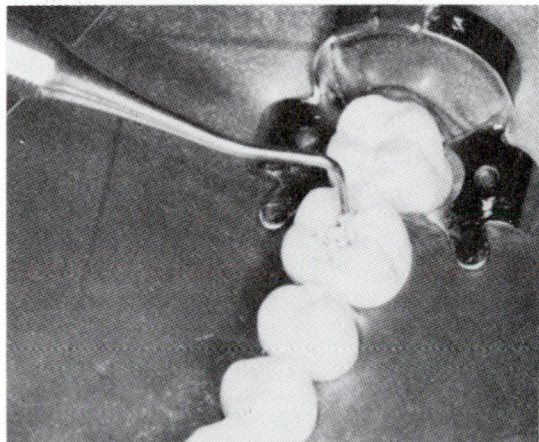

Fig. 34-67. Force of condensation directed perpendicular to pulpal wall.

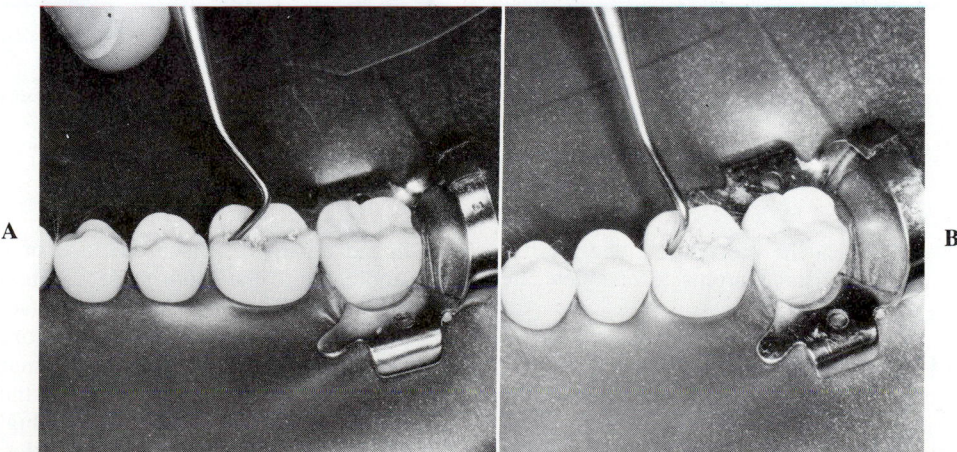

Fig. 34-68. **A,** Angle of condenser when directed toward the mesial wall and internal line angles. **B,** Angle of condenser when directed toward the lingual wall.

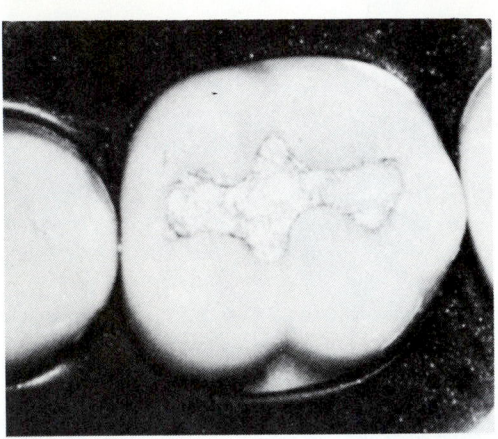

Fig. 34-69. Thoroughly condensed first increment of amalgam.

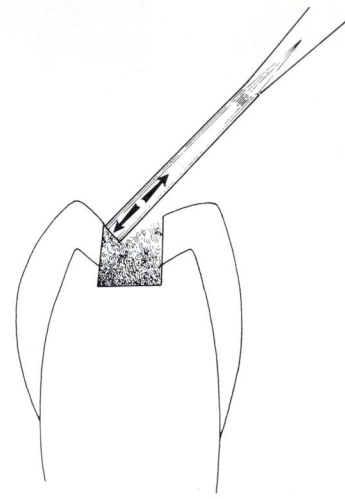

Fig. 34-70. Angle of condenser nib directed toward the internal walls during condensing of the second increment of amalgam.

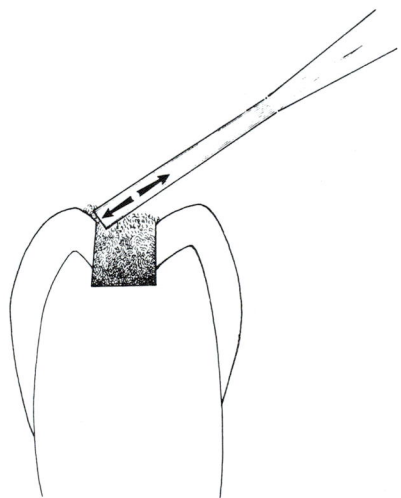

Fig. 34-71. Condensing the amalgam at the cavosurface margin. The nib is approximately perpendicular to the margin.

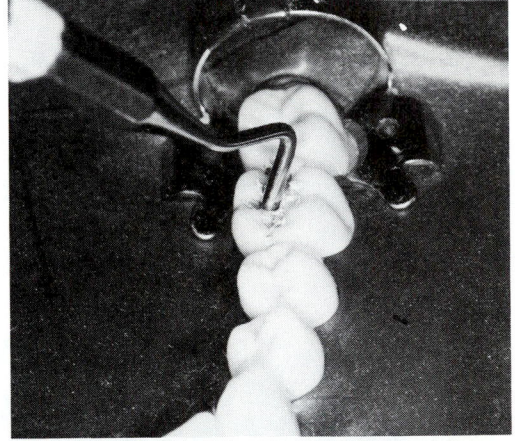

Fig. 34-72. Large condenser nib directed at an angle to the cavosurface margin.

light strokes. Repeat the procedure along the lingual, mesial, and distal margins to complete the burnishing.

Carving the restoration

The instrument commonly used for carving the occlusal surface is the cleoid-discoid carver. Position the rounded (discoid) end at the distal aspect of the facial surface with the side resting on both tooth and amalgam. Place the face of the blade perpendicular to the tooth surface. Move the instrument parallel to the faciocavosurface margin (Fig. 34-74) using short shaving strokes to remove the excess amalgam from the margin. Reposition the instrument and repeat the strokes along the linguocavosurface margin (Fig. 34-75). The instrument should be guided by the contours of the tooth to produce similar contours in the

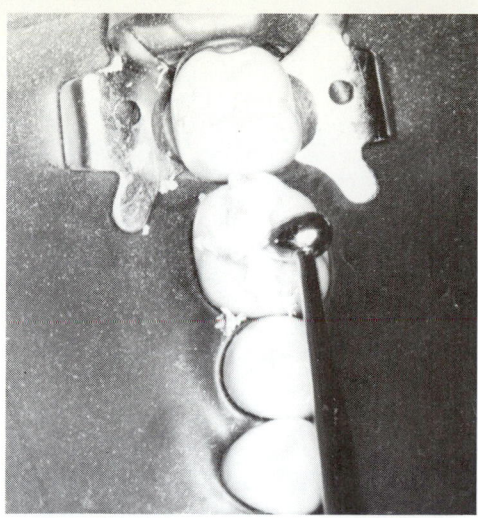

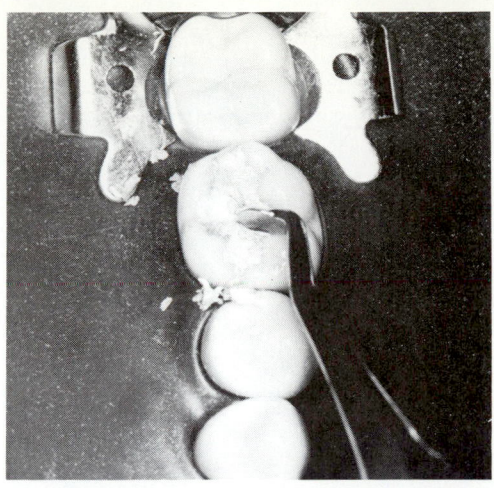

Fig. 34-73. Adapting the football-shaped burnisher along facial margin.

Fig. 34-74. Large discoid carver adapted on tooth surface and amalgam along the facial margin. The face of the blade is perpendicular to the tooth surface.

amalgam. Incorrect angulation will result in problems (Fig. 34-76).

Turn the instrument sideways to rest on the mesial marginal ridge (Fig. 34-77). Starting at the mesiolingual line angle, move the instrument towards the mesiofacial line angle. The instrument will follow the contour of the mesial marginal ridge, producing a concavity just inside the marginal ridge. This is the beginning of the mesial fossa. Repeat the same maneuver on the distal surface (Fig. 34-78). At this stage there should be little excess amalgam left on the occlusal surface.

Now concentrate on the details of the specific anatomy. Using the tip of the cleoid instrument, lightly mark the location of the central groove midway between the facial and lingual cusp tips. Starting approximately 1.5 mm from the distocavosurface margin,create a shallow groove extending to within 1.5 mm of the mesiocavosurface margin (Fig. 34-79).

Rest the cleoid carver on the most distal aspect of the faciocavosurface margin with the tip extended to the central groove. Pull the instrument mesially, allowing the blade to rise and fall as it is carried over triangular ridges and into fossae or grooves (Fig. 34-80). Repeat this movement along the linguocavosurface margin. The cusp ridges, central fossa, and central groove should be established.

Define the distocavosurface margin (Fig. 34-81). With the small discoid carver adapted against the distocavosurface enamel, move the in-

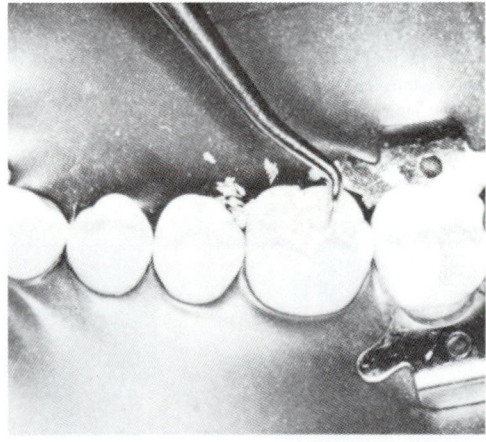

Fig. 34-75. Adaptation of large discoid carver along the lingual cavosurface margin. Amalgam is shaved away in thin layers.

strument from the facial to the lingual surface on a line parallel to the distal marginal ridge. Reverse the face of the instrument and repeat the stroke back from the lingual to the facial margin. Do the same to form the mesial fossa.

The remaining grooves and the central fossa are reproduced next. They need to be well defined but not deep. Place the small cleoid carver on the distofacial cusp ridge with the tip touching the central groove. Pull the instrument mesially until it reaches the area halfway between the distofacial

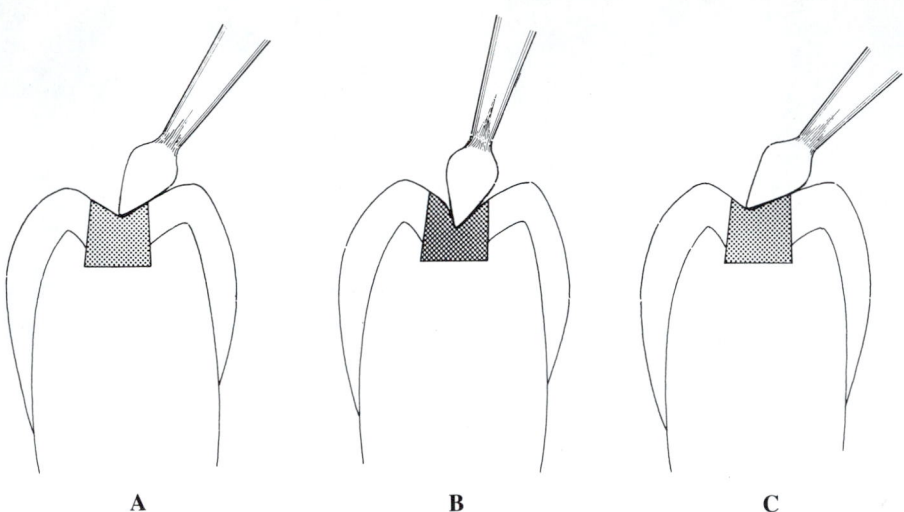

A B C

Fig. 34-76. **A,** Correct vertical angulation of the cleoid carver. The side of the blade is contacting tooth structure and amalgam. The tip is located in the central groove. **B,** Vertical angulation of the cleoid carver is too steep. **C,** Vertical angulation of the cleoid carver is too flat, and the tip is displaced too far toward the opposite cavosurface margin.

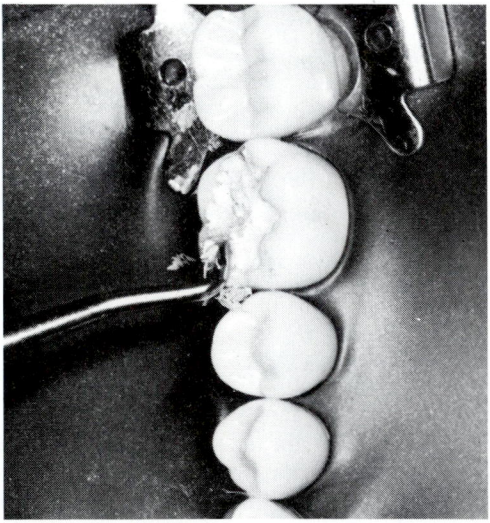

Fig. 34-77. Removing excess amalgam at the mesio-cavosurface margin.

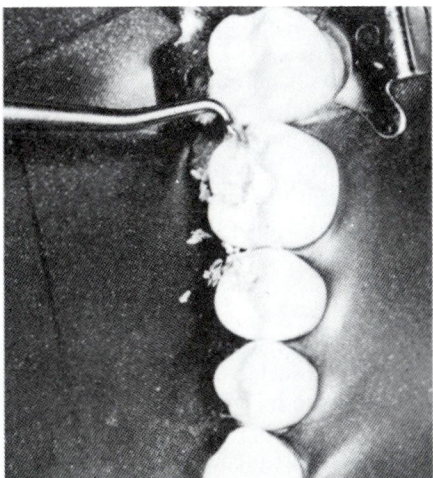

Fig. 34-78. The large discoid carver is adapted against the existing marginal ridge to aid in defining the distal margin and fossa.

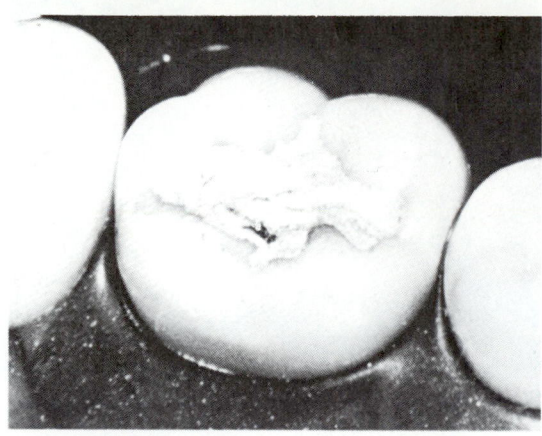

Fig. 34-79. The central groove is lightly defined in the surface of the amalgam. This serves as a reference point for placement of the tip of the cleoid carver.

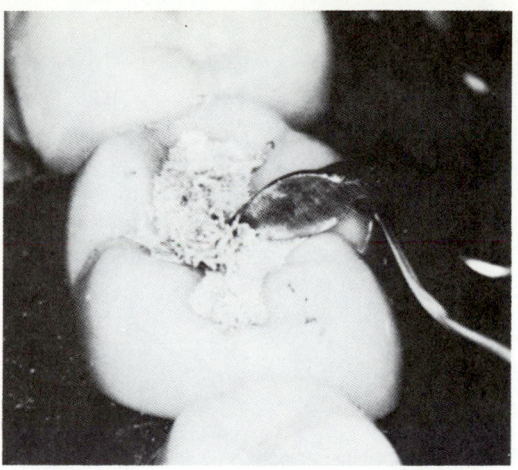

Fig. 34-80. The tip of the cleoid carver is maintained in the previously marked central groove as the excess amalgam is shaved away along the facial margin.

and mesiofacial cusp tips. Keep the blade at the same angle to the surface of the tooth by rotating the handle of the instrument as you move it from the height of the distal cusp ridge to the facial groove area. Reverse the steps just outlined, using the back of the cleoid carver as a pushing instrument to emphasize the contours as you move the instrument distally. The instrument does not carve as effectively when pushed rather than pulled, but access and hand placement may limit use of the pull stroke. Next, place the instrument on the mesiofacial cusp ridge. Use the same technique to shape the distal incline of the mesiofacial cusp as for the mesial incline of the distofacial cusp ridge. Repeat the process on the lingual aspects of the restoration.

If initial setting has occurred, use the tip of the cleoid carver for final definition of the grooves (Fig. 34-82). If the amalgam offers resistance to removal, place the the carver tip in the enamel groove and push the instrument from the enamel into the amalgam. Carry the stroke into the central groove or a fossa. This same action is carried out for the lingual groove and any supplemental grooves.

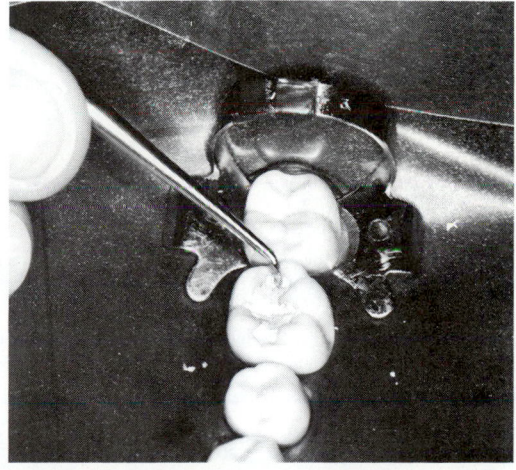

Fig. 34-81. The small discoid carver is used to define the distal fossa.

Check the restoration for the following criteria (Fig. 34-83):

1. Margins are flush with no open margins, submarginal areas, or flash.
2. Major anatomic contours such as cusp ridges, fossae, and major grooves are present.
3. All grooves and ridges present in the enamel are continued into the restoration.

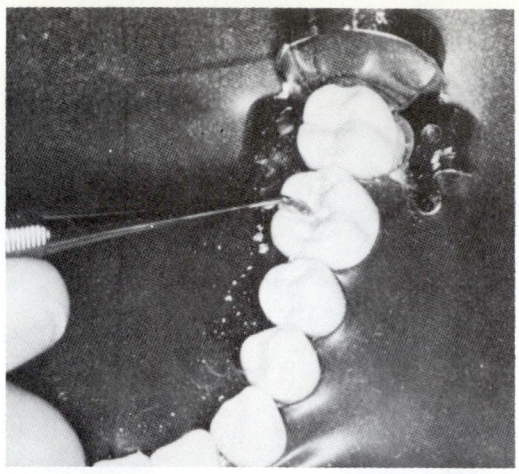

Fig. 34-82. Refining contours with the small cleoid carver adapted to the lingual margin. The tip is maintained in the central groove to avoid inadvertently creating grooves or scratches.

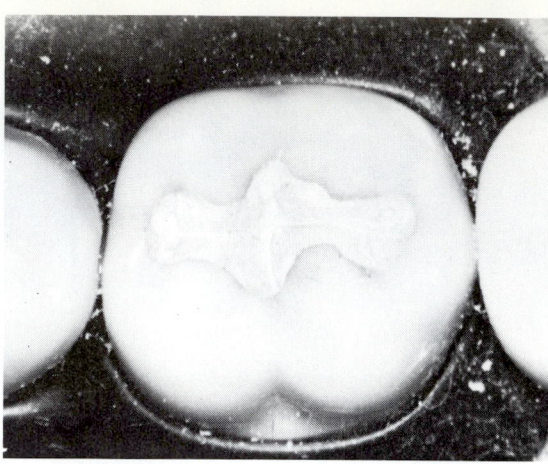

Fig. 34-83. Carving of the Class I restoration is complete. The outline of the restoration is smooth with no jagged edges.

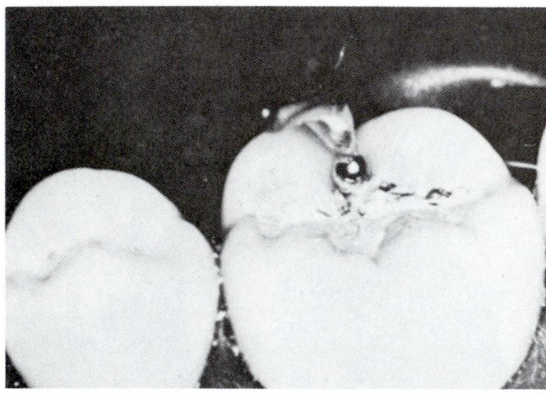

Fig. 34-84. The amalgam is burnished by moving the ball-shaped burnisher back and forth across the margins of the restoration.

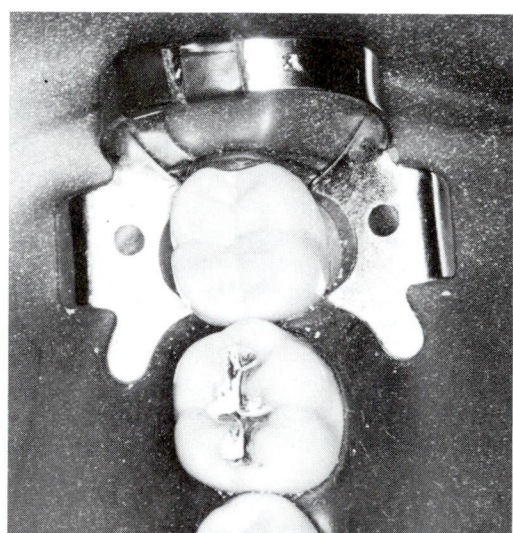

Fig. 34-85. The burnished restoration has a smooth, shiny appearance.

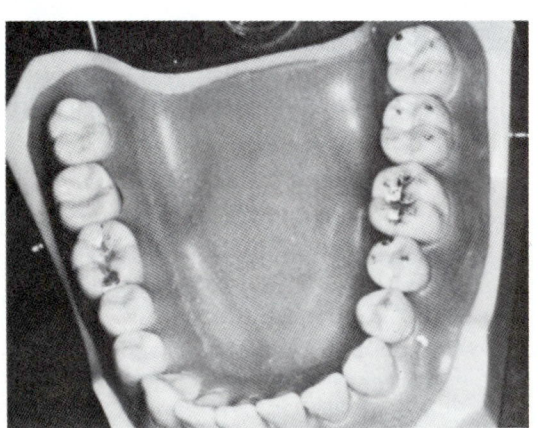

Fig. 34-86. Articulating-paper markings on the restoration must be of density equal to those on the surrounding tooth surface and adjacent teeth.

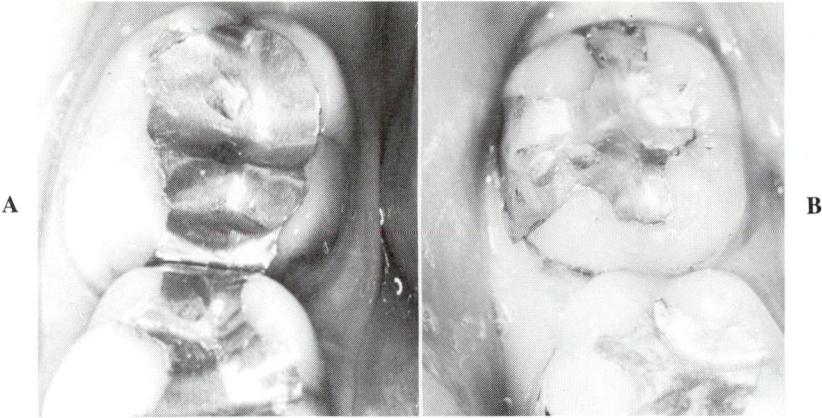

Fig. 34-87. Burnished spots on the amalgam surface.

Final burnishing

After initial set, burnish the contours using a small ball or football burnisher. Move the instrument back and forth from amalgam to tooth structure over the restoration with special emphasis on the margins. Use the tip to burnish in the fossae and down the grooves (Fig. 34-84) with enough force to create a shiny smooth appearance (Fig. 34-85). Wipe the surface of the restoration with a damp cotton roll. Rinse with a water spray and high-volume suction to remove debris. Remove the rubber dam.

Checking the occlusion

Check the patient's occlusion both visually and with the use of articulating paper. Before placing the articulating paper or (ribbon), dry both the maxillary and mandibular teeth. Use cotton pliers or Miller's holding forceps to insert the paper over the quadrant. Have the patient gently tap his or her teeth together. The marks on the restoration should be of the same density as those on the surrounding tooth structure and adjacent teeth (Fig. 34-86). Use a cleoid or discoid instrument to remove any area where markings indicate heavy contact. Have the patient close again on the marking articulating (paper) and then move the mandible from side to side and forward to check for premature contacts in lateral and protrusive movements. Remove areas indicating excessive contact. If the patient closes and moves without articulating paper in place, prematurities show as burnished or flattened spots on the amalgam sur-

face (Fig. 34-87). Ask the patient how the new restoration feels when he or she closes gently. If the patient notices any difference compared with before the restoration was placed, recheck for prematurities. After eliminating any prematurities, recheck that the restoration meets all of the criteria listed. (See criteria sheet at the end of the chapter.)

MATRIX FOR CONSERVATIVE CLASS II AMALGAM RESTORATIONS

The Class II cavity preparation removes the proximal surface as well as the occlusal grooves and fossae (Fig. 34-88). To create a "container" into which to condense the amalgam, a temporary wall is established (Fig. 34-89). The matrix that forms this wall creates a smooth external surface against which to condense the material.

The matrix is a thin metal band that is supported or stabilized, usually with a mechanical retainer, (e.g., the Tofflemire matrix retainer). A wedge adapts the band to the cervical region of the tooth and separates the teeth to ensure proper proximal contact in the completed restoration. Variations in Class II preparations affect the width of the band selected and the positioning of the matrix retainer (facial or lingual).

The commonly used matrix material is a thin stainless steel strip contoured to approximate the shape of the missing proximal tooth structure. Precut stainless steel matrix bands of various sizes are used with a Tofflemire retainer to accommodate variations in the location and size of the

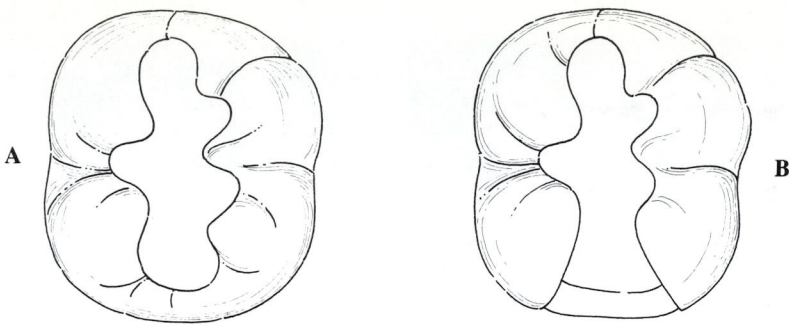

Fig. 34-88. Occlusal view of a Class I, **A**; and a Class II cavity preparation, **B**. A Class II cavity is the extension of a Class I cavity onto the proximal surface.

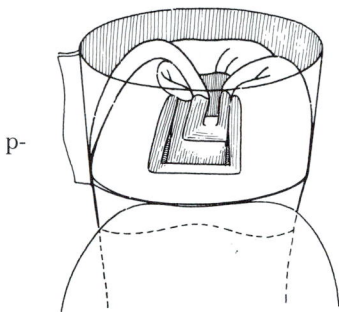

Fig. 34-89. Proximal view of the Class II cavity preparation with a matrix in place.

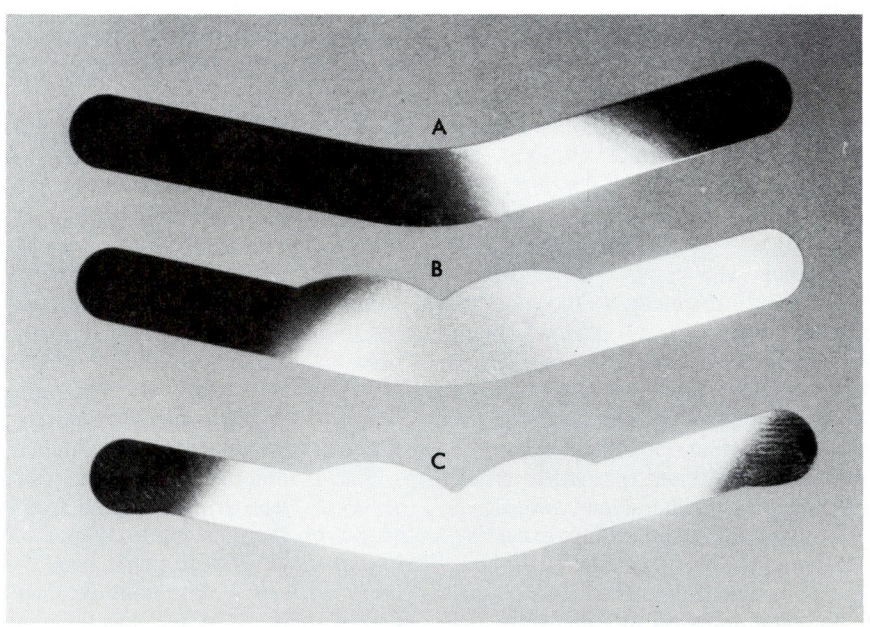

Fig. 34-90. Tofflemire matrix bands: **A**, universal band: **B** and **C**, variations of the extension band.

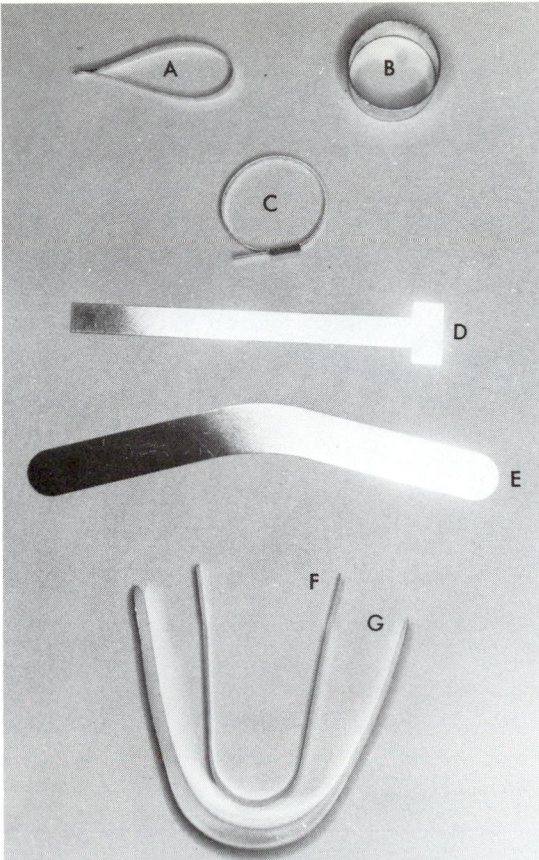

Fig. 34-91. Various forms of matrices: **A,** welded stainless steel; **B,** copper tube; **C,** T-band (assembled); **D,** T-band (unassembled); **E,** universal Tofflemire; **F** and **G,** precontoured stainless steel.

preparation. The two most commonly used bands are the universal and the MOD band (Fig. 34-90). The universal band is used for routine extension Class II preparations. The MOD band, which is elongated in the proximogingival areas, is used when the occlusogingival dimension of the preparation exceeds the height of the universal band. Other matrices are available for special applications (Fig. 34-91).

The band may need to be trimmed to fit variations in preparation design and size. In general, the principles for placement, wedging, and removal of the Tofflemire matrix will apply to all matrix systems.

The Tofflemire retainer is available in both straight (for application on the facial aspect) and

contraangled (for application on the lingual aspect) versions (Fig. 34-92). Sizes are available for both adult and deciduous dentitions. Fig. 34-93 demonstrates the placement of both the straight and contraangled retainers.

Armamentarium

The armamentarium suggested for the placement of the Tofflemire matrix is shown in Fig. 34-94. Cleanse and dry the preparation. Apply bases and liners before placing the matrix band. Examine the occlusogingival dimension to determine which size of band to use. It should extend 1 mm apical to the gingival wall(s) and 1 mm occlusal to the future marginal ridge(s). A band that extends too far occlusally obstructs the operator's mechanical and visual access to the preparation. A large facial extension of the preparation may require a contraangled retainer positioned from the lingual. Large lingual extensions call for a straight retainer applied from the facial.

Assembly of the retainer and band

Hold the retainer with the sliding body portion to the left and the slots opening towards the operator as shown in Fig. 34-95. Twist the outer knob counterclockwise to disengage the threaded set screw from the sliding body. The outer knob turns the set screw in the sliding body to wedge the matrix band in the slot. The inner knob moves the sliding body along the track toward or away from the head. Turn the inner knob counterclockwise until the sliding body resets against the retainer head (see Fig. 34-95). The retainer is now ready to receive the matrix band.

The matrix band is shaped like a shallow V with the base of the V downward. Place the ends together to create a loop with the smaller opening towards the operator. Place the ends into the slot of the sliding body, guiding the band through the first slot in the head. Then direct the band into the bottom slot (Fig. 34-96). Be certain that both ends have passed through the slots and have not been separated. Lock the band in place by turning the outer knob clockwise until the set screw is tight against the band.

In this arrangement, the band is ready for Class II preparations in the mandibular right or the maxillary left quadrants. Direct the band through the upper slot in the head for mandibular left or maxillary right quadrants (Fig. 34-97). Note that the smaller opening of the loop is facing in the

Text continued on page 761.

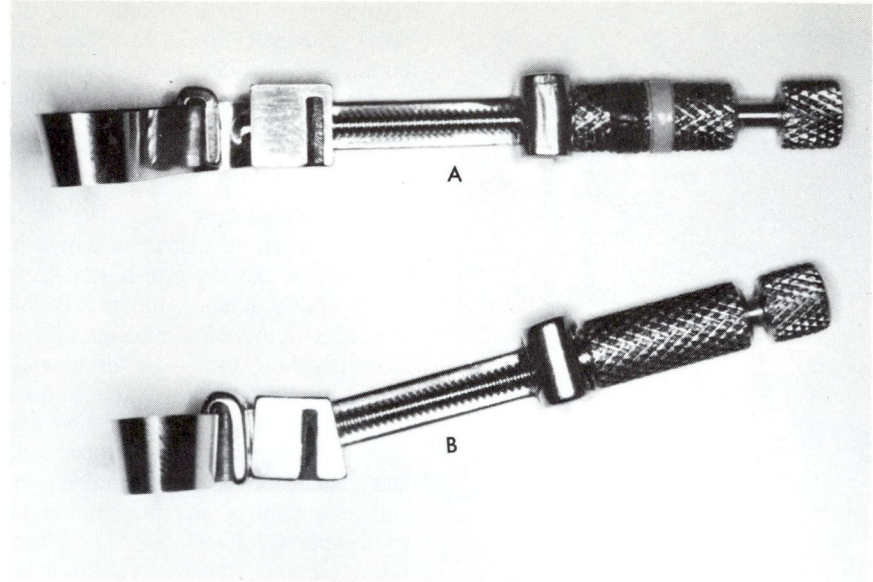

Fig. 34-92. Tofflemire matrix retainer and band assembled: **A,** straight; and **B,** contraangled.

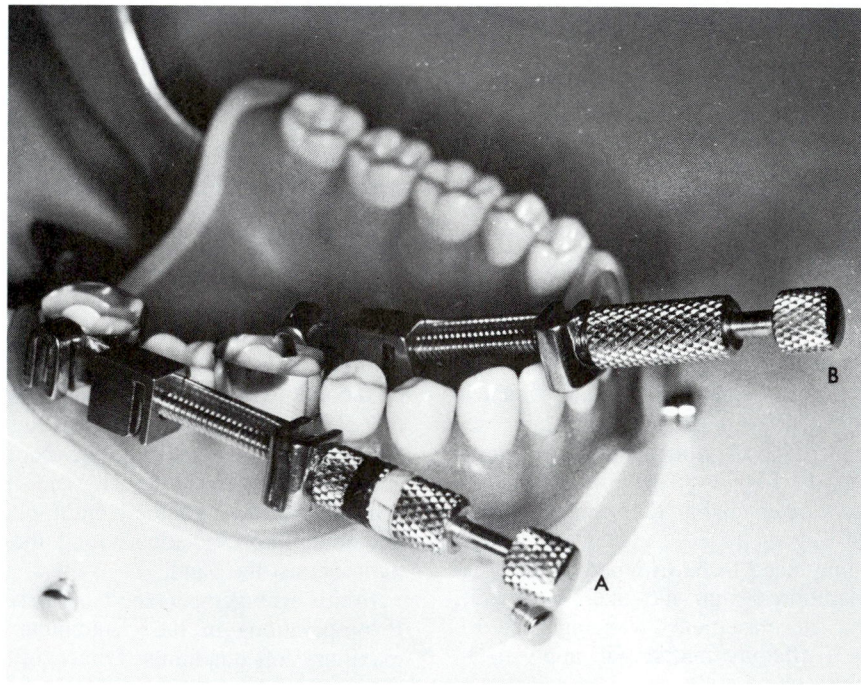

Fig. 34-93. Placement of the Tofflemire retainer and matrix band: **A,** straight retainer positioned from the facial aspect; and **B,** contraangled retainer positioned from the lingual aspect.

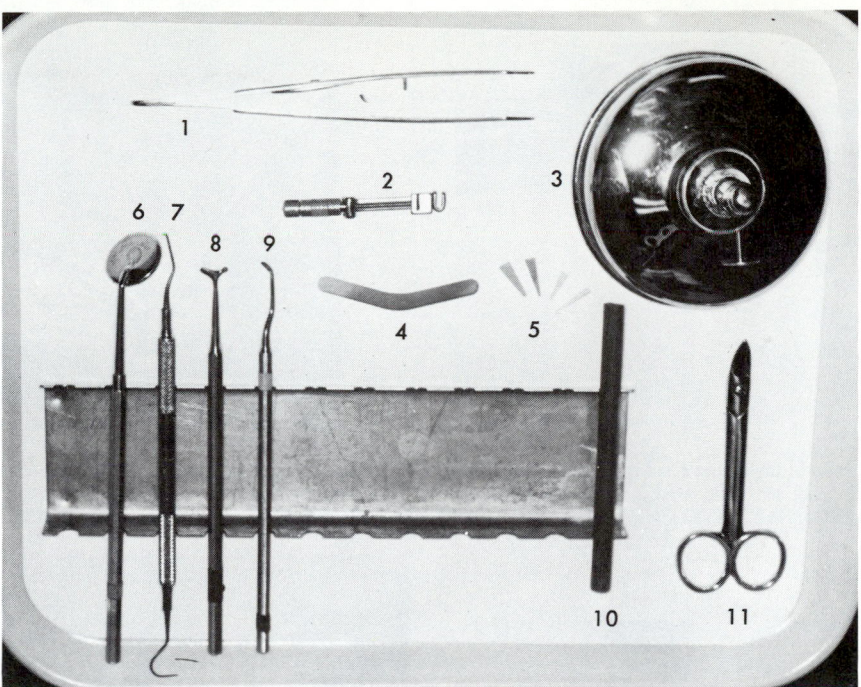

Fig. 34-94. The tray setup for placement of the Tofflemire matrix includes: *1*, locking cotton forceps; *2*, matrix retainer; *3*, alcohol lamp; *4*, matrix band; *5*, wooden wedges; *6*, mouth mirror; *7* shepherd's hook explorer; *8*, T-ball burnisher; *9*, gold knife; *10*, low-fusing dental compound stick; and *11*, crown and bridge scissors.

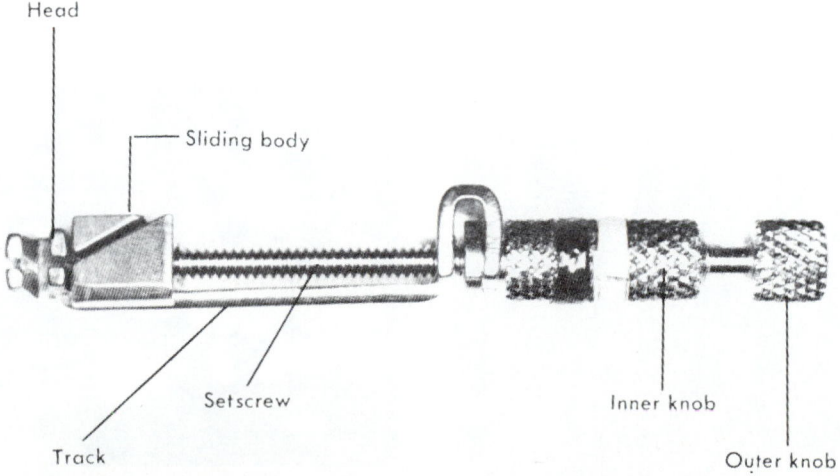

Fig. 34-95. The parts of the Tofflemire matrix retainer.

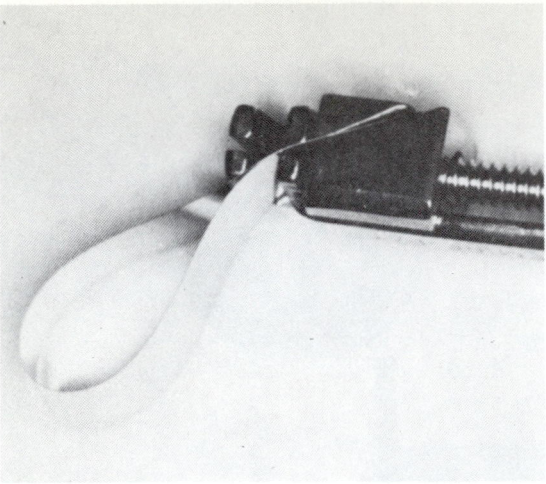

Fig. 34-96. The loop of the matrix band is passed through the bottom slot in the head. The band is positioned for application in the mandibular right or maxillary left quadrant.

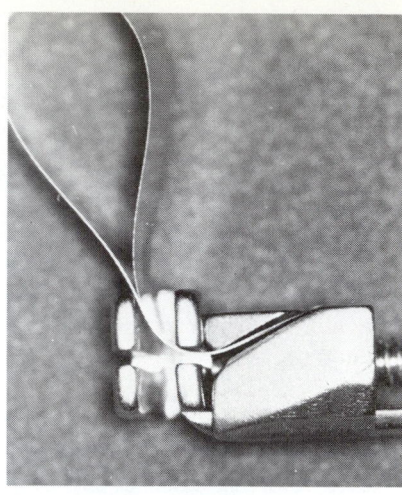

Fig. 34-97. The band is positioned for application in the mandibular left or maxillary right quadrant.

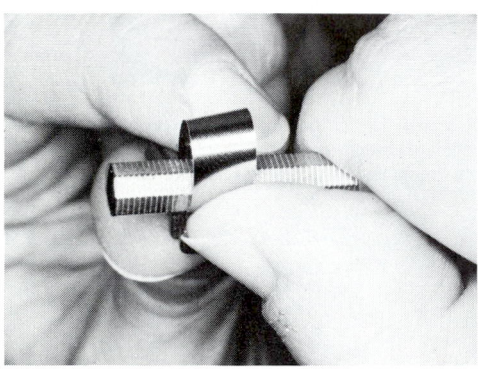

Fig. 34-98. Use an instrument handle to remove any creases in the band.

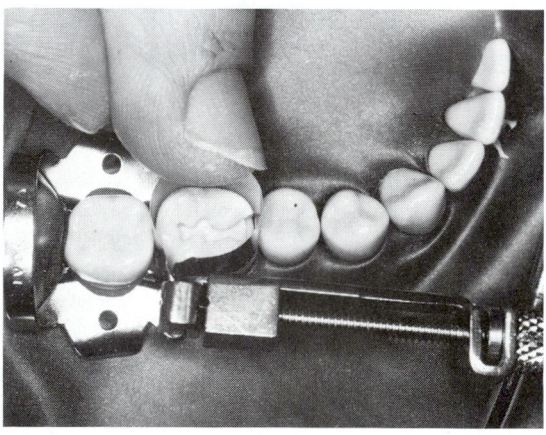

Fig. 34-99. Position the small opening of the band around the tooth.

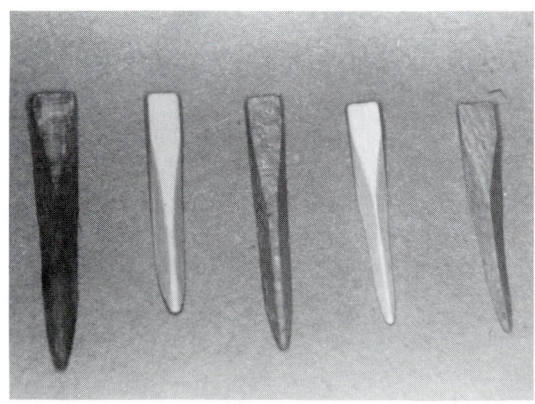

Fig. 34-100. Various sizes, shapes, and colors of precontoured wedges.

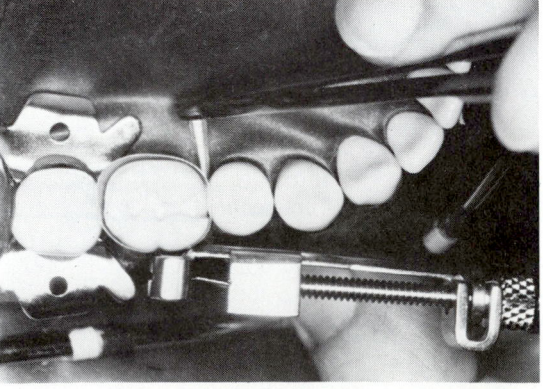

Fig. 34-101. Final positioning of the wedge with the handle of the forceps.

same direction as the slots of the head and body portions. This will be important for the removal of the matrix retainer.

After assembling the band and retainer, use a mirror handle to contour the band (Fig. 34-98). Press the band against the mirror handle to flatten any wrinkles or creases in the band. Avoid cutting your thumb on the sharp edge of the band.

Placement of the retainer and band on the prepared tooth

Position the retainer on the facial aspect of the tooth with the small opening toward the gingiva to adapt the band to the conical shape of the crown. Using your thumb or index finger against the occlusal edge, gently push the band gingivally through the contact areas. Seat the band until it extends approximately 1 mm beyond the gingival wall of the preparation. Avoid lacerating the gingival tissue with the edge of the band. Position the retainer parallel to the facial surfaces of the teeth (Fig. 34-99). While holding the band in position, twist the inner knob clockwise to tighten the band around the tooth. Tighten the knob until it offers moderate resistance. Turning the knob too tightly may flatten the proximal portion of the band, resulting in an undercontoured restoration. Insufficient tightening may result in an overcontoured restoration and poor adaptation along the margins.

Placement of the wedge

The wedge presses the band against the proximal surface apical to the gingivocavosurface margin to minimize amalgam being forced beyond the margin, which would create an overhang. The wedge also separates the teeth slightly to compensate for the thickness of the matrix band. This movement of the teeth, made possible by the compressibility of the periodontal ligament, ensures contact between the teeth after the band is removed and the teeth return to their normal position. Wedges are manufactured in various sizes and forms (precontoured and uncontoured) (Fig. 34-100). Precontoured wedges may not require any modifications for conservative class II preparations.

The wedge may need contouring to achieve the desired effect. Observe the height and width of the gingival embrasure, noting the level of the gingival margin and its relationship to the papilla. Note whether the faciolingual contour is broad and flat (most molars) or cylindrical (most premolars). Select the correct wedge and alter it to the

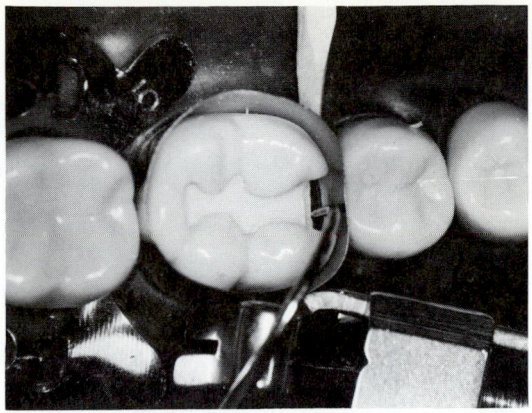

Fig. 34-102. Improper wedge selection or placement may result in the matrix band not being held against the tooth properly.

shape necessary to apply pressure to the band apical to the gingival margin.

Uncontoured wedges form a triangle with two longer sides of equal length. Place the base (shorter side) against the gingival tissue with a pair of locking forceps. Insert it into the lingual proximal embrasure. Angle the tip of the wedge to avoid injury to the papilla. Release the wedge from the locking forceps. Using moderate force with the handle, push the wedge into the embrasure until firmly placed (Fig. 34-101).

Evaluate the matrix and wedge. The band should be tightly adapted to the entire width at the gingival margin. To check this, place an explorer tip against the inside of the matrix at the gingival wall. If gentle force on the explorer tip creates an opening, the wedge is not holding the band against the tooth (Fig. 34-102). Either the wedge is too narrow or it has not been positioned far enough into the embrasure.

If the proximal portion is relatively flat, then little or no contouring of the wedge is necessary. If the tooth contour is cylindrical in shape, the wedge must be contoured.

If the wedge extends too far occlusally, trim it with a gold knife or scalpel (Fig. 34-103). Replace the wedge and re-evaluate it (Fig. 34-104). Burnish the matrix band using a small ball burnisher (Fig. 34-105). The contact area is at junction of the occlusal and middle thirds of the tooth. Burnish the metal to slightly stretch and contour the matrix in the contact area and ensure that contact with the adjacent tooth will be re-established.

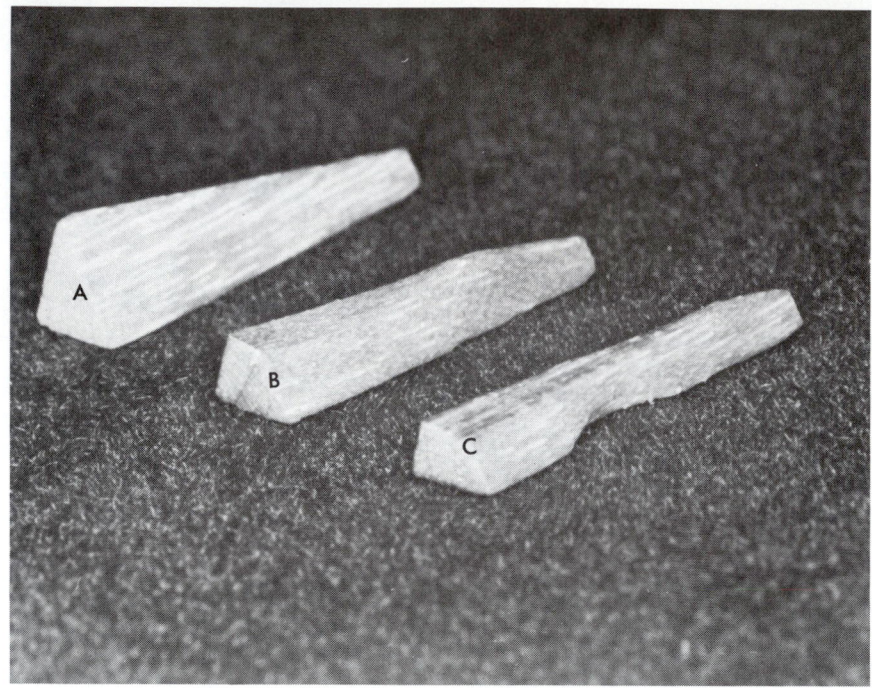

Fig. 34-103. The wedge trimmed for premolar application: **A,** untrimmed; **B,** occlusal height reduced; and **C,** proximal contour trimmed.

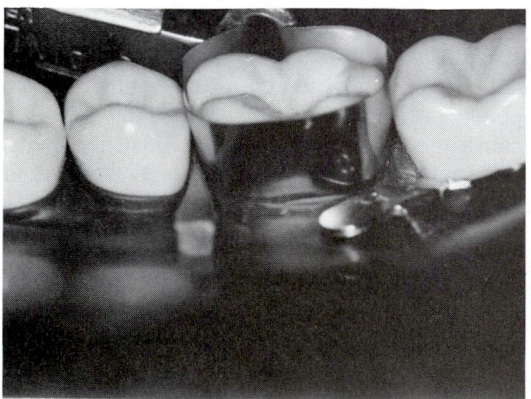

Fig. 34-104. Lingual view of a properly trimmed and positioned wedge.

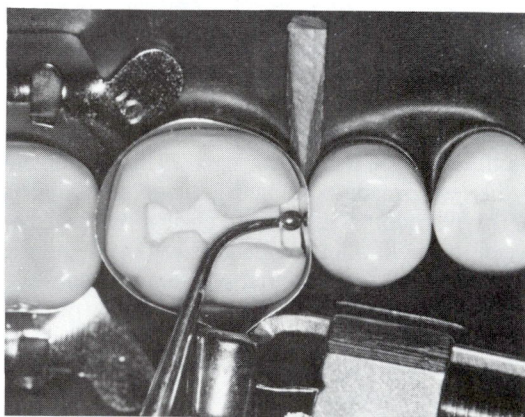

Fig. 34-105. The contact area is burnished before amalgam placement.

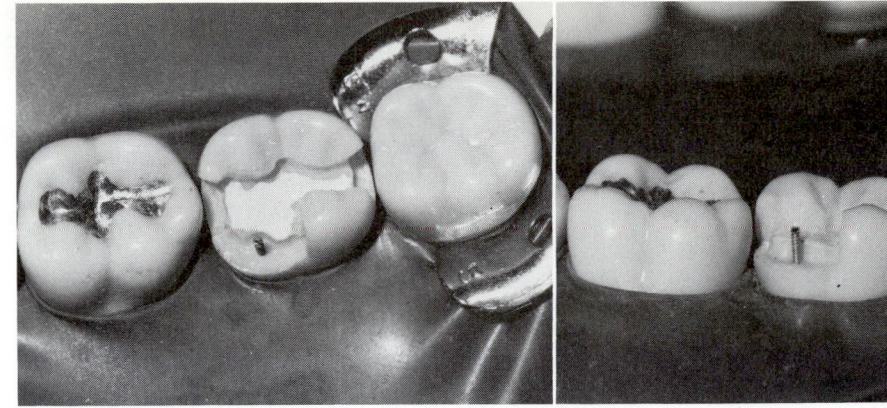

Fig. 34-106. **A,** Occlusal view of a complex Class II amalgam preparation with the mesiofacial cusp removed. A retentive pin has been placed. **B,** Facial view of the preparation.

Refer to criteria sheet at the end of the chapter.

A custom matrix may be required if the Tofflemire matrix does not provide adequate extension and/or support for placement of the amalgam. The functions, principles of application, and evaluation criteria for the custom matrix are basically the same as those for the Tofflemire matrix. A custom matrix may be indicated for cavity preparations involving:

1. Removal of one or more cusps
2. Teeth with unusually long clinical crowns
3. Teeth that have no contact with adjacent teeth
4. Interference with Tofflemire retainer placement by a rubber dam clamp
5. Adjacent class II preparations to be restored simultaneously

The Tofflemire matrix presents problems with large restorations. A gap occurs in the area where the band enters in the retainer head. The band does not provide a proper contour for this portion of the tooth. The matrix may collapse and lose proper contour when tightened if it is not sufficiently supported by the tooth. In general, the greater the extent of the preparation, the less satisfactory is the Tofflemire matrix system.

The application of the matrix and wedges is influenced by the location of the margins of the cavity preparation. Extensions of the proximal or occlusal walls onto the facial or lingual surfaces or the removal of a cusp(s) will determine which matrix will be placed and how it will be stabilized.

Fig. 34-106 illustrates a Class II preparation of the mesial, occlusal, distal, and facial surfaces. The mesiofacial cusp has been removed, and a threaded pin has been placed in this area. The gingival wall now extends from the linguoproximal wall to the distal wall on the facial surface. Because of lack of support for the matrix band in this area, dental compound will be used to provide support.

Several types of matrices are available, such as copper bands or tubes, brass T-bands, and stainless steel strips (bulk, roll, or precut) of various widths. The choice of the type of matrix is influenced by the clinical situation. Although these types are of different materials and handle somewhat differently, the basic principles for application described apply to all.

The copper band matrix is more rigid and self-supporting than the stainless steel band; these are advantages for very extensive preparations. If the restoration is a temporary one and a crown is to be placed later, re-creation of the exact anatomy is less critical. The copper band may be the matrix of choice because of the simplicity of adapting it to the cervical portion of the tooth and its strength.

The brass T-band matrix is available in both narrow and wide sizes. It is primarily used for the restoration of deciduous teeth but can be adapted and contoured for use on permanent teeth as well.

The thinness of the welded stainless steel custom matrix makes it more desirable for use when contact with the adjacent teeth must be re-established. Consult a current textbook of operative dentistry for more information.

RESTORATION OF THE CONSERVATIVE CLASS II AMALGAM PREPARATION
Review the preparation

Access to the proximal surfaces is limited by adjacent teeth, making it necessary to remove the marginal ridge. The occlusal portion is similar to the Class I preparation (Fig. 34-107). The proximal portion extends gingivally past the contact area near the gingival tissue and facially and lingually beyond the contact with the adjacent tooth (1 to 1.5 mm).

Retention of the restoration is provided by the parallel walls of the occlusal portion and the parallel or slightly convergent walls and retentive grooves of the proximal box (Fig. 34-108). Angulation of the walls resists occlusal displacement of the restoration. The retentive grooves are located in the proximal facioaxial and linguoaxial line angles, extending occlusally from the gingival wall to the dentinoenamel junction.

The proximal contact is important. If it is not correctly restored, the tooth may shift or drift, creating occlusion problems and upsetting the stability of other teeth in the arch. Inadequate contact and incorrect proximal contours may encourage food impaction and/or cause difficulty in maintaining adequate oral hygiene.

It is helpful to observe the occlusal relationships of the involved tooth before the rubber dam is placed. If the tooth or teeth have long or sharp cusps, marginal ridge discrepancies, or other variations from normal, changes in the anatomy of the planned restoration may be necessary.

Condensing the amalgam

Mix the amalgam as previously described. Place the first increment into the least accessible area along the gingival wall of the proximal box (Fig. 34-109). Extrude only one-half of the amalgam carrier load. Select a condenser that will fit easily into the proximal box.

Condense the amalgam against the gingival wall by holding the nib perpendicular to the gingival wall. Make overlapping strokes (Fig. 34-110) across the gingival wall from the facioproximal line angle to the linguoproximal line angle. Change the direction of the strokes to condense against the line angles. A 30- to 45-degree angle will ensure thorough condensation in these corners. Use the side as well as end of the condenser nib to condense the amalgam into the retentive grooves.

Condense the amalgam against the gingivocavosurface margin and the matrix band by directing the condenser against the side of the band and pushing gingivally. This ensures good condensation into the facial and lingual corners formed by the cavosurface margins and the band.

After the first increment is condensed, place the second increment (one-half carrier load) into the proximal box. Make each condensing stroke quickly and firmly, overlapping it with the previous stroke. Direct the strokes towards the gingival wall, the line angles, the retentive grooves, and the axial walls. If both proximal surfaces have been prepared, repeat the condensation process for the other proximal box. Remember that 2½ to 3 minutes is the maximum time before a new batch of amalgam must be mixed.

When the amalgam reaches the level of the pulpoaxial line angle (Fig. 34-111), spread it onto the pulpal floor. Place it in the same manner as for the Class I preparation. Focus attention on the marginal ridge area along the matrix band to ensure adequate filling. Be sure it is well condensed against the matrix band to a height of approximately 1 mm occlusal to the height of the marginal ridge of the adjacent tooth (Fig. 34-112).

The amalgam should now overfill the occlusal surface of the preparation by approximately 1.0 mm and extend 0.5 to 1.0 mm beyond the margins without pits or voids.

Initial burnishing

Burnish as for the class I amalgam. Avoid elimination of too much material in the area of the future marginal ridge. Use an explorer or Hollenback carver to round the outer portion of the marginal ridge area. Place the instrument on the tooth structure slightly facial to the marginal ridge at the juncture of the marginal ridge and the facial cusp. Hold the instrument at a 30-degree angle to the long axis with the tip touching the matrix band to guide the stroke. Move it lingually, ending the stroke about halfway between the facial and lingual margins. The marginal ridge should be rounded at a height equal to the adjacent marginal ridge. If it is too flat, increase the angulation of the explorer to approximately 45 degrees and repeat the stroke to round the marginal ridge. Place the instrument at the same angle and slightly lingual to the lingual margin. Move it facially to blend this area.

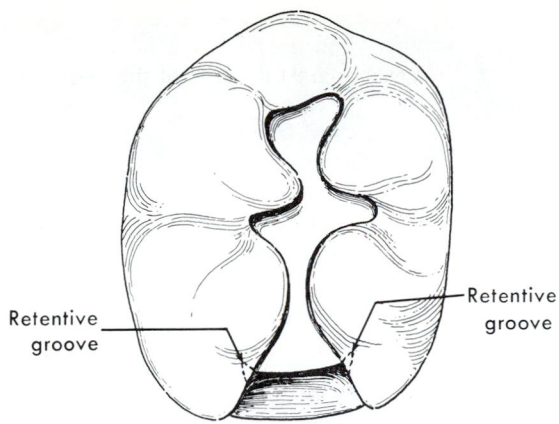

Fig. 34-107. The occlusal view of a Class II preparation shows the outline and extension. The retentive grooves in the facioaxial and linguoaxial line angles are indicated by the arrows.

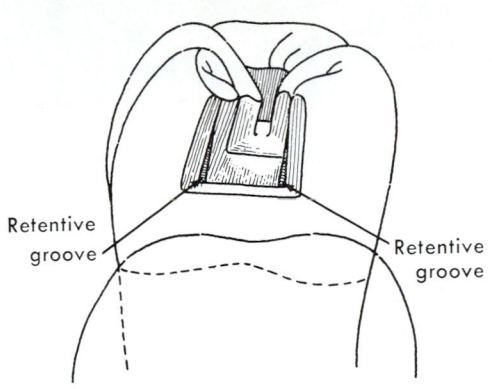

Fig. 34-108. The proximal view shows the proximal extension and the preparation's relationship to the gingival tissue. The retentive grooves are indicated by arrows.

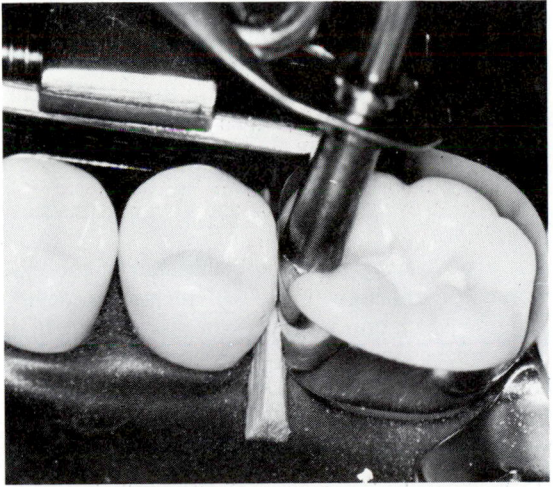

Fig. 34-109. Placing the first carrier load of amalgam into the proximal box enables the least accessible area to be condensed first.

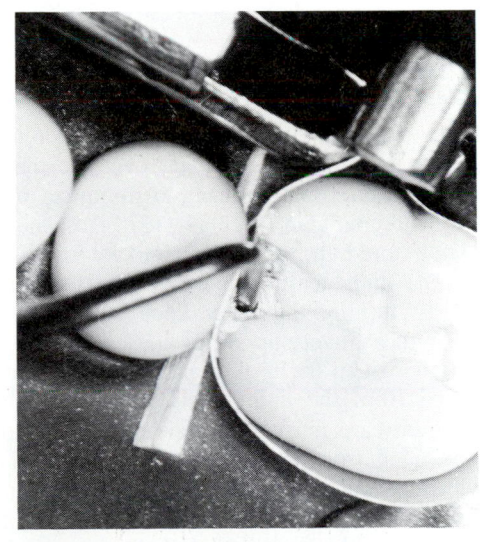

Fig. 34-110. The first condensing strokes are directed perpendicularly.

Remove the gross excess from the occlusal surfaces as described for the class I restoration. Initiate the carving of the mesial fossa with the large discoid carver. Because there is no marginal ridge to serve as reference, take care not to form the fossa too near the proximal surface. Observe the marginal ridge on the opposite proximal surface and/or the adjacent tooth. The fossa should be located just proximal to the facial and lingual triangular ridges. Be careful to preserve the marginal ridge area.

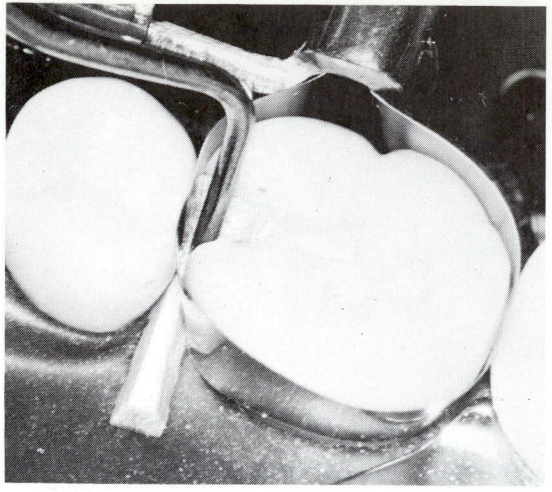

Fig. 34-111. The diamond-shaped nib can be used effectively to condense amalgam into the retentive grooves and the line angles formed by facial and lingual cavosurface margins and the matrix band.

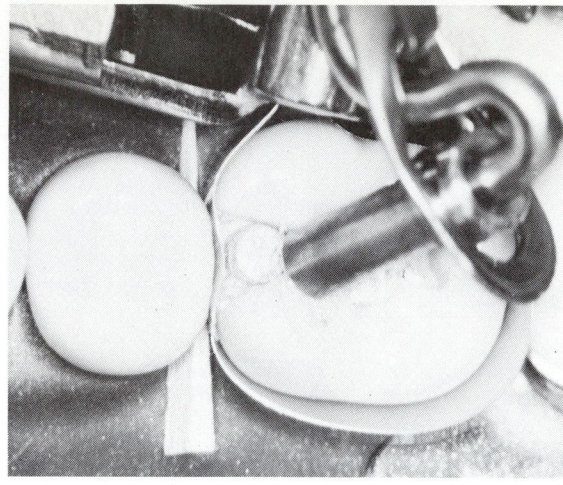

Fig. 34-112. The amalgam is placed onto the pulpal wall only after the proximal amalgam is condensed to the level of the pulpoaxial line angle.

Removal of the wedge, matrix band, and retainer

Pull the wedge lingually with the cotton pliers. Place the thumb or index finger over the matrix band at the proximal surfaces to minimize pressure on the amalgam (Fig. 34-113). Turn the inner knob one-half turn counterclockwise to increase the diameter of the loop. Release the set screw by turning the outer knob counterclockwise. With a finger supporting the band, remove the retainer in an occlusal direction. Then remove the band from the uninvolved proximal embrasure. Great care must be exercised when removing the band from the restored proximal area to avoid fracturing the marginal ridge. Grasp each end of the band a few millimeters from the tooth. If working with an assistant, have him or her place a large nibbed condenser on the marginal ridge area to counteract forces exerted when the band is pulled occlusally. Pull the band linguoocclusally until resistance is felt (Fig. 34-114). Change the direction of pull to a facioocclusal. Again, pull until resistance is felt (Fig. 34-115). Continue to pull and reverse direction when resistance is felt until the band is pulled free.

Carving of the proximal surface

Evaluate the gingival margin while the amalgam is still soft. Place the explorer tip into the gingival embrasure apical to the margin. Gently pass it over the margin to check for an overhang. Pass the explorer from the amalgam to tooth surface to check for a submarginal defect (Fig. 34-116). Repeat this from both the lingual and facial embrasures. Use the side rather than the tip of the explorer to prevent scratching or gouging the surface.

If an overhang exists, use the side of the explorer to burnish away excess. Recheck to determine if the margin is flush with the enamel. If it has hardened somewhat, insert the blade of an amalgam knife into the facial embrasure below the gingival margin and pull in an occlusofacial direction in a smooth shaving stroke (Fig. 34-117). As the proximal contact area is neared, decrease the carving pressure and pull the instrument out into the facial embrasure to avoid damaging the contact. Repeat the stroke from the lingual aspect, overlapping the stroke made from the facial direction. Recheck the margin using an explorer.

Remove any overcontoured areas or flash from the facial and lingual margins of the proximal surfaces. Hold the blade of the ½ Hollenback carver perpendicular to the facial margin of the preparation near the marginal ridge (Fig. 34-118). Angle the blade towards the adjacent tooth with the tip contacting it. Carve with the edge rather

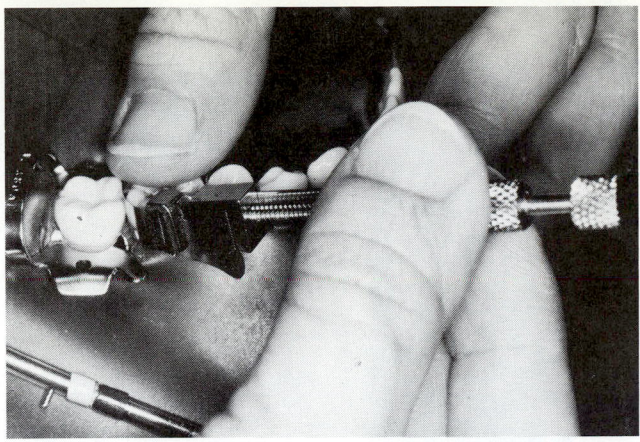

Fig. 34-113. Brace the matrix while turning the knob.

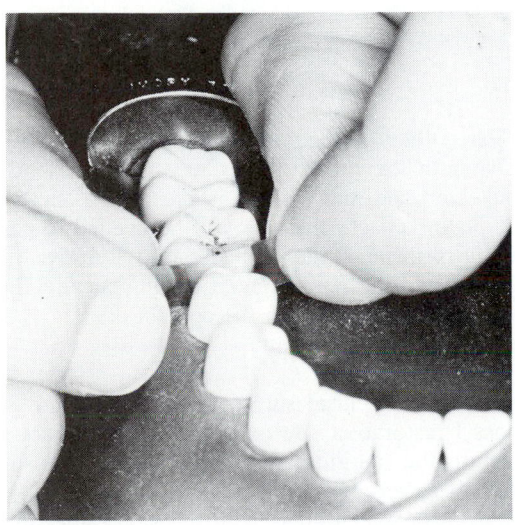

Fig. 34-114. The matrix band is pulled occlusolingually until resistance is felt.

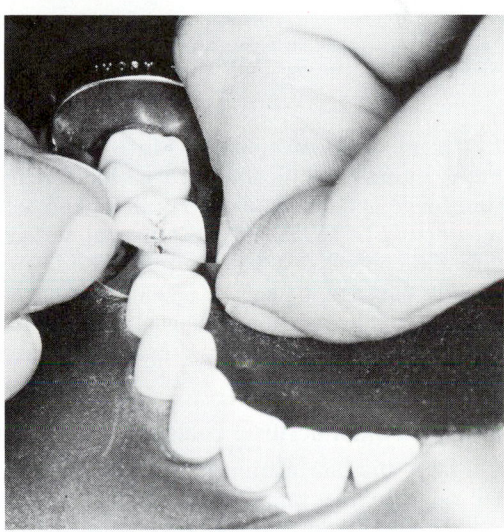

Fig. 34-115. The direction is changed to pull the band occlusofacially until resistance is felt.

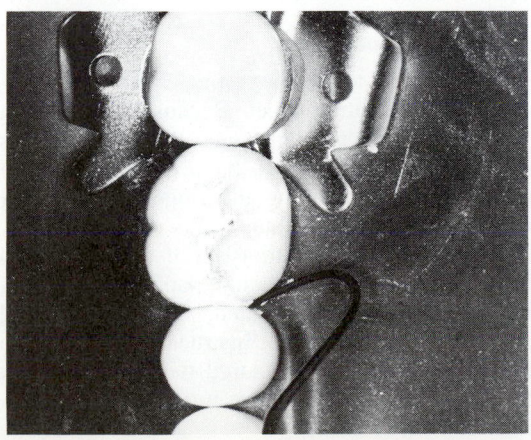

Fig. 34-116. Check for overextensions and submarginal areas with the explorer tip.

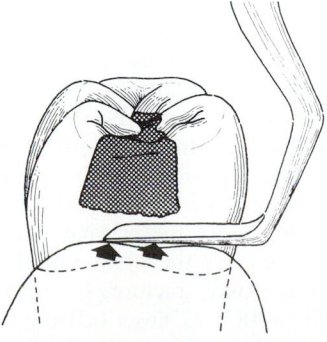

Fig. 34-117. The blade of the amalgam knife is inserted gingival to the gingival margin and is kept in contact with the tooth as it is moved occlusally past the margin. The amalgam is shaved away.

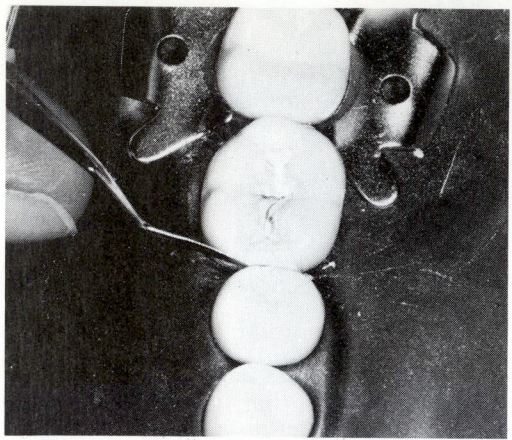

Fig. 34-118. Round the mesiofacial line angle with a ½ Hollenback carver. Use a shaving stroke to avoid the danger of fracturing the marginal ridge.

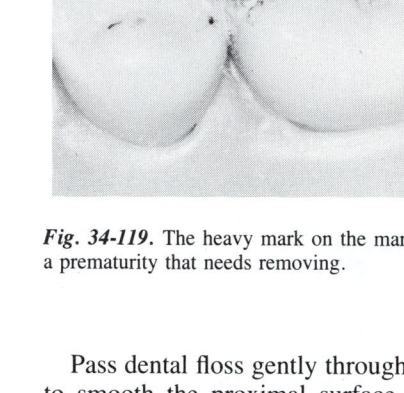

Fig. 34-119. The heavy mark on the marginal ridge indicates a prematurity that needs removing.

than the tip of the instrument. Move the instrument in a gingival direction to round the facioaxial line angle and open the embrasure without creating a ledge or corner on the proximal surface. Define the contour and the margin of the lingual portion in the same manner. Continue the shaving strokes until the facial and lingual surfaces are rounded and the embrasures are correctly contoured.

Carving the final occlusal contours

Use a large discoid instrument to adjust the marginal ridge to the same height as the adjacent tooth. Resting the instrument on the adjacent marginal ridge, move it from tooth to amalgam, stopping short of the opposite cavosurface margin. If the teeth are malaligned, supraerupted, or not correctly restored, there may be a discrepancy in marginal ridge height. The restored ridge height may be a compromise between matching the adjacent ridge and restoring the original anatomy of the tooth. After the marginal ridge is adjusted, redefine the adjacent fossa if necessary. Orient the small cleoid blade so the point rests in the central groove area and the side rests on enamel. Move the instrument in a mesial or distal direction. The tooth structure guides the carving to avoid overcarving. Do not carry the stroke into the marginal ridge; the ridge may fracture. Continue to carve the occlusal portion as described for the Class I restoration. Evaluate the carving by the criteria at the end of the chapter.

Pass dental floss gently through the contact area to smooth the proximal surface, remove debris, and determine that contact is present. If there is adequate contact, pressure will be needed to pass the floss through the contact area. Remove the floss by pulling it in a facial or lingual direction rather than back through the contact area.

Final burnishing

Burnish the occlusal surface as described for the Class I restoration. Be particularly careful not to fracture the marginal ridge by exerting pressure on it. If accessible, burnish the facioaxial and linguoaxial proximal areas with the side rather than the cutting edge of the Hollenback carver. Position the carver with the tip against the adjacent tooth to avoid creating a defect.

Checking the occlusion

After removing the rubber dam, check the occlusion with articulating paper. Because the marginal ridge is not well supported and the amalgam has not reached final strength, have the patient close gently to avoid breaking the ridge. Observe for burnish spots or dark blue spots (Fig. 34-119). Check the occlusal relationship of the unaffected teeth without the articulating paper in place. If prematurities are discovered, use the discoid carver to remove them. Instruct the patient to avoid chewing on the restored tooth for the next 24 hours. Indicate that there may be some sensitivity to heat or cold.

Evaluation criteria
Surface texture

1. The amalgam is smooth.
2. No pits or voids are present.
3. The amalgam has a dull luster; if the surface has been burnished, it is somewhat shiny.

Anatomic form

1. Triangular ridges of cusps extend to the central groove.
2. Fossae are the correct size, depth, and location.
3. Major grooves are distinct and correctly located.
4. Supplemental grooves present in the adjacent enamel extend into restoration.

Marginal integrity

1. No open margins are present.
2. No submarginal areas are present that cannot be smoothed during finishing and polishing.
3. Amalgam does not extend beyond cavosurface margin of the restoration.

Occlusal contacts

1. Articulating paper marks are of equal density on both restoration and tooth; contacts (indicated by marks) occur in fossae of the restoration if the relationship with opposing tooth or teeth permits.
2. Uninvolved teeth occlude as they did before procedure.
3. Patient reports that restoration does not feel "high."

Proximal contours and contact

1. Marginal ridge is rounded to form an occlusal embrasure.
2. Proximal contour is primarily convex faciolingually.
3. Occlusogingivally, the contact area is convex from the marginal ridge through the contact area.
4. From gingival border of the contact area to the cervical line, the contour is flat or slightly concave.
5. Lingual embrasure is slightly larger than facial embrasure.
6. Proximal contact with the adjacent tooth occurs facial to the midline faciolingually and in the gingival portion of the occlusal one-third occlusogingivally.

• • •

The procedures described provide the basic techniques for restoring a conservative Class II amalgam preparation. Larger preparations require more skill and the use of additional techniques.

For restoration of complex amalgam preparations, consult operative dentistry textbooks.

RECONTOURING AND FINISHING

It is important to recontour and finish both old and new restorations. If restorations are of questionable quality, they may need to be replaced. The decision depends on factors such as size of marginal discrepancies, uncorrectable overhangs, recurrent decay, and excessively deep occlusal anatomy.

Recontouring reduces or alters bulky and/or overextended areas to blend with the normal contours of the tooth. Finishing smooths the overall surface of the restoration and blends the specific details, such as margins, to the surrounding anatomy of the tooth. Polishing places a high shine or luster on the surface. Though polishing has been long advocated, research has not shown that it prolongs the life of high-copper amalgam, which is the type used in most dental offices and clinics. Recontouring, finishing, and polishing are not completely separate procedures but rather steps in a process. Amalgam is gradually removed in decreasing amounts to produce the desired results.

Overhangs are overcontours on proximal surfaces. One radiographic survey showed that 52% of class II restorations exhibit overhangs (Coxhead et al, 1978). Overhangs are associated with gingival and periodontal disease (Hakkarainen and Ainamo, 1980; Jeffcoat et al, 1980; Leon, 1977). Mechanical impingement on the soft tissues may be a problem but, more importantly, the overhang is a plaque-retentive area that complicates oral hygiene. Removal of overhangs and subsequent finishing and polishing of the area, in conjunction with plaque removal procedures by the patient, improve the health of the gingiva and supporting structures (Axelsson, 1981; Gorzo et al, 1979; Highfield and Powell, 1978; Rodriguez-Ferrer et al, 1980).

Armamentarium

A variety of instruments, including both hand and rotary instruments, are available for recontouring and finishing. Selection is based on accessibility of the area, amount of reduction required, and surface finish desired. Limit the number of instruments to keep the technique simple, speedy, and efficient. The rotary instruments commonly used for recontouring and finishing are burs, abrasive

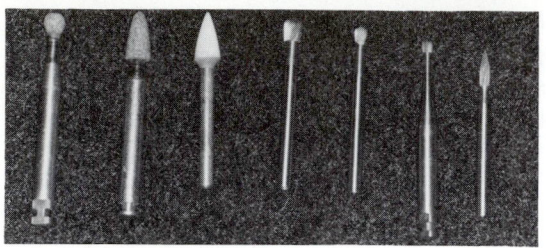

Fig. 34-120. Examples of burs and stones commonly used during finishing and polishing. *Left to right,* round and tapered green stones, white stone, plug-shaped, round-shaped, and flame-shaped finishing burs. Available for both friction-grip and latch-type handpieces.

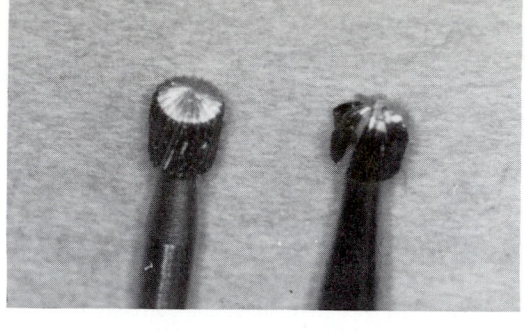

Fig. 34-121. The finishing bur on the left has more blades and produces a smoother surface than the cutting bur on the right.

stones, and finishing disks (Fig. 34-120).

Plain steel rather than carbide cutting burs are used for recontouring and finishing amalgam restorations (Fig. 34-121). Finishing burs have more and smaller cutting edges (18 to 20) which are designed to leave a smoother surface. Various shapes and sizes are needed for access. Flame-shaped burs recommended are for narrow areas such as embrasures, round or plug-shaped burs for fossae and grooves, and a pear-shaped or barrel-shaped bur for finishing cusp inclines. Rotary instruments with big circumferences contact more tooth structure and generate more heat. Take care to avoid overheating the tooth and restoration.

Stones can be long and tapered for occlusal or smooth surface restorations or rounded for use in fossae. Abrasiveness depends on the size and type of particles incorporated in the matrix of the stone. Particles in green stones are more abrasive than those in white stones. Green stones are used to remove excess amalgam. White stones are used to reduce small areas of enamel and/or amalgam around marginal discrepancies and for limited surface reduction.

Thin, flat discs can be adapted along broad, smooth surfaces. They are ideal for Class V restorations or facial and lingual extensions of Class II restorations. They are also used to recontour the interproximal surface in the occlusal embrasure areas. Discs are available in different sizes. Both snap-on and screw-in discs with correspondingly designed mandrels are available in a variety of grits (Fig. 34-122). The most commonly used are garnet (coarse) and cuttle (fine). In most instances

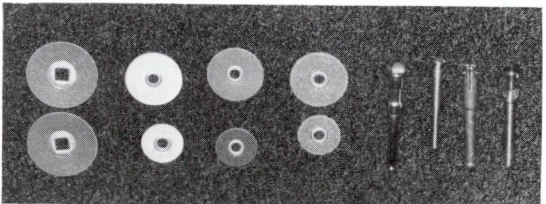

Fig. 34-122. Examples of the different types of mandrels and disks available.

fine garnet is the most abrasive disc used, followed by fine cuttle.

Hand instruments. Hand instruments used to remove overhangs on the gingival cavosurface margin are the amalgam knife, files, and curettes. The amalgam knife is usually the instrument of choice. Files are used when the amalgam knife is inadequate. Universal curettes can remove small amalgam extensions and, when necessary, smooth the amalgam after knives or files have been used.

Procedure

Because amalgam is not completely set until 24 hours after placement, recontouring and finishing should not be initiated until then. Premature attempts interfere with the crystalline structure of the hardening amalgam, resulting in a weakened restoration. Although there have been experiments with finishing high copper amalgams within 10 minutes of placement (Corpron et al, 1982; Creaven et al, 1980; Nitkin, 1979; Schemlitzer et al, 1982) it is presently recommended to wait at least 24 hours (Craig, 1989; Creaven et al, 1980; Schemlitzer et al, 1982).

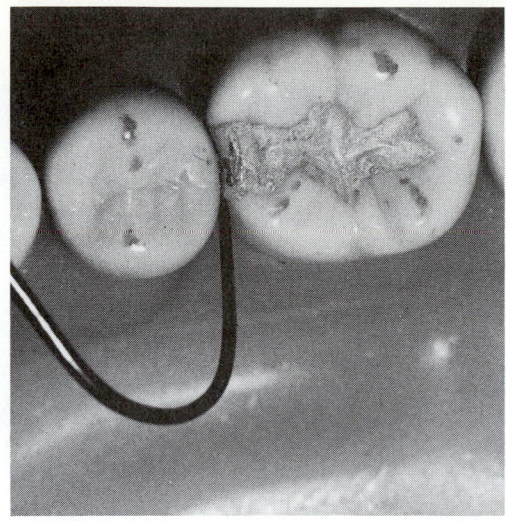

Fig. 34-123. Heavy occlusal contacts are detected with articulating paper. Note the darker marking on the mesial marginal ridge. The explorer points to an overextension along the mesiolingual margin.

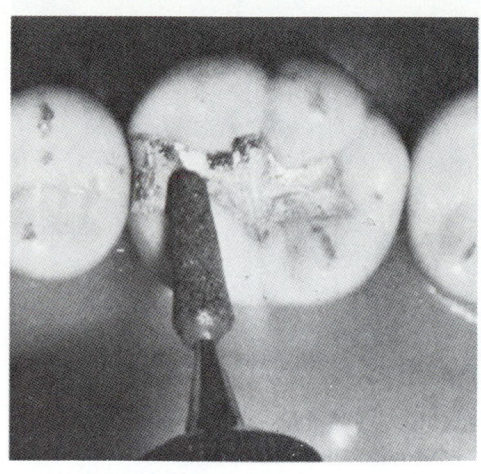

Fig. 34-124. The green stone removes excess amalgam rapidly. It is used only for recontouring because it leaves a rough finish.

Recontouring and finishing the occlusal surface

Evaluate the occlusal contours of the restoration. Mark the occlusion with articulating paper in centric and excursive movements. If the markings indicate prematurities, the areas must be reduced to prevent occlusal trauma (Fig. 34-123). Place the side of the tapered green stone against the amalgam and move it back and forth with light intermittent pressure until the excess is removed (Fig. 34-124). Recheck the occlusion and continue until the prematurity is eliminated.

Use a pointed white stone to smooth tarnished, corroded, and pitted surfaces or to eliminate any submarginal discrepancy less than 0.2 mm (Fig. 34-125). Place the side of the stone on the enamel, moving it back and forth at medium speed until the enamel is flush with the amalgam. Avoid excess heat and the possibility of removing too much enamel.

Finishing burs are used next to eliminate small excesses and to reshape and define the anatomy, producing a smooth finish. They are designed to cut when they are rotated either clockwise or counterclockwise. Smooth the occlusal margins with a round finishing bur. Place the side against both amalgam and tooth surface (Fig. 34-126). Use light, intermittent strokes as the bur is

moved along the entire margin. For larger restorations, a barrel- or pear-shaped finishing bur may be used.

It is possible to improve the occlusal anatomy by using a round finishing bur in the fossae (Fig. 34-127). The fossae should be extended only to a depth consistent with the rest of the occlusal anatomy. Define developmental grooves with a No. 1 round or flame-shaped finishing bur. As the bur is not resting on tooth structure, control it carefully (Fig. 34-128). Use the bur to make developmental and supplemental grooves distinct but not deep.

Recontouring and finishing facial and lingual surfaces

Recontour and smooth the facial and lingual surfaces with medium and fine finishing discs. Use light, sweeping strokes, moving the disk from the margin toward the center of the restoration (Fig. 34-129). Take care not to overreduce the restoration. After recontouring, further smooth the surface of the restoration with a very fine disc.

A flame-shaped bur also can be used to recontour and smooth the surface (Fig. 34-130). Adapt the side of the bur along the margins, contacting both tooth and amalgam. Use the same light,

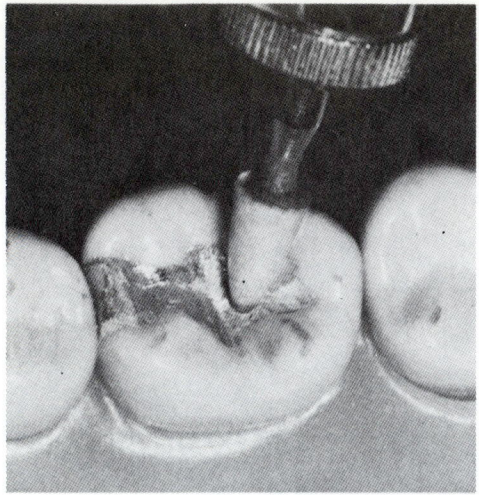

Fig. 34-125. The side of the stone is adapted to the enamel to correct marginal discrepancies of 0.2 mm or less.

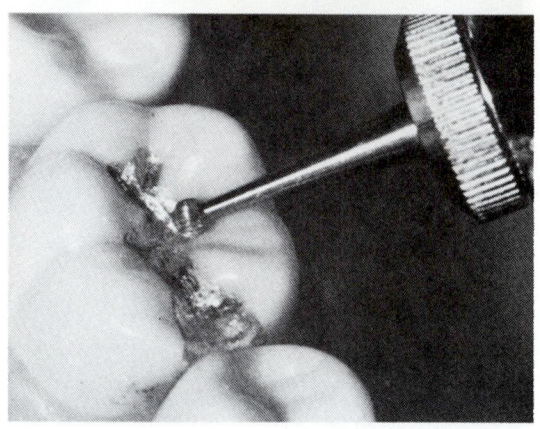

Fig. 34-126. The finishing burr is contacting both amalgam and tooth surface as it is moved along the entire cavosurface margin.

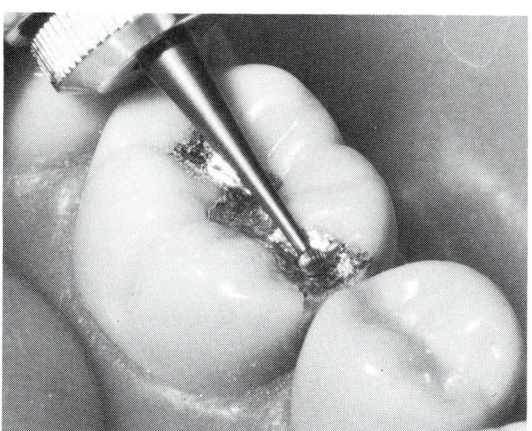

Fig. 34-127. Use the side of the plug-shaped finishing burr when defining mesial and distal fossae. Sweep the bur facio-lingually to create a convex area.

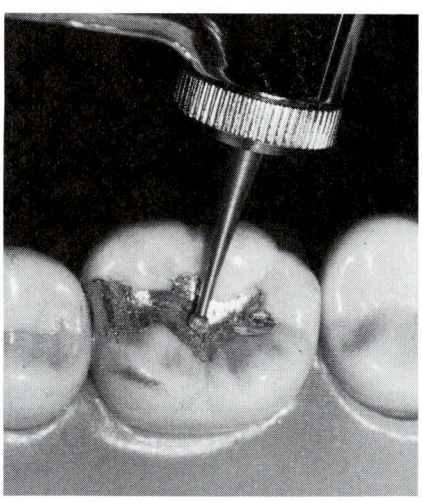

Fig. 34-128. A small finishing bur is used to define major developmental and supplemental grooves.

sweeping strokes over the entire margin. Use extreme caution along the gingival margins, especially those extending onto the root surface. Rotary instruments can damage the cementum and adjacent tissues. Use the side of the flame-shaped bur along the gingival margin, minimizing contact with the adjacent cementum. A gingival retractor may be needed to increase access.

Finish developmental grooves of the facial and lingual surfaces with round or flame-shaped burs. Select one that fits into the groove and use it in a manner similar to that used on the occlusal surface.

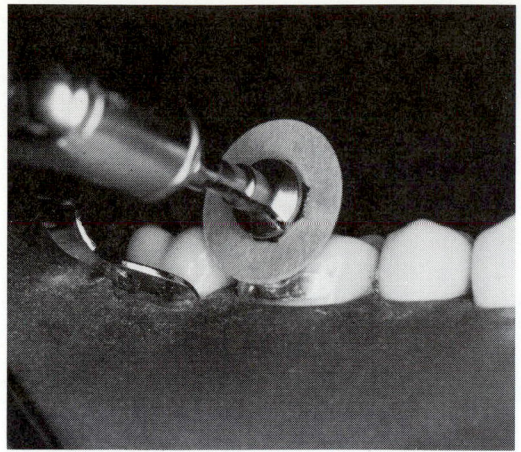

Fig. 34-129. The outer edge of the disc is adapted to the occlusal margin of a class V restoration.

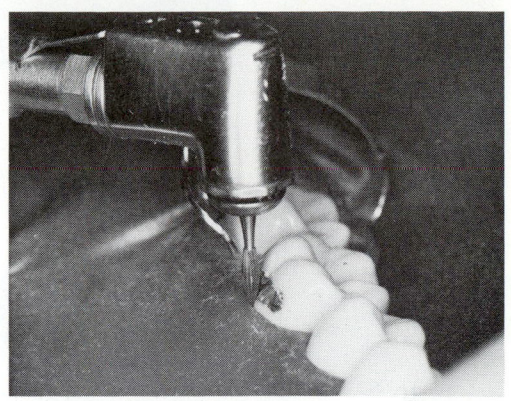

Fig. 34-130. The flame-shaped bur is adapted along the gingival margin of a Class V restoration. Caution is needed to minimize contact of the tip with cementum.

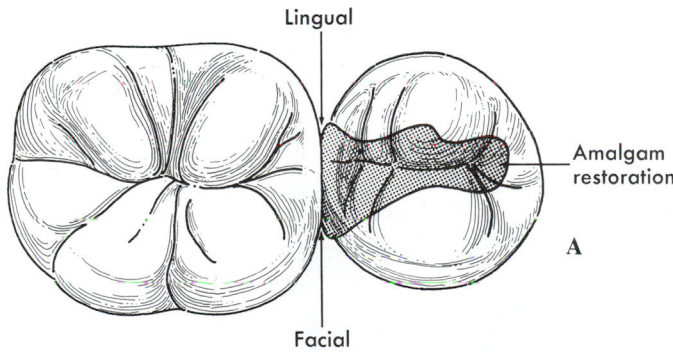

Fig. 34-131. **A,** This bulky, overcontoured occlusal embrasure may snag or tear dental floss. **B,** The finishing disc is adapted from the lingual aspect to contour the occlusal embrasure.

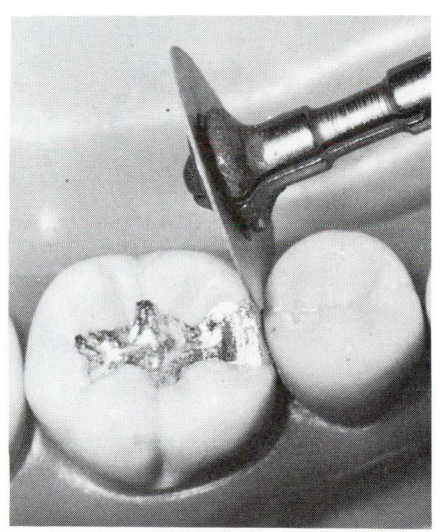

Recontouring and finishing the proximal surface

Excess amalgam located along the occlusal embrasure area can be removed with a fine finishing disc. Rotate the disc to fit into the facial or lingual aspects of the occlusal embrasure contacting the excess amalgam (Fig. 34-131). Move the disc into the embrasure in a sweeping motion. Stop frequently to evaluate the results, as amalgam can be abraded quickly. Repeat this step on the opposite surface if indicated. A garnet disc may be used for gross excess followed by a cuttle disc to remove flash from accessible facial and lingual margins. Adapt the edge of the disc using the same light, sweeping strokes to move it along the amalgam surface. Do not push the disc far enough into the embrasure to damage the contact area or the papilla.

A flame-shaped bur also can be used to finish the facial and lingual margins of the proximal area. Place the bur perpendicular to the facial or lingual margin with the point extending into the embrasure and the side of the bur contacting both

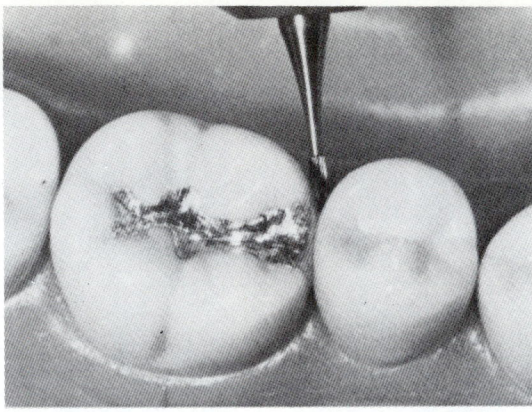

Fig. 34-132. The flame-shaped bur is held perpendicular to the lingual margin of the proximal box. Make sure the tip of the bur does not extend deep enough to affect the contact area.

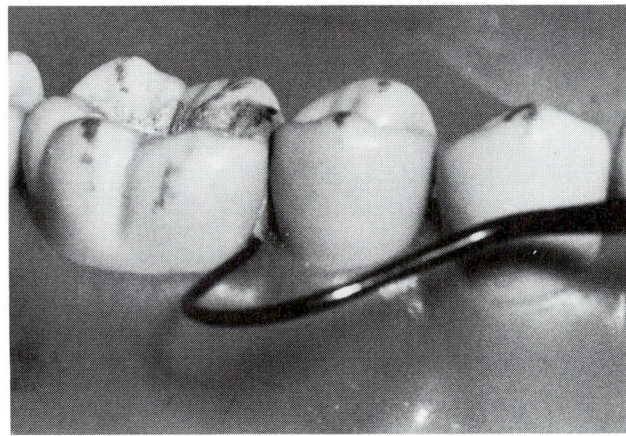

Fig. 34-133. An explorer can be used to detect an overhang, which is visible along the gingival margin.

amalgam and tooth surface (Fig. 34-132). Move the bur parallel to the margin from the gingival margin to the marginal ridge. Avoid placing pressure on the tip of the bur to prevent creating a ledge in the contact area.

Removing gingival overhangs

The proximal area should be evaluated visually from the facial and lingual aspects and tactilely by using floss and an explorer (Fig. 34-133). It may also be seen radiographically. If an overhang is detected, its location, size, and shape must be de-

termined, as with calculus deposits (Fig. 34-134).

Small overhangs often can be removed as part of scaling. Removal is most successful with small to moderate overhangs.

In cross-section, the amalgam knife looks like an upside-down sickle scaler. The apex of the triangle is the very sharp cutting edge. The instrument must be angled differently from a scaler (Fig. 34-135). The cutting edge is turned more toward the tooth than is the cutting edge of the sickle scaler. Some tissue displacement may be inevitable, but no damage to the epithelial attach-

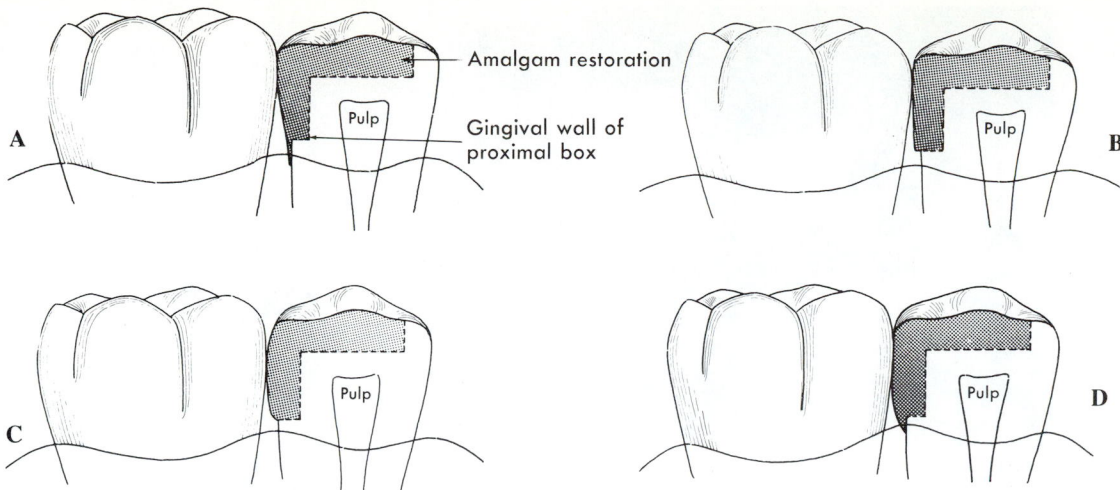

Fig. 34-134. Excess amalgam in the proximal box can occur in a variety of ways. **A,** Excess amalgam can extend in a thin layer on the cavosurface apical to the gingival margin. **B,** Excess amalgam can extend as an overhanging ledge beyond the cavosurface margin. This ledge would be difficult to clean with floss. **C,** An overhang may be combined with an overcontoured proximal surface. **D,** An overhang and a severely overcontoured proximal surface reduce the gingival embrasure space and impinge on the interdental papilla.

ment and papilla should occur. Removing an overhang is different from removing calculus because the amalgam is shaved away. The instrument is not placed under the entire overhang and activated to remove it in one stroke; if this is done the amalgam may fracture at the margin, necessitating placement of a new restoration.

Insert the tip of the knife at the faciogingival aspect of the proximal box until it catches on a definite ledge (Fig. 34-136). Increase the pressure on the blade as it is moved from the gingival margin to the contact area to begin removing amalgam. Move the blade farther into the proximal area while continuing the shaving strokes. On each stroke, insert the blade slightly deeper into the embrasure until the tip extends past the center of the proximal area. Avoid damaging the contact by bringing the instrument too far occlusally. Do not cut into too much amalgam, which might cause it to chip or fracture. Repeat the strokes until the excess is removed. Increased pressure may be needed on older restorations. Perform the same steps from the lingual, beginning at the linguogingival aspect of the proximal area.

Files are used when access is very limited or to produce a smoother surface after the amalgam

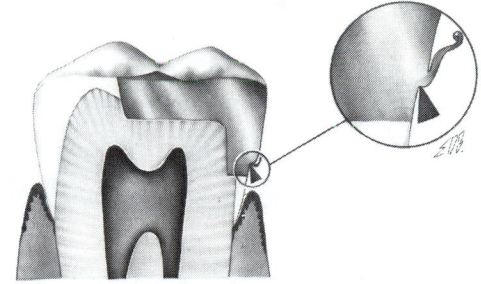

Fig. 34-135. Cross-section of amalgam knife being used to shave away an overhang.

knife has been used. Three sets of files can be used: heavy, medium, and finishing files (Figs. 34-137 and 34-138). Files are used in order of coarseness from heaviest to finest so that each successively finer file produces a smoother finish.

After the files, a universal curette can be used to smooth the interproximal surface further. As the amalgam is reduced, check the progress with an explorer to ascertain that the amalgam is flush with the tooth.

Overhang removal can also be accomplished with a reciprocating motor-driven tip designed for

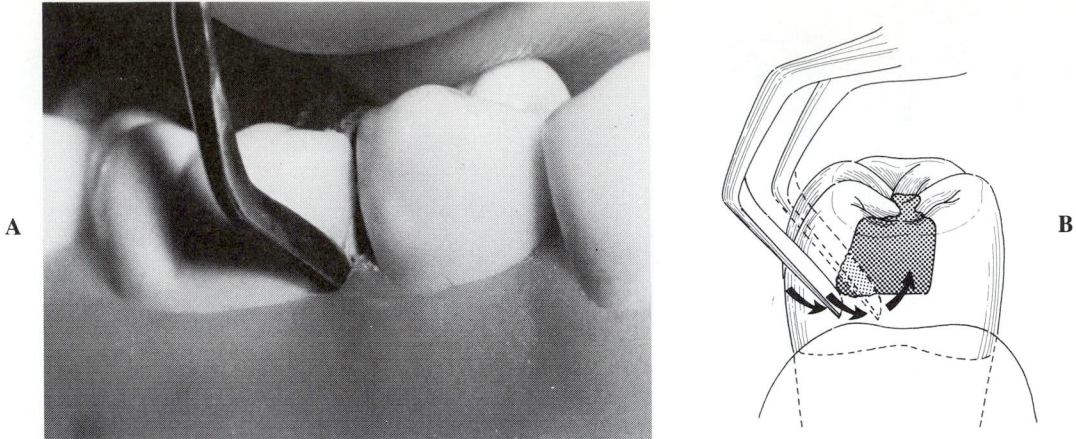

Fig. 34-136. **A,** Adaptation of the amalgam knife at the junction of the gingival and facioproximal cavosurface margins. **B,** Angle of the amalgam knife as it is inserted from the facial embrasure. The length of the stroke extends from the gingival margin to below the contact area.

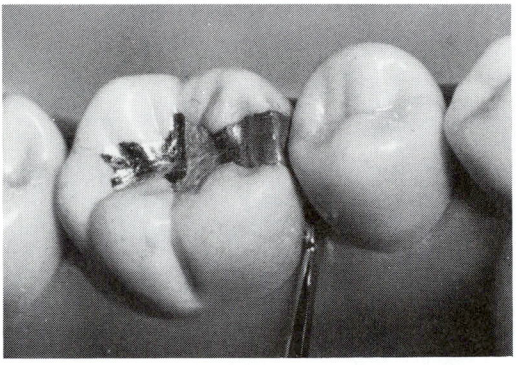

Fig. 34-137. The amalgam file is adapted flat against the gingival margin and adjacent tooth surface. The blades of the file shave the amalgam and produce a smoother margin.

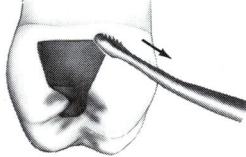

Fig. 34-138. File is placed on tooth and amalgam and is used with a pull stroke directed obliquely or horizontally.

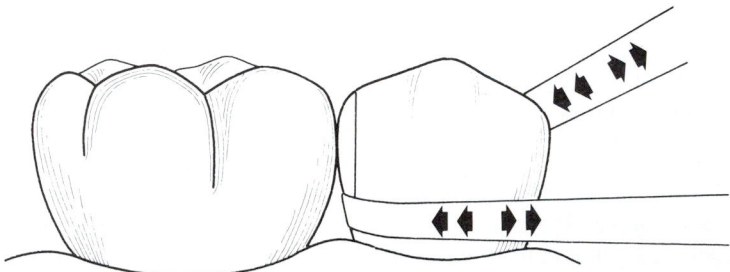

Fig. 34-139. The finishing strip is adapted against the gingival margin. As it is moved occlusally, avoid applying too much pressure, which may create an undercontoured surface.

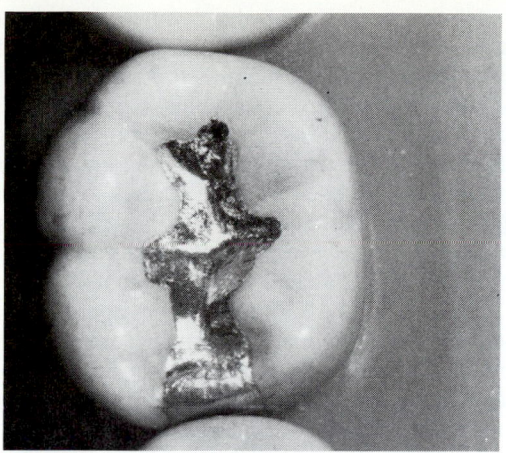

Fig. 34-140. The surface of the restoration after finishing and before polishing.

proximal surfaces (Profin Directional System, Wissman Technology). The triangular tips, embedded with diamond particles, can remove the overhangs efficiently and effectively (Axelsson, 1981; Gelsky, 1982; Vale and Caffesse, 1979). Axelsson (1981) has recommended that overhang removal be followed by recontouring the overhang, smoothing the surface, removing plaque completely, and applying fluoridated paste by means of a plastic tip.

Another approach is to use ultrasonic scaling equipment. High-frequency instrumentation using the heavier tips will easily remove overhangs (see Chapter 25).

The gingival margin of the restoration can be smoothed with a finishing strip (Fig. 34-139). If gapped strips are used, the nonabrasive-coated portion can be passed through the contact area to avoid abrading the amalgam. If ungapped strips are used, one end is cut into a point and threaded into the embrasure. Position the strip so that it is on both the tooth and the amalgam. Use a see-saw, back-and-forth motion to remove roughness. If the strip is on amalgam only, it could create a deficient or open margin.

At this point, carefully evaluate the restoration (Fig. 34-140). The margins should be flush with the adjacent tooth surface, contours should be consistent with the surrounding tooth structure, and the surface should be smooth with no scratches.

PROPERTIES OF COMPOSITE RESINS, ACID ETCHING OF ENAMEL, AND GENERAL PROCEDURES FOR PLACEMENT

Restoration of anterior teeth requires a material that can satisfy the esthetic demands of the patient. If an anterior restoration does not match the color, contour, and surface finish of the surrounding tooth structure, it is unsatisfactory no matter how well it is placed. Dental amalgam meets many of the criteria for desirable physical properties of dental materials but it fails in its esthetic characteristics. Researchers have sought to develop a material that has good chemical and physical qualities, is relatively easy to handle, is biologically compatible, and has an acceptable appearance. No material yet developed meets all of these criteria, although the tooth-colored materials now available come reasonably close.

Resins contain inorganic filler particles in the resin matrix. These materials are commonly called "filled" or "composite" resins to distinguish them from unfilled resins. Four classes of composite resin have evolved (Table 34-1). The first-developed composite resins were the *large-particle,* or *conventional,* composite resins.

These were followed in the late 1970s by the *microfilled* and more recently by the *small-particle* composite resins. Some composite resin systems now contain particles of varying sizes referred to as *hybrids*. These terms reflect the changes in filler particle size used in the material.

Composition

Composite resins are composed of two major components, an organic polymer resin matrix and inorganic filler particles. The basic molecule (monomer) of the resin is bisphenol A-glycidyl methacrylate (BIS-GMA). The particles of the conventional filler component are composed of

Table 34-1. Composite resin particle size

Type of composite	Particle size
Conventional (large-particle)	Above 5 μm
Microfilled (fine-particle)	
Silica filler	.05 μm
Prepolymerized particles	10–70 μm
Small particle	0.5 μm–5.0 μm
Blend (or hybrid): combination of microfilled and small particles	0.5 μm–5.0 μm

one of several inorganic materials, such as quartz, lithium aluminum silicate, barium aluminum silicate, or borosilicate glass. These filler particles are treated so that they chemically bond with resin during the setting reaction (Baum et al, 1985). Small amounts of inorganic pigments are added to provide variations in shades.

The reaction that causes BIS-GMA molecules to be linked together (polymerized) may be initiated chemically or by a special visible light source. The chemically activated product has two main components: a base (universal) portion and a catalyst (activator) portion. Both are supplied in paste form. When mixed together, the catalyst initiates polymerization of the molecules, resulting in hardening of the mass. The light-activated material has only one component, which contains both the resin monomer and the filler. When the material is exposed to visible light, polymerization is initiated and hardening occurs. Because there is a chemical reaction, new material may be added to previously set material. This chemical bond between the two materials permits repair of fractures and correction of defects in the restoration being placed or one that was previously placed.

The hardness and size of the particles in large-particle composite resins make it difficult to obtain a truly smooth surface. Microfilled resins can be truly polished to give a highly desirable surface finish. However, some of these resins may exhibit less desirable abrasion resistance. Microfilled composites are primarily indicated for areas not subject to heavy wear. Newer, small-particle and hybrid composites have been developed to combine the smooth surface of the microfilled resins with good wear resistance and strength. This is accomplished through higher proportions of filler particles; the undesirable characteristics of roughness and staining are minimized by using particles of smaller size.

Although the chemically-cured material is satisfactory, several advantages of the light-cured material have made it more popular. The one-paste, light-activated material does not require mixing. This avoids incorporation of air bubbles created when mixing the components. The material can be added in layers and shaped with hand instruments before curing. In contrast, the clinician must wait until the chemically cured material is set before contouring. The more commonly used light-activated small-particle and hybrid materials will be discussed.

All composite resins shrink somewhat as they cure. This shrinkage tends to pull the material away from walls and margins to which they were adapted. In turn, this contributes to microleakage, discoloration, and loss of the restoration. Chemically cured resin shrinks towards the greatest bulk of material. Light-cured resin shrinks towards the light source. To minimize the negative consequences of shrinkage, cure the material in small layers no thicker than 2 mm.

Manufacturers offer two different approaches to produce the desired surface finish. Some products include a glaze (resin without filler particles) to be coated over the surface to produce a very smooth finish that is bonded to the restoration. The glaze is susceptible to abrasion so its long-term benefits are limited. The other approach uses microfilled materials that can be polished to a more lustrous finish. This reduces plaque retention, which is especially important for class V restorations.

The composite resins may have adverse effects on the pulpal tissue because of free monomer molecules. A calcium hydroxide base is usually recommended under composite resin restorations in deep preparations.

Product packaging

The materials used for acid etching are usually supplied as a kit containing the acid, the instrument for application, and the bonding agent in addition to the composite resin. The acid (etchant) may be in gel form or a syringe with disposable applicator tips for direct placement (Fig. 34-141). Manufacturers may supply a disposable brush.

The bonding agent is commonly supplied in a squeeze bottle. One or two drops are dispensed onto a coated pad and picked up with a small

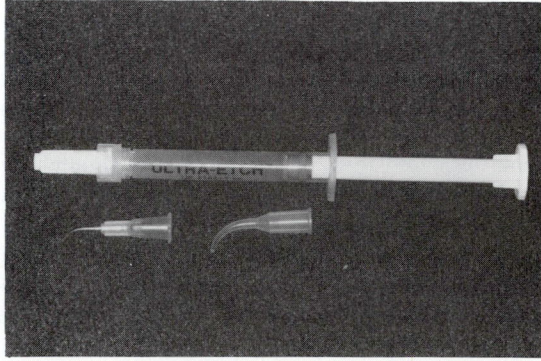

Fig. 34-141. Acid dispenser syringe and disposable applicator tips.

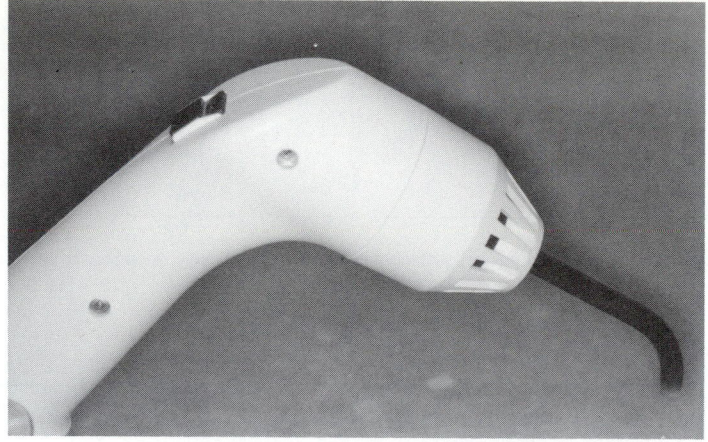

Fig. 34-142. An example of a visible light–projecting device.

brush or endodontic paper point for placement on the etched surfaces.

The composite resin comes in various shades of paste. It may be supplied in larger, multiple-application syringes from which the material is dispensed for insertion into the tooth. Alternatively, it may be supplied in single-application carpules, which load into a syringe for injection into the preparation. The carpules are color coded for easy identification.

The visible light–projecting devices used to cure the materials are available in several designs (Fig. 34-142). They all have the same objective: to project a bright blue light to which the ingredients in the resin react to begin the curing reaction. The light wands, or "guns," all have a timer so the period of exposure can be accurately timed. Curing lights should be checked regularly using a light meter designed to measure curing light output and determine that they are delivering the amount of light required. One study (Berry et al, 1992) determined that approximately 50% of the light wands in use in dental offices did not produce enough milliwatts per square centimeter of light to completely cure a 2 to 3 mm thickness of composite resin in the required time. Inadequate curing can result in a hard outer surface and soft, uncured resin in the deeper areas of the preparation. The scale used by the light meter may vary according to the type of meter used. Refer to the specific manufacturer's specifications to ensure that the output recorded for the light source is adequate for successful curing of the composite resin in the recommended time.

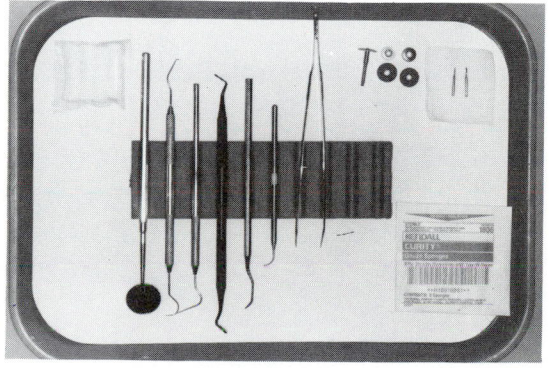

Fig. 34-143. Armamentarium for placement and finishing of a composite resin restoration includes: *1*, cotton rolls; *2*, mouth mirror; *3*, explorer; *4*, periodontal probe; *5*, placement instrument; *6*, gold knife; *7*, calcium hydroxide placement instrument; *8*, cotton pliers; *9*, mandrel; *10*, finishing discs; *11*, carbide finishing burs; *12*, gauze squares.

Armamentarium

The armamentarium suggested for composite resin restorations is shown in Fig. 34-143. Specific situations may require other instruments.

Acid etching

Excellent retention and a significant decrease in marginal leakage are provided by placing the composite resin over an etched enamel surface. Acid etching (conditioning) with 30% to 40% phosphoric acid selectively removes inorganic material from the enamel, leaving pits or micro-

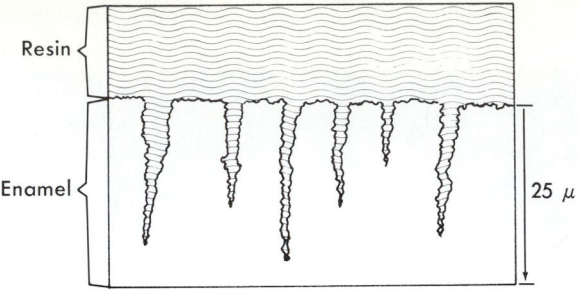

Fig. 34-144. The acid-etched enamel surface with resin applied. Note resin tags in the micropores.

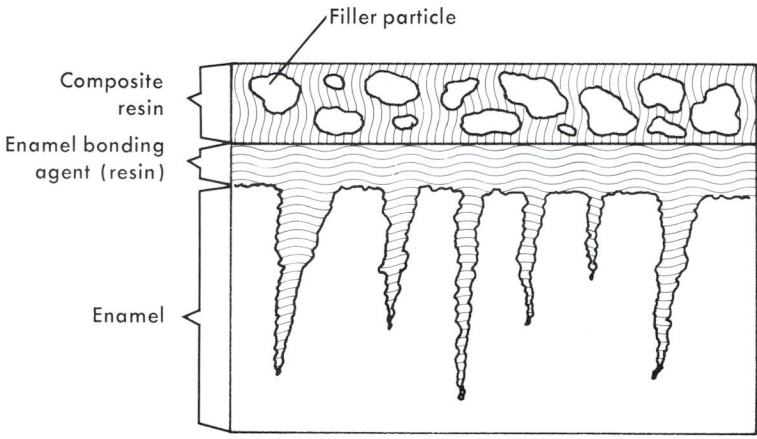

Fig. 34-145. The relationship of the acid-etched enamel, the enamel-bonding agent, and the composite resin.

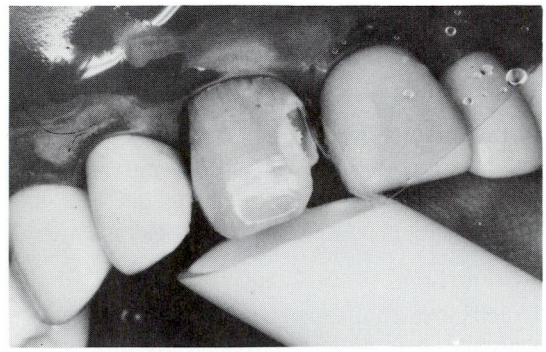

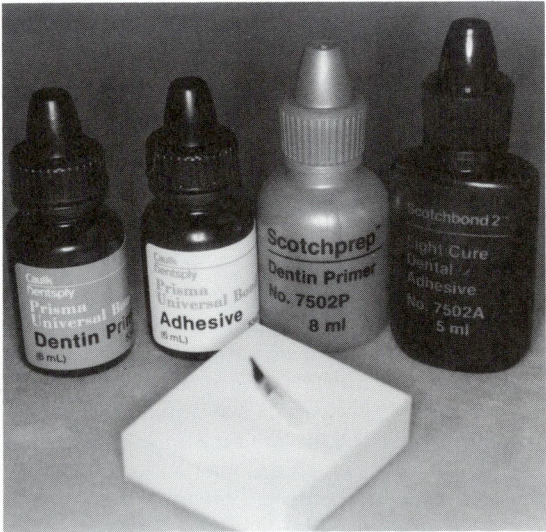

Fig. 34-146. The appearance of a Class IV preparation following acid etching and rinsing of beveled margins. Note matrix strip placed to protect adjacent tooth during acid etching procedure.

Fig. 34-147. Several types of dentin bonding agents are available. After mixing, they are applied with a small brush or an endodontic point.

pores approximately 25 μ in depth. Unfilled resin (bonding agent) is then flowed into the micropores, forming tiny fingers or tags into the enamel surface (Fig. 34-144). When set, it locks onto the surface. Composite resin then is chemically bonded to the bonding agent (Fig. 34-145). The cavosurface margins may be beveled at an angle of 30 to 45 degrees to add to the amount of enamel to which the material is bonded. This creates greater retention and, more importantly, less microleakage.

Fig. 34-146 shows a Class IV preparation with cavosurface margins that have been beveled and acid etched. The etched enamel appears chalky in contrast to the unetched surface.

Undercuts in dentin may be added to supplement the retention of the micropores. Two precautions about these retentive features are important. The calcium hydroxide base must not cover the enamel or undercuts. After the etching is completed, the enamel cannot be contaminated with saliva or other fluids, as this will significantly decrease retention (Knight, Barghi, and Berry, 1991).

In an effort to achieve greater adhesion to the tooth, researchers have developed techniques for bonding to dentin. Although the efficacy of enamel bonding is well documented, in many situations there is not enough enamel to provide an adequate bonding surface. This is especially true of Class V areas, which may have the gingival margin entirely on cementum or even have the incisal or occlusal margin where the enamel is very thin. To provide adequate retention and some degree of sealing, it is necessary to bond to dentin or cementum. Even where an adequate amount of enamel exists, dentin bonding offers supplemental retention and additional protection against microleakage.

Bonding to dentin presents a different situation from enamel bonding because dentin is structurally and chemically different. Enamel is 95% inorganic (hydroxyapatite), 4% water, and 1% organic (collagen) by weight. Etching dries the enamel leaving it with many microporosities that the hydrophobic (i.e., water-hating) resin can easily wet and flow into. Dentin, on the other hand, is 70% hydroxyapatite, 18% collagen, and 12% water by weight (ten Cate, 1989). It is hydrophilic (water-loving), has limited potential for creation of microporosities, and is full of tiny tubules through which moisture seeps. This requires a more elaborate surface conditioning regimen than for enamel.

Most dentin bonding agents require a multistep procedure that results in a combination of chemical and mechanical (micropores) bonding. Many dentin bonding systems are currently available. Each has its own set of directions to follow. It is absolutely necessary to follow the manufacturers' directions to ensure the maximum benefit from the specific dentin bonding process selected. Since there is no one universally accepted agent or technique, refer to the directions provided with the specific dentin bonding kit (Fig. 34-147).

Placing bonding agent

Bonding agent should be added carefully to avoid covering unconditioned areas. Preparations that involve the proximal surfaces usually require a matrix strip to protect the adjacent tooth from the liquid resin. Bonding agent cured over unconditioned enamel will not bond to the tooth. It will trap fluids between it and the enamel, allowing staining. It may fracture and leave jagged margins. Controlled placement of the bonding agent is best achieved using a small brush or an endodontic paper point. Wipe away any agent on unetched enamel with a small cotton pellet. Cure the agent by exposing it to the light for approximately 20 seconds. A large preparation may necessitate exposing segments to the light for 20 seconds each to ensure all sections cure adequately.

Placing and photocuring composite resin

Although manufacturers make a "universal shade" suitable for many situations, shade selection may be important. It must be done before the rubber dam is placed. For larger preparations, the darker shades generally are placed in the gingival section of the preparation with lighter and grayer ones placed towards the incisal edge of the restoration. Expose each layer of composite resin to the light for a minimum of 20 seconds. Then add the next segment and repeat the curing process. Segments thicker or deeper than 3 mm may not adequately cure completely. Do not add in layers thicker than 2 to 3 mm. Continue to add until the preparation is very slightly overfilled. Remove excess material before curing.

Composite resin needs careful adaptation into all areas of the preparation, with special attention to the retentive areas and the cavosurface margins. For a small or medium-sized preparation, place enough material to fill one half of the preparation and to ensure that it is pushed into all internal areas. A Teflon-coated instrument with a blade on one end and a small nib on the other is a good choice for placement. Use the blade to carry material to the preparation and the nib to adapt it the material into all areas.

A syringe may be used to completely fill all the areas of the preparation without undue entrapment of air bubbles. Special syringes that may be loaded with bulk material as well as prepackaged carpules with disposable syringe tips are available.

The materials generally are placed in the least accessible portion of the preparation first. This usually includes any retentive features within the preparation. The materials need to be carefully adapted to all walls to minimize the possibility of voids or defects at margins.

Place these materials in layers no thicker than 2.5 mm (less for darker shades) so that photocuring will cure the resin to its full depth. Hold the curing light 1 to 2 mm from the resin and expose it according to the manufacturer's recommendations (usually 20 seconds).

If a very thin outer layer of composite resin is not covered with a matrix strip, it will not cure completely because of exposure to air. This soft sticky surface must be removed to prevent excessive staining and premature wear. Once the uncured layer is removed, the remaining surface can be finished easily to a very smooth texture.

Use of matrices

Matrices for composite resins follow the same principles as those for amalgam restoration. The matrix is designed to confine the material to the preparation and to provide a smooth surface against which to adapt and cure the material. Class III or IV restorations require wedge placement to prevent flash along the gingival margin and to separate the teeth slightly to ensure contact after the restoration is placed. A matrix is not critical for the placement of a Class V restoration.

Finishing the composite resin restoration

Finishing of composite resin restorations removes excess material, contours, and smooths the surface. Rotary instruments such as discs, white stones, and carbide finishing burs are used. Coarse, medium, and fine discs of silicone carbide or zirconium silicate (Shofu Co.) are especially effective in shaping and smoothing the restorations. Carbide finishing burs specifically designed for composite resins produce a relatively smooth surface and are available in a variety of shapes. Do not confuse these with regular finishing burs, which are not as effective in cutting the material. A gold knife is useful when the margin of the restoration extends onto the cementum at the gingival margin. Abrasive strips also are very effective in finishing gingival and incisal proximal margins.

Start with the coarsest finishing material and progress to the finest one. Because of the hardness and size of the particles in the resin, the finishing process results in a smooth surface but may not reach a high luster.

THE CLASS V AND CLASS III COMPOSITE RESIN RESTORATIONS

The restoration must reproduce the form and match the color of the tooth. The outline of the preparation is usually similar to that of the Class V amalgam preparation (Fig. 34-148). It may have beveled margins and, retentive grooves in the occlusoaxial and gingivoaxial line angles (Fig. 34-149). Although retention may depend mostly on enamel and/or dentin bonding, it is important to take advantage of additional retentive features if present. Because the gingival margin of a Class V preparation is likely to be on cementum or in an area in which the enamel is very thin, dentin bonding may be a big advantage. If successfully accomplished, it will compensate for the lack of enamel bonding.

The preparation must be clean and dry. Before placing a rubber dam, select a shade of material that will match the color of the tooth (Fig. 34-150). Ensure that the preparation is well isolated and the soft tissue is protected. A correctly placed rubber dam with a 212 clamp for gingival retraction provides the best isolation.

Acid etching and bonding

The first step is acid etching to prepare the enamel for the bonding agent. In preparations with a thick layer of dentin, calcium hydroxide is not needed. Deep preparations may call for placement of a glass ionomer or calcium hydroxide layer to protect the pulp (Fig. 34-151). Apply acid to all areas of enamel to be covered by the restoration including the bevel. The acid should be left on the enamel for approximately 30 sec-

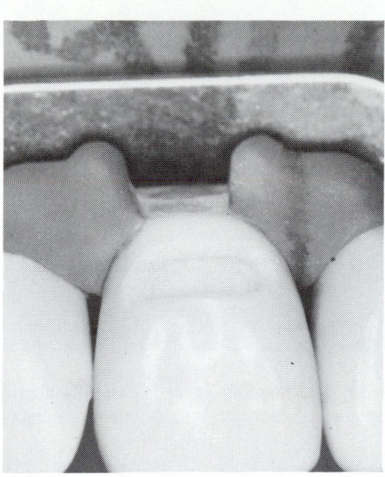

Fig. 34-148. Outline of Class V cavity preparation for a composite resin restoration.

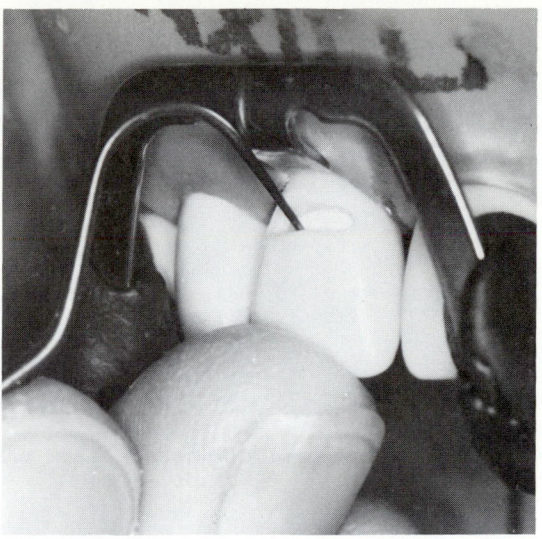

Fig. 34-149. Retention for the restoration may depend partly on retentive grooves cut into the incisoaxial and gingivoaxial line angles.

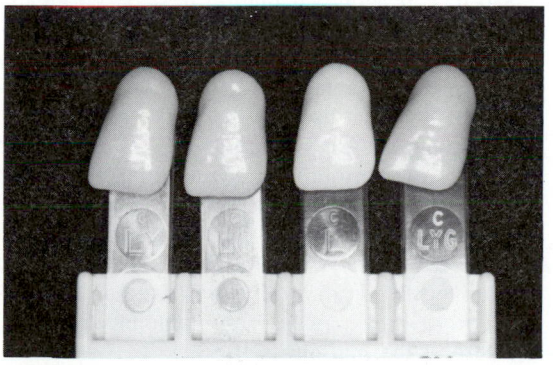

Fig. 34-150. The shade guide helps select the appropriate coloration of material.

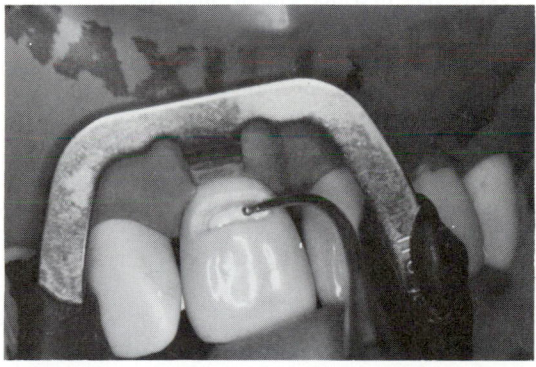

Fig. 34-151. Take care to place the calcium hydroxide on the dentin only. The dentin should be protected while the enamel is etched.

onds for permanent teeth (Fig. 34-152). Less than 30 seconds may inadequately etch the surface; a longer time may overetch, removing too much surface enamel. Either reduces the retentive characteristics of the surface. Note that deciduous teeth or teeth of patients in heavily fluoridated communities may require etching for longer periods. Rinse the surface thoroughly with water to stop the etching process. Dry and examine the etched enamel. A properly etched surface should be chalky white with a slightly rough texture. If it

is not, repeat the etching procedure.

Apply a thin layer of bonding material over the etched surfaces with a camel's hair brush or an endodontic paper point. It is important to coat all etched surfaces to achieve maximum retention and marginal seal (Fig. 34-153). If the etchant contacts the calcium hydroxide base, it is of little consequence. Polymerize the material with the curing light for the recommended time of 20 seconds. The surface is now ready for placement of the composite resin.

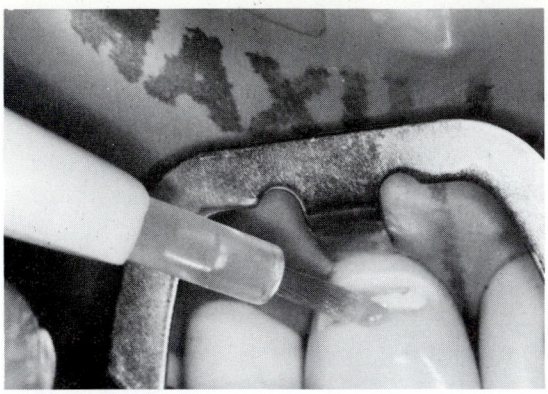

Fig. 34-152. The acid should be applied to the enamel walls and margins.

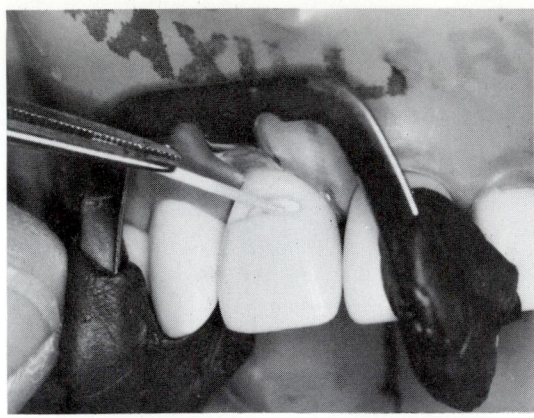

Fig. 34-153. The bonding agent is carefully applied to all of the etched surfaces but not onto the unetched enamel.

Placement and photocuring

With either the bladed instrument or a syringe, deposit the first increment into the preparation (Fig. 34-154). Do not fill the preparation with the first increment. Using the nib, adapt the material into all the line angles and retentive areas to completely cover the walls and to achieve maximum retention (Fig. 34-155). Expose the increment to the light for 20 seconds. Continue to add increments using the technique described. Completely cure each new increment. Place increments no more than 2 mm thick before curing. This is especially important with darker shades, which do not allow light to penetrate through the material as easily.

Evaluate the restoration visually and with an explorer. It should meet the following criteria:

1. Material extends 0.5 mm to 1.0 mm beyond the margins.
2. Enough excess exists to allow removal of the outer layer.
3. No voids, pits, or submarginal areas exist that are not correctable.

If voids or ditching exist, add more material to the uncontaminated surface.

Remove any excess from the incisal margin. Adapt the outer 1 mm edge of a medium disc to the area, using light sweeping strokes to contour the restoration (Fig. 34-156). Keep the disc adapted to the contours of the tooth by rotating it

slightly as it is moved from the distal to the mesial side. Avoid contact with the enamel.

Correct the gingival margin next. Even greater care is needed to avoid contacting the tooth structure. The cementum of the root surface is very susceptible to abrasion. Adapt the disc in a manner similar to that used on the incisal margin (Fig. 34-157). Direct the sweeping strokes towards the center of the restoration. Avoid contact with the rubber dam. The gold knife may be an effective instrument for removing flash from the gingival margin area. Shave layers away by pulling the blade incisally from tooth to restoration. Be careful not to break away larger amounts to avoid fracture of the margin itself.

Position the disc so only the outer edge is contacting first the mesial and then the distal margin. Use light sweeping strokes to contour these surfaces. Then contour the center of the restoration. To determine how much contouring is needed, examine the contour from both incisal and mesial viewpoints. At this stage, the middle of the restoration may be bulky. Adapt the disc to reduce the bulk and blend the contours. Be careful not to overreduce.

Check the margins with an explorer. Move the tip from restoration to tooth and back to ensure that there is no flash, ditching, or submarginal areas. If flash or bulk is noted at the gingiva, a flame-shaped carbide finishing bur may be helpful (Fig. 34-158). Its thin, tapered form lets it reach

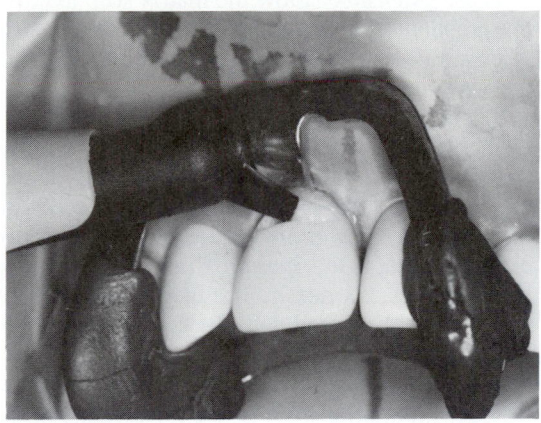

Fig. 34-154. Insert a layer of composite resin no thicker than 2 mm to ensure adequate curing.

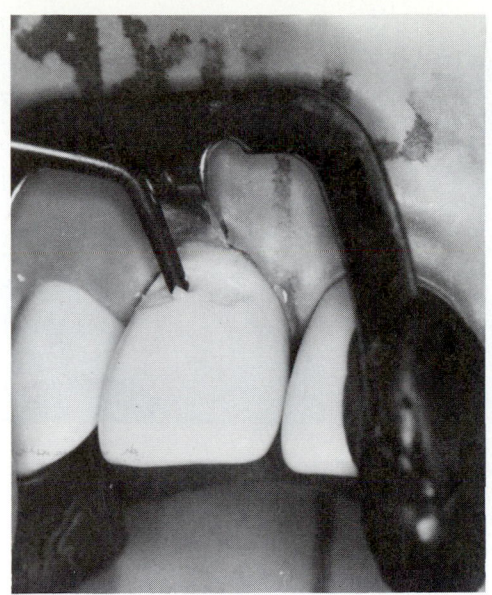

Fig. 34-155. Adapt the material into the incisoaxial line angle.

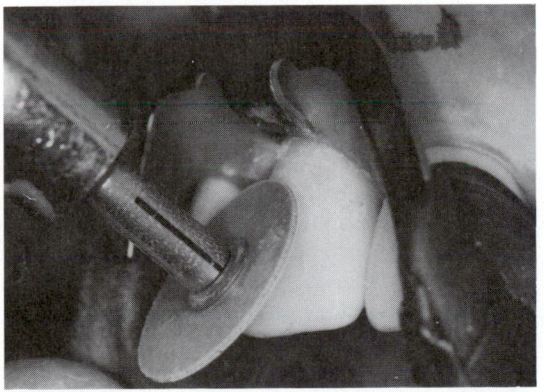

Fig. 34-156. Take care to adapt the disc carefully to the area to be reduced. Guard against abrading the enamel and overreducing the restoration.

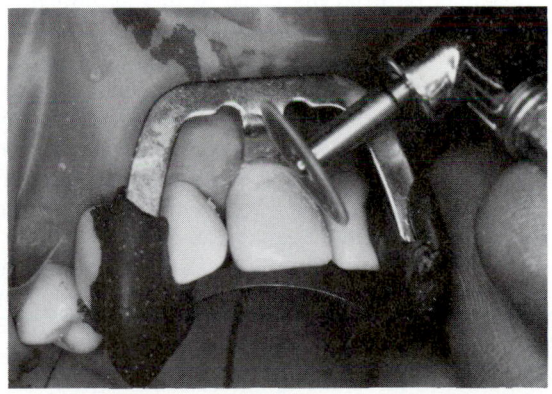

Fig. 34-157. The rest of the margins can be finished using the same careful adaptation of the disc.

places not accessible to a larger instrument. Use sweeping motions with the bur to avoid creating a rippled effect.

Once the basic contours have been established, change to a fine grit finishing disc and follow the same steps. After using the fine grit disc, evaluate the restoration according to the criteria listed for placement of composite resin restorations.

It is important to evaluate the restoration before removal of the rubber dam. If a problem is detected, it is better to correct it while the operating field is still isolated.

Remove the rubber dam. Re-evaluate the esthetic results after the dam has been removed and the teeth are beginning to rehydrate. Inform the patient that the color will not match completely until the tooth has regained its moisture.

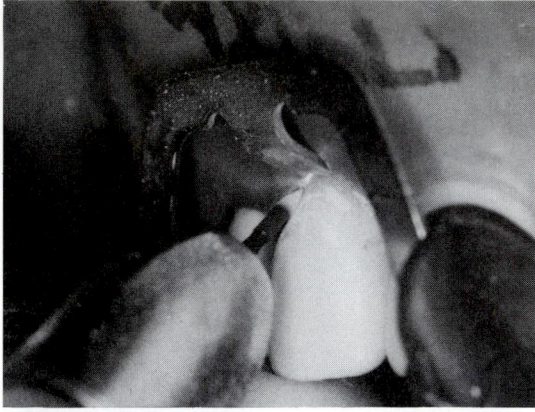

Fig. 34-158. The flame-shaped carbide finishing bur may be helpful to smooth the hard-to-reach areas along the gingival margin.

Class III composite resin

Because the Class III carious lesion occurs on the proximal surface, restoration of both the function and esthetics is necessary. Access to this preparation may be from the facial or lingual directions or both. The preparation usually is shaped like an egg or a Gothic arch (Fig. 34-159) if the access is from the facial. It is slot-shaped if access is from the lingual. Retention may be achieved both by retentive areas at the incisoaxial and gingivoaxial line angles and by acid etching of the enamel. The procedure that follows is for a preparation with facial access.

Visualize the outline to aid later in contouring and trimming the restoration. Determine whether a bevel has been placed around the cavosurface margins. Apply calcium hydroxide base, taking care not to leave any on the enamel.

Acid etching and enamel bonding

Place a Mylar strip interproximally to protect the adjacent tooth (Fig. 349-160). Acid etch and rinse the enamel. Replace the calcium hydroxide if needed. Place bonding agent on the etched enamel surfaces and photocure.

Place a matrix and wedge to confine the material within the preparation, prevent an overhang at the gingival margin, and provide a very smooth surface against which to cure the composite resin. Slide the matrix strip between the teeth. It should:

1. Extend gingivally past the gingival margin by 1.0 mm or more.

2. Extend 1.0 mm to 1.5 mm incisally beyond the incisal margin.
3. Extend far enough facially and lingually to be firmly grasped so the strip can be pulled tightly around the proximal surface.

These extensions allow the matrix strip to cover the preparation area completely. Pull on the strip to ensure it will fit tightly around the tooth without wrinkling or slipping.

Select a wedge to fit into the embrasure tightly enough to separate the teeth slightly and to press the strip against the tooth being restored. Direct the wedge into the lingual embrasure, as access to the preparation is from the facial. If the wedge extends through the interproximal far enough to hinder access, shorten it. The incisal height of the wedge should be level with the gingival margin of the preparation.

Using either the bladed instrument or a syringe, insert the first segment of composite resin into the preparation (Fig. 34-161). Use the nib to press the material into all areas carefully. To keep the material from being pushed out the lingual side, support the strip on the lingual surface with your finger. Reflect the strip away from the preparation on the facial with your middle or first finger. This way the strip is positioned to hold in the material on the lingual while allowing access from the facial.

Expose the composite resin to the light for 20 seconds. Even though the primary access is from the facial, expose the lingual aspect for 20 seconds also. Continue to add material until the preparation is very slightly overfilled. Check all areas facially and lingually to determine that contours are satisfactory and margins are completely covered. If so, carefully adapt the strip against the tooth on the lingual surface, holding it in place between the thumb and index finger of one hand. Expose the lingual surface to the light. Grasp the facial end of the strip between the thumb and index finger of your other hand. Slowly pull the strip across the facial surface toward the opposite proximal surface until the strip is tightly adapted. Pulling slowly allows excess composite resin to escape ahead of the strip as it closes. Once in place, use the thumb of the hand supporting the strip to hold the facial end in place. Expose the composite resin to the light to cure all marginal areas. During the curing process hold the matrix strip tightly in place. This produces an extremely smooth, well-shaped surface and greatly reduces finishing time.

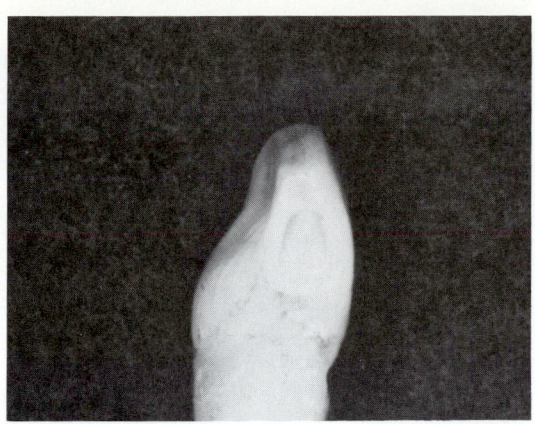

Fig. 34-159. Mesial view of a Class III preparation showing the gothic-arch shape.

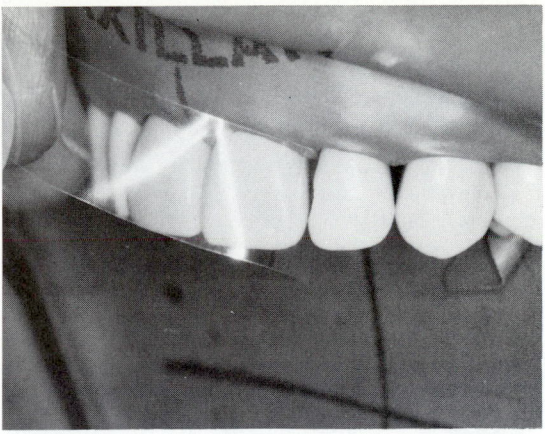

Fig. 34-160. A matrix strip will protect the adjacent teeth from the acid during the etching process.

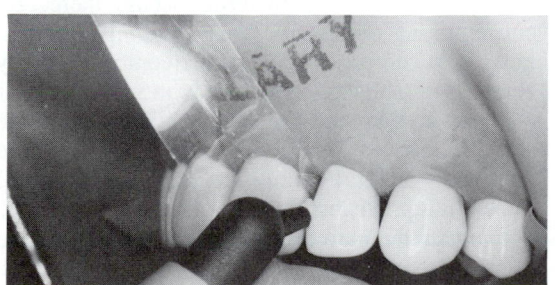

Fig. 34-161. Insert a limited amount to ensure adequate curing depth. Do not try to fill the preparation.

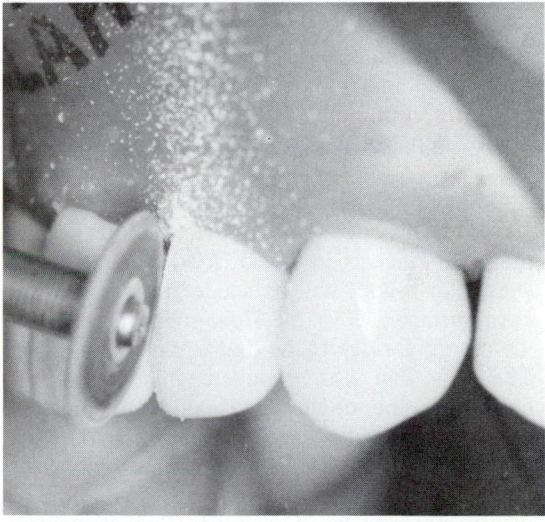

Fig. 34-162. Place the slowly rotating disc into the embrasure to shape and smooth the restoration.

After the restoration has set, remove the wedge and matrix to evaluate the restoration. The amount of contouring and finishing necessary determines which instruments to use. Remove thin layers of flash using a gold knife. Position the tip of the blade gingival to the flash and pull incisally. Cut away material up to within approximately 1.0 mm of the cavosurface margins. A stroke directed toward the gingiva may damage the soft tissue.

Reduce bulkier areas with rotary discs (Fig. 34-162). Place the slowly rotating disc into the facial embrasure contacting the restoration. Pull it in a facial direction, moving in an arc over the proximal line angle and past the facial margin, to produce a rounded line angle and to open the embrasure. Check the contours from a facial and incisal viewpoint. Make certain that the facioproximal contour is rounded and that no ledge is being formed. A ledge is usually created when the disc

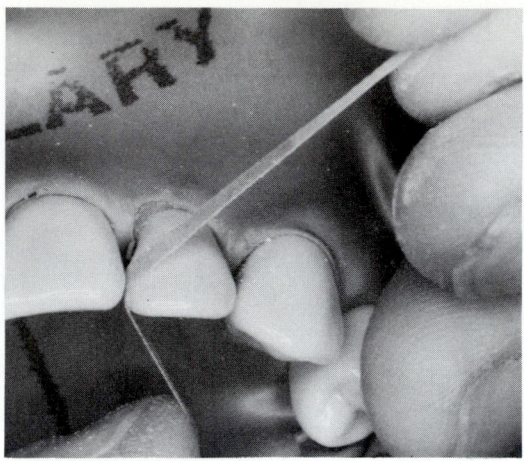

Fig. 34-163. A finishing strip, used with "shoeshine" motion, contours and smooths area that cannot be reached with a disc.

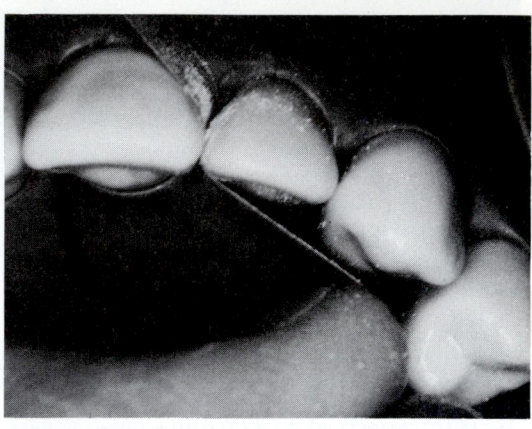

Fig. 34-164. When the strip is pulled in the direction shown, more pressure is applied to the lingual margins.

is moved straight back into the embrasure against the contact area without the rounding motion. The key is to apply pressure only as the rotating disc is moved out of the embrasure and onto the facial surface.

The lingual margin should be finished in the same manner. If a large section of the lingual marginal ridge is involved, a white stone (cone-shaped or round) will be needed to form the concave surface. Move the stone mesiodistally from the marginal ridge to the lingual margin and back. The stone can also be pulled gingivoincisally to help form the lingual incisogingival concavity. The marginal ridge should be of the same height and contour as of the adjacent tooth.

Once the contours are correct, use a fine-grit disc to produce the final finish. Repeat the same procedures used with the medium-grit disc. A finishing strip will contour areas such as the gingival margin that cannot be reached with the disc.

The finishing strip has a coarse abrasive on one end and medium abrasive on the other. Use the coarse end first. Slide the safe zone of a finishing strip through the contact area. If a tight contact prevents the insertion of the strip, place a wedge to separate the teeth slightly and allow insertion. Remove the wedge and slide the strip completely into place with its border located gingival to the gingival margin. Pull the strip back and forth in a shoeshine motion over the margin (Fig. 34-163).

Concentrate pressure on the area that most needs contouring. For instance, if the facial margin requires additional contouring, place an index finger lightly against the strip in the area of the margin and pull the strip mesiolingually with the thumb and forefinger of the other hand. This places more pressure on the facial margin so that greatest reduction of material occurs there. By concentrating on specific areas needing improvement, you can preserve the other contours already correctly established. The key is in using a finger to exert pressure in one area while drawing the strip through in a direction or at an angle that minimizes pressure in another area (Fig. 34-164). Repeat the procedures using a fine abrasive strip.

Evaluate the margins and the contours to ensure they are satisfactory (see criteria sheet). Remove the rubber dam to check the occlusion. Have the patient close on the articulation paper/ribbon in centric occlusion and evaluate for premature occlusion. Adjust prematurities if necessary, using the white stone. Have the patient perform excursive and protrusive movements. Reduce any prematurity with a white stone. Once the occlusion has been perfected, evaluate the restoration using criteria for placement of composite resin restorations.

The Class IV composite resin restoration involves replacement of the incisal angle of an anterior tooth. See textbooks of operative dentistry to acquire additional information about this restoration.

ACTIVITIES

1. Determine which states, provinces, and countries permit hygienists to perform restorative expanded-duty procedures.
2. Conduct a panel discussion with hygienists who practice both traditional and expanded duties in restorative dentistry to learn about the challenge of doing both in dental hygiene practice.
3. Research the history of expanded duties in restorative dentistry in your province or state. Investigate the process of changing the laws that govern the practice of dental hygiene.
4. Research the practice of dental therapists in Britain and New Zealand to determine how they provide dental care to schoolchildren.
5. Evaluate a classmate's performance and final product when placing an amalgam or composite resin restoration using the criteria stated.
6. Acid etch the surface of a natural tooth and observe through a low-power microscope.
7. Practice placement of conservative Class II amalgam restorations on maxillary and mandibular molars and premolar in a typodont. (A minimum of three acceptable restorations per quadrant is suggested.)
8. Conduct a survey among patients about their attitude towards auxiliary dental staff performing restorative procedures.

REVIEW QUESTIONS

1. List the walls and line angles of a Class III (lingual slot) preparation on the mesial surface of a maxillary central incisor.
2. When applying the rubber dam, how do you determine which is the anchor tooth?
3. Describe three methods for placing the rubber dam clamp and rubber dam on the anchor tooth.
4. True or false: Varnish is placed under all amalgam restorations but only under very deep composite resin restorations.
5. Describe the functions of the matrix band and wedge in the placement of a Class II amalgam restoration.
6. True or false: Each of the following situations would indicate the necessity of placing a calcium hydroxide base.
   a. Minimal depth amalgam preparation.
   b. Pulpal exposure.
   c. Deep subaxial extension in a Class III preparation.
   d. Minimal depth composite resin preparation.
7. Define an alloy.
8. Define an amalgam.
9. What is the chief ingredient of dental alloy?
10. Name the ingredients of most dental alloys.
11. What is trituration?
12. What are the characteristics of a correctly mixed amalgam?
13. Where should the first increment of amalgam be placed and condensed in a Class V preparation on tooth No. 14? A class II preparation involving both the mesial and distal surfaces of tooth No. 30?
14. What problem(s) occurs if the operator continues to add an amalgam after the approximately $2\frac{1}{2}$ minutes of working time for that mix has elapsed?
15. What occurs when any instrument or container with amalgam is subjected to heat?
16. What is a submarginal area?
17. True or false: During finishing and polishing procedures, the rotary instruments are most effective when applied with constant, medium pressure at a high speed.
18. True or false: When finishing composite resin restorations, discs are used in order of decreasing coarseness to produce a smooth surface finish.
19. Describe the procedure of acid etching enamel and how this allows the bonding of a composite resin to the tooth.
20. Describe the two ways that polymerization of composite resins occurs and the advantages and disadvantages of each in the clinical situation.
21. List two situations in which a temporary rather than a permanent restoration would be placed.
22. Explain the difference between the strokes used to remove calculus and those used to remove excess amalgam on an overhang.
23. How long should a composite resin be exposed to the curing light?
24. How thick an increment should be photocured at one time? What happens if a thicker layer is exposed to the curing light?
25. What are the main ingredients of a glass ionomer? What are the chief advantages using a glass ionomer base?

Rubber Dam Placement and Removal

Suggested check-off sheet

Mark **S** for satisfactory completion or **U** for unsatisfactory completion of each criterion in the appropriate space.

PERFORMANCE criteria	FACULTY	STUDENT
1. Assemble the necessary armamentarium		
2. Place the clamp properly		
a. Floss applied		
b. All four prongs contacting tooth		
c. Clamp stable		
d. Clamp centered on tooth		
e. Clamp does not impinge on gingiva		
3. Properly punch the dam		
a. Correct number of holes		
b. Position of holes modified for patient		
4. Place the dam properly		
a. Dam stretched over clamp first		
b. Most anterior tooth isolated and ligated		
c. Frame placed		
d. Dam carried through contact areas with tape		
e. Frame readjusted		
f. Clamp ligature pulled to outer surface		
g. Dam tucked into sulcus around each tooth		
h. Area rinsed and suctioned		
5. Remove the dam properly		
a. Ligature on most anterior tooth cut		
b. Interdental areas of dam pulled buccally and cut		
c. Lingual portion of dam freed interdentally		
d. Buccal portion of dam freed interdentally		
e. Clamp ligature held and clamp, dam, and frame removed		
f. Patient's mouth rinsed and suctioned		
g. Dam and patient's mouth checked for rubber dam debris		

Placement of Base and Varnish

Suggested check-off sheet

Mark **S** for satisfactory completion or **U** for unsatisfactory completion of each criterion in the appropriate space.

PERFORMANCE CRITERIA	FACULTY	STUDENT
1. Select the correct base		
2. Mix base correctly		
3. Place the calcium hydroxide properly		
a. Covers all subpulpal and subaxial areas		
b. Does not cover any enamel		
c. Applied in layer approximately 0.5 to 1.0 mm thick		
d. Does not fill retentive grooves		
4. Correctly place varnish for amalgam restorations		
a. Place over all walls including cavosurface margins		
b. No pooling or placement or varnish in thick layers		

Tofflemire Matrix Retainer and Band Placement and Removal

Suggested check-off sheet

Mark **S** for satisfactory completion or **U** for unsatisfactory completion of each criterion in the appropriate space.

PERFORMANCE CRITERIA	FACULTY	STUDENT
1. Assemble the necessary armamentarium		
2. Place the band in the retainer properly		
a. Occlusal opening of band faces curved portion of prongs		
b. Band held securely in retainer		
3. Place the band on the tooth properly		
a. Retainer on facial surface with knobs extending anteriorly		
b. Gingival portion of band around cervical area of tooth		
c. Retainer centered on buccal surface of tooth		
d. Band 1 to 2 mm above occlusal surface		
e. Band 1 to 2 mm below gingival margin		
f. Contact area burnished into band		
4. Place the wedge properly		
a. Inserted from lingual aspect		
b. Base of wedge place against gingiva		
c. Wedge not extending into preparation		
d. Band held against tooth tightly		
5. Remove the retainer, band, and wedge properly		
a. Retainer removed		
b. Wedge removed		
c. Band removed from unrestored area		
d. Band removed from restored area (lingual to buccal)		
e. Restoration undamaged		

Amalgam Restoration Placement

Suggested check-off sheet

Mark **S** for satisfactory completion or **U** for unsatisfactory completion of each criterion in the appropriate space.

PERFORMANCE CRITERIA	FACULTY	STUDENT
1. Assemble the necessary armamentarium		
2. Correctly mix the amalgam		
3. Place the amalgam and condense adequately		
a. Deposit first carrier load in least accessible area		
b. Thoroughly condense amalgam		
c. Condense into all areas of preparation		
d. Condense out over cavosurface margins		
e. Slightly overfill preparation		
4. Burnish the restoration		
a. Adapt amalgam to margins		
b. Smooth surface		
5. Establish occlusal anatomy		
a. Grooves, fossae, ridges, and cusps in the proper location		
b. Create stable occlusal contacts		
6. Establish proper proximal contours		
a. Establish proximal contact in the desired location		
b. Create the desired embrasure form and location		
c. Eliminate any amalgam overhang		
7. Adapt all amalgam margins to the surrounding enamel		
8. Burnish and smooth the entire restoration surface		
9. Completely remove all amalgam particles and other debris		

Amalgam Finishing and Polishing

Suggested check-off sheet

Mark **S** for satisfactory completion or **U** for unsatisfactory completion of each criterion in the appropriate space.

PERFORMANCE CRITERIA   FACULTY   STUDENT

1. Assemble the necessary armamentarium
2. Assess the amalgam
3. Check the occlusion and make necessary modifications
4. Isolate teeth
5. Observe the order of instrumentation
   a. Discs
   b. Finishing strips
   c. Pear-shaped bur
   d. Bud- or flame-shaped bur
   e. Round bur
   f. Pumice with brush
   g. Pumice with rubber cup
   h. Pumice with floss or tape
   i. Wet tin oxide with rubber cup
   j. Wet tin oxide with floss or tape
   k. Dry tin oxide with rubber cup
6. Finish and polish the amalgam restoration
   a. Lavage area after each abrasive
   b. Reproduce original contours of tooth
   c. All margins flush
   d. Amalgam smooth and shiny
   e. Remove dam and recheck occlusion
   f. Adjacent hard and soft tissues undamaged

Amalgam Overhang Removal (Margination)

Suggested check-off sheet

Mark **S** for satisfactory completion or **U** for unsatisfactory completion of each criterion in the appropriate space.

PERFORMANCE CRITERIA   FACULTY   STUDENT

1. Assemble the necessary armamentarium
2. Assess the overhang
3. Observe the order of instrumentation
   a. Amalgam knife
   b. Large files (e.g., Orban)
   c. Medium files (e.g., Hirshfeld)
   d. Fine file (e.g., Rhein 31/32)
   e. Universal curette
   f. Discs
   g. Finishing strips
   h. Dental tape with pumice
   i. Dental tape
4. Remove the overhang properly
   a. Area thoroughly lavaged
   b. Margins flush
   c. Amalgam smooth
   d. Contact present with adjacent tooth
   e. Interproximal contour of tooth reproduced
   f. Adjacent hard and soft tissues undamaged

Placement of Composite Resin Restorations

Suggested check-off sheet

Mark **S** for satisfactory completion or **U** for unsatisfactory completion of each criterion in the appropriate space.

PERFORMANCE CRITERIA	FACULTY	STUDENT
1. Assemble the correct armamentarium		
2. Select the desired shade(s) of material		
3. Correctly acid condition enamel		
a. Place acid on desired area only		
b. Leave acid no more than 30 to 60 seconds		
c. Completely rinse and dry the surface		
d. Correctly evaluate the adequacy of the etching process		
4. Place bonding agent		
a. Place on etched surfaces only		
b. Place without pooling resin		
c. Cure by exposing to the light source		
5. Correctly insert material		
a. Place first increment in least accessible area		
b. Place increments in layers 2 mm thick or less		
6. Expose all areas of material to light source for minimum of 20 seconds		
7. Slightly overfill preparation		
8. Contour the restoration before each exposure to the light source		
9. Confine the material to the preparation with the matrix (if present)		
10. Shape and smooth the restoration		
a. Establish the contours compatible with the general tooth contours		
b. Create proximal and/or occlusal contacts (when applicable)		
c. Create correct embrasure form (when applicable)		
d. Establish a margin that blends completely with surrounding enamel		
e. Produce a smooth, shiny surface free of pits and voids		

REFERENCES

Abrams H et al: Gingival sequela from a retained piece of rubber dam: report of a case, *J Ky Dent Assoc* 30:21, 1978.

Axelsson P: Concept and practice of plaque control, *Pediatr Dent* 3(special issue):101, 1981.

Baum L et al: *The textbook of operative dentistry,* ed 2, Philadelphia, 1985, WB Saunders.

Berry TG et al: Measurement of intensity of curing light units in dental offices, *J Dent Res* 71(special issue): 442(abstract, 1992.

Browne RM et al: Bacterial microleakage and pulpal inflammation in experimental cavities, *Int Endodont J* 16:147, 1983.

Charbeneau GT: Suggested technique for polishing amalgam restorations, *J Mich Dent Assoc* 47:420, 1965.

Charbeneau GT et al: *Principles and practice of operative dentistry,* ed 2, Philadelphia, 1981, Lea & Febiger.

Cohen S, Burns RC: *Pathways of the pulp,* St Louis, 1980, CV Mosby.

Corpron RE et al: A clinical evaluation of polishing amalgams immediately after insertion: 18 month results, *Pediatr Dent* 4:98, 1982.

Coxhead LJ et al: Amalgam overhangs—a radiographic study, *NZ Dent J* 74:145, 1978.

Craig RG, editor: *Restorative dental materials,* ed 6, St Louis, 1980, CV Mosby.

Creaven PJ et al: Surface roughness of two dental amalgams after various polishing techniques, *J Prosthet Dent* 43:289, 1980.

Eliasson ST: Compatibility of composite resins with pulp insulating materials, *J Dent Res* 58:397, 1979.

Farah JW et al: Cement bases under amalgam restorations: effect of thickness, *Operative Dent* 6(3):82, 1981.

Gelsky SC: Overhanging amalgam restorations: their prevalence, ramifications, and irradication, *Can Dent Hyg* 16:19, 1982.

Gilmore W et al: *Operative dentistry,* ed 4, St Louis, 1982, CV Mosby.

Gorzo I et al: Amalgam restorations, plaque removal, and periodontal health, *J Clin Periodontol* 6:98, 1979.

Hakkarainen K, Ainamo J: Influence of overhanging posterior tooth restorations on alveolar bone height in adults, *J Clin Periodontol* 7:114, 1980.

Highfield JE, Powell RN: Effects of removal of posterior overhanging metallic margins of restorations upon the periodontal tissues, *J Clin Periodontol* 5:169, 1978.

Hosoda H et al: Pulpal response to a new light cured composite placed in etched glass-ionomer lined cavities, *Operative Dent* 16:22, 1991.

Jeffcoat MK et al: Alveolar bone destruction due to overhanging amalgams in periodontal disease, *J Periodontol* 51:599, 1980.

Kanai S: Structural studies of amalgam. II. Effect of burnishing on margins of occlusal amalgam fillings, *Acta Odontol Scand* 24:46, 1966.

Kato S et al: Effect of burnishing on marginal seal of an amalgam restoration, *J Prosthet Dent* 19:393, 1968.

Klausner LH et al: Glass-ionomer cements in dental practice: a national survey, *J Operative Dent* 14:170, 1989.

Knight GT Barghi N, Berry TG: Comparing two methods of moisture control in bonding to enamel: a clinical study, *Operative Dent* 16:130, 1991.

Langeland K: Prevention of pulpal damage, *Dent Clin North Am* 16:709, 1972.

Laswell HR et al: High copper amalgam restorations at 11 years, *J Dent Res* 68:870, 1989 (abstract).

Lemmons PLM et al: Influences on the bulk fracture incidences of amalgam restorations: a 7-year controlled clinical trial, *Dent Materials* 3:90, 1987.

Leon AR: The periodontium and restorative procedures: a critical review, *J Oral Rehabil* 4:105, 1977.

Millstein PL, Nathanson D: Effect of eugenol and eugenol cements on cured composite resin, *J Prosthet Dent* 50:211, 1983.

Murray GA et al: Effect of four cavity varnishes and a fluoride solution on microleakage of dental amalgam restorations, *Operative Dent* 11:148, 1982.

Nitkin DA: Placing and polishing amalgam in one visit, *Quintessence Int* 10:23, 1979.

Osborne JW, Norman RD, Gale EN: *Quintessence Int* 22: 857, 1991.

Peters DD, Augsberger RA: In vivo cold transference of bases and restorations, *JADA* 102:642, 1981.

Rodriguez-Ferrer HJ et al: Effect on gingival health of removing overhanging margins of interproximal subgingival amalgam restorations, *J Clin Periodontol* 7:457, 1980.

Schemlitzer LD et al: A six month clinical evaluation of polishing techniques on the marginal integrity of a high copper alloy, *J Indian Dent Assoc* 61:17, 1982.

Stanley HR: Traumatic capacity of high-speed and ultrasonic dental instrumentation, *JADA* 63:749, 1961.

Stanley HR: Pulpal response to dental techniques and materials, *Dent Clin North Am* 15:115, 1971.

Svare CW, Chan KC: Effect of surface treatment on the corrodibility of dental amalgam, *J Prosthet Dent* 19:393, 1972.

ten Cate AR: *Oral histology: development, structure and formation,* St Louis, CV Mosby, 1989.

Tjan AH et al: The efficacy of resin-compatible cavity varnishes in reducing dentin permeability of free monomer, *J Prosthet Dent* 57:2, 1987.

Vale JD, Caffesse RG: Removal of amalgam overhangs, *J Periodontol* 50:245, 1979.

Yates JL et al: Cavity varnishes applied over insulation bases: effect on microleakage, *Operative Dent* 5:43, 1980.

SUGGESTED READINGS

Farah JW et al: Effect of cement base thickness on MOD amalgam restorations, *J Dent Res* 62:109, 1983.

Harper RH et al: In vivo measurements of thermal diffusion through restorations of various materials, *J Prosthet Dent* 43:180, 1980.

Hormati A, Fuller J: Fracture strength of amalgam overlying base materials, *J Prosthet Dent* 43:52, 1980.

Mount GJ: Adhesion of glass-ionomer cement in the clinical environment, *J Operative Dent*. 16:141 1991.

Reavis-Scruggs R: Comparing amalgam finishing techniques by scanning electron microscopy, *Dent Hyg* 56(9):30, 1982.

PART EIGHT	# EVALUATION

Chapters 35 to 38 address the need to *evaluate* the success, or at least the outcomes, of practice. Success is defined as the success of therapy (in terms of both short- and long-term goals) for the individual patient and also as the relative success that the health care provider experiences as a result of his or her participation as a dental professional.

Evaluation is discussed as the final stage of the project development cycle. However, because project development is a cycle and evaluation almost always prompts ideas for change, evaluation may blend in with a new phase of assessment and its subsequent phases. Evaluation then becomes not the end but the beginning.

35 STRATEGIES FOR CONTINUING CARE

Irene Woodall

LEARNING OUTCOMES

The dental hygienist will be able to

1. Adopt a philosophy of continuing care that incorporates the process of assessment, planning, treatment, and evaluation to help prevent the initiation or recurrence of disease.
2. Initiate and maintain a continuing care (recall) program.
3. Vigilantly watch for the risk factors and signs of oral disease and the manifestations of systemic disease.
4. Responsibly monitor patients who are candidates for referral and consult and make referrals promptly based on sound criteria.
5. Adopt the role of patient advocate in coordinating care among specialists and the generalist.

When the course of treatment is complete, a new phase of care commences. Completed treatment does not signal the end of the helping relationship in dentistry and dental hygiene. Rather, the patient should enter a phase of *continuing care*. The terms *recall*, *maintenance*, and *supportive therapy* also are used to describe continued monitoring. In a continuing care program, patients are scheduled at intervals that fit with the nature and severity of the disease for which they were treated and/or in relation to their risk of developing disease. Though some general and oral diseases are "cured" and require minimal continued monitoring, dental caries and periodontal disease are marked by the continual risk of recurrence. Both the patient and you will need to be aware of the importance of scheduling regular appointments to repeat the assessment, review oral hygiene procedures, identify and reduce roadblocks to health maintenance, and plan appropriate preventive or therapeutic care based on the findings.

RATIONALE AND RESEARCH

Several research studies have demonstrated that patients are more likely to resist disease recurrence if they adhere to an appropriate schedule for continuing care and maintain good oral hygiene. In two trials, postsurgical periodontitis patients were assigned to two groups: a well-maintained group who had professional care for plaque control every 2 weeks or a poorly maintained group who received care annually (Nyman, Lindhe, and Rosling, 1977; Rosling et al, 1976). The well-maintained group kept the good health they achieved postsurgically, while the poorly maintained patients lost periodontal attachment, regardless of the surgical technique used during active therapy. Though studies imposed an unrealistic timetable for professional plaque removal, similar results have been obtained in private practice using an interval of 3 to 4 months. Patients who did or did not follow prescribed continuing care in the practice (Becker, Becker, and Berg, 1984; Becker, Berg, and Becker, 1984) were followed for 1.6 to 9.7 years after treatment. Those who stopped maintenance had twice as much bone loss and tooth loss as those who continued regularly with the practice. Treatment without continuing care was of limited value.

One field study was done with Sri Lankans, who had no dental care and practiced no oral hygiene and who had remarkably similar patterns of diet and ecology within the group. This study showed that 11% of subjects never developed periodontitis and 8% had advanced disease with loss of most teeth by age 40. However, 80% of the population had moderately progressive periodontal disease, which matches the typical profile for adult periodontitis (Löe et al, 1986). Comparison of the Sri Lankans with Scandinavians who had received regular care showed similar percentages of patients with minimal, moderate, or advanced disease; however, the severity was lower in the Scandinavians, perhaps because of the interventions of oral hygiene and dental treatment (Löe et al, 1978a, 1978b). If these findings can be extrapolated to the population you will be seeing, it is likely that the 70% to 80% who have slowly or moderately advancing disease will benefit most from continuing care.

Other research (Hirschfeld and Wassermann, 1978; McFall, 1982; Meador, Lane, and Suddick, 1985; Suomi, 1971; Westfelt et al, 1983) shows that patients are less likely to experience disease if they are continuously monitored and that encouragement and assistance, as well as the regular disruption of the microbial flora, have a positive impact on overall health. Thus it is important for both the clinician and the patient to commit to a program that focuses on the continual monitoring of patient health.

APPROPRIATE CONTINUING CARE INTERVALS

Historically, the continuing care interval was 6 months—for everyone. This interval became the accepted norm during the 1950s because of television commercials that promoted "seeing your dentist twice a year" and using the toothpaste sponsoring the program. Twice-yearly dental visits fit well for the majority of patients when dental caries was the focus of assessment and treatment. Most dental caries developed sufficiently to be detected during that time yet did not progress to advanced stages. This interval was then applied to oral prophylaxis and oral hygiene instruction as well, because the regular examinations were tied to the routine of scaling, polishing, and educating. Radiographs and fluoride treatments were added to the routine, and soon the standard of care for dental hygiene was defined by those procedures. Much of the focus of visits was to detect new dental caries and schedule them for repair with the dentist.

As our focus has shifted from caries to periodontal disease, the recommended continuing care interval has shortened. Three- or four-month recall intervals have become the standard for patients with a history of periodontal disease and those with significant risk factors (Axelsson and Lindhe, 1978, 1981; Caffesse, 1990; Suomi et al, 1971; Westfelt et al, 1983). Driving this short-ened interval is research showing that the subgingival microflora will recolonize and reorganize in approximately 42 days after scaling and root planing (Mousques, Listgarten, and Phillips, 1980). With the 1980s' focus on disrupting periodontal pathogens on a regular basis, the 3-month interval has been a defensible choice. The expectation is that the disease can be prevented from fully recurring if the pathogens are disrupted before they reinstitute destruction.

The increasing focus on assessing each patient's health status and susceptibility patterns has produced a more individualized approach to selecting the interval. Patients who are susceptible to recurrence may be seen every 6 to 8 weeks, while others may be seen three times yearly. Patients with none of the risk factors for periodontal disease or caries may be asked to schedule assessments on an annual basis. Thus, the interval can and should be based on patient need rather than on tradition or a fixed pattern.

STRUCTURING A RECALL PROGRAM

Research shows that regardless of what interval you establish with the patient, the actual time lapse between visits will exceed the recommendation (Wilson, 1991). The patient who is supposed to appear again in 8 weeks will more likely have an appointment 3 to 4 weeks after the recommended time. This is because of the natural lapse between the initial contact to schedule the visit and the actual date that can be arranged. Appointments are forgotten or broken; the clinician needs to schedule a meeting or becomes ill and the appointments are moved back.

This factor should influence the methods used for scheduling visits and confirming appointments. There are many approaches that can be adopted, but the one you select should make it possible for you to (1) specify the individual's recall interval, (2) contact the person to schedule an appointment to occur at the designated interval, (3) easily identify when a patient is due for an appointment (patients may call and inquire which week or month is the anticipated time for scheduling), and (4) note when the continuing care visit has been scheduled and whether the appointment was kept. This system can be easily maintained by computer or by hand with a system of cards.

The simplest method is to schedule an appointment before the patient leaves. This means that the appointment book will be filling approximately 8 to 16 weeks in advance, depending on the number of continuing care patients in the practice. Each appointment should then be confirmed 1 week in advance and the day before to ensure that the long-range planning is still noted on the patient's calendar. Patients who must change or who miss an appointment should be rescheduled promptly, with one person designated to continue tracking patients who start to fall off the program. If the scheduling is computerized, it is easy to locate the appointment by searching for the patient's name. Often patients will call to inquire about when it was scheduled or to change an appointment. If scheduling is carried out by book and pencil, searching for the patient in the schedule is more troublesome. Another drawback is that the book will be scheduled so far in advance that it is difficult for the clinicians to adjust their workdays to attend professional meetings or take vacations.

Another method uses a card system for noting when a patient is due to be scheduled. One set of cards is arranged by the month the patient is due to return. There is one card for each patient. When the patient completes an appointment, the recall interval is determined and the card (with the patient's name and telephone number) is filed under the month in which the appointment should be scheduled. Approximately 3 weeks before the appropriate week, the card is pulled, the patient is called, and the appointment is scheduled. The scheduled time and date are noted on the card and it is clipped to the set of alphabetical cards (by last name) until the patient appears for care. Thus if the patient calls to find out when the appointment is scheduled, it can easily be located in the alphabetical file. At the time of the continuing care appointment, the card is pulled from the alphabetical file, the interval is (re)determined, and the card is refiled in the monthly file. The alphabetical file always maintains a card for the patient that is easily locatable. Therefore it is helpful to note the month or week in which the patient is next scheduled for a recall appointment. This way you can quickly determine approximately when a person is due to be scheduled without hunting through the monthly file. Names, addresses, telephone numbers for home and business, times of the day that work best for the patient, and the amount of time typically needed to perform the

reassessment and supportive therapy should be noted on both sets of cards.

Regardless of who is in charge of the continuing care system (it will probably be you), it is important to plan and take the time to call patients promptly for rescheduling, to maintain an up-to-date system, and to persist in scheduling patients so that the time between appointments does not slip from 3 to 6 to 9 months.

CONTINUING CARE PROCEDURES

Typically the continuing care appointment includes a reassessment of the patient's general and oral health (refer to Part Three). The medical history should be updated, vital signs recorded, and the intraoral and extraoral examinations repeated. For periodontal patients, sites that were active previously should be carefully assessed, along with an overall assessment of the rest of the mouth. The periodontal assessment should include microbiologic and/or host-response monitoring of the sites known to be at risk, followed by careful probing and comparison with previous readings. Bleeding on probing should be noted. Radiographs should be taken sparingly but when needed to confirm clinical findings.

Plaque should be disclosed using a fluoroscein dye (with PlakLite) so that the patient can see where his or her oral hygiene is effective and where it needs to be improved. The fluoroscein dye is preferable since it does not stain the soft tissues and lips. Follow the recommendations in Chapter 20 to help the patient identify ways to gain access to areas of chronic plaque retention. Work with the patient to find the proper method and adequate time and location for effective oral hygiene. Consider adding or changing antimicrobial agents for brushing, rinsing, and irrigating. Consider switching the patient to a different brush design or to an electric brush. Review the effectiveness of flossing and consider alternatives that will reach interdentally. Mention again to tobacco users that nicotine has a direct, negative impact on periodontal health and that there are programs to help them abandon the habit. Review the dietary recommendations from the last visit and see what is working and what is not.

For many patients, a light subgingival debridement at the recall visit is sufficient. This can be accomplished by using a curette or an ultrasonic instrument (low power) throughout the mouth to disrupt plaque. The instrument is moved lightly over the subgingival areas, concentrating on those sites which show signs of recurrent disease or in which the subgingival area is particularly difficult for the patient to maintain. The instrument is used to "scale" only when actual calculus deposits are encountered. This is important because subgingival scaling in healthy, shallow sites actually causes loss of attachment in those areas (Badersten et al, 1981; Knowles et al, 1980; Lindhe et al, 1982a, 1982b; Pihlstrom et al, 1981). The ultrasonic instrument or a Prophy-jet can be used to remove supragingival stain and other deposits that bother the patient. You can use subgingival irrigation as a final clinical procedure to introduce antimicrobial agents subgingivally and to create the same clean feeling that patients have traditionally associated with complete coronal polishing. If the patient is caries prone or has sensitive dentin, you can apply topical fluoride.

Products that deliver antibiotics to sites with advancing periodontal disease are likely to reach the market by the mid-1990s. These include vinyl acetate fibers impregnated with tetracycline that are wrapped around the tooth in the periodontal pocket and left in place for 10 to 14 days to slowly release the medication (Fiorellini and Paquette, 1992). Other products include subgingival chips, beads, or gels that can be placed in the pocket to release medications such as antibiotics or antiinflammatory agents over time. Some products may simply place a barrier between the tissue and the plaque endotoxin or actually neutralize the endotoxin as they resorb. With increasing knowledge of the role of the body's immune system in coping with a microbiologic challenge, we may soon be administering oral rinses or delivering local retroviruses to help monocytes and other cells function more effectively. Measures such as these will help to combat the microbiologic challenge or to more readily repair the damage caused by the challenge.

When these products are available it is conceivable that, other than a light, general debridement, continuing care therapy will focus on site-specific treatment that helps modify the local environment.

Regardless of the sophistication of the available technology, the continuing care appointment retains the same objective: to ensure that each individual is monitored and helped appropriately so that disease does not commence or recur, and, when it does, to institute the proper treatment to reverse the process.

REFERRAL

Patients with recurring or persistent problems may be considered for referral for specialized care. You will not be able to eliminate all disease in all patients, but you should be able to recognize those patients for whom your joint efforts are insufficient.

Establish guidelines for referring patients for specialized care and adhere to them so that patients do not slide along for a year or more with unmanaged destructive disease. Patients with physical problems that are not being treated by a physician should be referred to one for help. This includes high blood pressure; signs that suggest diabetes or nutritional deficiencies; skin lesions, persistent pain, malaise, chronic headaches, and a host of other signs that suggest physical problems.

Patients who are under stress or who have substance abuse problems or eating disorders can be guided to a competent counselor or psychologist.

Central to the area of oral health, periodontal sites that do not improve or that tend to worsen need the attention of a periodontist. Otherwise the attachment loss becomes so advanced that repair is greatly compromised. Two recall visits with a 2 to 3 month interval that show persistent disease are more than enough to suggest that your initial therapy has not succeeded. You and your employer- or coworker-dentist should agree on the specific criteria you will use for considering and recommending a referral.

Other oral health needs, such as orthodontic care, replacement of missing teeth, restoration of caries, endodontic therapy, intraoral or extraoral lesions, and tooth extraction should be referred to the general dentist for a dental diagnosis and treatment plan.

You will play a critical role in (1) explaining the need for special care, (2) ensuring that the appointment is scheduled with a competent clinician once the patient agrees to the referral, (3) communicating with the specialist regarding the diagnosis and recommended treatment, (4) discussing those plans with the patient to determine his or her attitude and intentions, and (5) maintaining contact with the patient and the specialist during and after treatment so that the patient can be reentered in the continuing care program when appropriate. Your overall role is to be the coordinator of referred care and to serve as the patient's advocate when more than one health care provider is involved in treatment. This requires excellent communication skills with both the professionals and the patient and a commitment to helping the-patient through the sometimes complex process of multiple diagnoses and (un)coordinated care.

RETRIEVING THE PATIENT FOR CONTINUING CARE

Often when a patient is referred for periodontal therapy, the periodontist will opt to enroll him or her in that practice's continuing care program. Though this approach helps the periodontist monitor the periodontal tissues, the evaluation may not include a complete review of the other risk factors and disease patterns that require attention. As a result, and to ensure that the generalist does not "lose" the patient to the specialist, many practices have a policy of alternating continuing care appointments with the periodontist (Caffesse, 1990). When the patient visits the generalist, a complete review of all oral health needs is conducted, including periodontal health. These findings should be transmitted to the periodontist for inclusion in their records, in the form of either a letter or a charting plus ancillary information. Likewise, when the patient visits the periodontist, the generalist should receive at least a summary of the patient's periodontal condition at that visit.

To help with such frequent communication, standard letters of referral and information regarding patient care can be developed and stored in a word processing program. Then you can enter the specifics regarding each patient in the alternating recall program and ensure that such information is mailed on a daily basis. Copies should be placed in the patient's record or the information noted on the recall record.

SUMMARY

Rounding out the cycle of dental hygiene care is the "continuing care" appointment that will characterize much of your working day in a practice with a large pool of patients who have been treated and are hoping to avoid further problems. This area of care equals thorough assessment, careful planning, oral health instruction, and therapy in importance. In fact, the continuing care appointment repeats the complete cycle of care to ensure that the patient is maintaining health. It also forms the basis for determining whether the care you provide is successful and is helping improve your patients oral health.

ACTIVITIES

1. Invite local dental hygienists to describe the recall systems they use in private practice and to discuss the ways in which they monitor patient progress over several continuing care visits.
2. Given any recall system, identify the ways in which it provides opportunities for the patients to miss being scheduled for care or to otherwise slip away from regular continuing care.
3. Investigate the status of new "site-specific" treatments entering the market: research findings, regulatory approval, marketing claims, ease of use, and likely benefits in clinical practice.

REVIEW QUESTIONS

1. Why is continuing care important?
2. On what was the traditional 6-month continuing care interval based?
3. On what is the 3 or 4 month interval based?
4. What percentage of patients is:
    a. Likely to be healthy regardless of regular care?
    b. Likely to have advancing disease that responds minimally to professional care?
    c. Likely to respond to professional care but needs careful monitoring?
5. Identify four essential characteristics of a sound recall system.
6. What clinical procedures are typically included at the continuing care appointment?
7. What is your role in coordinating care for patients who have been referred to a specialist?

REFERENCES

Axelsson P, Lindhe J: Effect of controlled oral hygiene procedures on caries and periodontal disease in adults, *J Clin Periodontol* 5:133, 1978.

Axelsson P, Lindhe J: Effect of controlled oral hygiene procedures on caries and periodontal disease in adults, *J Clin Periodontol* 8:281, 1981.

Badersten A et al: Effect of nonsurgical periodontal therapy I. Moderately advanced periodontitis, *J Clin Periodontol* 8:45, 1981.

Becker W, Becker B, Berg L: Periodontal treatment without maintenance: a retrospective study in 44 patients, *J Periodontol* 55:505, 1984.

Becker W, Berg L, Becker B: Long-term evaluation of periodontal treatment and maintenance in 95 patients, *Int J Periodont Rest Dent* 4(2):54, 1984.

Caffessee RG: Maintenance therapy: preventing recurrence of periodontal diseases. In Genco RJ, Goldman HM, Cohen DW: *Contemporary periodontics,* St Louis, 1990, Mosby–Year Book

Fiorellini JP, Paquette DW: The potential role of controlled release delivery systems for chemotherapeutic agents in periodontitis, *Current science: periodontology and restorative dentistry,* 63-79, 1992.

Hirschfeld L, Wasserman B: A long term survey of tooth loss in 600 treated periodontal patients, *J Periodontol* 49:225, 1978.

Knowles J et al: Comparison of results following three modalities of periodontal therapy related to tooth type and initial pocket depth, *J Clin Periodontol* 7:32, 1980.

Lindhe J et al: Healing following surgical/non-surgical treatment of periodontal disease, *J Clin Periodontol* 9:115, 1982.

Lindhe J et al: Scaling and root planing in shallow pockets, *J Clin Periodontol* 9:415, 1982.

Löe H et al: The natural history of periodontal disease in man: the rate of periodontal destruction before 40 years of age, *J Periodontol* 49:607, 1978a.

Löe H et al: The natural history of periodontal disease in man: tooth mortality before 40 years of age, *J Periodont Res,* 13:563, 1978b.

Löe H et al: The natural history of periodontal disease in man: rapid, moderate and no loss of attachment in Sri Lankan laborers 15 to 45 years of age, *J Clin Periodontol* 13:431, 1986.

Meador HL, Lane JJ, Suddick RP: The long term effectiveness of perioodntal therapy in a clinical practice, *J Periodontol* 56: 253, 1985.

McFall WT: Tooth loss in 100 patients with periodontal disease—a long term study, *J Periodontol* 53:539, 1982.

Mousques T, Listgarten MA, Phillips RW: Effect of scaling and root planing on the composition of the human subgingival microbial flora, *J Periodont Res* 15:144, 1980.

Nyman S, Lindhe J, Rosling B: Periodontal surgery in plaque-infected dentitions, *J Clin Periodontol* 4:240, 1977.

Pihlstrom BI et al: A randomized four-year study of periodontal therapy, *J Periodontol* 52:227, 1981.

Rosling B et al: The healing potential of the periodontal tissues following different techniques of periodontal surgery in plaque free dentitions: a 2-year clinical study, *J Clin Periodontol* 3:233, 1976.

Suomi JD et al: The effect of controlled oral hygiene procedures on the progression of periodontal disease in adults: results after the third and final year, *J Periodontol* 42:152, 1971.

Westfelt ES et al: Significance of frequency of professional tooth cleaning for healing following periodontal surgery, *J Clin Periodontol* 10:148, 1983.

Wilson T: *Dental maintenance for patients with periodontal diseases,* Surrey, England, 1991, Quintessence.

36 CASE DOCUMENTATION

Irene Woodall
Bonnie Dafoe

LEARNING OUTCOMES

The dental hygienist will be able to

1. Discuss the value and uses of case documentation in relation to record keeping.
2. Develop and present a case documentation, using either a written or verbal format.

Case documentation refers to a thorough record of the patient's dental therapy. This record is both visual and written. The visual record is composed of intraoral photographs, radiographs, and study models. The written information includes examination notes, diagnostic chartings, and recordings of treatment. A comprehensive documentation is composed of initial assessment data, the treatment outcome, and an evaluative summary of the therapy.

A lengthy record of each patient or each phase of care may not always be necessary. However, some patients with particular needs are well suited for case documentation. Patients who require extensive reconstructive therapy that includes home care instruction, initial hygiene periodontal preparation, and major restorative and periodontal procedures are candidates for documentation. In such cases, care is delivered in phases over an extended period. Thorough records of each phase reflecting the actual therapy are important for following care to completion. Occasionally a patient may expect an outcome that cannot be achieved. Records documenting the steps of therapy may help the patient or other professionals to evaluate the appropriateness of care.

Another patient may need to realize that even with impeccable home care procedures, fibrotic tissue from chronic inflammation will not change over several months. With the condition documented, the decision for a minor surgical procedure can be made with the patient. A patient with a condition such as acute necrotizing ulcerative gingivitis, for which dental therapy will dramatically improve the gingival conditions, is also well suited for documentation.

Documentation of treatment enhances the accuracy of the patient's record. Too often, when records are reviewed, pertinent details on specific patient conditions and treatment procedures are lacking.

In addition to improving record keeping, case documentation has several educational benefits.

For the clinician, the components of a documentation allow practice in almost all skill areas. Putting it all together in such a way is helpful for the clinician (especially a student) in appreciating and evaluating total care for the patient.

For the patient, involvement in case documentation creates a particular commitment to the goals of treatment. The patient is motivated by participating in the data collection and seeing the results of therapy. At the completion of care, the patient takes pride in his or her role in therapy and wants to maintain the successful outcome.

For colleagues and other patients, the case documentation can be presented as an example from which to learn. Documentation of the success (or failure) of a particular treatment plan or mode of therapy is helpful to other clinicians. The comparison of actual cases is an excellent format for discussion and professional sharing.

For the lay person, the prospect of a significant amount of dentistry may be overwhelming. Examples of completed cases may be helpful in proposing or convincing a patient of the need for specific therapy. Seeing examples of the course of care may be reassuring to the patient.

Showing patients the successful results of prevention-oriented dental therapy is one of the best motivators for preventive home care methods (Figs. 36-1 to 36-4).

Text continued on page 808.

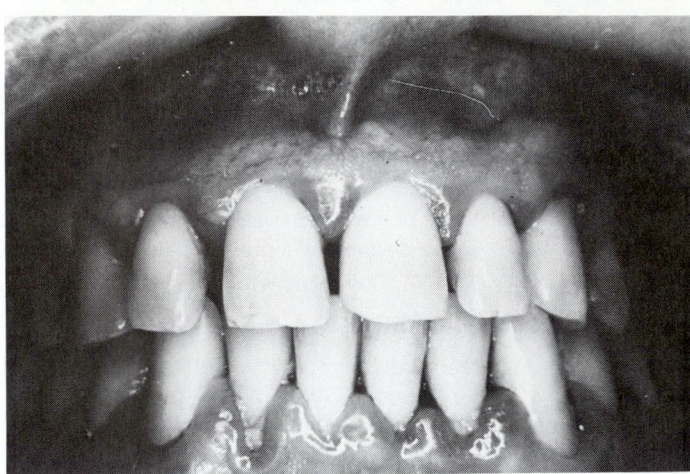

Fig. 36-1. Initial photograph. This 40-year-old man had multiple periodontal abscesses, one of which is clearly seen in mandibular right cuspid area. There are no systemic etiologic factors. Tissue bleeds readily and is swollen and edematous. Papillae are separated from lingual soft tissue. Maxillary and mandibular incisors are mobile, diastemas are present, and there is fremitus of anterior teeth in excursive movements.
(From Corn H, Marks M: *Contin Dent Educ* 1:10, 1978.)

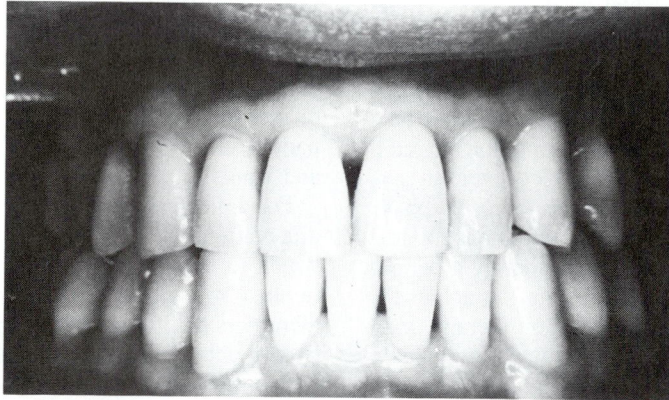

Fig. 36-2. This 12-year result clearly shows that reinforcement of plaque control procedures along with secondary preventive dentistry therapy has enabled patient to achieve this aesthetic result. Sequence of treatment was *(1)* successful completion of plaque control program and its reinforcement, *(2)* complete periodontal debridement, *(3)* occlusal adjustment in centric relation, *(4)* minor tooth movement to retract maxillary anterior teeth, and *(5)* occlusal adjustment to gain group function in excursive movements and eliminate fremitus patterns. Result shows how stability of tooth position as well as a healthy gingival attachment can be achieved once dental disease has been arrested.
(From Corn H, Marks M: *Contin Dent Educ* 1:10, 1978.)

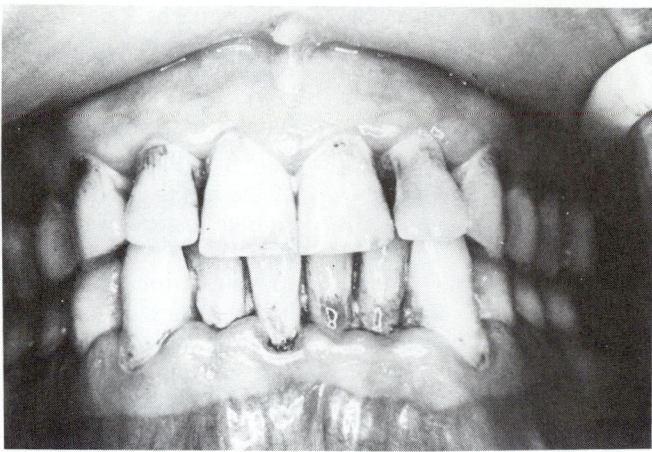

Fig. 36-3. This 50-year-old man had never been to a dentist and had no understanding of the benefits of preventive dentistry care. His treatment consisted of initial therapy and restoration of carious areas.
(From Corn H, Marks M: *Contin Dent Educ* 1:10, 1978.)

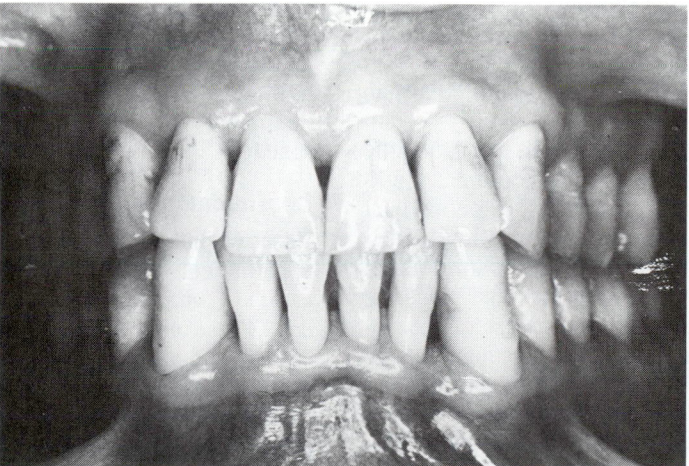

Fig. 36-4. Results of periodontal debridement along with extensive soft tissue curettage have provided this 14-year postoperative result. It is important to ensure that patients not be discouraged at the initial examination, since it is likely that they are unaware of the benefits that preventive dentistry can provide. Secondary preventive procedures enabled this man to have renewed pride and enthusiasm for aesthetics that were achieved during periodontal therapy.
(From Corn H, Marks M: *Contin Dent Educ* 1:10, 1978.)

DOCUMENTATION PROCEDURES

There is no doubt that documentation of care is time consuming. As a clinician approaches case documentation, the key word is *organization*.

The components of a case documentation are as follows:

1. Review of the comprehensive health history.
2. Initial clinical findings (intraoral and extraoral examination).
3. Chartings (periodontal survey and indices-gingival, plaque, bleeding).
4. Radiographs.
5. Diagnostic study casts.
6. Photographs.
7. Treatment considerations (goals, treatment plan).
8. Record of treatment.
9. Posttreatment findings (review components 2 to 6).
10. Evaluation summary.

The consistent quality of diagnostic aids is important. Periodontal records, radiographs, study models, and photographs are necessary to show changes in the patient's tissues as therapy progresses. Instruction for each of these procedures is given in earlier chapters.

Documentation involves making detailed notes of the dental appointment.

Sample chart note: 2/6/93—Prophylaxis with fluoride

A record entry this general tells us very little about what actually occurred. A record entry noting the plaque index, results of a periodontal screening, indications of trouble spots in the dentition, preventive education, the patient's response to care, the care rendered, and plans for future therapy documents the content of the appointment more specifically. Three months from the date of the appointment, the detailed chart notes will facilitate patient follow-up.

Documentation procedures are completed throughout treatment. Planning, with particular attention to the time needed to complete necessary documentation procedures, is recommended to avoid frustration during appointments or with the results of poor documentation.

PRESENTATION OF CASE DOCUMENTATION

The format for a case documentation presentation can be either written or oral. An oral presentation is most common. One format for presentation is described; however, many formats are acceptable. The prospective audience, the facilities for presentation, and the purpose of the presentation each play a part in determining the most appropriate approach. Refer to Figs. 36-5 through 36-14 and the accompanying case description as you review the componenets of a case documentation.

Patient assessment

Introduce the patient profile. Provide a summary of the health history, stating the chief complaint and the history of the present condition. Summarize the clinical findings and present pertinent information from the intraoral and extraoral examination. Show the initial intraoral photographs (slides), study casts, periodontal charting, indices, and radiographs. Describe the dental health education assessment. Use an order of presentation that emphasizes the important aspects of the individual case.

When extensive information is to be presented, a handout is helpful to complement the verbal presentation. The audience is able to take notes during the presentation so that important aspects can be reviewed later.

Patient planning

At this point, general concerns about the patient and reasons for selecting the case for documentation may be presented. State the goals of the treatment, and outline the proposed treatment schedule.

Implementation phase

Describe the treatment actually rendered at each appointment. Provide photographs and other indicators of ongoing care, such as periodontal indices. These aids support the treatment being described and allow the audience to follow the healing and restorative process.

Detailed slides of particular instrumentation procedures are excellent for educational purposes. A series illustrating ultrasonic scaling or other procedures may illustrate a particular technique. This allows the presenter to discuss instrument selection, the choice of materials, or the sequence of therapy.

In this phase, implementation of the preventive education plan is presented. In what area was oral health instruction given? What motivational appeal was used? How was the patient involved in learning? What positive reactions or roadblocks were encountered?

Treatment plans often are changed. Revisions are easily pointed out as the implementation phase is presented.

Posttreatment evaluation

The posttreatment evaluation allows for comparison of initial assessment data and follow-up data. Present the follow-up series of intraoral photographs, periodontal charting, indices, study models, and radiographs (if appropriate). When facilities allow, showing before and after slides simultaneously on two screens is effective.

Discuss or summarize the outcome in relation to the stated goals. If the outcome was not as anticipated, present the factors that may have influenced it. Alternative approaches to care may be included in the discussion also.

With a written presentation, the main consideration is organizing and including all the pertinent information. Present the case with objective comments. Use information as it was found in chartings and as reflected by photographs, models, and radiographs. Detail the posttreatment data to demonstrate the effectiveness of the clinical course.

It is appropriate to make judgments and evaluations after presenting the objective data. Provide the rationale for therapy, and summarize the treatment outcome in relation to expected goals.

SAMPLE CASE

Case Documentation

PATIENT PROFILE: Ms. Smith is a 23-year old African-American woman. She lives in Philadelphia. She originally came to the dental school for pain in the maxillary left area. The patient presented with large occlusal caries in No. 16, which was eventually extracted.

CHIEF COMPLAINT: Ms. Smith came to the dental hygiene clinic because she felt her "gums were in bad shape."

PAST DENTAL HISTORY: The patient was seen by a private dentist about 4 years ago to have her teeth cleaned. She has not been to a dentist since except for the emergency care in which No. 16 was extracted.

MEDICAL HISTORY SUMMARY: Ms. Smith reports having had mumps and chickenpox when she was a child. No residual effects were reported. She had a cyst removed from her left cheek 2 years ago on an outpatient basis. No complications were reported. The patient has broken her right leg and left arm in sports-related accidents. Both these accidents occurred more than 5 years ago, and the patient has recovered full function in both limbs.

The patient takes no prescribed medications at the current time. She does take a daily multivitamin. The patient does not take aspirin, because it upsets her stomach.

The patient's family history reveals that her father died of heart trouble when he was 52 years old. Her mother is alive and has high blood pressure. She has one sister who is alive and well. The patient is obese and follows a diet and exercise schedule prescribed by her physician. In the past 6 months she has lost 75 pounds.

SAMPLE CASE

Case Documentation—cont'd

REVIEW OF SYSTEMS:

HEENT: Wears glasses; recent sore throat

Skin, appendages: Reports her skin becomes dry when she diets

Bones, joints, muscles: Denies any related symptoms

CV: Denies chest pains, palpitations, syncope; blood pressure 130/86

Resp: Reports having bronchial trouble now and then, usually related to sore throats; quit smoking 2 months ago; denies excessive coughing

GI: When patient was taking liquid protein, she experienced gastrointestinal discomfort; no symptoms currently reported

GU: Drinking a great deal of water with the diet; states that this causes more frequent urination

Hemo: Denies excessive bruising or bleeding during extraction

Endo: Denies symptoms related to diabetes, thyroid disorder, and hormone function

CNS: Denies dizziness, restlessness, and hallucinations

CLINICAL FINDINGS:

Extraoral examination: The patient's facial symmetry, lips, TMJ, and larynx were within normal limits. Submandibular and posterior cervical lymph nodes were palpable.

Radiographic findings: Horizontal and vertical bone loss present between all mandibular anterior teeth. Radiographic calculus is apparent, expecially on mandibular anterior teeth. Caries was detected on the distal of No. 29.

Intraoral examination: The patient presented with generalized periodonitis, most severe in the mandibular anterior area. The posterior pharyngeal wall appeared inflamed. Tonsils were present and appeared enlarged. Bilateral mandibular tori were present. Calculus was generalized throughout the mouth with the heaviest deposits located on the lower anterior teeth. The gingiva was inflamed and edematous with some suppuration evident in the lower anterior area. Except for the lower anterior section, the tissue was generally scalloped with normal pigmentation. Tooth No. 9 had mesioincisal fracture, and occlusal caries was detected on Nos. 2, 20, and 29 by exploration.

Periodontal examination: To document reduction in periodontal pocket depth, only the chartings of the maxillary left buccal and of the mandibular anterior facial are noted.

Maxillary left

9	10	11	12	13	14	15	16	(Tooth number)
423	334	435	625	524	335	424	X	Pocket depth in mm (mesial buccal distal)

Mandibular anterior

323	335	544	535	534	533	(Pocket depth)
27	26	25	24	23	22	(Tooth number)

DENTAL-HEALTH EDUCATION:

1. The patient brushed her teeth once a day but did not floss. A random scrubbing method was used for cleaning the teeth and gingiva.
2. Initial bleeding index: 22
3. Initial plaque index: 30 (on a 30-point scale)

INITIAL ASSESSMENT: See Figs. 36-5 to 36-8 for initial assessment.

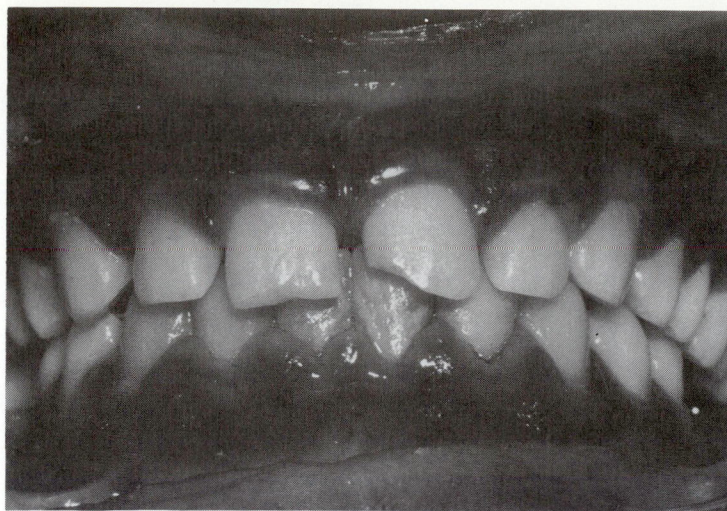

Fig. 36-5. Patient appeared for treatment with generalized periodontitis more severe in lower anterior area. Gingiva is edematous with suppuration evident.

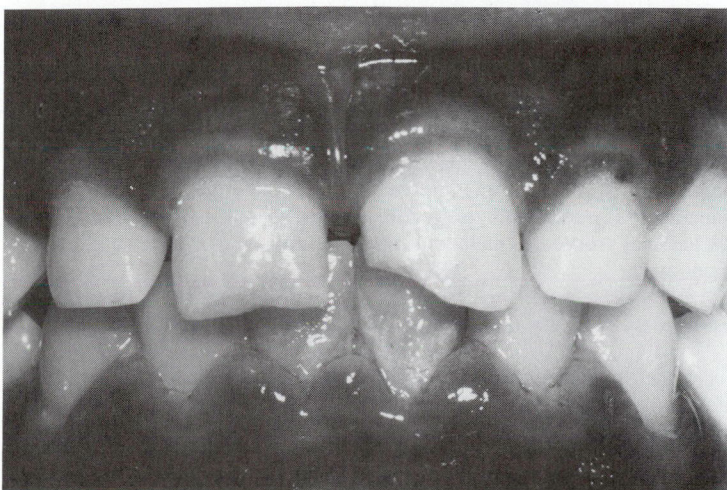

Fig. 36-6. Calculus is generalized but appears heaviest on facial and lingual aspects of mandibular anterior teeth. Several 4- to 5-mm pocket depths were noted on examination.

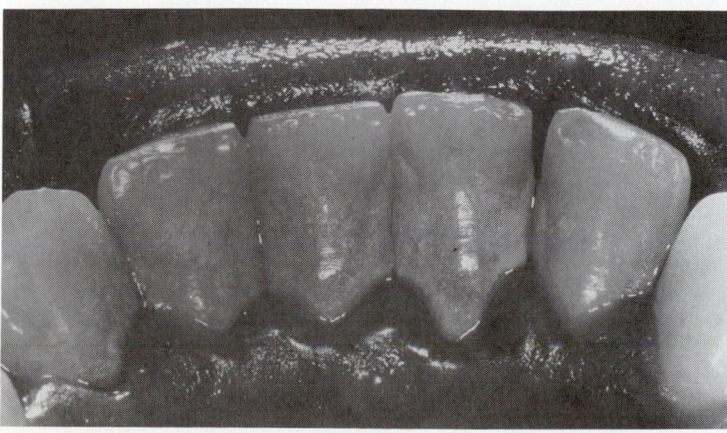

Fig. 36-7. Initial photograph of lingual tissue and heavy calculus deposits on lower anterior teeth. Note tissue contours due to inflammation.

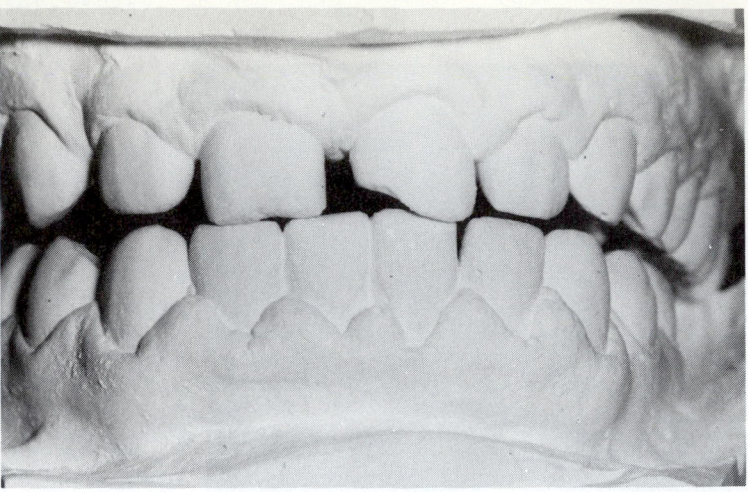

Fig. 36-8. Close-up of initial study models shows fractured maxillary central incisor and topography of gingival tissue.

Case Documentation—cont'd

PLANNING:

Rationale for case selection: Because of the nature of the calculus deposits, the depth of the periodontal pockets, and the patient's willingness to improve her oral conditions, I feel this patient will benefit by participating in documentation procedures. I anticipate that with proper home care instruction and periodontal procedures including thorough ultrasonic debridement, the patient's tissue will respond well.

Goals:

1. Improve the health status of the gingiva, teeth, and supporting ligaments, especially in the lower anterior area.
2. Remove all hard deposits so that the patient can effectively clean her own mouth.
3. Have the patient adopt an oral hygiene regimen to effectively disrupt and remove plaque.
4. Reduce the depth of periodontal pockets.

Initial treatment plan:

Appointment 1: Medical history; intraoral, extraoral examination

Appointment 2: Complete series of radiographs; initial study casts

Appointment 3: Complete periodontal charting; initial series of intraoral photographs

Appointment 4: Dental health education: emphasis on brushing technique; perform ultrasonic scaling for the entire mouth

Appointment 5: Dental health education: review brushing skills; emphasis on flossing and daily irrigation with antimicrobial agent; perform thorough ultrasonic debridement augmented by antimicrobial (two quadrants)

Appointment 6: Dental health education: review flossing and irrigation; assess for possible periodontal aids; complete ultrasonic debridement (two quadrants)

Appointment 7: Dental health education: review all home care procedures; apply stannous fluoride for root sensitivity; follow-up intraoral photographs

Appointment 8: Extension if necessary

IMPLEMENTATION: The treatment proceeded as planned. The patient was receptive to documentation procedures. No skill roadblocks were encountered with dental health education. The patient was able to demonstrate adequate skills with a modified sulcular brushing and loop flossing technique and to irrigate twice daily with dilute antimicrobial solution. The plaque index decreased steadily. Hygiene procedures were accomplished with a minimum of difficulty. Photographs were taken immediately after the ultrasonic scaling at appointment 4 (Figs. 36-9 and 36-10).

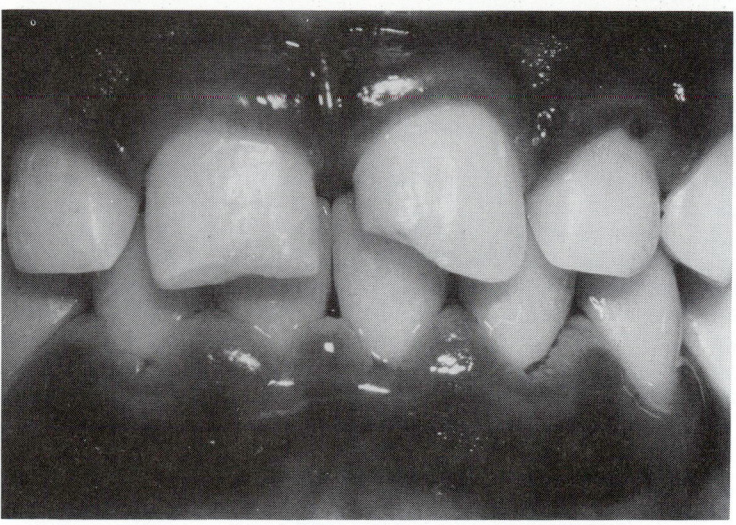

Fig. 36-9. Appointment 4. Following dental health education emphasizing brushing technique, entire mouth was ultrasonically scaled. Facial aspect of mandibular anterior teeth immediately following ultrasonic procedure.

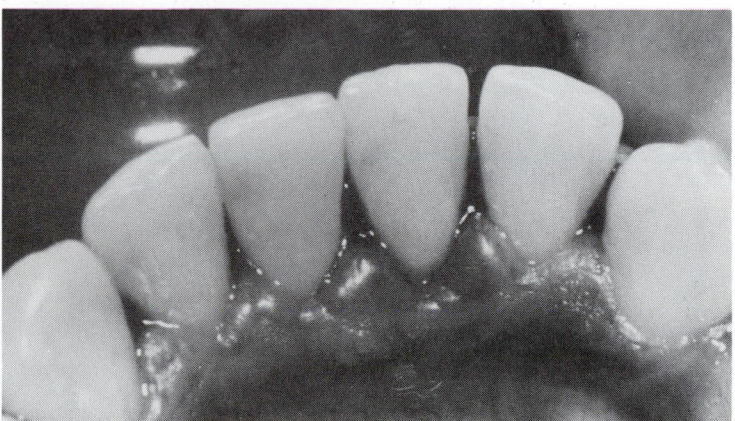

Fig. 36-10. Lingual aspect of mandibular anterior teeth following ultrasonic procedure. Compare with initial photograph, Fig. 35-7.

SAMPLE CASE

Case Documentation—cont'd

Treatment revisions:

Appointment 8: Observed healing of lower anterior tissue; administered maxillary infiltration between Nos. 9 and 10, using approximately one-fourth Carpule (0.5 cc) or 14 mg mepivacaine (Carbocaine) 3% anesthetic solution; dentist placed a composite resin on mesioincisal edge of No. 9

Appointment 9: Dental health education reinforcement; completed follow-up photographs and study models

Appointment 10: Follow-up periodontal charting; discussed recall and further restorative treatment needs

EVALUATION: Ms. Smith was treated in the dental hygiene clinic for a period of 2 months. The follow-up photographs and study models indicate that the tissue in the lower anterior area responded well to thorough debridement (Figs. 36-11 to 36-14). The patient can demonstrate an adequate technique for brushing and flossing. She effectively removes plaque and values her newly acquired skills and the appearance of her tissue. Continued home care has been reinforced to maintain this area. The final plaque index was 4, and the final bleeding index was 1. Following are the chartings of pocket depth after treatment in the areas originally noted.

Maxillary left

9	10	11	12	13	14	15	16	(Tooth number)
323	333	323	413	313	325	323	X	(Pocket depth in mm mesial buccal distal)

Mandibular anterior

323	323	223	322	223	332	(Pocket depth)
27	26	25	24	23	22	(Tooth number)

The patient and I are pleased that our goals for this phase of treatment have been accomplished. Ms. Smith will continue with restorative treatment and will be seen for periodontal recall in 2 months.

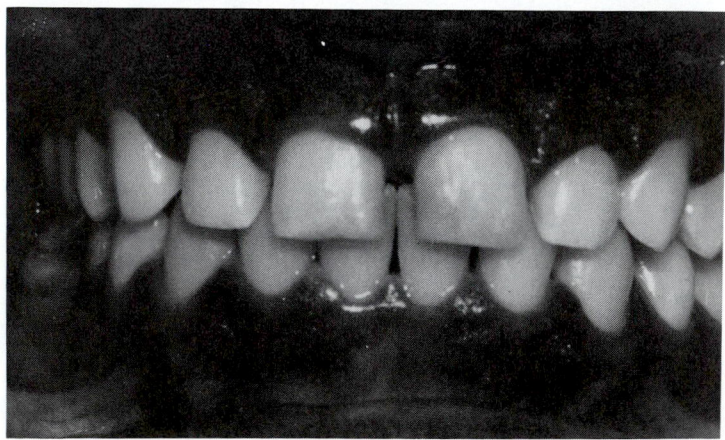

Fig. 36-11. Appointment 9. Composite resin was placed on maxillary left central incisor.

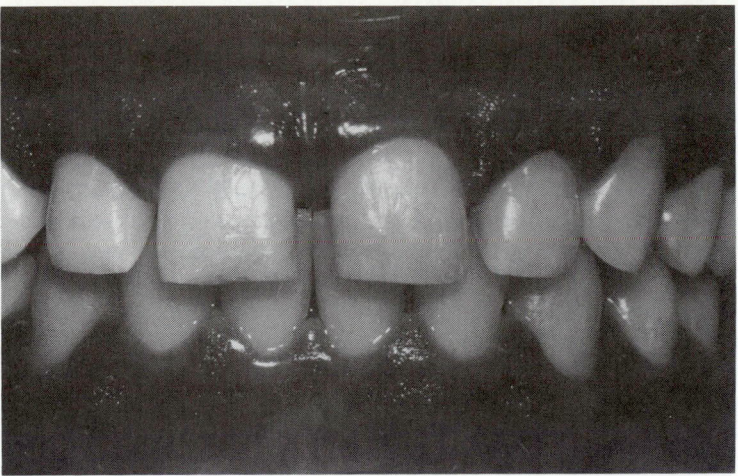

Fig. 36-12. Ten days after treatment, healing process in lower anterior area is evident. Deepest pocket depth noted in this area was 3 mm.

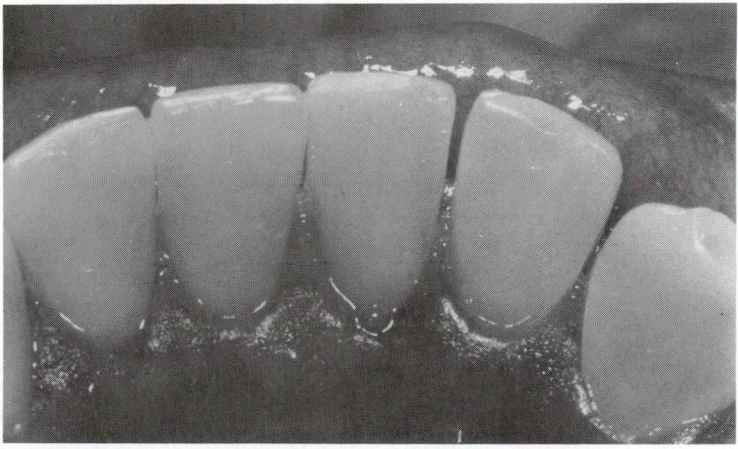

Fig. 36-13. Follow-up photograph of mandibular lingual anterior tissue reveals much improved gingival contour after debridement. Note papillae edge and stippled texture as compared with that in Fig. 35-7.

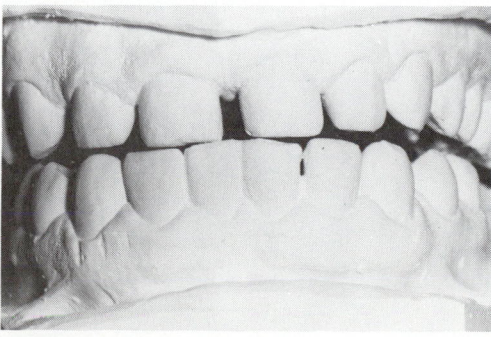

Fig. 36-14. Follow-up study models document healing process that occurred in mandibular anterior region and restoration of maxillary central incisor.

ORTHODONTIC CASE DOCUMENTATION

Orthodontic specialization for dental hygienists is an exciting career option. The skills a hygienist uses are varied, and he or she has a tremendous influence on the patient during the course of treatment.

The following case is presented to illustrate some of the ways in which a hygienist participates in orthodontic care. Figs. 36-15 through 36-26 document the case visually and suggest the components of care that should be photographed. Accompanying written descriptions of each phase of the case complete the documentation. Although not every educational program for hygienists includes all of these skills, the basic foundation of anatomic sciences, traditional clinical preventive services, and patient management skills can be enhanced through special courses and on-the-job training. State laws that provide for a full scope of practice and general supervision have made it possible for hygienists to become active in orthodontic care.

The hygienist's involvement begins with the pretreatment evaluation. This includes gathering information about the patient's medical and dental history and learning about his or her oral habits and home care practices. Photographic records can be completed by the hygienist. These include extraoral photographs, radiographs, cephalometric studies, temporomandibular joint views, and intraoral views. The patient is examined clinically to determine the health of the teeth and the periodontal tissues. The hygienist is able to complete plaque scores, and periodontal and restorative chartings. Following this, impressions and study models are completed. These initial records are used to prepare a treatment plan. Hygienists with an educational background in craniofacial growth and development may be involved in preparing parts of the treatment plan and presenting it to the patient. The hygienist will be able to help the patient and his or her family understand the proposed treatment and to answer questions during treatment.

As treatment moves to the active phase of removable or fixed orthodontic appliances, the hygienist will be the one who sees the patient the most during the frequent checks at the dental office. During this phase of care, modifying home care techniques, debriding the teeth, applying fluoride treatments, and adjusting the appliances will become the hygienist's responsibility. The ability to communicate with the patient about personal oral care, attention to diet, compliance with recommended hours for wearing various appliances, and so forth will be important for keeping the treatment plan on target and supporting the patient through the changes.

The hygienist can participate in removing and replacing various appliances and in keeping the records current by repeating photographs and chartings if necessary during treatment. When treatment is completed, new photos, radiographs, and models will be made to document the results of care. As the patient is usually followed for a period, the hygienist will stay involved with a recall schedule to monitor the posttreatment care. The opportunity to use skills in many clinical areas and to be an understanding friend throughout the years is a rewarding part of delivering primary care.

This orthodontic case documentation shows the value of written and photographic records. In actuality, many more records make up the patient's portfolio. This sample covers the essential aspects of the patient's care.

SAMPLE CASE
Orthodontic Case Documentation

PATIENT PROFILE: A 10-year, 2-month-old caucasian male. Resident of a Cleveland suburb. Patient came to orthodontist from referral of neighbor.

CHIEF COMPLAINT: Crowded teeth.

PAST DENTAL HISTORY: Patient involved in regular recall with primary care dentist. Patient experienced trauma to upper anterior teeth, resulting in fracture of both upper central incisors.

MEDICAL HISTORY: Negative, other than usual childhood disease; no complications or hospitalization.

CLINICAL FINDINGS: (Fig. 36-15): The patient appeared for treatment with a facial profile characterized by a slightly turned up nose with obtuse nasolabial angle, a long upper lip, retrognathic chin, and a sublabial crease which is indicative of a strong mentalis muscle. A slight midopening click of the left temporomandibular joint was noted. Several deciduous teeth were present; several were loose.

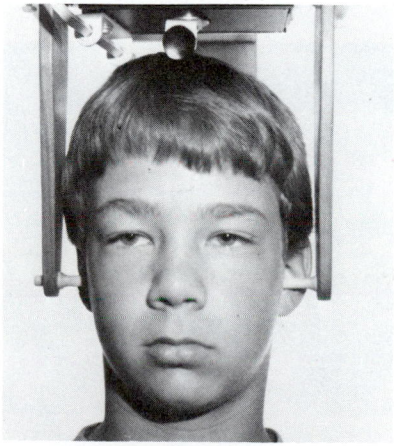

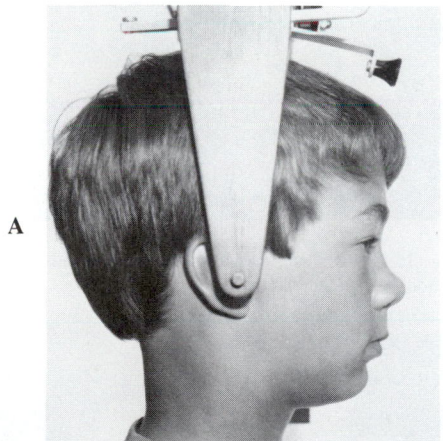

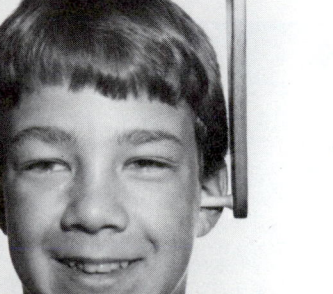

Fig. 36-15. Facial photographs before orthodontic treatment. **A,** Profile. **B,** Frontal. **C,** Smile.

SAMPLE CASE

Orthodontic Case Documentation—cont'd

INTRAORAL FINDINGS (Figs. 36-16 to 36-19): Patient exhibited excessive protrusion with a deep bite and crowded upper and lower teeth. Molars were in an approximate Class I bilateral occlusion. Generalized gingivitis was noted.

INITIAL TREATMENT: A recommendation was made by the orthodontist to the parents requesting the patient have several deciduous teeth extracted. The patient was seen at 9-month intervals until the permanent teeth erupted.

After approximately 18 months of observation, the orthodontist requested the patient be evaluated for full orthodontic treatment. The parents consented. A complete series of diagnostic records was gathered and processed by the dental hygienist. The diagnostic series of records taken included the following: panographic x-ray; frontal x-ray; lateral cephalometric x-ray; hand-wrist x-ray; facial photographs, including frontal, lateral, and smile; a series of intraoral 35 mm slides; impressions for diagnostic casts; and a maxillary intercuspation bite registration. A request was made for a complete series of periapical x-rays, which was to be obtained from the primary care dentist and forwarded to the orthodontist.

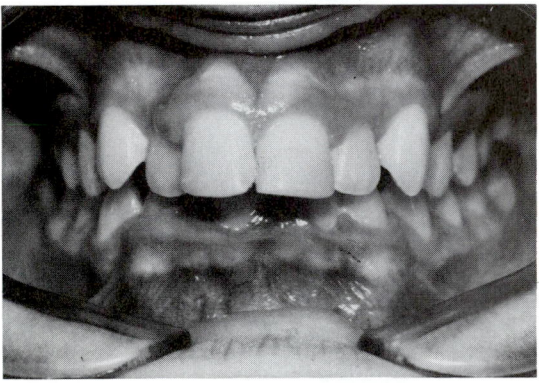

Fig. 36-16. Direct anterior view of teeth in occlusion before orthodontic treatment.

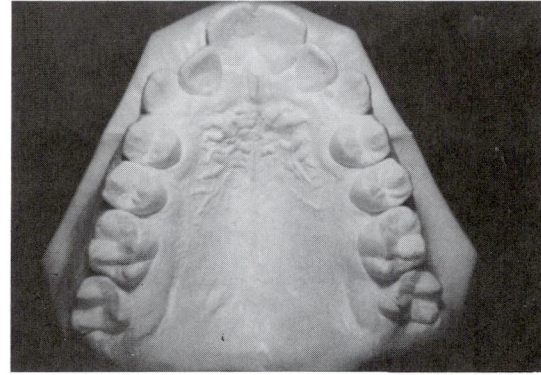

Fig. 36-17. Occlusal view of maxillary diagnostic cast before orthodontic treatment.

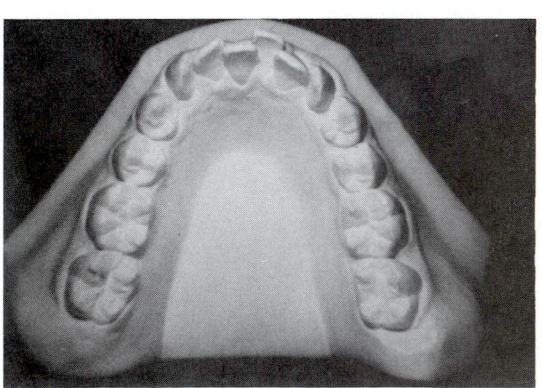

Fig. 36-18. Occlusal view of mandibular diagnostic cast before orthodontic treatment.

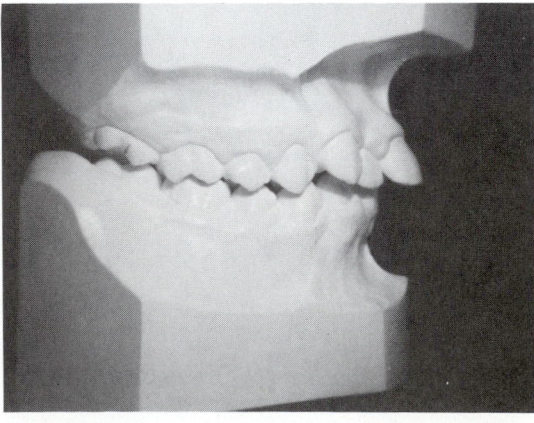

Fig. 36-19. Right lateral view of diagnostic casts in occlusion before orthodontic treatment.

SAMPLE CASE

Orthodontic Case Documentation—cont'd

REVIEW OF DIAGNOSTIC RECORDS AND TREATMENT PLAN: Confirmed the clinical observations and suggested the need for the removal of permanent teeth to relieve the crowding and advance the mandible to improve skeletal balance and the soft tissue profile. The treatment plan that would best accomplish these goals and work toward rehabilitation of the temporomandibular joint included the removal of all four permanent second molar teeth. This would create space for the relief of crowding and allow the full unhampered development of the third molars. Functional jaw orthodontics would accomplish mandibular advancement and improve the functional relationships in the temporomandibular joint.

TREATMENT CONSULTATION WITH PARENTS: Parents met with the dental hygienist for review of treatment recommendations made by the orthodontist. Parents consented to treatment.

SAMPLE CASE

Orthodontic Case Documentation—cont'd

TREATMENT: The patient met with the dental hygienist at a special patient orientation appointment for discussion and demonstration of proper oral hygiene and appliance care.

The four second molar teeth were removed by an oral surgeon. Removable functional appliances (sagittal appliance followed by an orthopedic corrector) were worn by the patient for approximately 2 years (Figs. 36-20 and 36-21). The patient wore the appliances 24 hours daily. He had recall appointments at 3- to 6-week intervals for adjustments to the appliances and monitoring of treatment progress and oral hygiene evaluation. During this time, he was advised to see his primary care dentist for his routine dental health care.

Retainers were placed after the 2 years of removable appliance treatment. The patient was monitored for another 18 months while the third molars erupted.

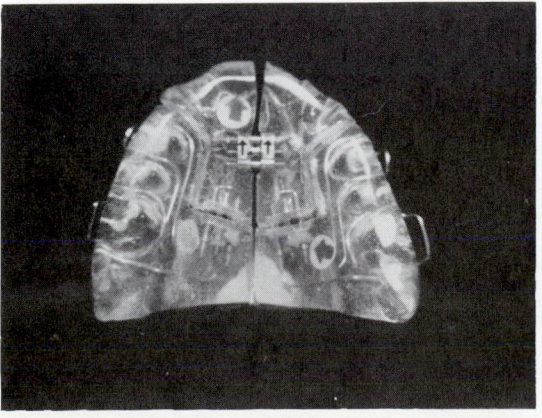

Fig. 36-20. Removable sagittal appliance.

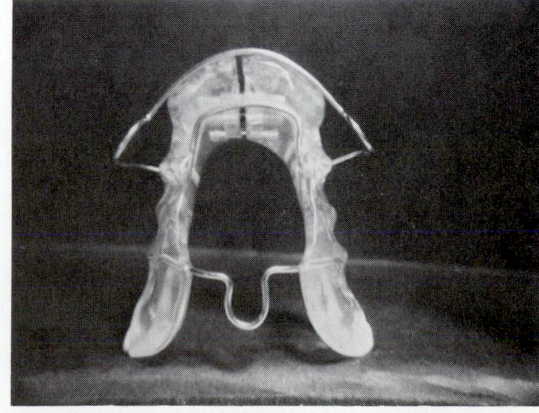

Fig. 36-21. Removable orthopedic corrector appliance.

Orthodontic Case Documentation—cont'd

Final treatment records were gathered by the hygienist for review by the orthodontist (Figs. 36-22 to 36-26). The orthodontist dismissed the patient from treatment.

EVALUATION: Stable treatment results were obtained during the growth years. The third molars erupted without incident. The patient and parents were delighted that treatment results could be accomplished without fixed appliances.

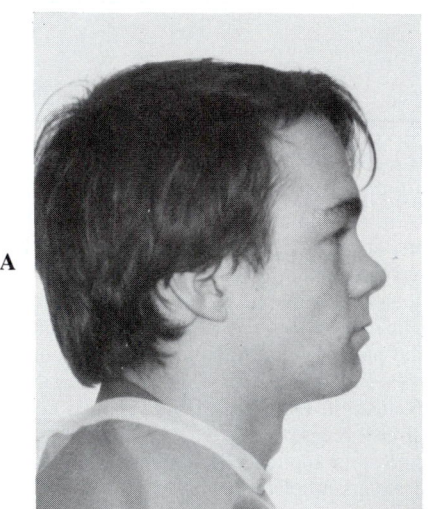
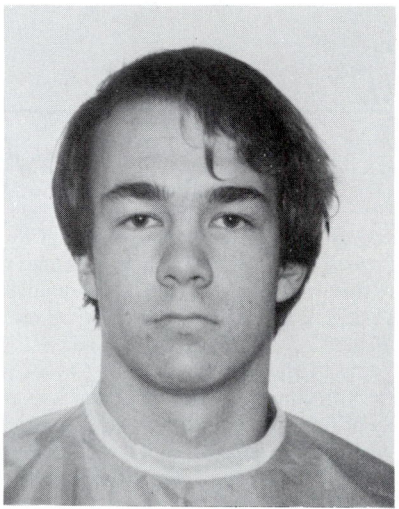

Fig. 36-22. Facial photographs following orthodontic treatment. **A,** Profile. **B,** Frontal. **C,** Smile.

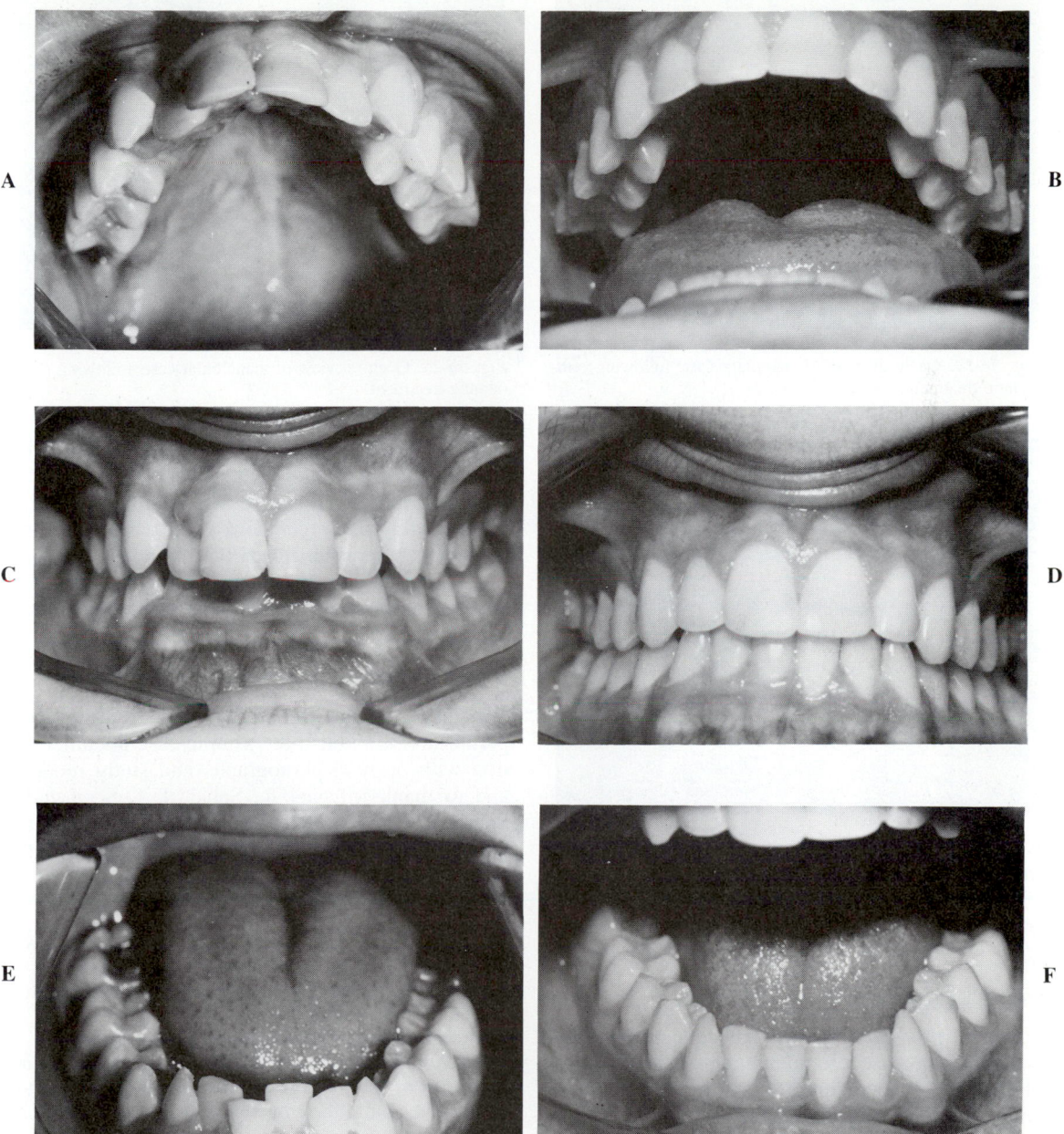

Fig. 36-23. Documentation of position of patient's teeth before and after orthodontic treatment. **A,** Initial maxillary occlusal view. **B,** Final maxillary occlusal view. **C,** Initial facial view of teeth in occlusion. **D,** Final direct anterior view of teeth in occlusion. **E,** Initial mandibular occlusal view. **F,** Final mandibular occlusal view.

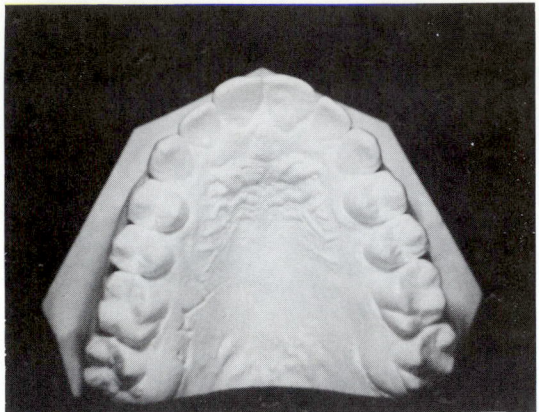

Fig. 36-24. Occlusal view of maxillary cast, following orthodontic treatment.

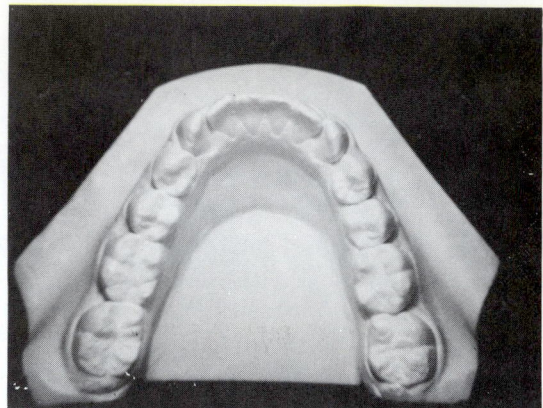

Fig. 36-25. Occlusai view of mandibular cast, following orthodontic treatment.

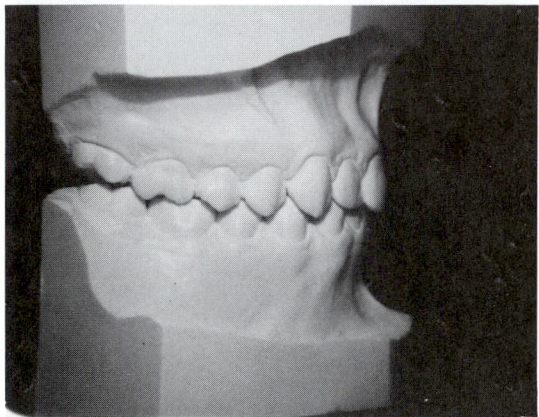

Fig. 36-26. Right lateral view of casts in occlusion following orthodontic treatment.

Practicing presenting a case documentation will be valuable experience as the student clinician enters the professional world. Maintaining standards for recording comprehensive quality care will become the responsibility of the clinician. Beyond this, sharing cases with others will be a primary area for professional contact and postgraduate education.

ACKNOWLEDGEMENTS
We wish to thank Deborah Drazek, R.D.H., for permission to publish the sample case documentation with original photographs and study models and to thank Michael R. Sabat, D.D.S., Lynda Sabat, R.D.H., and their patient for permission to publish the orthodontic case documentation with original photographs and study models.

ACTIVITIES
1. Listen to case documentations presented by faculty, visiting clinicians, or more advanced students.
2. Create a format for presentation to suit specific clinic needs if necessary.
3. Prepare and present a case documentation.*
4. According to class size, present documentations in groups of five or six. Select one documentation to be presented to the entire class and/or junior class.*

REVIEW QUESTIONS
1. List the components of a case documentation.
2. Describe how case documentation:
   a. Enhances record keeping.
   b. Can be used in patient education.

* Identify a patient (one or more) who presents conditions in which observable tissue changes will occur. Ten weeks to a full semester may be necessary to complete the documentation.

CONCLUSION
Student peers and professional colleagues enjoy learning from case documentations. This situation places the clinician or observer in a position to empathize with the care being delivered. Treatment options may be explored and discussed in an environment conducive to sharing past experiences and new ideas.

The clinician who presents a case documentation has the opportunity to display an aspect of his or her patient care. Fellow clinicians learn from observing the type and quality of care provided to the patient.

37 EVALUATING SUCCESS OF DENTAL HYGIENE CARE

Irene Woodall

LEARNING OUTCOMES

The dental hygienist will be able to

1. Explain how a philosophy of accountability for professional practice can affect a person's overall approach to providing care.
2. Identify several ways in which a dental hygienist can take account of the effectiveness of his or her professional practice, including the following:
   a. The degree to which prevention is emphasized in each day's routine.
   b. The overall effect on health levels of the population group he or she serves.
   c. The degree to which clinical protocols approximate nationally accepted standards and align with new research developments.
   d. Approach behaviors of patients to dental hygiene care.
   e. Personal gratification and health.
   f. Cost-effectiveness.
   g. Participation in professional advancement.
3. Integrate mechanisms for personally evaluating the quality and effectiveness of care that he or she provides as a student and as a graduate clinician.
4. Share personal convictions regarding the goals of professional practice, personal goals regarding professional life, and the future outcomes of an "accountable" approach to health care delivery.

A sound system of accountability will include ways to answer these and other questions: (1) Why am I doing what I am doing? (2) Do I make life better for each patient who seeks care? (3) Is the care I recommend justified? (4) Do I charge reasonable, just fees for care? (5) Do I listen to the wants and needs of my patients? (6) Does the care I deliver meet up-to-date protocols? (7) Could another hygienist review my care and find it to be of impeccable quality? and (8) How do I know the answers to these questions?

DEFINING GOALS

At the base of every system of accountability lies a series of goals, statements of what seems to matter in regard to achievement. These goals exist whether or not they are ever written down or expressed aloud. The process of defining and actually writing out these personal and professional goals or values can help clarify what needs to be evaluated to determine success or achievement. An exercise at the conclusion of this chapter provides one way in which you can clarify and delineate goals for yourself.

Once you have defined a series of goals, you can project ways to measure or at least examine your achievement. The following areas of evaluation are suggested for beginning a comprehensive program of self-evaluation.

PREVENTION ORIENTATION

Most of the literature that discusses the relative merits of prevention and treatment in eradicating disease supports prevention as the logical area of emphasis. Health care providers will be forever behind in keeping up with disease unless they can prevent it from occurring. Public health emphasizes prevention on a large scale. Clinical practice can emphasize it on a smaller scale with greater attention to the needs of individuals rather than groups.

If you believe that preventing dental disease is an essential goal for professional practice, then you may wish to document and evaluate the degree to which that orientation is apparent in daily practice. Some relatively simple measures can include recording and assessing the percentage of time spent in helping patients to care for themselves by removing plaque, routinely performing oral cancer self-examination, and adopting nutritional patterns that promote health. How many minutes per hour are spent educating the patient to prevent disease? Is time provided for measuring blood pressure to detect hypertension? Is the medical history updated at each visit? Are patients routinely evaluated for fluoride therapy and sealants? Have you integrated a tobacco use cessation program in daily practice?

If the vast percentage of the day is spent removing hard and soft deposits that reappear soon after the recall visit, has the clinician's goal of prevention been actualized or is it a value not yet integrated into behavior?

Effect on health levels

A more long-term measure of disease prevention is to evaluate the pattern of health needs of each patient while receiving care. If prevention efforts are successful, disease prevalence should decrease in the clinician's patient population. If the patient avoids or controls the primary etiologic factors in dental disease, the incidence of advanced dental caries, periodontal disease, and oral cancer should decrease. Patients who do not respond to preventive care should be referred for evaluation of their systemic health and immune system.

A historic overview of the patient's progress in oral health each year will reveal whether he or she is developing little or no dental disease, is showing a steady recurrence of problems, or is on a rapid downhill course to tissue destruction and tooth loss.

This overview can be accomplished at a recall visit when new assessment data are gathered. Sharing the findings with the patient can provide evidence of the effectiveness of the health partnership between you and patient. Observing health levels rise and remain high over the years, or at least noting the absence of signs of diseases provides a long-term evaluation of the quality of a preventive program. You can use the case documentation procedures described in Chapter 36 to track patient health.

COMPARISONS WITH NATIONAL STANDARDS AND INTEGRATING NEW RESEARCH FINDINGS

Regardless of whether the daily clinical procedures are oriented towards prevention or treating active disease, you may find it particularly helpful to compare your approach to practice and specific procedures with those published as national standards.

Standards regarding acceptable treatment practices are (1) published by professional associations, (2) discussed and reported in journals and other professional literature, and (3) presented at professional meetings and continuing education sessions. This becomes particularly important as the number of years since graduation increases.

One method is to join a professional study club or a peer group who investigate, test, and validate clinical protocols and assist their peers in integrating the agreed-on procedures into their daily practices. Being recognized as an open, up-to-date, competent clinician among one's peers can carry great personal reward and satisfaction.

APPROACH BEHAVIORS OF PATIENTS

Regardless of the strength of a preventive program and the degree to which national protocols are challenged or observed, the clinician can claim little overall success if the patient does not continue to seek care. If patients appear and disappear, you need to assess the way patients are viewed in the overall health process. Is the patient a means to an end, whether it be clinical requirements or a reasonable income? Is the patient an object of care? Does the patient feel that the health care provider respects, values, and looks forward to seeing him or her?

If the treatment files show large numbers of long-term patients who have continued to seek care over the years, relationships have developed that the patients see as helpful and worth maintaining.

The other point of view might be examined also. What are your approach behaviors to patients? Do you have a preconceived notion of what a patient ought to be? Do you reject patients who do not meet the expected standards of behavior, or do you see each person as valuable and worthy of care, regardless of their initial compliance or noncompliance with the criteria for the "ideal" patient?

PERSONAL GRATIFICATION AND HEALTH

An annual physical examination can be a way of measuring success. If the health professional's own health includes such elements as varicose veins; slumped shoulders; chronic headaches; regular use of drugs for indigestion, anxiety, insomnia, or "pep"; fatigue; and hostility, the "health" professional may need to carefully examine the relationship of clinical practice to these problems. Successful practice should allow time for relaxation, pleasure, exercise, and a broadening understanding of life and the surrounding world. It should be a source of pleasure rather than a daily drudgery. Physical and mental health reflect the degree to which the day's focus and activities stimulate gratification or anxiety.

The very process of annually evaluating the success of the preventive program, short- and long-term health progress of patients, compliance with accepted standards of practice, and approach behaviors of patients can produce a picture of gratification or dissatisfaction. One bottom-line question is: Do the process and outcome of what I am doing with my life bring me gratification? If the answer is yes, it can bring a renewed spirit to continue practice. If the answer is no, you may need to identify what kind of change is necessary.

COST-EFFECTIVENESS

In an economy that is based on competition, one element that is not easily ignored is the evaluation of the cost-effectiveness of practice. Providing the highest-quality health care services at a cost that is greater than the income they generate guarantees a short-lived practice. The basic costs of a health care facility (rent, insurance, utilities, supplies, salaries, etc.) must be covered by generated income. Therefore a complete evaluation of success should include an analysis of the ledger. A practice that does not break even or generate profit needs professional analysis of its operation and suggestions for change.

Cost-effectiveness implies more than generating sufficient income. Its primary connotation in terms of accountability to the profession and the public is the degree to which the expended health dollar actually improves health. Do patients pay money every 6 months for a slow immersion into advanced periodontal disease or eventual full-mouth reconstruction, or does the money they pay ensure the restoration and maintenance of health over the years? The answer to this question brings the health care provider back to the evaluation of prevention effectiveness.

PARTICIPATION IN PROFESSIONAL ADVANCEMENT

Professional advancement is closely tied to monetary success. Many people see their profession as a career ladder. Over the years following gradua-

tion, they acquire experience and advanced education so that they can assume new responsibilities and meet new challenges, either in the same job setting or in a series of different jobs. Goals can be set and measured along a pathway for advancement and opportunities.

A second aspect of professional advancement is tied to ensuring that the profession of dental hygiene is nurtured and guided as it changes over the decades. This usually involves a commitment to association activities at the local, state, national, or international levels. It is easy to acquire a degree and use it for personal advancement. However, in a "loner" profession such as dental hygiene—in which interaction with other hygienists is frequently sparse—it also is easy to lose track of what is happening to the profession through educational, regulatory, political, and legal changes. Five or ten years after graduation, the profession can look quite different in terms of the security it provides, its attractiveness to new applicants, and its ability to provide high-quality care. An accountable dental hygienist should be able to point to specific contributions he or she has made to help guide and sustain the profession.

CONCLUSION

Each area of evaluation helps you assess your individual contribution to the quality of life—your own life, the profession's, and of course that of each patient and thus of society.

A well-planned, thoughtful approach to the evaluation process may make dental hygiene a truly rewarding career and a source of lifelong fulfillment, or it may be a means for planning career changes and personal growth in new areas.

A format that can be used to generate personal and professional goals and to display evaluation findings for each year is shown in the box on p. 826.

ACTIVITIES

1. Using the evaluation of success format presented on p.— define personal and professional practice goals that are, in your opinion, signs of success. Then form groups of three to share those goals. Note similarities and differences in goals and values among the members of the small groups. Suggest ways in which these goals could be evaluated in practice on a regular basis.
2. Analyze the degree to which prevention-oriented procedures make up the clinical efforts in your daily practice as a student.

3. As a student, conduct a year-long or a semester-long system of accountability that measures the extent to which you have approximated or achieved personal and professional goals.
4. Invite representatives of the local or state dental hygienists' association to discuss how its members and leaders contribute to improving the profession.

REVIEW QUESTIONS

1. How can a philosophy of accountability of professional practice affect one's overall approach to providing care?
2. Identify seven ways in which a health professional can measure effectiveness or success in practice.
3. What can a health care provider do if he or she sees little evidence of success or gratification in his or her professional or personal life?

Defining and Evaluating Personal and Profession Goals

Use the following format for recording your response to questions 1 to 7

Question						
1	2	3	4	5	6	7
PROFESSIONAL GOALS:						
PERSONAL GOALS:						

1. List each goal that is important for your sense of success (short- and long-term).
2. Rank each goal you have listed according to its relative importance and significance in your determination of success.
3. Give the earliest date you will be able to evaluate your progress toward each goal.
4. How will you know progress has been achieved (what is your measure)?
5. How will you know when each goal has actually been achieved?
6. When do you expect that each goal will be achieved?
7. What roadblocks to achievement of each goal can you identify? How can you reduce them?

38 EXPECTATIONS, ACTUALITIES, AND STRATEGIES FOR CHANGE IN DENTAL HYGIENE PRACTICE

Irene Woodall

LEARNING OUTCOMES

The dental hygienist will be able to

1. Recognize the need to systematically apply the philosophy and procedures of dental hygiene care to a practice setting.
2. Identify strategies for integrating dental hygiene care into a practice setting in which:
   a. The practice has never had a dental hygienist on the team.
   b. The practice has had a hygienist for many years who has established well-accepted procedures.
   c. The practice has had a series of dental hygienists over the years who have integrated a variety of different approaches in varying degrees.
3. Set personal priorities for integrating various aspects of dental hygiene care into dental practice.
4. Describe the positive and negative aspects of developing a dental hygiene practice.

Many dental hygienists find their first employment in a private practice or group clinic. You may encounter an ideal situation that makes the transition from school to work an easy one. Such a practice would ensure that you can provide the broadest range of responsibilities, tapping to the fullest extent what you have learned. Ideal protocols may be followed, helping you feel confident about how care is delivered and the practice is managed. You may feel appreciated, welcome, involved, and respected.

It is more likely, however, that any employment situation will be less than ideal. Even a carefully selected site will have surprises and disappointments. How can you work well within a practice that could adopt more up-to-date protocols? How can you work with other employees who present interpersonal challenges? How can you get along with your employer and office manager? Some of these challenges or difficulties emerge the first day on the job. Others can occur after months, years, or even decades.

The main purpose of this chapter is to help you be aware of potential problems that can occur when you attempt to "fit in" or when an ideal employment situation begins to go sour. A second

purpose is to provide possible strategies to make the best of every situation. This chapter consists of four scenarios. They are stories of successes, of learning experiences, of disappointment, and of resolution. Read them carefully. Discuss them with fellow students and faculty. Identify alternative responses that might improve the outcome or that could be fruitless.

After years in practice, the needs of a dental hygienist may change, bringing difficult decisions. A hygienist may decide to assume more responsibility for the business aspects of a practice and adopt a situation where he or she works with a dentist as an independent contractor. Or the hygienist may be placed in a situation in which working unsupervised appears to be the best option. Though the legality of each of these situations differs from state to state, it is important to assess the opportunities and problems associated with each.

"REAL LIFE" SCENARIOS

To offer suggestions for addressing these possibilities, four scenarios or monologues are provided for review and discussion. Although each of the monologues is fictitious, together they represent the collective experiences and suggestions of dental hygienists who have returned to the educational environment to discuss their successes and their failures, their values, and their commitment. A helpful sequel to this chapter may be to invite recent graduates and dental hygienists who have had years of experience, preferably in a variety of practice settings, to discuss what they encountered in dental hygiene practice and to answer questions regarding the implementation of dental hygiene care in dental practice.

Scenario 1: I remember the first weeks of practicing in the office of Dr. J. It felt so good to be out of school and really working in a dental practice as a dental hygienist. Dr. J. gave me a great deal of freedom to schedule my patients so that I could build up speed and ensure that each patient received high-quality care. Quality was a very big item with Dr. J. I also had a great deal of freedom in selecting instruments, so one of my first official acts was to order six sets of curettes and ultrasonic tips so that I could improve on the few instruments that were left from the previous dental hygienist. The bill for the instruments was quite a shock to both the employer and to me, but Dr. J. seemed more than willing to go along with my suggestions as long as it would help ensure "smooth, calculus-free teeth."

For the first month Dr. J. checked every patient with a probe and explorer, looking for calculus deposits. It was clear that this was a focal point of care for him. It reminded me a great deal of the early days in school, and I found myself praying that my clinical skill had developed sufficiently so that he would find little if anything. There were, of course, a few problems, but soon it appeared that I had met the dentist's standards of excellence. Soon the careful checks of each surface were reduced to spot checks and a friendly conversation with the patient about the progress of care. Occasionally Dr. J. asked the patient directly for his or her opinion of me as a clinician.

The message became clear that the highest priority for this dentist was clean teeth at the end of the dental hygiene appointment. As my speed picked up, I decided that instead of reducing the time of the dental hygiene appointments, I would begin to integrate other kinds of dental hygiene procedures into this new free time. I wanted to move the practice from focusing on scaling and polishing to a more comprehensive approach. I decided to polish all the amalgams over a series of recall visits so that eventually they would be smooth and less likely to retain plaque and stain. I began to institute a much more thorough plaque control program, as the patients regularly returned with high plaque counts and seemed more willing to have me clean it off than to remove it themselves on a daily basis. I started teaching all the patients the oral cancer self-examination to round out the prevention program

in the practice. I even dared to discuss the possibility of reducing tobacco use with some heavy smokers to reverse some of the beginning signs of tissue change, such as nicotine stomatitis and to help curb their advancing periodontitis. I looked into smoking cessation programs for those who responded to the discussion.

It never occurred to me that the dentist might not agree that this series of decisions was appropriate or desirable. I had wanted to integrate this new approach as a sort of surprise for the dentist that would make for an even better feeling about my performance. I think what triggered the negative reaction was the complaint of a long-standing patient that he did not have time to sit around and practice flossing in a mirror or feeling the inside of his own cheeks. The patient hadn't seemed hostile during the appointment; I noticed nervousness but thought that was just because it was a new procedure. Anyway, the patient complained to the dentist, who wasn't fully aware of what I was doing. The dentist seemed to join sides with the patient and basically told me to cut out all that frivolous stuff and get back to scaling teeth. The dentist wanted to know whether I was charging the patients for all this "prevention"; I had to tell him I wasn't because I hadn't wanted anything to block the patient's acceptance of the procedure.

That decision and my decision to forego discussing my plans with Dr. J. were grave errors. The dentist decided I was giving away my time, which could be used to clean and plane teeth and which would generate income for the office. The dentist also, it turned out, really didn't have much faith in prevention as a reasonable approach to dental disease. The philosophy that emerged in the somewhat heated discussion of how I was spending my time was that dental disease was basically inevitable, that all the dental health education in the world wouldn't reverse that trend, and that the most efficient way to spend time was to clean the teeth every 6 months. The final comment was that the practice could not afford to lose patients such as the one who had complained and that I was to cease and desist from my fancy prevention techniques and get back to basics.

Back to basics it was. My appointment times were reduced to 45 minutes. I was allowed to bring patients back for additional scaling or other technical procedures, but not for extensive plaque control. There was a lot less agitation in the office with this edict, but somehow I felt as though I had missed an opportunity to integrate some prevention into an otherwise (in my opinion) fine clinical practice by having made some critical mistakes in integrating the changes. The two basic mistakes seemed to be the unilateral decision I made to include those procedures and ignoring the possibility that the patients' and the dentist's philosophies might be quite different from mine. The other contributing factor I had ignored was the financial implications of my decision.

Confronting this same kind of situation, what do you think could have been done differently to make the change more positive? What do you think could be done now to help improve the situation? Would you continue in this practice?

Scenario 2: My first position as a dental hygienist was in a practice where the dentist valued dental hygiene care and very much wanted a competent, caring person to take over that role and do well. It was a very busy restorative practice in a community where prevention had been lacking for most of the people. The dentist had no time to perform routine prophylaxes but definitely wanted that kind of care available for the patients.

A highlight of the practice was that I was involved in the initial examination of the patient. The dentist was quite willing to delegate the complete head and neck examination and the preparation of all dental chartings and radiographic series. All new patients were given a full 30-minute initial visit for the preparation of these assessment findings, which did not seem like much at first. As I picked up speed, I realized that the time was ample as long as I was fairly efficient in my procedures. After having talked with some of my classmates who were expected to fit the assessment into 10 minutes, I began to see how generous my time allotment was. I really enjoyed performing the initial procedures as well as completing periodontal debridement. I was expected to spend considerable time on preventive education, which definitely fit with the needs of this group.

Ironically, with all the freedom and opportunity to use my education, I felt the need to change some components of what I was expected to do. I did not believe that every recall patient needed to have every surface scaled or that complete polishing of the dentition was an appropriate procedure. It was clear at the interview and during my first few days that both the dentist and the patients were convinced that scaling and polishing defined the recall appointment, and that changing the orientation would upset them a great deal. Still, I needed to create a new way of thinking and to alter the standard appointment. I considered simply ignoring the expectations and doing scaling and polishing only where it was definitely needed. I also thought I might do better to work out the strategy over time by talking it through with the dentist and other staff members.

I suppose I could have chosen the former option and just gone ahead, but I knew better. I think it was the certainty in the voice of the dentist when she spoke with the patients about the importance of regular "cleanings." She had been a dental hygienist before she became a dentist, and she had all the characteristics of one who had been educated to value scaling and polishing every surface as a way of halting or preventing disease. Simply changing what I believed needed to be improved would have elicited a strong, negative re-

sponse. My decision to discuss it in increments, over time, was wise. At the end of my third week in the practice, I asked to speak with my employer. Dr. P. expressed confidence in my work, which I appreciated, and said that she really hoped I would stay with the practice and help her keep a prevention program running. I said that I looked forward to a long working relationship. I felt the beginning of closure in our conversation and decided to take the first step in easing in change: "I know you learned in dental hygiene school, and perhaps even in dental school, that scaling and polishing are important procedures for preventing disease and that they should be applied universally. But a newer view of prevention is that we subgingivally debride or disturb the microflora of the pocket without actually scaling unless we detect calculus. I also learned in school that polishing is not a particularly therapeutic procedure and that it should be restricted to obvious stains that affect the patient's esthetics. I'd like to show you some of the research and see what you think."

The dentist replied: "You're kidding. The research shows that subgingival instrumentation is extremely effective. Why would we want to abandon it? Whose idea was this? Did you really learn this in school?"

I decided to back off from the confrontation by saying: "How about if I bring in some of the studies we reviewed and show you the results? I realize that this may seem inconsistent with the research you are familiar with, but actually it is an extension of what you learned. We know subgingival instrumentation is effective. The question now is whether we need to do as much vigorous root planing in diseased pockets and scaling in healthy pockets. Would you like to go through the research with me?"

She agreed, although she seemed very skeptical. The first session lasted about 2 hours. We reviewed the literature about lipopolysaccharide and whether it was "cementum bound" or not. She was amazed. I suggested that we might want to discuss it with the rest of the staff. I thought they might want to know the research, too, especially since implementing any change based on it would affect scheduling and billing and the way we work with patients at each visit. We had three more lengthy review periods together and then introduced the "news" to the staff. Dr. P. took responsibility for presenting the data to them. I could tell from her voice that her skepticism was waning.

Two more weeks passed. She called me into her office and told me she had called some of her former professors. A couple seemed unaware of the indications of the literature, but her periodontics professors were fully aware. They agreed that instrumentation should be selective and that the focus is on debridement without loss of tooth structure. She asked me for ideas on how to introduce the change to the patients.

Ultimately, the staff, Dr. P., and I collaborated on an approach that slowly introduced patients (approximately three per day) to the new concept. We agreed on a strategy for patients who objected, and we brainstormed ways to handle scheduling and billing procedures to accommodate the change.

Now I use that assessment time, in part, to determine what periodontal needs each recall patient has and to explain carefully to each patient what their treatment needs are for that appointment and subsequent visits. It has been months since we started phasing in the program, and about 25% of the patients are fully into the change. We will step up the program now and hope that 100% of the patients will be treated in the new style by the end of the year.

I'm glad I took the slower route and that I worked with the dentist and staff to implement change. We're doing it together.

What would you have done in this situation?

Scenario 3: I was really lucky to find a practice in which the dentist was young and interested in adding a dental hygienist as the practice grew. I had all kinds of ideas about integrating dental hygiene into a clinical practice and really did not want to have to follow in the footsteps of a dental hygienist who had established all kinds of patterns and expectations over the years that might conflict with my ideas. I was certain that because the dentist was young there would be great opportunity for innovation, especially in performing expanded functions such as local anesthesia and placement of restorations. I wanted to add myofunctional therapy and conduct a mini-research study of the efficacy of using a behavioral approach to modification of the swallowing habit. Somehow I felt that such therapy often failed because the educational techniques failed, and that this was true for dental health education in general. A small clinical study performed over many years could provide answers to those questions.

I remember having big plans and being excited about my new position. My first letdown was seeing the operatory in which I was to work. The equipment was ancient. There was an old belt-driven engine that squeaked relentlessly. There was no high-speed evacuation and no stool to sit on. The comforting factor was that the dental chair had been partially converted from the prehistoric style to a lounge-type chair. However, I still had to pump it up with my foot and figure out all the levers for adjusting the back! My first reaction was one of grief and then of anger. The dentist had said he would equip an operatory for me, but I never thought it would be with this kind of equipment. I decided to confront Dr. W. with the problem of my expectations versus his. At first, he was a bit defensive, saying he couldn't imagine how such equipment would be a problem. When I discussed how difficult it would be to work without evacuation and without a stool, he admitted that he simply could not go any deeper into debt to buy modern dental equipment. He wanted to add a den-

tal hygienist to the team but couldn't add the new equipment that was necessary for ideal practice. What surprised me the most was how little he seemed to know about the needs of a dental hygienist in providing services for patients. The idea of a high-speed evacuation system for dental hygiene care was a new one to him. Also, he hadn't seemed to generalize what he had learned about sit-down dentistry to dental hygiene. It seemed as though he thought all the guidelines for efficient, relatively comfortable practice were not applicable to a dental hygienist.

Overcoming that first shock took quite a while. Plus there was the need to set up a reasonable recall system, to order appropriate supplies (sparingly to help balance the budget), to develop a system for making patient appointments, and to set down even basic protocols regarding when a dental hygienist becomes involved in dental treatment. The dentist and I spent long hours discussing whether a dental hygienist *could* record the medical history and then whether a dental hygienist *should* record the medical history, even if the skill was well developed.

Procedure by procedure, we worked out the protocols. I was glad that I had a solid rationale for each of the procedures I was to perform and that I had good skills in performing them. Step by step, we integrated dental hygiene into the practice. It required almost 1 year to accomplish this. The actual procedures were moved into place very slowly. The dentist did not wish to rush into anything, and he was very concerned about the patients' acceptance of a dental hygienist. He himself had never had dental care from a dental hygienist.

Through all of these slow developments, I could see progress, but I couldn't help remembering my dream to use all the functions I had learned and to begin my small clinical study of myofunctional therapy.

I first discussed my hopes with the dentist after I had been there for 18 months. He did seem to trust me now. I decided to inquire about beginning the myofunctional therapy study first, as that would be slow to start and he didn't seem to have much problem with detecting malocclusion and referring patients to orthodontists for care. I described what I wanted to do. The reply was a solid no. His rationale was basically that he didn't trust those kinds of efforts, that he had been taught in school that the only way to modify swallowing habits was with long-term orthodontic treatment, and that even then the techniques seemed to fail. It became apparent that there was no point in discussing it as an appropriate project—the idea was ludicrous to him.

I returned to traditional practice for another few months and decided to approach the topic of giving my own anesthesia as needed before periodontal debridement. So far, the dentist had been performing the pain control procedures at the beginning of appointments for which local anesthesia was indicated. I had learned and practiced local anesthesia in school and had received high praise from the dental hygiene, oral surgery, and periodontics faculty who had witnessed my technique and who had quizzed me on rationale, anatomy, pharmacology, and complications. I was careful to keep my skills up-to-date on all the expanded functions, including anesthesia, by taking every refresher course that was available at the local university and through my local dental hygiene component. I served as a clinical instructor 4 hours per week, working with the course director demonstrating and observing these procedures. I really knew my stuff.

Again I tried to approach the topic as a suggestion for modifying my functions in the practice. I pointed out to Dr. W. that my performing the anesthesia procedure would make scheduling for his patients a good deal easier. He commented that it was really essential that a specially trained person be ready to respond in case of an emergency involving local anesthesia procedures. I pointed out to him that he routinely left patients who had received an injection to be monitored by a dental assistant and that it is in the first few moments following an injection that an untoward response such as toxic or allergic reaction is most likely to occur. I told him about my background and my abilities and suggested that I would certainly be as able as the dental assistant to monitor signs and symptoms. I told him that I had had a full course in emergency procedures, including CPR. My defense was offensive. There was no further discussion.

I retreated to traditional dental hygiene procedures. Fortunately, there was a great deal of diversity in the procedures I could perform, and I derived satisfaction from the manner in which I had been able to integrate so much into a practice, even if it had taken months and months to do so. Based on the two previous reactions to my requests, I was, of course, hesitant to ask about restorative procedures. I wanted to be able to place the rubber dam and the matrix, place temporary restorations as needed, and place and carve amalgam and tooth-colored restorations. The dental practice was building, and the appointment book was filled for 3 weeks in advance. The practice was making a better income, and I was rewarded with new equipment for my operatory. I was asked to select the kind I wanted from three basic designs. Still, somehow I wanted to be able to practice expanded functions. I kept thinking that if I could add restorative functions to my list of procedures, perhaps I could eventually add local anesthesia. When I inquired, I was informed that the dental assistant would be the one to perform those skills if the dentist ever decided to delegate them. Dr. W. did not feel it was within the scope of dental hygiene practice to become involved with restorative procedures. He felt it was imperative that the dental hygienist perform preventive procedures, as was originally intended.

I am still practicing traditional dental hygiene in an efficient, well-designed, modern clinical practice in which dental hygiene procedures as they have been defined for decades are valued and fully integrated into daily routines. I know I will probably never have the freedom to do the things I had hoped to do in research projects and with anesthesia and restorative procedures. If that day ever does arrive, it will have been so long since I used those skills that I will probably not be able to prove my ability. I have to make a decision regarding whether I should stay or try to find a position in which I can do what I really want to do. I keep remembering what my boss said regarding the matter of local anesthesia: "If you really want to do all these things, why don't you go to dental school?"

How do you answer that final question? What can you do when faced with the prospect of a clinical practice that has many positive elements but where the care you deliver is limited by the dentist even more than by the law? How can practicing dentists learn more about what hygienists can do and what they know?

Scenario 4: My choice was a difficult one. I was forced after 26 years of clinical practice in a dental office to look for alternatives. I had worked for the same dentist from the day I passed my licensure examinations. I knew every patient by name and watched babies grow up to be young adults. I went to patients' funerals and weddings. I knew those people, and I thought I knew the dentist.

Things were going more slowly in the practice. The new children did not need extensive restorative care—something for which we were genuinely grateful. It looked as though we were winnning the prevention battle. But as the practice aged, Dr. S.'s appointment book was not booked as far ahead and his days were quite easy compared to the humming activity of the 1970s. It was a gradual change, but it happened. My salary was not increased for 3 years, and I was required to take my vacation when he took his—which became less frequent and of shorter duration. Then we dropped medical insurance. I kept hoping that Dr. S. would try some new ideas to bring life to the practice. It seemed that his colleagues were fresher in their approaches to drawing patients to the practice. Finally he went to a practice management seminar that was coming to town. I breathed a sigh of relief and wished him well.

When he returned, he was full of ideas for the practice, including some clever ways to attract patients. He seemed incredibly happy, but something was different in the way he approached me and the office manager. One week after his return he left the office without saying goodbye. The next day was Saturday, and I was greeted by a special delivery letter. In it was a check for 2 weeks' pay and a brief typed note that thanked me for my years of service. It added that he could no longer afford to pay me my salary and that he had opted to hire a dental hygienist right out of school who was willing to work for $20 less per day. This apparently was one of the fine ideas he learned at the seminar.

It was impossible to find a job as a hygienist without working for peanuts. I tried to swallow my pride and say I could take a 30% cut in my salary. But the thought brought tears of rage to my eyes. How was I going to live? I filed for unemployment and collected it while I sorted out my anger and my plans. At least Dr. S. did not contest the unemployment. But I still felt like a discarded piece of dental equipment. I missed my patients in that practice, and I resented that they would be receiving care from someone new. I hoped I would never lay eyes on the new hygienist or ever again on Dr. S. I was betrayed. I seemed to have counted for nothing.

I took stock of my savings and visited a business management consultant. I told her I wanted to set up my own practice—a few blocks from Dr. S. There was a small office suite with two treatment rooms available. With her help, I developed a business plan, and I was able to secure a sizable loan that helped me buy used dental equipment. I placed announcements in the local newspapers and used all of my connections in the community to ensure that people knew I was setting up my own business and would love to provide them with dental hygiene care. I used the idea of the "gentle first step" in seeking dental care to attract patients who have the financial means (usually through insurance) to obtain care but who are frightened of the prospect of visiting the dentist.

I lost money for 8 months. I watched my loan and my savings dwindle as I worked as hard as I could to draw in sufficient numbers of patients to pay the rent, utilities, a competent staff person, and the supply bill. It was very difficult to compete with the low fees dentists charge for dental hygiene care. The amount of time needed to provide complete dental hygiene care is clearly worth more than we were charging at Dr S.'s. There is no "flexible fee" associated with restorative care to make up the difference in a practice that relies on dental hygiene services for its income. For 2 months I broke even. I kept working to draw in patients, to give them the best care possible with the most flexible appointment times, and to develop reasonable relations with the local dental community.

Putting all my energy into building the practice actually helped me get over the anger of my dismissal. It also helped that so many of the patients I treated at Dr. S.'s felt as strongly about me as I did about them. They came to me for dental hygiene care, even though nearly all of them went to him for annual dental examinations and whatever other dental care they needed. A few went to other dentists, saying that they just didn't feel the same way about him after what he had done. One even described it as unethical for him to fire me.

Relations with area dentists were not so easy. I can understand how they would want to be cohesive and protect the right of a dentist to fire an employee. They also wanted to help protect Dr. S.'s good reputation and, by extension, their own. At first, they tried just about everything to keep me from opening my practice, including putting pressure on the bank to turn down my loan and trying to influence the State Board to say I could not see any of Dr. S.'s patients. They even tried to say I could not legally expose radiographs or use fluoride (a prescription agent) in the care of my patients. Fortunately, another hygienist who footed most of the legal costs had won decisions regarding those issues within the past 6 months. My financial costs in fighting off these efforts were relatively minor. But the emotional costs were high, and it was a very hard time for me.

The way I overcame the problem was to meet with one dentist at a time, usually over lunch. I would take the dentist to a nice restaurant near my practice, introduce him or her to my philosophy of dental hygiene care, present the forms I would use for data gathering and for transmitting information to the dentist after each visit, and discuss what special information he or she would like from me when I referred a patient. I tried to be disarmingly charming and impeccably professional. I made certain that the care I would deliver would be "by the book," meeting all accepted standards based on current research. I tried to be confident and sincere in my request for suggestions. I ended up by asking how the dentist felt about my treating patients from his or her practice. I then asked if he or she would like to receive new patients from me.

I worked hard to draw in people who had been unwilling to visit the dentist, and I made certain that they were referred promptly for their dental care. I spread around the referrals among the dentists whose work I knew was good. I complimented dentists on the quality of dental work I saw when one of their patients visited me. I worked hard to develop a supportive relationship. That was what pushed me from losing money to eventually making money. I don't think I will ever really prosper financially in my practice, but I certainly have much higher job security than I did as an employee. I am not at another person's mercy. I do, however, have to work very hard and concentrate continually on building the practice and making it even better than it is. I "stick to the knitting," ensuring that the practice gets all the attention it needs.

I also am more aware of how I treat my staff. I am careful to remember to give them the same respect and consideration I had hoped for in my employment situation. I have a strong sense of pride in what I have accomplished. I'll probably finish my years in dental hygiene in this, my own, practice. The irony is that I never intended to be an independent businessperson when I selected dental hygiene. I wanted to work with a dentist. But I also expected commitment from my employer and a sense of self-worth, nurtured by people who respect me for what I do well. Probably the hard times of the early 1980s had more to do with Dr. S.'s decision to fire me, but there should have been more between us than financial considerations. If I ever am in a position to work "for" a dentist, I'm going to be mighty careful to find one who seems to value me as a person and as a contributor to the good will of the office. I'll still give my very best; I'll just be more cautious.

How do you feel about the hygienist's experience with her employer dentist? What would you have done in her situation? What risks did the hygienist take in setting up her own practice? What are the problems she continues to face? Would you feel comfortable in this situation?

ACTIVITIES

1. Discuss each of the scenarios, analyzing the choice of actions the dental hygienist had in each of the situations andthe appropriateness of the action selected. Focus on the likely outcomes of alternative choices of action. Place yourself in the position of the dentist in each case, and project how the dentist may be seeing the actions and attitudes of the dental hygienist.
2. Were the dentists in the scenarios male or female? Is it confusing to picture a dentist as a woman? Did you picture the dental hygiensts as women? Which

hygienist might have been a male? Why would you make that assumption? How does sex role bias affect the way we interpret and anticipate behavior, regardless of their professional role?
3. Set personal priorities for what you hope to accomplish and what you expect to find in the "ideal" dental practice. Share your expectations with a small group of classmates. Explain how you will choose whether to try to change or to agree to live with less than ideal conditions. Ask others in the group how they would feel if they had a dental practice and you were to implement the approaches to change that you feel would work best in solving the less than ideal conditions.
4. Role-play a variety of encounters with hypothetical employers and patients regarding attempts to change the following:
   a. Integration of preventive measures into a practice.
   b. Integration of additional assessment procedures into the scope of practice of the dental hygienist.
   c. Changing outmoded clinical procedures.
   d. Procedures regarding sterilization, instrument purchase, office cleanliness, and nonfunctional equipment.
5. Invite hygienists from the area to discuss how they succeeded or struggled to integrate comprehensive dental hygiene care into their work settings.
6. Search back issues of *RDH* magazine for articles about independent contracting and independent practice and how hygienists breaking new ground in these areas felt they had succeeded or struggled.

SUGGESTED RESPONSES

CHAPTER 1

1. The patient is viewed as a partner in care, involved extensively in decision making and in the self-care components necessary for health.

2. A faculty member has had an opportunity to compare expectations with reality and to develop an educational approach that blends the ideal with the real. Individual faculty members differ according to their clinical, conceptual, and futuristic perceptions of practice.

3. a. Dental practice acts define the scope and limitations of dental practice and dental hygiene practice in each jurisdiction (usually defined by state boundaries). In many instances they differ widely from one another, resulting in significantly different roles and responsibilities for dental hygienists, depending on the jurisdictions in which they reside.

   b. The practice acts often limit programs within their jurisdiction to include only those skills that are legally allowable for practice in that jurisdiction. Thus programs differ widely in the functions and responsibilities they may legally include.

4. Legalization of independent dental hygiene practice would allow entrepreneurial hygienists to open their own practices and perform the full array of legal dental hygiene services learned in dental hygiene school. It would open practice opportunities for hygienists currently unable to find work as employees in solo dental practices, where only 42% of dentists use dental hygiene services. It could perhaps extend dental hygiene, and eventually dental care, to a population group that currently does not seek care because of fear.

5. *Professional culture* refers to those characteristics that are unique to a given profession. It refers to the attitudes, knowledge base, functions, demographics, and other features that make that profession distinct from others.

CHAPTER 2

1. Should; turning the light on and off wears out the switch and causes the lamp to burn out more quickly.

2. a. Begin in an upright position.
   b. Tilt chair back.
   c. Lower back of chair to supine position.
   d. Raise chair as necessary to proper height.
   e. Rotate chair if necessary.

3. To direct a stream of water; to direct a stream of air; and to spray air and water in an area.

4. The angle needs cleaning to remove abrasive and other foreign elements from the gears.

5. The clinician's feet are flat on the floor and thighs are parallel to the floor; the back rest supports the lumbar region.

6. The assistant's eye level is approximately 5 inches above the clinician's eye level and thighs are parallel to the floor; the abdominal rest should fit snugly below the rib cage as the clinician inclines forward.

7. Ultrasonic cleaner for removing debris and autoclave or any one of the following for sterilizing: dry heat oven, unsaturated chemical vapor sterilizer, or rapid heat transfer sterilizer.

CHAPTER 3

1. Except for surgeons, few other health professionals come in closer contact with patients for longer periods of time than the dental clinician. The oral cavity is abundant in organisms that are potentially pathogenic. The close physical contact with the patient, the nature of the work performed, and the instruments used all contribute to the clinician's susceptibility to infectious disease. The air, saliva, blood, and aerosols from instrumentation or breathing are potentially dangerous. The clinician must be aware of sources of infection and take precautions to protect himself or herself, the operatory environment, and patients from the spread of infectious organisms.

2. a. *Mycobacterium tuberculosis:* Tuberculosis; indirect transmission from inanimate sources or respiratory droplets.

   b. *Treponema pallidum:* Syphilis; indirect contact, break in skin, or contact with lesion.

   c. *Clostridium tetani:* Tetanus; airborne transmission by means of dust-carried spores.

   d. Respiratory virus (e.g., adenovirus): Respiratory tract infection; respiratory droplets, aerosol.

   e. Hepatitis B virus: Serum hepatitis; saliva or respiratory droplets, or direct transmission by contact with contaminated blood.

   f. Rubeola virus: Measles; respiratory secretions, saliva, or blood.

   g. HIV or human immunodeficiency virus: AIDS; transmitted by sexual contact, IV drug abuse, or contact with contaminated body fluids.

3. a. True
    b. False
    c. True
    d. False
    e. True
    f. True
    g. True
    h. True
    i. False
    j. True

4. Sanitation: The mechanical and/or chemical cleaning of an object.
    Disinfection: The destruction of bacteria and other microorganisms by means of chemicals or heat.
    Sterilization: total destruction of all forms of microbial life.

5. Start with an initial scrub that includes a thorough lathering of all surfaces using an antibacterial soap and copious amounts of running water; all jewelry should be removed; the initial scrub should be a series of three latherings, each followed by a thorough rinsing; the initial scrub should last 2 to 3 minutes.

6. Steam under pressure, dry heat, ethylene oxide gas, chemical vapor sterilizer, and chemical solution (glutaraldehyde only).

7. Steam under pressure: 121° C (250° F) at 15 to 20 psi for 15 to 20 minutes.
    Dry heat: 160° C (320° F) for 1 hr.
    Ethylene oxide gas: 49° C (120° F) for 2 to 3 hours *or* room temperature for 12 hours.
    Chemical vapor sterilizer: 127° C (260° F) at 20 to 25 psi for 30 minutes.
    Chemical solution (glutaraldegyde): Room temperature for 6¾ to 10 hours, assuming that the chemical concentration is optimal, manufacturer's instructions are followed, and the instruments have been properly prepared.

8. Trisyringe: Sterilize tips.
    Handpiece: Sterilize.

CHAPTER 4

1. The complete dental record is a medicolegal record that provides the information necessary to safely and knowledgeably treat a patient and provides protection for both the patient and the dental health care provider in a court of law.

2. a. Demographic data (name, address, and so on): To include the patient's identifying and emergency information.
    b. Medical and dental histories: To identify the patient's past and present needs.
    c. Examination findings and diagnosis: To identify the patient's present status and needs.
    d. Treatment goals and treatment plan: To clarify expected outcomes and sequence of care for both clinician and patient.
    e. Treatment performed with dates: To promote continuity of care and to protect the patient and the health care provider in a legal proceeding.
    f. Results of treatment: To provide follow-up, especially if the result was unexpected or unusual.
    g. Radiographs: To provide a diagnostic aid to charting, examinations, and tests.
    h. Fees charged and paid: As part of legal financial records.
    i. Correspondence: To protect the patient and the health care provider in a legal proceeding.

3. The primary difference is that the problem-oriented approach includes a problem list that is not included in the treatment-oriented approach.

4. The purpose of a chart audit is to ensure that the health care providers are maintaining complete, thorough, and accurate dental records.

5. A complete format would include the date, subjective findings, objective findings, medications administered, treatment, results, the patient's reaction, whether treatment is complete or incomplete, treatment to be performed at the next appointment, and the signature of the health care provider.

CHAPTER 5

1. If the hygienist ignores the patient's request to have her teeth polished, the patient will probably go elsewhere for polishing or try it herself at home with a strong abrasive. If the hygienist is willing to simply polish at the first visit (after at least a medical history), the patient will be more likely to return for further care (as explained by the hygienist) *after* the big event. The mother of the groom wants white teeth now, not sore gums. In some instances in which no harm can result, a patient can be satisfied in this manner, with long-term positive results for both the hygienist and the patient.

2. It is difficult to determine whether the patient is dependent on the dentist—believing that he will retain his teeth as long as he returns periodically for care—or if he does not really care if he keeps his teeth but does not want to experience pain (thus the necessity of dental visits). The hygienist might do well to point out the string of appointments for restorations and simply ask the patient if he expects to retain his teeth. Mentioning rather objectively that soon the restorative material will be all that is holding the teeth up may make an impression on the patient. Often a follow-up of "If you decide you really *do* want to keep them, let me know. I think there might be a couple of things you can do to prevent losing them over a period of time" will move the patient to ask for help. The hygienist can always resort to blatant fear tactics to awaken such a patient, but they are usually less effective than a calm inquiry and suggestion. Different degrees of subtlety and different opening lines are appropriate for each person—no key phrase works for all. In any case, the hygienist is unwise to proceed with a speech about flossing and diet. The patient will tune him or her out if possible.

3. Such a statement might imply a great deal of trust in the dental hygienist. It may also imply a dependency relationship in which the patient has transferred responsibility for oral health to the dental hy-

gienist. Rarely do such patients have a thorough program of preventive self-care.

4. a. Excessive familiarity.
   b. Professional closeness.
   c. Professional closeness (but worthy of discussion).
   d. Professional aloofness.

5. There are several possible actions, including refusing to provide care for the patient, having the patient sign a disclaimer for risks resulting from the omitted procedure, or working around the missing procedure until trust is increased and the need for the procedure becomes more apparent to the patient.

6. These are *possible* replies. The key to a *listening* response is to rephrase the *content* of the message and to reflect the *affect* or emotion behind the statement.
   a. "It sounds like you're worried about what I'm going to see in there."
   b. "You don't feel as comfortable lying down for your dental work."
   c. "You sound a little disturbed that you can feel this more than you could with other hygienists."
   d. "You sound upset that the dentist has hired someone else to treat you. You think the dentist is the person who should do it."
   e. "You clearly must enjoy having your teeth polished. Or perhaps you just expect that it will be done because we have always done it."

7. a. Although it is reassuring, this response cuts off a message the patient is trying to give: there is some reason the hygienist will be unhappy. It may be very important for the patient to say this before the hygienist looks. It also sounds like the patient may feel guilty. The patient may feel he or she is reporting in to the hygienist for judgment. A glib, nonlistening comment shuts off the patient's next statement and any exploration of what is behind the opening comment.
   b. This statement also shuts off communication because the hygienist is presenting a logical argument in favor of reclining chairs. The patient and the hygienist are both right, but the hygienist is actually denying the validity of the patient's statement by presenting an argument.
   c. Problem solving immediately after a comment closes off communication. The hygienist is closing out a great deal of information that the patient might have revealed if the hygienist had saved problem solving for later.
   d. No matter how tempting it may be to lecture, the patient should be listened to *first* so that his or her perceptions are clear. Information to enlighten the misinformed should follow the reflection and listening. The patient then knows the hygienist understands and the patient is more likely to listen. Also, the hygienist may have misunderstood the patient and given information that is irrelevant to his or her concerns.
   e. This statement shows frustration and giving in to the demands of the patient rather than understanding what he or she is concerned about. Even if the patient speaks strongly and in anger, either verbally or nonverbally, it is better to talk through the person's biases about a given procedure and to fully understand what is driving the statement before complying with or refusing a request.

CHAPTER 6

1. An appropriate response would be: "It sounds like you think this health history procedure is unnecessary. [Pause for verification.] Maybe it will help if I explain why we place so much value on it. I realize this is time consuming, but it is important for us to discuss your general health before I check your teeth. Certain medical conditions and medications patients may be taking may affect their dental treatment. For example, some patients with specific types of heart problems actually need to take an antibiotic before we treat them to prevent serious complications. The health history is the foundation for your total care. All this information is kept confidential. If some of the questions puzzle you, I'll be happy to explain why they are significant. My concern is that you receive safe and proper treatment. The few minutes we take at this point to get to know you and complete a thorough record are necessary to ensure that 'checking your teeth' stays as simple as it sounds."

2. All of the above (e) is the correct answer.
   a. Rheumatic heart disease: Consult the physician to determine if damage to heart valves makes antibiotic premedication necessary.
   b. History of myocardial infarction: Consult the physician to obtain a history of the most recent heart attack and to determine the severity of disease; the physician may advise on the patient's tolerance to stress and on the advisability of vasoconstrictors in local anesthetics.
   c. Blood pressure reading of 160/100 (hypertension): Consult the physician to determine if medication is required for the patient.
   d. Hemophilia: Consult the physician to determine the extent of the bleeding disorder, the need for transfusion before treatment, and other possible contraindications to treatment.

3. Antibiotic premedication is necessary for patients who report a history of rheumatic heart fever with valve damage, surgical replacement of a heart valve or a joint, and, depending on the physician's decision, the following conditions: (a) surgical replacement of a heart valve or joint, (b) congenital heart defect repair, and (c) pacemaker implant.

4. Communication principles:
   Ask direct but open questions.
   Follow a logical order.
   Guide but do not dominate the interview.
   Show support and empathy.
   Reflect the patient's response to clarify meaning.
   Avoid "yes" and "no" questions.
   Avoid "why" questions.
5. As part of the review of a patient's health status, the dental hygienist must be aware of the medication a patient is taking. The *Physicians' Desk Reference* is helpful in identifying medications and providing information on drug composition, action, dosage, precautions, and side effects that may affect dental treatment.

CHAPTER 7

1. Dental visits often are likely to create anxiety for patients. Patients who have a propensity for syncope (fainting) or other physical responses to anxiety are more likely to respond this way in the dental environment. Also the drugs used in dentistry, including local anesthetics, may cause an emergency situation. The dental hygienist may be the first person to recognize and respond to the situation.
2. Primary drugs
   Noninjectable drugs
   Oxygen
   Nitroglycerin (spray perferably)
   Injectable drugs
   Epinephrine (allergy)
   Chlorphenexamine (antihistamine)
   Diazepam (anticonvulsant)
   Naloxone (narcotic antagonist)
   Equipment
   Oxygen delivery system for portable oxygen
   Suction and suction tips
   Syringes for drug administration
   Tourniquets
3. All emergency equipment should be readily available and functioning. Drugs maintained in the kit should be up to date. All members of the team should be able to recognize signs of patient distress, and they should be prepared to respond appropriately. Rehearsing the proper procedures for any kind of emergency can be critically important if quick, responsible action is to occur. Emergencies can be prevented by the use of medical histories, fire and accident prevention devices, and by careful monitoring of the patient.
4. a. Move instruments and other dental equipment away from the patient, place the patient in a full supine position (a patient in the late stages of pregnancy should be turned on her side), place a cool cloth on the patient's forehead, alert another team member, prepare an ammonia ampule for wafting under the patient's nose if he or she loses consciousness, and administer oxygen until the patient is recovered.

b. Place the patient in an upright position, send a team member to call for emergency assistance, administer oxygen, place a nitroglycerin tablet under the tongue, monitor vital signs, and begin CPR in the event of cardiac arrest. If the pain is associated with angina, the nitroglycerin will relieve the discomfort. If it is associated with heart failure or myocardial infarction, the pain will persist.

c. Place the patient in a supine position and check for vital signs. Begin CPR if breathing and a heartbeat are absent and have a team member send for emergency assistance. If the patient is breathing and has a heartbeat, waft an ammonia ampule under his or her nose and administer oxygen. Continue monitoring vital signs until the patient is fully recovered. An awareness of the patient's medical history should help determine if there are causes other than syncope that could account for the loss of consciousness, such as hypoglycemia, hyperglycemia, cardiovascular problems, or acute adrenal insufficiency.

5. The unconscious patient does not possess protective reflexes; therefore a head tilt/chin lift maneuver must be maintained to prevent the tongue from causing airway obstruction and producing respiratory arrest. The unconscious patient must be monitored in case respiratory arrest occurs. In this event, oxygen would be delivered by positive pressure on an Ambu bag. The patient's airway would be maintained by the head tilt/chin lift maneuver.
   The conscious victim still possesses protective reflexes and, unless an obstruction occurs, is capable of inhaling and exhaling without assistance. The patient should be closely monitored in case the situation deteriorates.

6. Determine if the Ambu bag in your clinic is disposable, autoclavable, or subject to disinfection only. If you are unsure, contact the manufacturer and follow the guidelines.

CHAPTER 8

1. To gather assessment data for diagnosis and treatment planning; to provide early detection of disease, thus improving the prognoisis for recovery; to detect contraindications to dental treatment; to provide baseline and continuing data on the patient's health status; and to provide descriptions of the patient's health status for use as legal records.
2. Pulse, respiration rate, temperature, and arterial blood pressure.
3. a. Adult pulse: 60 to 80 beats per minute.
   b. Adult respiration rate: 14 to 20 breaths per minute.
   c. Adult temperature: 98.6° F (37° C).
   d. Adult blood pressure: 120/80 mm Hg.
   e. Borderline temperature for fever: 99.6° F.

f. Borderline blood pressure for hypertension: 160/95 mm Hg.

4. a. Pulse rate: Rest the patient's arm in a comfortable position. Place the index and second fingers on the radial artery found on the thumb side of the wrist. Compress this area gently and count the beats for 1 minute.

   b. Blood pressure: Rest the patient's arm in a comfortable position. Roll up the patient's sleeve. Place the sphygmomanometer on the patient's arm about 1 inch above the bend on the arm. Feel the radial pulse and inflate the cuff until the pulse is no longer felt. This provides an estimate of the systolic pressure. Release the air in the cuff. Let the patient's circulation return to normal. Place diaphragm of stethoscope over the brachial artery, 1 inch below the bend in the arm. Inflate the cuff 20 to 30 mm Hg higher than that previously noted. Slowly deflate the cuff. Note the point at which the first sound is heard with the stethoscope and the point at which the sound completely disappears. Record the first sound as systolic pressure and the last sound as diastolic pressure. Confirm this recording. Remove the cuff.

5. a. Inspection: A visual examination of each of the structures before they are palpated for signs of abnormal color, texture, or consistency.

   b. Palpation: Feeling or pressing on structures of the body, used for examining most intraoral and some extraoral structures.

   c. Ausculation: Listening for sounds produced within the body, used for examining the temporomandibular joint and larynx.

   d. Percussion: Striking tissues with the fingers or with an instrument to hear the resulting sounds and patient response; not previously described as a method used during the intraoral examination but often used as a means of assessing pulpal disease in individual teeth.

6. a. Submandibular lymph nodes: Standing behind the patient, push the soft tissues from one side of the submandibular area over to the other side, grasp these tissues with the cupped fingers of the hand, and roll tissues over bone of the mandible. Repeat for the other side.

   b. Floor of the mouth: Place the fingers of one hand intraorally in the floor of the mouth and the fingers of the other hand extraorally beneath the same area. Use bimanual palpation to examine the entire floor area.

   c. Buccal mucosa: Place one hand or several fingers intraorally and the other hand extraorally. Use bimanual palpation to examine the entire area from the labial mucosa back to the retromolar area.

7. a. To prevent the clinician from touching lesions in the mouth that might be contagious; to identify conditions that for the patient's well-being would contraindicate dental treatment, such as strep throat; and to prevent patient discomfort due to palpation of painful lesions such as ulcers.

8. a. Auricular chain.
   b. Cervical chain.
   c. Occipital chain.
   d. Submandibular (posterior) and submental (anterior) chains.

CHAPTER 9

1. To retract tissue, to reflect light, for indirect vision, and for transillumination.

2. To detect root irregularities and hard deposits; to measure the depth of the gingival sulcus or periodontal pocket; to trace the topography of the soft tissue attachment of the tooth; and to measure recession, masticatory mucosa, and the size of lesions.

3. To explore the teeth for caries and to explore the teeth for irregularities such as calculus deposits, root roughness, anatomic defects, and margins of restorations.

4. a. True
   b. False. If the first 1 to 2 mm are used, detection can identify the specific location and less soft tissue trauma is likely to occur.
   c. True
   d. False. The terminal shank should be parallel to the long axis of the tooth.

5.

Clinician position	Patient's head position
Right-handed	
a. 11 o'clock	Straight
b. 9 o'clock	Away from clinician
c. 9 o'clock	Away from clinician
d. 11 o'clock	Toward clinician
e. 11 o'clock	Toward clinician
f. 9 o'clock	Away from clinician
g. 9 o'clock	Away from clinician
Left-handed	
a. 1 o'clock	Straight
b. 3 o'clock	Toward clinician
c. 1 o'clock	Toward clinician
d. 3 o'clock	Away from clinician
e. 3 o'clock	Away from clinician
f. 1 o'clock	Toward clinician
g. 1 o'clock	Toward clinician

CHAPTER 10

1. This recall patient presented with several small carious lesions, changed oral hygiene status, and symptoms of third molar eruption. Considering these findings, selected periapical films or a panoramic radiograph for third molar evaluation and posterior bitewings for caries evaluation would be appropriate.

2. Zygomatic process, coronoid process, tuberosity, and sinus cavity.
3. Mental foramen.
4. Amalgam.
5. Saucer-shaped radiolucency below the CEJ.
6. Class III advanced lesion.
7. Tooth mobility, presence or absence of periodontal pockets, incipient bone loss, and morphology of bone deformities.
8. CEJs of adjacent teeth.
9. True
10. Widened periodontal ligament space.
11. Fig. 10-55 description: This is a large, single lesion of the left posterior mandible involving tooth No. 17. It extends from the first molar area to the coronoid process and involves the ramus, mandibular canal, lower border of the mandible, and angle of the mandible. It is an irregularly shaped unilocular radiolucent lesion with a continuous corticated border; it is well defined on the anterior and posterior aspects, less so in the superior and inferior aspects. The third molar had been displaced and had lost the periodontal ligament space, lamina dura, and part of the mesial root structure. The bone has been thinned and expanded with perforation of the alveolar ridge and lower border of the mandible. (This lesion was diagnosed as a dentigerous cyst. As you can see, without intervention these lesions can become quite large.)
12. Reduce exposure levels, image enhancement features, immediate image display; conventional processing eliminated.

CHAPTER 11

1. Legal record of the patient's initial condition and changes in oral status over a period of time; helpful in preparing a treatment plan; useful in cross-checking financial records; combines radiographic and clinical findings into a comprehensive record for diagnosis.
2. a. Anatomic: Most precise replica of tooth characteristic.
   b. Geometric: Stylized version of teeth and findings; usually makes charting neater and easier to read.
   c. Numerically coded: Provides a complete time line of oral conditions and changes on a single piece of paper.
   d. Computerized: Minimizes cross contamination, less prone to error, more time efficient.

	Universal	Palmer's notation	International	Description
3. a.	3	6⌋	16	Maxillary right first permanent molar
b.	29	5⌉	45	Mandibular right second premolar
c.	16	⌊8	28	Maxillary left third molar
d.	n	⌊b	72	Mandibular left primary lateral
e.	13	⌊5	25	Maxillary left second premolar

4. a. Class II
   b. Class III
   c. Class V
   d. Class I
   e. Class VI
   f. Class IV
5. a. A, amalgam
   b. T, temporary
   c. TC, tooth-colored restoration
   d. FGC, full gold crown
   e. GF, gold foil
   f. C, caries
   g. SSC, stainless steel crown
   h. DGO, defective gold onlay
6. a. Tooth anomaly: Mark with an asterisk and describe the condition elsewhere on the page, preceded by the asterisk.
   b. Pontic: Mark the root as missing, fill in the crown with the appropriate restoration, and draw horizontal bars to connect it to the adjacent pontic or abutment.
   c. Drifting: Draw a horizontal arrow parallel with and above the occlusal table, pointing in the direction of the drift.
   d. Rotation: Begin an arrow on the proximal side of the proximal surface of the tooth that is rotated facially and arc the arrow across the facial aspect of the tooth to suggest the direction of rotation.
   e. Attrition: Draw a horizontal line through the facial view of the teeth to indicate the amount of tooth lost because of mastication.
   f. Unerupted teeth: Circle.
   g. Overhang: Place an *O* in the appropriate box.

CHAPTER 12

1. Establishes baseline data on the patient; aids in establishing diagnosis; serves as a resource during treatment planning; aids in implementation of the treatment plan; as a reference for evaluating treatment success; as a source of legal evidence; used in forensic dentistry.

2. The amount of masticatory mucosa on the buccal surface of the tooth minus the buccal pocket depth of the same tooth equals the amount of attached gingiva.

3. a. Ledge: A ring or part of a ring that encircles the tooth, projecting from the tooth toward the gingiva, thus appearing like a ledge.
   b. Veneer: Thin sheet of burnished calculus that marks the location of a deposit incompletely removed by either an improperly adapted instrument or a dull instrument.
   c. Crustaceous: Chalky, white amorphous mass usually appearing supragingivally on the lingual aspect of the mandibular anterior teeth and on the facial surfaces of the maxillary molars. It may be afforded some shape by the action of the tongue and other musculature.
   d. Fingerlike projections: Projections that dip into the pockets formed during the advancement of periodontal disease.

4. Although research continues on the etiology of periodontal disease, it is accepted that calculus is a less important factor than plaque in disease initiation and progression. Calculus is usually covered with masses of microorganisms (plaque).

5. a. True
   b. True
   c. True
   d. False. While it is important to be able to locate and remove deposits of calculus, other functions such as prevention education, diagnostic testing, application of new therapies, and monitoring disease progression or status are equally important.
   e. True
   f. True
   g. False. AST is an enzyme released from human cells during severe inflammation and tissue destruction. It reflects the body's response.
   h. False. Their most important use will likely be at the conclusion of therapy to determine the treatment endpoint, to target patients with progressive disease for referral to a periodontist, and to monitor continuing care (recall) patients for sites at risk for periodontal breakdown.

6. Overangulate. The consequence of overangulation in a given area is that the reading may be slightly higher than the actual pocket depth. This would alert the hygienist or dentist to a potential problem area before it existed to that degree. If the probe is underangulated, the clinician runs the risk of assuming that an area is healthier than it actually is, and it may be overlooked in the dentist's diagnosis and treatment plan. Which would be worse for the patient?

7. No. Pocket depths are essentially meaningless unless the height of the gingival margin is also known. The depth of the pocket must be viewed in the context of whether or not there has been abnormal enlargement of the tissues or apical migration of the junctional epithelium. Without this context the clinician would not know whether a 3 mm pocket could be interpreted as normal, the result of gingival inflammation, or the result of periodontal destruction.

8. a. False. The probe should be adapted as close to parallel as possible as long as the clinician is certain that the tip is closely adapted to the tooth; the parallel relationship will exist for buccal and lingual adaptation, but the probe should be angled slightly for best assessment of the interproximal areas.
   b. False. In situations in which calculus prevents the clinician from adapting the probe to the base of the sulcus or pocket, it is often necessary to perform some scaling before accurate pocket depths can be determined.
   c. False. Although pocket readings are usually taken in six prescribed areas, it is the deepest point within each area that is recorded. This may not necessarily occur at exactly the same point on every tooth; in fact, it is unlikely that that would be true. In addition, if two distinctly separate vertical defects are detected within the same area of the tooth, the clinician may choose to include an extra reading to further define the bony morphology around that tooth.

CHAPTER 13

1. Bleeding; color change.

2. a. To initially evaluate the oral health status of the patient and provide a baseline record to compare changes.
   b. To periodically evaluate the patient's progress as well as the effectiveness of the clinical treatment.
   c. To monitor the patient's oral health status during the maintenance period to detect need for additional treatments.

3. Loe and Silness Gingival Index: Limitations: (in research) gingival sulcus is stimulated during the evaluation period and may promote a change in health when performed frequently; (in clinical practice) although a probe is used, it cannot be combined with a full mouth periodontal probing because the index calls for a sweeping of the sulcus.
   Lobene Gingival Index: Limitations: (for research and practice) the index is subjective and, for accuracy, the examiner must be calibrated.
   Bleeding on probing: Limitation: lack of control of probing force and sequence.

4. Turesky Modification of the Quigley-Hein Index: Limitation: it does not evaluate plaque thickness, only presence or absence of plaque; it does not take into account the proximal surfaces, which can provide important information regarding plaque control practices, such as flossing.

Modified Navy Plaque Index: Limitation: it is complex because it determines the plaque area accumulation by dividing the tooth into nine sections.

Silness-Loe Plaque Index: Limitation: plaque is disrupted during evaluation by periodontal probe, causing difficulty in calibration and re-examination.

5. Assessment: To evaluate present condition.
Implementation: To check progress.
Evaluation: To monitor health status.

CHAPTER 14

1. a. Overbite: The vertical distance that the maxillary teeth overlap the mandibular teeth.
   b. Occlusal trauma: Forces that cause damage to the supporting structures.
   c. Occlusal traumatism: Damage caused by abnormally arranged forces.
2. Tooth position, tooth-to-tooth habits, foreign object-to-teeth habits, oral musculature habits, and iatrogenic factors.
3. Subjective: Aching muscles, teeth that move, pain when biting, or pain with temperature changes. The patient may report grinding or clenching teeth or a habit of holding a pipe with the teeth or chewing or sucking a foreign object.
   Clinical: Mobility; wear patterns; changes in tooth position; poorly contoured restorations; plunger cusps; severe overbite or overjet; overdevelopment of the muscles of mastication; clicking, pain, or improper movement of the temporomandibular joint; and tooth sensitivity.
   Radiographic: Widened periodontal ligament space, necrosis of the periodontal ligament, cemental tears, loss of the lamina dura, bone resorption, and root resorption.
4. a. False. There must be damage to the supporting structures caused by occlusal trauma for the condition to be considered occlusal traumatism.
   b. False. Occlusal trauma does not cause periodontal pockets. Periodontitis is an inflammatory disease that affects the supporting structure; occlusal traumatism is a *non*inflammatory disease that affects the supporting structure.
   c. True in most cases.

CHAPTER 15

1. Permanent records, diagnostic aid, educational aid, and fabrication of temporary appliances.
2. Water-to-powder ratio, water temperature, and method of manipulation.
3. The tray should be large enough to permit ¼ inch (6 mm) of alginate to flow between the tray and oral structures without impinging on the soft tissues and without causing pain.
4. Fill the tray to the level of the beading wax; smooth alginate with wet fingers; retract one cheek with the fingers; retract the other cheek with the

side of the tray as it is being inserted; loosen the cheek and insert the other side of the tray; center the tray, place the posterior border of the tray first, and then the rest of the tray; muscle mold; and hold the tray gently.

5. Border molding is forming pliable materials (i.e., alginate) to conform to the muscle attachments of soft tissues so that the attachments are included in the cast for diagnostic and fabrication purposes.
6. The clinician can try to divert the patient's attention, reassure the patient, and/or ask the patient to breathe through the nose. If the patient reports a history of a gagging problem, the clinician can ask the patient to hold an ice cube in the mouth before inserting the tray or rinse the mouth with an anesthetic mouthwash.
7. Distortion and/or ripping of the alginate.
8. To permit the dental personnel to correctly relate the mandibular cast to the maxillary cast during the trimming procedure.
9. Initially, the gypsum is flowed into the tray in small increments to coat the tooth surfaces, and the excess is allowed to run out of the impression tray. Gradually, larger increments are added and flowed around the impression.
10. Use a sterile, disposable tray or a sterilized, reusable tray. Have patient use antiseptic mouthwash prior to making the impression. Soak impression in disinfecting solution prior to pouring.

CHAPTER 16

1. Intraoral photography has become an important communication tool in dentistry. For communicating ideas to patients and other professionals, intraoral images enhance everything from the clinical examination and basic patient identification to preparing a professional seminar. For treatment planning, intraoral video provides an immediate look at oral conditions, and video simulation allows the patient to see alternatives in treatment. Photos improve the thoroughness and accuracy of record-keeping. Other answers could include references to photography as a diagnostic aid, in case presentation, in case documentation, or as useful in education/motivation, instruction, and peer review.
2. a. 9
   b. 10
   c. 5
   d. 2
   e. 1
   f. 8
   g. 7
   h. 6
   i. 4
   j. 3
3. a. Wet the cheek retractor.
   b. Ask the patient to relax the lips and open the mouth slightly.

c. Place the rim of the retractor onto the edge of the lower lip.
d. Rotate the handle of the retractor until it is parallel to the corner of the mouth.
e. Instruct the patient to bite down. Pull the retractors out laterally and forward.

4. a. Mandibular anterior lingual: A lingual view of the mandibular anterior teeth and gingiva from the distal of the right cuspid to the distal of the left cuspid.
b. Buccal of right side: A direct buccal view of the right maxillary and mandibular teeth in occlusion from the distal of the right cuspid to the retromolar or maxillary tuberosity area.
c. Anterior direct: A direct view of the maxillary and mandibular teeth in occlusion from the distal of the right cuspid to the distal of the left cuspid.
d. Maxillary occlusal: A view of the maxillary occlusal surfaces and palatal tissues.

5. Criteria for above average photographic slide:
a. Inclusion of all desired oral structures.
b. Excellent photographic detail; excellent focus.
c. Excellent lighting and color.
d. No extraneous material.
e. Structures well centered.
f. Slide properly labeled.

CHAPTER 17

1. Dental hygiene diagnosis is defined as a formal statement of the dental hygienist's decision regarding the actual or potential problems of a patient that are amenable to treatment through the dental hygiene process of care.

2. Traditionally, dentists have assumed responsibility for diagnosing patient conditions. However, with the advances made in dental hygiene and the differences between dental and dental hygiene services, it is the dental hygienist's professional obligation to develop a dental hygiene diagnosis for each patient. This concept is new to dentistry and has yet to be widely embraced.

3. The components of the diagnostic-making process are initial review, hypothesis formulation, inquiry strategy, problem synthesis, diagnostic decision making, and learning from the process.

4. Resources that can be used as part of the initial review phase of diagnostic decision making include data obtained about the patient from the patient, parent, relatives, school personnel, social worker, director of a community agency, nursing home or other center, nurse, physician, physical therapist, occupational therapist, or any other person with knowledge of the patient.

5. Resources that can be used as part of the inquiry strategy phase of diagnostic decision making include follow-up questions related to the history of the problem as well as the medical and dental histories, extraoral and intraoral examinations, occlusal examination, periodontal charting, restorative charting, radiographs, blood assays, urinalysis, laboratory cultures, and excisional and incisional biopsies.

6. The significane of the dental hygiene diagnosis is that it enables the dental hygienist and the patient to focus on restoring total patient health and well-being.

CHAPTER 18

1. The nature of the patient's condition; a suggested plan of treatment; discussion of likely outcomes of treatment; risks involved in treatment; the likely outcome of not proceeding with care; and alternative treatment approaches.

2. Technical assault or technical battery.

3. The final treatment plan is more likely to be acceptable to the patient, and it will reflect a blending of the needs as seen by the patient and the dental hygienist, which will facilitate a partnership relationship and will increase the probability of cooperation in care and achievement of health goals.

4. Emergency.

5. The dental hygienist should perform thorough, reliable assessments; draw preliminary conclusions from the data, including proposed treatment and scheduling; use the dentist as a resource and arbiter of decisions regarding the patient's status and proper treatment; and follow through with high-quality care, providing status reports as care progresses.

CHAPTER 19

1. False. An attempt should be made to provide some service for the child, even if it is just counting teeth with a mouth mirror. The child may be more willing to cooperate if all procedures are carefully explained in simple terms that attract the patient rather than create fear.

2. Carefully explain each procedure, perhaps showing how pieces of equipment to be used function. Child patients may be allowed to manipulate some of the simpler pieces of equipment such as the air-water spray or the dental chair. A child may be allowed to feel the rubber cup. Encourage the patient to ask questions regarding the care he or she will receive so that he or she does not build up unnecessary fears.

3. For the patient who is visually handicapped, the hygienist can communicate by way of the other functioning senses. If the patient can hear, describe the procedures to be performed. Let the patient touch the equipment and hear it work before attempting an intraoral procedure. Guide the patient with a gentle touch and support his or her cooperation. Verbally introduce each step of care.

Concerning home care techniques, allow the patient to feel the method for brush and floss manipulation, in addition to feeling it intraorally. Repeat each step of instruction as necessary. Emphasize the feel of clean, plaque-free teeth.

4. Implements for delivery of safe dental care: physical restraints, mouth props (bite blocks), steel mirrors, rubber dam application, instruments secured with floss, and thimbles modified for finger protection.

5. The patient's sensory abilities and ability to communicate should be assessed before treatment begins so that appropriate modifications can be made. Manipulation of tissue should be kept to a minimum to avoid unnecessary trauma and resultant slower healing. Medical history assessments should be thorough because complicated medical histories may be encountered when older patients are treated. Appropriate modification based on medical histories should be made.

6. At age 6 months if the child has a developmental disorder or if the parents have poor oral health; other children should be seen between the ages of 18 and 24 months.

7. Only if stains are present. Preferred practice is to have the child (or parent) deplaque the teeth with a brush and fluoride paste, practicing proper technique and checking results with a disclosant. Topical fluoride can then be applied.

8. Depending on the limitation and the patient's ability to use his or her hand, wrist, and fingers, a brush could be modified by heating the plastic handle to turn the brush head in a way that would be more useful. The brush handle could be enlarged or elongated by attaching the brush to an object such as a ball or a wooden dowel. If the patient has head and neck mobility, an electric toothbrush could be mounted on a surface so that the patient could place the mouth on the brush and move the head position. It is important to evaluate the patient's abilities before helping select or create a modified tool.

9. The answer should include at least three of the following responses:
   a. Inform the patient when dentistry should be provided and what to avoid (radiographs, medications, treatment in the first and third trimesters).
   b. Dispel any myths the patient may have about dentistry and pregnancy.
   c. Stress the need for plaque control to prevent gingival inflammation.
   d. Stress the need for a balanced diet and nutrient supplements.
   e. Explain the role of sugar and decay and baby bottle syndrome.
   f. Discuss fluorides, the development of teeth, and/or eruption dates.

10. Xerostomia, rampant caries, and osteoradionecrosis.

11. Use of artificial saliva preparations, more frequent rinsing; preparation of foods that are easy to chew and swallow; use of sugarless mints, gum, or candies; use of lubricants on lips; or modifications in the living environment (e.g., vaporizor, air filter).

12. Patients should apply topical fluoride gel using customized fluoride trays once a day during treatment and continuing indefinitely. Choice of gel depends on patient's tolerance of an acidic pH; APF and SnF gels have lower (more acidic) pHs than sodium fluoride gels. Brush-on application may be appropriate for patients with good oral hygiene and minimal mouth dryness.

13. Dental care providers can use a drug history to identify medical conditions that exist; it allows them to research oral side effects of prescribed drugs and potential interactions with drugs used for dental treatment; it also provides an opportunity for care providers to assess whether or not the individual is complying with prescribed drug therapy.

14. Periodontal disease, root caries, oral cancer, edentulism.

15. Provider of direct patient treatment services, educator of patients and other care providers, dental coordinator or consultant.

16. Treatment is provided in bed with the patient propped up slightly; use of fluids for rinsing or use of a foaming dentifrice may be contraindicated because of danger of aspiration of fluids into the lungs; use of portable suction devices is helpful; mouth props may be needed.

CHAPTER 20

1. The first task is to help the patient understand and accept the importance of a total assessement at the first visit. If that assessment reveals minimal oral health problems, a routine oral prophylaxis may be indicated. However, if the assessment data reveals more important issues than removing calculus and stain or debriding the teeth, those procedures may be delayed for a subsequent visit.

2. If the patient is healthy and does not seem to be at risk of developing disease, reinforce the current procedures. It is not necessary to improve on success. However, it is wise to mention to the patient that although current techniques are working, a different approach may be needed if health begins to be compromised.

3. The roll method previously recommended by the American Dental Association.

4. A popularly recommended technique is the Bass method, which focuses on brushing the sulcular area and enhances access to proximal areas.

5. Floss has been shown to be effective in improving

gingival health interdentally. Used properly, it disrupts plaque in those areas. Interdental sticks and rubber tips can also disrupt proximal plaque, but they do not reduce plaque at contact points. Oral irrigation can also affect interdental plaque by detoxifying and reducing the pathogenic microflora.

6. Lecturing to an individual patient or to a group ensures that you have taught the lesson, but the patient or group members may not have learned the lesson. Lecture provides minimal feedback regarding what is being heard, understood, believed, and adopted. Discussion helps reveal attitudes, values, wants, needs, and expectations. It is more likely to result in adoption of the desired behaviors.

7. Avoiding nicotine in any form is a good behavior for general health but also for periodontal health specifically. Research shows that smoking increases the risk of periodontal disease, inhibits healing after treatment, and can mask poor periodontal health.

CHAPTER 21

1. *Streptococcus mutans*.
2. a. True
   b. True
   c. True
   d. True
   e. True
   f. False. The optimal concentration is 1 ppm.
3. Dental fluorosis is a change in the porosity of the enamel that occurs during tooth formation from the ingestion of too much fluoride. The white, chalky appearance of the enamel is due to a loss of normal translucency, while the brown discoloration is due to extrinsic stains in the porous areas.
4. After the teeth erupt, fluoride and other minerals that are in saliva further mineralize the enamel surface, adding to its ability to resist caries.
5. a. Once- daily rinsing.
   b. Twice- daily rinsing.
   c. Once- weekly rinsing.
   Read the manufacturer's directions for amount and duration of rinsing. Typically, 10 ml of the rinse is swished for 60 seconds and then expectorated. The rinses are not to be given to persons who cannot control the swallow reflex or who cannot thoroughly expectorate.
6. No. Laboratory and clinical trials have demonstrated that it makes no difference whether the teeth are polished, brushed, or left without intervention before fluoride is administered. However, dental hygiene procedures emphasize clean teeth; therefore, it is recommended that selective polishing, combined with the patient demonstrating proper plaque removal with a brush and floss, precede fluoride application. This procedure is intended to reinforce good at-home oral hygiene rather than to enhance fluoride uptake.

7. The Grand Rapids/Muskegon and Kingston/Newburg trials were instituted to determine whether or not fluoride in the water creates measurable changes in dental caries. Two of the cities contained insignificant amounts of fluoride and two were fluoridated to optimal levels of 1 ppm. The decayed, missing, and filled surfaces were significantly fewer in the fluoridated communities than in the nonfluoridated communities at the evaluation points, paving the way for widespread communal fluoridation of water supplies.

8. See the check-off sheet (p. 476) for each step.
9. c. All teeth to be treated must be covered by the fluoride gel or solution before the 4-minute timing begins.
10. Adults: 5 to 10 g.
    Children: 32 mg/kg body weight.
    The amount of fluoride gel or solution applied is somewhere in the range of 125 to 200 mg.
11. d. All three are acceptable antidotes for acute fluoride poisoning. Seek immediate emergency care if symptoms persist or if the amount ingested is more than 3.5 mg/kg body weight or is unknown.
12. The total fluoride dose would be about 192 to 195 mg.
13. This dosage would not be above the CLD (certainly lethal dose) for a 2-year-old child, which is estimated to be 320 mg.
14. Yes, hospitalization is indicated for this level of overdose. The total ingested dose of 192 to 195 mg is well beyond both the STD and the PTD estimates and is equivalent to a dose of 19 mg/kg body weight for a 2-year-old.

CHAPTER 22

1. The acid-etching process (conditioning) is the most critical part of the sealant technique. An acidic gel or solution is painted on the occlusal surface for 60 seconds. This removes inorganic material from the occlusal enamel and leaves a reactive porous surface. The increased surface area allows the sealant resin to penetrate the enamel and form a mechanical lock for the sealant. As a result of etching, a strong bond can be formed between the enamel and the sealant material that is highly resistant to bacterial leakage and occlusal wear.

2. This patient is at a caries-prone age and shows a history of restorations in commonly susceptible teeth. The patient's susceptibility may be exaggerated, as she previously lived in a nonfluoridated area. Clinically, the patient appears for treatment with good home care and a good preventive attitude reinforced by the parents. The newly erupted teeth are sound, and radiographic data reveal that there are no interproximal caries. These factors indicate

that the patient is a good candidate for sealant protection. In a consultation among the hygienist, dentist, patient, and family, information about the sealant procedure, the benefits, risks and responsibilities should be discussed and a decision made. (We would elect to seal teeth No. 18 and No. 31 and recommend that the patient return when teeth No. 2 and No. 15 erupt if this occurs before the next regularly scheduled visit.)

3. Steps in the sealant application procedure: (a) remove hard and soft deposits, (b) polish with pumice, (c) rinse thoroughly, (d) isolate and dry teeth, (e) condition the teeth, (f) rinse and examine (recondition if necessary), (g) reisolate and dry teeth, (h) apply sealant, (i) polymerize sealant, and (j) rinse and examine.

4. Possible reasons:
   a. New ideas are accepted slowly.
   b. The public was unaware of the benefits of sealants so did not demand this service.
   c. Employer attitudes about new techniques and delegation of sealants have changed slowly.
   d. Not all insurance carriers have recognized sealants as a service to be covered in their dental plans.

CHAPTER 23

1. c and d
2. c
3. b
4. False
5. *Candida albicans*
6. Clean dentures regularly, soak in diluted vinegar overnight when calculus first forms; never scrape a denture surface—bring it in for professional cleaning instead.
7. Wear mask, gloves, and glasses; isolate denture and solution in sealed plastic bag during cleaning; never reuse solution.
8. Clean over a sink partially filled with water or with a rubber mat or towel placed in the bottom; hold denture firmly.

CHAPTER 24

1. Carbohydrates, fats, and proteins.
2. Any of the three nutrients consumed in excess can cause weight gain. Their total contribution to daily caloric intake determines fat deposition (if it is in excess of expended calories) or fat use (if it is less than expended calories).
3. a. 6   h. 13
   b. 7   i. 1
   c. 5   j. 4
   d. 9   k. 3
   e. 10 l. 12
   f. 14 m. 2
   g. 11

4. Often the patient is fully aware of what he or she *ought* to include in the daily diet. Information about what to do and what not to do may not be what is needed. After the patient demonstrates his or her level of knowledge about diet and nutrition, it is easier to decide what kind of information still needs to be provided in the follow-up discussion. The self-assessment process itself may cause the patient to develop a need to know or a need to change.

5. The RDAs and the four food groups provide a guideline or standard for evaluating the appropriateness and healthfulness of a person's diet. With these guidelines, missing elements in a person's diet can be readily identified and suggestions for change can be made.

6. Plaque provides a matrix for absorbing fermentable carbohydrates, which are converted by bacteria into acid, which demineralizes the tooth structure. Plaque promotes smooth-surface caries, providing an attachment to the teeth that maintains acid contact.

7. Nutrition plays a role in the development, maintenance, and resistance of the periodontium. Poor nutrition may compromise the integrity of the periodontal tissues and impair the immune response, altering the host's resistance to disease.

8. A firm, fibrous diet stimulates salivary flow, increases circulation in the periodontium, strengthens the periodontal ligament, and may increase alveolar bone density. A soft diet may contribute to bacterial growth and plaque formation.

9. Saturated and unsaturated fats; salt-cured, smoked, and salt-pickled foods; alcohol, and food contaminants, including additives; alcohol in combination with tobacco promotes oral cancer.

10. Fruits and vegetables, especially dark-green leafy and deep orange and yellow varieties and cruciferous vegetables (cabbage, cauliflower, brussel sprouts, and broccoli).

CHAPTER 25

1. b and c are true. Scaling is less effective than other methods in removing plaque and endotoxin because it does not employ methodical coverage of the tooth surface with the instrument; therefore residual amounts of plaque and endotoxin will remain following treatment.

2. e. Closed debridement has been shown to be effective at all levels of periodontal disease.

3. a and c

4. c. Neither of the other measures provides reliable evidence that the tooth surface is biologically acceptable to the soft tissues as the actual healing response of the tissues does.

5. b. only

6. d. The ultrasonic action of the tip does the work so

less stress is placed on hand and arm muscles to remove difficult deposits. Also, because debridement is accomplished more quickly, fewer repetitive hand and wrist motions are required, thereby reducing the potential for occupational-related injury, such as carpal tunnel syndrome.

7. False. It has been shown that healing can occur in the presence of veneered residual calculus.
8. False. Bacterial plaque is the primary cause of periodontal disease. The presence of calculus is a contributory factor in that it provides a porous surface to which bacterial plaque and its by-products readily adhere.

CHAPTER 26

1. Angulation and working stroke are two principles that are necessary for use of cutting instruments but do not apply to use of explorers and probes.
2. a. False
   b. True
   c. True
   d. False
   e. False
   f. True
3. b, d, f, h.
4. Supragingival: Any hand instrument may be used; will probably require fewer strokes because calculus is less firmly attached and other methods can assist in debriding soft deposits (e.g., air polishing, rubber cup polishing, brushing, etc.); direction of strokes includes push and pull strokes; probably less pressure because of the nature of attachment of calculus (b, d, f, h).
   Subgingival: curettes preferred; more strokes needed to thoroughly debride root surfaces; all directions, with pull stroke used for all strokes; pressure depends on nature of deposits—light for finishing and removal of soft deposits, heavier for removal of tenacious subgingival calculus deposits.
5. Gracey curettes: Narrower blades for access to deep, tight pocket areas; only one cutting edge is used, offset blade design; multiple shank designs for area-specific use, multiangled shanks for posterior areas.
   Universal curettes: may have heavier, larger blades; both cutting edges used, cutting edges are parallel, not offset; simpler shank design to facilitate adaptation to all areas of the mouth.

CHAPTER 27

1. All three methods are acceptable.
2. a. False. The Arkansas stone is a natural stone.
   b. True. Cutting edges of good quality stainless steel instruments are not dulled by steam sterilization (Parkes and Kolstad, 1981—see references for Chapter 27).
   c. False. Only the lower cutting edge of Gracey curettes is used for periodontal procedures.

Therefore only that cutting edge should be sharpened.
3. The internal angle of 70 to 80 degrees forms a complementary angle with the sharpening stone, which is applied at 100 to 110 degrees.
4. Both the rounded toe and the rounded back of the curette design must be preserved during sharpening procedures.
5. a. Pressure is applied only to the downstroke to minimize formation of wire edges.

CHAPTER 28

1. a. False; it changes the quality of the plaque and reduces gingivitis.
   b. True
   c. True
   d. False; it is a blunt needle used primarily by the clinician to deliver agents subgingivally.
   e. True
   f. False; a number of antibiotics, generally given systemically, do supress bacterial proliferation. Recent research also shows slow-release agents delivered subgingivally are effective against bacteria.
   g. True
2. a. Essential oils
   b. Sanguinaria extract
   c. Stannous ion
   d. Chlorhexidine digluconate

CHAPTER 29

1. A periodontal dressing protects the area from irritants, protects newly exposed root surfaces, stabilizes mobile teeth, protects sutures, maintains the position of repositioned tissue, and helps control bleeding.
2. Either one can be used, depending on clinician preference. The eugenol pack is believed by some practitioners to soothe the tissues; other practitioners believe that eugenol irritates the tissues. Other factors to be considered are storage time, mixing time, consistency of the pack, and ease of manipulation of each material.
3. Refer to Fig. 29-15 for the suggested response.
4. If the sutures were tied on the facial surface, then the lingual pack should be removed first. The sutures can be cut on the lingual portion, and then they can be removed from the buccal portion at the same time the pack is removed. The clinician must be sure *never* to pull the knot through the tissue.
5. Dressings may promote the accumulation of plaque and associated inflammation, resulting in prolonged wound healing; dressings also may contribute to patient discomfort.

CHAPTER 30

1.a. Exogenous: Stains that originate outside the tooth.

b. Endogenous: Stains that develop within the tooth.

c. Extrinsic: Exogenous stain on the exterior of the tooth; removable by the patient or professioanl.

d. Intrinsic: Within the tooth structure, not removable by the patient or by basic polishing or scaling.

2. It removes and prevents formation of stains and/or discolorants (pellicle).

3. Essentially the same abrasives are used in both; higher concentrations are present in professional products.

4. Abrasive hardness; particle size, shape, concentration; and the pressure and speed used.

5. The type and amount of stain present and the patient's health status regarding allergies are important in selecting the appropriate abrasive.

6. Operate at a low speed (minimal speed at which the attachment can be applied to the tooth without stalling); use *moderate intermittent* pressure on the tooth; and use sufficient amounts of abrasive to minimize direct contact of rubber and brush with the tooth.

7. Advantages: Portability, provides gentle massage, can reach surfaces obscured by malposed teeth, generates minimal frictional heat, generates minimal noise, is easily cleaned and sterilized, and generates minimal aerosol.
Disadvantages: It is slow and tedious and requires considerable hand effort.

8. The presence of stains that cannot be readily removed by the patient.

9. Air pressure and water force a slurry of sodium bicarbonate against the tooth structure, loosening stain and polishing the tooth.

10. The air-powder polisher is indicated for use on patients with stain, orthodontic appliances, and for debridment of exposed and unexposed root surfaces. Use of the air-powder polisher is contraindicated on most restorative materials. Its use on patients with high blood pressure and dental implants is still controversial. Angulation of the spray into periodontal pockets and onto nonkeratinized tissues should be avoided. Because of the aerosols emitted, universal barrier precautions are required.

11. Polishing of unexposed root surfaces detoxifies or debrides the root of toxins or lipopolysaccharides (LPS) that can cause an inflammatory response.

12. Cosmetic polishing removes stains for esthetic purposes. Therapeutic polishing removes disease-causing toxins, antigens, and enzymes, thereby assisting the body in maintaining health.

CHAPTER 31

1. Areas in which dentin is exposed, primarily as a result of enamel and/or cementum being eroded, abraded, or planed away.

2. Root surface scaling, gingival surgery (causing gingival or root exposure recession), cavity preparation, and placement of crowns.

3. Mechanical, thermal, and chemical.

4. Depositing of precipitating insoluble materials into the dentinal tubules to occlude the opening and prevent fluid movement within the tubules from a stimulus.

5. a. True
   b. True
   c. True

6. a. Differences: Fluoride is applied more frequently; can be burnished on very sensitive areas.
   b. Similarities: Teeth should be clean (scaled and polished) and dry before application. The same preparations can be used. If the entire mouth is treated, the same mode of application (tray, painted on dry teeth) can be used.

7. The hydrodynamic theory states that pain-producing stimuli cause a movement of the fluids in the tubules in either an outward or an inward direction, depending on the pressure variations in the surrounding tissue. This movement stimulates the nerve processes in the pulpal dentin and the pulp.

CHAPTER 32

1. Refer to Fig. 32-4.

2. a. Hard tissue: Second and third molars and the first, excluding the mesiobuccal root and the associated supporting structures. Soft tissue: Overlying facial tissue.
   b. Hard tissue: None. Soft tissue: Palatal tissue from the margin of the gingiva to the midline and from the distal aspect of the posterior-most molar to the cuspid.
   c. Hard tissue: None. Soft tissue: Buccal tissue of mandibular molars.
   d. Hard tissue: Premolars, cuspid and incisors to the midline and the associated supporting structures. Soft tissue: Overlying tissue facial to premolars, cuspid, incisors, excluding molars, including lips.

3. a. Inferior alveolar, lingual, and buccal.
   b. Posterior-superior alveolar, middle-superior alveolar, and greater palatine.
   c. Infiltration facial to the incisors.

CHAPTER 33

1. Conscious sedation refers to a state of relaxation or central nervous system depression in which the patient remains conscious at all times. A conscious patient is defined as one who is capable of rational response to command and has all protective reflexes, such as maintenance of an airway and the cough reflex, intact.

2. a'. Inorganic inhalation agent, sweet smelling, and nonflammable.

b'. Has a low blood gas solubility compared with oxygen.

c'. Eliminated unchanged from the lungs.

d'. A mildly potent anesthetic when administered with oxygen.

e'. Affects the person's psychologic reaction to pain perception.

3. a. The patient with emphysema has a compromised respiratory system. Various concentrations of oxygen may decrease this person's ability to function. Expiration is difficult and may affect elimination of nitrous oxide from the bloodstream.

b. Generally the patient with an upper respiratory tract infection experiences difficulty breathing through the nose. Because such breathing is necessary to permit effective inhalation sedation, the patient will not benefit from the procedure.

4. $\dfrac{4}{4+6} = \dfrac{4}{10} = 40\%$

This is higher than the recommended optimal level for sedation (30% to 35%). Although patient responses vary, close observation is necessary to avoid an adverse response to too high a concentration. Although nitrous oxide and oxygen conscious sedation raises the pain threshold, the body perceives the pain and reacts to it. In the case of a tooth extraction, local or regional anesthesia is necessary.

5. Any three of the following: The patient appears lethargic, falls asleep, begins to perspire, complains of nausea, moves in an uncoordinated fashion, becomes uncooperative, and/or reports dreaming. See Table 33-1 for other responses.

CHAPTER 34

1. Walls: Gingival, axial, facial, and incisal.
   Line angles: Incisoaxial, facioaxial, gingivoaxial, faciogingival, facioincisal, linguoaxial.

2. Generally, for posterior teeth, the anchor tooth is the most distal tooth in the quadrant to provide maximum visibility and access to the operating field. Minimal access is obtained by clamping one tooth distal to the teeth being restored.

3. The clamp and dam can be applied by placing the clamp on the tooth and stretching the dam over the clamp onto the tooth; the dam can be placed over the bow of the clamp, the clamp placed on the tooth, then the dam stretched over the tooth; or the dam can be stretched over the wings of the clamp and both the clamp and wings placed together.

4. False. Varnish is indeed placed under all amalgam restorations; however, it interferes with the setting reaction of composite resin material.

5. The matrix band forms the missing wall(s) to complete the "container" into which the amalgam can be condensed. It also restores the proximal anatomic contours and contact areas to the tooth. The wedge adapts the matrix band to the cervical region of the tooth. It also separates the teeth to ensure proximal contact for the restored tooth.

6. a. False. There is no indication for placing calcium hydroxide because calcium hydroxide is effective as a pulp stimulator only when in direct contact with the pulp.

b. True. Calcium hydroxide would stimulate the pulp to form secondary dentin.

c. True. Calcium hydroxide would protect the pulp from possible irritation from the monomer in the composite resin material.

d. False. There is sufficient thickness of remaining dentin to protect the pulp from potential chemical irritation from the monomer.

7. An alloy is any combination of metals.

8. An alloy of any metal(s) with mercury is referred to as an amalgam.

9. It is silver—42% to 69%.

10. They are silver, copper, tin and zinc.

11. It is the process of mixing mercury with an alloy.

12. It should be in one pellet or mass that holds together without crumbling, has a slightly dull shine, and does not appear dry or grainy.

13. In a Class V preparation, the first increment should be placed and condensed along the axial wall at the distogingival line angle. In a Class II MOD preparation, the first increment is placed and condensed against the gingival wall of the distal box.

14. The amalgam is more difficult to load, place, and condense. It will not adhere well with the previously placed loads and will be subject to fracture/flaking.

15. Mercury vapor is released, resulting in potential mercury poisoning of those present.

16. It is an area at the cavosurface where the amalgam is not at the same height as the cavosurface enamel; either too little amalgam was added originally or too much amalgam has been carved away.

17. False. Light intermittent pressure is used to avoid heat production, which would bring mercury to the surface of the amalgam.

18. True. Finishing with the least coarse disk leaves the smoothest finish on the surface of the restoration.

19. Phosphoric acid in concentrations of 30% to 40% is applied to the enamel for 30 seconds to 1 minute. The phosphoric acid selectively removes inorganic material from the enamel surface leaving micropores or pits in the surface. The resin component of the composite resin flows into these countless pits to form resin tags that hold tightly by mechanical means to the surface. The many, many tags provide great retention.

20. The setting reaction can be initiated chemically by mixing a reactor with the base material, or it can

be activated by exposing the material to a visible light in the blue spectrum. The chemically cured composite resins require no special, expensive light and can be cured in a large mass. The light-cured resins allow methodic shaping of the restoration before curing. They also come in one paste, which requires no mixing and thus avoids incorporation of air bubbles.

21. A temporary restoration would be placed in situations where the vitality of the pulp is questionable, a tooth has been painful and is awaiting definitive diagnosis, there was insufficient time to place a permanent restoration, or the tooth is awaiting the placement of a cast intracoronal restoration.

22. When removing the calculus, the instrument is placed under the deposit and then activated to remove as much of the deposit as possible. When removing excess amalgam, the amalgam is shaved off in layers to avoid fracturing the amalgam and creating an open margin.

23. Depends on size of restoration. Each increment needs a minimum of 20 seconds from mesial and distal and/or facial and lingual aspects.

24. Should be increments no thicker than 2 to 3 ml. If thicker, the bottom layer may not achieve optimal curing.

25. Silicate glass powder and polyacrylic acid. It adheres to the dentin, releases fluoride, has biocompatability, and is a good thermal insulator.

CHAPTER 35

1. Dental disease, particularly periodontal disease, is not easily "cured." The patient continues to be at risk for recurrence, and, even in healthy patients, disease can appear when the body's immune response is compromised. Further, continuing care helps the patient maintain a focus on proper oral hygiene to help prevent initiation or recurrence of disease.

2. It was a logical interval for detecting dental caries that was promoted by the dental products industry via television advertising during the 1950s.

3. It is based on research suggesting that periodontal pathogens repopulate the subgingival pocket in approximately 12 weeks. It is believed that if the flora can be regularly disrupted, the disease will be less likely to advance.

4. a. 6%
   b. 9%
   c. 85%

5. The system you select should make it possible for you to (a) specify the individual's recall interval, (b) contact the person to schedule an appointment to occur at the designated interval, (c) easily identify when a patient is due for an appointment (patients may call and inquire which week or month is the anticipated time for scheduling), and (d) note when the continuing care visit has been scheduled and whether the appointment was kept.

6. All assessment procedures, with a special focus on sites that have had active disease and those areas at risk of developing disease; assessment of oral hygiene effectiveness and further guidance; application of light subgingival debridement with an ultrasonic or hand instrument; and administration of site-specific treatments, depending on specific patient need and as products become available.

7. You will play a critical role in (a) explaining the need for special care, (b) ensuring that the appointment is scheduled with a competent clinician once the patient agrees to the referral, (c) communicating with the specialist regarding his or her diagnosis and recommended treatment, (d) discussing those plans with the patient to determine his or her attitude and intentions, and (e) maintaining contact with the patient and the specialist during and after treatment so that the patient can be re-entered into the continuing care program when appropriate. Your overall role is to be the coordinator of referred care and to serve as the patient's advocate when more than one health care provider is involved in the treatment.

CHAPTER 36

1. Components of a case documentation: health history review, initial clinical findings, chartings, radiographs, study casts, photographs, treatment plan, record of actual treatment, posttreatment findings, and evaluation summary.

2. a. Case documentation enhances record keeping by ensuring that accurate data are available for the clinician to follow the patient's care. Documentation of before-and-after treatment establishes the initial condition and treatment outcome. Such information may be useful and necessary for reference and comparison at a later date.

   b. Participating in case documentation procedures motivates the patient because he or she is able to realize the changes that have occurred throughout the course of treatment. Examples of other patient documentations demonstrate potential modes of therapy and may aid the patient in making a decision for personal treatment.

CHAPTER 37

1. A system of accountability defines goals that can provide a direction or a target for the daily activities of practice. Such a system can add meaning to a lifetime of clinical practice. Accountability can also develop a support system for encounters with malpractice or third-party payer investigations.

2. The degree to which prevention is emphasized in each day's routine (i.e., the amount of time or effort spent on prevention and preventive educational activities); the overall effect on health levels of the

population (maintenance, improvement, or loss of health over time); the degree to which clinical protocols approximate nationally accepted standards through comparison with published protocols, reviews of the literature, and participation in peer group study clubs; approach behaviors of patients to dental hygiene care through the development of a long-term patient population; personal gratification and health; cost effectiveness; and participation in professional advancement.

3. Decide to live with the dissatisfaction or develop a plan for change.

INDEX

Page numbers in *italics* indicate boxes and illustrations. Page numbers followed by *t* indicate tables.